P9-CQI-618

Student Pharmacology CD-ROM Contents*

PART ONE

Multiple-Choice Review Questions

- Nursing Process and Drug Therapy
- Basic Pharmacology Principles
- Pediatric, Maternal, and Geriatric Considerations
- Legal, Ethical, and Cultural Considerations
- Over-the-Counter Medications and Herbal Therapy
- Medication Administration and Dosage Calculation
- Analgesics
- Anaesthetic and Neuromuscular Blocking Agents
- Central Nervous System Depressants
- Anticonvulsants (Anti-Epileptic Drugs)
- Antiparkinsonian Drugs
- Psychiatric Drugs
- Central Nervous System Stimulants
- Adrenergic Agents
- Adrenergic-Blocking Agents
- Cholinergic Drugs
- Anticholinergic Agents
- Inotropic Agents
- Antidysrhythmic Agents
- Anti-Anginal Agents
- Antihypertensive Agents
- Diuretic Agents
- Fluids and Electrolytes
- Coagulation Modifier Agents
- Antilipemic Agents
- Pituitary Agents
- Thyroid and Antithyroid Agents
- Antidiabetic and Hypoglycemic Agents
- Adrenal Agents
- Women's Health Agents
- Men's Health Agents
- Antihistamines, Decongestants, Antitussives, and Expectorants
- Bronchodilators and Other Respiratory Agents
- Antibiotics
- Antiviral Agents
- Antitubercular Agents
- Antifungal Agents
- Antimalarial, Antiprotozoal, and Anthelmintic Agents
- Antiseptic and Disinfectant Agents
- Anti-Inflammatory, Antirheumatoid, and Related Agents
- Immunosuppressant Drugs
- Immunizing Agents
- Antineoplastic Agents
- Immunomodulating Agents
- Acid-Controlling Agents
- Antidiarrheals and Laxatives
- Anti-Emetic Agents
- Vitamins and Minerals
- Nutritional Supplements
- Blood-Forming Agents
- Dermatological Agents
- Ophthalmic Agents
- Otic Agents

PART TWO

Pharmacology Animations

- Nursing, Medical, and Pharmacology Domains
- Patient Non-Adherence
- Agonists/Antagonists
- Receptor Interaction
- Passive Diffusion
- Impact of Surface Area
- Overview of Pharmacokinetics: Oral Administration
- Distribution: Fat- vs. Water-Soluble Drugs
- Cytochrome P-450 Drug Metabolism
- Half-Life of Intravenously Administered Ampicillin
- Drug Movement Through the Body
- Normal Electrophysiology
- Renin-Angiotensin in Control of Blood Pressure
- Time to Steady State
- Time to Steady State: Starting and Stopping Drug
- Pharmacokinetic Profiles: Normal, Renal Failure, and Hemodialysis

PART THREE

Medication Administration Checklists

- Interpreting Medication Orders
- Transcribing Medication Orders
- Reviewing Medication Orders
- Administering Medications to Prevent Medication Errors
- Preparing Medications
- Assessing Client Response
- Appropriate Documentation of Medication Administration
- Procedural Safeguards
- Reporting Medication Errors

PART FOUR

IV Therapy Checklists

- Administering Bolus Medication Through Continuous IV
- Administering Medication Through an Intermittent IV (Saline) Lock
- Adding Medication to an Intravenous Bag, Bottle, or Volume Control Set
- Administering Medication via a Piggyback or Secondary Set
- Changing the Container of an Existing Intravenous Solution

*Student CD-ROM content prepared by Dorothy Mathers, RN, MSN, and Beth Swart, BScn, MES. Pharmacology animations prepared by Ed Tessier, PharmD, MPH, BCPS.

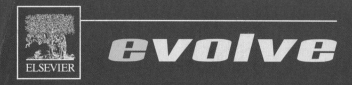

To access your Student Learning Resources, visit:

http://evolve.elsevier.com/Lilley/pharmacology/

Evolve® Student Learning Resources for *Lilley: Pharmacology and the Nursing Process in Canada, First Canadian Edition,* offers the following features:

Student Resources

- **Student Worksheets**
  Review exercises, including answers, provided for each chapter.

- **Learning Tips and Content Updates**
  The latest content updates from the authors to keep you current with recent developments in pharmacology.

- **WebLinks**
  An exciting resource that lets you link to hundreds of Web sites carefully chosen to supplement the content of the textbook. The WebLinks are regularly updated, with new ones added as they develop.

- **Answer Key**
  Answers to the Multiple-Choice Examination Review Questions, Critical Thinking Activities, and Case Studies in the text.

- **Mosby/Saunders ePharmacology Update newsletter**
  An online newsletter released twice each semester.

- **Supplemental Resources**
  Additional information on generic versus trade names; common formulas, weights, and equivalents; and more!

Pharmacology
and the Nursing
Process in
Canada

FIRST CANADIAN EDITION

Linda Lane Lilley, RN, PhD
Associate Professor and University Professor
School of Nursing
Old Dominion University
Norfolk, Virginia

Scott Harrington, PharmD
Harrington Health Informatics, LLC
Tucson, Arizona;
Director of Pharmacy, Northern Cochise
    Community Hospital
Willcox, Arizona

Julie S Snyder, MSN, RN, C
Adjunct Faculty
School of Nursing
Old Dominion University
Norfolk, Virginia

Canadian Editor:

Beth Swart, BScN, MES
School of Nursing
Ryerson University
Toronto, Ontario

With Study Skills content by:
Richard E Lake, BS, MS, MLA
Director, Center for Student Success
Professor, Reading Department
St. Louis Community College at Florissant Valley
St. Louis, Missouri

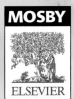

MOSBY

ELSEVIER

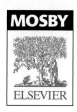

NOTICE

Pharmacology is an ever-changing field. Standard safety precautions must be followed, but as new research and clinical experience broaden our knowledge, changes in treatment and drug therapy may become necessary or appropriate. Readers are advised to check the most current product information provided by the manufacturer of each drug to be administered to verify the recommended dose, the method and duration of administration, and contraindications. It is the responsibility of the licensed prescriber, relying on experience and knowledge of the patient, to determine dosages and the best treatment for each individual patient. Neither the publisher nor the author assumes any liability for any injury and/or damage to persons or property arising from this publication.

Library and Archives Canada Cataloguing in Publication

Lilley, Linda Lane
Pharmacology and the nursing process in Canada / Linda Lilley,
Scott Harrington, Julie S. Snyder; Beth Swart, editor. -- 1st ed.
Includes bibliographical references and index.
ISBN 0-7796-9971-8
1. Nursing--Canada. 2. Pharmacology. I. Harrington, Scott
II. Snyder, Julie S. III. Swart, Beth , 1948– IV. Title.

RM301.L54 2006   615'.1   C2005-907582-1

Publisher: Ann Millar
Managing Developmental Editor: Martina van de Velde
Developmental Editor: May Look
Managing Production Editor: Lise Dupont
Project Manager: Tricia Carmichael
Editorial Assistant: Kim Armstrong
Copy Editor: Gilda Mekler
Interior Design: Teresa McBryan
Cover Design: Sonya V. Thursby, Opus House, Inc.
Typesetting and Assembly: Graphic World, Inc.
Cover Printing: Phoenix
Printing and Binding: Transcontinental Inc.

Elsevier Canada
905 King Street West, 4th Floor, Toronto, ON, Canada M6K 3G9
Phone: 1-866-896-3331
Fax: 1-866-359-9534

For illustration credit information for the illustrations in Chapter 9, please refer to the illustration credits listed at the end of the chapter.

Printed in Canada

1 2 3 4 5 11 10 09 08 07

About the Authors

LINDA LANE LILLEY, RN, PhD

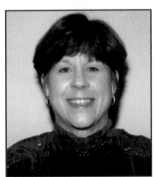

Linda Lilley received her diploma from Norfolk General School of Nursing, her BSN from the University of Virginia, her Master of Science (Nursing) from Old Dominion University, and her PhD in Nursing from George Mason University. Her teaching experience spans more than 25 years, with the last 18 years at Old Dominion University School of Nursing. As an Associate Professor, Linda's areas of teaching expertise include pharmacology, adult nursing, physical assessment, fundamentals, oncology nursing, nursing theory, and trends in health care and nursing. She also has mentoring and teaching responsibilities within the Master of Science in Nursing program – education track. Linda has over 12 years of experience teaching RNs returning for their BSN via the "distance learning" mode. Areas of research interest include retention of minority students in baccalaureate schools of nursing and human needs of patients with cervical or uterine cancer. Dr. Lilley's professional service is varied; she acts as a consultant with the school nurses in the city of Virginia Beach, is a member of the City of Virginia Beach's Health Advisory Board, and sits on the national advisory panel on medication errors prevention with the U.S. Pharmacopeia in Rockville, Maryland. In August, 1999, Linda received Old Dominion University's most prestigious award of teaching excellence for tenured faculty members with the title of University Professor. She has also been a two-time university nominee for the State Council of Higher Education in Virginia award for excellence in teaching, service, and scholarship.

SCOTT HARRINGTON, PharmD

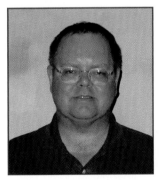

Scott Harrington received his Associate of Science in Pharmacy Technology with High Honors from Pima Community College, Tucson, Arizona, in 1991. He then worked as both an outpatient and inpatient pharmacy technician while completing his Doctor of Pharmacy degree at the University of Arizona College of Pharmacy, which he received in 1997. He then completed two post-doctoral residency training programs. The first was a specialty residency in Pharmacocybernetics at Creighton University in Omaha, Nebraska, which he completed in 1998. The second was an additional specialty residency in Drug Information and Pharmaceutical Informatics at the University of California San Francisco Medical Center and First DataBank in San Bruno, California, which he completed in 1999. Since that time he has worked in a variety of settings, including outpatient retail pharmacy, where he also compounded customized prescriptions. He has since worked in hospital pharmacy and has served as a proofreader and content reviewer for Mosby beginning in 1999. He is now Director of Pharmacy for Northern Cochise Community Hospital in Willcox, Arizona. He serves as a relief pharmacist for Bob's IGA Food and Drug grocery store pharmacy in Willcox, Thrifty Pharmacy in Safford, Arizona, and Willo Compounding Pharmacy in Phoenix. He is also a regular part-time clinical pharmacist at Hu Hu Kam Memorial Hospital in the Gila River Indian Reservation in Sacaton, Arizona. Scott regularly offers public education regarding medication use in mental illness during public outreach support groups at the office of the National Alliance for the Mentally Ill of Southern Arizona in Tucson. He also offers public medication education on various topics for the citizens of Willcox through his hospital position. Scott's professional affiliations include the American Society of Health-System Pharmacy, the American Society for Consultant Pharmacists, the American Pharmacists Association, the Society for Technical Communicators, the American Medical Informatics Association, and the American College of Clinical Pharmacy, which invited Scott to lead a discussion on the topic of whistle-blowing in healthcare organizations in November of 2003. Scott is a member of American MENSA.

JULIE S. SNYDER, MSN, RN, C

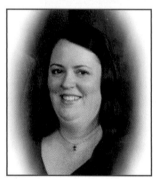

Julie Snyder received her diploma from Norfolk General Hospital School of Nursing, and her BSN and MSN from Old Dominion University. After working in medical-surgical nursing for over ten years, she began working in nursing staff development and community education. After eight years, she transferred to teaching in a school of nursing, and over the past seven years has taught fundamentals of nursing, pharmacology, physical assessment, gerontological nursing, and adult medical-surgical nursing. She has been certified by the ANCC in Nursing Continuing Education and Staff Development, and currently holds ANCC certification in Medical-Surgical Nursing. She is a member of Sigma Theta Tau International, and was inducted into Phi Kappi Phi as Outstanding Alumna for Old Dominion University. She has worked for Mosby/Elsevier as a reviewer and ancillary writer since 1997. Julie's professional service has included serving on the Virginia Nurses' Association Continuing Education Committee, writing items for the ANCC, working with a local hospital educators' group, and serving as a consultant for the School at Work program, a workforce development program.

BETH SWART, BScN, MES

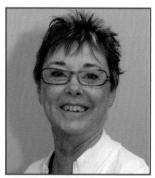

Beth Swart, RN, MES, is a professor in the School of Nursing, Ryerson University. She received her diploma in nursing from the Hospital for Sick Children School of Nursing, her BScN from the University of Toronto, and her MES from York University. For more than 30 years, Beth has taught nursing students at the baccalaureate level. She has also been a mentor to Masters students. Her areas of specialty are pathophysiology and epidemiology. Beth has also developed innovative Distance Education courses for RNs returning to university to pursue their degree. Research interests include differences in student learning between online and in-class teaching. Beth was for many years a board member of the Lambda-Pi Chapter-At-Large of Sigma Theta Tau International. She has served on the steering committee and the board of the National Immunization Education Initiative since 2003. In 2005, Beth received an award for teaching excellence in the faculty of Community Services. Beth has worked as a reviewer and author for Elsevier since 2004.

Reviewers

LINDA HOPPER COOK, RN, MN, PhD (Cand)
Faculty Member
Grant MacEwan College
Edmonton, Alberta

MARGARET HADLEY, RN, MN
Instructor
Grant MacEwan College
Edmonton, Alberta

MARGARET JOHNS, RegN, BScN, MScN (Cand)
Professor of Nursing
Northern College of Applied Arts and Technology
Schumacher, Ontario

LORI LABATTE, RN, BED, BScN
Faculty, Nursing Department
SIAST, Wascana Campus
Regina, Saskatchewan

KEN RENTON, PhD
Professor, Department of Pharmacology
Dalhousie University
Halifax, Nova Scotia

LINDA VON TETTENBORN, RN, BSc(Nu), MSN, Adv Dipl
Health Science
(Critical Care–Cardiac Surgery)
Faculty Member, Bachelor of Science in Nursing Program
Faculty of Health Sciences
Douglas College
New Westminster, British Columbia

BARBARA TURNER, RN, MN
Acting Associate Director, Curriculum
Western Regional School of Nursing
Corner Brook, Newfoundland

ANN-MARIE URBAN, RN, BSN, MN
Faculty, Nursing Education Program of Saskatchewan
SIAST, Wascana Campus
Regina, Saskatchewan

Preface

INTRODUCTION

This is the first edition of *Pharmacology and the Nursing Process in Canada*. This text provides the most current and clinically relevant information in an appealing, understandable, and practical format. The accessible size, readable writing style, and full-colour design are ideal for today's busy nursing student. This text takes a unique approach to the study of pharmacology by presenting study skills that will help students understand and learn this particularly demanding subject. Each part begins with a Study Skills Tips section, which features a discussion of researched and proven study skills and applies the discussion to the content in that part. Students are encouraged to use research-based study skills to enhance their study of pharmacology and nursing.

MARKET RESEARCH

The original authors incorporated suggestions from focus group participants composed of nursing instructors from 2-, 3-, and 4-year degree programs across the United States. These focus groups assessed changes that had occurred in the teaching of pharmacology and determined what was needed to better teach pharmacology to nursing students. Based on faculty descriptions of their courses and students, these general recommendations were made:

- Accommodate the reading styles and abilities of the growing number of non-traditional nursing students.
- Increase the use of tables, boxes, illustrations, graphics, and other visually oriented approaches.
- Use colour to increase interest and highlight important drug interactions and processes.

The Canadian edition maintains this philosophy of making a difficult subject approachable and easy to understand. A collaborative approach has been taken with this text. Many concerns raised by reviewers have been addressed, as have additional improvements suggested by faculty members who served as reviewers or consultants, either formally or informally, throughout the manuscript's development and by the author and editors of this text.

ORGANIZATION

This book includes 57 chapters presented in 10 parts organized by body system. The nine concept chapters in Part One lay a solid foundation for the subsequent drug units and address the following topics:

- Study skills applied to learning pharmacology
- The nursing process and drug therapy
- Pharmacological principles
- Lifespan considerations related to pharmacology
- Legal, ethical, and cultural considerations
- Medication errors: preventing and responding
- Client education and drug therapy
- Over-the-counter drugs and natural health products
- Substance use problems
- Photo atlas of medication administration techniques, including more than 100 illustrations

Parts Two through Ten present pharmacology and nursing management in a traditional body systems/drug function framework. This approach facilitates learning by grouping functionally related drugs and drug groups. It provides an effective means to integrate the content into medical-surgical or adult health nursing courses or for teaching pharmacology in a separate course.

The 48 drug chapters in these parts constitute the main portion of the book. Drugs are presented in a consistent format with an emphasis on drug groups and key similarities and differences among the drugs in each group. Each chapter is subdivided into two discussions; these begin with a complete, clear discussion of pharmacology, followed by a comprehensive yet succinct discussion of the nursing process. Pharmacology is presented for each drug group in a consistent format:

- Mechanism of Action and Drug Effects
- Indications
- Contraindications
- Side Effects and Adverse Effects
  - Toxicity and Management of Overdose
- Interactions
- Dosages

Drug group discussions are followed by Drug Profiles, or brief narrative capsules of individual drugs in the class or group, including Pharmacokinetics tables for each drug. Key drugs, or prototypical drugs within a class, are identified with the ➤➤ symbol for easy identification. These individual drug profiles are followed by a Nursing Process discussion relating to the entire drug group. The nursing content is covered in the following functional, six-step nursing process format:

- Assessment
- Nursing Diagnoses
- Planning
- Outcome Criteria
- Implementation
- Evaluation

At the end of each nursing process section is a Client Teaching Tips box that summarizes key points to cover in educating the client about the uses and effects of drugs within a given group. The role of the nurse as client educator continues to grow in importance, so this text emphasizes this key content.

Each part begins with a Study Skills Tips section that presents a study skills topic and relates it to the unit being discussed. Topics include time management, note taking, studying, test taking, and others. This unique approach to teaching pharmacology is intended to aid students who find pharmacology difficult and to provide a tool that may prove beneficial throughout their nursing education. Coverage of this study skills content is limited to the beginning of each part so that instructors who choose not to require their students to read this material can easily eliminate it. However, this arrangement of content may be beneficial to faculty members who teach pharmacology through an integrated approach because it helps the student identify key content and concepts. This arrangement also facilitates location of content for either required or optional reading.

Most importantly, the pharmacology and nursing content reflects the latest drug information and research. This includes current information on bioterrorism agents, the threat of avian flu, genetics, and hypertension, as well as drugs to treat HIV/AIDS, psychiatric conditions, diabetes, osteoporosis, Alzheimer's disease, cancer, infection, and much more. In addition to this, the following items are included:

- The **Student Pharmacology CD-ROM** features 400 multiple-choice review questions, pharmacology animations, and printable checklists on IV drug therapy and preventing medication errors.
- **Chapter 5: Medication Errors: Preventing and Responding** discusses the scope of the medication errors problem, specific nursing measures to prevent medication errors, possible consequences of medication errors to nurses, responses to errors, reporting and learning from mistakes, and other ethical issues.
- **Chapter 9: Photo Atlas of Medication Administration** provides an extensive coverage of drug admin-

istration routes and more than 100 full-colour illustrations.
- **Chapter 48: Gene Therapy and Pharmacogenomics** provides an overview of some major concepts in genetics, including genetic influences on disease and the development of gene-based therapies.
- **Natural Health Products** boxes cover commonly used natural health products, including Overview, Common Uses, Adverse Effects, Potential Drug Interactions, and Contraindications.

NEW TO THE CANADIAN EDITION

Pharmacology and the Nursing Process in Canada incorporates chapter-specific Canadian content that will ensure relevance to Canadian students and instructors and strengthen their knowledge of the field.

- Text refers to evidence-based (research-based) Canadian clinical practice guidelines produced or endorsed in Canada by a national, provincial, or territorial medical or health organization, or by a professional society, government agency or expert panel.
- Only generic drug names are used within the body of the text to promote the use of generic drug names in practice. Appendix B at the back of the book provides an extensive list of Canadian generic names and trade name equivalents.
- Ethnocultural examples reflect the varied and complex ethnodemographic diversity of Canada.

FEATURES

This book includes various pedagogical features that prepare the student for important content covered in each chapter and encourage review and reinforcement of that content. Chapter opener pedagogy includes the following:

- Learning Objectives
- e-Learning Activities box listing related content and exercises on the Student Pharmacology CD and Evolve Web site
- Summary box listing the Drug Profiles in the chapter with page number references
- Glossary of key terms with pronunciations and definitions

Glossary terms are bolded in the narrative to emphasize this essential terminology. In addition, included in Appendix C is a list of glossary terms with page numbers for quick reference.

The following features appear at the end of each chapter:

- *Client Teaching Tips* specific to the drug class or topic
- *Points to Remember* boxes summarizing key points
- *Examination Review Questions*, with answers provided on the Evolve Web site
- *Critical Thinking Activities*, with answers provided on the Evolve Web site
- Bibliography listing references for more information

Special features that appear throughout the text include the following:

- *Ethnocultural Implications* boxes
- *Community Health Points* boxes
- *Natural Health Product* boxes
- *Legal and Ethical Principles* boxes
- *Geriatric and Pediatric Considerations* boxes
- *Case Studies*, with answers provided on the Evolve Web site
- *Research* boxes
- Case-based *Nursing Care Plans* applying pharmacology to the nursing process
- Alphabetized *Dosages* tables listing drug generic names, pharmacological class, usual dosage ranges, and indications

For a more comprehensive listing of the special features, please refer to the final pages of the book.

An additional special feature in this book is the separate *Disorders Index* that references disorders in the text. This unique feature aids in integrating the text with medical-surgical or adult health nursing course content.

COLOUR

The first American edition of this book was the first full-colour pharmacology text for nursing students. Faculty members had suggested that colour be used in both a functionally and visually appealing manner to more fully engage students in this demanding yet important content. Full colour is used throughout this Canadian edition to do the following:

- Highlight important content
- Illustrate how drugs work in the body in numerous anatomic and drug process colour figures
- Improve the visual appearance of the content to make it more engaging and appealing to today's more visually sophisticated reader

The use of colour in these ways should significantly improve students' involvement and understanding of pharmacology.

SUPPLEMENTAL RESOURCES

A comprehensive ancillary package is available to students and instructors using *Pharmacology and the Nursing Process in Canada*. The following supplemental resources have been thoroughly revised and can significantly assist in the teaching and learning of pharmacology:

Study Guide

The carefully prepared student workbook includes the following:

- Study Tips Guide that reinforces the study skills explained in the text and provides a "how to" guide to applying test-taking strategies
- Chapter worksheets with a variety of learning activities, including multiple-choice questions, review exercises, critical thinking questions, and crossword puzzles
- In-depth case studies followed by related critical thinking questions
- A special Drug Calculations Overview with helpful tips for calculating doses, sample drug labels, practice problems, and a quiz
- Answers to all questions provided in the back of the book to enable self-study

Evolve Web site

Located at http://evolve.elsevier.com/Lilley/pharmacology/, the Evolve Web site for this book includes the following:

- Online Student Worksheets for each chapter, including answers, to provide additional review of challenging content and important concepts
- A variety of supplemental resources, including a list of Canadian trade names and generic equivalents; information on poisons and antidotes; and common formulas, weights, and equivalents
- Frequently Asked Questions, Content Updates, Learning Tips, and Teaching Tips
- An updated library of pharmacology WebLinks
- Answers to the Case Studies, Examination Review Questions, and Critical Thinking Activities in the textbook
- Bonus medication administration animations

Instructor's Resource (CD-ROM)

This CD product includes the following main components:

- Instructor's Manual, including Chapter Overviews, Key Terms, Chapter Outlines, Teaching Tips and Strategies, and open-book quizzes
- Test Bank with over 500 multiple-choice formatted questions coded for cognitive level, nursing process step, and client need categories. All answers include rationales. The test bank is provided in the user-friendly ExamView program, which allows the instructor to create new tests; edit, add, and delete test questions; sort questions by cognitive level; and administer and grade online tests.
- Image Collection with approximately 300 full-colour images from the book. The images can be viewed, printed, or imported into PowerPoint®.

PowerPoint® Presentations

This online product is available to instructors through the Evolve Web site. The expanded and updated presentations feature lecture outlines covering every chapter in the textbook. These outlines can be customized by adding or deleting text, as well as images from the Image Collection.

Mosby/Saunders ePharmacology Update

This online publication is available free to students who purchase and instructors who adopt this text. Released twice each semester, this newsletter helps students and instructors keep up to date on the latest new drugs, indications, warnings, and precautions. It also includes helpful questions and answers, information on common medication errors, and updates on herbal remedies.

Mosby's Drug Consult Internet Edition

Students and faculty members using this book are provided with basic-level access to this comprehensive database of the most current, unbiased, accurate, and reliable drug information available. It provides drug updates, free information on the top 200 drugs by prescription, and Online Extras, including new drug approvals, safety notices, new drug indications, and links to pharmaceutical manufacturers for more information.

Acknowledgements

My part in this book would not have been possible without the original efforts of the American authors who conceptualized and wrote the first four U.S. editions of *Pharmacology and the Nursing Process*, the fourth edition of which forms the core of *Pharmacology and the Nursing Process in Canada*. Linda Lane Lilley, RN, PhD; Scott Harrington, PharmD; and Julie S. Snyder, MSN, RN, C are to be commended for their thorough and expert handling of a vast and complex subject matter, and creating an excellent textbook over which the Canadian content could be easily laid.

I dedicate *Pharmacology and the Nursing Process in Canada* to my sons, Jeffrey I. and Derk, who are my strength; I could not have met the challenges of editing this pharmacology textbook without their support and understanding. To my students, both past and present, who are a never-ending source of inspiration and who constantly challenge me to make material relevant, fun, and interesting, I give heartfelt thanks for inspiring my writing in this book. I could not have accomplished the deadlines without the assistance of May Look, Developmental Editor, whose quirky sense of humour, dedication, attention to detail, and subtle reminders about deadlines kept me on track and made the task almost enjoyable! Many individuals at Elsevier Canada are responsible for this first Canadian edition. Thanks to Ann Millar, Publisher, who provided encouragement and ongoing support; Kim Armstrong, Editorial Assistant, who responded almost immediately to all my calls for help, pointed me in the right direction, and shared her love of chocolate; Martina van de Velde, Managing Developmental Editor; Tricia Carmichael, Project Manager, for handling all the details involved in the final production of the book; and, finally, Brenda Kirkconnell, Senior Sales Representative and Electronic Product Specialist, for her encouragement and friendship.

Thanks are also due to the Canadian reviewers who reviewed both the Canadian and U.S. content of this book and gave their invaluable comments, expertise, and editing suggestions on the draft manuscript.

As existing diseases and disorders and their treatments evolve, bringing with them new challenges and information in pharmacology, we will no doubt be looking forward to future editions of this textbook. Instructors and students are welcome to send comments to the publisher; your feedback will be invaluable to future editions.

Beth Swart

Contents

PART ONE

Pharmacology Basics: Study Skills Tips

- INTRODUCTION TO STUDY SKILLS CONCEPTS
- PURR
- PHARMACOLOGY BASICS

INTRODUCTION TO STUDY SKILLS CONCEPTS

What to study? When to study? How much to study? How to study? In the best of worlds, every student would have all the skills necessary to be effective in all academic areas. Unfortunately, many students do not know how to study effectively or have developed techniques that work well in some circumstance but not in others. The purpose of this Study Skills Tips is to introduce you to the steps to follow in learning text and maintaining focus on the appropriate material. This section also offers some specific examples for selected chapters in Part One to help you apply the study techniques and strategies discussed here.

Extensive study skills covering time management, note taking, mastering of the text, preparation for and taking of examinations, and development of vocabulary are presented in the *Study Guide* that accompanies this text. These tools are important to any student, but even more valuable in challenging technical areas such as nursing and pharmacology. The techniques described here and in the *Study Guide* will not necessarily make learning easy, but they will help you achieve your goals as a student.

PURR

PURR is a handy mnemonic device representing a four-step process that will lead to mastery of material:

- *Prepare*
- *Understand*
- *Rehearse*
- *Review*

PURR has positive and negative aspects. The negative is that it requires that you go through every chapter four times. The good news is that you are not going to actually *read* the chapter four times. You are only going to *go through* it four times. Only one of those times is a slow, careful, intensive reading. The other trips through the chapter are much quicker. The first time you go through the chapter should only take 5 or 10 minutes. Each time you go through the chapter, you are processing the information in distinctly different ways. The PURR approach will enhance your learning, and if you use it from the first assignment on, you will find that it takes you less time than you were spending before you adopted the PURR approach to learn what you need.

Prepare

Reading the text, like any complex process, is not something to dive into without thought and planning. *Pharmacology and the Nursing Process* is organized to help you learn the material, but you have to take advantage of what the authors have done for you to facilitate this. Preparing to read means setting goals and objectives for your own learning, but the tools you need to help you do this are already in place. Look at the opening pages of any chapter in the text and you will see a standard structure.

Every chapter begins with a **title.** Learn to use the title as the first step in preparing to learn. Chapter 4 is entitled "Legal, Ethical, and Ethnocultural Considerations." This instantly identifies what the chapter is about. Do not start reading immediately; instead think about the title for a few seconds. Are there any unfamiliar terms? If your answer is "no," great. If it is "yes," then you already have some focus for your reading because you know you will need to learn the unfamiliar terms and their meanings.

The next feature of every chapter is the **objectives.** You need objectives for learning, and the authors have anticipated this. Read the objectives actively. Do not just look at the words; think about the objectives. Ask yourself the following questions: What do I already know about this material? How do these objectives relate to earlier assignments? How do they relate to objectives the instructor has given? The chapter objectives identify things you should be able to do after you have read the material. Do not wait until you have read the chapter to start trying to respond. *Prepare* means getting the brain engaged from the beginning. Studying the chapter objectives establishes a direction and purpose for your reading. This will enable you to maintain concentration and focus while you read.

Another feature in the opening pages of each chapter is the **glossary.** This is one of the most valuable tools the authors have provided. They know that there are many terms to learn and are giving you a head start on learning them. Spend a few minutes with the glossary. Notice the terms that are also used in the chapter objectives. Go back and look at the objectives and think about what you have learned from the glossary. As you study the glossary, look for shared root words, prefixes, or suffixes. Words that share common elements usually also have a shared meaning. Learning the meaning of common word elements can simplify the whole process of learning vocabulary. Perhaps you remember in elementary school being told to "look for the little words in the big word." This is essentially the same technique—one that worked then and that will work now.

Now make a quick pass through the chapter or the assigned pages from the chapter. Focus on the text conventions, which are described later in this chapter. Look for anything that stands out in the chapter, such as boldfaced text, boxed material, and tables. This provides a quick overview of the chapter, which will make the next steps in the PURR process much more effective and efficient.

The **chapter headings** show the major points to be covered. Study them and notice the major headings (topics) and the subordinate headings (subtopics). This is essentially a picture of the chapter, and using the picture is an essential step in preparing to read. As you read through the chapter headings, turn the topic and subtopics into a series of questions that you want to be able to answer when you finish reading. Think about the objectives and how these headings relate to them. Finally, in the headings devoted to specific classes of agents, notice there are elements that are common to every one. The last two headings are always "Implementation" and "Evaluation." This tells you that these are two common elements you will be expected to know at the end of every chapter. The minutes you spend *preparing* will pay off in a big way when you start to read.

Preparing makes the whole approach to learning an active one. It may not make the chapters the most exciting reading you will ever do, but it will help you accomplish your personal learning objectives as well as those set by the authors.

On-the-run Action. Preparing is great to do during "found" time. It should not take more than 5 or 10 minutes. Time between classes, time spent waiting for the coffee water to boil, or any other small block of time that usually just slips away can be used to accomplish this step.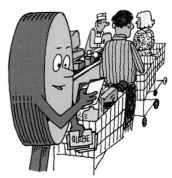

Understand

The time has now come to read the assignment. Go to your desk, the library, or wherever you have chosen for serious study. Reading the assignment is where all your preparation pays off. If you did the *Prepare* step earlier in the day, it is not a bad idea to spend a minute or two going through the chapter features again to get your focus. As you read the assignment, remember the chapter objectives and notice the chapter headings in the body of the chapter. As you read, rephrase the chapter headings as questions to help keep you focused on the task at hand. Because this is the first time you are really focusing on the concepts and the details, this is not the time to do any text notations. Read and, as you read, think. Terms from the glossary are repeated, and their meanings are often expanded and clarified in the body of the text. Pay attention to these terms as you read. Think about what they mean and how you would define them to someone else. Read for meaning. Read to *understand*. Do not read just to get to the end of the assignment. That is a passive action. Ask yourself questions. Analyze, respond, and react as you read.

Often reading assignments are too long to be read with complete understanding in one session. If you find that your concentration is flagging or you do not remember anything you read on the previous page, it is time to take a break. All too often students have only one objective—to finish the assignment. You might be able to force yourself to continue reading, but you will not learn much. Mark your place and take a 5- or 10-minute break. Take a walk, read the daily comic strips, get a cold drink or a cup of coffee, and then go back to reading. When you come back to the assignment, spend the first 3 or 4 minutes reviewing. Look back at the previous chapter heading and think about what you were reading before the break. The chapter can be broken down into many small reading sessions, but it is critical that you do not lose sight of the chapter as a whole. Spending these minutes in review may seem like time that could be better spent continuing with the reading, but this quick review will save time in the long run.

There is no quick way to read a chapter. You will not find an "on-the-run action" for this step because it cannot be done in this way. However, if you do the *Prepare* step first, you will be surprised at how much more easily you get the reading done and how much more learning you have achieved in the process.

Rehearse

Rehearsing is the third step in the process. It starts the process of consolidating your learning and establishing a basis for long-term memory. Rehearsal accomplishes two things. First, it helps you find out what you understand from the reading. Knowing what you know is really important. Second, it identifies what you do not understand, and this may be an even more important benefit. Knowing what you do not know before it comes to light during an examination is critical.

How to Rehearse. Everything you do in the *Prepare* and *Understand* steps comes into play in the *Rehearse* step. Rehearsal should begin with the features at the beginning of the chapter. Open the text to the beginning of the chapter. Start with the chapter title and begin to quiz yourself on what you have read. Compose three or four questions pertaining to the chapter title, and then try to answer them to your satisfaction. The questions you ask yourself should be both literal (asking for specific information presented in the chapter) and interpretive (testing your comprehension of concepts and relationships). An example of a literal question using the Chapter 4 title might be, "What are the definitions of *legal, ethical,* and *ethnocultural?*" This question would help you determine whether you can satisfactorily define these terms in your own words. Asking and answering such questions as this always serves to move learning from short-term to long-term memory. Literal questions are important to help you grasp the factual information and terminology contained in the reading assignment. However, it is

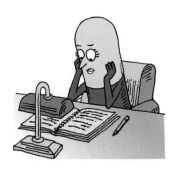

also necessary to ask questions that stimulate thought about the concepts and the relationships between the facts and concepts presented in the chapter. An example of an interpretive question regarding the Chapter 4 title might be: "What are the most important legal, ethical, and ethnocultural concepts pertaining to the use of drugs?" Sometimes you will find that, even though the question is interpretive, the authors have anticipated the question and the text does contain the direct answer to your question. Other times you will need to formulate your own response by pulling together bits and pieces of information from the entire reading assignment.

Once you have exhausted the question potential for the chapter title, move on to the chapter objectives. Use the same process here. Rephrase the objectives as questions and try to answer them. Remember that the object of rehearsal is to reinforce what you have learned and to identify areas where you need to spend additional time (review).

Go to the glossary. Cover the definitions, and try to define each term in your own words. Another method is to cover the term, and on the basis of the definition, name the term. Do not just memorize the definition, because you may find the information presented differently on an examination, and you will then be unable to respond.

Now proceed to the chapter or assigned pages. The chapter headings are the main tools for rehearsal. Apply the same question-and-answer technique used for the title and objectives to test what you may already know about the chapter content. Turn the headings into questions and answer them. Look at the text for boldfaced and italicized items, lists, and other text conventions. These too can become the basis for questions. The tables and diagrams should also be used for this purpose. Keep in mind the importance of asking both literal and interpretive questions. Some of the questions you ask yourself should also tie different topic headings together. Ask yourself how topic A relates to topic B.

As you proceed through the chapter, do not worry if you cannot answer the questions you ask. As stated earlier, one of the goals of the rehearsal process is to identify what you need to spend more time on. If you can give no response to a particular question, put a mark in 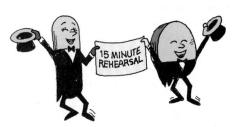 the margin of the pertinent place in the text to remind yourself to come back and spend more time on this material, but move on at this point. Rehearsal should be a relatively quick procedure. Once you become accustomed to the PURR method, it should take no more than 15 or 20 minutes to rehearse 15 pages after doing the *Prepare* and *Understand* steps.

As you reach the end of the chapter, skim the *Implementation* and *Evaluation* sections. Make sure that the relationship between these sections and the information in the rest of the chapter is clear. If you have questions or concerns, note them in the margins and ask your instructor to clarify these points. Although the objective is to master the chapter content as an independent learner, sometimes it is essential to ask questions of the instructor to facilitate the process.

When to Rehearse. Ideally rehearsal should take place almost immediately after you finish reading the material. Take a 10- to 15-minute break, and then start the process. The longer the gap between reading and rehearsal, the more you will forget and the longer it will take to rehearse. If you are breaking a reading assignment down into smaller segments, do the rehearsal for each segment before you begin reading the new material. This helps maintain the sense of continuity in the chapter. This seems like a lot of work to do in a study session, but with practice it will go quickly and you will be pleasantly surprised at the quality and quantity of your learning.

Review

Review is the fourth and final step in the PURR process, and it is an essential step. No matter how well you have learned material in the preceding steps, forgetting will always occur. Reviewing is the only way to store what you have learned in long-term memory. The good news is that, using the PURR model, the review can be done for small segments of material and can be done relatively quickly.

How to Review. The basic review process is essentially the same as the rehearsal process, with some limited rereading as the only difference. When you cannot immediately answer a question, read the pertinent material again. *This does not mean you should read the entire chapter again.* Often the answer to the question will pop into your mind after you have read only a few lines. When this happens, stop reading and go back to responding to your question. The idea is to reread only as much material as is necessary to make the answer clear. One or two words or one or two sentences may trigger personal recall, but it may also take two or three paragraphs for this to happen.

Frequency of Review. How many times should you review material in this way? This actually depends on many factors, such as the difficulty of the material, the length of the assignment, and your personal background. Only you can determine how often you need to review, but some guidelines will help you decide this for yourself.

First, consider the difficulty of the material. If it is complex, contains many new terms and difficult concepts, and seems difficult to grasp, then you should review frequently. On the other hand, if the material is straightforward and you are able to relate it well to what you have already learned, then less frequent reviews will serve to keep the material in your memory.

Second, consider how well the review went. If you had difficulty answering many questions to your satisfaction or had to do a lot of rereading, you should schedule another review soon (a day or two later at most).

Use the success of each review session to help you determine when to schedule another session. The review step is a means of monitoring the success of the learning process. If reviews go well, limited rereading is necessary, and you are able to give clear answers to your questions, this tells you that you can wait several days (4 or 5) before reviewing this material again. A mediocre review, more extensive rereading, and poor answers indicate that you should only let 2 or 3 days go by before reviewing the material again. If the review goes poorly, you should plan to review the material again the next day. It is up to you to judge the success of each review and to decide how often you need to review. The nice thing about PURR is that it enables you to monitor your success and to easily regulate the learning process.

Technique for Rehearsal and Review. Both rehearsal and review foster active learning, which helps you maintain interest in the material and strengthens your memory. For these benefits to occur, it is essential to review and rehearse orally. Simply talk aloud as you go through the material. Ask questions and give your answers out loud. This forces you to think about the material. It helps you organize it and translate it into your own words. The object is not to memorize everything you have read but to understand and be able to explain it. Eventually you will need to answer questions on an examination. Framing questions as a part of the learning process is a way to anticipate examination questions. The more questions you ask yourself during study time, the more likely it is that some of the questions on the examination will be ones you have asked yourself. Further, by doing the rehearsal and review orally, you will find it easier to recall the answers during the examination, because this oral model requires more than just remembering seeing the material; you will actually be able to hear the rehearsed answers in your mind. Another advantage of doing the rehearsal and review processes orally is, as stated earlier, that it helps to identify what needs further study. When your oral answer is fragmentary, contains many "uhs," and is really disorganized, then you know that you need to devote more time to learning this term, fact, or concept.

The PURR system may seem like a lot of work at first. The idea of going through a chapter four times understandably seems daunting. Add to this the need for several review sessions, and the first reaction is likely to be: "This won't work," or "I don't have the time to do this." Don't take that attitude. This system does work. It cultivates interest, aids concentration, fosters mastery of the material, and ensures long-term memory of the material, which is important not just for doing well on examinations but also for doing well as a nurse with the safe care of clients at stake. The PURR system will work if you use it. It may take 3 or 4 weeks to get comfortable with the system, but if you keep at it, pretty soon it will become a good habit. After a while you will not be able to imagine studying in any other way.

Like all study systems, the PURR method is a model. As you use it, you may discover ways of changing it that work better for you. That is okay. Do not hesitate to make adjustments that better suit your learning style and strategies. Just remember as you start out that *Preparation, Understanding, Rehearsal,* and *Review* are solid learning principles and cannot be ignored.

Study skills tips are included on the two pages at the beginning of each part. These hints are directly applied to the con- 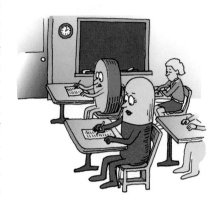 tent found within the chapters of the following unit. Detailed information on specialized study skills, such as time management, note taking, examination preparation, and vocabulary building, are present in the *Study Guide* that accompanies this text.

PHARMACOLOGY BASICS

Prepare

As you begin to work with individual chapters, consider how the first step in the PURR system can be used to help you set a purpose and become an active learner.

Chapter 1 Objectives

Consider Objective 1. *List the five phases of the nursing process as applicable to drug therapy.* Now turn the objective into a question. *What are the five phases of the nursing process?* Now move to Objective 2 and make it a question. *What are the components of the assessment process for clients receiving medications, including collection of subjective and objective data?* You might recognize that this question relates to Objective 1 because assessment is one phase of the nursing process. By putting Objective 2 into a question format you will begin to expand and extend on the focus of the first objective, and you will begin to focus on active learning with a clear purpose.

When you begin to read Chapter 1 you will discover that the five phases of the nursing process are repeated as topic headings, and you have the Objective 2 question on which to focus your reading. Begin now to develop the habit of applying this strategy to the objectives in every chapter assigned before you begin to read. Remember to look at the chapter headings at this point as well. It is amazing how much can be learned by using the text structures provided.

Vocabulary Development

Turn to Chapter 2. Objective 1 makes an important point. "Define common terms used in pharmacology." Success depends heavily on knowledge of the "language." The objective makes it clear that this chapter contains a number of terms that the author views as important to be mastered. This is only Chapter 2, and now is the time to be-

gin to apply yourself to mastering the language of this content. Look at the glossary. There are six terms that share the common element *pharmaco.* Although each of these six words will have different meanings, they will have something in common. *Pharmaco* is an example of a group word. No matter what prefixes, group words, and/or suffixes are added to it, a part of the meaning of any word containing *pharmaco* will be "drug" or "medicine." Look up *pharmaco* in any dictionary and you will find "drug" or "medicine" to be the definition. Although you probably already knew that, it is always beneficial to start working on a new technique with something that is familiar. Look at four of the words that begin with *pharmaco,* and consider the rest of the word:

dynamics   genetics   gnosy   kinetics

What do each of these word parts mean? The meaning of *pharmacodynamics* is simply the combination of the meaning of *pharmaco* and *dynamics.* The definition, according to the glossary, begins, "the study of the biochemical and physiological interactions of drugs." You could simply memorize this definition, which would seem to accomplish Objective 1. However, memorization does not always equal understanding. Try another approach. What does *dynamics* mean? Think about the word, and relate it to your own experience and background. It appears to deal with movement or action. After looking it up in the dictionary, all the meanings given seem to relate in some fashion to the idea of motion and/or action. A simplistic definition of *pharmacodynamics* would be "drugs in action." Certainly this is not a technical or medical definition, but it contributes a great deal to an un- 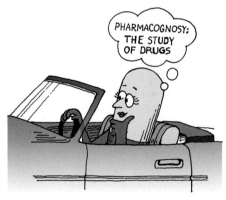 derstanding of the definition provided in the glossary. This is the object of learning vocabulary. Do not memorize words without understanding. Apply a little thought, and relate the term and definition in a way that makes the meaning personal for you. When you do that, you will find that you understand the glossary definition better, and your ability to retain the meaning will be significantly improved. This means that the test item that asks you to select the definition for *pharmacodynamics* from a list of similar definitions will be much easier, because you will remember action and movement and look for the choice that best represents that concept.

Apply this same strategy to *genetics.* You already know what genetics means. Now you must determine how to connect that to the meaning in the text. After you have the definitions of *gnosy* and *kinetics,* you can apply the same procedure. When you have done this with all four words, you will discover that you will not need to spend a great amount of time trying to memorize esoteric definitions. You will have personalized the meanings. Those meanings will stay with you much more readily than those learned by rote memorization. By the way, do you know what *biochemical* and *physiological* mean? These terms are used in the glossary definition of *pharmacodynamics.* You need to know what they mean to fully understand pharmacodynamics.

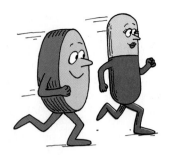

The Nursing Process and Drug Therapy

OBJECTIVES

After reading this chapter, the successful student will be able to do the following:

1 List the five phases of the nursing process as applicable to drug therapy.

2 Identify the components of the assessment process for clients receiving medications, including the collection of subjective and objective data.

3 Discuss the process of formulating nursing diagnoses for clients receiving medications.

4 Identify goals and outcome criteria as related to clients receiving medications.

5 Discuss the evaluation process as it relates to the administration of medications.

6 Apply all phases of the nursing process to the drug administration process.

7 Briefly discuss the "5 Rights" of drug administration and the professional responsibility to clients for safe medication practice.

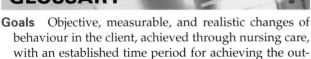

e-LEARNING ACTIVITIES

Student CD-ROM
- Review Questions: see questions 1–3
- Animations
- Medication Administration Checklists
- IV Therapy Checklists

evolve **Web site** (http://evolve.elsevier.com/Lilley/ pharmacology/)
- Online Chapter Worksheet • Frequently Asked Questions
- Learning Tips and Content Updates • WebLinks • Online Appendices and Supplements • Mosby/Saunders ePharmacology Update • Access to *Mosby's Drug Consult*

GLOSSARY

Goals Objective, measurable, and realistic changes of behaviour in the client, achieved through nursing care, with an established time period for achieving the outcome.

Medication error (ME) Failure to complete a planned action as it was intended, or when an incorrect plan is used, at any point in the process of providing medications to clients.

Nursing process An organizational framework for the practice of nursing. It encompasses all steps taken by the nurse in caring for a client: assessment, nursing di-

agnosis, planning (with outcome criteria), implementation of the plan (with client teaching), and evaluation. The rationale for each step is founded on nursing theory.

Outcome criteria Descriptions of client goals that are succinct and well thought out. They include behavioural expectations to be met by specific deadlines and are always developed with the ultimate goal of client safety.

OVERVIEW

The **nursing process** is central to all nursing care. It is flexible, adaptable, and adjustable to numerous situations, including the administration of medications. The nursing process has five specific phases: assessment, nursing diagnoses, planning (with **goals** and **outcome criteria**), implementation, and evaluation. Box 1-1 provides an example of the application of the nursing process to a particular client care situation and its specific use in the administration of medications.

ASSESSMENT

During the assessment phase of the nursing process, subjective and objective data on the client, drug, and environment are collected. The information on the client and

BOX 1-1
Nursing Process: Client Care and Medication Administration

Client Care Situation and the Nursing Process
Assessment
Objective Data
- 43-year-old Black male
- Family history of diabetes mellitus
- Vital signs within normal limits (BP 130/70, R20, P84)
- Fasting blood glucose 13.3 mmol/L
- Diminished pedal pulses

Subjective Data
Complains of frequent urination, increase in thirst, weight loss, headache, lethargy, confusion.

Nursing Diagnosis
Impaired urinary elimination (frequency) related to possible pathophysiological changes from diabetes mellitus, as evidenced by frequent trips to bathroom at night.

Planning/Outcome Criteria
Goal
Client will regain normal urinary patterns.

Outcome Criteria
Client will awaken to void no more than once per night and void per usual routine during the day.

Implementation
- Monitor fasting blood glucose as ordered and as deemed necessary.
- Monitor fluid intake and output daily for excessive output or any other imbalance.
- Assess skin turgor daily.
- Assess pre-illness urinary elimination patterns.
- Educate client about the disease process and management of symptoms once therapy is initiated.

Evaluation
- Sleeping most of the night; only gets up once during the night to void for the last few weeks since treatment.
- Has regained normal urinary patterns during the day, as noted by voiding in regular intervals (six times per day).

Medication Administration and the Nursing Process
Assessment
Objective Data
- 43-year-old male
- Recent diagnosis of type 1 diabetes mellitus
- New insulin regimen of rapid-acting (regular) and intermediate-acting (NPH) brands
- No history of previous illnesses
- No other health problems

Subjective Data
- States "uneasy with treatment plan"
- States "knows little about diabetes mellitus, its treatment and complications"
- States "fearful of giving self-injections"

Nursing Diagnosis
Deficient knowledge related to newly diagnosed diabetes mellitus and new treatment regimen with insulin, as evidenced by voicing fears and anxieties and asking many questions.

Planning/Outcome Criteria
Goal
Client adheres to new insulin treatment regimen without complications.

Outcome Criteria
- Client will state reasons for taking insulin therapy to help regulate blood sugars.
- Client will state importance of daily glucometer testing to maintain consistent blood sugar levels.
- Client will state the signs and symptoms of hypoglycemia and means of treatment.
- Client understands importance of follow-up with physician for close monitoring.
- Client demonstrates safe "drawing-up" of insulin and injection technique with rotation of sites of injection.

Implementation
- Educate client and family about diabetes mellitus, its treatment with insulin, and side effects of therapy.
- Use audiovisual aids, films, pamphlets for education about insulin therapy, injection sites, and storage.
- Monitor glucose levels as ordered.
- Assess client's response to diagnosis of diabetes mellitus and to its treatment.
- "5 Rights": right dose, right drug, right time, right client, right route.

Evaluation
- Has normal glucose levels and monitors blood sugar levels daily with glucometer.
- Able to continue insulin therapy at home.
- Has minimal-to-no complications related to insulin therapy.
- Able to treat signs and symptoms of hypoglycemia, should they occur.

BP, Blood pressure; *R,* respirations; *P,* pulse.

environment may be collected from the client, family, or significant other. Data regarding the drug may be collected from authoritative sources such as a current (less than 5 years old) reference textbook like the *Compendium of Pharmaceuticals and Specialties* (CPS; a subscription-based e-CPS is also available online), drug manufacturer's insert, drug handbook, licensed pharmacist, or reliable online resources such as Health Canada's Drug Product

Database (http://www.hc-sc.gc.ca/hpb/drugs-dpd/) or other Canadian Web sites such as http://www.rxfiles.ca/. All of the information obtained is synthesized and analyzed by the nurse so that appropriate nursing diagnoses and a plan of care may be developed.

Information regarding the client and environment (both objective and subjective) can be collected by completing a drug history, performing a nursing physical assessment, and creating a medication profile. Often nurses use standardized forms to collect this information. A drug history may include information such as the use of prescription and over-the-counter (OTC) medications, home remedies, and natural health products including vitamins and herbal and homeopathic treatments; intake of alcohol, tobacco, or caffeine; any current or prior use of street drugs (or illicit drug use); past and present health history; and family history. The nursing assessment should include a head-to-toe physical assessment and a collection of information in a holistic framework regarding religious preferences, health beliefs, socio-cultural profile, lifestyle, stressors, socio-economic status, educational level, motor skill abilities, cognitive ability, and sensory intactness (such as visual and hearing acuity). Objective data may be obtained through physical assessment and may include vital signs, weight, height, laboratory studies, and results of diagnostic tests. Creating a thorough medication profile is important to ensure clients' safe use of medications. The following list is an example of the type of information that would be collected:

- OTC medications (e.g., vitamins, dietary supplements, acetaminophen products [e.g., Tylenol], laxatives, cold preparations, sinus medications, antacids, acid reducers, antidiarrheals, minerals, elements)
- Prescription medications (e.g., birth control pills, hormone replacement therapy, drugs for sexual dysfunction)
- Street drugs (e.g., marijuana, cocaine, phencyclidine hydrochloride [PCP or "angel dust"], lysergic acid diethylamide [LSD], amphetamines, ecstasy, illegally obtained narcotics such as oxycontin)
- Natural health products including herbal and homeopathic substances, plant or animal extracts
- Problems with drug therapy in the past (e.g., allergies, adverse effects, side effects, diseases or injuries, organ pathology)
- Growth and development issues as related to the client's age and specific expectations (e.g., Erikson's stages) and tasks for each major age group

It is important for the nurse to have excellent interviewing skills to establish a therapeutic relationship with the client. Open-ended questions are more helpful in collecting thorough information than questions that may be answered with a simple "yes" or "no." Nurses can ask the client, significant other, caregiver, and others involved in the care of the client:

- What is the client's oral intake? How does the client tolerate fluids? Can the client swallow pills and liquids? If not, what difficulty does he or she have?
- What are the laboratory and diagnostic test values, such as renal and liver function studies, hemoglobin, hematocrit, and protein and albumin levels?
- What experiences has the client had with medicines, health-care professionals, or previous hospitalizations?
- What are the client's vital signs?

- What medications are ordered and what medications is the client already taking? How is the client taking and tolerating the medications?
- What emotional, physical, cognitive, ethnocultural, and socio-economic factors affect the client's drug therapy and the nursing process (for a holistic framework)?
- What are the drug's adverse effects, contraindications, appropriate dosages, routes of administration, toxicity, and/or any antidotes and therapeutic levels?
- What does the particular drug do? Is it really helping the client?
- What are the age-specific developmental concerns, issues, or implications related to the client?
- What are the client's ethnocultural origin and racial-ethnic group, and how do they influence drug therapy?

Information collection on the drug or medication must begin by obtaining a complete order from the physician or other licensed individual. The order contains the following six elements:

1 Client's name
2 Date order was written
3 Name of medication
4 Dosage (includes size, frequency, and number of doses)
5 Route of delivery
6 Signature of the prescriber

Once these six elements have been verified and transcribed appropriately, the medication should be researched. The use of a current drug handbook, pharmacology textbook, reference such as *Mosby's Drug Consult,* or other authoritative source is recommended for the review of drug information. Information to be reviewed includes classification, mechanism of action, dosage, routes, side effects, contraindications, drug incompatibilities, interactions, cautions, and nursing implications. If information is unavailable, the nurse may contact a registered pharmacist for information about the medication. The nurse should document the source of information, including the pharmacist's name. The nurse should never give a medication with which the nurse is unfamiliar until drug information has been researched and there is complete knowledge about its mechanism of action, cautions, contraindications, drug and/or food interactions, dosage ranges, and routes of administration. The nurse should always assess thoroughly by completing data collection about the client and the drug.

It is important during the assessment phase of the nursing process to consider the expanded and collaborative role of the nurse. Physicians and dentists are no longer the only health-care professionals prescribing and writing medication orders. Nurse practitioners have also gained the professional privilege of legally prescribing medications. Nurses should always be aware of and obtain a copy of their province's standards of nursing practice so that they are informed of role-related responsibilities, including responsibilities for any expanded roles (e.g., nurse practitioner).

Analysis of Data

Once all of the data regarding the client, environment, and drug have been collected and reviewed, the nurse must critically evaluate (analyze) the information to decide its importance and implications for the client. Effort should be made to ensure that all information is obtained and documented at this time.

NURSING DIAGNOSES

Nurses use nursing diagnoses as a means of communicating information about the client and the client experience. Nursing diagnoses are the result of critical thinking, analysis, creativity, and accurate data collection

BOX 1-2
Selected NANDA-Approved Nursing Diagnoses

Activity intolerance
Acute pain
Anticipatory grieving
Anxiety
Caregiver role strain
Constipation
Deficient fluid volume
Deficient knowledge
Diarrhea
Disturbed body image
Disturbed energy field
Disturbed sensory perception
Disturbed thought processes
Dysfunctional family processes: alcoholism
Excess fluid volume
Fatigue
Imbalanced nutrition, less than or more than body requirements
Impaired gas exchange
Impaired urinary elimination
Ineffective airway clearance
Ineffective breathing pattern
Ineffective coping
Ineffective health maintenance
Ineffective therapeutic regimen management
Ineffective tissue perfusion
Non-adherence
Powerlessness
Risk for aspiration
Risk for disuse syndrome
Risk for falls
Risk for impaired skin integrity
Risk for infection
Risk for injury
Sexual dysfunction
Situational low self-esteem
Sleep deprivation
Urinary retention

From NANDA International (2002). *NANDA Nursing Diagnoses: Definitions and Classification 2003–2004,* Philadelphia: NANDA.

about the client. Once the assessment has been completed, the next step is for the nurse to analyze the information before developing appropriate nursing diagnoses. Nursing diagnoses, as related to drug therapy, should be a judgement or conclusion, based on adequate knowledge, about actual client needs or problems and the risk for problems.

As mentioned earlier, the major tasks associated with the assessment phase include the collection of subjective and objective data. After assessment, the nursing diagnoses are formulated. Nursing diagnoses related to drug therapy will most likely develop out of data such as deficient knowledge; risk of injury; non-adherence; and various disturbances, excesses, or impairments.

The North American Nursing Diagnosis Association (NANDA) is the formal organization recognized by professional groups such as the Canadian Nurses Association (CNA) and the American Nurses Association (ANA) as a major contributor to the development of nursing knowledge and as the leader in the classification of nursing diagnoses. The purpose of NANDA is to increase the visibility of nursing's contribution to the care of clients and to further develop, refine, and classify information and phenomena related to nurses and professional nursing practice. In 1987, NANDA and the ANA developed and endorsed a model or framework for establishing nursing diagnoses. In 1990, *Nursing Diagnoses,* the official journal of NANDA, was published, which became *The International Journal of Nursing Terminologies and Classifications* in 1997. In 1998, NANDA celebrated its twenty-fifth anniversary. In 2001, and again in 2003, NANDA diagnoses were modified and updated by the organization. New nursing diagnoses are continually submitted for consideration to the Ad Hoc Research Committee within the NANDA organization. This committee articulates with other specialty groups about nursing diagnosis research and consults with NANDA members who wish to do research. One change in the format of nursing diagnoses is the replacement of the phrase "potential for" with the phrase "risk for." The phrase "risk for" represents the fact that a client, family, or community may be more vulnerable to developing a particular problem than others in the same situation. Terms in the NANDA Nursing Taxonomy II include *impaired, deficient, ineffective, decreased, increased,* and *imbalanced.* The terms *altered* and *alteration* are considered to be outdated. Box 1-2 provides a list of selected NANDA-approved nursing diagnoses.

PLANNING

After data are collected and nursing diagnoses formulated, the planning phase begins. Planning includes the identification of goals and outcome criteria.

The major aims of the planning phase are to prioritize the nursing diagnoses and to specify the goals and outcome criteria, including when these should be achieved. The planning phase provides time to get special equipment, review the possible procedures or techniques to be rendered, and gather information either for oneself or the client. This step leads to the provision of safe care if professional judgement is combined with knowledge about the client and the medication.

Goals and Outcome Criteria

Goals are objective, measurable, and realistic, with an established time period for achievement of the outcomes, which are specifically stated in the outcome criteria. Client goals are reflected in expected changes through nursing care. The outcome criteria (descriptions of client goals) should be succinct, well thought out, and client focused. They should include behavioural expectations to be met by certain deadlines. The ultimate aim of these criteria is the safe and effective administration of medications. They should relate to each nursing diagnosis and guide the implementation of the nursing care plan. Their formulation begins with the analysis of the judgements made about all of the client data and subsequent nursing diagnoses and ends with the development of a nursing care plan. Outcome criteria provide a standard of measure that can be used to move toward goals. They may address special storage and handling techniques, administration procedures, equipment needed, drug interactions, side effects, and contraindications. In this text specific time frames generally are not included in the goals and outcome criteria because the process of establishing a time frame must be individualized for each client situation and reflect individual and specific planning and nursing judgement.

Client-oriented outcome criteria must apply to any medications the client will receive. For example, in the sample situation described in Box 1-1, the outcome criteria of the 43-year-old man with diabetes mellitus were focused on the administration and general aspects of insulin therapy. In this situation, the client-oriented outcome criteria include specific client education about insulin, its side effects, contraindications to its use, and injection techniques. The nurse has the responsibility for being knowledgeable about the medication *before* it is to be administered. If there are any questions about the order, its appropriateness, or safety in a given client, the nurse should get answers to these questions and then use professional judgement in the implementation of the order. During the planning phase, if the client's condition is changing and could be worsened by the medication or if the physician's order is unclear or incorrect, the medication should be withheld, the physician should be contacted for clarification or further instructions, and the information should be documented. If the physician is unavailable, the nurse manager or nursing supervisor should be notified immediately about the problem. Nursing policy guidelines should also be checked to find out who else should be contacted.

IMPLEMENTATION

Implementation is guided by the earlier phases of the nursing process (assessment, nursing diagnoses, and planning). Implementation requires constant communi-

cation and collaboration with the client and with members of the healthcare team, as well as with any family, significant others, or other caregivers. Implementation consists of initiation and completion of the nursing care plan as defined by the nursing diagnoses and outcome criteria. When it comes to medication administration, the nurse also needs to know and understand all of the information about the client and each medication prescribed (see assessment questions on p. 9). It is also important for the nurse always to adhere to the "5 Rights" of medication administration: right drug, right dose, right time, right route, and right client. In addition, the nurse needs to be aware of the following client rights:

- The right to a double check and constant system analysis (e.g., the system of the drug administration process with regard to everyone involved, including the doctor, the nurse, the nursing unit, and the pharmacy department, and also with regard to client education)
- The right to proper drug storage and documentation
- The right to accurate calculation and preparation of the dosage of medication and proper use of all types of medication delivery systems
- The right to careful checking of the transcription of medication orders
- The right to client safety with correct procedures and techniques of medication administration
- The right to accurate routes of administration and specific implications
- The right to the close consideration of special situations (e.g., client with difficulty swallowing, client with a nasogastric tube, unconscious client)
- The right to have all measures taken with regard to the prevention and reporting of medication errors
- The right to individualized and complete client teaching
- The right to accurate and cautious client monitoring for therapeutic effects, side effects, and toxic effects
- The right to continued safe use of the nursing process, with accurate documentation in narrative form or in the SOAP (subjective, objective, assessment, planning) notes format
- The right of refusal of medication with proper documentation

Right Drug

An important component of the right drug begins with the nurse's valid licence to practise. In addition, the nurse must check all medication orders and/or prescriptions. To ensure that the right drug is administered, the nurse must pay attention to both the drug orders and the medication labels when preparing medications for administration. The nurse should also consider whether the drug is appropriate for the client. The nurse must always clarify the name and indication of the drug, as well as its dosage and route. These orders must be signed by the physician or healthcare provider within 24 hours or per the specific facility's protocol. Verbal and telephone orders are acceptable only in emergency situations. To be sure that the drug is appropriate, the nurse must obtain information about the client, such as the client's past and present medical history and a thorough and updated medication history, including OTC medications used. Pertinent laboratory studies should be considered. Information about the drug is also important. As stated earlier, authoritative sources of current (less than 5-year-old) information include drug reference books (e.g., the *Compendium of Pharmaceuticals and Specialties* [CPS]), electronic references including the Internet (e.g., Health Canada's Drug Product Database [DPD] Web site), drug inserts (manufacturer's information), and licensed pharmacists. It is important for nurses to be familiar with the generic (non-proprietary) drug name and the trade name (proprietary name that belongs to a specific drug manufacturer). The nurse must be careful not to rely on information from peers and co-workers because, as a professional nurse, he or she is responsible for administering the right drug. Therefore the nurse should always look to the appropriate and current authoritative sources. Before administering any drug by any route, the nurse must know the particulars about that drug as well. It is the nurse's professional responsibility to check the order and the label on the medication and check for *all* of the "5 Rights" at least three times *before* giving the medication to the client. If the nurse has any questions, the physician should be contacted to clarify the order. The nurse should never *assume* anything when it comes to drug administration.

Right Dose

Whenever a medication is ordered, a dosage is also identified and prescribed. The nurse must always check the dose and whether it is appropriate to the client's age and size and remember to always *recheck* any mathematical calculations. The nurse must pay careful attention to decimal points because an error could cause a tenfold or even greater overdosage. The client's age, sex, weight, height, or vital signs may indicate a different dosage. Remember, neonates, pediatric, and geriatric clients are more sensitive to medications than are younger adults and extra caution is warranted.

Right Time

Each healthcare agency or institution has a policy for routine medication administration times; therefore it is important that the nurse always check this policy. When it comes to the right time for medication administration, often the nurse will be confronted with a conflict between the pharmacokinetic and pharmacodynamic properties of the drugs prescribed and the client's lifestyle and likelihood of adherence. For example, the right time for the administration of antihypertensive agents may be four times a day, but for an active, working 42-year-old male client who is taking a medication associated with the side effect of impotence, a dosage schedule of four times a day may lead to decreased adherence. This emphasis on the right time for the administration of medications must be reflected in the nurse's own practice. The nurse must concentrate on each

client and assess each individually to identify any special time considerations.

In addition, for routine medication orders, medications must be given within ½ hour before or after the actual time specified in the physician's orders (i.e., if a medication is ordered to be given at 0900 every morning it may be given anytime between 0830 and 0930), except for stat ("to be given immediately") medications, which must be given within ½ hour of the order. The nurse should always check the hospital or facility policy and procedure for any other specific information concerning the "½ hour before or after" rule. Most healthcare facilities use international time when writing medication and other orders: 0100 (1 a.m.), 0200 (2 a.m.), 0300 (3 a.m.), 0400 (4 a.m.), 0500 (5 a.m.), 0600 (6 a.m.), 0700 (7 a.m.), 0800 (8 a.m.), 0900 (9 a.m.), 1000 (10 a.m.), 1100 (11 a.m.), 1200 (12 noon), 1300 (1 p.m.), 1400 (2 p.m.), 1500 (3 p.m.), 1600 (4 p.m.), 1700 (5 p.m.), 1800 (6 p.m.), 1900 (7 p.m.), 2000 (8 p.m.), 2100 (9 p.m.), 2200 (10 p.m.), 2300 (11 p.m.), and 2400 (12 midnight).

Nursing judgement may lead to some variations in timing, but the nurse should be sure to document any change and the rationale for it. If medications are ordered once every day, twice daily, three times daily, and/or even four times daily, the times of administration may be changed if this is not harmful to the client, if the medication and the client's condition do not require adherence to an exact schedule, and with physician approval or notification. For example, an antacid is ordered to be given three times daily at 0900, 1300, and 1700, but the nurse has misread the order and gives it at 1100. Depending on the hospital or facility policy, the medication, and the client's condition, this may not be considered an error. The dosing times may be changed to be given at 1100, 1500, and 1900 without harm to the client and without incident to the nurse. Medication orders that are prn (pro re nata) are for the administration of medications with special timing and circumstances.

There are other factors to be considered when it comes to the right time. These include multiple-drug therapy, drug–drug or drug–food compatibility, diagnostic studies, bioavailability of the drug (such as the need for consistent timing of doses around the clock to maintain blood levels), drug actions, and any biorhythm effects such as those that occur with steroids. It is also critical to client safety to avoid using abbreviations with any component of a drug order (i.e., dosing, time, route). The nurse should spell out all terms (e.g., "three times daily" instead of "tid").

Right Route

As previously stated, the nurse must know the particulars about each medication before administering it to ensure that the right drug, dose, and route are being used. A complete medication order includes the route for administration. If a medication order does not include the route, the nurse must ask the physician to clarify it. The nurse must never *assume* the route of administration.

Right Client

It is critical to the client's safety that the nurse checks the client's identity before giving each medication dose. The nurse should ask the client to state his or her own name and then check the client's identification band or bracelet to confirm the client's name, identification number, age, and allergies. With pediatric clients, the parents and/or legal guardians are often the ones who identify the client. This identification should then be checked against the client's identification band or bracelet. In the newborn nursery and labour and delivery units, the mother and baby have identification bracelets with matching numbers.

Other areas to be assessed in reference to the right client include the client's ethnocultural background, pre-existing ideas and attitudes, personal beliefs, and religious affiliation. Although the standard "5 Rights" of medication administration hold true for safe nursing practice, they do not include all of the variables that affect medication administration. Therefore it is important to also consider a possible sixth right—the process of system analysis. System analysis looks at more than just the "5 Rights." It also addresses the entire system of medication administration, including ordering, dispensing, preparing, administering, and documenting.

Medication Errors

When discussing the "5 Rights" of medication administration and system analysis, it is important to discuss medication errors. Medication errors are a major problem in all settings of health care today. The U.S. National Coordinating Council for Medication Error Reporting and Prevention (NCCMERP) defines **medication error** as

. . . any preventable event that may cause or lead to inappropriate medication use or client harm while the medication is in the control of the health-care professional, client, or consumer. Such events may be related to professional practice, health-care products, procedures, and systems including prescribing; order communication; product labelling, packaging, and nomenclature; compounding; dispensing; distribution; administration; education; monitoring; and use.

This definition of medication errors is important for the nurse to understand because it emphasizes that the nurse look not *only* at the "5 Rights" of medication administration as contributors to a medication error but also at various systems involved in the medication administration process. Systems may involve any part of the process, from the point at which the order is received to the point at which the medication is administered, and may include various healthcare professionals and ancillary personnel, as well as unit stocking, transcription of orders, and how the medication order is verified and interpreted. For further discussion of medication errors, as well as information on how they can be prevented, see Chapter 5.

EVALUATION

Evaluation occurs after the plan has been implemented, but it is actually an ongoing part of the nursing process and drug therapy. Evaluation in the context of drug therapy is the monitoring of the client's responses to the drug—the expected and unexpected responses, therapeutic effects (produced intended effects), side effects, and toxic effects. An example of both a therapeutic effect and an adverse effect is as follows: A client receives an antihypertensive agent to treat hypertension. A therapeutic effect results if the blood pressure decreases to within normal limits. An adverse effect results if the blood pressure decreases to *less* than 100/60 mm Hg with postural hypotension occurring. Documentation is an important component of evaluation; thus the therapeutic effects and/or adverse or toxic effects to a medication are identified and noted (see the Legal and Ethical Principles box).

Evaluation is also important in determining the status of educational goals and client care goals regarding medication administration. Several standards are in place to help in the evaluation of outcomes of care, such as those standards established by nursing provincial governing bodies and the Canadian Council on Health Services Accreditation (CCHSA). Within the CCHSA, guidelines are established for nursing services policies and procedures. There are even specific standards regarding medication administration, which are established to protect both the client and the nurse.

The nursing process is an ongoing and essentially circular process (see Box 1-1). The evaluation of the client's

LEGAL and ETHICAL PRINCIPLES

Charting "Don'ts"

- Don't record staffing problems (don't mention them in a client's chart but write a memo instead to the nurse manager).
- Don't record a peer's conflicts; for example, don't chart possible disputes between a client and a nurse.
- Don't mention incident reports in charting, because they are confidential and filed separately and not in the client's chart. You may document the facts of an incident, but don't mention the terms.
- Don't use the following terms: "by mistake," "by accident," "accidentally," "unintentional," or "miscalculated."
- Don't chart other clients' names, because this is a violation of confidentiality.
- Don't chart anything but facts.
- Don't chart casual conversations with peers, doctors, or other members of the healthcare team.
- Don't use abbreviations.
- Don't use negative language, because it may come back to haunt you!

Data from Institute for Safe Medication Practices: *ISMP medication safety alert,* Feb 20, 2003; and Medication & Prescription Errors available at http://www.injuryboard.com.

response to previous therapy and other components of his or her medical or surgical regimen is an important facet of safe and effective delivery of drug therapy. The documentation of any findings and cautions regarding medication use and the continual assessment of clients are critical aspects of safe and effective nursing care. The nursing process as it relates to drug therapy is the way in which the nurse organizes and provides drug therapy in the context of prudent nursing care. The nurse's ability to make astute assessments, formulate sound nursing diagnoses, establish goals and outcome criteria, correctly administer drugs, and continually evaluate the client's response to the drug increases with additional experience and knowledge.

POINTS to REMEMBER

▼ Nurses are entrusted with confidential information and with the lives of their clients during all facets of client care, including drug therapy.

▼ Safe, therapeutic, and effective medication administration is a major responsibility of professional nurses in the care of clients of all ages and in a wide variety of facilities.

▼ Nurses are responsible for safe and prudent decision making in the nursing care of their clients, including the provision of drug therapy, the use of the "5 Rights," and the adherence to legal and ethical standards related to medication administration and documentation.

EXAMINATION REVIEW QUESTIONS

1 Your 86-year-old client is being discharged to home on digitalis and has little information on the medication. Which of the following statements best reflects a realistic goal or outcome of client teaching activities?
   a. Include significant others in the teaching about the medication.
   b. Provide the client with only written instructions about the medication.
   c. Provide the client with instruction about monitoring at home with an electrocardiogram at least once monthly.
   d. The client will identify three parameters to use in assessing whether he or she needs to adjust the dosage.

2 What is the most appropriate response to a client who informs you that she does not want to share information about the drugs she takes at home?
   a. "Information about the types of prescription and over-the-counter medications, as well as any herbal agents, is important to the safe administration of other medications and will be kept confidential."
   b. "We really don't need to know detailed information about your medications because you won't need them while you are here in the hospital."
   c. "Drug interactions rarely occur today due to synthetically made drugs."
   d. "Information about drug allergies is really the only issue of any significance in the medication administration process."

3 Your client's chart includes an order that reads as follows: Lanoxin 0.025 mg once daily at 0900. What should the dosage route be for this drug?
   a. Transdermal is the only correct assumption about route.
   b. The drug should only be given orally.

   c. The drug can be given subcutaneously.
   d. Never assume the oral dosage route when an order is without a route.

4 Which of the following questions is most effective when compiling a drug history for a client?
   a. "Do you frequently take analgesics?"
   b. "Do you experience diarrhea when taking antibiotics?"
   c. "Have you ever had an allergic or anaphylactic reaction?"
   d. "What type of reactions have you experienced when taking either prescribed drugs or over-the-counter medications?"

5 Mr. H. is a 77-year-old male with newly diagnosed hypertension. His medical history includes a 2-year history of stroke and the use of warfarin sodium. He has smoked two packs of cigarettes a day for the past 15 years. He states to the nurse that he is "allergic" to penicillin. Which of the following would be the nurse's most appropriate response?
   a. "All unexpected reactions to medications are of an allergic nature."
   b. "This allergy is not of major concern because the drug is given so commonly."
   c. "Any drug allergy is important to know about, and documentation of it is even more important, to help decrease medication errors and injury to the client."
   d. "Drug allergies don't usually occur in older individuals because they have built up resistance."

CRITICAL THINKING ACTIVITIES

1 Because of the changes in the ordering, distribution, and administration of drugs; the advances in technology; and the increased potency of medications, what is the crucial responsibility of the nurse when implementing drug therapy?

2 On the night shift, a client refused to take his 0200 dose of an antibiotic, claiming that he had just taken it. What actions by the nurse would ensure sound decision making and maintain client safety?

3 What are the implications of biotransformation on drug therapy?

For answers see http://evolve.elsevier.com/Lilley/pharmacology/.

BIBLIOGRAPHY

Bruccoliere, T. (2000). How to make patient teaching stick. *RN, 63*(2), 34–38.

Canadian Pharmacists Association. (2003). *Therapeutic choices* (4th ed.). Ottawa, ON: Author.

Canadian Pharmacists Association. (2005). *Compendium of pharmaceuticals and specialties. The Canadian drug reference for health professionals.* Ottawa, ON: Author. [The subscription-based e-CPS is available at http://www.pharmacists.ca.]

Davies, J.M., Hébert, P., & Hoffman, C. (2003). *The Canadian patient safety dictionary.* Retrieved October 30, 2005, from http://rcpsc.medical.org/publications/PatientSafetyDictionary_e.pdf

Health Canada. (2005). *Drug product database.* Retrieved August 1, 2005, from http://www.hc-sc.gc.ca/hpb/drugs-dpd/

Hughes, R., & Edgerton, E.A. (2005). Reducing pediatric medication errors. *American Journal of Nursing, 105*(5), 79–84.

Lewis, S.M., Heitkemper, M.M., & Dirksen, S.R. (2004). *Medical-surgical nursing: Assessment and management of clinical problems* (6th ed.). St Louis, MO: Mosby.

McCaffery, M. & Pasero, C. (1999). *Pain: Clinical manual* (2nd ed.). St Louis, MO: Mosby.

NANDA International. (2005). *NANDA nursing diagnoses: Definitions and classification 2005–2006.* Philadelphia: NANDA.

Skidmore-Roth, L. (2006). *Mosby's 2006 nursing drug reference* (19th ed.). St Louis, MO: Mosby.

Smetzer, J. (2001). Take ten giant steps to medication safety. *Nursing, 31*(11), 49–53.

Wilkinson, A. (1998). Nursing malpractice. *Nursing, 6,* 34.

CHAPTER
2
Pharmacological Principles

OBJECTIVES

After reading this chapter, the successful student will be able to do the following:

1 Define common terms used in pharmacology.

2 Understand the role of pharmaceutics, pharmacokinetics, and pharmacodynamics in medication administration and in use of the nursing process.

3 Discuss the application of the four principles of pharmacotherapeutics to everyday nursing practice as related to drug therapy and with a variety of clients in different healthcare settings.

4 Apply the phases of pharmacokinetics to drug therapy and the nursing process.

5 Discuss the use of natural drug sources in the development of new drugs.

e-LEARNING ACTIVITIES

Student CD-ROM
- Examination Review Questions: see questions 4–15
- Animations
- Medication Administration Checklists
- IV Therapy Checklists

evolve Web site (http://evolve.elsevier.com/Lilley/ pharmacology/)
- Online Chapter Worksheet • Frequently Asked Questions
- Learning Tips and Content Updates • WebLinks • Online Appendices and Supplements • Mosby/Saunders ePharmacology Update • Access to *Mosby's Drug Consult*

GLOSSARY

Additive effect Result of a drug interaction that occurs when two drugs with similar actions are given together. Also called *synergistic effect.*

Adverse drug event (ADE) An injury caused by a medication or failure to administer an intended medication; may or may not be preventable (i.e., due to error); may or may not cause client harm; includes all adverse drug reactions (*ADRs*) but is not always caused by a medication error (*ME*) (see below); also includes expected or anticipated *side effects* (SE) of medications (see below).

Adverse drug reaction (ADR) Any unexpected, unintended, undesired, or excessive response to a medication; may or may not be preventable (i.e., due to error);

may or may not cause client harm; all ADRs are ADEs, but not all ADEs are ADRs.

Agonist A drug that binds to and stimulates the activity of one or more biochemical receptor types in the body, resulting in stimulatory or agonistic drug effects.

Antagonist A drug that binds to and inhibits the activity of one or more biochemical receptor types in the body, resulting in inhibitory or antagonistic drug effects. Antagonists are also called *inhibitors.*

Antagonistic effect A drug interaction that results in combined drug effects that are less than those that could be achieved if either drug were given alone.

Bioavailability Term used to quantify the extent of drug absorption.

Chemical name The name that describes a drug's chemical composition and molecular structure.

Contraindication Any condition, including any current or recent drug therapy, especially related to disease states or other client characteristics, that renders a particular form of treatment improper or undesirable.

Cytochrome P-450 General term for a wide variety of tissue enzymes (especially in the liver) that play a significant role in drug metabolism.

Dissolution The process by which solid forms of drugs disintegrate in the gastrointestinal tract, become soluble, and are absorbed into circulation.

Drug Any chemical that affects the physiological processes of a living organism.

16

Drug actions   The cellular processes involved in the drug and cell interaction (e.g., the action of a drug on a receptor).

Drug effect   The physiological reaction of the body to a drug. It is similar to a drug's *therapeutic effect* in that it constitutes how the function of the body is affected as a whole by the drug. The terms *onset, peak,* and *duration* are used to describe drug effects.

Drug-induced teratogenesis   (ter ə to jen' ə sis) The study of drug-induced congenital anomalies, which deals with the toxic effects that drugs can have on the developing fetus.

Drug interaction   Alteration of the pharmacological activity of a given drug by the presence of one or more additional drugs, usually due to effects on the activity of enzymes required for metabolism of all involved drugs.

Duration of action   The length of time that a drug concentration in the blood or tissues is sufficient to elicit a therapeutic response.

Enzyme   A protein molecule that catalyzes one or more of a variety of biochemical reactions, including those related to the body's own physiological processes as well as those related to drug metabolism.

First-pass effect   The initial metabolism in the liver of a drug absorbed from the gastrointestinal (GI) tract, before the drug reaches systemic circulation through the bloodstream.

Generic name   The name given to a drug approved by Health Canada. Also called the *non-proprietary name* or the *official name.* The generic name is much shorter and simpler than the chemical name and is not protected by trademark.

Iatrogenic hazard   (ī a trə jen' ik) Any potential or actual client harm that is caused by errant actions of healthcare staff members.

Idiosyncratic reaction   An abnormal and unexpected susceptibility to a medication, other than an allergic reaction, that is peculiar to an individual client.

Incompatibility   Reaction that occurs when two parenteral drugs or solutions are mixed together, resulting in chemical deterioration of at least one of the drugs.

Medication error (ME)   Failure to complete a planned action as it was intended, or the use of an incorrect plan, at any point in the process of providing medications to clients.

Medication misadventure (MM)   The broadest term for any undesirable medication-related event in client care that is usually *iatrogenic* in nature (i.e., usually caused by healthcare professionals but possibly by the client).

Medication use process   The administration, dispensing, monitoring, and prescribing of medications.

Metabolite   A chemical form of a drug that is the product of one or more biochemical metabolic reactions involving the parent drug (see *parent drug*). Active metabolites are those that have pharmacological activity of their own, even if the parent drug is inactive (see *pro-drug*). Inactive metabolites lack pharmacological activity and are simply drug waste products awaiting excretion from the body (e.g., via urinary, GI, or respiratory tract).

Onset of action   The time it takes for the drug to elicit a therapeutic response.

Parent drug   The chemical form of a drug before it is metabolized by the body's biochemical reactions into its active or inactive metabolites (see *metabolite*). A parent drug that is not pharmacologically active itself is called a *pro-drug* (see below), which is then metabolized to pharmacologically active metabolites.

Partial agonist   A drug that stimulates the biochemical receptors in the body poorly, resulting in lower stimulatory response than with a full agonistic drug effect alone.

Peak effect   The time it takes for a drug to reach its maximum therapeutic response in the body.

Pharmaceutics   The science of dosage form design (e.g., tablets, capsules, injections, patches, etc.).

Pharmacodynamics   (fahr mə ko di na' miks) The study of the biochemical and physiological interactions of drugs. It examines the physicochemical properties of drugs and their pharmacological interactions with suitable body receptors.

Pharmacogenetics   (fahr mə ko je ne' tiks) The study of genetic factors and their influence on drug response. It investigates the nature of genetic aberrations that result in the absence, overabundance, or insufficiency of drug-metabolizing enzymes (also called *pharmacogenomics*; see Chapter 48).

Pharmacognosy   (fahr mə kog' nə see) The study of drugs that are obtained from natural plant and animal sources. This science was formerly called *materia medica* (materials of medicines) and is concerned with the botanical or zoological origin, biochemical composition, and therapeutic effects of natural drugs, their derivatives, and their constituents.

Pharmacokinetics   (fahr mə ko ki ne' tiks) The study of drug distribution rates among various body compartments after a drug has entered the body. It includes the phases of absorption, distribution, metabolism, and excretion of drugs.

Pharmacology   The study or science of drugs.

Pharmacotherapeutics   (fahr mə ko ther ə pu' tiks) The treatment of pathological conditions through the use of drugs. The two forms of therapeutics are empirical and rational. In empirical therapeutics there is no suitable explanation for effectiveness of the drugs involved. In rational therapeutics the drugs have known mechanisms of action (also called *therapeutics*).

Pro-drug   An inactive drug dosage form that is converted to an active metabolite by various biochemical reactions once inside the body. Often a pro-drug is more readily absorbable than its active metabolite.

Receptor   A molecular structure within or on the outer surface of cells. Receptors are characterized by the binding of specific substances (e.g., drug molecules) and one or more corresponding cellular effects (drug effects) that occur as a result of this drug–receptor interaction.

Side effect Any undesirable effect of a medication that is expected or anticipated to occur in a predictable percentage of clients who receive a given medication. Side effects can range from mild to severe client responses but usually eventually resolve with completion of drug therapy.

Steady state The physiological state in which the amount of drug removed via elimination is equal to the amount of drug absorbed with each dose.

Substrate A substance (e.g., drug or natural biochemical in the body) on which an enzyme acts.

Synergistic effect (sin er jis' tik) A drug interaction that results from combined drug effects that are greater than those that could have been achieved if the drugs were given alone.

Syrup of ipecac An extract from the plant *Cephaelis ipecacuanha.* It is used to induce vomiting to clear the stomach of certain types of poisons.

Therapeutic effect The desired or intended effect of a particular medication.

Therapeutic index The ratio of a drug's therapeutic dose to its toxic dose.

Toxic Poisonous (i.e., injurious to health or dangerous to life).

Toxicology (tok si kol' ə jee) The study of poisons. It deals with the effects of drugs and chemicals in living systems, their detection, and the treatment to counteract their poisonous effects.

Trade name The final name given to a drug; also called the *proprietary name.* A trade name indicates that a particular drug is registered and that its production is restricted to the owner of the patent for that drug until the patent expires.

OVERVIEW

Any chemical that affects the processes of a living organism can broadly be defined as a **drug.** The study or science of drugs is known as **pharmacology.** This study may incorporate knowledge from a variety of areas:

- Absorption
- Biochemical effects
- Biotransformation
- Distribution
- Drug history
- Drug origin
- Excretion
- Mechanisms of action
- Physical and chemical properties

- Physical effects
- Therapeutic (beneficial) effects
- Toxic (harmful) effects

Study in any one of these areas can be defined as pharmacology. Knowledge of these various areas of pharmacology enables the nurse to better understand how drugs affect humans. Without a sound understanding of basic pharmacological principles, the nurse cannot appreciate the therapeutic benefits and potential toxicity of drugs.

Pharmacology is an extensive science that incorporates five interrelated sciences: pharmacokinetics, pharmacodynamics, pharmacotherapeutics, toxicology, and pharmacognosy. The various pharmacological agents discussed within each chapter of this text are described from the standpoint of these five sciences. Commonly used terms such as *therapeutic index, tolerance, dependence,* and *dose–response curves* are discussed within this chapter.

Throughout the process of development, a drug will acquire at least three different names. The **chemical name** describes the drug's chemical composition and molecular structure. The **generic name,** an official or non-proprietary name, is given to the drug and approved by Health Canada under the Food and Drugs Act and Food and Drug Regulations. It is often much shorter and simpler than the chemical name. The generic name is used in most official drug compendiums to list drugs. The **trade name,** or proprietary name, indicates that the drug has a registered trademark and that its commercial use is restricted to the owner of the patent for the drug. The company that researches and manufactures the drug retains sole rights to sell that drug for a specified number of years owing to patent protection (in Canada, 20 years) (Figure 2-1). After the patent period expires, other manufacturers may produce the drug. Generic drugs are identical in terms of active ingredients to brand name drugs and are usually much cheaper.

Three basic areas of pharmacology—pharmaceutics, pharmacokinetics, and pharmacodynamics—describe the relationship between the dose of a drug given to a client and the effectiveness of that drug in treating the client's disease. **Pharmaceutics** is the study of how various dosage forms (e.g., injection, capsule, controlled-release tablet) influence pharmacokinetic and pharmacodynamic properties. **Pharmacokinetics** is the study of what the body does to the drug. **Pharmacodynamics** is the study of what the drug does to the body. Figure 2-2 illustrates the three phases that affect drug activity, starting with the pharmaceutical phase, proceeding to the pharmacokinetic phase, and finishing with the pharmacodynamic phase.

Chemical name
(+/−)-2-(p-isobutylphenyl) propionic acid
Generic name
ibuprofen
Trade name
Motrin

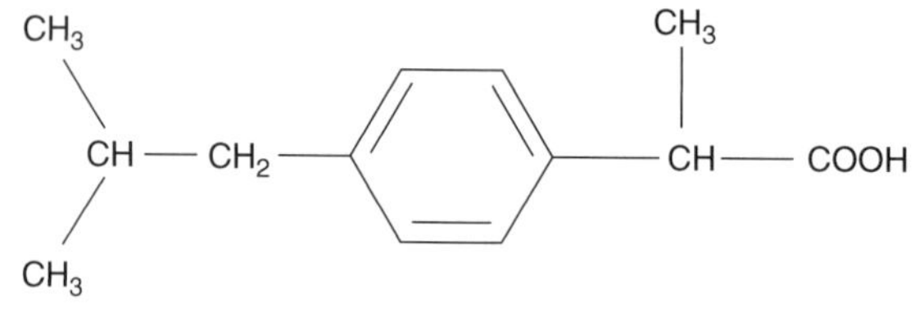

FIG. 2-1 The chemical, generic, and trade names for the common analgesic ibuprofen are listed next to the chemical structure of the drug.

Pharmacokinetics examines four phases of drugs in the body: absorption, distribution, metabolism, and excretion. These four phases and their relationship to drug and drug **metabolite** concentrations are then determined for various body sites over specified periods. The onset of action, the peak effect of a drug, and the duration of the effect of a drug are also studied by pharmacokinetics. Pharmacodynamics investigates the biochemical and physical effects of drugs in the body. More specifically, it determines a drug's mechanism of action. **Pharmacotherapeutics** focuses on the use of drugs and the clinical indications for drugs to prevent and treat diseases. It incorporates the principles of **drug actions;** therefore an understanding of pharmacotherapeutics is essential for nurses when implementing drug therapy. The study of the adverse effects of drugs on living systems is **toxicology.** Such toxicological effects are often an extension of a drug's therapeutic action. Therefore toxicology often involves overlapping principles of both pharmacotherapy and toxicology. Plants are the source for many drugs, and the study of these natural drug sources (both plants and animals) is called **pharmacognosy.**

Pharmacology is dynamic, incorporating several different disciplines (as mentioned earlier). Traditionally, chemistry was seen as the primary basis of pharmacology, but pharmacology also relies heavily on the physical, biological, and social sciences.

PHARMACEUTICS

Different drug dosage forms have different pharmaceutical properties. Drug dosage forms can determine the rate at which drug **dissolution** and thus absorption occurs in the body. Multiple pharmaceutical-related changes in a dosage formulation can affect drug dissolution. When a drug is ingested orally it may come in either a solid form (tablet, capsule, or powder) or a liquid form (solution or suspension). The process of dissolution describes how solid forms of drugs disintegrate, become soluble, and get absorbed into the bloodstream. Table 2-1 shows various drug preparations and the rate at which they are absorbed. Oral drugs that are liquids, elixirs, or syrups are already dissolved and are usually absorbed more quickly. Enteric-coated tablets, on the other hand, have a coating that prevents them from being broken down and therefore are not absorbed until they reach the lower pH of the intestines. This pharmaceutical property results in slower dissolution and therefore slower absorption. Sometimes the size of the particles within a capsule can make different capsules containing the same drug dissolve at different rates, get absorbed at different rates, and thus have different onsets of action. A prime example of this is the difference between micronized and non-micronized forms of glyburide. The micronized formulation of glyburide (not available in Canada) reaches a maximum concentration peak more quickly than does the non-micronized formulation.

A variety of dosage forms exist to provide both accurate and convenient drug delivery systems (Table 2-2). These delivery systems are designed to achieve a desired therapeutic response with minimal side effects. Many dosage forms have also been developed to improve client

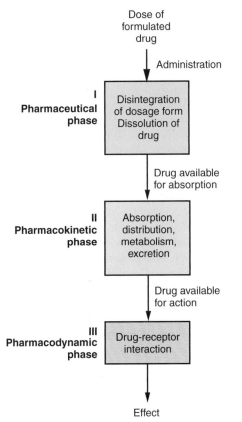

FIG. 2-2 Phases of drug activity. (From McKenry, L. M., & Salerno, E. (2003). *Mosby's pharmacology in nursing—revised and updated* (21st ed.). St Louis, MO: Mosby.)

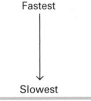

TABLE 2-1

DRUG ABSORPTION OF VARIOUS PREPARATIONS

Liquids, elixirs, and syrups	Fastest
Suspension solutions	
Powders	
Capsules	
Tablets	
Coated tablets	
Enteric-coated tablets	Slowest

TABLE 2-2

DOSAGE FORMS

Route	Forms
Enteral	Tablets, capsules, pills, timed-release capsules, sublingual or buccal tablets, elixirs, suspensions, syrups, timed-release tablets, emulsions, solutions, lozenges or troches, suppositories (rectal)
Parenteral	Injectable forms, solutions, suspensions, emulsions, powders for reconstitution
Topical	Aerosols, ointments, creams, pastes, powders, solutions, foams, gels, transdermal patches, inhalers

adherence, since adherence tends to be better when administration is convenient. Many of the extended-release oral dosage forms were designed with this in mind.

The specific characteristics of various dosage forms have a large effect on how and to what extent the drug is absorbed. If a drug is to work at a specific site in the body, it must either be applied directly at that site in an active from or it must have a way of getting to that site. A drug's dosage form influences this placement. Oral dosage forms rely on gastric and intestinal enzymes and pH to break them down into particles small enough to be absorbed into the circulation. Once absorbed through the mucosa of the stomach or intestines, the drug is then transported to the site of action by blood or lymph.

Many topically applied dosage forms work directly on the surface of the skin. Therefore when the drug is applied, it is already in a dosage form that allows it to work immediately. To other topical dosage forms the skin acts as a barrier through which the drug must pass to get to the circulation, which then carries the drug to the site of action.

Dosage forms that are administered via injection are called *parenteral dosage forms*. They must have certain characteristics to be safe and effective. The arteries and veins that carry drugs throughout the body can easily be damaged if the drug is too concentrated or corrosive. The solutions used in these dosage forms must be similar to the blood to be safely administered. Parenteral dosage forms that are injected intravenously or intra-arterially are already in solution and do not have to be dissolved in the body. Their absorption occurs immediately on injection.

PHARMACOKINETICS

A particular drug's onset of action, time to peak effect, and duration of action are all characteristics defined by pharmacokinetics. Pharmacokinetics is the study of what actually happens to a drug from the time it is put into the body until the **parent drug** and all metabolites have left the body. Therefore, drug absorption into, distribution and metabolism within, and excretion from a living organism represent the combined focus of pharmacokinetics.

Absorption
Process

Absorption is the rate at which, and the extent to which, a drug leaves its site of administration. A term used to quantify the extent of drug absorption is **bioavailability**. For example, a drug that is absorbed from the intestine must first pass through the liver before it reaches the systemic circulation. If the drug is metabolized in the liver or excreted in the bile, some of the active drug will be inactivated or diverted before it can reach the general circulation and its sites of action. This is known as the **first-pass effect**, and it reduces the bioavailability of the drug to less than 100 percent. Many drugs administered by mouth have a bioavailability of less than 100 percent, whereas drugs administered by the intravenous (IV) route are 100 percent bioavailable. If two medications have the same bioavailability, they are said to be *bioequivalent*.

Various factors affect the rate of drug absorption. These include the administration route of the drug, food or fluids administered with the drug, dosage formulation, status of the absorptive surface, rate of blood flow to the small intestine, acidity of the stomach, and status of gastrointestinal (GI) motility. Various administration routes and their effects on absorption are now examined in detail, followed by drug distribution, metabolism, and excretion.

Route

How a drug is administered, or its route of administration, affects the rate and extent of absorption of that drug. Although several dosage formulations are available for delivering medications to the body, they can all be broken down into three basic categories, or routes of administration: enteral (GI tract), parenteral, and topical. Absorption characteristics vary depending on the dosage form and category.

Enteral. In enteral drug administration the drug is absorbed into the systemic circulation through the oral or gastric mucosa, small intestine, or rectum. The rate of absorption of enterally administered drugs can be altered by many factors. When drugs are taken orally, they are absorbed from the GI tract into the portal circulation (liver). Depending on the particular drug, it may be extensively metabolized in the liver before it reaches the systemic circulation. Normally, orally administered drugs are absorbed from the intestinal lumen into the mesenteric blood system and conveyed by the portal vein to the liver. Once the drug is in the liver, the **enzyme** systems metabolize it, and it is passed into the general circulation. This initial metabolism of a drug and its passage from the liver into the circulation is called the *first-pass effect* (Figure 2-3). If a large percentage of a drug is metabolized into inactive metabolites in the liver, then a much less active drug will make it into circulation. The drug would have a high first-pass effect (e.g., oral nitrates).

When drugs with a high first-pass effect are administered orally, a large amount of drug may be metabolized before it reaches the systemic circulation. The same drug given intravenously will bypass the liver. This prevents the first-pass effect from taking place, and therefore more of the drug reaches the circulation. Parenteral doses of drugs with a high first-pass effect are much smaller than enterally administered oral doses, yet they produce the same pharmacological response.

Oral. Many factors can alter the absorption of orally (enterally) administered drugs. Acid changes within the stomach, absorption changes in the intestines, and the presence or absence of food and fluid can alter the rate and extent of absorption of drugs administered enterally. Stomach acidity is affected by the time of day; the age of the client; and the presence and types of any medications, foods, or beverages. Food in the stomach during the dissolution of an orally administered medication may interfere with its dissolution and absorption and delay its transit from the stomach to the small intestine, where most drugs are absorbed. On the other hand, food may enhance

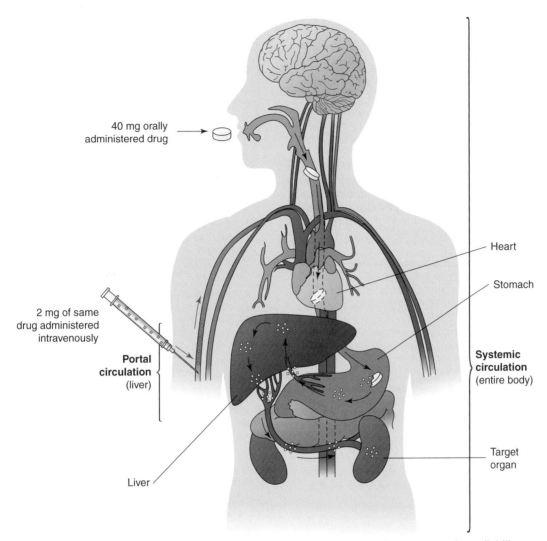

FIG. 2-3 First-pass effect is the metabolism of a drug by the liver before its systemic availability.

the absorption of some fat-soluble drugs or drugs that are more easily broken down in an acidic environment.

Before orally administered drugs pass into the portal circulation of the liver, they are absorbed in the small intestine, which has an enormous surface area. Drug absorption may be altered in clients who have had portions of their small intestine removed because of disease. Anticholinergic drugs may slow down the GI transit time, or the time it takes substances in the stomach to be dissolved and passed into the intestines. This may allow more time for an acid-susceptible drug to be in contact with the acid in the stomach and subsequently broken down, reducing the extent of drug absorption.

The stomach and small intestine are highly vascularized. When blood flow to that area is decreased, for example through sepsis or exercise, absorption may also be decreased. With both of these, blood tends to be routed to the heart and other vital organs, and in the case of exercise, the skeletal muscles.

Sublingual. Drugs administered by the sublingual route—for example, sublingual nitroglycerin—are absorbed into the highly vascularized tissue under the tongue (the oral mucosa). Sublingually administered

drugs are absorbed rapidly because the area under the tongue has a large blood supply, and such drugs bypass the liver. Drugs administered by the buccal, sublingual, vaginal, and intravenous routes bypass the liver. By doing so, drugs such as sublingual nitroglycerin are absorbed rapidly into the bloodstream and delivered to their site of action—in the case of nitroglycerin, to the coronary arteries. These same characteristics are true for rectally administered medications. Most enemas and suppositories (rectal and vaginal) are absorbed directly into the bloodstream, thus bypassing the liver and the first-pass effect. The various drug routes according to whether they are affected by first-pass effects in the liver are listed in Box 2-1.

Parenteral. With most medications, the parenteral route is the fastest route by which a drug can be absorbed, followed by the enteral and the topical routes. *Parenteral* is a general term that refers to any route of administration other than the GI tract. Most commonly it refers to injection by any method, though transdermal medications can also be considered parenteral dosage forms. Intravenous injections deliver the drug directly into the circulation, where it is distributed with the blood

Drugs To Be Taken on an Empty Stomach and with Food

Many medications are taken on an empty stomach with at least 180 mL of water. The nurse must give clients specific instructions regarding those medications *not* to be taken with food, that should be taken on an empty stomach. Examples include alendronate sodium and risedronate sodium.

Medications that are generally taken with food include carbamazepine (anticonvulsant), iron and iron-containing products (e.g., $FeSO_4$), hydralazine (antihypertensive), lithium (antimanic), propranolol (beta-blocker), spironolactone (potassium-sparing diuretic), NSAIDs (anti-inflammatory agents), and theophylline (xanthine bronchodilator).

Erythromycins, tetracyclines, and theophylline are often taken with food (although instructions indicate they should be taken with a full glass of water and on an empty stomach) to minimize the GI irritation associated with these agents.

Nurses also need to be aware of the many drugs that can interact adversely with certain foods or drinks. Grapefruit juice, for example, inhibits the liver enzyme cytochrome P450 3A4, resulting in blocked metabolism of several drugs and elevated serum drug levels; in severe cases death may occur. A 2004 article by A. Karch lists several drug classes and examples to be aware of when educating clients about drug–food interactions. If in doubt, consult your licensed pharmacist or a current authoritative drug resource. An Internet source to use is The Medication Library (Shopper's Drug Mart; http://www.shoppersdrugmart.ca/english/health_wellness/medication_library/index.html).

Karch, A. (2004). The grapefruit challenge. *American Journal of Nursing, 104*(2), 33–35.

NSAIDs, Non-steroidal anti-inflammatory drugs; *GI*, gastrointestinal.

BOX 2-1

Drug Routes and First-Pass Effects

First-Pass Routes
Hepatic artery
Oral
Portal vein
*Rectal

Non–First-Pass Routes
Aural (instilled into the ear)
Buccal
Inhalation
Intra-arterial
Intramuscular
Intranasal
Intra-ocular
Intravaginal
Intravenous
Subcutaneous
Sublingual
Transdermal

*Undergoes both first-pass and non–first-pass effects.

Subcutaneous and Intramuscular. Parenteral injections under the skin are referred to as *subcutaneous injections*, and parenteral injections into the muscle are referred to as *intramuscular injections*. Muscles have a greater blood supply than the skin does; therefore drugs injected intramuscularly are typically absorbed faster than ones injected subcutaneously. Absorption from either of these sites may be increased by applying heat to the injection site or by massaging the site. Both increase the blood flow to the area and therefore enhance absorption. Most intramuscularly injected drugs are absorbed over several hours. However, specially designed long-acting intramuscular dosage forms known as depot forms are designed for slow absorption and may be absorbed over a period of several days to a few months or longer. The intramuscular corticosteroid known as methylprednisolone acetate can provide anti-inflammatory effects for several weeks. The intramuscular contraceptive medroxyprogesterone acetate normally prevents pregnancy for 3 months per dose. With regard to subcutaneous administration, insulin glargine is a long-acting insulin product that is now in use.

Absorption can be decreased by administering cold packs to the site of injection. This is typically done to localize an injection; for example, when an intravenously administered vasopressor, such as epinephrine, has *extravasated*, or leaked out of the vein and into the surrounding tissue, and has begun to cause ischemia and tissue damage. Cool compresses produce vasoconstriction, which reduces cellular activity and in turn may limit tissue injury. Sometimes injections may be given with a vasoconstrictor such as epinephrine to confine an injected drug to the site of injection, thereby limiting its pharmacological action to that area. A similar principle applies when processes within the client's own body, such as

---

throughout the body. An intravenous drug formulation is absorbed the fastest. At the other end of the spectrum are transdermal patches, intramuscular (IM) injections, and subcutaneous (SC) injections. These drug formulations are usually absorbed over a period of several hours.

Parenterally administered drugs can be given intravenously, intradermally, subcutaneously, intramuscularly, intrathecally (into the spinal canal), and intra-articularly (into a joint). The medications that are commonly given by the parenteral route offer the advantage of bypassing the first-pass effect and are in general quickly absorbed. The parenteral route of administration offers an alternative route of delivery for those medications that cannot be given orally. The problems posed by acid changes within the stomach, absorption changes in the intestines, and the presence or absence of food and fluid are not then a concern. There are fewer obstacles to absorption in parenteral administration than in enteral administration of drugs. However, drugs that are administered by the parenteral route must still be absorbed into cells and tissues before they can exert their pharmacological effect.

hypotension or poor peripheral blood flow, compromise the circulation and therefore reduce drug activity.

Topical. Topical routes of drug administration involve the application of medications to various body surfaces, and several different drug delivery systems exist. Topically administered drugs can be applied to the skin, eyes, ears, nose, and lungs, to name but a few surfaces. As with the enteral and parenteral routes, there are both benefits and drawbacks to using the topical route of administration. A topically applied drug delivers a constant amount of drug over a long period, but the effects of the drug are usually slow in their onset and prolonged in their offset. This can be a problem if the client begins to experience side effects from the drug and there is already a considerable amount of drug in the subcutaneous tissues. Exceptions are some inhaled drugs such as aerolized albuterol for acute treatment of an asthma attack.

Topical ointments, gels, and creams are examples of topically administered drugs. They are commonly used for their local effects, and they include sunscreens, antibiotics, and nitroglycerin paste and ointment. The drawback to their use is that their systemic absorption is unreliable. Therefore topically applied ointments, gels, and creams are seldom used for the treatment of any systemic illnesses.

Topically applied drugs can also be used in the treatment of various illnesses of the eyes, ears, and sinuses. In such conditions, the required drug is commonly delivered topically to the actual site of illness and bypasses the first-pass effect in the liver.

Transdermal. Transdermal drug delivery through adhesive drug patches is a commonly used topical route of drug administration. Some examples of drugs administered by this route are fentanyl, nitroglycerin, nicotine, and estrogen. This method of drug delivery offers the advantage of bypassing the liver and its first-pass effects. It is suitable for clients who cannot tolerate orally administered medications or when it is a practical or convenient method for drug delivery. The various drug delivery systems of specific transdermal patches determine their length of effect. Although transdermal drug administration is considered a topical route, this is not an entirely accurate categorization. "Topical" suggests a localized effect near the site of administration; however, the transdermal route is often used for systemic drug delivery.

Inhalation. Inhaled drugs are delivered to the lungs as micrometre (μm)-sized drug particles. This small drug size is necessary to get the drug to the small airways within the lungs (alveoli). Once the small particle of drug is in the alveolus, drug absorption is fairly easy. At this site the thin-walled pulmonary alveolus is in contact with the capillaries, where the drug can be absorbed quickly. Many pulmonary-related diseases can be treated with such topically applied (inhaled) drugs. Examples of inhaled drugs include salbutamol sulphate, a bronchodilator used for the treatment of bronchial constriction in asthmatics; and zanamivir, an antiviral used to prevent influenza.

Distribution

Distribution is the transport of a drug in the body by the bloodstream to its site of action (Figure 2-4). Once a drug enters the bloodstream (circulation), it is distributed throughout the body. At this point it is also beginning to be eliminated by the organs that metabolize and excrete drugs—the liver and the kidneys. A drug can be freely distributed to extravascular tissue only if it is not bound to protein. If a drug is bound to protein, it is generally too large to pass through the walls of blood capillaries into tissues. There are three primary proteins that bind to and carry drugs throughout the body: albumin, alpha$_1$-acid glycoprotein, and corticosteroid-binding globulin. By far the most important of these is albumin. When a client has a low albumin level, for instance when he or she is malnourished or burned, more free, unbound drug results.

When an individual is taking two medications that are highly protein bound, the medications compete for binding to these proteins. This competition results in either less of both or less of one of the drugs binding to the proteins. Consequently, this leaves more free, unbound drug. This process can lead to an unpredictable drug response called a *drug–drug interaction*. A drug–drug interaction occurs when a drug decreases or increases the response of another drug that is concurrently administered (given at the same time). The areas where the drug is distributed first are those that are most extensively supplied with blood. Areas of rapid distribution are the heart, liver, kidneys, and brain. Areas of slower distribution are muscle, skin, and fat.

A theoretic volume, called the *volume of distribution,* is sometimes used to describe the various areas where drugs may be distributed. These areas, or compartments, can be the blood, total body water, body fat, or other body tissues and organs. Typically a drug that is highly water soluble will have a small volume of distribution and high blood concentrations. The opposite is true for drugs that are highly fat soluble. Fat-soluble drugs have a large volume of distribution and low blood concentrations. Drugs that are water soluble and highly protein bound are more strongly bound to proteins in the blood and less likely to be absorbed into tissues. Because of this, their distribution and onset of action can be slow. Drugs that are highly lipid (fat) soluble and poorly bound to protein are easily taken up into tissues and distributed throughout the body. They may even be resorbed back into the circulation from fatty tissue.

There are some sites in the body where it may be difficult to distribute a drug. These sites typically either have a poor blood supply (e.g., bone) or have barriers that make it difficult for drugs to pass through (e.g., the blood–brain barrier).

Metabolism

Metabolism is also referred to as *biotransformation* because it involves the biological transformation of a drug into an inactive metabolite, a more soluble compound, or a more potent metabolite. An inactive drug dosage form that is converted to an active metabolite by various biochemical chemical reactions once inside the body is called a **pro-drug**. Once administered, the pro-drug is metabolized to its more active and more readily absorbable form.

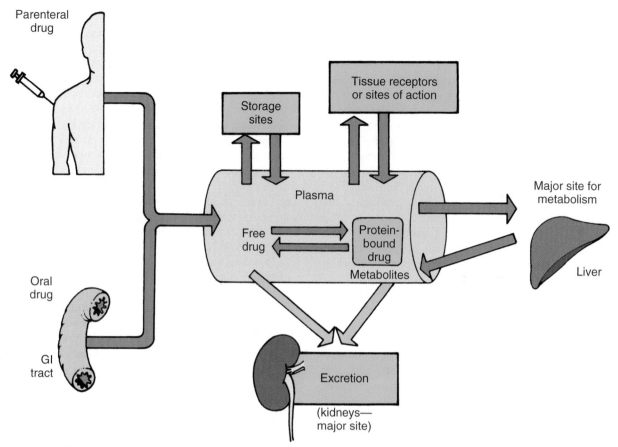

FIG. 2-4 Drug transport in the body. (From McKenry, L.M., & Salerno, E. (1995). *Mosby's pharmacology in nursing* (19th ed.). St Louis, MO: Mosby.)

TABLE 2-3

MECHANISMS OF BIOTRANSFORMATION

Type of Biotransformation	Mechanism	Result
Oxidation Reduction Hydrolysis	Chemical reactions	Increase polarity of chemical, making it more water soluble and more easily excretable. Often this results in a loss of pharmacological activity.
Conjugation	Combination with another substance (e.g., glucuronide, glycine, methyl, or alkyl groups)	

Biotransformation is the next step after absorption and distribution. The organ most responsible for the biotransformation or metabolism of drugs is the liver. Other tissues and organs that aid in the metabolism of drugs are skeletal muscle, kidneys, lungs, plasma, and intestinal mucosa.

Hepatic biotransformation involves the use of an enormous variety of enzymes known as **cytochrome P-450** enzymes (or simply P-450 enzymes) or microsomal enzymes. These enzymes control a variety of chemical reactions that aid in the biotransformation (metabolism) of medications and are targeted against lipid-soluble, nonpolar (no charge) drugs, which are typically difficult to eliminate. This includes the majority of medications. Those medications with water-soluble (polar) molecules may be more easily metabolized by simpler metabolic re-

actions such as hydrolysis (metabolism by water molecules). Some of the chemical reactions by which the liver can metabolize drugs are listed in Table 2-3. Drug molecules that are the metabolic targets of specific enzymes are said to be **substrates** of those enzymes. Specific P-450 enzymes are identified by standardized number and letter designations. Some of the most common P-450 enzymes and common drug substrates are listed in Table 2-4.

The biotransformation capabilities of the liver can vary considerably from client to client. Various factors, including genetics, diseases, conditions, and the presence of other medications that can alter biotransformation are listed in Table 2-5.

Delayed drug metabolism results in the accumulation of drugs and a prolonged action of the effects or responses

TABLE 2-4

COMMON LIVER CYTOCHROME P-450 ENZYMES AND CORRESPONDING DRUG SUBSTRATES

Enzyme	Common Drug Substrates
1A2	acetaminophen, caffeine, theophylline, warfarin sodium
2C9	ibuprofen, phenytoin
2C19	diazepam, naproxen, omeprazole, propranolol
2D6	clozapine, codeine, fluoxetine, haloperidol, hydrocodone, metoprolol, oxycodone, paroxetine, propoxyphene, risperidone, selegiline, tricyclic antidepressants
2E1	acetaminophen, enflurane, halothane, ethanol (ETOH)
3A4	acetaminophen, amiodarone, cocaine, cyclosporine, diltiazem, norethindrone, indinavir, lidocaine, macrolides, progesterone, spironolactone, sulfamethoxazole, testosterone, verapamil

TABLE 2-5

CONDITIONS AND DRUG-INDUCED CHANGES IN BIOTRANSFORMATION

Condition or Drug-Induced	Actual Disease or Drug	Biotransformation Increased	Biotransformation Decreased
Diseases	Cardiovascular dysfunction		X
	Renal insufficiency		X
Condition	Starvation		X
	Obstructive jaundice		X
	Genetics		
	Fast acetylator	X	
	Slow acetylator		X
Drugs	Barbiturates	X	
	rifampin	X	
	erythromycin		X
	ketoconazole		X

ETHNOCULTURAL IMPLICATIONS

Liver Cytochrome CYP2D6 Deficiency and Drug Metabolism

An alteration in drug metabolism can alter the efficacy, potency, and toxicity of a drug. Approximately 7 to 10 percent of the white population, 2 percent of the Black population, and 2 percent of the Asian population genetically lack the liver cytochrome CYP2D6, an enzyme that helps to convert codeine to morphine. When given codeine, these individuals do not get pain relief. CYP2D6 also helps break down certain other drugs. People who genetically lack CYP2D6 may not be able to cleanse their systems of these drugs and may be vulnerable to drug toxicity. CYP2D6 is currently under investigation for its role in pain.

to drugs. Stimulating drug metabolism can thus cause diminishing pharmacological effects. This is often the case with the repeated administration of some drugs, which may stimulate the formation of new microsomal enzymes.

Excretion

Excretion is the elimination of drugs from the body. Whether they are parent compounds or are active or inactive metabolites, all drugs must eventually be removed from the body. The primary organ responsible for this is the kidney. Two other organs that play an important role in the excretion of drugs are the liver and the bowel. Most drugs are metabolized or biotransformed in the liver by various glucuronidases and by hydroxylation and acetylation. Therefore by the time most drugs reach the kidneys, they have been extensively metabolized and only a small fraction of the original drug is excreted as the original compound. Other drugs may circumvent metabolism and reach the kidneys in their original form. Drugs that have been metabolized by the liver become more polar and water soluble. This makes elimination by the kidney much easier. The kidney itself is capable of forming glucuronides and sulphates from various drugs and their metabolites.

The actual act of excretion is accomplished through glomerular filtration, reabsorption, and tubular secretion. Free, unbound water-soluble drugs and metabolites go through passive glomerular filtration, which takes place between the blood vessels of the afferent arterioles and the glomeruli. Many substances present in the nephrons go through active tubular reabsorption. Reabsorption occurs at the level of the tubules, where substances are taken back up into the circulation and transported away from the kidney. This is an attempt by the body to retain needed substances. These substances are actively resorbed back into the systemic circulation. Some substances may also be secreted into the nephron from the vasculature surrounding it. The processes of filtration, reabsorption, and secretion are shown in Figure 2-5.

The excretion of drugs by the intestines is another common route of elimination. This is also referred to as *biliary excretion*. Drugs that are eliminated by this route are taken up by the liver, released into the bile, and eliminated in the feces. Once certain drugs, such as fat-soluble drugs, are in the bile, they may be resorbed into the bloodstream, returned to the liver, and again secreted into the bile. This process is called *enterohepatic recirculation*. Enterohepatically recirculated drugs persist in the body for much longer periods. Less common routes of elimination are the lungs and the sweat, salivary, and mammary glands. Depending on the drug, these organs and glands can be highly effective eliminators.

Half-Life

Another pharmacokinetic variable is the half-life of the drug. The half-life is the time it takes for one half of the original amount of a drug in the body to be removed and is a measure of the rate at which drugs are removed from the body. For instance, if the maximum level that a particular dosage could achieve in the body is 100 mg/L, and in 8 hours the measured drug level is 50 mg/L, the estimated half-life for that drug is 8 hours. The concept of

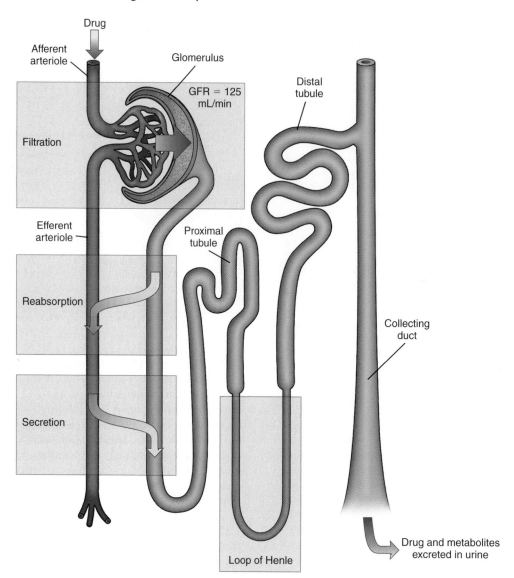

FIG. 2-5 Renal drug excretion. The primary processes involved in drug excretion and the approximate location that these processes take place in the kidney are illustrated.

TABLE 2-6

THE CONCEPT OF DRUG HALF-LIFE

Different Perspectives	Changing Values					
Drug concentration (mg/L)	100	50	25	12.5	6.25	3.125
Hours after peak concentration	0	8	16	24	32	40
Number of half-lives	0	1	2	3	4	5
Percentage of drug removed	0	50	75	88	94	97

drug half-life from several perspectives is illustrated in Table 2-6.

After about five half-lives, most drugs are considered removed from the body. At that time approximately 97 percent of the drug has been removed, and what little is remaining is too small to have any beneficial or toxic effects.

The concept of half-life is clinically useful for determining when a client taking a particular drug will be at steady state. **Steady state** blood levels of a drug refer to a physiological state in which the amount of drug removed via elimination (e.g., renal clearance) is equal to the amount of drug absorbed with each dose. This physiological plateau phenomenon typically occurs after four to five half-lives of administration of a drug. Therefore if a drug has an extremely long half-life, it will take much longer for the drug to reach steady state blood levels. Once an individual has reached steady state blood levels, there are consistent levels of drug in the body that correspond to maximum therapeutic benefits.

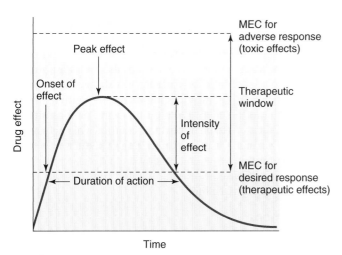

FIG. 2-6 Characteristics of drug effect and relationship to the therapeutic window. (From Hardman, J.G., & Limbird, L.E. (2002). *Goodman and Gilman's the pharmacological basis of therapeutics* (10th ed.). New York: McGraw-Hill. Reproduced with permission of The McGraw-Hill Companies.)

Onset, Peak, and Duration

The pharmacokinetic terms *absorption, distribution, metabolism,* and *excretion* are all used to describe the movement of drugs through the body. Drug actions are the cellular processes involved in the drug and cell interaction (e.g., a drug's action on a receptor). This is in contrast to **drug effects,** which are the physiological reactions of the body to the drug. The terms *onset, peak,* and *duration* are used to describe drug effects.

A drug's **onset of action** is the time it takes for the drug to elicit a therapeutic response. A drug's **peak effect** is the time it takes for a drug to reach its maximum therapeutic response. Physiologically, this corresponds to increasing drug concentrations at the site of action. The **duration of action** of a drug is the length of time that the drug concentration is sufficient to elicit a therapeutic response. These concepts are illustrated in Figure 2-6.

The timing of onset, peak, and duration of action often plays an important part in determining peak (highest blood level) and trough (lowest blood level). The Minimum Effective Concentration (MEC) is the plasma drug level that must be reached for a therapeutic drug effect. If the peak blood level is too high, then toxicity may occur. If the trough blood level is too low, then the drug may not be at therapeutic levels. (A common example involves antibiotic drug therapy with aminoglycoside antibiotics [see Chapter 37]). Therefore peak and trough levels are important monitoring parameters for some medications. The processes of drug absorption, distribution, metabolism, and elimination directly determine the duration of action of a drug.

PHARMACODYNAMICS

Pharmacodynamics is the study of the mechanism of drug actions in living tissues. Anatomy and physiology are the study of body structure and of why the body functions the way it does. Drug-induced alterations in these normal physiological functions are explained by the con-

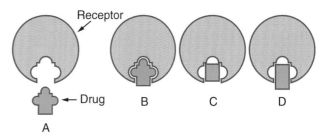

FIG. 2-7 **A,** Drugs act by forming a chemical bond with specific receptory sites, similar to a key and lock. **B,** The better the "fit," the better the response. Those with complete attachment and response are called *agonists.* **C,** Drugs that attach but do not elicit a response are called *antagonists.* **D,** Drugs that attach, elicit a small response, and also block other responses are called *partial agonists* or *agonist–antagonists.* (From Clayton, B.D., & Stock, Y.N. (2004). *Basic pharmacology for nurses* (13th ed.). St Louis, MO: Mosby.)

cept of pharmacodynamics. A positive change in a faulty physiological system is called the **therapeutic effect** of a drug. This is the goal of drug therapy. Understanding the pharmacodynamic characteristics of a drug can aid in assessing a drug's therapeutic effect.

Mechanism of Action

There are several ways by which drugs can produce mechanisms of action (therapeutic effects). The effects of a particular drug depend on the cells or tissue targeted by the drug. Once the drug is at the site of action, it can modify (i.e., increase or decrease) the rate at which that cell or tissue functions, or it can modify the function of that cell or tissue. A drug cannot, however, make a cell or tissue perform a function that it was not designed to perform.

There are three basic ways by which drugs can exert their mechanism of action: receptor, enzyme, and nonselective interactions.

Receptor Interaction

If the mechanism of action of a drug is the result of a receptor interaction, then the structure of the drug is essential. This type of drug–receptor interaction involves the selective joining of the drug molecule with a reactive site on the surface of a cell or tissue. This in turn elicits a biological effect. Therefore a **receptor** is a reactive site on the surface of a cell or tissue. Once a substance (drug or chemical) binds to and interacts with the receptor, a pharmacological response is produced (Figure 2-7). The degree to which a drug attaches and binds with a receptor is called its *affinity.* The drug with the best "fit" and strongest affinity for the receptor will elicit the greatest response from the cell or tissue. A drug becomes bound to the receptor through the formation of chemical bonds between receptors on the cell and the active site of the drug. Drugs that bind to receptors interact with receptors in different ways to either elicit or block a physiological response. Table 2-7 lists the different types of drug–receptor interactions and their definitions. Drugs that are most effective at eliciting a response from a receptor are those that most closely resemble the body's endogenous substances, which normally bind to that receptor.

TABLE 2-7

DRUG–RECEPTOR INTERACTIONS: DEFINITIONS

Interaction Term	Definition
Agonist	Drug binds to receptor; there is a response.
Partial agonist (agonist–antagonist)	Drug binds to receptor; there is a diminished response compared with that elicited by the agonist.
Antagonist	Drug binds to receptor; there is no response. Drug prevents binding of agonists.
Competitive antagonist	Drug competes with the agonist for binding to receptor. If it binds, there is no response.
Non-competitive antagonist	Drug combines with different parts of receptor and inactivates it; agonist has no effect.

Enzyme Interaction

Enzymes are substances that catalyze nearly every biochemical reaction in a cell. The second way drugs can produce effects is by interacting with these enzyme systems. For a drug to alter a physiological response this way, it must inhibit the action of a specific enzyme. To do this, the drug "fools" the enzyme into binding to it instead of its normal target cell. This protects these target cells from the actions of the enzymes. For example, angiotensin converting enzyme (ACE) causes an enzymatic reaction that results in the production of a substance called *angiotensin II*, which is a potent vasoconstrictor and mediator of several other processes. The group of drugs called *ACE inhibitors* suppresses the production of angiotensin II, the most vasoactive product of the renin-angiotensin system, by binding to the ACE and thus preventing the enzyme from binding to angiotensin I. This action causes vasodilation and helps reduce blood pressure.

Non-specific Interactions

Non-specific mechanisms of drug action do not involve a receptor or an enzyme in the alteration of a physiological or biological function of the body. Instead, cell membranes and various cellular processes such as metabolic processes are their main sites of action. Such drugs can either physically interfere with or chemically alter these cellular processes. Some cancer drugs and antibiotics have this mechanism of action. By incorporating themselves into the normal metabolic process, they cause the formation of a defective final product. This final product could be an improperly formed cell wall that results in cell death caused by cell lysis, or it could be the lack of a needed energy substrate that leads to cell starvation and death.

PHARMACOTHERAPEUTICS

Before the initiation of a drug therapy, an endpoint or expected outcome of therapy should be established. This desired therapeutic outcome should be client specific and should be established in collaboration with the client and, if appropriate, with other members of the healthcare team.

Outcomes must be clearly defined and be either measurable or observable by the client or caregiver. There should also be a specified timeline for these outcomes. Progress toward the targeted objective should also be monitored. These outcomes should be realistic and should be prioritized so that drug therapy begins with interventions that are essential to the client's acute well-being or those that the client perceives to be important. Examples of such outcomes are curing a disease, eliminating or reducing a pre-existing symptom, arresting or slowing a disease process, preventing a disease or other unwanted condition, or improving the quality of life.

Assessment

Client therapy assessment is the process whereby a practitioner integrates his or her knowledge of medical and drug-related facts with information about a specific client's medical and social history. Items that should be considered in the assessment are current medications (prescription, over-the-counter [OTC], and illicit), pregnancy and breastfeeding status, and concurrent illnesses that could contraindicate starting a medication. A **contraindication** to a medication is any characteristic about the client—especially disease state—that makes the use of the medication dangerous for the client. Careful attention to this assessment process helps to ensure an optimal therapeutic plan for the client.

Implementation

Implementing a treatment plan can involve several types and combinations of therapies. Therapy can be acute, maintenance, supplemental (or replacement), palliative, supportive, or prophylactic. Therapy may be based on theory or may be empirical.

Acute Therapy

Acute therapy often involves more intensive drug therapy and is implemented in the acutely ill client (one with a rapid onset of illness) or even critically ill client. It is often needed to sustain life. Examples are the administration of vasopressors to maintain blood pressure and cardiac output after open-heart surgery, the use of volume expanders in a client who is in shock, and the use of antibiotics in high-risk trauma clients.

Maintenance Therapy

Maintenance therapy typically does not eradicate problems but prevents progression of the disease. It is used for the treatment of chronic illnesses such as hypertension. Maintenance therapy maintains the client's blood pressure within certain limits, which prevents certain end-organ damage. Another example is the use of oral contraception for birth control.

Supplemental Therapy

Supplemental or replacement therapy supplies the body with a substance needed to maintain normal function. This substance may be needed either because it cannot be made by the body or because it is deficient in quantity. Examples are the administration of insulin to diabetic clients and of iron to clients with iron-deficiency anemia.

Palliative Therapy

The goal of palliative therapy is to make the client as comfortable as possible. It is typically used in the end stages of an illness when all possible therapy has failed. Examples are the use of high-dose opioid analgesics to relieve pain in the final stages of cancer and the use of oxygen in end-stage pulmonary disease.

Supportive Therapy

Supportive therapy maintains the integrity of body functions while the client is recovering. Examples are providing fluids and electrolytes to prevent dehydration in a client with influenza who is vomiting and has diarrhea; and giving fluids, volume expanders, or blood products to a client who has lost blood during surgery.

Prophylactic Therapy

Prophylactic therapy is drug therapy provided on a preventative or precautionary basis. For example, a surgeon knows that when an incision is made through the skin, skin bacteria may be present that can later infect that incision. The surgeon therefore administers an antibiotic before making the incision. Practical experience dictates which antibiotic is chosen. Prophylactic therapy is also used with dental procedures for clients with mitral valve prolapse or for a client with prosthetic valves or joints or Teflon grafts. Intravenous antibiotic therapy may also be used to prevent infection during a high-risk surgery and is considered prophylactic.

Empirical Therapy

Empirical therapy is therapy founded not on a theoretical understanding but on practical experience. The prescriber may not know exactly what is happening in the body or how the drug is acting, but simply knows from experience that the treatment generally works. For example, acetaminophen is given to a client who has a fever. The cause of the fever may not be known, but the client is given acetaminophen because it is expected to lower the body temperature.

Monitoring

Once the appropriate therapy has been implemented, the effectiveness of that therapy must be evaluated. This constitutes the clinical response of the client to the therapy. Evaluating this clinical response requires that the evaluator be familiar with both the drug's intended therapeutic action (beneficial effects) and its unintended but potential **side effects** (predictable adverse drug reactions).

All drugs are potentially **toxic** and can have cumulative effects. Recognizing these toxic effects and knowing their effect on the client are integral components of the monitoring process. A drug accumulates when it is absorbed more quickly than it is eliminated, or when it is administered before the previous dose has been metabolized or cleared from the body. Knowledge of the function of the organs responsible for metabolizing and eliminating a drug, combined with knowledge of how a particular drug is metabolized and excreted, enables the nurse to anticipate problems and treat them appropriately if they occur.

Therapeutic Index

The ratio of a drug's therapeutic dose to its toxic dose is referred to as the drug's **therapeutic index.** The safety of a particular drug therapy is determined by this index. A low therapeutic index means that the range between a therapeutically active dose and a toxic dose is narrow. Such a drug has a greater likelihood than other drugs of causing an adverse reaction and therefore requires closer monitoring. Two drugs with narrow therapeutic indexes are warfarin and digoxin.

Drug Concentration

Drug concentration in clients can be an important tool for evaluating the clinical response to drug therapy. Certain drug levels correspond to therapeutic responses, whereas others correspond to toxic effects. Toxic drug levels are typically seen when the body's normal mechanisms for metabolizing and excreting drugs are impaired. This commonly occurs when liver and kidney functions are impaired or in persons, such as neonates, who have an immature liver or immature kidneys. Dosages should be adjusted for these clients to appropriately accommodate their impaired metabolism and excretion.

Client's Condition

Another client-specific factor to be considered when monitoring drug therapy is the presence of concurrent diseases or other medical conditions. A client's response to a drug may vary greatly depending on his or her physiological and psychological demands. Disease, infection, cardiovascular function, and GI function are just a few of the physiological factors that can alter a client's therapeutic response. Stress, depression, and anxiety are some of the psychological factors.

Tolerance and Dependence

Monitoring drug therapy requires knowledge of tolerance and dependence and an understanding of the difference between the two. Tolerance is a decreasing response to repetitive drug doses, whereas dependence is a physiological or psychological need for a drug. Physical dependence is the physiological need for a drug (e.g., an opioid in a client with cancer-related pain). Psychological dependence is the desire for the euphoric effects of drugs and typically involves the recreational use of various drugs such as benzodiazepines, narcotics, and amphetamines.

Interactions

Drugs may interact with other drugs, foods, or agents administered as part of laboratory tests. Knowledge of drug interactions is vital for the appropriate monitoring of drug therapy. The more drugs a client receives, the more likely it is that a drug interaction will occur. This is especially true in older adults, who typically have an increased sensitivity to drug effects and are receiving several medications. In addition, OTC medications and natural health preparations, including herbal therapies, can interact significantly with prescribed medications.

The alteration of the action of one drug by another is referred to as **drug interaction.** A drug interaction can either increase or decrease the actions of another drug and can be either beneficial or harmful. Drug interactions increase in frequency with the number of concomitant drugs taken by a client. Careful client care combined with knowledge of all drugs being administered can decrease the likelihood of a harmful drug interaction.

Understanding the mechanisms by which drug interactions occur can help prevent them. Concomitantly administered drugs may interact with each other, altering the pharmacokinetics of one or both, during four phases: absorption, distribution, metabolism, and excretion. Table 2-8 provides examples of these mechanisms for drug interactions. It also illustrates how some drug interactions can be beneficial.

Many terms are used to describe these drug interactions. When two drugs with similar actions are given together, the result is an **additive effect.** Examples of this are the many combinations of analgesic products, such as acetylsalicylic acid and opioid combinations (acetylsalicylic acid and codeine) or acetaminophen and opioid combinations (acetaminophen and oxycodone). Often drugs are used together for their additive effects so that smaller doses of each drug can be given, thus avoiding toxic effects while maintaining adequate drug action.

Synergistic effects, in contrast, describe a drug interaction that results in combined effects greater than those that could have been achieved if either drug were given alone. The combination of hydrochlorothiazide with enalapril maleate for the treatment of hypertension is an example.

The term used to describe the drug effect that is nearly opposite of the synergistic effect is **antagonistic effect.** Antagonistic effects result when the combination of two drugs results in drug effects that are less than if the drugs were given separately. These effects are experienced when antacids are given with tetracycline, resulting in decreased absorption of tetracycline.

Incompatibility is a term most commonly used with parenteral drugs. An incompatibility occurs when two parenteral drugs or solutions are mixed together and the result is a chemical deterioration of one or both of the drugs. The combination of these two drugs usually produces a precipitate, haziness, or change in colour in the solution. The combination of parenteral furosemide and heparin is an example.

Drug Misadventures

Adverse client outcomes associated with medication use vary from mild discomfort to death. The most serious outcomes are life-threatening complications, permanent disability, and death. These outcomes are caused by **medication misadventures,** such as medication errors, drug interactions, drug allergies, and unknown causes. The two broad categories of drug or medication misadventures are **adverse drug events (ADEs)** and **adverse drug reactions (ADRs).** ADE is a more general term used to describe any adverse outcome of drug therapy in which a client is harmed in some way. The cause may be internal to the client or may be due to an external factor (e.g., staff error, malfunctioning equipment). **Medication errors (MEs)** are the most common type of ADE and occur during the administration, dispensing, monitoring, or prescribing of a medication, which together are known as the **medication use process** (for more information see Chapter 5).

An ADR is one type of ADE that is caused by factors inside the client's body (e.g., drug allergy, idiosyncratic reaction). ADRs may be less predictable than ADEs and, therefore, less preventable. However, a drug misadventure could be categorized as both ADR and ADE. For example, if a nurse gives a drug to a client who on admission reported an allergy to that drug, it might be considered both an ADR (by the client) and an ADE (by the failure of the nurse to heed the client's reported drug allergies). The main reason for an expansion in terminology is the growing realization that harmful consequences associated with medication use and misuse extend beyond ADRs and may be caused by therapeutic inappropriateness (or misuse), medication errors, lack of client adherence, and other problems that result in suboptimal outcomes. Both ADEs and ADRs may or may not be preventable depending on the clinical situation. Good institutional practice involves tracking all ADEs with the intention of preventing those judged to be preventable. (More information on prevention is presented in Chapter 5).

TABLE 2-8			
EXAMPLES OF DRUG INTERACTIONS AND THEIR EFFECTS ON PHARMACOKINETICS			
Pharmacokinetic Phase	**Drug**	**Mechanism**	**Result**
Absorption	Antacids with ketoconazole	Increases gastric pH, preventing the breakdown of ketoconazole	Decreased effectiveness of ketoconazole, resulting from decreased blood levels (harmful)
Distribution	warfarin with amiodarone	Both drugs compete for protein-binding sites	Higher free, unbound warfarin and amiodarone, increasing actions of both drugs (harmful)
Metabolism	erythromycin with cyclosporine	Both drugs compete for the same hepatic enzymes	Decreased metabolism of cyclosporine, possibly resulting in toxic levels of cyclosporine (harmful)
Excretion	amoxicillin with probenecid	Inhibits the secretion of amoxicillin into the kidneys	Elevates and prolongs the plasma levels of amoxicillin (can be beneficial)

An ADR occurs in the normal therapeutic use of a drug. An ADR is any reaction to a drug that is unexpected; is undesirable; occurs at doses normally used for prophylaxis, diagnosis, or therapy; and results in hospital admission, prolongation of hospital stay, change in drug therapy, initiation of supportive treatment, or complication of a diagnosed disease state. Some ADRs can be classified as side effects. Side effects are expected, well-known reactions resulting in little or no change in client management. They have predictable frequency, and intensity and occurrence are related to the size of the dose. Other ADRs lead to serious adverse events. Serious adverse events are defined as events that are fatal, life threatening, or permanently or significantly disabling; require or prolong hospitalization; cause congenital anomalies in the fetuses of clients given the medication; or require intervention to prevent permanent impairment or damage.

Two other more specific types of ADE are potential adverse drug events (PADEs) and adverse drug withdrawal events (ADWEs). A PADE is an elevated laboratory value of a narrow therapeutic index drug known to predispose a client to increased risk of death or injury but not resulting in an adverse event. A common example of a PADE is an elevated bleeding time (INR) in a client on warfarin that has not yet resulted in any adverse outcome. An ADWE is an adverse outcome associated with discontinuation of therapy. An example of an ADWE is hypertension after abrupt discontinuation of clonidine therapy.

Other terms used for ADE are *therapeutic misadventure* and *medication-related problem*. ADEs are also defined as injury resulting from medical intervention related to a drug.

The study of poisons and unwanted responses to therapeutic agents is commonly referred to as *toxicology*. ADRs can be classified as either side effects or harmful effects, and many are extensions of the drug's normal pharmacological actions. ADRs can be broken down into four basic categories: pharmacological reaction, idiosyncratic reaction, hypersensitivity reaction, and drug interaction.

Pharmacological ADRs are extensions of the drug's effects in the body. For example, a drug that is used to lower blood pressure in a client with hypertension causes a pharmacological ADR when it lowers the blood pressure to the point where the client becomes unconscious.

Idiosyncratic reactions are not the result of a known pharmacological property of a drug or client allergy but are peculiar to that client. Such a reaction is a genetically determined abnormal response to ordinary doses of a drug. Genetically inherited traits that result in the abnormal metabolism of drugs are universally distributed throughout the population. The study of such traits, which are revealed solely by drug administration, is called **pharmacogenetics** (see Chapter 48 for further information). Idiosyncratic drug reactions are usually caused by abnormal levels of drug-metabolizing enzymes (a complete absence, a deficiency, or an overabundance of the enzyme).

There are many pharmacogenetic disorders. A common one is glucose-6-phosphate dehydrogenase (G6PD) deficiency. This pharmacogenetic disease is transmitted as a sex-linked trait and affects approximately 100 million people worldwide. People who lack proper levels of G6PD have idiosyncratic reactions to a wide range of drugs. There are more than 80 variations of the disease, and all produce varying degrees of drug-induced hemolysis. Drugs capable of inducing hemolysis in such clients are listed in Box 2-2.

Hypersensitivity reactions involve the client's immune system. The client's immune system recognizes the drug, a drug metabolite, or an ingredient in a drug formulation as a dangerous foreign substance. This foreign substance is then attacked, neutralized, or destroyed by the immune system, causing a hypersensitivity reaction.

The final type of ADR is a drug interaction and results when two drugs interact and produce an unwanted effect. This unwanted effect can be the result of one drug either making the other more potent and accentuating its effects or diminishing the effectiveness of the other. As previously mentioned, in some instances drug interactions are intentional and beneficial.

Iatrogenic Hazards. An **iatrogenic hazard** is any potential or actual client harm that is caused by the errant actions of healthcare staff members. A variety of iatrogenic hazards may occur as a result of drug therapy:

- Treatment-induced dermatological responses (e.g., rash, hives, acne, psoriasis, erythema)
- Renal damage (from, e.g., aminoglycoside antibiotics, non-steroidal anti-inflammatory drugs [NSAIDs], contrast agents)
- Blood dyscrasias (e.g., a total destruction of all cells produced by the bone marrow, or just a particular cell line such as platelets; most common after therapy with antineoplastic agents)
- Hepatic toxicity (although not as common as the other iatrogenic responses, the hepatic response will take the form of elevated hepatic enzymes, presenting as a hepatitis-like syndrome)

BOX 2-2

Drugs to Avoid in Clients with Glucose-6-Phosphate Dehydrogenase Deficiency

acetylsalicylic acid
chloramphenicol
chloroquine
nitrofurantoin
oxidants (all)
primaquine
probenecid
sulfonamides
sulfones

Glucose-6-Phosphate Dehydrogenase Deficiency

G6PD is an enzyme found in abundant amounts in tissues in most individuals. It reduces the risk of hemolysis of red blood cells (RBCs) when they are exposed to oxidizing agents such as acetylsalicylic acid and Chinese remedies such as naphthalene, henna, and fava. There is an increased prevalence of G6PD deficiency in descendants of immigrants to Canada, particularly from Mediterranean and Southeast Asian countries and from India. When exposed to agents such as sulphonamides, antimalarials, and acetylsalicylic acid, clients with this deficiency may suffer life-threatening hemolysis of the RBCs, whereas individuals with the enzyme have no problems taking these drugs.

Other Drug Effects

Other drug-related effects that need to be monitored during therapy are teratogenic, mutagenic, and carcinogenic effects. These can result in devastating client outcomes and can be prevented in many instances by appropriate monitoring.

Teratogenic Effects. The teratogenic effects of drugs result in structural defects in the fetus. Such agents are called *teratogens*. There are three major categories of exogenous human teratogens: viral diseases, radiation, and drugs or chemicals. Fetal development involves a delicate programmed sequence of interrelated embryological events. Any significant disruption in embryogenesis can result in a teratogenic effect. Drugs that are capable of crossing the placenta can act as teratogens and cause **drug-induced teratogenesis**. Drugs administered during pregnancy can produce different types of congenital anomalies. The period when the fetus is most vulnerable to teratogenic effects begins with the third week of fetal development and usually ends after the third month.

Mutagenic Effects. Mutagenic effects are permanent changes in the genetic composition of living organisms and consist of alterations in the chromosome structure, the number of chromosomes, and the genetic code of the deoxyribonucleic acid (DNA) molecule. Agents capable of inducing mutations are called *mutagens*. Radiation, chemicals, and drugs can act as mutagenic agents in human beings. The largest genetic unit that can be involved in a mutation is a chromosome; the smallest is a base pair in a DNA molecule. Agents that affect genetic processes are active only during cell reproduction.

Carcinogenic Effects. The carcinogenic effects of drugs cause cancer, and such chemicals and drugs are called *carcinogens*. There are several exogenous factors that contribute to the development of cancer besides drugs, and the list grows daily. Some of the more notable ones are listed in Box 2-3.

Chemically induced carcinogenesis usually requires lengthy exposure to carcinogens. Even brief exposures to potent carcinogens will involve a long latent period before cancer develops.

Reassessment

The data collected during the assessment phase of the nursing process lead to the nursing diagnosis, planning, implementation, and evaluation phases. This dynamic process involves a constant reassessment and evaluation of the client as related to clinical symptoms in the context of drug therapy. This constant evaluation is ongoing during the entire medication administration process to always reflect the client's current status. As the client's condition improves or worsens, the treatment plan (pharmacotherapy) should be changed to accommodate the client's new therapeutic needs. Neglecting the reassessment component of pharmacotherapy heightens the risk for inappropriate and ineffective therapy.

PHARMACOGNOSY

The source of all early drugs was nature, and the study of these natural drug sources (plants and animals) is called *pharmacognosy*. Although many current drugs are synthetically derived, most were first isolated in nature. By studying the composition of the natural substance and its physiological effects in living systems, researchers can identify the exact chemical features of a substance that produce the desired response. Armed with this knowledge researchers can then go to the laboratory and produce that exact substance, making it devoid of the unwanted effects that many naturally occurring substances have. Although most new drug products are synthetic, the underlying principle of pharmacognosy is that an understanding of the actions and effects of natural drug sources is essential to new drug development. The principles of pharmacognosy have enabled isolation of the naturally occurring hormone insulin, determination of its exact genetic sequence, and synthesis of that exact sequence over and over again. This has enabled the production of synthetic human insulin.

The four main sources for drugs are plants, animals, minerals, and laboratory synthesis. An example of a plant from which a drug is derived is foxglove. It is the source of cardiac glycosides and has yielded the present-day drug digoxin. Plants also provide alkaloids, which are useful and potent drugs. Examples include atropine (belladonna), caffeine (coffee), and nicotine (tobacco). Animals are the source of many hormone therapies. Conjugated estrogen is derived from the urine of pregnant mares. Insulin available in Canada is of two types: porcine (pork) and human. Human insulin is either semi-synthetic (converting pork to human insulin by changing one amino acid) or is made by recombinant DNA techniques. Heparin is another commonly used drug that is derived from cows and pigs (bovine and

BOX 2-3
Exogenous Carcinogens

Dietary customs
Drug abuse
Environmental pollution
Food processing procedures
Food production procedures
Oncogenic viruses
Smoking

TABLE 2-9
COMMON POISONS AND ANTIDOTES

Poison	Antidote
acetaminophen	acetylcysteine
organophosphates (e.g., insecticides)	atropine
tricyclic antidepressants, quinidine	sodium bicarbonate
calcium channel blockers	IV calcium
iron salts	deferoxamine
digoxin and other cardiac glycosides	digoxin antibodies
ethylene glycol (e.g., automotive antifreeze solution), methanol	ethanol (same as alcohol used for drinking), given intravenously
benzodiazepines	flumazenil
beta-blockers	glucagon
opiate/opioid drugs	naloxone
carbon monoxide (by inhalation)	oxygen (high-concentration)

porcine heparin). Some common mineral sources of currently used drugs are acetylsalicylic acid, aluminum hydroxide, and sodium chloride. Recombinant DNA techniques provide many laboratory-derived drug products, such as recombinant human erythropoietin, granulocyte-colony stimulating factor (filgrastim), and human insulin (Humulin and Novolin).

TOXICOLOGY

Toxicology is the science of the adverse effects of chemicals on living organisms. Clinical toxicology deals specifically with the care of the poisoned client. Poisoning can result from a variety of mechanisms, ranging from prescription drug overdose, to ingestion of household cleaning agents, to snakebite. The most common types of poisonings involve ingestion of toxic substances such as prescription drugs, street drugs, and a variety of other chemicals. Poison control centres (PCCs) are healthcare institutions equipped with sufficient personnel and information resources to recommend appropriate treatment for the poisoned client. They are usually staffed with specially trained nurses who triage incoming calls. Telephone contact with a PCC is usually an important early step in aiding the poisoned client. Computerized drug and chemical information databases are often searched to quickly determine the most effective known treatment for a particular case of poisoning. Many cases can be managed over the telephone with advice from the PCC nurse. Treatment of more severe poisonings is overseen by clinical toxicologists, who are usually specially trained physicians.

Effective treatment of the poisoned client is based on a system of priorities, the first of which is to preserve the client's vital functions by maintaining airway, ventilation, and circulation. The next priority is to prevent absorption of the toxic agent and to speed its elimination from the body using a variety of clinical methods. These include adsorption of the agent from the stomach using activated charcoal, and cathartics (laxatives) to speed fecal elimination of the charcoal-toxin complex. **Syrup of ipecac** has been used for several decades as a means to induce vomiting to clear the stomach. However, there is currently a clinical trend away from its use in favour of other treatments for most types of poisoning because of frequent misuse by clients/caregivers and limited effi-

cacy. Whole bowel irrigation, using solutions of polyethylene glycol (PEG), for example, may also be helpful in eliminating some agents. In more severe cases, hemodialysis or peritoneal dialysis may be effective in removing certain types of drugs that have already been absorbed into the bloodstream. Hemoperfusion is similar to dialysis and involves pumping the client's blood through a charcoal column, clearing certain drugs from the blood by adsorption (as when it is used in the GI tract). Diuretic drugs may be administered to force renal elimination of the toxic substance. Acid or alkaline diuresis involves administering weak acids or bases to speed renal elimination of basic or acidic drugs, respectively, by altering the chemistry of the urine. Oral or intravenous solutions of ascorbic acid or sodium bicarbonate are often used for this purpose. In the case of snakebite, a drug product known as antivenin is often administered intravenously. This compound chemically binds venom molecules to reduce tissue damage. Radiation poisoning requires decontamination using specially trained personnel and equipment. Several common poisons with specific antidotes are listed in Table 2-9.

CONCLUSION

Having a thorough understanding of the interrelated pharmacological principles of pharmacokinetics, pharmacodynamics, pharmacotherapeutics, pharmacognosy, and toxicology is essential to understanding pharmacology and the nursing practice. Medications can be powerful and effective, but without the proper knowledge a useful treatment modality could become a harmful one in the nurse's hands. Having a thorough understanding of pharmacological principles enables the nurse to provide safe and effective drug therapy.

POINTS to REMEMBER

▼ It is important to be aware of the definitions and processes involved in drug therapy, such as the following:

Pharmacology: The study or science of drugs.

Pharmacokinetics: The study of drug distribution rates between various body compartments after a drug has entered the body. It includes the phases of distribution, metabolism, and excretion.

Pharmaceutics: The science of dosage form design.

▼ The nurse's role in drug therapy and the nursing process as related to all aspects of pharmaceutics,

pharmacokinetics, and pharmacodynamics requires more than just memorizing the names of pharmacological agents, their use, and associated interventions. It involves a sound comprehension and application of drug knowledge to a variety of clinical situations.

▼ Drug actions are the pharmacological, pharmaceutical, pharmacokinetic, and pharmacodynamic properties of a specific medication, with each of these having a specific effect on the overall way that a drug works within a client.

EXAMINATION REVIEW QUESTIONS

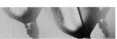

1 Which of the following is a pharmacological principle that is important for the nurse to understand?
   a. Drugs often need receptors with which to interact.
   b. Drugs produce only agonistic reactions in the body.
   c. Drugs result in effects that are not desirable.
   d. Drugs create all new responses in target organs or body systems.

2 Clients with cirrhosis or hepatitis may have abnormalities with which of the following?
   a. Liver function studies
   b. Renal function studies
   c. Hemoglobin or hematocrit
   d. Complete blood counts

3 Clients with disorders of the peripheral circulation would have problems with which phase of pharmacokinetics?
   a. Excretion
   b. Absorption
   c. Distribution
   d. Metabolism

4 Which of the following factors would contribute the most to a decreased client response to IM injections?
   a. Altered biliary functioning
   b. Altered glomerular filtration
   c. Diminished liver metabolism
   d. Diminished peripheral circulation

5 Your client just received a prescription for an enteric-coated stool softener. Instructions to the client should include which of the following statements?
   a. "Take the tablet with 60 to 90 mL of orange juice."
   b. "Avoid taking all other medications with any enteric-coated tablet."
   c. "Crush the tablet before swallowing if you have problems with swallowing."
   d. "To achieve maximal absorption, take the enteric-coated tablet with at least 180 to 240 mL of fluid."

For answers see http://evolve.elsevier.com/Lilley/pharmacology/.

CRITICAL THINKING ACTIVITIES

1 Your client is inquiring about the benefits that transdermal medication offers over the administration of some oral medications. In relation to the pharmacological principle of absorption, what is one major benefit of transdermal patches vs. oral medication administration?

2 Your client tells you during the nursing assessment that he experiences some "strange" problem with drug metabolism that he was born with, so he is not to take certain medications. What type of disorder do you think this client is referring to, and what problems can it cause in the client when taking specific medications?

3 Mr. L. is admitted to the burn trauma unit with multisystem injuries from an automobile accident. He presented to the unit with multiple abnormal findings including shock, decreased cardiac output, and less than 30 mL/h urinary output. Which route of administration would be indicated for any medications in this client? Explain your rationale.

4 Explain the difference between a medication's action and its effect.

5 Explain the importance of each phase of pharmacokinetics.

For answers see http://evolve.elsevier.com/Lilley/pharmacology/.

BIBLIOGRAPHY

Canadian Pharmacists Association. (2003). *Therapeutic choices* (4th ed.). Ottawa, ON: Author.

Canadian Pharmacists Association. (2005). *Compendium of pharmaceuticals and specialties. The Canadian drug reference for health professionals.* Ottawa, ON: Author. [The subscription-based e-CPS is available at http://www.pharmacists.ca]

Canadian Pharmacists Association. (2004). *Guide to drugs in Canada.* Toronto, ON: Dorling Kindersley.

Hardman, J.G., & Limbird, L.E. (2002). *Goodman and Gilman's the pharmacological basis of therapeutics* (10th ed.). New York: McGraw-Hill.

Health Canada. (2005). Canadian adverse drug reaction monitoring program (CADRMP) adverse reaction database. Retrieved July 14, 2005, from http://www.hc-sc.gc.ca/hpfb-dgpsa/tpd-dpt/cadrmp-pcseim/index_e.html

Karch, A. (2004). The grapefruit challenge. *American Journal of Nursing, 104*(2):33–35.

Katzung, B.G. (2004). *Basic and clinical pharmacology* (9th ed.). New York: McGraw Hill.

Lehne, R.A. (2004). *Pharmacology for nursing care* (5th ed.). St Louis, MO: Saunders.

McKenry L.M., & Salerno, E. *Mosby's pharmacology in nursing* (21st ed.). St Louis, MO: Mosby.

Mosby. (2005). *Mosby's drug consult 2005: The comprehensive reference for generic and brand name drugs* (15th ed.). St Louis, MO: Mosby.

Sgro, M., Shah, V., & Campbell, D. (2005). The challenge of early discharge. Newborn assessment for jaundice. Canadian Pediatric Society. Retrieved July 1, 2005, from http://www.cps.ca/english/CPSP/Resources/NHS.htm

Skidmore-Roth, L. (2006). *Mosby's 2006 nursing drug reference* (19th ed.). St Louis, MO: Mosby.

CHAPTER

3

Lifespan Considerations

OBJECTIVES

After reading this chapter, the successful student will be able to do the following:

1 Discuss the influence of a client's age on the effects of medications.

2 Identify medication-related concerns during pregnancy and the physiological basis for these concerns.

3 Identify age-related considerations specific to the drug administration process.

4 Discuss the process of pharmacokinetics in relation to lifespan considerations as well as related physiological concerns.

5 Calculate a drug dosage for a pediatric client using a variety of formulas.

6 Identify the importance of a body surface area (BSA) nomogram in pediatric clients.

7 Develop a nursing care plan for the administration of medications appropriate to lifespan considerations.

e-LEARNING ACTIVITIES

Student CD-ROM
- Review Questions: see questions 16–19
- Animations
- Medication Administration Checklists
- IV Therapy Checklists

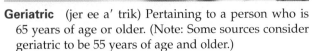 **Web site** (http://evolve.elsevier.com/Lilley/pharmacology/)
- Online Chapter Worksheet • Frequently Asked Questions
- Learning Tips and Content Updates • WebLinks • Online Appendices and Supplements • Mosby/Saunders ePharmacology Update • Access to *Mosby's Drug Consult*

GLOSSARY

Geriatric   (jer ee a' trik) Pertaining to a person who is 65 years of age or older. (Note: Some sources consider geriatric to be 55 years of age and older.)

Pediatric   (pee dee a' trik) Pertaining to a person who is 12 years of age or younger.

Polypharmacy   (pol ee fahr' mə see) The use of many different drugs in treating a client who may have one or several health problems.

Most of our experience with drugs and pharmacology has been gained from the adult population, and by far the greater majority of drug studies and articles on drugs have focused on the population between the ages of 13 and 65 years. To further compound the problem, it has been estimated that fewer than 30 percent of currently approved drugs have been appropriately tested and deemed suitable for pediatric use by Health Canada's Food and Drugs Directorate. The majority of drugs therefore lack specific dosage guidelines for use in neonates and children. Drug usage, however, extends far beyond clients between the ages of 13 and 65 years. Most drugs are also effective in younger and older clients, but drugs often behave differently in these clients at the opposite ends of the age spectrum. It is therefore vitally important from the standpoint of safe and effective drug administration to understand what these differences are and how to adjust for them.

During the time from the beginning to the end of life, the human body changes in many ways. These changes have a dramatic effect on the four phases of pharmacokinetics (drug absorption, distribution, metabolism, and excretion). Newborn, pediatric, and geriatric clients each have special needs, which are discussed in this chapter. Drug therapy at the two ends of the spectrum of life is more likely to result in adverse effects and toxicity. This is especially true if certain basic principles are not understood and followed. However, response to drug therapy changes in a reasonably predictable manner in younger and older clients. Knowing the effect that age has on the pharmacokinetic factors of drugs helps predict these changes.

36

DRUG THERAPY DURING PREGNANCY

Exposure to drugs occurs across the entire lifespan, which begins before birth. A fetus is exposed to many of the same substances as the mother, including drugs. Women, on average, take at least four drugs during a pregnancy. Therefore it is important to know and understand drug effects during gestational life. The first trimester of pregnancy is the period of greatest danger for drug-induced developmental defects.

Transfer of drugs and nutrients to the fetus occurs primarily by diffusion across the placenta. Active transport plays a lesser role. The factors that contribute to the safety or potential harm of drug therapy during pregnancy can be broadly broken down into three areas: drug properties, fetal gestational age, and maternal factors.

Drug properties that affect drug transfer to the fetus are a drug's chemical properties and dosage. The important chemical properties are molecular weight, protein binding, lipid solubility, and chemical structure. Important drug dosage variables are dose, duration of therapy, and concomitantly administered drugs.

Fetal gestational age is an important factor in determining the potential for harmful drug effects to the fetus. During the first trimester of pregnancy the fetus is at the greatest risk for drug-induced developmental defects. During this period the fetus undergoes rapid cell proliferation, and the skeleton, muscles, limbs, and organs are developing most rapidly. Self-treatment of any minor illness should be strongly discouraged anytime during pregnancy, but especially during the first trimester. Gestational age is also important in determining when a drug can most easily cross the placenta to the fetus. During the last trimester the greatest percentage of maternally absorbed drug gets to the fetus.

Maternal factors can also play a role in determining drug effects on the fetus. Any change in the mother's physiology that could affect absorption, distribution, metabolism, or excretion can also affect the amount of drug to which the fetus may be exposed. Maternal kidney and liver function play a major role in drug metabolism and excretion and are critical factors, especially if the drug crosses the placenta. Impairment in either kidney or liver function may result in higher drug levels than normal and/or prolonged drug exposure. Maternal genotype may also affect how and to what extent certain drugs are metabolized, which in turn affects the fetus's drug exposure. The lack of certain enzyme systems, as seen in the pharmacogenetic disease glucose-6-phosphate dehydrogenase (G6PD) deficiency, may result in adverse drug effects to the fetus when the mother is exposed to a susceptible drug.

Although drug exposure to the fetus is most detrimental during the first trimester, drug transfer to the fetus is more likely during the last trimester. This is the result of enhanced blood flow to the fetus, increased fetal surface area, and an increased amount of free drug in the mother's circulation.

As important as it is to judiciously use drugs during pregnancy, certain situations require their use. Without

TABLE 3-1	
FDA PREGNANCY SAFETY CATEGORIES	
Category	**Description**
Category A	Studies indicate no risk to the human fetus.
Category B	Studies indicate no risk to animal fetus; information in humans is not available.
Category C	Adverse effects reported in animal fetus; information in humans is not available.
Category D	Possible fetal risk in humans reported; however, considering potential benefit vs. risk may, in selected cases, warrant the use of these drugs in pregnant women.
Category X	Fetal abnormalities reported and positive evidence of fetal risk in humans is available from animal and/or human studies. These drugs should not be used in pregnant women.

FDA, U.S. Food and Drug Administration.

drugs, such maternal conditions as hypertension, epilepsy, diabetes, and infection could seriously endanger both the mother and the fetus.

The United States Food and Drug Administration (FDA) classifies drugs according to their safety for use during pregnancy. The potential fetal risk of a drug is determined by comparing the drug category listed on the drug label with the FDA's pregnancy safety categories, listed in Table 3-1. The basis for this system of drug classification is rooted primarily in animal studies and limited human studies. This is due in part to ethical dilemmas surrounding the study of potential adverse effects in fetuses. We have also learned from some unfortunate mistakes, such as thalidomide-induced birth defects and maternal use of diethylstilbestrol (DES), which causes a high occurrence of gynecological malignancy in female offspring.

Canada does not have a specific category list of drugs that are safe to use during pregnancy, so Canadian healthcare providers refer to the FDA categories. However, Motherisk, a Canadian organization based in The Hospital for Sick Children, Toronto, Ontario, is considered an international authority in maternal-fetal toxicology. Since 1985, this program has provided evidence-based research and education about the safety or risk for the developing fetus of maternal exposure to drugs. A hotline is available to give women and healthcare providers information on risk or safety of prescription or over-the-counter drugs, as well as natural health products, including herbal products. Their Web site is http://www.motherisk.org/.

DRUG THERAPY DURING BREASTFEEDING

Breastfed infants are also at risk for exposure to drugs consumed by the mother. A wide variety of drugs easily cross from the mother's circulation to the breast milk and subsequently to the breastfeeding infant. Drug characteristics similar to those discussed in the previous section on drug therapy during pregnancy apply to drugs taken by a breastfeeding mother. Drugs are more likely to end up in the breast milk if they are fat soluble, of low molecular weight, non-ionized, and present in high concentrations.

In general, breast milk is not the primary route for maternal drug excretion. Drug levels in breast milk are usually lower than those in the maternal circulation. The actual amount of drug that a breastfeeding infant is exposed to depends largely on the volume of milk consumed. The ultimate decision as to whether a breastfeeding mother should take a particular drug depends on the risk-to-benefit ratio. The risks of transfer of maternal medication to the infant vs. the benefits of continuing breastfeeding and the therapeutic benefits to the mother must be considered on a case-by-case basis.

NEONATAL AND PEDIATRIC CONSIDERATIONS

In medical terms, a child is a person between the ages of 1 and 12. Neonates and infants should not be referred to as *children*. Table 3-2 gives the terminology for young clients. This classification applies throughout this chapter.

Physiology and Pharmacokinetics

The anatomy and physiology unique to **pediatric** clients accounts for most of the differences in the pharmacokinetic and pharmacodynamic behaviour of drugs in their bodies. The immaturity of organs is the physiological factor most responsible for these differences. The various physiological characteristics of the neonatal population also apply to the total pediatric population, but to a lesser extent. In both groups, anatomic structures and physiological systems and functions are still in the process of developing. The Pediatric Considerations box lists those physiological factors responsible for altering the pharmacokinetic properties of drugs.

Pharmacodynamics

As previously mentioned, drug actions (or pharmacodynamics) are altered in young clients, and the maturity of various organs plays a role in how drugs act in the body. In young clients certain drugs may be more toxic than they are to adult clients and others less toxic. Drugs that are more toxic in children include phenobarbital, morphine, and acetylsalicylic acid. Drugs that children tolerate as well as or better than adults include atropine, codeine, digoxin, and phenylephrine. The sensitivity of receptor sites may also vary with age; thus higher or lower doses are required depending on the drug. In addition, rapidly developing tissues may be more sensitive to certain drugs and therefore smaller

doses are required. Certain drugs are contraindicated during the growth years. For instance, tetracycline may discolour and/or mottle teeth; corticosteroids may suppress growth if given systemically; and fluoroquinolone antibiotics may damage cartilage, leading to deformities in gait.

Dose Calculations for Pediatric Clients

Many drugs commonly used in adults have not been sufficiently investigated to ensure their safety and effectiveness in children. Most drugs administered in pediatrics are given on an empirical basis. Because pediatric clients (especially premature infants and neonates) are small and have immature organs, they are particularly susceptible to drug interactions, toxicity, and unusual drug responses

---

PEDIATRIC CONSIDERATIONS ◆▲◆▪

Pharmacokinetic Changes in the Neonate and Pediatric Client

Absorption
- Gastric pH is less acidic because acid-producing cells in the stomach are immature until approximately 1–2 yr of age.
- Gastric emptying is slowed because of slow or irregular peristalsis.
- First-pass elimination by liver is reduced because of immaturity of liver and reduced levels of microsomal enzymes.
- Topical absorption is faster because of a proportionally greater BSA and thin skin.
- Intramuscular absorption is faster and irregular.

Distribution
- In infants, TBW is 70–80 percent in full-term infants, 85 percent in premature newborns, and 64 percent in children 1–12 yr of age.
- Fat content is less in young clients because of greater TBW content.
- Protein binding is decreased because of decreased production of protein by immature liver.
- More drugs enter the brain because of an immature blood–brain barrier.

Metabolism
- Levels of microsomal enzymes are decreased because the immature liver has not yet started producing enough.
- Older children may have increased metabolism and require higher doses once hepatic enzymes are produced.
- Many variables affect metabolism in premature infants, infants, and children, including the status of liver enzyme production, genetic differences, and what the mother has been exposed to during pregnancy.

Excretion
- Glomerular filtration rate and tubular secretion and resorption are all decreased in young clients because of kidney immaturity.
- Perfusion to the kidneys may be decreased and results in reduced renal function, concentrating ability, and excretion of drugs.

BSA, Body surface area; *TBW,* total body water.

TABLE 3-2
CLASSIFICATION OF YOUNG CLIENTS

Age Range	Classification
<38 wk gestation	premature or pre-term infant
<1 mo	neonate or newborn infant
1 mo–<1 yr	infant
1 yr–<12 yr	child

and therefore require different dosage calculations. Characteristics of pediatric clients that play a significant role in dosage calculation include the following:

- Skin is thin and permeable.
- Stomach lacks acid to kill bacteria.
- Lungs lack mucous barriers.
- Body temperatures are poorly regulated and dehydration occurs easily.
- Liver and kidneys are immature and so drug metabolism and excretion is impaired.

Many formulas for pediatric dose calculation have been used throughout the years. Formulas involving age,

weight, and body surface area (BSA) are most commonly used as the basis of calculations. BSA is the most accurate of these dosage formulas. To use the BSA method, the nurse needs the following information:

- Drug order with drug name, dosage, route, time, and frequency
- Pediatric client's height in centimetres (cm) and weight in kilograms (kg)
- BSA nomogram for children (e.g., West nomogram [Figure 3-1], which uses a child's height and weight for determining the BSA)
- Recommended adult drug dosage

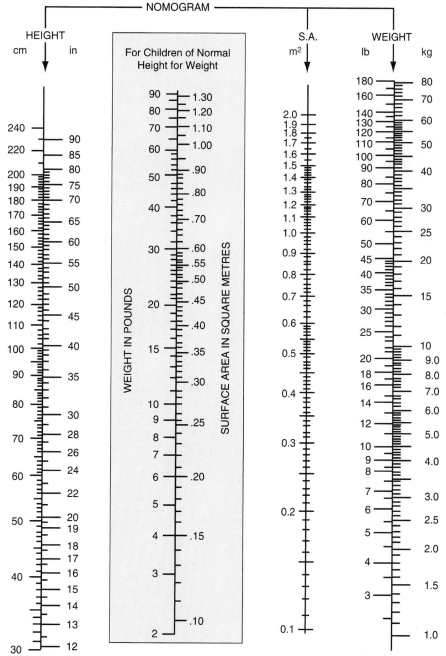

FIG. 3-1 West nomogram for infants and children. (Modified from data by Boyd, E., & West, C.D. (2004). In R.E. Behrman, R.M. Kliegman, & H.B. Jensen (Eds.) *Nelson textbook of pediatrics* (17th ed.). Philadelphia: Saunders.)

Calculating the drug dosage according to body weight is appropriate when the child is of usual stature, and most drug references recommend dosages based on "mg/kg" of body weight. The following information is needed to calculate the pediatric dosage:

- Drug order (as discussed previously)
- Pediatric client's weight in kilograms (1 kg = 2.2 pounds)
- Pediatric dosage as per manufacturer or drug formulary guidelines
- Information regarding dosage forms available

At the end of the drug calculation process, the nurse does the following:

- Determines the pediatric client's weight in kilograms.
- Uses a current drug reference to determine the usual dosage range per 24 hours for mg/kg.
- Determines the dose parameters by multiplying the weight by the minimum and maximum daily doses of the drug.
- Determines the total amount of the drug to administer per dose and per day.

- Compares the drug dosage ordered with the calculated "safe" range.
- If the drug dosage raises any concerns or varies from the "safe" range, contacts the healthcare provider or prescriber immediately.

The West nomogram (see Figure 3-1) uses a child's height and weight to determine the specific BSA. This information is then applied to the BSA formula to obtain a drug dosage for a specific pediatric client. See the following example:

$$\frac{\text{BSA of child}}{\text{BSA of adult}} \times \text{adult dose} = \text{estimated child's dose}$$

$$\text{BSA of child (m}^2) \times \frac{\text{dose}}{\text{m}^2} = \text{estimated child's dose}$$

The nurse should never underestimate the importance of organ maturity along with BSA and age in the process of pediatric dosage calculation. If all of these factors are considered, the likelihood of safe and effective drug administration is increased. Developmental considerations must also be a part of the decision-making process in drug therapy with pediatric clients (Box 3-1).

BOX 3-1

Age-Related Considerations for Medication Administration

General Interventions
- Always come prepared for procedure with all equipment and assistance necessary.
- Ask the parent and/or child if the parent should or should not remain for procedure (for in-hospital administration).
- Assess comfort methods appropriate before and after administration.

Infants
- While maintaining safe and secure positioning of the infant (e.g., parent holding, rocking, cuddling, soothing), perform procedure swiftly and safely.
- Allow self-comforting measures as age appropriate (e.g., use of pacifier, fingers in mouth, self-movement).

Toddlers
- Offer a brief, concrete explanation of procedure. Hold child securely and administer medication.
- Accept aggressive behaviour, within reasonable limits, as a healthy response.
- Provide comfort measures immediately after procedure (e.g., touching, holding).
- Help the child understand the treatment and his or her feelings through puppet play, stuffed animals, or play with hospital equipment such as needleless syringes and water.
- Provide ways to release aggression, such as hammering or water play.

Preschoolers
- Offer brief, concrete explanation of procedure.
- Provide comfort measures after procedure (e.g., touching, holding).
- Accept aggressive responses and provide outlets for them.

- Make use of magical thinking (e.g., using "ointments" or "special medicines" to make discomfort go away).
- Note that the role of the parent is important for comfort and understanding.

School-Age Children
- Explain procedure, allowing for some control over body and situation.
- Provide comfort measures.
- Explore feelings and concepts by therapeutic play, drawings of own body and self in hospital; use books and realistic hospital equipment.
- Set appropriate behaviour limits (e.g., okay to cry or scream, but not bite).
- Provide activities for releasing aggression and anger.
- Use opportunity to teach about relation of getting medication to body function and structure (e.g., what a seizure is and how medication helps prevents the seizure).
- Offer the complete picture (e.g., need to take medication, relax with deep breaths, medication will help prevent pain).

Adolescents
- Prepare in advance for procedure.
- Allow for expression in a way that does not cause "losing face," such as giving the adolescent time alone after the procedure (once the seizure is controlled) and, if he or she wants to verbalize feelings, giving time to discuss discomfort.
- Explore current concepts of self, hospitalization, and illness, and correct any misconceptions.
- Encourage self-expression, individuality, and self-care.
- Encourage participation in procedure to an agreed-upon extent. Increased participation should be discussed after procedure.

From McKenry, L.M., & Salerno, E. (2003). *Mosby's pharmacology in nursing—revised and updated* (21st ed.). St Louis, MO: Mosby.

GERIATRIC CONSIDERATIONS

Between the beginning and end of life, the human body changes in many ways. These changes have a dramatic effect on the pharmacokinetics of drugs. The geriatric client has special needs due to pharmacokinetic changes and decline in organ function; therefore drug therapy at this end of the lifespan is much more likely to result in adverse effects and toxicity. This is especially true if certain basic principles are not understood and followed.

For the sake of this discussion, a **geriatric** client is defined as a person who is 65 years of age or older. This segment of the population is growing at a dramatic pace (see the Geriatric Considerations). At the beginning of the twentieth century, geriatric persons constituted a mere 5 percent of the total population in Canada. At that time more people died of infections than of degenerative, chronic illnesses such as heart disease, cancer, and diabetes. As medical technology has advanced, so has the ability to prolong life, often by treating and controlling, or even curing, illnesses that people commonly died from in the past. This has resulted in a growing population of older adults. According to the 2001 Canada Census, seniors over 65 years of age constituted 13 percent of the population. Life expectancy is currently approximately 75 years for men and 82 years for women, and it is estimated that by the year 2026, 21 percent of the population— 7.8 million—will be 65 years of age or older. Older adults represent the fastest growing segment of the population. Interestingly, the fastest growing group is seniors aged 80 years and over. This trend is expected to continue as new disease prevention and treatment methods are developed.

Polypharmacy and Drug Use

The growing geriatric population consumes a larger proportion of all medications than other populations. The geriatric client population consumes anywhere between 25 and 30 percent of all prescription drugs and over 40 percent of over-the-counter (OTC) drugs. Commonly prescribed drugs include antihypertensives, beta-blockers, digitalis, diuretics, insulin, and potassium supplements. The most commonly used OTC drugs include analgesics, laxatives, and nonsteroidal anti-inflammatory drugs (NSAIDs). Therefore older adults are at greater risk for adverse drug reactions and drug interactions than younger adults. Not only do geriatric clients consume a greater proportion of prescription and OTC medications, they commonly take multiple medications daily. In the United States, one in three geriatric clients takes more than eight different drugs each day, and some take as many as 15. More than 80 percent of these clients have

one or more chronic illnesses. In Canada, according to the 1996/7 National Health Survey, 80 percent of seniors aged 65–69 years used prescription drugs, while 88 percent over the age of 80 years used prescription drugs. Expenditures on prescription-drug coverage for seniors are one of the fastest rising components of Canadian healthcare spending.

According to the National Population Health Survey, conducted by Statistics Canada, multiple medication use is more common for seniors, and the proportion of seniors that report using five or more drugs is increasing. Studies have also shown increasing prevalence of conditions for which drug therapies are widely used, such as cancer, depression, cardiac conditions, and asthma.

In this age of medical specialization, clients may see several physicians for their many illnesses. These specialists may all prescribe medications for the illness(es) they are treating, which explains why a client could be taking eight to 15 prescription medications as well as OTC drugs. This practice is called **polypharmacy.** The risk of drug interactions, adverse reactions, and potentially a hospitalization (possibly prolonged) is far greater in this situation. As the number of medications a person takes increases, so does the risk of drug interaction (Table 3-3). For example, a client receiving two medications has a 6 percent chance of suffering a drug interaction. This risk dramatically increases as the number of drugs the client is taking increases. A client taking five medications has a 50 percent chance of having a drug interaction. This chance rises to 100 percent if the client is taking eight medications. According to Health Canada's Adverse Drug Reaction database, as many as 3300 seniors die every year because of adverse drug reactions.

Along with the risk of drug interaction come other risks: more hospitalizations for the treatment of adverse drug effects; greater likelihood of drug-induced falls that lead to hip fractures; and heightened risk of addiction are just a few. All of these are preventable. Recognizing polypharmacy in a client and taking steps to reduce it by seeing to it that drugs are eliminated (excreted) or changed (metabolized) or that the dosages are altered can dramatically reduce the incidence of these undesirable drug effects.

Physiological Changes

The physiological changes that geriatric persons undergo also affect how drugs may act. Having an understanding of these physiological changes and how they affect pharmacokinetics and pharmacodynamics (drug actions) helps ensure the provision of safe and effective drug therapy.

GERIATRIC CONSIDERATIONS

Percentage of Population Over 65 Years of Age

Year	Percentage >65 Years
1900	5%
2001	18%
2021	20%

TABLE 3-3

RISK OF POLYPHARMACY-INDUCED DRUG INTERACTIONS

Number of Drugs	Risk
2	6%
5	50%
8	100%

TABLE 3-4
PHYSIOLOGICAL CHANGES IN THE GERIATRIC CLIENT

System	Physiological Change
Cardiovascular	↑ Cardiac output = ↓ absorption and distribution ↓ Blood flow = ↓ absorption and distribution
Gastrointestinal	↑ pH (alkaline gastric secretions) ↓ Peristalsis = delayed gastric emptying
Hepatic	↓ Enzyme production = ↓ metabolism ↓ Blood flow = ↓ metabolism
Renal	↓ Blood flow = ↓ excretion ↓ Function = ↓ excretion ↓ Glomerular filtration rate = ↓ excretion

The functions of several organ systems slowly deteriorate after many years of wear and tear. The collective physiological changes associated with the aging process have a major effect on the disposition of drugs. Table 3-4 lists some of the body systems most affected by the aging process.

These and other physiological changes that take place in older adults directly affect drug action. The sensitivity of the geriatric client to many drugs is altered as a result of these physiological changes; therefore drug usage should be adjusted to accommodate these changes. For instance, with aging there is a general decrease in body weight. However, the drug doses administered to geriatric clients are often the same as those administered to younger adults. The criteria for drug doses in older adults therefore should include consideration of "kg of body weight" and organ functioning, with emphasis on liver, renal, cardiovascular, and central nervous system function (similar to the criteria for pediatric doses).

It is important for the nurse to monitor the laboratory values that have been ordered in geriatric clients. These values may serve as a gauge of organ function. The most important organs from the standpoint of how drugs are broken down and eliminated are the liver and the kidneys. Assessment of kidney function is done by testing urine for levels of blood urea nitrogen (BUN) and serum creatinine. Assessment of liver function is done by testing liver enzymes for levels of aspartate aminotransferase (AST) and alanine aminotransferase (ALT). These laboratory values can help in the assessment of an older client's ability to metabolize and eliminate medications and would help to anticipate risks of toxicity and/or drug accumulation.

Pharmacokinetics

What happens during the pharmacokinetic phases of absorption, distribution, metabolism, and excretion may be different in the older adult than in the younger adult. An awareness of these changes helps in the appropriate administration of drugs and monitoring of geriatric clients. The Geriatric Considerations box at top right lists the four pharmacokinetic phases and summarizes how they are altered by the aging process.

GERIATRIC CONSIDERATIONS

Alzheimer's Disease

In 2005, the predicted prevalence of Alzheimer's disease is expected to affect approximately 280 000 Canadians over the age of 65 years. This figure is anticipated to reach 480 000 by the year 2031. It is presently the fourth leading cause of death in adults, behind heart disease, cancer, and strokes. Approximately 1 in 4 families in Canada has a loved one with Alzheimer's disease. This disease process has a major impact on the client's mental and physical abilities. Owing to deterioration of mental status and a chronic state of physical decline, these clients need assistance with activities of daily living (ADLs), including assistance with medication administration. Caregivers and family members need to be informed of the short-term and long-term nature of the illness and resources need to be provided, either in a private care setting or through special needs units in assisted living settings or nursing homes.

Absorption

Absorption in the older person can be altered by many mechanisms. Advancing age results in reduced absorption of both drugs and nutrients from the diet. Several physiological changes account for this. There is a gradual reduction in the ability of the stomach to produce hydrochloric acid, which results in a decrease in gastric acidity and may alter the absorption of weakly acidic drugs such as barbiturates and acetylsalicylic acid. In addition, the combination of decreased cardiac output and advancing atherosclerosis results in a general reduction in the flow of blood to major organs, including the stomach. By 65 years of age there is an approximate 50 percent reduction in blood flow to the gastrointestinal (GI) tract. Absorption, whether nutrient or drug, is dependent on good blood supply to the stomach and intestine. Once the drug is absorbed, it must be carried by the bloodstream to its eventual site of action.

GI motility is important not only for moving substances out of the stomach but also for moving them throughout the GI tract. Muscle tone and motor activity in the GI tract are reduced in older adults. This often results in constipation, for which older adults frequently take laxatives. This use of laxatives may accelerate GI motility and reduce the absorption of drugs. One particular category of laxatives, bulk-forming laxatives, has been shown to reduce the absorption of certain medications such as cardiac glycosides (digoxin). Bran and high-fibre foods may have the same effect.

Two other consequences of aging that affect absorption are (1) an overall reduction in the absorptive surface area of the gastrointestinal (GI) tract, and (2) a flattening and blunting of the villi. These changes reduce overall GI absorptive capabilities.

Distribution

The distribution of medications throughout the body is vastly different in older adults than in younger adults. There seems to be a gradual reduction in the total body water (TBW) content with aging. Therefore the concen-

GERIATRIC CONSIDERATIONS ❯❮❯❮❯

Pharmacokinetic Changes in the Geriatric Client

Absorption
- Gastric pH is less acidic because of a gradual reduction in the production of hydrochloric acid in the stomach.
- Gastric emptying is slowed because of a decline in smooth muscle tone and motor activity.
- Movement throughout the gastrointestinal (GI) tract is slower because of decreased muscle tone and motor activity.
- Blood flow to the GI tract is reduced by 40–50 percent because of decreased cardiac output and decreased blood flow.
- The absorptive surface area is decreased because the aging process blunts and flattens villi.

Distribution
- Total body water (TBW) in adults 40–60 years of age is 55 percent (male) and 47 percent (female); for those >60 years of age, 52 percent (male) and 46 percent (female).
- Fat content is increased because of decreased lean body mass.
- Protein (albumin) binding sites are reduced because of decreased production of proteins by the aging liver and reduced intake.

Metabolism
- The levels of microsomal enzymes are decreased because the capacity of the aging liver to produce them is reduced.
- Liver blood flow is reduced by approximately 1.5 percent/yr after 25 years of age, decreasing hepatic metabolism.

Excretion
- Glomerular filtration rate is decreased by 40–50 percent, primarily because of decreased blood flow.
- Number of intact nephrons is decreased.

TABLE 3-5

PROBLEMATIC GERIATRIC MEDICATIONS

Medication	Common Geriatric Complications
Analgesics	
Opioids	Confusion, constipation, urinary retention, nausea, vomiting, respiratory depression, decreased level of consciousness (LOC), falls
NSAIDs	Edema, nausea, abdominal distress, gastric ulceration, bleeding
Anticoagulants (heparin, warfarin)	Major and minor bleeding episodes, many drug interactions, dietary interactions
Anticholinergics	Blurred vision, dry mouth, constipation, confusion, urinary retention, tachycardia
Antihypertensives	Nausea, hypotension, diarrhea, bradycardia, heart failure, impotence
Cardiac glycosides (digoxin)	Visual disorders, nausea, diarrhea, dysrhythmias, hallucinations, decreased appetite, weight loss
Sedatives and hypnotics	Confusion, daytime sedation, ataxia, lethargy, forgetfulness, increased risk of falls
Thiazide diuretics	Electrolyte imbalance, rashes, fatigue, leg cramps, dehydration

Metabolism

Metabolism declines with advancing age. The transformation of active drugs into inactive metabolites is primarily performed by the liver, but the liver slowly loses its ability to metabolize drugs effectively because the production of microsomal enzymes is reduced. There is also a reduction in blood flow to the liver because of reduced cardiac output and atherosclerosis. A reduction in the hepatic blood flow of approximately 1.5 percent per year occurs after 25 years of age. All of these factors contribute to prolonging the half-life of many drugs, which can potentially result in drug accumulation if drug intervals are not closely monitored.

Excretion

The excretion of drugs is reduced in the geriatric population. A reduction in the glomerular filtration rate of 40 to 50 percent in older adults, combined with a reduction in blood flow (for the same reasons that apply to the liver) can result in extremely delayed drug excretion and hence drug accumulation. To prevent drug accumulation in geriatric clients, renal function should be monitored frequently through laboratory blood work such as BUN and creatinine. Appropriate dose and interval adjustments can be made easily based on a client's renal function, and potentially dangerous complications can thereby be prevented.

Problematic Geriatric Medications

Drugs in certain classes are more likely to cause problems in geriatric clients because of many of the physiological alterations and pharmacokinetic changes already discussed. Table 3-5 lists the drugs most commonly problematic.

---

trations of highly water-soluble drugs may be higher in geriatric clients because they have less body water in which the drugs can be diluted. The composition of the body also changes with aging. As the lean muscle mass decreases, body fat increases. In both men and women there is an approximate 20 percent reduction in muscle mass between the ages of 25 and 65 years and a corresponding 20 percent increase in body fat. Drugs such as hypnotics and sedatives that are primarily distributed to the fat will therefore have a prolonged effect.

Many drugs distributed by means of the blood are carried by proteins. By far the most important of these is albumin. Reduced protein concentrations, including reduced albumin concentrations, result from aging. This may be due in part to reduced liver function (which produces many of these proteins), to decreased intake or poor absorption despite adequate intake, or to a combination of these factors. Whatever the cause, a reduced number of protein-binding sites for highly protein-bound drugs results in higher levels of unbound drug. Drugs that are not bound to proteins are active. Therefore the effects of highly protein-bound drugs may be enhanced if their doses are not adjusted in keeping with the albumin concentrations.

Knowledge of the physiological changes in older adults, combined with an understanding of the various pharmacokinetic changes that occur, is extremely useful in the management of geriatric clients. It can lead to improvements in drug therapy and thereby the prevention of unwanted consequences of inappropriate dosing.

NURSING PROCESS

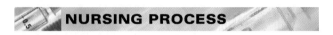

■ Assessment

Before administering any medication to a pediatric client, a thorough health and medication history must be obtained (often from parents or caregivers) that includes the following:

- Age
- Age-related concerns about organ functioning
- Allergies to drugs and food
- Baseline vital signs
- Fears
- Head-to-toe assessment findings
- Height
- Level of growth and development
- Medical and medication history (including adverse drug reactions); medication and related dosage forms and routes and the client's tolerance of the forms and/or routes
- State of anxiety
- Use of prescription and OTC medications
- Usual method of medication administration, such as use of a calibrated spoon or syringe (no needle!)
- Usual response to medications
- Weight (important because many doses are calculated per kilogram of body weight)

The prescriber's orders should be triple-checked by the nurse because there is no room for error when working with pediatric clients (or any client). The medication dosage should be calculated and rechecked for safety purposes.

General assessment data to be gathered in the geriatric client include the following:

- Age
- Allergies to drugs and food
- Dietary habits
- Limitations (sensory, visual, hearing, cognitive/motor skills)
- List of all physicians
- Present and past medical and medication history (especially prescription and OTC medications currently taken)
- Results of renal and liver function studies
- Self-medication practices
- Use of natural health products, including herbal preparations
- Use of home remedies
- Use of polypharmacy

Just because clients appear to be alert does not mean that they understand what the nurse is saying or can self-administer medications without difficulty or without causing themselves harm. It is important for the nurse to realize that although most geriatric clients are able to provide their own information, some might be confused or poorly informed about their medications. In this case, it is recommended that the nurse seek additional information or confirm information with significant others, family, or friends. Geriatric clients may also have difficulty with sensory deficits that may require the nurse to speak slowly, loudly, and more clearly while facing the client.

With both pediatric and geriatric clients, the nurse should assess the family support system and the client's ability to take medications safely or to have medications given safely by the caregiver. Whenever possible, unless ordered otherwise, opt to use a non-pharmacological approach to treatment in pediatric and geriatric clients.

Other information the nurse needs to have about pediatric and geriatric clients includes any chronic illnesses, nutritional problems, or GI tract disorders; attitudes toward medical treatment; and the ability of the client or family to understand information about the medication, instructions concerning its use, and the importance of medication adherence.

■ Nursing Diagnoses

Nursing diagnoses related to the administration of medications to pediatric and geriatric clients include the following:

- Risk for injury related to side effects of medications or to the method of medication administration
- Imbalanced nutrition, less than body requirements, related to age or medication therapy and possible side effects
- Risk for injury related to idiosyncratic reactions to medications due to age-related drug sensitivity
- Deficient knowledge related to information about medications and their side effects or about when to contact the physician

■ Planning

Goals related to the pediatric or geriatric client include the following:

- Client is free of complications associated with the adverse effects of medications.
- Client remains adherent (or takes medication as prescribed with assistance) until medication is discontinued by physician.
- Client (or parent, legal guardian, or caregiver) contacts physician when appropriate (such as with unusual effects).

■ *Outcome Criteria*

Outcome criteria related to the administration of medications to the pediatric (or the parent, legal guardian, or caregiver) or geriatric client include the following:

- Client (or parent, legal guardian, or caregiver) will state the importance of taking medication as prescribed (e.g., improved condition, decreased symptoms) and use return demonstration when applicable.

- Client (or parent, legal guardian, or caregiver) will follow instructions specific to the administration of the medication ordered (e.g., the special application of an ointment, taking of liquid, and dosage).
- Client (specifically the geriatric client) will state why he or she is taking a specific medication, as well as identify what the drug looks like and when the drug is to be taken.
- Client will show improvement in condition related to adherence and successful medication therapy.
- Client will take or receive medications safely and without injury to self.
- Client (or parent, legal guardian, or caregiver) will state specific situations when the physician must be contacted (e.g., fever, pain, vomiting, rash or diarrhea, worsening of condition, bronchospasms, dyspnea, intolerable side effects, signs of major adverse effects).

■ Implementation

In general, it is always important to emphasize and practise the "5 Rights" (right drug, right dose, right time, right route, and right client) and to follow the label and medication instructions. Clients should be encouraged to take medications as directed and not to discontinue them, double up on doses, or take any OTC medications unless prescribed by the healthcare provider. In general, when it comes to pediatric or geriatric clients, be sure that the client, parent, legal guardian, or caregiver understands instructions specific to the medication and understands that all medications should be kept out of the reach of small children. Provide written and oral instructions concerning the drug name, action, purpose, dose, time of administration, route, side effects, safety of administration, storage, interactions, and any cautions or contraindications. Specific guidelines for medication administration for various routes and dosage forms are presented in this textbook. The Community Health Points box lists some home health points for the pediatric client.

■ Evaluation

In general, when dealing with pediatric or geriatric clients, the nurse should be constantly watching for expected and therapeutic effects of medication. The client should also be monitored for side effects (frequently and as needed), possible toxic effects, and overdosage. The client, parent, legal guardian, or caregiver should also be aware of these points of monitoring.

COMMUNITY HEALTH POINTS

Pediatric Client

- Avoid disguising medications in essential foods such as milk, orange juice, or cereal because the child may develop a dislike for the food in the future. Do not add medication to fluid in a cup or bottle because the amount consumed may be difficult to calculate.
- Always document what is successful so that the method may be communicated to others (e.g., a Popsicle before administration of an unpleasant tasting pill or liquid).
- Unless contraindicated, adding small amounts of water to elixirs may help the child to tolerate the medication. Be cautious with this practice, however, because it is essential that the child take the entire volume.
- Avoid using the word "candy" in place of "medication." Medications should be called medicines and their dangers made known to children.
- Keep all medications out of the reach of children of all ages. Secure medications, including natural health products (vitamins and herbal remedies), at all times to prevent accidental poisoning.
- Request child-resistant medication containers when children are in the home.
- Most medications are better tolerated and absorbed when 180 to 240 mL of fluid such as juice, water, or milk follows the medication dose.
- Always ask about how the pediatric client is used to taking medications (e.g., liquid vs. pill or tablet dosage forms).

POINTS to REMEMBER

- ▼ There are many age-related pharmacokinetic effects, with dramatic differences in drug absorption, distribution, metabolism, and excretion.
- ▼ At one end of the lifespan there is the pediatric client and at the other end there is the geriatric client, both of whom are sensitive to the effects of drugs.
- ▼ Classifications of pediatric client: premature or preterm = <38 weeks; neonate or newborn = <1 month; infant = 1 month to <1 year; child = 1 year to <12 years.
- ▼ Most common dosage calculations use the mg/kg formula related to age; however, BSA is also used for drug calculations, as is consideration of organ maturity.
- ▼ The percentage of the population over the age of 65 years continues to increase, meaning that nurses will be exposed to increasing numbers of geriatric clients.

- ▼ Polypharmacy (use of more than one drug in a client, usually geriatric), which stems from the fact that the client is often taking several drugs for one or many illnesses, increases the client's risk for drug interactions, adverse reactions, hospitalization due to adverse effects, and possible toxicity.
- ▼ The nurse's role is to act as a client advocate as well as to be informed about growth and development principles and the effects of various drugs during the lifespan and in various phases of illness.
- ▼ Always follow the "5 Rights" of medication administration to prevent drug errors and harm to clients of all ages.
- ▼ Thorough client education for *all* involved in the client's care includes both written and oral instructions.

EXAMINATION REVIEW QUESTIONS

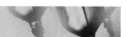

1 Which of the following pharmacokinetic factors puts the neonatal client at risk as related to drug therapy?
   a. Immature renal system
   b. Hyperperistalsis in the GI tract
   c. Functional temperature regulation
   d. Dysfunctional musculoskeletal movement

2 Physiological differences between pediatric and adult clients affect the amount of drug needed to produce a therapeutic effect. Which of the following is one of the main differences in infants?
   a. An immature organ status.
   b. Fat composition less than 0.001 percent.
   c. Greater body muscular composition.
   d. Water composition of approximately 75 percent.

3 The nurse encourages Mr. Y., a 76-year-old client, to keep a journal of side effects experienced from his medications. Which of the following alterations in pharmacokinetics best explains why this intervention may be critical to the geriatric client?
   a. Increased renal excretion of protein-bound drugs
   b. More alkaline gastric pH, resulting in more side effects

   c. Decreased liver blood perfusion with altered metabolism
   d. Less adipose tissue and therefore more distribution of fat-soluble drugs

4 Of the following medications that this same 76-year-old client is taking, which may result in hypotension, postural orthostatic blood pressures, and possible syncope?
   a. NSAIDs
   b. Adrenaline
   c. Epinephrine
   d. Antihypertensives

5 Which of the following is an important nursing intervention with the geriatric client?
   a. Communicate with patience, empathy, dignity, and understanding.
   b. Suggest to the family that the client needs to be institutionalized.
   c. Refer the client to several healthcare providers for a multi-provider plan.
   d. Develop a plan for self-medication administration with detailed instructions.

For answers see http://evolve.elsevier.com/Lilley/pharmacology/.

CRITICAL THINKING ACTIVITIES

1 Select either phenytoin or tetracycline and discuss its potential risks to the fetus or breastfeeding newborn in relation to the needed benefits to the mother.

2 A 73-year-old nursing home resident is experiencing problems that the nurse thinks are indicative of absorption problems with his oral medications (he is currently taking warfarin sodium). Specifically, the nurse notices that he has been experiencing unusual "bleeding" tendencies over the past few days; however, he tolerated the medication "very well" over the "last 3 years." Which of

the following physiological changes is *most* likely the basis of his untoward reaction to the warfarin?
   a. Increased cardiac output and cardiac volume
   b. Increased glomerular filtration and renin excretion
   c. Decreased GI pH with increased peristalsis
   d. Decreased hepatic enzyme production and altered liver perfusion

3 List medications that are high risk for causing adverse effects or toxicity for the geriatric client. Discuss the problems or complications associated with these drugs or drug classifications.

For answers see http://evolve.elsevier.com/Lilley/pharmacology/.

BIBLIOGRAPHY

Alzheimer Society of Canada. (2005). Alzheimer disease statistics. Retrieved July 3, 2005, from http://www.alzheimer.ca/english/disease/stats-people.htm

Briggs, G.G., Freeman, R.K., & Yaffe, S.J. (2005). *Drugs in pregnancy and lactation. A reference guide to fetal and neonatal risk* (7th ed.). Philadelphia: Lippincott, Williams & Wilkins.

Canadian Institutes of Health Research. (2004). Alzheimer's disease. Retrieved July 14, 2005, from http://www.cihr-irsc.gc.ca/e/24936.html

Canadian Pediatric Society. (2003). Position statement. Drug investigation for Canadian children. The role of the Canadian Pediatric Society. [Electronic version] *Pediatric Child Health, 8*(4), 231–234. Retrieved July 2, 2005, from http://www.cps.ca/english/statements/DT/dt03-01.pdf

Health Canada. (2005). Canadian adverse drug reaction monitoring program (CADRMP) adverse reaction database. Retrieved

July 14, 2005, from http://www.hc-sc.gc.ca/dhp-mps/medeff/databasdon/index_e.html

Hockenberry, M.J., Wilson, D., Winkelstein, M.L., & Kline, N.E. (2003). *Wong's nursing care of infants and children* (7th ed.). St Louis, MO: Mosby.

Lehne, R.A. (2004). *Pharmacology for nursing care* (5th ed.). St Louis, MO: Saunders.

McKenry, L.M., & Salerno, E. (2003). *Mosby's pharmacology in nursing—revised and updated* (21st ed.). St Louis, MO: Mosby.

Mosby. (2005). *Mosby's drug consult 2005. The comprehensive reference for generic and brand name drugs* (15th ed.). St Louis, MO: Mosby.

Motherisk. (2005). Drugs in pregnancy. Retrieved July 14, 2005, from http://www.motherisk.org/drugs/index.php

Statistics Canada. (2005). Canadian statistics. Accessible at http://www.statscan.ca

Taketomo, C.K., Hodding, J.H., & Kraus, D.M. (2002). *Pediatric dosage handbook* (9th ed.). Hudson, OH: Lexi-Comp.

Legal, Ethical, and Ethnocultural Considerations

GLOSSARY

Benzodiazepines and Other Targeted Substances Regulations   Implemented in 2000, these regulations specify the requirements for producing, assembling, importing, exporting, selling, providing, transporting, delivering, or destroying benzodiazepines and other targeted substances.

Blinded investigational drug study   A research method in which the subject taking the drug under study is purposely unaware of a key element or elements in the study (e.g., whether an administered substance is the drug under study or a placebo). This method eliminates bias on the part of the subject.

Canada Health Act   Canada's federal legislation for publicly funded healthcare insurance.

Controlled Drug and Substances Act (CDSA)   In 1997, replaced the Narcotic Control Act and parts III and IV of the Food and Drugs Act. This act makes it a criminal offence to possess, traffic, produce, import, or export controlled substances.

Double-blind, placebo-controlled study   A research method in which both the investigator and subject are purposely unaware of key elements in the study (e.g., whether an administered substance is the drug under study or a placebo). This method eliminates bias on the part of both the investigator and the subject.

Drug Identification Number (DIN)   A number, assigned by the Drugs Directorate, to be placed on the label of prescription and over-the-counter drug products that have been evaluated by the Therapeutic Products Directorate (TPD) and approved for sale in Canada.

Drug polymorphism   (pol ee mor'fizm) Variation in response to a drug because of a client's age, sex, size, and body composition.

Food and Drugs Act   Amended many times since its inception in 1953, this act is the main piece of drug legislation in Canada. It protects consumers from contaminated, adulterated, and unsafe drugs and labelling practices and addresses appropriate advertising and selling of drugs, foods, cosmetics, and devices.

Food and Drug Regulations   An adjunct to the Food and Drugs Act, the regulations clarify terms used in the act, and state the processes that companies must carry out to comply with the act in terms of importing, preparing, treating, processing, labelling, advertising, and selling foods, drugs, cosmetics, natural health products including herbal products, and medical devices.

Informed consent   Permission obtained from a client consenting to the performance of a specific test or procedure. Informed consent is required before most invasive procedures can be performed and before a client can be admitted into a research study. The document must be written in a language understood by the client and be dated and signed by the client and at least one witness. Included in the document are clear, rational descriptions of the procedure or test. Should the client decide *not* to participate in the research at any time, the client should be informed that this decision will not have an adverse or negative effect on his or her nursing or health care. Informed consent is voluntary. By law, informed consent must be obtained more than a given number of days or hours before certain procedures are performed and must always be obtained when the client is fully mentally competent.

Investigational new drug (IND)   A drug not yet approved for marketing by Health Canada's Therapeutic Drugs Directorate (TDD) but available for clinical evaluation to determine its safety and efficacy prior to approval for use and sale.

Marihuana Medical Access Regulations   Implemented in 2001, these regulations clearly define the circumstances and the manner in which access to marijuana for medical purposes is permitted.

Narcotic Control Act   This act addressed the possession, sale, manufacture, production, and distribution of narcotics. It was enacted in response to increasing misuse and abuse of drugs in the middle to late 1960s.

New drug submission (NDS)   Once a drug successfully completes the first three phases of an IND study, the drug manufacturer may submit a new drug submission to the Therapeutic Products Directorate (TPD) of Health Canada. If this application is approved, the company may sell the drug exclusively.

Notice of compliance (NOC)   When Health Canada decides that the drug and the manufacturing process are safe and effective, an NOC is issued to the drug company. The NOC allows the company to sell the product by prescription to the Canadian population.

Over-the-counter (OTC) drugs   Drugs that are available to consumers without a prescription. Also called *non-prescription drugs*.

Patent Act   Canada's drug price regime is based on factors established in the Patent Act. This act was created in 1987 to allow pharmaceutical companies intellectual property and a time frame in which a drug could be marketed without competition from generic drugs.

Patented Medicine Prices Review Board (PMPRB)   Created in 1987 to protect consumers and to contribute to Canadian health care. The independent tribunal limits the prices set by manufacturers for all patented medicines, prescription or over-the-counter, to ensure that both existing and new drugs are not sold at excessive prices in Canada.

Placebo   An inactive (inert) substance (e.g., saline, distilled water, starch, sugar); used in experimental drug studies to compare the "effects" of the inactive substance with the bona fide effects of the experimental drug. Placebos are also prescribed to satisfy the requests of clients who cannot be given the medication they request or who, in the judgement of the healthcare provider, do not need this medication.

Precursor Control Regulations (PCRs)   A scheme intended to allow Canada to fulfill its international obligations and meet its domestic needs with respect to the monitoring and control of precursor chemicals such as methamphetamine, gamma hydroxybutyrate (GHB), and other drugs listed in Schedules I, II, and III of the Controlled Drugs and Substances Act, across Canadian borders and within Canada.

Romanow Commission   A commission on the future of health care in Canada, Romanow's report focuses on healthcare reform.

Special Access Programme (SAP)   A hastening of the usual IND approval process by Health Canada's TPD and Biologics and Genetic Therapies Directorate (BGTD). SAP allows practitioners to apply for access to drugs currently unavailable for sale in Canada. The access is limited to individuals who have life-threatening conditions and may require experimental drugs for compassionate reasons or on an emergency basis when other conventional therapies have failed. Drugs showing promise in Phase I and Phase II clinical trials are given to qualified clients, and the drug approval process is shortened if the drug continues to show promise.

CANADIAN DRUG LEGISLATION

In Canada, concerns over the sale and use of foods, drugs, cosmetics, and medical devices began long before these concerns arose in the United States. Canadian drug legislation began in 1875 when the Parliament of Canada passed an act to prevent the sale of adulterated foods, drinks, and drugs. Since that time foods and drugs have been controlled on a national basis. Two acts form the underlying foundation for the drug laws in Canada: the Food and Drugs Act and the Controlled Drugs and Substances Act. The Therapeutic Products Directorate (TPD) is responsible for administering these acts. Currently, there are more than 22 000 human drug products and 40 000 medical devices available on the Canadian market.

Food and Drugs Act

The **Food and Drugs Act** is the primary piece of legislation concerning drugs in Canada. The act has been amended several times since its inception in 1953 and has two main purposes:

1. To protect the consumer from drugs that are contaminated, adulterated, or unsafe for use
2. To address drugs that are labelled falsely and those with misleading or deceptive labelling

With regard to the first purpose, this legislative act recognizes several pharmacopoeias and formularies to be used as references. These are listed in Schedule B, and include the following:

- European Pharmacopoeia
- Pharmacopoeia Internationalis
- The United States Pharmacopoeia/National Formulary
- The British Pharmacopoeia
- Pharmacopée française
- The Canadian Formulary
- The National Formulary
- The Pharmaceutical Codex: Principles and Practices of Pharmaceuticals

The second purpose of the Food and Drugs Act is to address appropriate advertising and selling of drugs, foods, cosmetics, and devices. The act stipulates that no food, drug, cosmetic, or device is to be advertised or sold to the general public as a treatment, preventive, or cure for certain diseases listed in Schedule A of the act. Some examples of these diseases are alcoholism, arteriosclerosis, and cancer. When a drug meets these standards it is labelled with the legend Canadian Standard Drug, or CSD, on its inner and outer labels.

This act has many amendments, or schedules, that have been added over the years. Some of the more important ones are listed in Table 4-1.

Narcotic Control Act

The first **Narcotic Control Act**, passed in 1961, was enacted in response to the growing use and misuse of drugs in the middle and late 1960s. It replaced the previous act, the Canadian Opium and Narcotic Act of 1952. The Narcotic Control Act and parts III and IV of the Food and Drugs Act prohibited activities such as possession; possession for the purpose of trafficking; trafficking; importing and exporting; and cultivation of narcotics, controlled, and restricted drugs.

Controlled Drug and Substances Act (CDSA)

The **Controlled Drug and Substances Act (CDSA)** was passed in 1997, replacing the Narcotic Control Act and parts III and IV of the Food and Drugs Act. The regulations that address the possession, sale, manufacture, disposal, production, import, export, and distribution of certain drugs, their precursors, and other substances classified as controlled are covered in the CDSA. Interestingly, not *all* possession and use of illicit drugs is prohibited. For example, the regulations of the CDSA allow the use of methadone, heroin, and marijuana for medical purposes.

TABLE 4-1

ADDITIONS TO THE FOOD AND DRUGS ACT

Schedule	Description
Schedules C and D	Drugs in these schedules must list where the drug was manufactured and the process and conditions of manufacturing.
Schedule F	List of drugs that can be sold and refilled only on prescription; refills cannot exceed 6 months; labels on these drugs are marked *Pr,* or prescription required. *Examples:* Antibiotics, hormones, and tranquilizers.
Part G	These drugs, also known as controlled drugs, affect the central nervous system (CNS); labels on these drugs are marked *C*. Controlled drugs are categorized into three parts. Part I: designated controlled drugs with misuse potential that may be used for designated medical conditions outlined in Food and Drug Regulations. *Examples:* Amphetamines, methylphenidate, pentobarbital, and preparations containing one controlled drug and one or more active non-controlled drug. Part II: controlled drugs with misuse potential prescribed for medical conditions. *Examples:* Sedatives such as barbiturates and derivatives (secobarbital), thiobarbiturates (pentothal sodium). Part III: controlled drugs with misuse potential. *Examples:* Anabolic steroids (androstanolone), weight reduction drugs (anorexians).
Narcotic Drugs and Preparations	Drugs with high misuse potential. *Examples:* Morphine, codeine >8 mg, amidones (methadone), coca and derivatives (cocaine), benzazocines (analgesics such as pentazocine), fentanyls
Part J	These are restricted drugs with high misuse potential, dangerous physiological and psychological side effects, and no recognized medical use. *Examples:* lysergic acid diethylamide (LSD), mescaline (peyote), harmaline, psilocin and psilocybin (magic mushrooms).
Benzodiazepines and Other Targeted Substances Regulations	A "targeted substance" is either a controlled substance that is included in Schedule 1, or a product or compound that contains a controlled substance that is included in Schedule 1. These are drugs with misuse potential. *Examples:* Benzodiazepine tranquilizers such as diazepam, lorazepam, flumitrazepam, zolpidem

The **Food and Drug Regulations** (Parts G and J) outline similar regulations for controlled and restricted drugs respectively. The Narcotic Control Regulations apply to narcotics, defined as "any substance set out in the schedule or anything that contains any substance set out in the schedule." The CDSA is based on eight schedules that list controlled drugs and substances in order of misuse or harm potential. Schedule I contains the most dangerous drugs, including heroin and cocaine. Schedule II contains cannabis (marijuana) and its derivatives. Schedule III contains the more dangerous drugs such as amphetamines and lysergic acid diethylamide (LSD). Schedule IV contains drugs, such as barbiturates, which are dangerous but have therapeutic uses. Schedules V and VI contain precursors required to produce controlled substances. Schedules VII and VIII contain amounts of cannabis and cannabis resin required for charge and sentencing purposes. The factors that determine which schedule a controlled substance should be placed under are international requirements, the dependence potential and likelihood of abuse of the substance, the extent of its abuse in Canada, the danger it represents to the safety of the public, and the usefulness of the substance as a therapeutic agent. The **Benzodiazepines and Other Targeted Substances Regulations** specify similar restrictions with regards to benzodiazepines, their salts and derivatives, and other targeted substances mentioned in Schedules I and II. The **Precursor Control Regulations**, introduced in 2003, address the need for the control of essential and precursor chemicals routinely used in clandestine labs for the production of methamphetamine, ecstasy, and other Schedule III (chemical) drugs. The **Marihuana Medical Access Regulations** deal with the production, distribution, sale, destruction, record keeping, and licensing issues concerning marijuana for medical use. The Controlled Drugs and Substances Act (Police Enforcement) Regulations apply to the members of a police force. The Royal Canadian Mounted Police (RCMP) are responsible for enforcing the CDSA and related sections of the Criminal Code.

NEW DRUG DEVELOPMENT

The research into and development of new drugs is an ongoing process. The pharmaceutical industry is a multibillion-dollar industry, and pharmaceutical companies must continuously develop new and better drugs to maintain a competitive edge. The research required for the development of new and better drugs may take several years. Hundreds of substances are isolated that never make it to market. Once a potentially beneficial drug has been isolated, the pharmaceutical company must go through a specific process before the drug can be used in the open market. This highly sophisticated, systematic process is regulated and carefully monitored by Health Canada. The primary purpose of Health Canada's TPD is to ensure clients the safety, efficacy, and quality of the drug.

This system of drug research and development is one of the most stringent in the world, and there are many benefits and drawbacks to it. It was developed out of concern for client safety and drug efficacy. To ensure that these two important objectives are met with some degree of certainty requires much time and paperwork. This is the downside to the system. Many drugs are marketed and used in foreign countries long before they get approval for use in Canada. However, drug-related tragedies are more likely to be avoided by this more stringent drug approval system. For example, thalidomide was a widely used sedative-hypnotic that was originally marketed in Europe and made available for distribution in Canada in 1961. It was later found to cause severe deformities in the babies of mothers who took the drug during pregnancy. It was never approved in the United States because a Canadian pharmacologist working for the U.S. Food and Drug Administration (FDA) as a medical officer convinced authorities that the drug was not proven to be safe for use during pregnancy. As a result of the thalidomide tragedy, many governments, including Canada's, tightened their drug approval process. It now takes approximately five years of animal and human testing for a drug to be approved in Canada.

There must be a balance between making new lifesaving therapies available and protecting consumers from potential drug-induced adverse effects. While in the United States the FDA still does not have any significant regulatory authority over vitamins and herbal and homeopathic products, in 2003 Canada introduced the Natural Health Products Regulations. The Regulations cover natural health products such as vitamins and minerals, herbal remedies, homeopathic medicines, traditional medicines (e.g., traditional Chinese medicines), probiotics, and other products like amino acids and essential fatty acids (e.g., omega-3). Before these regulations, the usual stringent system of biological research did not apply to such products. One reason was that many of these products were considered to be dietary supplements rather than medications. The manufacturers' primary obligation regarding such products was to not make "false or misleading" claims regarding their efficacy. For example, a product label may read "For depression," but cannot read "Known to cure depression." Reliable, objective information about these kinds of products was limited but is now growing as more formal research studies are conducted. Consumer demand for and interest in these "alternative medicine" products was the driving force behind the new regulations.

Investigational New Drug Application

A pharmaceutical company must prove both the safety and efficacy of a newly isolated drug before it can be used in the general population. It has been noted that on average approximately 12 years are needed for a drug to go from application to actually being available for prescribing. The new medication must be tested for its pharmacological use in treating the disease or disorder, optimum dosage ranges, and possible side or toxic effects. After extensive laboratory and animal testing, if the results of these preclinical trials are promising, the pharmaceutical company can then submit an application for an **investigational new drug (IND)** to Health Canada to begin clinical trials. Only after the Health Products and Food Branch Inspectorate of Health Canada reviews and approves this application can the pharmaceutical company proceed with investigational studies of the IND in human subjects. There are four phases to this clinical evaluation process in human subjects. The collective goal of these phases is to provide information on the safety, toxicity, efficacy, potency, bioavailability, and purity of the IND. The informed consent of all clients must be obtained before they can be enrolled in an IND study.

Informed Consent

Informed consent involves the careful explanation of the purpose of the study, procedures to be used, possible benefits, and risks involved. The principles of medical ethics dictate that participants in experimental drug studies (research subjects) should be informed volunteers and not be uninformed or coerced to participate in a given study in any way. Some clients may have unrealistic expectations of the IND's usefulness. Often they have the misconception that because an investigational drug is new it must automatically be better than existing forms of therapy. Other volunteers may be reluctant to enter the study because they think they will be treated like "guinea pigs." Whatever the circumstances of the study, the research subjects must be informed of all potential hazards as well as the possible benefits of the new therapy. It should be stressed that involvement in IND studies is truly voluntary and that the subject can quit the study at any time. To enhance objectivity, many studies are designed to incorporate a placebo. A **placebo** is an inert substance that is not a drug (e.g., normal saline). The rationale for administering a placebo to a portion of the research subjects is to separate out real benefits of the investigational drug from those apparent benefits arising out of researcher or subject bias regarding expected or desired results of the drug therapy. A study incorporating a placebo is called a **placebo-controlled** study. In most studies neither the

LEGAL and ETHICAL PRINCIPLES

Administering Placebo Therapy

It is important to remember that the nurse cannot legally administer any medication without a prescriber's order, even in the case of placebo therapy. Even though a placebo is usually physically harmless, and may help a client feel better, its administration should never be taken lightly. Typically placebos are ordered for unusual situations, where there are limited options available. Most prescribers who honour an open and honest relationship with their clients will write a placebo order only when it is absolutely necessary, and when they have explained the rationale for the decision. This can present an ethical dilemma for the nurse. Nurses usually agree and choose to administer the placebo after all other viable alternatives have been used and do so for the client's well-being.

research staff nor the subjects being tested know which subjects are being given the real drug and which the placebo. This further enhances the objectivity of the study results and is known as a **double-blind, placebo-controlled study** because both the researcher and the subject are "blinded" to the actual identity of the substance given to the subject.

Health Canada Drug Approval Process

The Therapeutic Products Directorate (TPD) of Health Canada is responsible for approving drugs for clinical safety and efficacy before they are brought to the market. The process begins with preclinical testing phases and includes *in vitro* studies (using tissue samples and cell cultures) and animal studies. Clinical testing continues throughout Phases I, II, and III to determine safety, dose, and efficacy in human clients. The drug is then put on the market after Phase III if a **new drug submission (NDS)** submitted by the manufacturer is approved by the TPD. Phase IV consists of post-marketing studies as listed in the section "Phase IV" later in this chapter.

Preclinical Investigational Drug Studies

Current medical ethics still require that all new drugs undergo laboratory testing using both *in vitro* (cell or tissue) and animal studies before any testing in human subjects can be done. *In vitro* studies include testing the response of various types of mammalian (including human) cells and tissues to different concentrations of the investigational drug. Various types of cells and tissues for this purpose are originally collected from living or dead animal or human subjects (e.g., surgical or autopsy specimens). These cell samples may then be grown synthetically in the laboratory for several generations of continuous research. These *in vitro* studies help researchers to determine early on if a substance might be too toxic for human clients. Many prospective new drugs are ruled out for human use by this preclinical phase of drug testing. However, a small percentage of the many drugs tested in this manner are referred on for clinical testing in human subjects. At this stage, an application is made to Health Canada with a protocol of the objectives, methods, and rules under which the sponsor will operate during the trial. Clinical trials are normally done in four phases, with each successive phase involving a larger number of individuals.

Four Clinical Phases of Investigational Drug Studies
Phase I: Safety

Phase I studies usually involve small numbers (normally fewer than 100) of healthy volunteers. An exception might involve a toxic drug for a life-threatening illness when administration of the drug to healthy volunteers is not ethical. In this case the only study subjects might be those who already have the illness and for whom other viable treatment options are not available. The purpose of Phase I studies is to determine the drug's side effects, safe dosage range, and the pharmacokinetics (i.e., absorption, distribution, metabolism, and excretion). These are

LEGAL and ETHICAL PRINCIPLES

Client Access to and Costs of Prescription Drugs

The twenty-first century in Canada has seen rapid growth in prescription drug use and costs. In 2004, prescription drugs for Canadians cost $562 per capita (not including drugs provided in hospital). Almost half of this cost (approximately $268) was paid directly out of clients' pockets. Prescription drug costs are increasing at 9 percent annually. In 2004, Canadian pharmacists filled 381 million retail prescriptions. According to the Canadian Institute for Health Information, costs of prescription-only medicines accounted for $18 billion in 2004, more than double the 1996 figure of $7.6 billion. The increased costs are attributed not only to the increase in numbers of prescriptions but also to more costly drugs. Costs of prescription drugs are determined by ingredient costs (manufacturer cost), pharmacy retail mark-up, and the dispensing fee. Dispensing fees are the additional fee pharmacists charge for dispensing prescription drugs to clients. Such costs can vary from $2 to over $10, depending on the pharmacy.

Prescription drugs are not covered under the **Canada Health Act**. Clients must pay for a drug unless the drug is covered by a private drug plan or a federal, provincial, or territorial (F/P/T) drug plan. Most provincial plans provide for the costs of drugs to the poor, the elderly, those with catastrophic drug costs, and those with certain conditions (e.g., cancer, HIV/AIDS). The federal government provides coverage for aboriginal peoples. Each Canadian province and territory has a formulary committee that decides which drugs are "listed" on a provincial formulary and reimbursed by the drug benefit health plan, which have restricted access, and which are not covered. There is a wide variety of access to prescription drugs across the country: provincial and territorial drug plans vary in eligibility criteria, drugs covered, and financing. Provinces base the decision to list a drug on a variety of factors such as effectiveness analyses, cost, government priorities, and client advocacy. Some drugs may be restricted if they require special monitoring or if the cost is high.

Because of discrepancies in drug coverage among F/P/T drug plans, the Common Drug Review Directorate was established in 2002 at the Canadian Coordinating Office for Health Technology Assessment. An independent advisory body, the Canadian Expert Drug Advisory Committee (CEDAC), has members from all jurisdictions except Quebec. CEDAC makes evidence-based recommendations regarding the listing of drugs to the F/P/T formularies. This process is intended to provide equal access to all drugs, to reduce duplication between formularies, and to streamline the review process for new drugs. However, the drug plans make the decision on which drugs will make the final formulary listing.

In 2002, Roy Romanow, the head of the **Romanow Commission**, presented a report, *Building on Values: The Future of Health Care in Canada,* that recommended extensive changes to protect the long-term sustainability of the Canadian healthcare system. One recommendation was to establish a national pharmacare program. One aspect of the national program would be the Catastrophic Drug Transfer Program (CDTP), under which the federal government would assist the provinces to cover those who have extremely high drug costs. In addition, a national formulary administered by a National Drug Agency would be formed in an effort to control costs and to evaluate safety and cost-effectiveness of all new and existing prescription drugs. Romanow also recommended a review of the Canadian patent legislation regarding new prescription drugs and better access to generic drugs. A full discussion of the report is available at http://www.hc-sc.gc.ca/english/care/romanow/hcc0086.html.

---

determined through blood tests, urinalyses, assessments of vital signs, and specific monitoring tests. These trials usually last a few days to a few weeks.

Phase II: Effectiveness

Phase II studies involve larger numbers of volunteers (usually around 100 to 500) who have the disease or ailment that the drug is designed to diagnose or treat. This is usually a randomized control study composed of clients of similar age, sex distribution, and medical history. Volunteers are divided randomly into two groups. The experimental group receives the experimental drug; the control group receives a placebo or standard treatment. These studies may be "blind," meaning that the volunteers do not know which drug they are receiving (called **blinded investigational drug study**), or "double blind," meaning that neither the volunteers nor the researchers are aware who is receiving the drug (called **double-blind, placebo-controlled study**). Study participants are closely monitored for the drug's effectiveness and any side effects. This is also the phase for refining therapeutic dosage ranges. Phase II trials normally last six months to one year. If no serious side effects occur, the study can progress to Phase III.

Phase III: Duration and Longer Term Impacts

Phase III studies involve larger numbers of clients (normally 500 to 2500), who are followed by medical research centres and other types of healthcare facilities. The clients may be treated at the centre itself or be spread over a wider geographic area and followed at a local inpatient or outpatient facility. The purpose of this larger sample size is to provide more in-depth information about the drug's efficacy, benefits, and full range of possible adverse effects. Information obtained during this clinical phase helps identify any risks associated with the new drug. Most Phase III studies are randomized and blinded. The length of Phase III can vary but generally lasts from two to four years. After Phase III is completed, the drug's sponsor can submit an NDS to Health Canada's TPD and BGTD for a thorough review. The NDS contains detailed information about the drug's safety (including any anticipated side effects), efficacy, and quality; results of the preclinical and clinical trials; and packaging and labelling information. The review process for an NDS drug takes an average of 18 months.

Once the drug is proven to have a health benefit (efficacy), a **notice of compliance (NOC)** and a **drug identification number (DIN)** are issued, which pave the way for the pharmaceutical company to market the new drug exclusively.

Phase IV: Post-marketing Studies

Phase IV studies are studies voluntarily conducted by pharmaceutical companies after the new drug has gone onto the market to obtain further proof of its therapeutic effects and safety. Additional clinical studies may determine alternative uses for the drug (e.g., other health conditions). Data from such studies are usually gathered for at least two years after commercial release. Often these studies compare the safety and efficacy of the new drug with that of another drug in the same therapeutic category. An example would be a comparison of a new nonsteroidal anti-inflammatory drug (NSAID) with ibuprofen in the treatment of osteoarthritis. Some medications make it through all phases of clinical trials without any problems. However, when they are used in the general population, sometimes severe adverse effects show up. If a pattern of severe reactions to a newly marketed drug begins to emerge, Health Canada may request that the manufacturer of the drug issue a voluntary recall. If the drug manufacturer refuses to recall the medication, and if the number and/or severity of reactions reaches a certain level, then the Health Products and Food Branch Inspectorate of Health Canada will seek court action to condemn the product and allow it to be seized by legal authorities. Such an action, in effect, becomes an involuntary recall on behalf of the manufacturer.

Health Canada may issue a recall, alert, or warning about a drug. Notification by Heath Canada may take the form of press releases, Web site announcements (http://www.hc-sc.gc.ca/dhp-mps/medeff/advisories-avis/index_e.html), and "Dear Health Professional" letters.

Special Access Programme

Health Canada has attempted to make life-saving investigational drug therapies available on an individual basis through the **Special Access Programme (SAP)**. The SAP provides compassionate access to drugs not approved for sale in Canada and is limited to those with serious or life-threatening conditions such as intractable depression, epilepsy, transplant rejection, hemophilia and other blood disorders, terminal cancer, and AIDS. It can also respond to an emergency health crisis. One example is when the drinking water in Walkerton, Ontario became contaminated with *Escherichia coli* 0157:H7. Doctors in Walkerton applied to Health Canada for access to a drug not yet approved for use for seriously ill clients with *Escherichia coli* bacteria infections. Because of the urgent need, Health Canada approved the application.

This program is not intended to get around the clinical trial approval process. The physician is responsible for initiating the request on the client's behalf and for ensuring that the request is supported by reliable evidence. Health Canada then reviews the request and upon approval delivers a Letter of Authorization to both the drug manufacturer and the physician. The drug company makes the final decision whether and under what conditions the client may receive the drug. The physician is responsible for informing the client of all possible risks and benefits of the drug.

Patent Act

The Patent Act originated in 1987 and was revised in 1993. A patent allows brand-name drug companies to extend their exclusive market rights of patented medicine to 20 years from the previous time frame of 17 years. Regulations also link the issuing of notices of compliance for generic drugs to the expiry of the patent protection period for the innovator drug. The Act also established the **Patented Medicine Prices Review Board (PMPRB)** to monitor and control the price of patented medicine. Twice yearly, patentees must file price and sales information for all patented medicine. If a price is deemed excessive, the PMPRB can order it reduced (this has only happened eight times since 1999). When patents expire, competing pharmaceutical companies can manufacture and sell generic forms of the drug.

Generic Drugs

A generic drug is a chemically identical equivalent of a brand name drug. A manufacturer will develop a generic version in about two to three years, with a cost of approximately $1 million. Once developed, the generic manufacturer submits an Abbreviated New Drug Submission (ANDS) to Health Canada TPD, with evidence that the generic formulation is bioequivalent to the brand formulation.

The consumer cost of a generic drug is generally about 45 percent less than the brand name equivalent drug. Generic drug (and all non-patented drugs) prices are not regulated by the PMPRB but are determined provincially. For example, in Ontario, the Ontario Drug Benefit Act and the Ontario Drug Interchangeability and Dispensing Fee Act allow the Ontario government to establish generic drug prices for the drugs that it will reimburse. Basically there is a "70/90" rule. A new generic drug is priced at no higher than 70 percent of the price of the brand name; succeeding generic drugs are priced no higher than 90 percent of the price of the initial generic drug. Generic and existing or revised drugs do not have to go through the Common Drug Review to receive a listing recommendation as new drugs do, but are submitted directly to the various drug plans to request listing.

Drug Advertising in Canada

Drug advertising in Canada is regulated by Health Canada. Direct-to-consumer advertising (such as ads in consumer magazines and on subways) is restricted to simply giving the names of prescription drugs, but these ads do not make claims for product effectiveness. (This is not the case in the United States). Advertising in professional healthcare journals contains claims and prescribing information. Advertising Standards Canada (ASC) and the Pharmaceutical Advertising Advisory Board (PAAB) review and clear advertisements according to standards set by the Food and Drugs Act. Although the clearance procedure is voluntary, most companies follow it.

NURSING IMPLICATIONS

Legal Issues

In Canada, nursing is a self-regulated profession. Nurses' roles and responsibilities are defined within the framework of the Code of Ethics for Registered Nurses and provincially and territorially established nursing practice standards. Besides these standards, nurses must be familiar with specific institutional policies and procedures to fulfill their legal obligation and responsibility to their clients. Some of the legal issues and concepts are listed and defined in the box below. The "5 Rights" of medication administration and the law provide necessary standards for safe client care and should never be ignored (see Chapter 1). The law should be viewed as a helpful framework for practice, not as an impediment to care. Standards of care, nurse practice acts, federal and provincial/territorial legislation, and institutional policies should also be examined and put into practice with drug therapy as related to the nursing process.

BOX 4-1

Canadian Nurses Association *Code of Ethics for Registered Nurses*

The Canadian Nurses Association *Code of Ethics for Registered Nurses* provides guidance for decision-making processes about clients and ethical matters of professional nursing practice. It serves as a means of self-evaluation and reflection about ethics and nursing practice and also provides peer review initiatives. This code educates nurses, other healthcare providers, and the lay public about moral obligations and commitment. It is revised periodically to address societal needs, values, and conditions impacting ethical nursing practice. This code is applicable to all nurses and in all settings. This code also defines and briefly discusses the following: values, safe and competent nursing care, health, well-being, choices, dignity, confidentiality, accountability, and quality practice environments. The code views the client as someone deserving of respect and who has individual needs and values. The client is also to have his or her control respected at all times; confidentiality of all information about the client is demanded. The client's dignity is of utmost importance in nursing care, as is the role of the nurse as an advocate. Regarding the health team, all clients should be treated in a comprehensive and individualized approach. Clients are treated with the assistance of experts around the nurse, who should acknowledge his or her own limitations when appropriate. The social context of nursing means that nurses should work in a setting that contributes to client care and to their own professional satisfaction. The responsibilities of the profession hold that nurses are to always sustain ethical conduct and remain true to the client and his or her rights, needs, and interests.

Data from Canadian Nurses Association. (2002). *Code of ethics for registered nurses*. Ottawa, ON. Complete Code available online at http://www.cna-nurses.ca/cna/documents/pdf/publications/CodeofEthics2002_e.pdf.

Ethical Practice

Ethical nursing practice is based on basic ethical principles such as beneficence, autonomy, justice, veracity, and confidentiality. The Canadian Nurses Association Code of Ethics (Box 4-1) should be a familiar framework of practice to all nurses and serve as an ethical guideline for nursing care. These ethical principles and codes of ethics ensure that the nurse is acting on behalf of the client and with the client's best interests at heart.

As professionals, nurses are responsible for providing safe nursing care to clients regardless of the setting, person, group, community, or family involved. Although it is not within nurses' realm of ethical and professional responsibility to impose their own values or standards on the client, it is within their realm to provide information and to help clients face healthcare decisions.

Nurses have the right to refuse to participate in any treatment or aspect of a client's care that violates their personal ethical principles. However, this should be done without deserting the client. Should this situation arise, it is the nurse's responsibility to inform the appropriate persons about the conflict and to transfer the client to the safe care of another professional nurse before the start of treatment. However, the nurse should always be a client advocate, and this includes being non-judgemental.

It is a nurse's responsibility to always provide the highest quality nursing care and practice within the standards of care. The CNA Code of Ethics (Box 4-1), standards of nursing practice, federal and provincial codes, and the previously mentioned ethical principles should constitute the framework for the professional practice of nursing. Another relevant document is the *ICN Code of Ethics for Nurses*. The ICN (International Council of Nurses), located in Geneva, Switzerland, was founded in 1899 and published its first version of a code of ethics for nurses in

---

LEGAL and ETHICAL PRINCIPLES

Common Legal and Ethics-Related Terms

Autonomy: Self-determination and ability to act on one's own; implications include promoting a client's decision-making process, supporting informed consent, and assisting in decisions or making a decision when a client is posing harm to himself or herself.

Beneficence: The doing or active promotion of good; implications include determining how the client can best be served.

Confidentiality: The duty to respect privileged information about a client; implications include not talking about a client in public or outside the context of the healthcare setting.

Justice: Being fair or equal in one's actions; implications include the fair distribution of resources for the care of the client and determination of when to treat.

Non-maleficence: The duty to do no harm to a client; implications include avoiding doing any deliberate harm while rendering nursing care.

Veracity: Duty to tell the truth; implications include telling the truth with regard to placebos, investigational new drugs, and informed consent.

1953. The code has been revised many times, and the last revision was in 2000. A new code is forthcoming. For more information, visit the International Council of Nurses Web site at http://www.icn.ch/ethics.htm.

ETHNOCULTURAL CONSIDERATIONS

Canada is a tremendously ethnoculturally diverse nation. With a healthcare system emphasizing cure, prescribed drugs are often a major part of a client's therapeutic regimen. The Canadian healthcare system often advocates a "one size fits all" approach to treatment; however, a more multicultural, holistic approach to alterations in health status would help in meeting the needs of such a diverse client population. Canadian demographics continue to change. In 2001, 18 percent of Canada's population was foreign born. The number of visible minorities is growing, with more than 200 ethnic groups listed in the 2001 Canada Census. The three largest visible minorities, which account for approximately two-thirds of the visible minority population, are Chinese, South Asians, and Blacks. They are followed by Filipinos, Arabs and West Asians, Latin Americans, Southeast Asians, Koreans, and Japanese. Aboriginal people account for 3.3 percent of Canada's total population. In addition, the white majority not only is shrinking but also is aging, whereas the Aboriginal and immigrant populations not only are growing but also are young. It is estimated that by 2017, one in every five Canadian residents will be a member of a visible minority. These changes in the nation's demographics will continue to demand a holistic, individualized, and ethnoculturally competent approach to health care, with both non-pharmacological and pharmacological treatment regimens.

Ethnocultural factors are important to holistic nursing care because they affect the client's health, health beliefs, and healthcare practices, including drug therapy. To prevent conflict from between the goals of nursing and health care and the dictates of a client's ethnocultural background, the nurse needs to acknowledge and accept the influences of a client's ethnocultural beliefs, values, and customs. Some examples of ethnocultural influences are presented in the Ethnocultural Implications box at right.

Influence of Ethnicity and Genetics

In reference to specific drug therapy and a client's response, the concept of polymorphism is critical to further understanding how the same drug can result in a different response. For example, why does a Chinese client require lower doses of an anti-anxiety drug than a Caucasian client? Why does a Black Canadian respond differently to antihypertensives than a Caucasian does? **Drug polymorphism** refers to the effect of a client's age, sex, size, body composition, and other variables with associated changes in how an individual absorbs or metabolizes specific drugs. Factors contributing to drug polymorphism may be loosely categorized into environment (e.g., diet and nutritional status), ethnicity, and genetics (inherited factors).

Medication response depends greatly on the client's adherence level with the therapy. Adherence may vary depending on a client's ethnocultural beliefs, experiences with medications, personal expectations, family expectations, family influence, and level of education. However, adherence is not the only issue. Healthcare providers also need to be aware that some clients subscribe to other therapies, such as herbal and homeopathic remedies, that can inhibit or accelerate drug metabolism and therefore alter a drug's response.

Environmental considerations that play an important part in drug responses include factors such as diet. For

ETHNOCULTURAL IMPLICATIONS

Common Practices of Selected Ethnocultural Groups

Ethnoculture	Common Practices
Blacks and Caribbeans	Practise folk medicine; reluctant to seek health care unless seriously ill; spiritual beliefs influence
Chinese	Believe in and practise humoral medical system involving a balance of life forces; various parts of the body respond to yin and yang; use physicians, acupuncturists, acupressurists, and herbalists in their health care
Hispanic	View health as a balance of hot/cold and strong/weak; external influences such as curses, spirits, "bad wind" are believed to have an effect
European	Traditional health beliefs are held; some still practise folk medicine
Aboriginal people	Healing practices to promote mental, spiritual, and emotional well-being, which may include herbal and other remedies, ceremony, counselling, and the wisdom of elders; healers may be herbalists, medicine men, and shamans; believe in harmony with nature; ill spirits are seen as disease-causing
Filipino	Believe in and practise traditional and Western medicine; illness results from an imbalance in the body
South Asian	Healing practices used to restore imbalance in body humours, bile, wind, phlegm. Dietary imbalance often seen as source of illness. Use traditional medicines, vows, rituals, and bio-medicine; elderly women may suggest home remedies.
Western	Increased participation in health care; demand more explanation about diseases and treatment, as well as the prevention of diseases

Note: The above are generalizations. It is important for the nurse to conduct a thorough assessment of individual clients.

example, a diet high in fat has been documented to increase the absorption of the agent griseofulvin (an antifungal agent). Malnutrition with deficiencies in protein, vitamins, and minerals may alter the functioning of metabolic enzymes and the body's ability to absorb or eliminate a medication.

Genetic factors also influence how different racial or ethnic groups may respond to drugs. Some clients of European and African descent are "slow acetylators" and metabolize drugs at a slower rate, resulting in elevated drug level concentrations because of these changes in metabolism. Some clients of Japanese and Inuit descent are more "rapid acetylators" and metabolize drugs more aggressively, resulting in decreased drug concentrations. Chinese, Japanese, Malaysians, and Thais are "poor metabolizers" of debrisoquine; therefore agents such as codeine are likely to be *more* effective at lower dosages in these clients than in those of European descent. Several major drug classifications are relatively well researched with regard to responses in different genetic backgrounds; these are outlined in Table 4-2.

Individuals throughout the world often share common views and beliefs regarding health practices and medication use. However, specific ethnocultural influences, beliefs, and practices related to medication administration do exist. In an increasingly diverse Canada, nurses need to be alert to and concerned with each client's ethnocultural background to ensure safe, high-quality nursing care.

Specifically, some people in the Black and Caribbean communities believe in spiritual influences on prevention and treatment and follow health practices such as proper diet and rest; the use of herbal teas, laxatives, and protective bracelets; and the use of folk medicine, prayer, and the "laying on of hands." Varied home remedies also can be an important component of their health practices.

Some Asians, especially the Chinese, believe in the yin and yang, which are opposing forces that lead to health when balanced and to illness when out of balance. The yin represents the female and the negative energies of darkness and cold; the yang represents the male and the positive energies of light and warmth. Beliefs in yin and yang must be respected by all who participate in the care of Chinese clients. Some Cambodians may believe in the traditional practice of coin rubbing, in which an area of the body is rubbed with a coin or spoon until the skin becomes red. Vietnamese clients may believe that illness results from excesses of hot or cold, bad wind, and cool water. Bad wind is thought to be released by creating small bruises on the body or by "cupping." In cupping, a cup is heated and then placed on the skin, usually on the forehead or abdomen; as it cools, it contracts, drawing the skin and what is believed to be excess energy or "air" into the cup; a circular bruise is left on the skin. All of these beliefs and practices need to be considered—especially when a client strongly believes in their use versus the use of medications. Many of these beliefs are strongly grounded in religion, and similar beliefs may be held by other Asian communities, including Thais, Koreans, and Japanese.

Some Aboriginal Canadians hold a belief in maintaining health by seeking harmony with nature or keeping a balance between the body and mind and the environment. The traditional healer for this culture is the medicine man. "Smudging" is a common ceremony used to cleanse the body spiritually and physically. A herb such as sage or sweetgrass is burned and the smoke is rubbed or brushed over the body

Some individuals of South Asian descent follow a variety of traditional health practices. Illness is seen as an imbalance in the body humours, bile, wind, and phlegm, and treatment is seen to restore these imbalances. Treatment may consist of home remedies, dietary regimens, prayers, rituals, and consultation with hakims, veds, babajis, pundits, homeopaths, and jyotshis.

However, it is important to remember that these beliefs still vary from client to client; therefore the nurse should always consult with the client first. Barriers to adequate health care for the ethnoculturally diverse Canadian client population include language, poverty, access, pride, and beliefs regarding medical practices. Medications may represent different meanings to different ethnocultures, as would any form of medical treatment.

TABLE 4-2		
EXAMPLES OF VARYING RESPONSES		
Racial or Ethnic Group	**Drug Classification**	**Response**
Blacks and Caribbeans	Antihypertensive agents	Blacks and Caribbeans respond better to diuretics than to beta-blockers and ACE inhibitors.
		Blacks and Caribbeans respond less effectively to beta-blockers.
		Blacks and Caribbeans respond best to calcium channel blockers, especially diltiazem.
		Blacks and Caribbeans respond less effectively to single-drug therapy.
Asian and Hispanic	Antipsychotic and anti-anxiety agents	Asians need lower doses of certain drugs such as haloperidol.
		Japanese and Chinese are more prone to rapid build-up of mephenytoin and so are at risk for sedation and overdosage.
		Asians and Hispanics respond better to lower doses of antidepressants.
		Chinese require lower doses of antipsychotics.
		Japanese require lower doses of antimanic agents.

Note: The comparative group with these responses is whites. *ACE*, Angiotensin converting enzyme.

Therefore, before any medication is administered, a thorough ethnocultural assessment should be completed, including questions regarding the following:

- Health beliefs and practices
- Past uses of medicine
- Folk remedies
- Home remedies
- Use of over-the-counter (OTC) drugs, and natural health products including herbal remedies
- Usual responses to illness
- Responsiveness to medical treatment
- Religious practices and beliefs (e.g., many Christian Scientists believe in taking no medications at all)
- Dietary habits

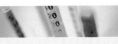

POINTS to REMEMBER

▼ Various pieces of federal legislation, as well as provincial law, provincial practice acts, and institutional policies, are there to support the safety and efficacy of drug therapy and the nursing process.

▼ Nurses should refer to authoritative resources, such as Health Canada and the *Compendium of Pharmaceuticals and Specialties* to expand their knowledge base on official standards for therapeutic use, client safety, quality, purity, strength, packaging safety, and dosage forms.

▼ The Food and Drugs Act and the Controlled Drugs and Substances Act provide nurses and other healthcare providers with information on those drugs that cause little to no dependency and those with a high level of abuse and dependency and include agents such as narcotics and central nervous system depressants.

▼ Informed consent should always be implemented and will help nurses understand their responsibilities to their clients as client advocates.

▼ A nurse's role in the IND process should be one of adhering to the research protocol while also being a client advocate.

▼ The "5 Rights" of medication administration include the right drug, dose, time, route, and client. There are other rights to consider, such as the right to a "system analysis" (see Chapter 1), the right to proper functioning of equipment for administration of specific medications (i.e., intravenous [IV] pump, client-controlled analgesia [PCA]), the right to know about the medications for safe and efficient use, and the right to documentation.

▼ Legal guidelines, ethical principles, and the CNA Code of Ethics ensure that the nurse is acting from a solid foundation of practice through these various standards and policies.

EXAMINATION REVIEW QUESTIONS

1 Your client states that she has been taking six or more acetylsalicylic acid tablets per day for her "bad bones." The nurse continues with a thorough assessment and makes the decision to double up on the prescribed dose to help minimize this client's "bad bones." Which of the following statements correctly describes this scenario?
a. The nurse is planning to give medications with a certain level of professional autonomy such as deciding on a dose not ordered.
b. The nurse is making the decision to change the specific dosage of the drug.
c. The nurse is following one of the "5 Rights" of drug administration, specifically the right to fairly safe standards of care.
d. The "right" to the right dosage of drug is being violated in this situation.

2 Barriers to health care for your 59-year-old female Chinese client would most likely include which of the following?
a. X-rays are seen as a break in the soul's integrity.
b. Hospital diets are interpreted as being healing and healthful.
c. Being hospitalized is a source of peace and socialization for this ethnoculture.
d. Intrusive procedures are seen as contrary to holding the body in high regard and respect.

3 A 39-year-old Muslim woman was just admitted to the labour and delivery unit for pre-term labour. Perceived barriers to health care for this client with regard to self-care include which of the following? Individuals of this religious faith or belief system
a. cannot consume pork.
b. do not believe in self-help.
c. do not believe in self-discipline.
d. cannot value good health because of their beliefs.

4 The same 39-year-old Muslim woman is diagnosed as having type 1 diabetes mellitus. Which of her beliefs may pose a problem for her because of pork allergy?
a. The pork allergy is not problematic because insulin is made only from beef.
b. She cannot consume pork, so she cannot take this type of insulin and needs to know about her other options.
c. Her belief of not helping herself because it may be perceived as weakness will not allow her to take insulin.
d. She does not believe in self-help, so she will not inquire about other options available to her for treatment.

5 Some clients are poor metabolizers of medications. Which of the following is the racial-ethnic group most commonly associated with this characteristic?
a. Whites
b. Hispanics
c. Chinese
d. Blacks and Caribbeans

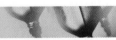

For answers see http://evolve.elsevier.com/Lilley/pharmacology/.

CRITICAL THINKING ACTIVITIES

1 Discuss the impact of ethnocultural practices as they relate to safe and effective drug therapy.

2 Medication errors have been occurring with increasing frequency in the unit where you are employed. A committee has been appointed to look at why the medication errors occur and how to resolve the problem. In consideration of this and of the drug administration process, is it always safe to go by only the guidelines of using the "5 Rights" of drug administration? Why or why not? Explain your answer.

3 One of your psychiatric clients is an Aboriginal youth with a problem of alcohol abuse. He is 17 years old and has a history of repeated problems with being drunk, coming to school with alcohol detected on his breath, and acting as if under the influence. What is of particular concern for this client and why?

For answers see http://evolve.elsevier.com/Lilley/pharmacology/.

BIBLIOGRAPHY

Bon Bedard, C. (2003). Cross-cultural profiles. Updated by Health Care Interpreters, Calgary Health Region. Calgary, AB: Multicultural Awareness Program, Peter Lougheed Centre.

Canada Gazette. (2003). Order amending schedule III to the controlled drugs and substances act. Retrieved July 17, 2005, from http://canadagazette.gc.ca/partII/2003/20031231/html/sor412-e.html

Canadian Institute for Health Information. (2005). *Drug expenditure in Canada 1985 to 2004.* Ottawa, ON: Source. Retrieved July 17, 2005, from http://secure.cihi.ca/cihiweb/dispPage.jsp?cw_page=AR_80_E

Canadian Institute for Health Information. (2005). *Exploring the 70/30 split: how Canada's health care system is financed.* Retrieved November 4, 2005 from http://secure.cihi.ca/cihiweb/dispPage.jsp?cw_page=PG_469_E

Canadian Nurses Association. (2002). *Code of ethics for registered nurses.* Ottawa, ON: Author. Available online at http://www.cna-nurses.ca/

Canadian Pharmacists Association. (2003). *Therapeutic choices* (4th ed.). Ottawa, ON: Author.

Canadian Pharmacists Association. (2005). *Compendium of pharmaceuticals and specialties. The Canadian drug reference for health professionals.* Ottawa, ON: Author. [The subscription-based e-CPS is available at http://www.pharmacists.ca.]

Department of Justice Canada. (2004). *Narcotic control regulations.* Retrieved July 17, 2005, from http://laws.justice.gc.ca/en/C-38.8/C.R.C.-c.1041/76122.html

Health Canada. (2002). Commission on the future of health care in Canada. Retrieved October 31, 2005 from http://www.hc-sc.gc.ca/english/care/romanow/hcc0403.html

Health Canada. (2003a). Natural health products regulations. *Canada Gazette* 137(13). Ottawa, ON: Author. Retrieved July 17, 2005, from http://canadagazette.gc.ca/partII/2003/20030618/html/sor196-e.html

Health Canada. (2003b). Clinical trials. Retrieved July 17, 2005, from http://www.hc-sc.gc.ca/english/media/releases/2000/2000_11ebk1.htm

Katzung, B.G. (2004). *Basic and clinical pharmacology* (9th ed.). New York: McGraw Hill.

Kudzma, E.C. (1999). Culturally competent drug administration. *American Journal of Nursing* 99(8), 46–51.

McKenry, L.M., & Salerno, E. (2003). *Mosby's pharmacology in nursing—revised and updated* (21st ed.). St Louis, MO: Mosby.

Lehne, R.A. (2004). *Pharmacology for nursing care* (5th ed.). St Louis, MO: Saunders.

Morgan, S. (2005). Canadian prescription drug costs surpass $18 billion. [Electronic version]. *Canadian Medical Association Journal* 172(10). Retrieved July 17, 2005, from http://www.cmaj.ca/cgi/content/full/172/10/1323

Saul, D. (2004). National pharmacare: A pill not easily swallowed. *University of Toronto Medical Journal* 82, 14–15.

Skidmore-Roth, L. (2006). *Mosby's 2006 nursing drug reference* (19th ed.). St Louis, MO: Mosby.

Statistics Canada. (2004). Canada's ethnocultural portrait: The changing mosaic. Retrieved July 17, 2005, from http://www12.statcan.ca/english/census01/products/analytic/companion/etoimm/canada.

Medication Errors: Preventing and Responding

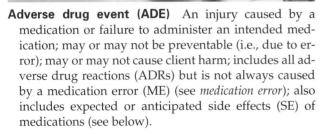

OBJECTIVES

After reading this chapter, the successful student will be able to do the following:

1 Define the terms *adverse drug event* (ADE), *medication error* (ME), and *medication misadventure* (MM).

2 Discuss the various MEs common to nurses and other healthcare professionals.

3 Discuss nursing measures to prevent MEs.

4 Identify possible consequences of MEs to clients and to nurses.

5 Discuss the possible impact and consequences of MEs on a client's physiological and psychological well-being.

6 Identify the impact of MEs on the cost of health care.

7 Discuss the ethical issues of medication administration as related to the nursing process.

8 Analyze the need for political action from professional nurses as related to drug therapy and the prevention of MEs.

e-LEARNING ACTIVITIES

Student CD-ROM
- Animations
- Medication Administration Checklists
- IV Therapy Checklists

evolve Web site (http://evolve.elsevier.com/Lilley/pharmacology/)
- Online Chapter Worksheet • Frequently Asked Questions
- Learning Tips and Content Updates • WebLinks • Online Appendices and Supplements • Mosby/Saunders ePharmacology Update • Access to *Mosby's Drug Consult*

GLOSSARY

Adverse drug event (ADE) An injury caused by a medication or failure to administer an intended medication; may or may not be preventable (i.e., due to error); may or may not cause client harm; includes all adverse drug reactions (ADRs) but is not always caused by a medication error (ME) (see *medication error*); also includes expected or anticipated side effects (SE) of medications (see below).

Adverse drug reaction (ADR) Any unexpected, unintended, undesired, or excessive response to a medication. It may or may not be preventable (i.e., due to error) and may or may not cause client harm. All ADRs are ADEs, but not all ADEs are ADRs.

Allergic reaction An immunological hypersensitivity reaction resulting from an unusual sensitivity of a client to a particular medication.

Iatrogenic hazard Any potential or actual client harm that is caused by errant actions of healthcare staff members.

Idiosyncratic reaction An abnormal and unexpected susceptibility to a medication, other than an allergic reaction, that is peculiar to an individual client.

Medical error Broad term commonly used to refer to any error in any phase of clinical client care that causes or has the potential to cause client harm; may involve wrong medications or medical or surgical procedures (error of commission), or the failure to implement any of these interventions when they would normally be indicated (error of omission).

Medication error (ME) Failure to complete a planned action as it was intended, or the use of an incorrect plan, at any point in the process of providing medications to clients.

Medication misadventure (MM) The broadest term for any undesirable medication-related event in client care that is usually *iatrogenic* in nature (i.e., caused by healthcare professionals, not by the client) but is sometimes caused by the client's actions (e.g., unintentional or intentional overdose).

Side effect Any undesirable effect of a medication that is expected or anticipated to occur in a predictable percentage of the population of clients who receive a given medication. Side effects can range from mild to severe client responses but usually eventually resolve with completion of drug therapy.

INTRODUCTION

General Impact of Errors on Clients: Overview

In 2004, The World Health Organization launched the World Alliance for Patient Safety to learn more about why adverse events occur and to find ways to prevent them. According to a landmark study of adverse events in Canadian hospitals, between 9000 and 24 000 clients die each year because of adverse events or errors. Although the term **medical error** is often used as an umbrella term in the published literature, errors can occur during all phases of healthcare delivery and involve errant actions by all categories of health professionals. Some of the more common types of errors include misdiagnosis, client misidentification, wrong-site surgery, and medication errors (MEs). Intangible losses resulting from such adverse outcomes include loss of client trust in, and dissatisfaction with, the healthcare system. This chapter focuses on the issues related to MEs and how to prevent and respond to these errors. Included is an overview of various institutional, educational, and sociological issues that may contribute to such errors.

Medication Errors

As mentioned in Chapter 2, a more general term that includes **medication errors (MEs)** is **medication misadventures (MMs)**. Figure 5-1 illustrates the various classes and subclasses of MMs and highlights the following facts:

- MMs include *all* types of clinical problems with medications. These include MEs, **adverse drug events (ADEs)**, and **adverse drug reactions (ADRs)**.
- All ADRs are by definition also ADEs, but not all ADEs are ADRs. For example, a client suffers a toxic reaction due to a mistaken overdose of medication by a nurse. If this client's body would normally tolerate the same medication at a therapeutic dose (instead of an overdose), then his toxic reaction is not an ADR, per se. However, this situation still represents an ADE, and in this case an ME as well. Two major types of ADRs include **allergic reactions** and **idiosyncratic reactions**. The latter of these is normally unpredictable, whereas the former may or may not be predictable. **Side effects** are usually predictable and are usually not thought of as ADRs, but are still ADEs.
- MEs may or may not lead to ADEs, including ADRs. For example, a nurse may give an unintended medication to a client without causing the client any harm; however,

this situation still constitutes an ME because the medication was not ordered by the prescriber and not intended for the client. Even if the medication was ordered by the prescriber, it could represent an ME on the part of the prescriber. A nurse who administers such an incorrectly prescribed medication may also commit an ME if a "reasonably prudent" nurse would normally be expected to have sufficient knowledge to at least question a given prescriber order. **Iatrogenic hazard** refers to client harm caused by any healthcare personnel.

It is important to consider the medication administration and system analysis processes when discussing MEs. Identifying, responding to, and ultimately preventing MEs requires more than utilizing the "5 Rights" of drug administration or consideration of the nurse. All persons involved in the medication administration process must be considered, including the prescriber, the transcriber of the order to the chart, nurses, pharmacy staff, and any other ancillary staff involved in this process. A system analysis takes the "5 Rights" one step further and examines the entire healthcare system, the healthcare professionals involved, and any other factor that has an impact on the error.

MEs are a particularly important segment of MMs in general because, by definition, any error is preventable. MEs are a common cause of adverse healthcare outcomes and can range in severity from having no significant effect on the client to directly causing client disability or death. The pediatric population and the elderly are particularly vulnerable. U.S. figures estimate MEs as the eighth leading cause of death. Approximately five MEs occur for every 100 medication administrations, and an estimated 30% of clients with drug-related injuries are disabled for more than six months or die. MEs can occur with any type of drug, but certain classifications of medications are associated with a higher likelihood of adverse outcomes because of pharmacological properties or narrow therapeutic indices or simply because of the frequency of prescribing. Top causative agents for drug-induced disability are chemotherapeutic agents, narcotic analgesics, antibiotics, and vaccines. The non-profit Institute for Safe Medication Practices Canada (ISMP Canada) independently reviews voluntary reports of MEs and regularly composes a list of "high-alert" medications (Box 5-1) that have a

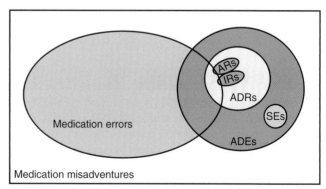

FIG. 5-1 Diagram illustrating the various classes and subclasses of medication misadventures. *ADEs,* Adverse drug events; *ADRs,* adverse drug reactions, *ARs,* allergic reactions; *IRs,* idiosyncratic reactions; *SEs,* side effects.

narrow margin of safety and the greatest potential for significant client harm when misused.

Many preventable ADRs begin at the ordering stage with the prescriber. Many of these errors result from the increasing number of drugs on the market to keep track of, some of which have names that look or sound alike. It is most dangerous when two drugs from different therapeutic classes have similar names. This can result in effects on the client that are grossly different from those intended. Generally in Canada the use of generic drug names is advocated, trade names can be included as an error prevention strategy. For instance, to avoid confusion between diphenhydramine and dimenhydrinate, the prescriber could include the commonly used trade names: diphenhydramine (Benadryl) and dimenhydrinate (Gravol). Other strategies can also include storing medications in functional groupings rather than in alphabetical order, and buying from different manufacturers when there are issues of look-alike packaging. Another strategy is "tall man lettering": using capital letters for se-

quences of letters that distinguish a drug name from its look-alike (see Table 5-1). In addition, prescribers in practice may continue to order medications according to certain well-known trade names such as "Tylenol" for acetaminophen (personal communication, Thursday,

BOX 5-1

Common Classes of Medications Involved in Serious Errors

- Analgesics
- Antibiotics
- Anticoagulants
- Antidiabetic agents (particularly insulin)
- Cardiovascular agents
- Chemotherapeutic (anticancer) agents
- Vaccines

TABLE 5-1

SELECTED EXAMPLES OF COMMONLY CONFUSED GENERIC DRUG NAMES

Drug Products	Recommended Revision/Comments
acetohexamide vs. acetazolamide	acetoHEXAMIDE (oral antidiabetic, not available in Canada) acetaZOLAMIDE (carbonic anhydrase inhibitor)
clomiphene vs. clomipramine	clomiPHENE (estrogen agonist–antagonist) clomiPRAMINE (norepinephrine reuptake inhibitor)
chlorpropamide vs. chlorpromazine	chlorproPAMIDE (oral antidiabetic) chlorproMAZINE (phenothiazine)
chlorpromazine vs. prochlorperazine	chlorproMAZINE (phenothiazine) prochlorPERAZINE (phenothiazine)
Claritin-D 24-Hour vs. Claritin-D	24-hr vs. 12-hr duration of action
Cytovene vs. Cytosar	Antiviral agents vs. antineoplastic (anticancer) agent
daunorubicin vs. doxorubicin	Two different antineoplastic agents with possibly different indications for use
Depo-Estradiol vs. Depo-Testadiol	Female vs. male hormonal injection
Elavil vs. Plavix	Antidepressant vs. antiplatelet agent
enoxaparin vs. erythropoietin	Anticoagulant vs. antibiotic
Epivir vs. Combivir	Single-drug anti-HIV agent vs. double-drug combination anti-HIV agent
fentanyl vs. sufentanil	Both are injectable anesthetics but with a significant difference in potency and duration of action
glipizide vs. glyburide	Two different antidiabetic agents
gliclazide vs. glimepiride or glyberide	Immediate-release vs. sustained-release antidiabetic agent (different duration of action and thus different effect on blood sugar levels)
Lacrilube vs. Surgilube	Ophthalmic lubricant vs. skin/orifice lubricant
Micronase vs. Micro-K	Antidiabetic agents vs. potassium supplement
Narcan vs. Norcuron	Opiate antidote vs. skeletal muscle paralyzing agent for use in operating rooms
Ocuflox vs. Ocufen	Ophthalmic antibiotic vs. ophthalmic anti-inflammatory agent
paclitaxel vs. Paxil	Antineoplastic agent vs. antidepressant
Paxil vs. Plavix	Antidepressant vs. antiplatelet agent
quinine vs. quinidine	Antimalarial agent vs. cardiac antidysrhythmic agent
Reminyl vs. Amaryl	Cholinesterase inhibitor for mild to moderate Alzheimer's disease vs. antidiabetic agent for type 2 diabetes
Soma Compound vs. Soma	Combination muscle relaxant with acetylsalicylic acid vs. muscle relaxant alone
Tamiflu vs. Theraflu	Prescription antiviral agent vs. nonprescription (OTC) cold remedy
Tegretol vs. Toradol	Anticonvulsant vs. anti-inflammatory agent
TobraDex vs. Tobrex	Combination ophthalmic antibiotic and anti-inflammatory agent vs. ophthalmic antibiotic alone
Vancenase vs. Vanceril	Nasal steroid inhaler vs. oral steroid inhaler
Viagra vs. Allegra	Male sexual stimulant vs. antihistamine allergy drug
Xanax vs. Zantac	Anti-anxiety agent vs. anti–stomach acid agent
Zocor vs. Cozaar vs. Zoloft	Anticholesterol agent vs. antihypertensive agent vs. antidepressant
Zofran vs. Zyban	Antiemetic agent vs. smoking cessation aid

October 27, 2005 1:28 PM, Christine Koczmara, Nurse Educator, Institute for Safe Medication Practices Canada).

Nursing Measures to Prevent Medication Errors

Nurses can reduce the likelihood of MEs by taking the following precautions:

- Minimize verbal/telephone orders, but when necessary repeat the order to confirm with prescriber, spell the drug name aloud, and speak slowly and clearly.
- List the indication (reason for use) next to each drug order.
- Avoid medical shorthand, including abbreviations and acronyms, which can cause confusion and miscommunication (see the Legal and Ethical Principles box below). This is especially true with abbreviations for

LEGAL and ETHICAL PRINCIPLES

Use of Abbreviations

Medication errors often occur as a result of misinterpretation of abbreviations. The Institute for Safe Medication Practices (ISMP) recommends that the following be written out *in full* and the abbreviation avoided.

Abbreviation	Intended Meaning	Common Error
U	Units	Mistaken as a zero (0), a four (4), and cc.
mcg (μg)	micrograms	mistaken for mg (milligrams)*
Q.D.	Latin abbreviation for "every day"	The period after the abbreviation "Q" has been mistaken for an "I" and results in medications being given "QID" (4 times daily) vs. once daily.
Q.O.D.	Latin abbreviation for "every other day"	Misinterpreted as "QD" (daily) or QID. If "O" is poorly written it may look like a period or "I."
D/C	Discharge or discontinue	Medications have been prematurely discontinued when D/C (intended to mean "discharge") was misinterpreted as "discontinue" because it was followed by a list of drugs.
HS	Half strength	Misinterpretation as the Latin abbreviation "HS" (hour of sleep).
cc	Cubic centimetres	Mistaken as "U" (units) when written poorly.
AU, AS, AD	Both ears, left ear, right ear	Misinterpreted as the Latin abbreviation "OU" (both eyes), "OS" (left eye), or "OD" (right eye).

*In Canada, the trend is now towards using mcg in practice so it is important to note the difference between mcg and mg in orders.

medications, which can be ambiguous and can result in the administration of an unintended drug (e.g., CPZ can be interpreted as Compazine, an anti-emetic, or chlorpromazine, an antipsychotic agent).

- Never assume anything, including medication routes or anything else not specified in a drug order.
- If questioning a medication order for any reason (e.g., dose, drug, indication), don't assume that the prescriber is correct. Resist any fear of challenging prescriber authority when in doubt or when the situation clearly warrants such action. Prescribers may and often do make errors. The nurse should remember also his or her important role as client advocate and seek support from colleagues and superiors wherever available and whenever appropriate.
- Don't try to decipher illegibly written orders. The nurse should contact the prescriber for clarification and report prescribers who habitually write illegible orders to appropriate authorities within or even outside of the institution (e.g., College of Physicians and Surgeons). Illegible orders fall below applicable standards for quality medical care and can endanger client well-being.
- When in doubt about the correctness of even a legibly written order, always double-check with the prescriber, a pharmacist, or the literature (e.g., reference books).
- Check the medication order and what is available, while using the "5 Rights" of medication administration.
- Always read the label three times and check it against the medication order before administering the medication.
- *Never* use trailing zeros with medication orders and/or their transcription (e.g., do not use 1.0 mg). *Always* use a leading zero for decimal dosages (e.g., do use 0.25 mg). Otherwise, unintended overdoses or underdoses may result. For example, .25 mg digoxin could be misread as 25 mg digoxin, a potentially lethal dose, and 1.0 mg warfarin could be misread as 10 mg warfarin, a tenfold dose increase with possible risk of hemorrhage.
- Carefully read all labels for the "5 Rights" of medication administration: drug, dose, time, route, and client.
- Take time to learn the nuances of unusual dosage forms (e.g., the need to "prime" the salmeterol xinafoate-fluticasone propionate Diskus or salmeterol xinafoate Diskus inhalers before dosing; proper application of transdermal medication patches, which can vary among different drug products). If in doubt, consult a pharmacist or other knowledgeable colleague.
- Encourage the use of both trade names and generic names with orders for medications.
- Listen to and honour any concerns expressed by clients. Check with the prescriber if the client states, "That isn't what I usually take," "I already had that pill today," or "The doctor said he was changing my medication or dosage."
- Check client allergies and update the client's chart and wristband whenever needed.
- Strive to always be alert. Never be too busy to stop, learn, and inquire.
- If working conditions are a problem, join organizations with other nurses to advocate for improved working conditions (see Political Action on p. 65).

Possible Consequences to Nurses of Medication Errors

As mentioned earlier, the possible effects of an ME on a client range from no significant effect to permanent disability and even death in the most extreme cases. However, MEs can also affect healthcare professionals, including nurses and student nurses, in a number of ways. An error that involves significant client harm or death may take an extreme emotional toll on the nurse involved in the error. Nurses may be named as defendants in malpractice litigation, with possibly serious consequences. Many nurses choose to carry personal malpractice insurance for this reason, although nurses working in institutional settings are usually covered by the institution's liability insurance policy. Nurses should obtain clear written documentation of any provided institutional coverage before deciding whether to carry individual malpractice insurance. Administrative responses to MEs vary from institution to institution and depend on the severity of the error. Possible responses include directives to obtain continuing education or refresher training and disciplinary action, including suspension or termination of employment. Nurses who have violated regulations of their provincial Standards of Nursing Practice may also be counselled or disciplined by their provincial governing body, including suspension or permanent revocation of their nursing registration. Student nurses, given their lack of clinical experience, should be especially careful to avoid MEs, as well as errors in general. When in doubt about the correct course of action, students should consult with clinical instructors or more experienced staff nurses. Nonetheless, if a student nurse realizes that he or she has committed an error, the student should notify the responsible clinical instructor immediately. The client may require additional monitoring or medication, and the prescriber may also need to be notified. Though no-one wants to see errors occur, they can ultimately be useful, though stressful, learning experiences for the student nurse. However, student nurses who commit sufficiently serious errors or display a pattern of errors can expect more severe disciplinary action. This can range from required extra clinical time or repeating of a clinical course to suspension or expulsion from the nursing school program (see the information on Educational System Issues in the next section).

PSYCHOSOCIAL ISSUES THAT CONTRIBUTE TO ERRORS

Organizational Issues

Research strongly suggests that errors are not due primarily to the actions of habitually errant individuals or of a single subgroup; rather, they result from a failure at the *system* level. Vindictive disciplinary action or finger pointing is now generally recognized as counterproductive in the long run. An institutional culture of safety that fosters non-punitive reporting of MEs, near misses, and ADEs will facilitate safer practices and promote change. MEs can occur at many different stages in the administration process, and although nurses are often blamed for the errors, about half the time the source of the error can be traced back to the medication ordering (prescriber) stage. Interdisciplinary collaboration and communication are key to an environment that promotes a culture of safety. The value of collaborative relationships cannot be overestimated. Such relationships can be especially helpful when approaching prescribers regarding questionable orders or when advocating for workplace improvements that can benefit both clients and staff.

The Human Factors (HF) concept in organizational functioning is important because of the impact of workplace interpersonal relationships on performance. Especially important is the need to recognize the limits of human performance in any system and to plan accordingly. Examples include safe nurse-to-client staffing ratios; a higher proportion of professional nurses in the staff mix; having two nurses double-check high-risk medications before administering these medications to the client; and contacting prescribers regarding any questionable medication orders. Effective responses to health system errors are the result of an open, proactive approach in which the healthcare team works together to prevent errors from occurring and to report, analyze, and learn from actual MEs. Nurses need to be active on committees within their employment setting that focus on quality assurance issues, that help to promote safety with high-risk drugs and practice areas, and that look at the medication administration process in its entirety. Pharmacy, medical, nursing, and other technical staff should *always* have regular input with regard to safety measures and client care.

Educational System Issues

Because of the rigorous cognitive and even physical challenges of healthcare study and practice, the health professions tend to attract strong-willed, intelligent people. However, the constant expectation to be "smart" and "on top of things" with regard to clinical knowledge often leads to denial, fear, or shame about being wrong or simply not remembering a piece of information. Instead of making guesses in clinical situations about medications, nurses need to stop and check the order and be sure to have a thorough knowledge about the drug, route, dosage, and indications *before* giving the drug. Authoritative sources for finding information about drugs include current (<5 years old) drug reference guides such as *Mosby's Drug Consult*, the *Compendium of Pharmaceuticals and Specialties, Drug Formulary (DF)*, and others written by legitimate experts. Even the most capable healthcare provider cannot know everything nor have every fact ever read available for immediate recall. This is especially true given the increasing complexity of healthcare practice. Forward-thinking faculty members recognize that learning is a lifelong process. Endorsing a philosophy of "no question is a stupid question" helps clinical instructors teach error prevention habits. In contrast, berating or otherwise penalizing a student for not immediately recalling a given fact or for asking questions instills fear and shame. It also discourages dialogue that would otherwise promote and enhance student learning and mastery of concepts.

Related Sociological Factors

Healthcare practice has a longstanding and ingrained tradition of disparate social and economic class structures among different categories of professionals. The most recognized differences are those among nurses, physicians, and administrators. At their worst, these differences have fostered maltreatment of nurses, especially by physicians, whose behaviour has often not been challenged or corrected by administrators. A 2005 study published in the *American Journal of Nursing* (Rosenstein & O'Daniel) assessed nurses' perceptions of the effects of disruptive behaviour on relationships between disciplines and on client care. Disruptive behaviour is defined in this study as "any inappropriate behaviour, confrontation, or conflict, ranging from verbal abuse to physical or sexual harassment" (p. 55). This survey revealed a significant level of disruptive behaviour among nurses as well as physicians, suggesting a sobering problem within and across disciplines. The respondents reported that disruptive behaviour contributed to levels of stress, frustration, and concentration and undermined team collaboration, information transfer, communication, and nurse–physician relationships. Respondents felt that disruptive behaviour decreased both staff morale and the quality of client care. In addition, they identified a strong correlation between disruptive behaviour and the occurrence of adverse events and errors.

Communication between prescribers and other members of the healthcare team has improved somewhat over the years with newer generations of physicians. This is due in large part to more progressive approaches in medical education that emphasize a team-oriented approach—a more realistic approach, given the ever-increasing complexities of healthcare delivery and the undeniable fact that no one team member can master every fact and skill.

PREVENTING AND RESPONDING TO ERRORS

Reporting and Responding to Medication Errors

Reporting MEs is a professional responsibility that is shared by nurses and all members of the healthcare team. To prevent and respond to MEs, nurses should
- Assess and document all relevant client parameters (e.g., vital signs, latest laboratory values).
- Assess the client for effects of the drug and consult reference materials or colleagues as needed.
- Complete ME reporting forms after contacting the physician, charge nurse, or nurse supervisor. If a student nurse, contact the client's nurse and the instructor.
- Monitor the client's condition closely.
- Think and act critically; modify nursing practice to prevent further errors.
- Conduct detailed root cause analyses (RCAs) to learn from errors and avoid error repetition.

- Analyze methods to reduce the complexity of drug administration and develop consistent, easy-to-read procedures related to medication administration.
- Suggest changes in policy and procedures to ensure safe medication administration; propose simple medication error-related policies.
- Join political efforts to advocate for safer "nurse-to-client" staffing ratios and for improved quality assurance protocols in the handling of MEs.

Effective use of technology such as computerized prescriber order entry (CPOE) and bar coding of medication packages has also been shown to reduce MEs. Error reporting systems that offer the option of anonymity can also improve practice safety. Internal, facility-based systems of error tracking may generate data to help customize policy and procedure development. Most institutional pharmacies in Canada have an internal ADE system. Nurses should be aware of this system and comfortable with reporting suspected ADEs to this department for evaluation and follow-up. Additionally, there are nationwide confidential reporting programs that collect and disseminate safety information on a larger scale. One such program is the Canadian Medication Incident Reporting and Prevention System (CMIRPS), which collects national data on medical incidents to "strengthen the Canadian healthcare system's capacity to report, analyze, and manage medication incident data on a national basis, while mounting comprehensive prevention and education programs for healthcare practitioners" (Health Canada). Saskatchewan has become the first jurisdiction in Canada to require health districts to report all medical errors to the province.

The Canadian Adverse Drug Reaction Monitoring Program (CADRMP) is another useful program provided by Health Canada's Therapeutic Products Directorate. A member of the public or a health professional can report problems with medications or medical devices via telephone, mail, or online at the Health Canada Web site. The Institute for Safe Medication Practices Canada (ISMP Canada) and The Canadian Council on Health Services Accreditation (CCHSA) also provide useful information and reporting services to healthcare providers aimed at safety enhancement. Table 5-2 contains Web site addresses of these and other helpful organizations.

OTHER ETHICAL ISSUES

Notification of Client Regarding Errors

A 2001 article (McCleave) published in the *Journal of Clinical Outcomes Management* recognizes the obligation of institutions and healthcare providers to notify clients when errors have occurred in their care. The article not only emphasizes the ethical basis for this practice but also addresses the legal implications. Clients who seek lawyers are often motivated primarily by a perceived imbalance in power between themselves and their healthcare providers, and also by fear of financial burden. Healthcare organizations that apologize, accept responsibility for obvious errors, and even offer needed financial

TABLE 5-2

ORGANIZATIONS AND WEB SITES WITH INFORMATION PERTAINING TO MEDICATION SAFETY

Name of Organization	Internet Address
Institute for Safe Medication Practices (ISMP) Canada	http://www.ismp-canada.org/
Canadian Medication Incident Reporting and Prevention System (CMIRPS)	http://www.ismp-canada.org/cmirps.htm
Medication Error Report: Voluntary Medication Incident and Near Miss Reporting Program	https://www.ismp-canada.org/err_report.htm
Canadian Council on Health Services Accreditation	http://www.cchsa.ca/
Canadian Institutes of Health Research	http://www.cihr-irsc.gc.ca/e/193.html
Canadian Institute for Health Information	http://www.hc-sc.gc.ca/hppb/healthcare/health_research.htm
Health Canada: Health Care Network	http://www.hc-sc.gc.ca/dhp-mps/medeff/
Health Canada: Canadian Adverse Drug Reaction Monitoring Program (CADRMP) Adverse Reaction Database	databasdon/index_e.html
Canadian Safety Patient Institute National Steering Committee on Patient Safety (NSCPS)	http://www.patientsafetyinstitute.ca
Safer Health Care Now!	http://www.saferhealthcarenow.ca/

support (e.g., for travel expenses, temporary loss of wages) are more likely to avoid litigation and potentially much larger financial settlements.

Whistle-blowing

In clinical settings, whistle-blowing refers to a disclosure of client care errors made outside a healthcare facility when the organization's internal chain of command has failed to correct significant problems. Such a disclosure may be made to a regulatory or investigative agency or to the public through the news media. One theory is that whistle-blowing results from a failure of organizational ethics. Virtually all practising nurses will eventually witness lapses in client care. Though a student or inexperienced nurse may not realistically be in a viable position to challenge an institution's hierarchy, every nurse should consider, preferably in advance, how he or she might choose to respond to such a situation. The *Code of Ethics for Registered Nurses* (see Box 4-1 on p. 54) makes clear several moral imperatives that may ultimately justify blowing the whistle, even at the risk of losing one's job. All healthcare providers should familiarize themselves with their institution's usual procedures for error reporting, including

how and when to approach levels of leadership above their immediate supervisor. When the usual systems fail, disclosure may be the most ethical course of action.

POLITICAL ACTION

An Ounce of Prevention: Nurse Advocacy for Safer Healthcare Organizations

From its foundation in 1908 (as the Canadian National Association of Trained Nurses), the CNA has advocated for legislation on behalf of nurses and their clients. A 2001 Canadian study (Baumann et al.) found that nurses are stressed, vulnerable to injury, and have one of the highest professional absentee and disability rates, undermining quality of client care and overall client satisfaction. Almost two-thirds of the 17 000 Canadian nurses participating in the study saw an increase in their workloads. Thirty percent said they were confident that their discharged clients were not capable of managing their own care. Almost half said the quality of care in their workplace had deteriorated in the last year. This is a major reason that nurses choose to leave the profession or practice setting.

One of the earliest studies to address the modern problem of hospital nursing shortages was published in 1989 in the *New England Journal of Medicine* (Hartz et al.). The study found that hospitals with fewer registered nurses tended to have higher client mortality rates. In the 1990s massive illegal strikes by nurses in Alberta, Saskatchewan, Quebec, and Nova Scotia protested working conditions and cuts to healthcare spending. Provincial governments refused to negotiate and nurses were legislated back to work. Canada's Office of Nursing Policy was developed in 1999 in an attempt to bring more attention to nursing issues. One of the current initiatives is to develop *Healthy Work Environment Best Practice Guidelines (BPG)*. Two specific areas of focus are workload and staffing and workload and safety of the nurse. In addition, the Canadian Institute for Health Information in collaboration with Statistics Canada and Health Canada is undertaking a national survey on the health of nurses. *Building the Future: An integrated strategy for nursing human resources in Canada* (2005), the first national nursing study endorsed and led by nursing stakeholder groups, is gathering input from nurses across Canada to identify and develop long-term solutions to current and future challenges.

Nurses as Legislators

Another significant way that nurses can advocate for themselves and for quality client care is to run for election to public office and to support nurse members of parliament at the provincial and federal levels. An important strategy is to be knowledgeable of the healthcare issues and to vote for the party that supports and promotes nursing. Nurses in Canada are approximately 260 000 strong, and united are a major force that can advocate for change.

SUMMARY

The increasing complexity of nursing practice also increases the risk for MEs. Widely recognized and common causes of errors include misunderstanding of abbreviations, illegible prescriber handwriting, miscommunication during verbal or telephone orders, and confusing drug nomenclature. The structure of various organizational, educational, and sociological systems surrounding healthcare delivery may also contribute directly or indirectly to the occurrence of MEs. Understanding these factors can help the nurse take proactive steps to im-prove these systems. Such actions can range from fostering improved communication with other healthcare team members, including students, to advocating politically for safer conditions for both clients and staff. The first priority when an error does occur is to protect the client from further harm whenever possible. All MEs should serve as red flags that warrant further reflection, detailed analysis, and future preventive actions on the part of nurses, other healthcare professionals, and possibly even clients themselves.

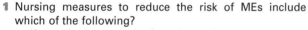

POINTS to REMEMBER

▼ ADEs may or may not cause client harm. They include all ADRs and expected side effects of medications.
▼ *Medical error* is a broad term used to address any error that occurs within any phase of clinical client care. Medical errors *may* involve medications.
▼ MEs may or may not lead to ADEs. MEs include giving the drug to the wrong client; confusing sound-alike and look-alike drugs; giving the wrong drug or the wrong dose; and giving a drug by the wrong route or at the wrong time.
▼ To help prevent MEs, nurses should be prepared and knowledgeable and always take the time to perform the three checks of the "5 Rights" of medication administration. It is also important for the nurse to always be aware of the entire medication administration process and of the system analysis approach to preventing MEs.

▼ Nurses should always encourage clients to ask questions about their medications and to let their healthcare provider know if they are questioning the drug or any component of the medication administration process.
▼ Nurses should encourage clients to always keep drug allergy information on their person and a current list of medications in their wallet or purse and on their refrigerator with the following information:
• Drug name
• Why the drug is being used
• Usual dosage range and what dose the client is taking
• Expected side effects and toxic effects of the drug
• Physician's name and phone number

EXAMINATION REVIEW QUESTIONS

1 Nursing measures to reduce the risk of MEs include which of the following?
a. If questioning an order for a drug, always assume that the prescriber is correct.
b. Never question the order a board-certified surgeon has prescribed for a client.
c. Always double-check sound-alike and look-alike drug names due to high risk of error.
d. Always go with your gut reaction and if you think a drug route has been incorrectly prescribed, go ahead and use the oral route.

2 It is important with the medication administration process to remember which of the following?
a. When in doubt about an order, ask a colleague about the drug.
b. Contact the client and ask what they know about the medication and if they have taken it prior to this hospitalization.
c. If too busy, stop, ask the charge nurse, and be sure to research the drug once you have given it to the client at the right time.
d. List and honour any concerns expressed by the client.

3 If a student nurse realizes that a drug error has been committed, it is important—in the student's educational process—to emphasize which of the following?
a. The student bears no legal responsibility when giving medications.
b. The major legal responsibility is on the healthcare institution where the student is placed for clinical and therefore the school and faculty are not legally liable.
c. Student nurses lack the needed knowledge for medications and therefore should never give drugs to their clients.
d. Once the student has committed a medication error, his or her responsibility is to the client and to being honest and accountable. Responsibility continues from there with constant monitoring of the client and his or her physiological and emotional responses to the error.

4 Which of the following is an acceptable authoritative resource for information about medication?
a. An experienced and well-qualified professional nurse colleague.
b. The faculty person supervising the student during clinical rotations.
c. Drug information pulled from Internet sites.
d. Fellow colleagues, students, or the physician in charge.

CRITICAL THINKING ACTIVITIES

1 Discuss the medication administration process related to prevention of MEs with the inclusion of some actual suggestions for implementing this process on a nursing unit.

2 You are a charge nurse at a small community hospital. The physician ordered a stat IV vancomycin infusion, but when the bag comes up from the pharmacy, you notice that the dosage is incorrect. It takes 2 hours for the pharmacy to send up an IV bag with the correct dose. As you check the medication, you note that it is the right drug, right dose, etc., yet it has been 2 hours since it was ordered stat. What, if anything, should you do before you give this medication?

3 List several Internet sources for medication safety and briefly discuss how this information could be shared with clients in a community outpatient setting that includes mostly indigent clients.

For answers see http://evolve.elsevier.com/Lilley/pharmacology/.

BIBLIOGRAPHY

Baker, G.R., Norton, P.G., Flintoft, V., Blais, R., Brown, A., Cox, J. et al. (2004). The Canadian adverse events study: The incidence of adverse events among hospital patient in Canada. [Electronic version]. *Canadian Medical Association Journal, 170* (11).

Baumann, A., O'Brien-Pallas, L., Armstrong-Stausser, M., Blythe, J., Bourbonnais, R., Cameron, S. et al. (2001). Commitment and care. The benefits of a healthy workplace for nurses, their patients, and the system. Retrieved July 20, 2005, from http://www.chsrf.ca/funding_opportunities/commissioned_research/polisyn/pdf/pscomcare_e.pdf

Benner, P., Sheets, V.J.D., Uris, P., Malloch, K., Schwed, K.J.D., & Jamison, D. (2002). Individual, practice, and system causes of errors in nursing: A taxonomy. *Journal of Nursing Administration, 32*(10), 509–523.

Bournes, D.A., & Flint, F. (2003). Mis-takes: Mistakes in the nurse-person process. *Nursing Science Quarterly, 16*(2), 127–130.

Building the Future. (2005). *Building the future: An integrated strategy for nursing human resources in Canada.* Retrieved July 20, 2005, from http://www.buildingthefuture.ca/

Canadian Institute for Health Information. (2004). *Health care in Canada.* Ottawa, ON: Author.

Canadian Nurses Association. (2002). Code of ethics for registered nurses. Retrieved July 20, 2005, from http://www.cna-nurses.ca/cna/documents/pdf/publications/CodeofEthics2002_e.pdf

CBC Health and Science News. (2004). Hospital goes high-tech to prevent medication errors. Retrieved July 19, 2005, from http://www.cbc.ca/storyview/AOL/2004/06/24/scitech/rx_automate040624

CBC News. (2004). Faint warning. From coloured tabs to computerized signals: How Canada tracks dangerous drugs. Retrieved July 19, 2005, from http://www.cbc.ca/news/adr/

College of Nurses of Ontario. (2004). Best practices in disclosing health care error. Retrieved July 19, 2005, from http://www.cno.org/new/nptices/disclosing_error.htm

Cook, A. F. (2004). An error by any other name. *American Journal of Nursing, 104*(6), 32–43.

Ehman, A.J. (2004). Mandatory error reporting in Saskatchewan. [Electronic version]. *Canadian Medical Association Journal, 171*(10).

Fletcher, J.J., Sorrell, J.M., & Silva, M.C. (1998). Whistleblowing as a failure of organizational ethics. *Online Journal of Issues in Nursing.* Retrieved July 19, 2005, from http://nursingworld.org/ojin/topic8/topic8_3.htm

Hall, L. M., Doran, D., & Pink, G. (2004). Nurse staffing models, nursing hours, and patient safety outcomes. *Journal of Nursing Administration, 34*(1), 41-45.

Harding, J., & Lefebvre, P. (2002). Medication incidents. Retrieved July 19, 2005, from http://www.lillyhospitalsurvey.ca/HPC2/Content/rep_2002_Medincidents.asp

Hartz, A.J., Krakauer, H., Kuhn, E.M., Young, M., Jacobsen, S.J., Gay, G. et al. (1989). Hospital characteristics and mortality rates. [Electronic version]. *New England Journal of Medicine, 321* (25): 1720–1725.

Health Canada. (2004). Canadian medication incident reporting and prevention system (CMIRPS). Retrieved February 3, 2006, from http://www.hc-sc.gc.ca/dhp-mps/medeff/advers-react-neg/fs-if/cmirps-scdpim_e.html

Hughes, R. (2004). Are you tired? Sleep deprivation compromises nurses' health and jeopardizes patients. *American Journal of Nursing, 104*(3), 36–38.

Hughes, R. (2005). Medication errors: Why they happen, and how they can be prevented. *American Journal of Nursing, 105*(2), 14–24.

Institute for Safe Medication Practices Canada. (2003). High alert medications. No room for error. Retrieved July 19, 2005, from http://www.ismp-canada.org/download/HNews0308.pdf

Institute for Safe Medication Practices. (2005). Do not use these dangerous abbreviations or dose designations. Retrieved July 19, 2005, from http://www.ismp.org/Newsletters/acutecare/articles/20030220_2.asp

Johnston, L., & Conly, J. M. (2004). Patient safety: What does it all mean? [Electronic version]. *Infectious Diseases & Medical Microbiology, 15*(2).

Koczmara, C., Jelincic, V., & Dueck, C. (2005). Dangerous abbreviations: "U" can make a difference! *Canadian Association of Critical Care Nurses, 16*(3), 11–15. Retrieved November 5, 2005, from http://www.ismp-canada.org/publications.htm

Kozer, E., Scolnik, D., Macpherson, A., Keays, T., Shi, K., Luk, T. et al. (2002). Variables associated with medication errors in pediatric emergency medicine. *Pediatrics, 110*(4), 737–742.

McCleave, S.H. (2001). How to respond to a formal patient complaint. *Journal of Clinical Outcomes Management, 8*(10), 35–42.

McRoberts, S. (2005). The use of bar code technology in medication administration. *Clinical Nurse Specialist, 19*(2), 55–56.

National Association of Pharmacy Regulatory Authorities. (2002). Minimizing medication errors. Retrieved July 19, 2005, from http://www.napra.org/docs/0/95/157/166.asp

Orser, B. (2000). Reducing medication errors. [Electronic version]. *Canadian Medical Association Journal, 162*, 1150–1151.

Rich, V. (2005). How we think about medication errors: A model and a change. *American Journal of Nursing, 105*(3), 10–11.

Richardson, W.C., Berwick, D.M., Bisgard, J.C., Bristow, L.R., Buck, C.R., Cassel, C.K. et al. (1999). *To err is human: Building a safer health system.* Washington, DC: National Academy Press.

Rosenstein, A.H., & O'Daniel, M. (2005). Original research: Disruptive behavior and clinical outcomes: Perceptions of nurses and physicians: Nurses, physicians, and administrators say that clinicians' disruptive behavior has negative effects on clinical outcomes. *American Journal of Nursing, 105*(1), 54–64.

Wong, J. (2005). Medication awareness key to catching errors: Study. Retrieved July 19, 2005, from http://www.news.utoronto.ca/bin6/050228-1038.asp

World Health Organization. (2005). World alliance for patient safety. Retrieved July 19, 2005, from http://www.who.int/patientsafety/worldalliance/en/

Client Education and Drug Therapy

OBJECTIVES

After reading this chapter, the successful student will be able to do the following:

1. Discuss the importance of client education in the safe and efficient administration of medications, including application of the nursing process.

2. Discuss some of the teaching–learning principles related to client education and drug therapy and the nursing process in any healthcare setting and with clients of any age.

3. Identify the effect of the various developmental phases (as per Erikson) on client education and drug therapy.

4. Develop a comprehensive client teaching care plan for medication administration.

e-LEARNING ACTIVITIES

Student CD-ROM
- Animations
- Medication Administration Checklists
- IV Therapy Checklists

evolve Web site (http://evolve.elsevier.com/Lilley/pharmacology/)
- Online Chapter Worksheet • Frequently Asked Questions
- Learning Tips and Content Updates • WebLinks • Online Appendixes and Supplements • Mosby/Saunders ePharmacology Update • Access to *Mosby's Drug Consult*

With the ever-changing arena of health care and the increasing emphasis on consumer awareness, the role of nurses as educators is expanding. Because more clients are being managed in the home setting, client education is an essential component of health care. Without it, high quality client care could not be provided. Client education is crucial to help clients adapt to illness, prevent illness, maintain wellness, and provide self-care. It is identified as a process, similar to the nursing process, whereby clients are assisted to learn and to assimilate healthy behaviours into their lifestyle. Learning is defined as a change in behaviour and teaching as a sharing of knowledge. Although nurses can never be certain that clients will take medications as prescribed, they can be sure to carefully assess, plan, implement, and evaluate the teaching they provide to clients about their medications.

ASSESSMENT OF LEARNING NEEDS RELATED TO DRUG THERAPY

As in the nursing process, a thorough assessment of learning needs must be completed before clients are educated about their medications. A thorough assessment includes gathering subjective and objective data about the following:

- Adaptation to any illnesses
- Cognitive abilities
- Coping mechanisms
- Ethnocultural background
- Emotional status
- Environment at home and work
- Family relationships
- Financial status
- Growth and development level as per Erikson's stages of development (Box 6-1)
- Health beliefs
- Information the client understands about past and present medical condition, medical therapy, and medications
- Language(s) spoken
- Level of education
- Limitations (physical, psychological, cognitive, and motor)
- Medications currently taken (including over-the-counter [OTC] drugs, prescription drugs, and herbal products)
- Mobility
- Nutritional status

Erikson's Stages of Development

American psychoanalyst Erik Erikson (1902–1994) believed that the interaction between internal drives and cultural demands causes people to develop through eight crises, or psychosocial stages (Erikson, 1959).

Infant (birth–1 year of age): Trust vs. mistrust. Infant learns to trust himself or herself, others, and the environment; learns to love and be loved.

Toddler (1–3 years of age): Autonomy vs. shame and doubt. Toddler learns independence; learns to master the physical environment and maintain self-esteem.

Preschooler (3–6 years of age): Initiative vs. guilt. Preschooler learns basic problem solving; develops conscience and sexual identity; initiates activities, as well as imitates.

School-age child: Industry vs. inferiority. School-age child learns to do things well; develops a sense of self-worth.

Adolescent: Identity vs. role confusion. Adolescent integrates many roles into self-identity through role models and peer pressure.

Young adult: Intimacy vs. isolation. Young adult establishes deep and lasting relationships; learns to make commitment as spouse, parent, partner.

Middle-aged adult: Generativity vs. stagnation. Adult learns commitment to community and world; is productive in career, family, civic interests.

Older adult: Integrity vs. despair. Older adult appreciates life role and status; deals with loss and prepares for death.

- Past health behaviours
- Self-care ability
- Sensory status
- Social support

The nurse needs to also inquire about any drug misinformation and use of folk medicine, home remedies, and natural health products, including herbal treatments. Other questions may need to focus on the client's beliefs about his or her illness, its treatment, past experiences with healthcare regimens, adherence history, and barriers to learning (language, finances, ethnocultural beliefs, previous negative or limited experiences with the healthcare system/team, and denial of illness or need for healthcare intervention). During the assessment of learning needs, the nurse must be astutely aware of the client's verbal and non-verbal communication. Often a client does not tell the nurse how he or she truly feels. A seeming discrepancy is an indication that the client's emotional or physical state may need to be further assessed in relation to his or her readiness for learning and/or motivation to learn. The nurse should use open-ended questions when assessing clients because this type of question encourages more clarification and discussion. Closed-ended questions that require only a "yes" or "no" answer provide limited information and insight.

ETHNOCULTURAL IMPLICATIONS

Client Education

The nurse must research various ethnocultures to enhance his or her individualized approach to nursing care. For example, with the Somali client all aspects of nursing care need to be approached in a sensitive manner with strong consideration for the family, communication needs, and religion. Respect for ethnocultural beliefs and values, which are linked to the Muslim religion, is paramount in establishing rapport. Attitudes, social customs, and gender roles in Somalia are based primarily on Islamic tradition. Married Somali women cover their bodies and veil their faces in a hijab. Elders are treated with respect. Somalis believe that spirits reside within each individual. When the spirits become angry, illnesses such as fever, headache, dizziness, and weakness can result. The cure involves a healing ceremony including reading from the Koran, eating special foods, and burning incense. During Ramadan, people pray, fast, and refrain from drinking during the day, and will eat and take medicines only at night. Because of prohibitions against interactions between adult men and women, Somali women have a strong preference to work with female interpreters and healthcare providers. Somalis often expect to receive medication when they are ill, so if no medications are given, providers should explain why.

NURSING DIAGNOSES APPROPRIATE TO DRUG THERAPY

Some of the most common nursing diagnoses related to client education and drug therapy include deficient knowledge, ineffective health maintenance, ineffective therapeutic regimen management, risk for injury (self), impaired memory, and non-adherence. Deficient knowledge means that the client (or caregiver, significant other) lacks or has limited understanding of the medication, its action, side effects, or cautions, and any related administration techniques, or lacks the motor skills needed to safely self-administer the medication. Non-adherence means that the client does not take the medication as prescribed, or does not take it at all—in other words, the client does not adhere to the instructions given. The condition or symptoms for which the medicine was prescribed have reoccurred or were never resolved because the client did not take the medication per the physician's orders. Other nursing diagnoses, as listed by the North American Nursing Diagnosis Association (NANDA) (see Chapter 1), may also be used.

PLANNING RELATED TO LEARNING NEEDS AND DRUG THERAPY

The planning phase of the teaching–learning process occurs as soon as a learning need has been identified in a client or caregiver. With mutual understanding, the nurse and client identify goals and outcome criteria related to the specific medication the client is taking as associated with the identified nursing diagnosis. An example of a measurable goal with outcome criteria related to a nursing diagnosis of deficient knowledge follows:

A client who is self-administering an oral antidiabetic agent has many questions about the medication.

Goal: The client safely self-administers the prescribed oral antidiabetic agent.

Outcome criteria: The client remains without signs and symptoms of overmedication with oral antidiabetic agents, such as hypoglycemia with tachycardia, palpitations, diaphoresis, hunger, and fatigue.

When drug therapy goals and outcome criteria are developed, appropriate time frames for outcome criteria should be identified (see Chapter 1 for more information on the nursing process and related phases). Measurable verbs such as list, identify, demonstrate, self-administer, state, describe, and discuss should be used. Goals and outcome criteria should be realistic and stated in client terms related to drug therapy.

IMPLEMENTATION RELATED TO DRUG THERAPY

After the nurse has completed the assessment phase, including identifying nursing diagnoses and creating a plan of care, the implementation phase of the teaching–learning process begins, which includes conveying specific information about the medication to the client. Teaching–learning sessions should include clear, simple, concise written instructions; oral instructions; and pamphlets, films, or any other learning aids that will help ensure client learning. It may be necessary for the nurse to conduct several short teaching–learning sessions, depending on the needs of the client. (Table 6-1 lists educational strategies for changes related to aging that may influence learning.) It may also be necessary for the nurse to identify aids to help in the safe administration of medications at home, such as medication day and time calendars, "pill reminder" stickers, daily medication containers with alarms, and/or a method of documenting doses taken to avoid overdosage or omitting doses.

Special considerations must be made for clients who speak little or no English. The nurse should communicate in the client's native language if at all possible. If the nurse is not able to speak the client's native language, an appropriate translator should be made available—if at all possible—to prevent communication problems, minimize errors, and improve the client's level of trust and understanding. The translator available is often a lay family member (maybe even a child) or a non-clinical staff member. The nurse should keep in mind that these individuals may not be competent at or comfortable with communicating technical clinical information.

In response to the rapidly growing population of non-English-speaking Chinese in Canada, a number of publications have appeared containing client education mate-

rials printed in both English and Chinese. Similar materials for other languages may also be available. These publications may enable the nurse to speak a sufficient amount of the client's language to effectively educate the client and can be given to the client and family members to read on their own. The publishers of these client education materials have granted permission to photocopy them for educational purposes.

Healthcare professionals who work in a geographic area where a variety of languages are widely spoken should consider learning one or more languages. Adult foreign language education is available in many Canadian cities, often at colleges or universities. Many classes are designed for working professionals and are scheduled at a variety of convenient times during the day and evening to accommodate demanding work schedules. Many employers will pay for job-related courses, and some courses may be used as professional continuing education (CE) credits. Language courses provide a means for networking and developing friendships with other highly motivated, empathetic individuals, both within and outside the healthcare profession.

Note that native English speakers may also have problems learning about their medications and treatment regimen as a result of learning deficits and/or difficulties, hearing and speech deficits, lack of education, or minimal previous exposure to treatment regimens and medication use.

Teaching manual skills for specific medication administration is also part of the teaching–learning session. Each client has different needs; sufficient time should be allowed for the client to become familiar with any equipment and to perform several return demonstrations to the nurse. Family members, significant others, or caregivers should also be included in this session or sessions for reinforcement purposes. Audiovisual aids may be incorporated.

Resources for information about medications may also be shared with the client, such as the Shopper's Drug Mart medication library, which provides information for the public. This type of resource may be helpful to the client when inquiring about a medication, including its purpose, side effects, and method of administration.

To ensure the effectiveness of the teaching–learning session, the nurse should

- Individualize the teaching session.
- Use rewards or reinforcement for accurate return demonstration of the procedure and/or technique during teaching session.
- Complete a medication calendar with medications to take and dosage schedule.
- Use audiovisual aids.
- Involve family members or significant others.
- Keep the teaching on a level that is most meaningful to that client.*

---

*In general, for adults it is recommended that materials be written at a Grade 8 reading level.

TABLE 6-1

EDUCATIONAL STRATEGIES FOR COMMON CHANGES RELATED TO AGING

Changes Related to Aging That May Influence Learning	Educational Strategy
DISTURBED THOUGHT PROCESSES	
Slowed cognitive functioning	Slow the pace of the presentation, and use verbal and non-verbal client cues for validation.
Decreased short-term memory	Provide smaller amounts of information at one time. Repeat information frequently. Provide written instructions for home use.
Decreased ability to think abstractly	Use examples to illustrate information. Use a variety of methods, such as audiovisuals, props, videos, large-printed materials, vivid colour use, return demonstrations, and practice sessions.
Decreased ability to concentrate	Decrease external stimuli as much as possible. Always allow sufficient time.
Increased reaction time (slower to respond)	Allow more time for feedback.
DISTURBED SENSORY PERCEPTION	
Hearing	Baseline hearing assessment. Use tone- and volume-controlled teaching aids; use bright, large-printed material to reinforce.
Decreased ability to distinguish sounds (e.g., words beginning with S, Z, T, D, F, and G)	Speak distinctly and slowly, and articulate carefully.
Decreased conduction of sound	Sit on side of learner's "best" ear.
Loss of ability to hear high-frequency sounds	Do not shout; speak in a normal voice, but lower the pitch.
Partial to complete loss of hearing	Face the client so that lip reading is possible. Use visual aids to reinforce verbal instruction. Reinforce teaching with easy-to-read materials. Decrease extraneous noise. Use community resources for the hearing impaired.
Vision	
Decreased visual acuity	Ensure that glasses are clean and in place and that the prescription is current.
Decreased ability to read fine detail	Use large-print, clear, brightly coloured material.
Decreased ability to discriminate: all colours tend to fade, with red fading the least	Use high-contrast materials, such as black on white. Avoid using blue, violet, and green in type or graphics; use red instead.
Thicker and yellowed lenses of eyes, with decreased accommodation	Use non-glare lighting and avoid contrasts of light (e.g., darkened room with single light).
Decreased depth perception	Adjust teaching to allow for the use of touch to gauge depth.
Decreased peripheral vision	Keep all teaching materials within the client's visual field.
Touch and Vibration	
Decreased sense of touch	Increase time for the teaching of psychomotor skills, repetitions, and return demonstrations.
Decreased sense of vibration	Teach client to palpate more prominent pulse sites (e.g., carotid and radial arteries).

Modified from Weinrich, S.P., Boyd, M., & Nussbaum, J. (1989). Continuing education: Adapting strategies to teach the elderly. *Journal of Gerontology Nursing, 15*(11), 17. In McKenry, L.M. & Salerno, E. (2003). *Mosby's pharmacology in nursing* (21st ed.). St Louis, MO: Mosby.

Box 6-2 lists some general teaching and learning principles.

After completing the teaching–learning process, the nurse should document what was taught (content), strategies used, client response, and evaluation of learning. Client teaching should begin with admission to the healthcare setting and should be documented in the nurse's notes of the client's chart (see the Legal and Ethical Principles box on p. 73). Throughout this textbook,

Client Teaching Tips boxes are specific to a particular class of medications or a particular drug.

EVALUATION RELATED TO DRUG THERAPY

Evaluating client learning is crucial to safe client drug administration. Nurses should always validate whether learning has occurred by asking the client questions

BOX 6-2
General Teaching and Learning Principles

- Make learning client-centred and individualized to each client's needs, including his or her learning needs. This includes assessment of the client's ethnocultural beliefs, educational level, previous experience with medications, level of growth and development (to best match a teaching–learning strategy), age, gender, family support system, resources, ability to learn and learning style, and level of sophistication with regard to health care and the client's own healthcare treatment.
- Assess motivation and readiness to learn.
- Assess the client's ability to use and interpret label information on medication containers.
- Remember that a client's ability to interpret drug instructions is more ethnoculturally based and therefore somewhat consistent regardless of age, sex, or educational background.
- Some studies have shown that as much as 22% of the Canadian population is functionally illiterate. Therefore ensure that educational strategies and materials are at a level that the client is able to understand, while taking care to not embarrass the client.
- An illiterate client still needs to be instructed on safe medication administration. Use pictures to re-emphasize instructions.
- Consider, assess, and appreciate language and ethnicity during client teaching. Make every effort to educate non-English-speaking clients in their native language. Ideally the client is instructed by a health professional familiar with the client's clinical picture who also speaks the client's native language. At the very least, provide the client detailed written instructions in his or her native language, if possible.
- Assess the family support system for adequate client teaching. Family living arrangements, financial status, resources, communication patterns, the roles of family members, and the power and authority of different family members should always be considered.
- Make the teaching–learning session simple, easy, fun, thorough, effective, and not monotonous. Make it applicable to daily life and schedule it at a time when the client is ready to learn.
- Remember that learning occurs best with repetition and periods of demonstration and with the use of audiovisuals and other educational aids.

LEGAL and ETHICAL PRINCIPLES

Discharge Teaching

The safest documentation practices for discharge teaching include the following:

- Always follow the healthcare facility's policy on discharge teaching regarding how much information to impart.
- Do not assume that any client has received adequate teaching before interacting with you.
- Always begin discharge teaching as soon as possible, when the client is ready.
- Minimize any distractions during the teaching session.
- Evaluate any teaching with the client and significant others by having individuals repeat any instructions.
- Contact the institution's social service department or the discharge planner if there are any concerns regarding the learning capacity of the client.
- Document what you have taught, who was present with the client, any specific written instructions, responses by the client or significant other or caregiver, and your own nursing actions, such as specific demonstrations or referrals to community resources.
- Document teaching–learning strategies, such as use of videos and pamphlets.

suggests non-adherence or an inadequate level of learning, a new plan of teaching should be developed and implemented.

SUMMARY

Client education is a critical part of client care, and medication administration is no exception. From the time of initial contact with the client throughout the time the nurse works with the client, the client is entitled to all information about the medication as well as all aspects of his or her care. Evaluation of learning and adherence to the medication regimen should be a continual process, and the nurse should always be willing to listen to the client about any aspects of his or her drug therapy. The Institute of Safe Medication Practices (ISMP) Canada and the Canadian Patient Safety Institute advocate for client safety and medications, while the Canadian Patient Safety Institute is taking on the challenge of reducing injuries and deaths due to medication errors. These organizations are also a tremendous resource for client information. Client education is a means of enhancing client safety as well as decreasing medication errors in the hospital setting or at home. Healthcare professionals must continue to be client advocates and take the initiative to plan, design, create, and implement discharge teaching for drug therapy and other parts of their therapy regimen.

related to the teaching session and having the client provide a return demonstration of skills. Most important, the client's behaviour is the key to whether the teaching was successful and learning occurred—behaviour such as adherence to a schedule for medication administration with few or no complications of therapy. If a client's behaviour

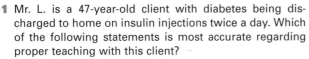

CLIENT TEACHING TIPS

▲ Teaching may need to focus on the cognitive, affective, or psychomotor domain or a combination of all three.
  • The cognitive domain refers to thought processes and problem-solving abilities and may involve recall for synthesis of facts.
  • The affective domain refers to values and beliefs and may involve responding, valuing, and organizing.
  • The psychomotor domain refers to gross motor movements, speech, and non-verbal communication and may involve learning how to perform a procedure.

▲ A thorough assessment of the client and/or the client's spouse, significant others, family members, caregivers and their readiness to learn is crucial to effective client education.
▲ Realistic client teaching goals should be established and the client should be involved in establishing these goals.
▲ The importance of knowing about his or her medications to prevent errors and maximize therapeutic benefits should be emphasized to the client.

POINTS to REMEMBER

▼ Client teaching is an important and necessary part of the nursing function during the implementation phase of the nursing process to ensure safe and cautious drug therapy.
▼ Client teaching should occur after the nurse has thoroughly assessed the client's readiness to learn and should take a comprehensive, holistic approach.
▼ Clients need to receive information through as many senses as possible, such as aurally and visually (as

with pamphlets, videos, diagrams), to maximize learning. Information should also be on the client's reading level, in the client's native language (if possible), and on the client's level of cognitive development (see Erikson's stages in Box 6-1).
▼ The client and any significant others should always be involved in the teaching process.

EXAMINATION REVIEW QUESTIONS

1 Mr. L. is a 47-year-old client with diabetes being discharged to home on insulin injections twice a day. Which of the following statements is most accurate regarding proper teaching with this client?
  a. Begin teaching at the time of diagnosis or admission and individualize teaching to the client's reading level.
  b. Assume that because the client is in his forties he will be able to read any written or printed documents you provide.
  c. Send home with the client any pamphlets that he can share with family members.
  d. Develop a thorough and comprehensive teaching plan based on a Grade 11 reading level.

2 Which of the following strategies for discharge teaching about medication therapy is correct? It should
  a. always be done right before the client leaves the hospital or doctor's office.
  b. be reserved for when the client is comfortable or after narcotics are administered.
  c. include videos, demonstrations, and instructions written at least at a Grade 8 level.
  d. be individualized and based on the client's level of cognitive development.

3 A nurse finds herself responsible for preoperative teaching for a client who is mildly anxious about receiving narcotics post-operatively. Which of the following is a possible effect of this level of anxiety?
  a. Impeded learning because no anxiety is helpful
  b. Major unsteadiness of emotional status
  c. Learning by increasing one's willingness to learn
  d. Reorganizing one's thoughts with inadequate potential for learning

4 How do you, as a professional nurse, most accurately assess a client's learning needs?
  a. Quiz the client daily on all medications.
  b. Begin with validation of the client's present level of knowledge.
  c. Assess the family's knowledge of the medication even if they are not involved in the client's care.
  d. Question other caregivers about their level of experience with the drug regimen and assume lack of interest if no answers are given.

5 Which of the following techniques would be most appropriate for teaching clients with a potential language barrier?
  a. Speak slowly and clearly.
  b. Use detailed and lengthy explanations.
  c. Always assume that if no questions are asked the client understands all information.
  d. Use any type of jargon to help explain the specific type of medication regimen.

CRITICAL THINKING ACTIVITIES

1 Develop a teaching plan for a client who is 65 years old and is to begin treatment for diabetes mellitus with insulin injections. Your task is to develop a 10-minute teaching plan on the basics of self-administration of subcutaneous insulin.

2 Develop a teaching plan for a 69-year-old male client who has experienced a left-sided stroke, is aphasic, and is paralyzed on the right side. He is going to be returning home to have his wife care for him. Your discharge teaching will take place with the client and his wife, and you are to teach them about safety measures for a client with slight

difficulty in swallowing who is going to be sent home on oral medications. He tolerates liquids, soft foods, and thickened liquids fairly well.

3 Your client does not speak English or understand any of your communication techniques thus far. Develop a plan of care that addresses the client's need for medication information on the cardiac drug digoxin and focus also on the potential for toxicity. (Note: You may need to look the drug up in the textbook if you are not familiar with it.)

For answers see http://evolve.elsevier.com/Lilley/pharmacology/.

BIBLIOGRAPHY

Bass, L. (2005). Health literacy: Implications for teaching the adult patient. *Journal of Infusion Nursing, 28,* 15–22.

Canadian Pharmacists Association. (2003). *Therapeutic choices* (4th ed.). Ottawa, ON: Author.

Canadian Pharmacists Association. (2004). *Guide to drugs in Canada.* Toronto, ON: Dorling Kindersley.

Canadian Pharmacists Association. (2005). *Compendium of pharmaceuticals and specialties. The Canadian drug reference for health professionals.* Ottawa, ON: Author. [The subscription-based e-CPS is available at http://www.pharmacists.ca.]

Canobbio, M.M. (2000). *Mosby's handbook of patient teaching* (2nd ed.). St Louis, MO: Mosby.

Erikson, E.H. (1959). *Identity and the life cycle.* New York: Norton. Reissued 1980.

Health Canada (2005). *Drug product database.* Retrieved July 21, 2005, from http://www.hc-sc.gc.ca/hpb/drugs-dpd/

Heath Canada. (2005). Medication matters. How you can help seniors use medications wisely. Retrieved July 21, 2005, from http://www.phac-aspc.gc.ca/seniors-aines/pubs/med_matters/pdf/med_matters_e.pdf

Koelling, T.M., Johnson, M.L., Cody, R.J., & Aaronson, K.D. (2005). Discharge education improves clinical outcomes in patients with chronic heart failure. *Circulation, 111,* 179–185.

McKenry, L.M. & Salerno, E. (2003). *Mosby's pharmacology in nursing* (21st ed.). St. Louis, MO: Mosby.

Potter, P.A., & Perry, A.G. (2006). *Fundamentals of nursing* (6th ed.). St Louis, MO: Mosby.

Public Health Agency of Canada. (2005). Beyond words. The health-literacy connection. Retrieved July 21, 2005, from http://www.canadian-health-network.ca/

Redman, B.K. (2001). *The practice of patient education* (9th ed.). St Louis, MO: Mosby.

Shopper's Drug Mart. (2005). HealthWATCH medication library. Retrieved July 21, 2005, from http://www.shoppersdrugmart.ca/english/health_wellness/medication_library/index.html#

Skidmore-Roth, L. (2006). *Mosby's 2006 nursing drug reference* (19th ed.). St Louis, MO: Mosby.

Statistics Canada. (2005). Adult literacy and life skills survey. Retrieved July 21, 2005, from http://www.statcan.ca/Daily/English/050511/d050511b.htm

Winslow, E.H. (2001). Patient education materials. Can patients read them or are they ending up in the trash? *American Journal of Nursing, 101*(10), 33–38.

7 Over-the-Counter Drugs and Natural Health Products

OBJECTIVES

After reading this chapter, the successful student will be able to do the following:

1 Discuss the differences between prescription drugs, over-the-counter (OTC) drugs, and natural health products, including the legal implications.

2 Explain the differences in federal legislation that govern the promotion and sale of prescription vs. OTC drugs and natural health products.

3 Describe the advantages and disadvantages of OTC drugs and natural health products.

4 Explain the proper use of OTC drugs and natural health products.

5 Discuss the potential dangers associated with OTC drugs and natural health products.

6 Develop a nursing care plan for the client who is self-administering OTC drugs or natural health products.

e-LEARNING ACTIVITIES

Student CD-ROM
- Review Questions: see questions 23–24
- Animations
- Medication Administration Checklists
- IV Therapy Checklists

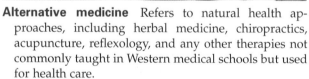 **Web site** (http://evolve.elsevier.com/Lilley/pharmacology/)
- Online Chapter Worksheet • Frequently Asked Questions
- Learning Tips and Content Updates • WebLinks • Online Appendices and Supplements • Mosby/Saunders ePharmacology Update • Access to *Mosby's Drug Consult*

GLOSSARY

Alternative medicine Refers to natural health approaches, including herbal medicine, chiropractics, acupuncture, reflexology, and any other therapies not commonly taught in Western medical schools but used for health care.

Compendium of Monographs Comprehensive published herbal recommendations from Health Canada's Natural Health Products Directorate.

Conventional medicine The practice of medicine as taught in a Western medical school.

Herbal medicine The practice of using herbs to heal.

Herbs Refers not only to herbaceous plants but also to bark; roots; leaves; seeds; flowers and fruit of trees,

shrubs, and woody vines; and extracts of the same that are valued for their savoury, aromatic, or medicinal qualities.

Iatrogenic effects Unintentional adverse effects that are induced by a physician or healthcare professional or by treatment.

Marihuana Medical Access Regulations Allow special access to marijuana for medical purposes.

Natural health products (NHPs) Also referred to as complementary medicines or traditional remedies; an umbrella term that includes supplements, vitamins and minerals, herbal remedies, homeopathic remedies, and sports nutrition.

Over-the-counter (OTC) drugs Medications that are legally available without a prescription from a licensed prescriber (e.g., physician or nurse practitioner).

Phytochemicals The pharmacologically active ingredients in an herbal remedy.

OVER-THE-COUNTER DRUGS

Healthcare consumers are becoming increasingly involved in the diagnosis and treatment of common ailments. This has led to a great increase in the use of non-prescription, or **over-the-counter (OTC)**, drug products. In Canada, there are three categories of non-prescription drugs that limit their sale. A restricted access drug "kept behind the counter" is physically controlled by a pharmacist; consumers have to ask a pharmacist for such a drug,

product, correct dosing, common side effects, and drug interactions with other medications.

For specific information on various OTC drugs, see the appropriate drug chapters later in this text (see Table 7-3 for a cross-reference to these chapters).

THE USE OF NATURAL HEALTH PRODUCTS, INCLUDING HERBAL PRODUCTS

History

Herbs have been an integral part of society since the beginning of human civilization. The use of plants for healing purposes dates back to Neanderthals. Herbs are valued for their culinary and medicinal properties, and herbal medicine has made many contributions to current commercial drug preparations (Table 7-4). About 30 percent of all modern drugs are derived from plants. In the early nineteenth century, scientific methods became more advanced and preferred, and the practice of botanical healing was dismissed as quackery. **Herbal medicine** lost ground to new synthetic medicines as the development of patent medicines took off in the early part of the twentieth century. These new synthetically derived medicines were touted by scientists and physicians to be more effective and reliable.

In the 1960s concerns were expressed over the **iatrogenic effects** of **conventional medicine**. These concerns, along with a desire for more self-reliance, led to a renewed interest in "natural health" and as a result the use of **natural health products (NHPs)**, including herbal products, increased. In 1974 the World Health Organization (WHO) encouraged developing countries to use traditional plant medicines to fulfill a need unmet by modern systems. In

1978 the German equivalent of Health Canada published a series of herb recommendations known as the *Commission E Monographs* (Blumenthal, Goldberg, & Busse, 2001). These monographs focus on herbs that are supported by literature as effective for specific indications. Worldwide use of NHPs, including herbal products, again became popular.

Recognition of the rising use of herbal medicines and other non-traditional remedies, known as **alternative medicine,** and concerns over the accessibility and regulation of all NHPs led the Health Canada Directorate to establish the Advisory Panel on Natural Health in 1997. After consultations with interested stakeholders, the Minister of Health tabled *Natural Health Products: A New Vision*, which provided the framework for the development of the Office of Natural Health Products. This office would later be renamed the Natural Health Products Directorate (NHPD). In January 2004, the Natural Health Products Regulations came into effect, allowing for a transitional time period for site licensing and acquiring a valid Natural Product Number (NPN). Manufacturers must obtain a product license from Health Canada to sell their products in Canada. Health Canada assesses the product and if it deems it to be safe, effective, and of high quality, will issue a NPN. Homeopathic medicines (HMs) receive a DIN-HM followed by a product number. Extensive product labelling must meet specific requirements regarded as essential to risk management. Based on information from the World Health Organization, European Scientific Cooperative on Phytotherapy, and the German Commission E, NHPD developed the **Compendium of Monographs**. The NHPD classifies NHPs into six risk categories from highest to lowest:

Level 1: Risk NHPs on TPD's Listing of Drugs Currently Regulated as New Drugs

---

TABLE 7-3

COMMON OTC DRUGS DISCUSSED IN THIS BOOK

Type of OTC Drug	Examples	Where Discussed in This Book
Acid-controlling agents (H_2 blockers) and antacids	cimetidine, famotidine, nizatidine, ranitidine; aluminum- and magnesium-containing products (Maalox, Mylanta), calcium-containing products (Tums)	Chapter 49: Acid-Controlling Agents
Allergy drugs, including nasal sprays and H_1 blockers	desloratadine (Aerius) fexofenadine (Allegra)	Chapter 36: Bronchodilators and Other Respiratory Agents
Anti-asthma drugs	epinephrine	Chapter 36: Bronchodilators and Other Respiratory Agents
Antifungal agents (topical)	butoconazole (Gynazole), clotrimazole (Canesten), miconazole (Monistat)	Chapter 55: Dermatological Agents
Antihistamines and decongestants	brompheniramine (Dimetapp), Novo-Pheniram (Contac), clemastine (Tavist), diphenhydramine HCL (Benadryl), guaifenesin (Robitussin), loratadine (Claritin), pseudoephedrine (Sudafed)	Chapter 35: Antihistamines, Decongestants, Antitussives, and Expectorants
Eye drops	Artificial tears (Murine)	Chapter 56: Ophthalmic Agents
Hair growth drugs (topical)	minoxidil (Rogaine)	Chapter 55: Dermatological Agents
Pain-relieving drugs (analgesics)	acetaminophen	Chapter 10: Analgesic Agents
Pain-relieving drugs (NSAIDs)	acetylsalicylic acid, ibuprofen	Chapter 43: Anti-Inflammatory, Antirheumatic, and Related Agents

Level 2: Risk Isolates, amino acids, fatty acids, concentrated volatile (essential) oils indicated for internal use, and extracts other than those prepared by traditional methods

Level 3: Risk Algal, bacterial, probiotic, fungal, and non-human animal materials

Level 4: Risk Plants, plant materials, extracts prepared by traditional methods, and volatile (essential) oils other than those that are concentrated and indicated for internal use

Level 5: Risk Vitamins and minerals

Level 6: Risk Homeopathic medicines

In the United States, dietary supplements are considered food products under the Dietary Supplements Health Education Act (DSHEA) of 1994 and claims may not be made about the use of a dietary supplement to diagnose, prevent, mitigate, treat, or cure a specific disease. However, the DSHEA requires no proof of efficacy or safety and sets no standards for quality control for products labelled as supplements. The burden lies with the FDA to prove a product unsafe rather than with a manufacturer to prove its product safe. The FDA posts recent warnings on herbal products on its Web site (http://www.fda.gov). With its new regulations, Canada, like Germany, France, and the United Kingdom, enforces standards of natural products quality and safety assessment.

Consumer Use of Natural Health Products

In general, more than 50 percent of Canadian consumers use NHPs. The umbrella term NHPs under the *Natural Health Products Regulations* includes vitamins and minerals, herbal remedies, homeopathic medicines, traditional medicines such as traditional Chinese medicines, and probiotics and related products such as amino acids and essential fatty acids. They are used as therapeutic agents for the treatment and cure of diseases and pathological conditions, as prophylactic agents for long-term prevention of disease, and as proactive agents to maintain health and wellness and "boost" one's immune system (e.g., reduce cardiovascular risk factors, increase liver and immune system functions, increase feelings of wellness). Additionally, herbs and phytomedicinals can be used as adjunct therapy to support conventional pharmaceutical therapies. The latter use is usually found in societies in which phytotherapy, the use of herbal medicines in clinical practice, is considerably more integrated with conventional medicine, such as in Germany. Box 7-2 lists resources for more information on NHPs.

TABLE 7-4 CONVENTIONAL MEDICINES DERIVED FROM PLANTS

Medicine*	Plant
acetylsalicylic acid	*Salix alba*
atropine	*Atropa belladonna*
capsaicin	*Capsicum frutescens*
cocaine	*Erythroxylon coca*
codeine, morphine	*Papaver somniferum*
digoxin	*Digitalis purpurea*
ipecac	*Cephaelis ipecacuanha*
quinine	*Cinchona officinalis*
reserpine	*Rauwolfia serpentina*
scopolamine	*Datura fastuosa*
senna	*Cassia acutifolia*
taxol	*Taxus brevifolia*
vincristine	*Catharanthus roseus*

*Includes both over-the-counter and prescription drugs.

BOX 7-2 Resources for Information on Natural Health Products

Canadian College of Naturopathic Medicine
1255 Sheppard Ave. E.
Toronto, ON M2K 1E2 Canada
Toll free: 1-866-241-2266
http://www.ccnm.edu

American Botanical Council
6200 Manor Rd.
Austin, TX 78723
Tel: 512-926-4900
Fax: 512-926-2345
http://www.herbalgram.org/

Canadian Health Network
Complementary and Alternative Health
Public Health Agency of Canada
http://www.canadian-health-network.ca/

American Herbalists Guild
1931 Gaddis Rd.
Canton, GA 30115
Tel: 770-751-6021
Fax: 770-751-7472
http://www.americanherbalistsguild.com/

Canadian Holistic Nurses' Association
50 Driveway
Ottawa, ON K2P 1E2
Tel: (613) 237-2133
Toll-free: 1-888-910-9998
Fax: (613) 237-3520
http://mypage.direct.ca/h/hutchings/chna.html

Health Canada Natural Health Products Directorate Compendium of Monographs
A database listing evidence-based information on the available scientific data underlying the use of natural products for health. Each monograph includes information on the proper name, common name(s), source(s), route of administration(s), dosage form(s), use or purpose(s), dose(s), duration of use, risk information, specifications, and non-medicinal ingredients.
http://www.hc-sc.gc.ca/dhp-mps/prodnatur/applications/licen-prod/monograph/list_mono1_e.html

NCCAM, National Institutes of Health
Bethesda, Maryland 20892 USA
http://nccam.nih.gov

Other NHPs may be used to treat minor conditions and illnesses (e.g., coughs, colds, stomach upset) in much the same manner as conventional OTCs approved under the Food and Drugs Regulations. As the number of NHPs in the market increases, nurses will have more opportunities for client education about these products.

Safety

Herbal medicines are often perceived as being natural and therefore harmless; however, this is not the case. Many examples exist of allergic reactions, toxic reactions, drug interactions, and adverse effects related to herbs. Herbs have been shown to have possible mutagenic effects. Cases have also been reported in which whole plants or parts of plants have not been identified properly and thus are mislabelled. Because of underreporting, our present knowledge may well be just the tip of the iceberg.

Little is known about the relative safety of herbal remedies compared with synthetic drug treatments. Recent examples of some of the growing concerns with herbal remedies include Health Canada warnings about possible liver toxicity with the use of kava and possible cardiovascular and stroke risks with the use of ephedra. In July 2005, Health Canada warned consumers to avoid the use of certain Ayurvedic medicinal products because they contain high levels of heavy metals such as lead, mercury, and/or arsenic. Healthcare providers should be on constant watch for literature about the safe and effective use of herbal remedies, as well as reported side effects or problems. For some herbal remedies the risk may be less than that for conventional drugs. The discriminate and proper use of some herbal products is safe and may provide some therapeutic benefits, but the indiscriminate or excessive use of herbs can be unsafe and even dangerous. Health Canada has established the Canadian Adverse Drug Reaction Monitoring Program (CADRMP), which has a toll-free number (866-234-2345) consumers can call to report adverse effects of herbs, drugs, or medical devices.

Medical Use of Marijuana

Marijuana is an herb with a long history of use for its therapeutic and medicinal qualities. In Canada, marijuana remains an illegal and controlled substance. In 2003, Health Canada implemented the **Marihuana Medical Access Regulations** to allow access to and possession of marijuana for individuals suffering from specific grave and debilitating illnesses. Marijuana seeds and dried product are made available to those authorized to use marijuana for medicinal purposes from a company under contract to Health Canada, which produces marijuana for clinical trials to determine the safety and efficacy of marijuana for medical purposes.

Epidemiology

In Canada natural health remedies include not only traditional herbal medicines but traditional Chinese, Ayurvedic (East Indian), and Native North American medicine, homeopathic preparations, and vitamin and mineral supplements. Natural health remedies are increasingly popular in Canada, with as many as one in three using herbal remedies to improve their health. The many different herbs that make up these herbal remedies contain a wide variety of active **phytochemicals** (plant compounds). Some of the more common are listed in Box 7-3. A great deal of public interest exists in the use of natural health remedies. According to a 2005 Health Canada survey, among those who use NHPs, approximately 38 percent use them daily, 37 percent do so "only during certain seasons," and 11 percent have weekly usage. The most common NHPs are vitamins (57 percent), echinacea (15 percent), herbal remedies, and algal and fungal products (11 percent). However, almost 45 percent of Canadians state that they are unfamiliar with NHPs.

Herbal medicine is based on the premise that plants contain natural substances that can promote health and alleviate illness. Some of the more common ailments and conditions treated with herbs are anxiety, arthritis, colds, constipation, cough, fever, headache, infection, insomnia, intestinal disorders, premenstrual syndrome (PMS), stress, ulcers, and weakness.

United States figures estimate that the use of herbal products is growing at a rate of 20 to 25 percent a year, far exceeding growth in the conventional drug category. Twelve of the most commonly used herbal remedies are aloe, echinacea, feverfew, garlic, ginkgo, ginseng, goldenseal, hawthorn, kava, St. John's wort, saw palmetto, and valerian. These products are covered in more detail in the Natural Health Therapies boxes that appear throughout the drug chapters, where the main indications are discussed (see p. 1034 for a complete listing of these boxes with page numbers).

NURSING PROCESS

■ Assessment

■ *Over-the-Counter Drugs*

Assessment of clients taking any type of OTC drugs should include consideration of allergies to any of the ingredients. A medication history is needed documenting *all* medications used (including prescription, OTC, NHPs, and vitamins and minerals, plus alcohol use and smoking habits). Also needed is a past and present medical history to identify possible drug interactions, contraindications, and cautions. Clients should be screened carefully before an OTC drug is recommended. They should realize that OTC status does *not* mean a drug is safe and without negative consequences. With all OTC drugs, the client's level of education and understanding needs to be assessed so

---

BOX 7-3

Common Phytochemicals in Herbal Remedies

- Carotenoids
- Coumarins
- Curcumins
- Flavonoids
- Lignans
- Phthalides
- Plant sterols
- Polyphenolics
- Saponins
- Sulphides
- Terpenoids

that information may be shared with the client as necessary, and at an appropriate reading level.

Other important assessment data include the client's knowledge about the medication, frequency of use, and long-term vs. short-term use. Many clients perceive (incorrectly) that OTCs are not harmful even if taken over a long period. Assessment of a client's level of knowledge and circumstances of self-medication with OTCs is crucial to the client's safety. Overuse and overdosage could lead to serious complications. The client's level of readiness for learning should be assessed so that teaching may be individualized.

Generally speaking, OTC drugs are self-administered and self-monitored, and are not taken in response to laboratory values. Individuals at greater risk of adverse reactions to OTC drugs include older adults; children; frail persons; those with medical problems, who are in poor health, or who are immunocompromised; and anyone with a history of renal, hepatic, cardiac, or circulatory disorder. These factors are important to assess in clients for safe use of OTC drugs.

For specific assessment information on various OTC drugs, see Table 7-3.

■ *Herbal Products*

Many herbal products can be obtained OTC in drug, health food, and grocery stores and may also be found in gardens, kitchens, and medicine cabinets. Commonly used herbal products discussed here are aloe, echinacea, garlic, ginkgo, ginseng, St. John's wort, saw palmetto, and valerian.

Assessment of system functions in the client allows the healthcare provider to be sure that a client is taking herbal products in as safe a manner as possible. Many herbal products may cause dermatitis when used topically. Nephritis has been reported with systemic use; therefore clients with kidney dysfunction should seek medical advice before using any herbal product. Contraindications for some herbal remedies include renal, liver, or cardiac disorders; platelet or clotting disorders; stroke or cerebral bleeding of any nature; hypertension; peptic ulcers; gastrointestinal (GI) bleeding; and any other type of abnormal bleeding (e.g., hematuria, hematemesis, hematomas). Ginseng may cause hypertension and is contraindicated in clients with hypertension, cardiovascular diseases, and irregular heart rhythms. St. John's wort may precipitate seizures, particularly in seizure-prone clients; therefore it is contraindicated in those clients. Cautious use is recommended in those clients taking any herbal product who are also taking multiple drugs because of the increased risk for problems and interactions caused by polypharmacy.

Drug interactions associated with the use of herbal agents include the following:

Aloe: Digitalis drugs, antidysrhythmics, diuretics, and steroids.

Echinacea: Drugs altering the immune system and anabolic steroids. Note: Tachyphylaxis may develop in those clients using echinacea for more than eight weeks; therefore assessment of the duration of self-administration is important.

Garlic: Antiplatelets, anticoagulants, non-steroidal anti-inflammatory drugs (NSAIDs), and acetylsalicylic acid. *Note:* When using garlic, it is best to avoid any other agents that may interfere with platelet and clotting function.

Ginkgo: Acetylsalicylic acid, NSAIDs, anticoagulants, anticonvulsants, and tricyclic antidepressants.

Ginseng: Anticoagulants, acetylsalicylic acid, and NSAIDs.

St. John's wort: Fluoxetine, monoamine oxidase inhibitors (MAOIs), selective serotonin reuptake inhibitors (SSRIs), other psychoactive drugs, sympathomimetics, tetracyclines, and tyramine-containing foods (e.g., nuts, beer, avocados, cheeses, wines). Note: Allergic reaction to acetylsalicylic acid indicates that the client is most likely allergic to St. John's wort.

Saw palmetto: Estrogen hormone replacements and oral contraceptives.

Valerian: Central nervous system (CNS) depressants, narcotics, sedatives, hypnotics, antidepressants, and barbiturates.

■ Nursing Diagnoses

Nursing diagnoses appropriate for the client who is taking an OTC drug or NHP include the following:
- Acute pain related to various disease processes
- Chronic pain related to tissue injury
- Impaired physical mobility related to disease processes or injury
- Deficient knowledge related to first-time drug therapy with OTC drugs and/or NHPs
- Risk for injury related to potential drug interactions and adverse reactions of OTC drugs and NHPs
- Risk for injury to self related to possible nicotine withdrawal (applies to clients using a smoking deterrent system)

For specific nursing diagnoses related to various OTC drugs, see the appropriate drug chapters later in this text (see Table 7-3 for a cross-reference to these chapters).

■ Planning

Goals pertinent to clients using an OTC drug or NHP include the following:
- Client is able to describe the use of the agent as related to symptoms or complaints.
- Client experiences pain relief or relief of the symptoms of the disease process or injury within the expected time period.
- Client reports both adverse effects and therapeutic responses to the appropriate healthcare professional.
- Client states the rationale for and proper use of the agent.
- Client states the adverse effects, cautions, and contraindications associated with the use of the agent.
- Client has minimal complaints and experiences minimal side effects related to use of the agent.
- Client remains free from injury caused by improper use of the agent.
- Client avoids detrimental effects of nicotine withdrawal due to proper self-administration. (Applies to clients using a smoking deterrent system.)

For specific planning information related to the various OTC drugs, see the appropriate drug chapters later in this text (see Table 7-3).

■ *Outcome Criteria*

Outcome criteria for clients taking an OTC drug or NHPs include the following:

- Client states the actions of the agent and how it decreases the intended symptoms.
- Client identifies factors that aggravate or alleviate symptoms.
- Client describes non-pharmacological approaches to treatment of symptoms, such as the use of hot or cold packs, physical therapy, massage, relaxation therapy, biofeedback, imagery, and hypnosis.
- Client states the importance of immediately reporting any severe side effects or complications associated with the agent.
- Client maintains standard precautions while self-administering an OTC drug or NHP (particularly with any type of topical application).
- Client experiences relief of symptoms (the actual indication for the use of OTC or NHP).
- Client takes the OTC drug or NHP as indicated, using proper dosing (no more than directed) and technique, and knows to stop medication if untoward effects occur.
- Client contacts healthcare provider or local poison control hotline should toxicity or complications occur.
- Client demonstrates correct technique for route of administration ordered.

For specific outcome criteria related to the various OTC drugs, see the appropriate drug chapters later in this text (see Table 7-3).

■ Implementation

With OTC drugs the most important determinant of safe client self-administration is whether the client receives thorough and individualized client education. Clients need to receive as much information as possible and should understand that just because these drugs are non-prescription does *not* mean they are completely safe and without toxicity. Instructions should include information about safe use, frequency of dosing and dosage, specifics about how to take the medication (e.g., with food or at bedtime), and how the client may help to prevent complications and toxic effects.

For clients using NHPs (as with other OTC medications), education is of utmost importance for safe and effective use. The healthcare provider must inform the client that Health Canada now requires the manufacturers of all NHPs, including herbal remedies, to provide evidence of safety and effectiveness. Unfortunately many clients believe that no risks exist if a medication is herbal and "natural." It is important for clients to realize that "natural" products need to be taken as cautiously as any other medication. Health Canada requires standard labelling of all NHPs with the product name, the quantity of product in the bottle, recommended conditions of use (including such things as its recommended use or purpose, dosage form, route of administration, recom-

mended dose, and any cautionary statements, warnings, contraindications, and possible adverse reactions associated with the product), as well as any special storage conditions.

Just because an agent is an NHP or a "dietary supplement" does not mean that it can be safely administered to children, infants, pregnant or lactating women, or clients with other conditions that increase risks.

Clients using a transdermal nicotine smoking deterrent system should be informed that they are to apply the patch to a non-hairy site on the upper part of the body or upper outer arm daily as instructed and to rotate sites to prevent skin irritation. Once the protective covering is removed, the client needs to apply the patch immediately to prevent a decrease in the strength of the patch. All nicotine patches and gums should be kept out of the reach of children and pets. Clients must be aware that these systems (patch and gum) are just as toxic as cigarettes and should be used only to deter smoking. Dosages for the transdermal systems range from 7 mg/day to 21 mg/day; other patches range from 5 mg/day to 15 mg/day; and some are available in 11 mg/day to 22 mg/day dosages. Dosages and recommendations vary depending on the specific system used. The manufacturers of the Nicoderm system recommend that if a client weighs less than 45 kg or smokes less than 10 cigarettes a day, he or she should begin with the 14 mg/day patches. The nicotine gum dosage is 2 or 4 mg (1 piece of gum) as needed, and generally the initial requirement is 20 mg/day of the 2-mg strength or 80 mg/day of the 4-mg strength. The amount of gum that is needed is individually based and on a fixed schedule of every 1 to

2 hours. The gum should be chewed slowly until a tingling sensation is felt, and then it is placed between the gums and cheek without chewing until the tingling sensation disappears, which usually takes about 1 minute. Nicotine via inhalation is also available in Canada. Each inhaler contains 10 mg of nicotine released in the form of a vapour when inhaled and continuously puffed for 20 minutes. The initial dose is individualized and may be titrated to the level needed to reduce abstinence symptoms. Regardless of the system used (patch, gum, or inhaler), clients should avoid overuse of the product and follow the instructions closely.

For specific nursing implementation information related to the various OTC drugs, see the appropriate drug chapters later in this text (see Table 7-3).

Client teaching tips for OTC drugs and herbal remedies are presented below.

■ Evaluation

To prevent overuse, clients taking OTC or NHPs should carefully monitor themselves for unusual or adverse reactions and for therapeutic responses. The range of therapeutic responses will vary, depending on the specific agent and the indication for which it is used. These may include decreased pain, decreased stiffness and swelling in joints, increased ability to carry out activities of daily living (ADLs), the ability to move around with more ease, increased hair growth, decreased symptoms (asthma-related, GI, or allergic), decreased vaginal itching and discharge, increased healing, increased sleep, decreased fatigue, or improved energy.

For specific evaluation information related to the various OTC drugs, see the appropriate drug chapters later in this book (see Table 7-3).

CLIENT TEACHING TIPS

▲ The client should be provided with verbal and written information about how to choose an appropriate OTC drug or NHP (e.g., correct dosing, common side effects, possible interactions with other medications).

▲ The healthcare provider must inform the client that Health Canada requires manufacturers of herbal remedies to provide evidence of safety and effectiveness.

▲ Many clients believe that no risks exist if a medication is herbal and "natural" or if it is sold OTC. Therefore education about the pros and cons of these agents is crucial to client safety.

▲ The client should be instructed on how to read OTC and NHP labels. Clients should ask questions of their pharmacist or healthcare provider about specific agents.

▲ The client should take all natural health and OTC medications with caution and contact his or her healthcare provider if adverse effects occur.

▲ The client taking natural health or OTC products should monitor himself or herself for both improvement in symptoms and adverse effects.

▲ The client should be instructed to read directions on all OTC products carefully with particular attention to drug interactions, cautions and contraindications, and specific instructions for self-administration.

▲ The client should be instructed to keep all OTC products out of the reach of children and pets.

▲ The client should be instructed to apply transdermal medications to any non-hairy site on the upper part of the body or upper outer arm daily. Rotation of sites is encouraged to prevent skin irritation. All old patches should be removed and the date and time the patch has been applied should be noted.

POINTS to REMEMBER

▼ Consumers use NHPs as therapeutic agents for treatment and cure of diseases and pathological conditions, as prophylactic agents for long-term prevention of disease, and as proactive agents to maintain health and wellness.

▼ Health Canada has established the Canadian Adverse Drug Reaction Monitoring Program (CADRMP), with a toll-free number (866-234-2345) for reporting adverse effects of herbs and other natural products; their Web site is at http://www.hc-sc.gc.ca/dhp-mps/medeff/report-declaration/index_e.html.

▼ The term *phytotherapy* refers to the use of herbal medicines in clinical practice.

▼ Some of the more commonly used herbal remedies are aloe, echinacea, garlic, ginkgo, ginseng, kava, St. John's wort, saw palmetto, and valerian.

▼ NHPs are approved by Health Canada with specific labelling requirements to provide adequate instructions for use and warnings.

▼ That an agent is an NHP, "dietary supplement," or OTC medication is no guarantee that it can be safely administered to children, infants, pregnant or lactating women, or clients with other conditions that increase risk.

EXAMINATION REVIEW QUESTIONS

1 The most commonly used OTC products currently available include which of the following drugs?
   a. Mild antihypertensives
   b. Topical anti-infective agents
   c. Acetaminophen with codeine 30 mg
   d. Ibuprofen mixed with low doses of codeine and 65 mg of caffeine

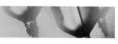

2 Which of the following points is important for the nurse to tell clients using natural health products?
  a. Natural health and OTC products are approved by Health Canada and under strict regulation.
  b. These products are scrutinized for safety and tested repeatedly by Health Canada.
  c. No side effects are associated with these agents because they are "natural" and may be purchased without a prescription.
  d. Labelling is not reliable for the provision of proper instructions or warnings, and the products should be taken with caution.

3 Natural health products are often used to do which of the following?
  a. Prevent the use of any prescription drugs in the general population
  b. Increase lipoproteins and cholesterol for increasing fat in the elderly
  c. Increase feelings of wellness and strengthen the immune system
  d. Improve cardiac, cerebral, and central nervous system functioning and increase sex hormones

4 Ginseng may exacerbate which of the following conditions?
  a. Sedation and low energy levels
  b. Mental slowness
  c. Decreased ability to exercise
  d. Hypertension

5 Which of the following characteristics is associated with current legislation about herbal products?
  a. Herbals were regulated in the early 1900s in reference to their efficacy and toxicity.
  b. Natural Health Products Directorate (NHPD) permits the sale of herbal remedies as dietary supplements.
  c. The Marihuana Medical Access Regulations allow access to and possession of marijuana for individuals.
  d. The NHPD was specifically designed to control the safety and efficacy of OTC and herbal agents.

For answers see http://evolve.elsevier.com/Lilley/pharmacology/.

CRITICAL THINKING ACTIVITIES

1 Is the following statement true or false? Explain your answer:
  OTC agents and natural health products may be safely taken in the recommended amounts without concern about adverse effects.

2 From which law have current laws regulating OTC medications evolved?

3 Discuss some important points to include when teaching clients about analgesia and pain control for at-home management with OTC products.

For answers see http://evolve.elsevier.com/Lilley/pharmacology/.

BIBLIOGRAPHY

Be Medwise. (2005). Survey on Canadians' use of OTC medications. Retrieved July 21, 2005, from http://www.bemedwise.ca/english/usagesurvey.html

Blumenthal, M., Goldberg, A., & Busse, W.R. (2001). The complete German Commission E Monographs: therapeutic guide to herbal medicines. New York, NY: Thieme.

Canadian Pharmacists Association. (2003). Therapeutic choices (4th ed.). Ottawa, ON: Author.

Canadian Pharmacists Association. (2005). Compendium of Pharmaceuticals and Specialties. The Canadian drug reference for health professionals. Ottawa, ON: Author. [The subscription-based e-CPS is available at http://www.pharmacists.ca.]

Canadian Institute for Health Information. (2005). Drug expenditure in Canada 1985 to 2004. Ottawa, ON: Author. Retrieved July 21, 2005, from http://www.cihi.ca

Harkness, R., & Bratman, S. (2003). Mosby's handbook of drug-herb and drug supplement interactions. St Louis, MO: Mosby.

Health Canada. (2003). Marihuana medical access regulations. Retrieved March 15, 2006, from http://www.hc-sc.gc.ca/dhp-mps/alt_formats/hecs-sesc/pdf/marihuana/marihuana-reg_e.pdf

Health Canada. (2003). Natural health products regulations. Retrieved March 15, 2006, from http://www.hc-sc.gc.ca/dhp-mps/prodnatur/legislation/acts-lois/prodnatur/regs_cg2_e.html

Health Canada. (2004). Compendium of monographs. Retrieved July 21, 2005, from http://www.hc-sc.gc.ca/dhp-mps/prodnatur/applications/licenprod/monograph/list_mono1_e.html

Health Canada. (2005). Health Canada baseline natural health products survey among consumers. Retrieved January 9, 2006, from http://www.hc-sc.gc.ca/dhp-mps/pubs/natur/eng_cons_survey_e.html

Kline and Company. (2004). Growth for Canadian OTC industry remains modest in 2004. Retrieved July 22, 2005, from http://www.klinegroup.com/6_20050414.htm

Millar, W. (2004). Patterns of use—alternative health care practitioners. [Electronic version]. Health Reports 13(1). Retrieved July 22, 2005, from http://www.statcan.ca/english/studies/82-003/feature/hrar2001013001s0a01.pdf

Mosby (2005). Mosby's drug consult 2005: The comprehensive reference for generic and brand name drugs (15th ed.). St Louis, MO: Mosby.

National Association of Pharmacy Regulatory Authorities. (2002). Information Ephedra/Ephedrine. Retrieved July 22, 2005, from http://www.napra.ca/docs/0/310/315.asp

Novey, D.W. (2000). Clinician's complete reference to complementary and alternative medicine. St Louis, MO: Mosby.

Proud, K. (2004). History of Canadian regulatory affairs. Retrieved July 22, 2005, from http://www.raps.org/s_raps/docs/24100/24058.pdf

Ross, M. (September 5, 2000). Jumping over the counter. Medical Post, 36(29). Retrieved August 1, 2005, from http://www.medicalpost.com/mpcontent/article.jsp?content=/content/EXTRACT/RAWART/3629/26A.html

Skidmore-Roth, L. (2004). Mosby's handbook of herbs and natural supplements (2nd ed.). St Louis, MO: Mosby.

Skidmore-Roth, L (2006). Mosby's 2006 nursing drug reference (19th ed). St Louis, MO: Mosby.

Wren, K.R., & Norred, C.L. (2003). Real world nursing survival guide: Complementary and alternative therapies. St Louis, MO: Saunders.

8 Problematic Substance Use

OBJECTIVES

After reading this chapter, the successful student will be able to do the following:

1 Define problematic substance use.

2 Discuss the significance of problematic substance use in health care.

3 Identify the major drug categories for problematic substance use and the major individual agents in each category.

4 Identify the signs and symptoms of and drugs used for opioid or opiate withdrawal.

5 Identify the commonly misused/abused stimulants and treatment regimens.

6 Describe the signs and symptoms of depressant misuse/abuse and the treatment process for benzodiazepine and barbiturate withdrawal.

7 Describe alcohol abuse syndrome and its treatment.

8 Identify the signs and symptoms of ethanol withdrawal, ranging from mild to severe, and medications used to treat the various stages of withdrawal.

9 Develop a nursing care plan with all phases of the nursing process, for the client being treated for chemical dependency and/or problematic substance use.

10 Identify the various resources, including Web sites, for information on problematic substance use.

e-LEARNING ACTIVITIES

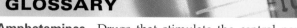

Student CD-ROM
- Animations
- Medication Administration Checklists
- IV Therapy Checklists

evolve Web site (http://evolve.elsevier.com/Lilley/pharmacology/)
- Online Chapter Worksheet • Frequently Asked Questions
- Learning Tips and Content Updates • WebLinks • Online Appendices and Supplements • Mosby/Saunders ePharmacology Update • Access to *Mosby's Drug Consult*

GLOSSARY

Amphetamines Drugs that stimulate the central nervous system (CNS).

Enuresis Urinary incontinence.

Illicit drug use The use of a drug or substance that is not intended to be used in the manner in which it is be-ing used, or the use of a drug that is not legally approved for human consumption.

Micturition Urination, the desire to urinate, or the frequency of urination.

Narcolepsy A sleep disorder characterized by sleeping during the day, disrupted nighttime sleep, cataplexy, sleep paralysis, and hypnagogical hallucinations.

Narcotic Any agent that produces insensibility or stupor (narcosis); applies most commonly to the opioid analgesics.

Opioid analgesics Synthetic pain-relieving substances that originated from the opium plant. Naturally occurring opium derivatives are called *opiates*.

Physical dependence A condition characterized by physiological reliance on a substance; usually indicated by tolerance to the effects of the substance and withdrawal symptoms that develop when use of the substance is terminated.

Psychoactive properties Properties having a tendency to affect mood, anxiety levels, behaviour, cognitive processes, and mental state.

Psychological dependence   A condition characterized by behaviours related to obtaining and using a substance.

Raves   Increasingly popular all-night parties that typically involve dancing, drinking, and the use of various illicit drugs.

Roofies   Pills that are classified as benzodiazepines. They have recently gained popularity as a recreational drug; chemically known as flunitrazepam.

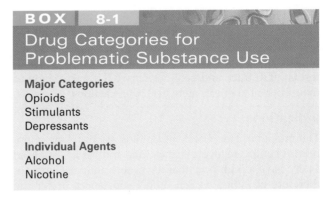

Substance use problems affect people of all ages, sexes, and ethnic and socio-economic groups. Health Canada regards problematic substance use as a serious health issue that often results in social, economic, and public safety consequences for Canadians. According to Health Canada, "problematic substance use" best captures the range of consequences that can result from drug use. Any psychoactive substance, whether legal (such as alcohol and prescription medication) or illegal (such as marijuana, cocaine, or heroin) may result in problematic use. **Physical dependence** and **psychological dependence** on a substance are chronic disorders with remissions and relapses such as with any other chronic disorder. Exacerbations should not be seen as failures but as times to intensify treatment. Recognizing physical or psychological dependence and understanding the basis and various guidelines for treatment are important skills for the individual caring for these clients. Assessment, intervention, prescription of medications, participation in specific addiction treatment strategies, and monitoring of recovery are essential to the care of this client population.

The use and misuse of alcohol, tobacco, and drugs is associated with a wide variety of adverse health, social, and economic consequences. The Canadian Addiction Survey (CAS), conducted in 2004, revealed that use of alcohol, cannabis, and other drugs has increased in Canada since the previous study, conducted in 1994.

This chapter focuses on three major classes of commonly misused/abused substances and two individual agents that are commonly misused/abused at this time (Box 8-1). Each is described, with a discussion of possible effects, signs and symptoms of intoxication and withdrawal, peak period and duration of withdrawal symptoms, and agents used to treat withdrawal.

The specific agents used to treat withdrawal are discussed with the major category or the individual agent for which they are used to treat. Pharmacological therapies are indicated for use in clients with addictive disorders to prevent life-threatening withdrawal complications, such as seizures and delirium tremens, and to increase adherence with psychosocial forms of addiction treatment.

OPIOIDS

Opioid analgesics are synthetic pain-relieving substances that originated from the opium plant. Similar substances that occur in nature are called *opiates*. More than 20 different alkaloids are obtained from the unripe seed of the opium poppy plant, only a few of which are clinically useful. Morphine and codeine are the only two that are useful as analgesics. The multitude of other opioid analgesics that are currently used in medical practice are synthetic or semi-synthetic derivatives of these two agents.

Diacetylmorphine (better known as *heroin*) and opium are also opioids. Heroin and opium are covered by the Controlled Drugs and Substances Act (CDSA) and the Food and Drug Regulations (FDR) and are not available in Canada for therapeutic use. Heroin was banned in 1908 because of its high potential for misuse/abuse and the increasing number of heroin addicts. Heroin addiction afflicts an estimated 60 000 to 90 000 Canadians.

Some of the other commonly misused/abused substances in the opioid category are codeine, hydromorphone, meperidine, morphine, opium, oxycodone, and propoxyphene.

Currently heroin remains the most misused/abused drug after marijuana in Canada and often is used in combination with the stimulant drug cocaine (discussed in the section on stimulants in this chapter). When heroin is injected ("mainlining" or "skin-popping"), sniffed ("snorted"), or smoked ("chasing the dragon"), it binds with opiate receptors found in many regions of the brain. The result is intense euphoria, often referred to as a "rush." This rush lasts only briefly and is followed by a couple of hours of a relaxed, contented state. In large doses, heroin can reduce or eliminate respiration.

Mechanism of Action and Drug Effects

Opioids are agonists that work by binding to specific protein receptors in the pain pathways of the central nervous system (CNS), blocking the perception of pain. Opioids bind to four main receptor types: mu, kappa, sigma, and delta. These receptors and their physiological effects when stimulated are discussed in Chapter 10. The unique mixture of receptor affinities that a specific opioid possesses determines the therapeutic and toxic effects. Euphoria is produced by a mu-receptor response to stimulation.

The drug effects of opioids are primarily centred on the CNS. Opioids produce analgesia, drowsiness, euphoria, tranquility, and other alterations of mood. The mechanism by which opioids produce these effects is not entirely clear. Such effects can be collectively referred to as *narcosis* or *stupor*, which involves reduced sensory response, especially to painful stimuli. For this reason, opioid analgesics, along with other classes of drugs that produce similar effects, are also referred to as **narcotics,** especially by the law enforcement authorities. However, opioids also act outside the CNS, on areas including the skin, gastrointestinal (GI) tract, and genitourinary (GU) tract. Many of their unwanted effects stem from these actions.

Indications

The intended drug effects of opioids are to relieve pain, reduce cough, relieve diarrhea, and induce anaesthesia. Many have a high potential for problematic use and are therefore classified as Schedule I substances under the CDSA, with restrictions on and consequences for possession, and as narcotic drugs or preparations under Part G of the FDR. However, the relaxation and euphoria that accompany these effects can lead to problematic use and psychological dependence. Oxycodone is one example of an opioid narcotic that is controversial because it is often overprescribed, misused, and grossly abused (see Research box below).

RESEARCH ▶ ◀ ◀

Problematic Use Considerations for Oxycodone, a Narcotic Opioid Agonist

In July 2004 Health Canada issued an awareness warning of increasing concerns about the possible problematic use of oxycodone-based products in Canada, especially Atlantic Canada. Three years earlier the U.S. FDA had reported increased concerns regarding the problematic use of oxycodone. Oxycodone is an analgesic indicated for an extended period of pain relief associated with chronic illness (e.g., cancer pain, chronic severe low back pain) and is *not* intended for "as needed" (prn) use. Many healthcare professionals are concerned about its potential for physical dependence, and even more about the tendency for clients to overuse and misuse it—even when it is prescribed by a physician or other healthcare provider. Controversy increases when this type of narcotic opioid is ordered for pain that could be treated effectively with other narcotics that are less addictive and associated with less physical dependence. The other concern with this drug is that fatal drug interactions can occur if it is misused and taken along with alcoholic beverages. Dosage concerns are important to note. "Opioid naïve" clients (i.e., those not used to taking narcotics) can only safely tolerate lower dosages; yet opioid-tolerant clients often need higher dosages. However, the greatest concern is that Oxycodone is often ordered in situations for which it is not indicated. This leads to addiction/dependence and the street sale of the drug because of its associated euphoric effects.

Data from Health Canada News Release. (2004). *Misuse and abuse of Oxycodone-based prescription drugs.* Retrieved July 24, 2005, from http://www.hc-sc.gc.ca/english/media/releases/2004/oxycodone.htm; and Canadian Centre on Substance Abuse. (2004). *OxyContin (Oxycodone hydrochloride).* Retrieved July 24, 2005, from http://www.ccsa.ca/NR/rdonlyres/982C25CB-125F-4611-826A-3999C6B889B6/0/ccsa0100512004.pdf *FDA,* U.S. Food and Drug Administration.

Contraindications

Contraindications to the therapeutic use of opioid medications include known drug allergy, pregnancy (in high or prolonged doses), respiratory depression or severe asthma without available resuscitative equipment, and paralytic ileus (bowel paralysis).

Side Effects and Adverse Effects

The side effects and adverse effects of opioids can be broken down into two areas: CNS and all other. The primary side effects and adverse effects of opioids are related to their actions in the CNS. The primary CNS-related side effects and adverse effects are diuresis (increased urination), miosis (constriction of the pupil of the eye), convulsions, nausea, vomiting, and respiratory depression. Many of the side effects and adverse effects that occur outside the CNS are secondary to the release of histamine caused by opioids. This histamine release can cause vasodilation leading to hypotension; spasms of the colon leading to constipation; increased contractions of the ureter resulting in decreased urine flow; and dilation of cutaneous blood vessels leading to flushing of the skin of the face, neck, and upper thorax. This release of histamine is also thought to cause sweating, urticaria (hives), and pruritus (itching).

TOXICITY AND MANAGEMENT OF OVERDOSE

Box 8-2 lists the signs, symptoms, and timing of opioid drug withdrawal. (See Chapter 10 for a detailed discussion of physical dependence and the management of acute intoxication.) Withdrawal symptoms include nausea, dysphoria, muscle aches, lacrimation (watering eyes) or rhinorrhea (runny nose), pupillary dilation, piloerection ("goose bumps") or sweating, diarrhea, yawning, fever, and insomnia. The medications listed in Box 8-3 are intended to help reduce the severity of these withdrawal symptoms and of opioid cravings.

BOX   8-2

Signs and Symptoms of Opioid Drug Withdrawal

Peak Period
1–3 days

Duration
5–7 days

Signs
Drug seeking, mydriasis (prolonged dilation of the pupil), piloerection, diaphoresis (sweating), rhinorrhea, lacrimation, diarrhea, insomnia, elevated blood pressure and pulse

Symptoms
Intense desire for drugs, muscle cramps, arthralgia, anxiety, nausea, vomiting, malaise

---

Medications are sometimes used to prevent relapse to drug use once an initial remission is secured. These medications are only useful when used with concurrent counselling and provide additional insurance against return to **illicit drug use.** For opioid abuse or dependence, naltrexone, an opioid antagonist, is used (50 mg/day) orally or by implant inserted under the skin. Naltrexone works by blocking the opioid receptors so that use of opioid drugs does not produce euphoria. When euphoria is eliminated, the reinforcing effect of the drug is lost. The client should be free from opioids for at least 1 week before beginning this medication, because naltrexone can produce withdrawal symptoms if given too soon. Naltrexone is also approved for use with alcohol-dependent clients. The same dose of naltrexone used with opioid-dependent clients, 50 mg/day, decreases craving for alcohol and reduces the likelihood of a full relapse if a slip occurs.

STIMULANTS

Some of the effects of stimulants that have led to their problematic use are elevation of mood, reduction of fatigue, a sense of increased alertness, and "invigorating aggressiveness." One stimulant drug that produces strong CNS stimulation and is commonly misused/abused is **amphetamine.** Chemically, three classes of amphetamine exist: salts of racemic amphetamine, dextroamphetamine, and methamphetamine. These classes vary with respect to their potency and peripheral effects. Another misused/abused stimulant drug is cocaine, which also produces strong CNS stimulation. According to Health Canada, cocaine is the second most commonly misused/abused illicit drug in

Canada. The Proprietary or Patent Medicines Act in 1909 banned the use of "narcotics" such as cocaine and opium in medicines; cocaine was legally restricted in the Opium and Drug Act of 1911. In legal terminology, and in rules of secured storage, cocaine is classified as a narcotic. However, unlike the opioid analgesics, cocaine does not normally induce a state of narcosis or stupor and is therefore more correctly classified pharmaceutically as a stimulant agent. Other commonly misused/abused substances within this category include benzedrine, butyl nitrite, and methylphenidate (Ritalin).

One of the most commonly misused/abused CNS stimulants is methamphetamine. Multiple slight chemical derivations of methamphetamine exist. Table 8-1 lists common forms of amphetamine (and cocaine) and their street names. These "designer drugs" have **psychoactive properties** along with their stimulant properties, further enhancing their problematic use potential.

Methamphetamine is a stimulant drug chemically related to amphetamine, but it has a much stronger effect on the CNS than the other two classes of amphetamine. Methamphetamine is generally used in pill form or in powder form by snorting or injecting. Crystallized methamphetamine, known as "ice," "crystal," "glass", "jibb," or "tina" is a smokable and more powerful form of the drug. Methamphetamine users who inject the drug and share needles are at risk for acquiring HIV/AIDS. Methamphetamine is an increasingly popular drug at **raves** (all-night dance parties) and is one of several drugs used by college age students. Marijuana, ecstasy, ketamine, and alcohol are also commonly used by methamphetamine users. Methamphetamine use is not well documented in Canada but usage appears to be increasing, particularly in Western Canada. In British Columbia, deaths from methamphetamine have increased each year since 2000 (Nordeste, 2004). More recently "crystal meth" has become a drug of choice for abuse because it is inexpensive and for its immediate "rush" or "surge" when smoked or injected. Crystal meth is easily produced from pseudoephedrine, an ingredient in cold

BOX 8-3
Medications for Treatment of Opioid Drug Withdrawal

North American Opiate Medication Initiative
The North American Opiate Medication Initiative (NAOMI), a clinical trial where pharmaceutical heroin will be prescribed to addicted street-heroin users, began in Canada in 2005. NAOMI is intended to determine if this harm reduction approach will reduce death, disease (particularly HIV/AIDS and hepatitis C), criminal activity, and suffering associated with illicit heroin use.

Methadone Substitution
The sale and manufacture of methadone is controlled by the Office of Controlled Substances within Health Canada. To prescribe methadone, physicians must receive an exemption under the Controlled Drugs and Substances Act. The initial dose of methadone is 15 to 30 mg per day given orally (usually diluted in juice) for the first three days in order to reach a steady state. Dose adjustments (stabilization) are in the 5 to 15 mg range every five days and are based on specific criteria including signs and symptoms of withdrawal. Maintenance doses are in the 5 to 15 mg range. An optimum dose of under 120 mg is usually achieved in two to six weeks of methadone initiation.

TABLE 8-1
VARIOUS FORMS OF AMPHETAMINE AND COCAINE WITH STREET NAMES

Chemical Name	Street Names
Dimethoxymethylamphetamine	DOM, STP
methamphetamine (crystallized form)	Ice, crystal, glass, jibb, tina
methamphetamine (powdered form)	Speed, meth, crank
Methylenedioxyamphetamine	MDA, the "love drug"
Methylenedioxymethamphetamine	MDMA, Ecstasy or E, "blue lips", "blue kisses," "white dove," "XTC"
cocaine (powdered form)	coke, dust, snow, flake, blow, girl
cocaine (crystallized form)	crack, crack cocaine, freebase rocks, rock

medicines readily available from pharmacies. It is combined with red phosphorous and iodine, but also other chemicals including ammonia, paint thinner, ether, Drano, and lithium from batteries. Crystal meth is highly addictive and the initial energy and confidence may eventually, in regular users, lead to an amphetamine psychosis that includes hallucinations, delusions, paranoia, and violent behaviour. Health Canada is currently investigating strategies to prevent easy access to pseudoephedrine.

Another illicit drug use problem is the use of cocaine. Cocaine is a white powder that comes from the leaves of the South American coca plant. The powder is either snorted through the nasal passages or injected intravenously. Cocaine tends to give a temporary illusion of limitless power and energy that, when it ends, leaves the user feeling depressed, edgy, and craving more. Crack is a smokable form of cocaine that has been chemically altered. Cocaine and crack are highly addictive. The psychological and physical dependence can erode physical and mental health and can become so strong that these drugs dominate all aspects of an addict's life.

Mechanism of Action and Drug Effects

Stimulants work by releasing biogenic amines from their storage sites in the nerve terminals. The primary biogenic amine released is norepinephrine. This release results in stimulation of the CNS. The drug effects of stimulants are typically cardiovascular stimulation resulting in increased blood pressure and heart rate and possible cardiac dysrhythmias. The effect on smooth muscle is primarily seen in the urinary bladder, resulting in contraction of the sphincter. This is helpful in treating **enuresis** (urinary incontinence) but otherwise results in pain and difficulty in **micturition** (voiding or urination). Stimulants, particularly amphetamines, are potent CNS stimulants. This CNS stimulation commonly results in wakefulness, alertness, and a decreased sense of fatigue; elevation of mood, with increased initiative, self-confidence, and ability to concentrate; often elation and euphoria; and an increase in motor and speech activity. Physical performance in athletes may be improved due to both enhanced alertness and reduction of fatigue. This quality leads to problematic use of these agents by many athletes, especially those under in-

tense pressure to perform. However, these performance enhancement effects may reach a plateau and even result in a personal or professional crisis for an athlete who uses these agents on a long-term basis.

Indications

Many therapeutic uses of stimulants exist. Stimulants may be used to prevent or reverse fatigue and sleep, such as when they are used to treat **narcolepsy** (episodes of acute sleepiness). They also have a slight analgesic effect and may be used to enhance the analgesic effects and limit the CNS-depressant effects of stronger analgesics, such as opioids. Another therapeutic effect of amphetamines is their ability to stimulate the respiratory centre. Occasionally they are used after anaesthesia in individuals whose respirations are slowed. Stimulants are also used to reduce food intake and treat obesity. This therapeutic effect is limited because of rapid development of tolerance. Stimulants have also shown benefits in the treatment of attention deficit disorders.

Contraindications

Contraindications to the therapeutic use of stimulant medications include drug allergy, diabetes, cardiovascular disorders, states of agitation, hypertension, known history of problematic drug use, and Tourette's syndrome.

Side Effects and Adverse Effects

The side effects and adverse effects of stimulants are commonly an extension of their therapeutic effects. The CNS-related side effects are restlessness, dizziness, tremor, hyperactive reflexes, talkativeness, tenseness, irritability, weakness, insomnia, fever, and sometimes euphoria. Confusion, aggression, increased libido, anxiety, delirium, paranoid hallucinations, panic states, and suicidal or homicidal tendencies occur, especially in mentally ill clients. Fatigue and depression usually follow the CNS stimulation. Cardiovascular effects are common and include headache, chilliness, pallor or flushing, palpitations, cardiac dysrhythmias, anginal pain, hypertension or hypotension, and circulatory collapse. Excessive sweating can also occur. GI effects include dry mouth, metallic taste, anorexia, nausea, vomiting, diarrhea, and abdominal cramps.

Toxicity and Management of Overdose

Box 8-4 lists the signs, symptoms, and timing of withdrawal from stimulants. Fatal poisoning, or death due to toxic levels, usually occurs because of convulsions, coma, or cerebral hemorrhages and may occur during periods of intoxication or withdrawal.

BOX 8-4
Signs and Symptoms of Stimulant Withdrawal

Peak Period
1–3 days

Duration
5–7 days

Signs
Social withdrawal, psychomotor retardation, hypersomnia, hyperphagia (excessive appetite)

Symptoms
Depression, suicidal thoughts and behaviour, paranoid delusions

DEPRESSANTS

Depressants are drugs that relieve anxiety, irritability, and tension when used as they are intended. They are also used to treat seizure disorders and induce anaesthesia. The two main pharmacological classes of depressants are benzodiazepines and barbiturates. Benzodiazepines are relatively safe. They offer many advantages over older agents used to relieve anxiety and insomnia. However, they are often intentionally and unintentionally misused. Benzodiazepines co-ingested with alcohol can be lethal.

A benzodiazepine that has recently gained popularity as a recreational drug is flunitrazepam. Flunitrazepam is not legally available for prescription in Canada, but it is legal in more than 60 countries for treatment of insomnia. The drug, known as **roofies** among young people, creates a sleepy, relaxed, drunk feeling that lasts 2 to 8 hours. A single dose costs from $2.00 to $6.50 in Canada. Roofies are commonly used in combination with alcohol as an "alcohol extender." They are sometimes taken to enhance a heroin high or to mellow or ease the experience of coming down from a cocaine or crack high. Used with alcohol, roofies produce disinhibition and amnesia.

Roofies have recently gained a reputation as the "date rape drug." Girls and women around the country have reported being sexually assaulted after being involuntarily sedated with roofies, which were often slipped into their drink by an attacker. The drug has no taste or odour, so the victims do not realize what is happening. About 10 minutes after ingesting the drug, the woman may feel dizzy and disoriented, simultaneously too hot and too cold, and nauseous. She may experience difficulty speaking and moving and then pass out. Such a victim will have no memories of what happened while under the influence of the drug.

Flunitrazepam is sold under the trade name Rohypnol, from which the street name "Rophy" is derived. Street names include "circles," "Mexican valium," "rib," "roach-2," "roofies," "roopies," "rope," "ropies," and "ruffies." Being under the influence of the drug is referred to as being "roached out." Flunitrazepam is similar in appearance to an acetylsalicylic acid tablet and has 10 times the potency of diazepam.

Mechanism of Action and Drug Effects

Benzodiazepines and barbiturates work by increasing the action of gamma-aminobutyric acid (GABA). GABA is an inhibitory amino acid in the brain that functions to inhibit nerve transmission in the CNS. The alteration of GABA in the CNS results in relieved anxiety, sedation, and muscle relaxation. The effects of depressants are primarily limited to the CNS. Their CNS effects include sedation, amnesia, muscle relaxation, unconsciousness, and reduced anxiety. They have moderate effects outside the CNS, causing slight blood pressure decreases.

Indications

Many therapeutic uses of depressants exist. Benzodiazepines are more widely used and misused/abused than barbiturates, and they are more commonly prescribed because they are felt by many to be safer than barbiturates. Benzodiazepines are used primarily to relieve anxiety, to induce sleep, to sedate, and as anticonvulsants. Barbiturates are used as hypnotics, as sedatives, as anticonvulsants, and to induce anaesthesia.

Contraindications

Contraindications to the therapeutic use of depressant medications include known drug allergy, dyspnea or airway obstruction, narrow-angle glaucoma, and porphyria.

Side Effects and Adverse Effects

The most common undesirable effect of benzodiazepines and barbiturates is an overexpression of their therapeutic effects. The CNS is the primary area of the body adversely affected by these drugs. Drowsiness, sedation, loss of coordination, dizziness, blurred vision, headaches, and paradoxical reactions (insomnia, increased excitability, hallucinations) are the primary CNS side effects. Occasional GI effects include nausea, vomiting, constipation, dry mouth, and abdominal cramping. Other possible side effects include pruritus and skin rash.

Toxicity and Management of Overdose

Box 8-5 lists the signs, symptoms, and timing of withdrawal from depressants. Fatal poisoning is unusual with benzodiazepines when they are ingested alone. However, when benzodiazepines are ingested with ethanol or barbiturates the combination can be lethal. Death is typically due to respiratory arrest. Abrupt withdrawal of benzodiazepines that have been taken for several months to years has resulted in autonomic withdrawal symptoms, seizures, delirium, rebound anxiety, myoclonus (involuntary twitching or jerking), myalgia (muscle pain), and sleep disturbances.

BOX   8-5

Signs, Symptoms, and Treatment of Depressant Withdrawal

Peak Period
2–4 days for short-acting agents
4–7 days for long-acting agents

Duration
4–7 days for short-acting agents
7–12 days for long-acting agents

Signs
Increased psychomotor activity; agitation; muscular weakness; hyperpyrexia (high fever); diaphoresis; delirium; convulsions; elevated blood pressure, pulse, and temperature; tremors of eyelids, tongue, and hands

Symptoms
Anxiety; depression; euphoria; incoherent thoughts; hostility; grandiosity; disorientation; tactile, auditory and visual hallucinations; suicidal thoughts

Treatment of Benzodiazepine Withdrawal
7- to 10-day taper (10- to 14-day taper with long-acting benzodiazepines). Treat with diazepam (Valium) 10–20 mg orally qid on day 1, then taper until the dosage is 5–10 mg orally on last day. Avoid giving the drug "as needed." Adjustments in dosage according to the client's clinical state may be indicated.

Treatment of Barbiturate Withdrawal
7- to 10-day taper or 10- to 14-day taper. Calculate barbiturate equivalence and give 50 percent of the original dosage (if actual dosage is known before detoxification); taper. Avoid giving the drug "as needed."

TABLE 8-2

BARBITURATE EQUIVALENCIES

Drug	Dose (mg)	Phenobarbital Dose (mg)	Conversion Factor
BARBITURATES			
butalbital	600	180	0.3
phenobarbital sodium	600	180	0.3
phenobarbital sodium	180	180	1
OTHERS			
meprobamate	2400	180	0.075

Table 8-2 should be used for conversion from various barbiturates to phenobarbital, which is less addicting and easier to withdraw from. To use this table, the nurse determines the total dose of the barbiturate that the client is dependent on, takes this dose and multiplies it by the conversion factor to get the equivalent dose of phenobarbital, and then tapers from there as described in Box 8-5.

Flumazenil can be used to acutely reverse the sedative effects of benzodiazepines. Flumazenil antagonizes the action of benzodiazepines on the CNS by directly competing with them for binding at the benzodiazepine receptor in the CNS. However, flumazenil has a stronger affinity for the receptor and knocks the benzodiazepine off the receptor, reversing the sedative action of the benzodiazepine. The dosage regimen to be followed for the reversal of conscious sedation or general anaesthesia induced by benzodiazepines and the management of suspected benzodiazepine overdoses are summarized in Table 12-6 on p. 193.

Limiting depressant misuse/abuse is important. Barbiturates and benzodiazepines are commonly implicated in suicides, especially when combined with alcohol. None of the depressants should be regularly prescribed over a long period. Relatively safe hypnotic agents such as benzodiazepines should be preferentially used whenever possible, especially in emotionally disturbed clients. Combinations of sedative–hypnotic compounds and the single use of these drugs with alcohol should be avoided. Chronic hypnotic drug use leads to ineffective control of insomnia, decreased rapid eye movement (REM) sleep, dependence, and drug withdrawal symptomatology.

ALCOHOL

Alcoholic beverages have been used since the beginning of human civilization. Individuals of Arab descent introduced the technique of distillation to Europe in the Middle Ages. Alcohol has been termed the "elixir of life" and has been a remedy for practically all diseases, which led to the term *whisky*, Gaelic for "water of life." It has been determined that the therapeutic value of ethanol is extremely limited, and chronic ingestion of excessive amounts is a major social and medical problem.

Mechanism of Action and Drug Effects

Alcohol, more accurately known as *ethanol* (abbreviated as ETOH), causes CNS depression by dissolving in lipid membranes in the CNS. The latest hypothesis is that ethanol causes a local disordering in the lipid matrix of the brain. This has been termed *membrane fluidization.* Some also believe that ethanol may augment GABA-mediated synaptic inhibition and fluxes of chloride. Enhancing GABA, an inhibitory neurotransmitter in the brain, leads to CNS depression. Many drug effects of ethanol exist. The CNS is continuously depressed in the presence of ethanol. Moderate amounts of ethanol may stimulate or depress respirations. Effects of ethanol on the circulation are relatively minor. In moderate doses, ethanol causes vasodilation, especially of the cutaneous vessels, and produces warm, flushed skin. Ingestion of ethanol causes a feeling of warmth because alcohol enhances cutaneous and gastric blood flow. Increased sweating may also occur. Heat is therefore lost more rapidly, and the internal temperature consequently falls. The acute ingestion of ethanol, even in intoxicating doses, probably produces little lasting change in hepatic function. Ethanol exerts a diuretic effect by virtue of its inhibition of antidiuretic hormone (ADH) secretion and the resultant decrease in renal tubular reabsorption of water.

Indications

Few legitimate medical uses of ethanol and alcoholic beverages exist. Ethanol is an excellent solvent for many drugs and is commonly employed as a vehicle for medicinal mixtures. When applied topically to the skin ethanol acts as a coolant. Ethanol sponges are therefore used to treat fever. Ethanol may also be used in liniments. Applied topically, ethanol is the most popular skin disinfectant. It is a common ingredient in hand lotions, after-shave lotions, cosmetics, and other pharmaceuticals. More commonly, however, the type of alcohol used on the skin is isopropyl alcohol, which is similar in structure to ethanol but is more toxic and not drinkable.

Ethanol is still widely employed for its hypnotic and antipyretic effects in various cold and cough products. Dehydrated alcohol is injected in the close proximity of nerves or sympathetic ganglia for the relief of the long-lasting pain that occurs in trigeminal neuralgia, inoperable carcinoma, and other conditions. Systemic uses of ethanol are primarily limited to the treatment of methyl alcohol and ethylene glycol intoxication.

Side Effects and Adverse Effects

Chronic excessive ingestion of ethanol is directly associated with serious neurological and mental disorders. These neurological disorders can result in seizures. Nutritional and vitamin deficiencies, especially of the B vitamins, can occur, resulting in Wernicke's encephalopathy, Korsakoff's psychosis, polyneuritis, and nicotinic acid deficiency encephalopathy.

Moderate amounts of ethanol may stimulate or depress respirations. Large amounts produce dangerous or

BOX 8-6
Treatment of Ethanol Withdrawal

Mild Withdrawal

Signs and Symptoms

Systolic blood pressure >150 mm Hg, diastolic blood pressure >90 mm Hg, pulse >110 beats/min, temperature >37.7°C, tremors, insomnia, agitation

Treatment
- diazepam, 5–10 mg PO prn
- lorazepam, 1–2 mg PO q4–6h prn for 1–3 days

Moderate Withdrawal

Signs and Symptoms

Systolic blood pressure 150–200 mm Hg, diastolic blood pressure 100–140 mm Hg, pulse 110–140 beats/min, temperature 37.7–38.3°C, tremors, insomnia, agitation

Treatment
- diazepam
  Day 1: 15–20 mg PO qid
  Day 2: 10–20 mg PO qid
  Day 3: 5–15 mg PO qid
  Day 4: 10 mg PO qid
  Day 5: 5 mg PO qid
- lorazepam
  Days 1 and 2: 2–4 mg PO qid
  Days 3 and 4: 1–2 mg PO qid
  Day 5: 1 mg PO bid

Severe Withdrawal (Delirium Tremens)*

Signs and Symptoms

Systolic blood pressure >200 mm Hg, diastolic blood pressure >140 mm Hg, pulse >140 beats/min, temperature >38.3°C, tremors, insomnia, agitation

Treatment
- diazepam, 10–25 mg PO prn q1h while awake until sedation occurs
- lorazepam, 1–2 mg IV prn q1h while awake for 3–5 days

*Monitoring in an intensive care unit is recommended for cardiac and respiratory function, fluid and nutrition replacement, vital signs, and mental status. Restraints are indicated in clients who are confused or agitated to protect the client from self and others (DTs can be a terrifying and life-threatening state). Thiamine (100 mg IM or PO qd for 3–7 days), hydration, and magnesium replacement may be indicated according to the severity of the withdrawal state. *PO*, orally; *IV*, intravenously; *IM*, intramuscularly; *DTs*, delirium tremens.

TABLE 8-3
ACETALDEHYDE SYNDROME

Body System Affected	Body System Result
Cardiovascular	Vasodilation over the entire body, hypotension, orthostatic syncope, chest pain
Central nervous	Intense throbbing of the head and neck leading to a pulsating headache, sweating, marked uneasiness, weakness, vertigo, blurred vision, confusion
Gastrointestinal	Nausea, copious vomiting, thirst
Respiratory	Difficulty breathing

(FAS) and often results in craniofacial abnormalities, CNS dysfunction, and both pre- and postnatal growth retardation in the infant. Pregnant women should therefore be strongly advised not to consume alcohol during pregnancy, and appropriate treatment and counselling should be arranged for pregnant women addicted to alcohol or any other drug of problematic use.

Toxicity and Management of Overdose

Box 8-6 lists the common signs and symptoms of ethanol withdrawal. Signs and symptoms may vary depending on the individual's usage pattern, his or her preferred type of ethanol, and the existence of other concurrent disorders.

One pharmacological option for the treatment of alcoholism is disulfiram, more commonly know by its trade name Antabuse. Disulfiram is not a cure for alcoholism; it helps a client who has a sincere desire to stop drinking. The rationale for its use is that clients know that if they are to avoid the devastating experience of the acetaldehyde syndrome (Table 8-3), they cannot drink for at least 3 or 4 days after taking disulfiram. These side effects are obviously uncomfortable and even potentially dangerous for someone with any other major illnesses. For this reason, disulfiram is usually reserved as a last resort for the "hard core" alcoholic client who has failed other treatment options (e.g., Alcoholics Anonymous, psychotherapy) but who still hopes to avoid continued alcohol abuse. A less noxious drug therapy option is the use of naltrexone, as mentioned previously in the section on opioids in this chapter.

Disulfiram works by altering the metabolism of alcohol. When ethanol is given to an individual previously treated with disulfiram, the blood acetaldehyde concentration rises five to ten times higher than in an untreated individual. Within about 5 to 10 minutes of ingesting alcohol, the face feels hot, and soon afterward it is flushed and scarlet in appearance. After this, throbbing in the head and neck, nausea, copious vomiting, diaphoresis, dyspnea, hyperventilation, vertigo, blurred vision, and confusion appear. As little as 7 mL of alcohol will cause mild symptoms in a sensitive person. The effects last from 30 minutes to several hours. After the symptoms wear off, the client is exhausted and may sleep for several hours. Most of the signs and symptoms observed after the ingestion of disulfiram plus alcohol are attributable to

lethal depression of respiration. Although circulatory effects of ethanol are relatively minor, acute severe alcoholic intoxication may cause cardiovascular depression. Long-term excessive use of ethanol has largely irreversible effects on the heart, such as cardiomyopathy.

When consumed on a regular basis in large quantities, ethanol produces a constellation of dose-related negative effects or serious sequelae, such as alcoholic hepatitis or its progression to cirrhosis. Teratogenic effects can be devastating and are due to a direct action of ethanol inhibiting embryonic cellular proliferation early in gestation. This condition is known as *fetal alcohol syndrome* the resulting increase in the concentration of acetaldehyde in the body. The usual dosage of disulfiram is 250 mg per day, or 125 mg per day in clients who experience side effects such as sedation, sexual dysfunction, and elevated liver enzymes.

NICOTINE

Nicotine was first isolated from the leaves of tobacco by Posselt and Reiman in 1828. The medical significance of nicotine lies in its toxicity, its presence in tobacco, and its potential for dependence. The chronic effects of nicotine and the untoward effects of the chronic use of tobacco are considerable. Although many people smoke because they believe cigarettes calm their nerves, smoking releases epinephrine, a hormone that creates physiological stress in the smoker rather than relaxation. The use of tobacco is addictive. Most users develop tolerance for nicotine and need greater amounts to produce a desired effect. Smokers become physically and psychologically dependent and will suffer withdrawal symptoms. Smoking is particularly dangerous in adolescents because their bodies are still developing and changing. The 4000 chemicals in cigarette smoke, including 200 known poisons, can adversely affect this process. One-third of young people who are just "experimenting" end up being addicted by the time they are 20 years old.

Mechanism of Action

Nicotine works by directly stimulating the autonomic ganglia of the nicotinic receptors. Its site of action is the ganglion itself rather than the preganglionic or post-ganglionic nerve fibre. These receptors are so named because they were originally tested with nicotine to measure their response. Nicotine can have multiple, unpredictable, and dramatic effects on the body because the nicotinic receptors are found in several organ systems, including the adrenal glands, skeletal muscle, and the CNS.

Drug Effects

The major action of nicotine is initially transient stimulation, followed by more persistent depression of all autonomic ganglia. Small doses of nicotine stimulate the ganglion cells directly and facilitate the transmission of impulses. When larger doses of the drug are applied, the initial stimulation is followed quickly by a blockade of transmission.

Nicotine markedly stimulates the CNS. Respiratory stimulation is also common. This stimulation of the CNS is followed by depression. Nicotine can have dramatic effects on the cardiovascular system as well, resulting in increases in heart rate and blood pressure. The GI system is generally stimulated by nicotine, resulting in increased tone and activity in the bowel. This often leads to nausea and vomiting and occasionally diarrhea.

Therapeutic Uses

Nicotine has no therapeutic uses. It has significance primarily because of its medical significance secondary to its toxicity.

Side Effects and Adverse Effects

Nicotine primarily affects the CNS. Large doses can produce tremors and even convulsions. Respiratory stimulation is also common. The initial stimulation of the CNS induced by nicotine is quickly followed by depression. Death can even result from respiratory failure, which is thought to be due to both central paralysis and peripheral blockade of respiratory muscles.

The cardiovascular effects of nicotine are an increase in heart rate and blood pressure. Nicotine stimulates sympathetic ganglia with the discharge of catecholamines from the sympathetic nerve endings.

The effects of nicotine on the GI system are largely due to parasympathetic stimulation, which results in increased tone and motor activity of the bowel. Nicotine induces vomiting by both central and peripheral actions. Centrally, nicotine's emetic effects are due to stimulation of the chemoreceptor trigger zone (CTZ).

Toxicity and Management of Overdose

Smoking cessation is the primary cause for nicotine withdrawal, although discontinuation of any tobacco product can lead to this syndrome. An important and often overlooked problem in hospitalized clients is nicotine withdrawal, which manifests largely as cigarette craving. Irritability, restlessness, and a decrease in heart rate and blood pressure occur. Cardiac symptoms resolve over 3 to 4 weeks, but cigarette craving may persist for months or even years.

The nicotine transdermal system (patch), nicotine polacrilex (gum), and nicotine inhaler can be used to provide nicotine without the carcinogens in tobacco and are now available over the counter (OTC). The patch uses a stepwise reduction in subcutaneous delivery to gradually decrease the nicotine dose and appears to have greater client adherence than the gum. Acute relief from withdrawal symptoms is most easily achieved with use of the gum because rapid chewing releases an immediate dose of nicotine. However, the dose is approximately half the dose the average smoker receives in one cigarette and the onset of action is 30 minutes, vs. 10 minutes or less from smoking. These pharmacological changes in delivery minimize the reinforcement and self-reward effects that are prominent with the rapid nicotine delivery of cigarette smoking.

A sustained-release form of bupropion, better known as Zyban, has been approved as first-line therapy to aid in smoking cessation treatment. Zyban is an innovative treatment because it is the first nicotine-free prescription medicine to treat nicotine dependence. Table 8-4 lists the currently available agents for nicotine withdrawal. Box 8-7 lists helpful resources containing information on problematic substance use.

NURSING PROCESS

■ Assessment

The nurse must include questions about problematic substance use in any medication history or assessment process to identify problems or the potential for withdrawal. The nurse must assess thoroughly clients who are suspected of or diagnosed with problematic substance use and be attentive to every detail so as to avoid withdrawal symptoms, assist with appropriate medications as ordered, and determine and develop an appropriate plan of care. Clients with problematic substance use may not be honest about their drug use; therefore the nurse should use open-ended questions and maintain a non-judgemental approach. All current medications should be listed on the medication history (OTC, prescription, illegal, herbal, etc.), including names of drugs, dosages, and frequency and duration of dosing. When a client states that he or she has multiple prescribed drugs or multiple prescribers, this may be a sign of problematic drug use. The nurse must always be alert to the client's behaviour and mental status for cues.

The most dangerous substances for withdrawal are CNS depressants, which include alcohol, barbiturates, and benzodiazepines. Delirium tremens (DTs) may begin with tremors and agitation and may progress to hallucinations and sometimes death. Careful assessment of vital signs and mental status is once again critical to the safe care of these clients because early withdrawal symptoms may include an increase in blood pressure and pulse with an alteration in mental status.

▮ Nursing Diagnoses

Nursing diagnoses related to the individual with problematic substance use are as follows:

- Risk for injury and falls related to problematic substance use and abrupt withdrawal
- Situational low self-esteem related to the influence of problematic chemical and/or substance use on the person and his or her physiological and emotional functioning
- Disturbed thought processes related to biochemical changes as a result of the problematic chemical use
- Deficient knowledge about abusive, addictive behaviours and their long-term management

▮ Planning

Goals related to management of the client with problematic substance use include the following:

- Client remains without injury during treatment for problematic substance use.
- Client gains an improved self-esteem during treatment.
- Client discusses problematic drug use problem and its management openly with the healthcare team.

TABLE 8-4
NICOTINE WITHDRAWAL THERAPIES

Drug	Dosage Per Patch	Recommended Duration of Use
TRANSDERMAL NICOTINE SYSTEMS		
Habitrol Sustained-Release Disc	7 mg/24 h, 14 mg/24 h, 21 mg/24 h	2–4 wk, 2–4 wk, 4–8 wk
Nicoderm	7 mg/24h, 14 mg/24 h, 21 mg/24 hr	2–4 wk, 2–4 wk, 4–8 wk
Nicotrol Transdermal Patch	5 mg/16 h, 10 mg/16h, 15 mg/16h	2–4 wk, 2–4 wk, 4–12 wk
Prostep Transdermal Patch	15 mg/24 h, 30 mg/24 h	2–4 wk, 4–8 wk
NICORETTE GUM/NICORETTE GUM PLUS		
	When the client has a strong urge to smoke, a stick of gum is chewed; gradually reducing over a 2- to 3-mo period.	
NICORETTE INHALER		
	6–12 cartridges/day up to 12 weeks; gradual tapering over 6–12 weeks	
ANTIDEPRESSANT		
Bupropion HCL (Zyban)	150 mg sustained release tabs	150 mg once daily for 3 days, then 150 mg bid for 7–12 wk

BOX 8-7
Resources for Information on Problematic Substance Use

Canadian Centre on Substance Abuse
75 Albert Street, Suite 300
Ottawa, ON K1P 5E7
Tel: 613-235-4048
Fax: 613-235-8101
http://www.ccsa.ca/CCSA/EN/TopNav/Home/

Canadian Psychiatric Association (CPA)
141 Laurier Avenue West, Suite 701
Ottawa, Ontario K1P 5J3
Tel: 613-234-2815
Fax: 613-234-9857
http://www.cpa-apc.org/index.asp

International Nurses Society on Addictions
PO Box 10752
Raleigh, NC 27605
Tel: 919-821-1292
Fax: 919-833-5743
http://www.intnsa.org/

Health Canada National Native Alcohol and Drug Abuse Program
http://www.hc-sc.gc.ca/fnih-spni/substan/ads/nnadap-pnlaada e.html

Substance Abuse and Mental Health Services Administration (SAMHSA)
Room 12–105 Parklawn Building
5600 Fishers Lane
Rockville, MD 20857
Tel: 301-443-4795
http://www.samhsa.gov/

Outcome Criteria

Outcome criteria related to problematic substance use are as follows:

- Client is safely withdrawn from drugs with stabilization of physical state that was aggravated by the problematic substance use (see the specific drug and related signs and symptoms).

GERIATRIC CONSIDERATIONS ▶◀▶◀

Problematic Substance Use in Older Adults

- Approximately 58 percent of women and 75 percent of men over 65 years of age use alcohol.
- Problematic alcohol use occurs in approximately 6 to 10 percent of people over 65 years of age and leads to significant alcohol-related hospitalization.
- Alcohol may alter the effects of other medications (such as CNS depressants) that geriatric clients are taking, with effects of lethargy, confusion, hypotension, and dizziness. This interaction may occur even with OTC alcohol-containing products such as cough and cold syrups.
- Nicotine addiction from lifelong smoking is problematic in older adults. It may alter drug metabolism and cause increased peripheral vasoconstriction, stimulation of antidiuretic hormone (ADH), and increased gastric acid.
- Caffeine use is found in older adults with the following implications: GI irritation, medication-induced changes in drug metabolism, increased lithium excretion, increased CNS stimulation, and cardiac irregularities.

- Client has appropriate referrals and humane treatment for the problematic substance use problem in a safe, non-threatening, healthy environment.

Implementation

Nurses working with problematic substance use clients need a special understanding and empathy, beginning with the nurse's knowledge about the problematic substance use process and understanding of the client's lifestyle. Once a therapeutic rapport has been established, the client may then need to have information about the drug being misused/abused, its characteristics, and problems associated with the use of the drug and its withdrawal. The withdrawal process also needs to be discussed with the client if appropriate. The nurse closely monitors the client through the parameters of vital signs and mental status. Family members and significant others should be encouraged to lend their support and assistance during treatment. Lifelong treatment is often indicated, and support for the long-term process of recovery should be emphasized and recommended. Education about the particular recovery process and medication regimen for promoting abstinence (if recommended) should be thorough and reinforced to the client and family members or significant others. Client teaching tips are presented below.

Evaluation

The client should feel safe and secure during treatment and should understand the symptoms that he or she may experience during withdrawal of the drug and associated treatment. Any change in mental status or in any parameter (vital sign) should be reported to the physician or healthcare provider immediately.

CLIENT TEACHING TIPS

- ▲ The client and family members or significant others must receive current and accurate information about the treatment regimen to make a more informed and individualized decision about the treatment plan.
- ▲ Education of family members or significant others about support groups and community resources is important for success during and after a treatment program.
- ▲ The healthcare provider should include information about any medication the client may be receiving, with

an emphasis on timing and amount of doses, consequences of missed doses, and side or toxic effects. For example, many over-the counter drugs such as acetaminophen and dimenhydrinate are incorrectly believed to be safe. However, problematic use of these drugs such as in suicide attempts can result in catastrophic outcomes because of the toxic effects.
- ▲ The healthcare provider should emphasize the danger of multiple drug use and of combining drugs with alcohol.

POINTS to REMEMBER

- ▼ Nurses and all other healthcare providers continually encounter a variety of problematic substance use problems and may play a significant part in the client's recovery.
- ▼ A thorough assessment of a client's past and present medical history with a medication history is crucial to the successful treatment of clients with problematic substance use.
- ▼ Withdrawal symptoms are characteristic of the drug class and may be opposite to the drug's action, such as

with alcohol (a CNS depressant), which produces withdrawal symptoms that are typically characterized by hyperactivity.
- ▼ The nurse must understand the pathology of problematic substance use and how dependent behaviours dominate all aspects of the client's life as the client "lives for the drug" every minute of the day.
- ▼ Including family members or other supportive persons in the treatment regimen results in a more successful treatment.

EXAMINATION REVIEW QUESTIONS

1 Your client in the emergency room has been diagnosed with an opioid overdose. Which of the following is most commonly associated with acute overdosage of opioids and opioid-like drugs?
   a. Flushing of the face
   b. Polyuria
   c. Hypertension
   d. Dysphagia with water
2 Which of the following medications may be used for opioid drug withdrawal?
   a. methamphetamine
   b. methadone
   c. diazepam
   d. GABA
3 One of your clients coming from the emergency room is a young female adolescent of unknown age. She is being transferred to the intensive care unit after a suicide attempt. Your initial assessment shows the following: blood pressure 80/40 mm Hg, pulse 118 beats/min, and respiratory rate 8 breaths/min; thought processes are al-

tered, and she is only responsive to some verbal commands. Which of the following agents did she probably take?
   a. Alcohol
   b. Adrenaline
   c. Barbiturates
   d. Amphetamines
4 Acetaldehyde syndrome is manifested by which of the following?
   a. Vasoconstriction
   b. Dry skin
   c. Hypertension
   d. Copious vomiting
5 Which of the following would you find while assessing an individual for possible use of amphetamines?
   a. Lethargy and fatigue
   b. Vomiting and incontinence of urine
   c. Cardiovascular depression
   d. Aggressiveness and euphoria

For answers see http://evolve.elsevier.com/Lilley/pharmacology/.

CRITICAL THINKING ACTIVITIES

1 Your client has been admitted to labour and delivery. She has a history of heavy use of alcohol and appears to be intoxicated. What are the potential complications of alcohol on a fetus, and what would be some concerns during the first few months of the newborn's life?
2 Explain how any substance ingested or misused/abused by the pregnant female can affect the fetus.

3 Your client arrives at the emergency room with symptoms of weakness, tremulousness, restlessness, anxiety, insomnia, orthostatic hypotension, and a variety of GI complaints. What do you think is occurring with this client?

For answers see http://evolve.elsevier.com/Lilley/pharmacology/.

BIBLIOGRAPHY

Arcangelo, V.P., & Peterson, A.M. (2005). *Pharmacotherapeutics for advanced practice: A practical approach* (2nd ed.). Philadelphia: Lippincott Williams & Wilkins.

Canadian Institutes of Health Research. (2005). North America's first clinical trial of prescribed heroin begins today. Retrieved July 23, 2005, from http://www.cihr-irsc.gc.ca/e/26516.html

College of Physicians and Surgeons of Ontario. (2001). Methadone maintenance guidelines. [Electronic version]. Retrieved July 24, 2005, from http://www.cpso.on.ca/Publications/methguide.htm

Health Canada. (2004). Preventing and addressing problematic use. Retrieved November 6, 2005 from http://www.hc-sc.gc.ca/dhp-mps/substan/index_e.html

Health Canada. (2000). Straight facts about drugs and drug abuse. [Electronic version]. Ottawa, ON: Author. Retrieved August 12, 2005, from http://www.hc-sc.gc.ca/ahc-asc/pubs/drugs-drogues/straight_factsfaits_mefaits/index_e.html

Health Canada. (2004). Misuse and abuse of oxycodone-based prescription drugs. [Electronic version]. Ottawa, ON: Health Canada. Retrieved July 24, 2005, from http://www.hc-sc.gc.ca/english/media/releases/2004/oxycodone.htm

Lehne, R.A. (2004). *Pharmacology for nursing care* (5th ed.). St Louis, MO: Saunders.

McKenry, L.M., & Salerno, E. (2003). *Mosby's pharmacology in nursing*—revised and updated. (21st ed.). St Louis, MO: Mosby.

Mosby. (2005). *Mosby's drug consult 2005: The comprehensive reference for generic and brand name drugs* (15th ed.). St Louis, MO: Mosby.

Nordeste, B. (2004). The potential expansion of methamphetamine product and distribution in Canada. A background study. [Electronic version]. Retrieved July 25, 2005, from http://www.carleton.ca/cifp/docs/nordestemethreport.pdf

Skidmore-Roth, L. (2006). *Mosby's 2006 nursing drug reference* (19th ed.). St Louis, MO: Mosby.

Statistics Canada. (2004). The Canadian addiction survey. [Electronic version]. Ottawa, ON: Statistics Canada. Retrieved August 12, 2005, from http://www.ccsa.ca/pdf/ccsa-004804-2004.pdf

Sullivan, P. (2001). OxyContin abuse appears limited to US. [Electronic version]. *Canadian Medical Association Journal, 165* (5). Retrieved August 12, 2005, from http://www.cmaj.ca/cgi/content/full/165/5/624

Tjepkema, M. (2002). Alcohol and illicit drug dependence. [Electronic version]. Ottawa, ON: Statistics Canada. Retrieved August 12, 2005, from http://www.statcan.ca/english/freepub/82-003-SIE/2004000/pdf/82-003-SIE20040007447.pdf

9 Photo Atlas of Drug Administration

PREPARING FOR DRUG ADMINISTRATION

Note: This photo atlas is designed to illustrate general aspects of drug administration. For detailed instructions, please refer to a nursing fundamentals or skills book.

When giving medications, the nurse must remember safety measures and correct administration techniques to avoid errors and to ensure optimal drug actions. Keep in mind the "5 Rights":

1 Right drug
2 Right dose
3 Right time
4 Right route
5 Right client

Refer to Chapter 1 for additional rights regarding drug administration. Other things to keep in mind when preparing to give medications:

- Remember to wash your hands before preparing or giving medications.
- If unsure about a drug or dosage calculation, do not hesitate to double check with a drug reference or with a pharmacist. **DO NOT** give a medication if you are unsure about it!
- Be punctual when giving drugs. Some medications must be given at regular intervals to maintain therapeutic blood levels.
- Figure 9-1 shows an example of a computer-controlled drug dispensing system. To prevent errors, the nurse should obtain the drugs for one client at a time.
- Remember to check the drug at least three times before giving it. The nurse is responsible for checking medication labels with the transcribed medication order. In Figure 9-2, the nurse is checking the drug against the medication administration record (MAR) after taking it out of the dispenser drawer. The drug should also be checked before opening it, and again after opening but before giving it to the client.
- Check the expiration date of all medications. Medications used past the expiration date may be less potent or even harmful.
- Before administering any medication, check the client's identification bracelet. In addition, the client's

drug allergies should be assessed (Figure 9-3). Some hospitals use a bar code system, shown in Figure 9.4.
- Be sure to take the time to explain to the client the purpose of each medication, its action, possible side effects, and any other pertinent information, especially drug–drug or drug–food interactions.
- Open the medication at the bedside into the client's hand or into the medicine cup. Try not to touch the drugs with your hands. Leaving them in their packaging until you get to the client's room helps to avoid contamination and waste should the client refuse the drug.
- Discard any medication that falls to the floor or becomes contaminated by other means.
- Chart the medication on the MAR as soon as it is given and before going to the next client (Figure 9-4). Be sure to also document therapeutic responses, adverse effects (if any), and other concerns in the nurse's notes.
- Return to evaluate the client's response to the drug within 30 minutes.

ENTERAL DRUGS

Administering Oral Drugs

Always begin by washing your hands, and maintain Standard Precautions (see Box 9-1). When administering oral drugs, keep in mind the following points:

Oral Medications

- Healthcare facilities have various means of checking the MAR when a new one is printed, so before giving the oral medication be sure that you are working from a MAR that has been checked or verified. If the client's MAR has a new drug order on it, the best rule of practice is to double check that order against the client's chart.
- Some oral medications (and medications by other routes) require special assessments. For example, the apical pulse should be auscultated for 1 full minute before any digitalis preparation is given (Figure 9-5). Other oral medications may require blood pressure monitoring. Be sure to document all parameters on the MAR. Do not forget to check your client's identification

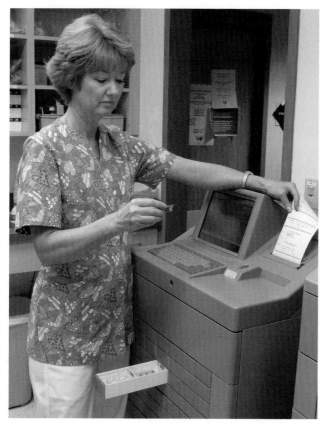

FIG. 9-1 Using a computer-dispensing system to remove unit-dose medication.

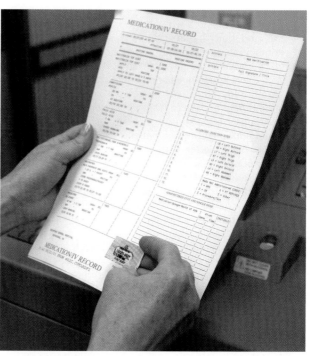

FIG. 9-2 The nurse checks the medication against the order on the MAR.

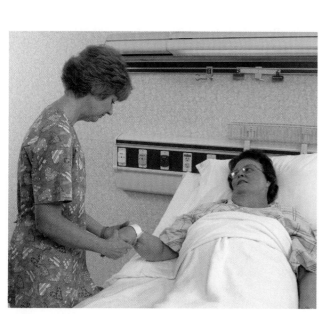

FIG. 9-3 Always check the client's identification and allergies before giving medications.

FIG. 9-4 Example of a medication administration record (MAR).

TTH / PMH / OCI	Run from 06/03/17 07:31 to 06/03/18 07:30		

24 Hour Check Done	*Location:* TEST	*Physician:* Doctor, John Q.	
Date: _____	*Name:* Test, Patient	*MRN #:* 0012457	*Age:* 49
Time: _____	*Diagnosis:*	*Visit #:* 000012457	
RN: _____	*Allergies:* No Known Allergy		

US/RN	START STOP	MEDICATION		07:31 – 19:30	19:31 – 07:30
		***** ROUTINE MEDS *****			
/	06/03/16 07/03/16	ENOXaparin Sodium Inj 80 MG/0.8 ML SYRINGE 80 MG = 0.8 ML SC every 12 hours	Q12H	10:00	22:00
/	06/03/16 07/03/16	Famotidine Inj 20 MG in Dextrose Inj 5% 50 ML Baxter Batch Infuse IV over 15–30 min	Q12H	10:00	22:00
/	06/03/16 07/03/16	Mycophenolate Susp 1000MG/5ML 1000 MG = 5 ML PO/NG 2 times a day	BID	10:00	22:00
		***** PREMEDS *****			
/	06/03/16 07/03/16	Acetaminophen Tab 325 MG 650 MG = 2 Tab orally as directed (For Tylenol) pre platelets infusion	UD		
		***** ANTIMICROBIAL PREMIXED INJECTABLES *****			
/	06/03/16 06/04/15	Ampicillin Inj 1 GM Sodium Chloride Inj 0.9% Infuse IV over 15 min	Q6H	12:00 18:00	00:00 06:00
		***** CHEMO & MISC. INJECTABLES *****			
/	06/03/16 06/03/18	Doxorubicin HCl Inj 100 MG For IV use **VESICANT** Total number of syringes: ____ Each syringe contains: ____MG per ____mL	Q24H	17:00	–
/	06/03/16 06/03/18	Granisetron HCl Inj 1 MG in Dextrose Inj 5% 25 ML Baxter Batch Infuse IV over 5 min	Q24H	15:00	
		***** PRN ORDERS *****			
/	06/03/16 07/03/16	Docusate Sodium Cap 100 MG 100 MG = 1 Cap orally 2 times a day as needed (For Colace) Give with plenty of water	BIDPO		

Standard Precautions

Always adhere to Standard Precautions, including the following:

- Wear clean gloves when there is potential exposure to blood, body fluids, secretions, excretions, and any items that may contain these substances. Always wash hands immediately when there is direct contact with these substances or any item contaminated with blood, body fluids, secretions, or excretions. Gloves should be worn when giving injections but there are exceptions (e.g., gloves may not need to be worn when administering vaccines).
- Wash hands after removing gloves and between client contacts.
- Wear masks, eye protective gear, and face shields during any procedure or client care situation with the potential for splashes or spraying of blood, body fluids, secretions, or excretions. A gown may also be indicated for these situations.
- While administering medications, once the exposure or procedure is completed and exposure risk is eliminated, remove soiled protective garments or gear.
- Never remove, recap, cap, bend, or break any used needle or needle system. Be sure to discard any disposable syringes and needles in the appropriate puncture-resistant container.
- In the case of a needle-stick injury, flush the area affected or wash it. The area can be swabbed with alcohol or betadene or some other disinfectant. Report the injury to Occupational Health, or to the Emergency Department if off hours. Most Emergency and most Occupation Health Departments now have a plan for managing exposure to blood and body fluids.
- If during drug administration you are handling or transporting soiled and contaminated items from the client, dispose of them in the appropriately labelled containers for contaminated wastes.

and allergies before giving any medication (or medication by any other route).
- If your client is experiencing difficulty swallowing (dysphagia), some tablets can be crushed with a clean mortar and pestle (or other device) (Figure 9-6). Crush one type of pill at a time because if you mix together all of the medications and then spill some, there is no way to tell which drug has been wasted. Also, if all are mixed together, you cannot check the "5 Rights" three times before giving the drug. Mix the crushed medication in a small amount of soft food, such as applesauce or pudding. Be sure that the pill-crushing device is clean before and after you use it.
- CAUTION: Be sure to verify whether a medication can be crushed by consulting a drug reference book or a pharmacist. Some oral medications, such as capsules, enteric-coated tablets, and sustained-release (SR) or long-acting drugs, should *not* be crushed, broken, or

chewed (Figure 9-7). These medications are formulated to protect the gastric lining from irritation or protect the drug from destruction from gastric acids, or designed to break down gradually and slowly release the medication. If these drugs, designated with labels such as SR or extended-release (XR), are crushed or opened, then the intended action of the dosage form is destroyed. As a result, gastric irritation may occur, the drug may be inactivated by gastric acids, or the immediate availability of a drug that was supposed to be released slowly may cause toxic effects. Check with the healthcare provider to see if an alternate form of the drug is needed.

- Be sure your client is sitting or side-lying to make it easier to swallow oral medications and to avoid the risk of aspiration (Figure 9-8). Provide measures as needed to prevent aspiration.
- Offer the client a full glass of water; 120 to 180 mL of water or other fluid is recommended for the best dissolution and absorption of oral medications. If the client prefers another fluid, be sure to check for interactions between the medication and the fluid of choice.
- If the client requests, you may place the pill or capsule in his or her mouth with your gloved hand.
- Lozenges should not be chewed unless specifically instructed.
- Effervescent powders and tablets should be mixed with water and then given immediately after they are dissolved.
- Remain with the client until all medication has been swallowed. If you are unsure whether a pill has been swallowed, ask the client to open his or her mouth so that you can inspect to see if it is gone. Assist the client to a comfortable position after the medication has been taken.

Sublingual and Buccal Medications

The sublingual and buccal routes prevent destruction of the drugs in the gastrointestinal (GI) tract and allow for rapid absorption into the bloodstream through the oral mucous membranes. These routes are not often used. Be sure to provide instruction before giving these medications.

- Sublingual tablets should be placed under the tongue (Figure 9-9). Buccal tablets are placed between the upper or lower molar teeth and cheek area.
- Be sure to wear gloves if you are placing the tablet into the client's mouth. Adhere to Standard Precautions (see Box 9-1).
- Instruct the client to allow the drug to dissolve completely before swallowing.
- Fluids should not be taken with these drug forms. Instruct the client not to drink anything until the tablet has dissolved completely.
- Be sure to instruct the client not to swallow these tablets.
- When using the buccal route, alternate sides with each dose to reduce possible irritation of the oral mucosa.

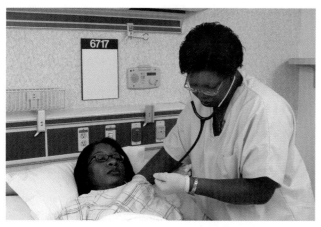

FIG. 9-5 Some medications require special assessment before giving, such as taking an apical pulse.

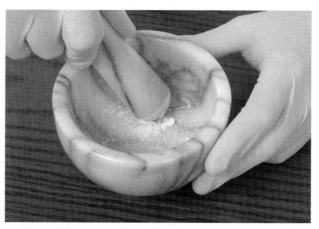

FIG. 9-6 Crushing tablets with a mortar and pestle.

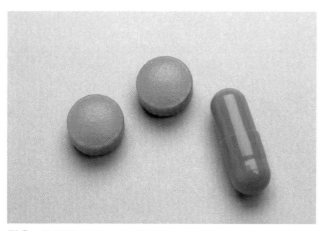

FIG. 9-7 Enteric-coated tablets and long-acting medications should not be crushed.

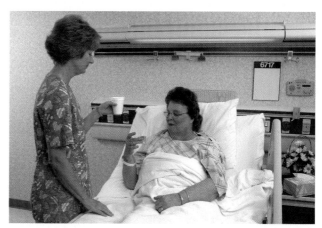

FIG. 9-8 Giving oral medications.

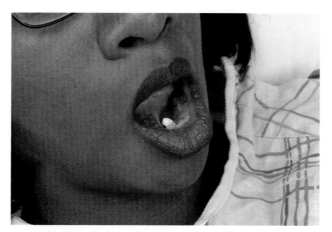

FIG. 9-9 Proper placement of a sublingual tablet.

Liquid Medications

- Liquid medications may come in a single dose (unit dose) package, be poured into a medicine cup from a multi-dose bottle, or be drawn up in an oral-dosing syringe (Figure 9-10).
- When pouring a liquid medication from a container, first shake the bottle gently to mix the contents if indicated. Remove the cap and place it on the counter, upside down. Hold the bottle with the label against the palm of your hand to keep any spilled medication from altering the label. Place the medication cup at eye level and fill to the proper level on the scale (Figure 9-11). Pour the desired amount of liquid so that the base of the meniscus is even with the line measure on the medicine cup.
- If you overfill the medication cup, discard the excess in the sink. Do not pour it back into the multi-dose bottle. Before replacing the cap, wipe the rim of the bottle with a paper towel.
- Liquid medication doses under 5 mL should be drawn up in a sterile syringe, without a needle. If possible, use an oral-dosing syringe that is made for this purpose.

Oral Medications and Infants

- Because infants cannot swallow oral pills or capsules, liquids are usually ordered.
- A plastic disposable oral-dosing syringe is recommended for measuring small doses of liquid medications. Using an oral-dosing syringe prevents the inadvertent parenteral administration of a drug once it is drawn up into the syringe.
- Position the infant so that the head is slightly elevated to prevent aspiration. Not all infants will be co-operative, and many may need to be partially restrained (Figure 9-12).
- Place the plastic dropper or syringe inside the infant's mouth, beside the tongue, and administer the liquid in small amounts while allowing the infant to swallow each time.
- Take great care to prevent aspiration. A crying infant can easily aspirate medication.
- Do not add medication to a bottle of formula; the infant may refuse the feeding or may not drink all of it.
- Make sure that all of the oral medication has been taken, and then return the infant to a safe, comfortable position.

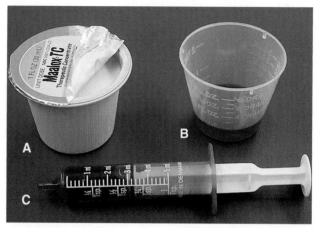

FIG. 9-10 **A,** Liquid medication in a unit-dose package. **B,** Liquid measured into a medicine cup from a multi-dose container. **C,** Liquid medicine in an oral-dosing syringe.

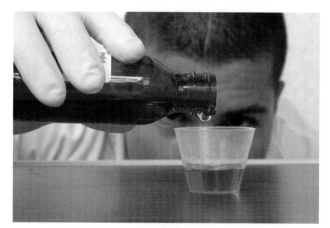

FIG. 9-11 Measuring liquid medication.

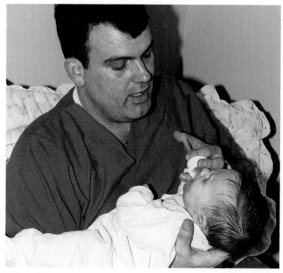

FIG. 9-12 Administering oral liquid medication to an infant.

Administering Drugs Through a Nasogastric or Gastrostomy Tube

Always begin by washing your hands, and maintain Standard Precautions (see Box 9-1). Gloves should be worn for these procedures. When administering drugs via these routes, keep in mind the following points:

- Before giving drugs via these routes, position the client in a semi-Fowler's or Fowler's position, and leave the head of the bed elevated for at least 30 minutes afterward to reduce the risk of aspiration (Figure 9-13).
- Assess whether fluid restriction or overload is a concern. It will be necessary to give water along with the medications to flush the tubing.
- Check to see whether the drug should be given on an empty or full stomach. If the drug should be given on an empty stomach, the feeding may need to be stopped before and/or after giving the medication.
- Whenever possible, give liquid forms of the drugs to prevent clogging the tube.
- If tablets must be given, crush the tablets, individually, into a fine powder. Administer the drugs separately (Figure 9-14). Keeping the drugs separate allows for accurate identification if a dose is spilled. Be sure to check whether the medication should be crushed; enteric-coated and sustained-release tablets or capsules should not be crushed. Check with a pharmacist if unsure.
- Before administering the drugs, follow the institution's policy for verifying tube placement and checking gastric residual. Re-instill gastric residual per institutional policy, and then clamp the tube (Figure 9-15).

- Dilute a crushed tablet or liquid medication in 15 to 30 mL of warm water. Some capsules may be opened and dissolved in 30 mL of warm water; check with a pharmacist.
- Remove the piston from an adaptable-tip syringe and attach to the end of the tube. Unclamp the tube and pinch the tubing to close it again. Add 30 mL of warm water and release the pinched tubing. Allow the water to flow in by gravity in order to flush the tube, and then pinch the tubing closed again before all the water is gone to prevent excessive air from entering the stomach.
- Pour the diluted medications into the syringe, and release the tubing to allow it to flow in by gravity. Flush between each drug with 15 to 30 mL of warm water (Figure 9-16). Be careful not to spill the medication mixture.
- If water or medication does not flow freely you may apply gentle pressure with the plunger of the syringe or the bulb of an Asepto syringe. Do not try to force the medicine through the tubing.
- After the last drug dose, flush the tubing with 30 mL of warm water, then clamp the tube. Resume the tube feeding when appropriate.
- Have the client remain in a high Fowler's or slightly elevated right-side-lying position to reduce the risk of aspiration.
- Document the medications given on the MAR, the amount of fluid given on the client's intake and output record, and the client's response.

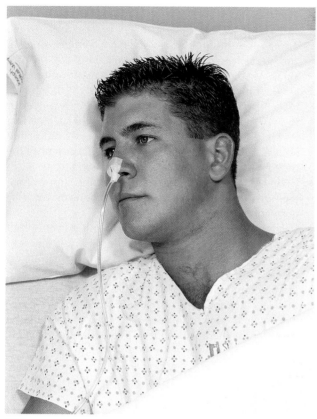

FIG. 9-13 The head of the bed should be elevated before administering medications through a nasogastric tube.

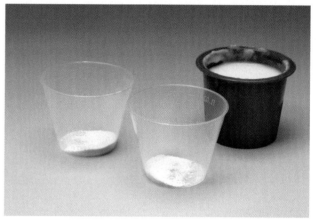

FIG. 9-14 Medications given through gastric tubes should be administered separately.

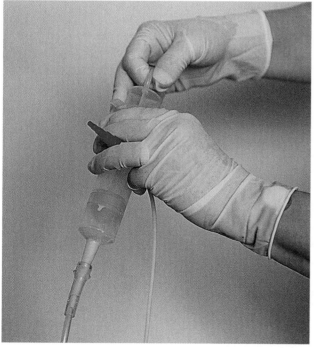

FIG. 9-15 Checking gastric residual before administering medications.

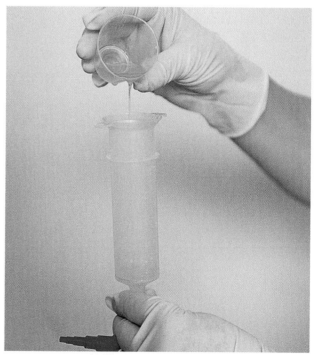

FIG. 9-16 Pour liquid medication into the syringe, then unclamp the tubing and allow it to flow in by gravity.

Rectal Administration

Always begin by washing your hands, and maintain Standard Precautions (see Box 9-1). Gloves should be worn for these procedures. When administering rectal drugs, keep in mind the following points:

- Assess the client for the presence of active rectal bleeding or diarrhea, which generally are contraindications for rectal suppositories.
- Suppositories should not be divided to provide a smaller dose. The active drug may not be evenly distributed within the suppository base.
- Position the client on his or her left side, unless contraindicated. The uppermost leg should be flexed toward the waist (Sims' position). Provide privacy and drape.
- The suppository should not be inserted into stool. Gently palpate the rectal wall for presence of feces. If possible, have the client defecate. DO NOT palpate the client's rectum if the client has had rectal surgery.
- Remove the wrapping from the suppository and lubricate the rounded tip with water-soluble jelly (Figure 9-17).

- Insert the tip of the suppository into the rectum while having the client take a deep breath and exhale through the mouth. With your gloved finger, quickly and gently insert the suppository into the rectum, alongside the rectal wall, at least 2.5 cm beyond the internal sphincter (Figure 9-18).
- Have the client remain lying on his or her left side for 15 to 20 minutes to allow absorption of the medication. With children it may be necessary to gently but firmly hold the buttocks in place for 5 to 10 minutes until the urge to expel the suppository has passed.
- If the client prefers to self-administer the suppository, the nurse should give specific instructions on the purpose and correct procedure.
- Use the same procedure for medications administered by a retention enema, such as sodium polystyrene sulfonate (see Chapter 26). Drugs given by enemas are diluted in the smallest amount of solution possible. If possible, retention enemas should be held for 30 minutes to 1 hour before expulsion.
- Document the medication on the MAR and monitor the client for the therapeutic effects of the rectal medication.

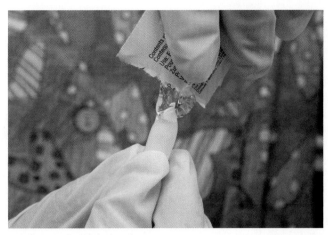

FIG. 9-17 Lubricate the suppository with a water-soluble lubricant.

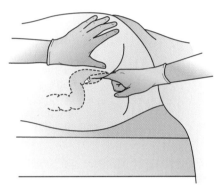

FIG. 9-18 Inserting a rectal suppository.

PARENTERAL DRUGS

Preparing for Parenteral Drug Administration

Figures 9-19 through 9-30 show equipment used for parenteral drugs.

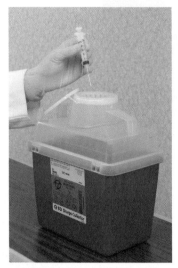

FIG. 9-19 NEVER RECAP A USED NEEDLE! Always dispose of *uncapped* needles in the appropriate sharps container. Refer to Box 9-1 for Standard Precautions.

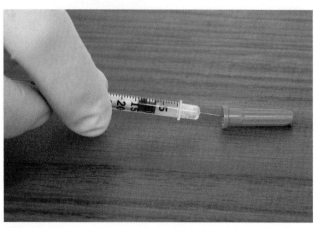

FIG. 9-20 An UNUSED needle may need to be recapped before the medication is given to the client. The "scoop method" is one way to recap an unused needle safely. Several devices are also available for recapping needles safely. Be sure not to touch the needle to the counter top or to the outside of the needle cap.

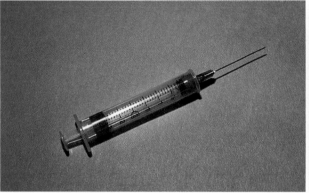

FIGS. 9-21 AND 9-22 There are several types of needle-stick prevention syringes. This example (Fig. 9-21) has a guard over the unused syringe. After the injection, the nurse pulls the guard up over the needle until it locks into place (Fig. 9-22).

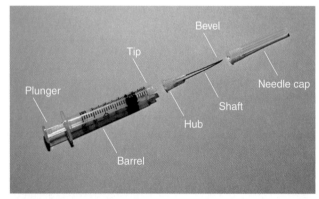

FIG. 9-23 The parts of a syringe and hypodermic needle.

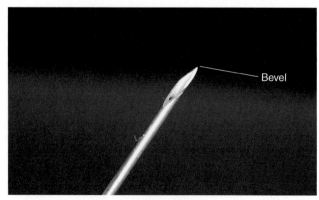

FIG. 9-24 Close-up view of the bevel of a needle.

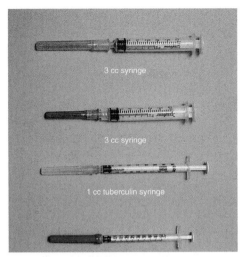

FIG. 9-25 Be sure to choose the correct size and type of syringe for the drug ordered.

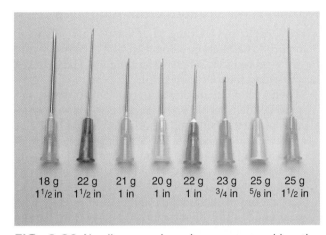

18 g   22 g   21 g   20 g   22 g   23 g   25 g   25 g
1¹/₂ in   1¹/₂ in   1 in   1 in   1 in   ³/₄ in   ⁵/₈ in   1¹/₂ in

FIG. 9-26 Needles come in various gauges and lengths. The larger the gauge, the smaller the needle. Be sure to choose the correct needle—gauge and length—for the type of injection ordered.

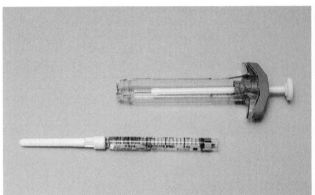

FIGS. 9-27 AND 9-28   Some medications come in a prefilled, sterile medication cartridges that fit into a syringe. Figures 9-27 and 9-28 show the Carpuject prefilled cartridge and syringe system. Follow the manufacturer's instructions for assembling prefilled syringes. After use, the syringe is disposed of in a sharps container.

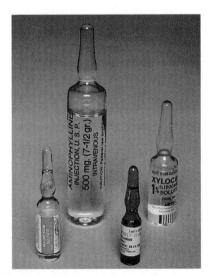

FIG. 9-29 Ampoules containing medications come in various sizes. These ampoules must be broken carefully to withdraw the medication.

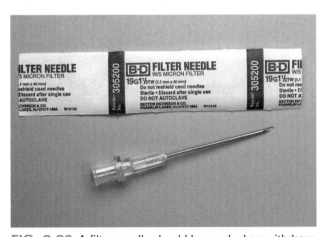

FIG. 9-30 A filter needle should be used when withdrawing medication from an ampoule. Filter needles help to remove minute glass particles that may result from the ampoule breakage. DO NOT USE A FILTER NEEDLE for injection into a client! Filter needles should be used to withdraw medications from a vial, too, if a needleless system is not used.

Removing Medications From Ampoules

Always begin by washing your hands, and maintain Standard Precautions (see Box 9-1). Gloves may be worn for these procedures. When performing these procedures, keep in mind the following points:

- When removing medication from an ampoule, use a sterile filter needle (see Figure 9-30). These needles are designed to filter out glass particles that may be present inside the ampoule after it is broken. The filter needle IS NOT intended for administering the drug to the client.
- Medication often rests in the top part of the ampoule. Tap the top of the ampoule lightly and quickly with your finger until all fluid moves to the bottom portion of the ampoule (Figure 9-31).
- Place a small gauze pad or dry alcohol swab around the neck of the ampoule. Snap the neck quickly and firmly (Figures 9-32 and 9-33).
- To draw up the medication, either set the open ampoule on a flat surface or hold the ampoule upside down. Insert a needle (attached to a syringe) into the centre of the ampoule opening. Do not allow the needle tip or shaft to touch the rim of the ampoule (Figure 9-34).
- Gently pull back on the plunger to draw up the medication. Keep the needle tip below the fluid within the vial; tip the ampoule to bring all of the fluid within reach of the needle.
- If air bubbles are aspirated do not expel them into the ampoule. Remove the needle from the ampoule, hold the syringe with the needle pointing up, and tap the side of the syringe with your finger to cause the bubbles to rise toward the needle. Draw back slightly on the plunger, and slowly push the plunger upward to eject the air. Do not eject fluid.
- Dispose of excess medication in the sink. Hold the syringe vertically with needle tip up and slanted toward the sink. Slowly eject the excess fluid into the sink, then recheck the fluid level by holding it vertically.
- Remove the filter needle and replace with the appropriate needle for administration.
- Dispose of the glass ampoule pieces and the used filter needle into the appropriate sharps container.

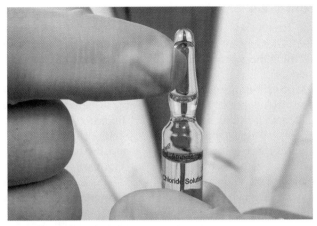

FIG. 9-31 Tapping the ampoule to move the fluid below the neck.

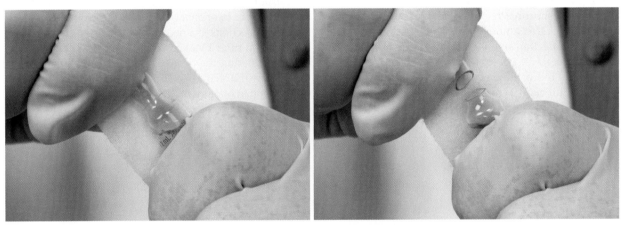

FIGS. 9-32 AND 9-33 Breaking an ampoule.

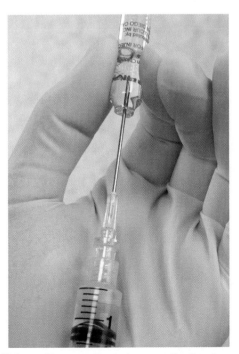

FIG. 9-34 Using a filter needle to draw medication from an ampoule.

Removing Medications From Vials

Always begin by washing your hands, and maintain Standard Precautions (see Box 9-1). Gloves may be worn for these procedures. When performing these procedures, keep in mind the following points:

- Vials can contain either a single dose or multiple doses of medications. Follow the institution's policy for using opened multi-dose vials. Many facilities require that vials be marked with the date and time of opening and that they be discarded within a specified time frame. If you are unsure about the age of an opened vial of medication, discard it and obtain a new one.
- Check institutional policies regarding which drugs should be prepared using a filter needle.
- If the vial is unused, remove the cap from the top of the vial.
- If the vial has been previously opened and used, wipe the top of the vial with an alcohol swab.
- Air must first be injected into a vial before fluid can be withdrawn. The amount of air injected into a vial should equal the amount of fluid that needs to be withdrawn.
- Determine the volume of fluid to be withdrawn from the vial. Pull back on the syringe's plunger to draw the amount of air into the syringe that is equivalent to the volume of medication to be removed from the vial. In-

sert the syringe, preferably using a needleless system. Figure 9-35 shows a needleless system of vial access. Inject the air into the vial.

- While holding onto the plunger, invert the vial and remove the desired amount of medication (Figure 9-36).
- Gently but firmly tap the syringe to remove air bubbles (Figure 9-37). Excess fluid, if present, should be discarded into a sink.
- Some vials are not compatible with needleless systems and therefore require a needle for fluid withdrawals (Figures 9-38 and 9-39).
- When an injection requires two medications from two different vials, begin by injecting air into the first vial (without touching the fluid in the first vial), then inject air into the second vial. Immediately remove the desired dose from the second vial. Change needles (if possible), then remove the exact prescribed dose of drug from the first vial. Take great care not to contaminate the drug in one vial with the drug from the other vial.
- For injections, if a needle has been used to remove medication from a vial, always change the needle before administering the dose. Changing needles ensures that a clean and sharp needle is used for the injection. Medication that remains on the outside of the needle may cause irritation to the client's tissues. In addition, the needle may become dull if used to puncture a rubber stopper.

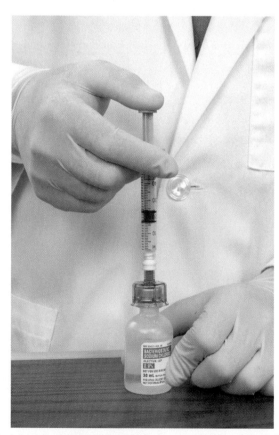

FIG. 9-35 Insert air into a vial before withdrawing medication (needleless system shown).

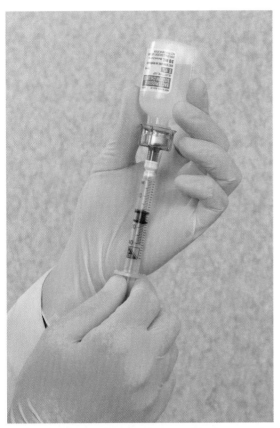

FIG. 9-36 Withdrawing medication from a vial (needleless system shown).

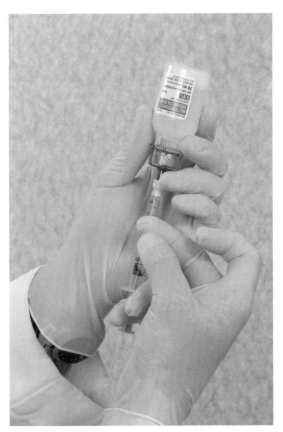

FIG. 9-37 Remove air from the syringe with gentle tapping.

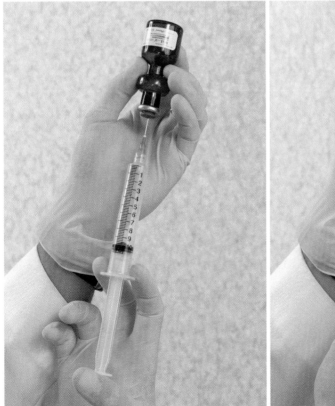

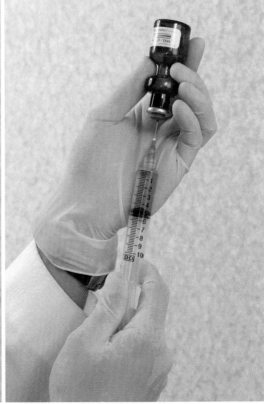

FIG. 9-38 AND 9-39 Using a needle and syringe to remove medication from a vial.

Injections Overview

Needle Insertion Angles for Intramuscular, Subcutaneous, and Intradermal Injections

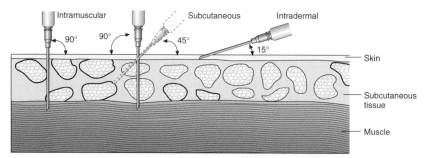

FIG. 9-40 Various needle angles.

- Intramuscular (IM) injections are inserted at a 90-degree angle (see Figure 9-40). Intramuscular injections deposit the drug deep into muscle tissue, where the drug is absorbed through blood vessels within the muscle. The rate of absorption with an intramuscular medication is slower than with the intravenous (IV) route but faster than the subcutaneous route. Intramuscular injections require a longer needle to reach the muscle tissue, but older clients, children, and adults who are malnourished may need shorter needles. In general, use a 21- to 25-gauge, 1½-inch needle.
- Subcutaneous (SC or SQ) injections are inserted at either a 90- or 45-degree angle. Subcutaneous injections deposit the drug into the loose connective tissue under the dermis. This tissue is not as well supplied with blood vessels as is the muscle tissue; as a result, drugs are absorbed more slowly than drugs given intramus-

cularly. In general, use a 25-gauge, ½- to ⅝-inch needle. A 90-degree angle is used for an average-sized client; a 45-degree angle may be used for thin, emaciated, and/or cachectic (weak) clients and for children. The following rule is sometimes used: If about 2.5 cm of tissue can be grasped, the needle is inserted at a 45-degree angle; if 5 cm can be grasped, the needle is inserted at a 90-degree angle.
- Intradermal (ID) injections are given into the outer layers of the dermis in small amounts, usually 0.01 to 0.1 mL. These injections are used mostly for diagnostic purposes, such as testing for allergies or tuberculosis, and for local anaesthesia. Little of the drug is absorbed systemically. In general, choose a tuberculin or 1-mL syringe with a 26- or 27-gauge needle that is ¼ to ½ inch long. The angle of injection is 5 to 15 degrees.

Z-Track Method

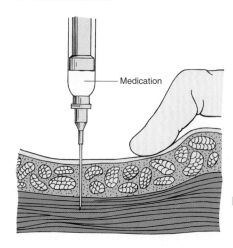

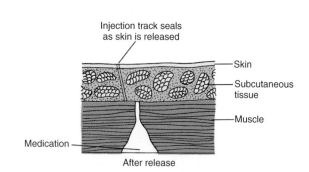

FIGS. 9-41 AND 9-42 The Z-track method for intramuscular injections.

- The Z-track method (Figures 9-41 and 9-42) is used for irritating substances such as iron dextran and hydroxyzine injections. The technique reduces pain, irritation, and staining at the injection site.
- After choosing and preparing the site for injection, pull the skin laterally down and hold in this position

while giving the injection. After injecting the medication, wait 10 seconds before withdrawing the needle.
- Release the skin immediately after withdrawing the needle in order to seal off the injection site. This technique forms a "z-track" in the tissue that prevents the medication from leaking through to the more sensitive subcutaneous tissue from the muscle site of injection.

Air-Lock Technique

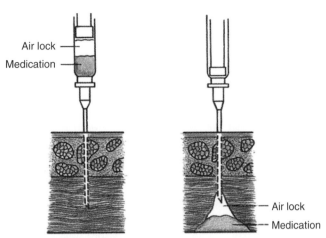

FIG. 9-43 Air-lock technique for intramuscular injections.

- Some facilities recommend administering intramuscular injections by the air-lock technique (Figure 9-43). Check institutional policies.
- After withdrawing the desired amount of medication into the syringe, withdraw an additional 0.2 mL of air. Be sure to inject using a 90-degree angle. The small air bubble that follows the medication during the injection may help prevent the medication from leaking through the needle track into the subcutaneous tissues.

Intradermal Injection

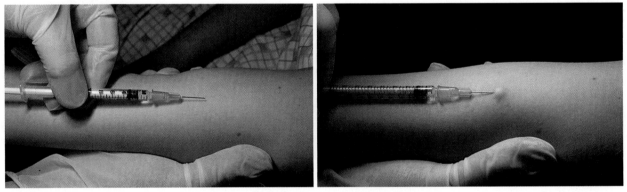

FIGS. 9-44 AND 9-45 Intradermal injection.

Always begin by washing your hands, and maintain Standard Precautions (see Box 9-1). Gloves should be worn for these procedures. When giving an intradermal injection, keep in mind the following points:

- Be sure to choose an appropriate site for the injection. Avoid areas of bruising, rashes, inflammation, edema, or skin discolorations.
- In general, the preferred location on the forearm is three to four finger-widths below the antecubital space and one hand-width above the wrist. If the forearm is not appropriate, areas on the back are suitable for subcutaneous injections.
- After cleansing the site with an alcohol swab and allowing it to dry, stretch the skin over the site with your non-dominant hand.
- With the needle almost against the client's skin, insert the needle, bevel UP, at a 5- to 15-degree angle (Figure 9-44) until resistance is felt, and then advance the needle through the epidermis, approximately 3 mm. The needle tip should still be visible under the skin.
- Do not aspirate. This area under the skin contains few blood vessels.
- Slowly inject the medication. It is normal to feel resistance, and a bleb that resembles a mosquito bite should form at the site (Figure 9-45).
- Withdraw the needle slowly while gently applying an alcohol swab or gauze at the site, but do not massage the site.
- Dispose of the syringe and needle in the appropriate container. DO NOT RECAP the needle. Wash your hands after removing gloves.
- Provide instructions to the client as needed for a follow-up visit for reading the skin testing.
- Document in the MAR the date of the skin testing and the date that results should be read, if applicable.

Subcutaneous Injections

Always begin by washing your hands, and maintain Standard Precautions (see Box 9-1). Gloves should be worn for these procedures. When giving a subcutaneous injection, keep in mind the following points:

- Be sure to choose an appropriate site for the injection. Avoid areas of bruising, rashes, inflammation, edema, or skin discolorations (Figure 9-46).
- Ensure that the needle size is correct. Grasp the skin fold between your thumb and forefinger and measure from top to bottom. The needle should be approximately half this length.
- Cleanse the site with an alcohol or antiseptic swab (Figure 9-47), and let the skin dry (occurs almost immediately).
- Tell the client that a "sting" or a "prick" will be felt as you insert the needle.
- For an average-sized client, pinch the skin with your non-dominant hand and inject the needle quickly at a 90-degree angle (Figure 9-48).
- For an obese client, pinch the skin and inject the needle at a 90-degree angle. Be sure the needle is long enough to reach the base of the skin fold.
- For a thin client or a child, pinch the skin gently, and then inject the needle at a 45-degree angle.
- Injections given in the abdomen should be given at least 5 cm away from the umbilicus owing to the surrounding vascular structure (Figure 9-49).
- After the needle enters the skin, grasp the lower end of the syringe with your non-dominant hand. Move your dominant hand to the end of the plunger—be careful not to move the syringe.
- Some institutions recommend aspirating the medication to check for blood return before giving a subcutaneous injection. Check institutional policy. Heparin injections and insulin injections are NOT aspirated before injection.

- With your dominant hand, slowly inject the medication.
- Withdraw the needle quickly and place a swab or sterile gauze pad over the site.
- Apply gentle pressure but do not massage the site. If necessary, apply a bandage to the site.
- Dispose of the syringe and needle in the appropriate container. DO NOT RECAP the needle. Wash your hands after removing gloves.
- Document the medication given on the MAR and monitor the client for a therapeutic response, as well as for adverse reactions.
- For heparin or other subcutaneous anticoagulant injections, follow manufacturers' recommendations for injection technique as needed. DO NOT ASPIRATE before injecting, and DO NOT massage the site after injection. These actions may cause a hematoma at the injection site.

Insulin Syringes

- Always use an insulin syringe to measure and administer insulin. When giving small doses of insulin, use a syringe that is calibrated for smaller doses. Figure 9-50 shows two different calibrations of insulin syringes. Note that in the 100-unit syringe, each line represents 2 units; in the 50-unit syringe, each line represents 1 unit. Note: A unit of insulin is NOT equivalent to 1 mL of insulin.
- Figure 9-51 shows several examples of devices that can be used to help the client self-administer insulin. These devices feature a multi-dose container of insulin and easy-to-read dials for choosing the correct dose. The needle is changed with each use.
- When drawing up two different types of insulin in the same syringe, always draw up the clear, rapid-acting insulin into the syringe first (Figure 9-52). See page 112 about mixing two medications in one syringe.

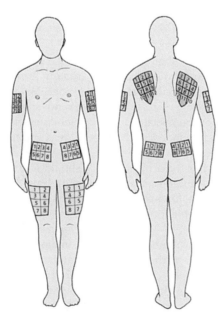

FIG. 9-46 Potential sites for subcutaneous injections.

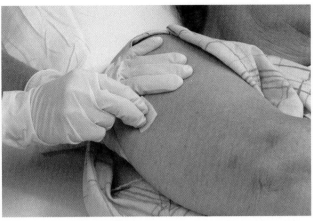

FIG. 9-47 Before giving an injection, cleanse the skin with an alcohol or antiseptic swab.

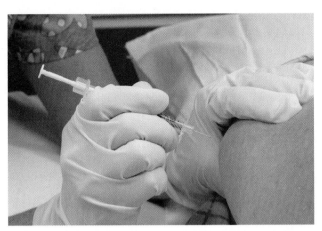

FIG. 9-48 Giving a subcutaneous injection at a 90-degree angle.

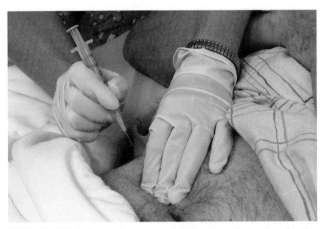

FIG. 9-49 When giving a subcutaneous injection in the abdomen, be sure to choose a site at least 5 cm away from the umbilicus.

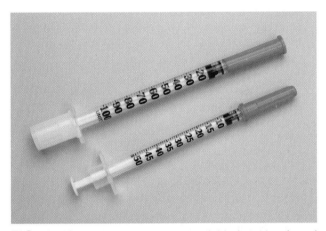

FIG. 9-50 Insulin syringes are available in 100-unit and 50-unit calibrations.

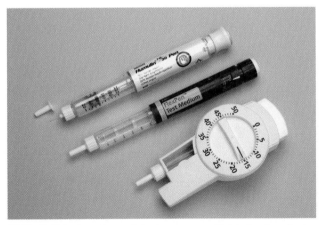

FIG. 9-51 A variety of devices are available for insulin injections.

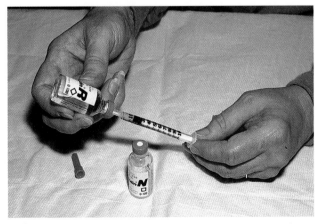

FIG. 9-52 Mixing two types of insulin in the same syringe.

Intramuscular Injections

Always begin by washing your hands, and maintain Standard Precautions (see Box 9-1). Gloves should be worn for these procedures. When giving an intramuscular injection, keep in mind the following points:

- Choose the appropriate site for the injection by assessing not only the size and integrity of the muscle but the amount and type of injection. Palpate potential sites for areas of hardness or tenderness, and note the presence of bruising or infection.
- Assist the client to the proper position and ensure his or her comfort.
- Locate the proper site for the injection and cleanse the site with an alcohol swab. Keep the swab or a sterile gauze pad nearby, and allow the alcohol to dry before injection.
- With your non-dominant hand, pull the skin taut. Follow the instructions for the Z-track method (see page 114) if appropriate.
- Hold the syringe with your dominant hand, as if holding a dart, and hold the needle at a 90-degree angle to the skin. Tell the client that a "sting" or "prick" will be felt as you insert the needle.
- Insert the needle quickly and firmly into the muscle. Hold the syringe and aspirate with one hand for at least 5 to 10 seconds.
- If no blood appears in the syringe, inject the medication slowly, at the rate of 1 mL every 10 seconds. After the drug is injected, wait 10 seconds, then withdraw the needle smoothly.
- Apply gentle pressure at the site and watch for bleeding. Apply a bandage if necessary.
- If blood does appear in the syringe, remove the needle, dispose of the medication and syringe, and prepare a new syringe with the medication.
- Dispose of the syringe and needle in the appropriate container. DO NOT RECAP the needle. Wash your hands after removing gloves.
- Document the medication given on the MAR and monitor the client for a therapeutic response, as well as for adverse reactions.

Ventrogluteal Site

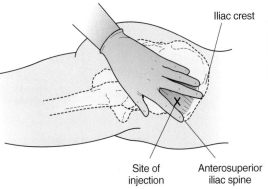

Iliac crest

Site of injection

Anterosuperior iliac spine

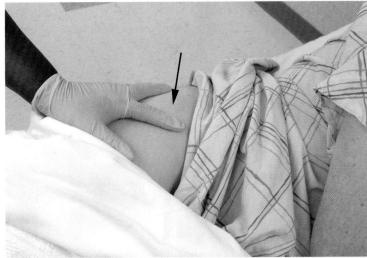

FIGS. 9-53, 9-54, AND 9-55
Ventrogluteal intramuscular injection.

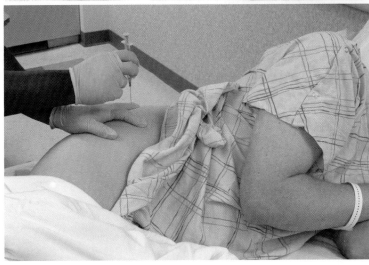

• The ventrogluteal site is the *preferred* site for adults and for children over age 18 months. Infants over age 7 months may also receive large volumes of immune globulin injections at this site; however, it is recommended to check the institutional policy for recommended sites and age guidelines. It is considered the safest of all the sites because the muscle is deep and away from major blood vessels and nerves (Figure 9-53).

• The client should be positioned on one side, with knees bent and upper leg slightly in front of the bottom leg. If necessary, the client may remain in a supine position.

• Palpate the greater trochanter at the head of the femur and the anterosuperior iliac spine. As illustrated in Figure 9-54, use the left hand to find landmarks when injecting into the client's right ventrogluteal, and use the right hand to find landmarks when injecting into the client's left ventrogluteal site. Place the palm of your hand over the greater trochanter and your index finger on the anterosuperior iliac spine. Point your thumb toward the client's groin and fingers toward the client's head. Spread the middle finger back along the iliac crest, toward the buttocks, as much as possible.

• The injection site is the centre of the triangle formed by your middle and index fingers (see arrow in Figure 9-54).

• Before giving the injection you may need to switch hands so that you can use your dominant hand to give the injection.

• In general, the total volume for an intramuscular injection is not to exceed 5 mL in adults of average weight. Volumes in excess of 5 mL should be administered in divided doses at different sites. The maximum volume for infants (birth to 1 year) is 0.5 mL; for children 1–2 years, 1 mL; for children 2–12 years, 2 mL. Check the institutional policy on age-related guidelines prior to administering intramuscular injections.

• Follow the general instructions for giving an intramuscular injection (Figure 9-55).

Vastus Lateralis Site

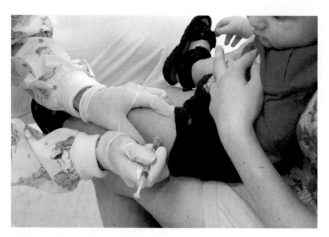

FIG. 9-56 Vastus lateralis intramuscular injection in an infant.

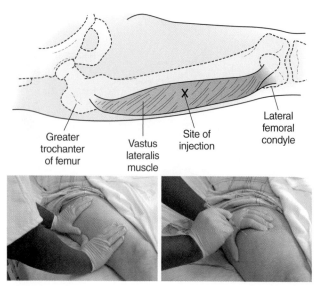

FIGS. 9-57, 9-58, AND 9-59 Vastus lateralis intramuscular injection.

- Generally this muscle is well developed and not located near major nerves or blood vessels. It is the preferred site of injection for infants under 18 months of age (Figure 9-56).
- The client may be sitting or lying supine; if supine, have the client bend the knee of the leg in which the injection will be given.

- To find the correct site of injection, place one hand above the knee and one hand below the greater trochanter of the femur. Locate the midline of the anterior thigh and the midline of the lateral side of the thigh. The injection site is located within the rectangular area (Figures 9-57, 9-58, and 9-59).

Dorsogluteal Site

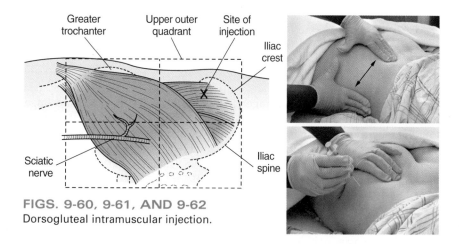

FIGS. 9-60, 9-61, AND 9-62 Dorsogluteal intramuscular injection.

- The dorsogluteal is not the preferred site for intramuscular injections because of the proximity of the sciatic nerve. It may be necessary to use this site, but extreme care should be taken when choosing the site for injection (Figure 9-60).
- Have the client lie on the abdomen with toes pointed in. Or, if preferred, the client may lie on one side with the upper leg bent and anterior to the lower leg.

- Palpate the greater trochanter of the femur and the posterosuperior iliac spine. Draw an imaginary line (Figure 9-61) between these landmarks.
- The injection should be given in the muscle above and outside this imaginary line (Figure 9-62).

Deltoid Site

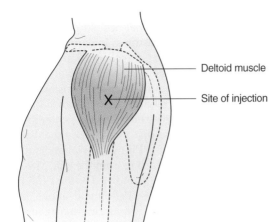

Deltoid muscle

Site of injection

FIGS. 9-63, 9-64, AND 9-65
Deltoid intramuscular injection.

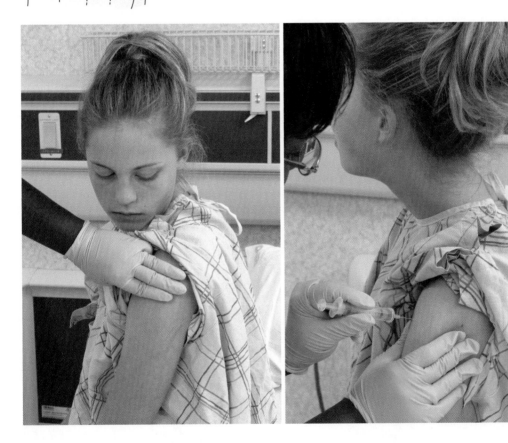

- The deltoid injection site is easily accessible but should only be used for small volumes of medication (0.5 to 1 mL). Assess the site carefully—this muscle may not be well developed in some adults (Figure 9-63). Always check medication administration policies because some facilities do not use deltoid intramuscular injections.
- The client may be sitting or lying down. Remove clothing to expose the upper arm and shoulder. Tight-fitting sleeves should not be rolled up. Have the client relax his or her arm and slightly bend the elbow.
- Palpate the lower edge of the acromion process. This edge becomes the base of an imaginary triangle (Figure 9-64).

- Place three fingers below this edge of the acromion process. Find the point on the lateral arm in line with the axilla. The injection site will be in the centre of this triangle, 3 finger-widths (3 to 5 cm) below the acromion process.
- In children and smaller adults it may be necessary to bunch the underlying tissue together before giving the injection and/or use a shorter (1-inch) needle (Figure 9-65).
- To reduce anxiety, have the client look away before giving the injection.

Preparing Intravenous Medications

Always begin by washing your hands, and maintain Standard Precautions (see Box 9-1). Gloves should be worn for most of these procedures. When administering intravenous drugs, keep in mind the following points:

- The intravenous route for medication administration provides for rapid onset and faster therapeutic drug levels in the blood than other routes. However, the intravenous route is also potentially more dangerous. Once an intravenous drug is given, it begins to act immediately and cannot be removed. The nurse must be aware of the drug's intended effects and possible side or adverse effects. In addition, hypersensitivity (allergic) reactions may occur quickly.

- Some institutions now use a needleless system for all infusion lines.

- Before giving an intravenous medication, assess the client's drug allergies, assess the intravenous line for patency, and assess the site for signs of phlebitis or infiltration.

- If more than one intravenous medication is to be given, check with the pharmacy for compatibility if medications are to be infused at the same time.

- Check the expiration date of both the medication and infusion bags.

- In many institutions, the pharmacy provides the intravenous piggyback (IVPB) admixtures for administration. If you are mixing the IVPB medications, be sure to verify the correct type of fluid and the correct amount of solution for the dosage.

- Most IVPB medications are provided with a system that allows the intravenous medication vial to be attached to a small-volume minibag for administration. Figure 9-66 shows two examples of IVPB medications attached to small-volume infusion bags.

- These IVPB medication setups allow for mixing of the drug and diluent immediately before the medication is given. If the seals are not broken and the medication is not mixed with the fluid in the infusion bag, then the medication stays in the vial! As a result, the client does not receive the ordered drug dose; instead, he or she receives a small amount of plain intravenous fluid.

- One type of IVPB that needs to be activated before administration is illustrated in Figure 9-67. To activate this type of IVPB, snap the connection area between the intravenous infusion bag and the vial (Figure 9-68). Gently squeeze the fluid from the infusion bag into the vial and allow the medication to dissolve (Figure 9-69). After a few minutes, rotate the vial gently to ensure that all of the powder is dissolved. When the drug is fully dissolved, hold the IVPB by the vial and squeeze the bag; fluid will enter the bag from the vial. Make sure that all of the medication is returned to the IVPB bag.

- When hanging these IVPB medications, take care NOT to squeeze the bag. Squeezing may cause some of the fluid to leak back into the vial and alter the dose given.

- Always label the IVPB bag with the client's name and room number, the name of the medication, the dose, the date and time mixed, your initials, and the date and time it was given.

- Some intravenous medications must be mixed using a needle and syringe. After checking the order, and the compatibility of the drug and the intravenous fluid, wipe the port of the intravenous bag with an alcohol swab (Figure 9-70).

- Carefully insert the needle into the centre of the port and inject the medication (Figures 9-71 and 9-72). Note how the medication remains in the lower part of the intravenous infusion bag. To infuse an even concentration of medication, gently shake the bag after injecting the drug (Figure 9-73).

- Always label the intravenous infusion bag when a drug has been added (Figure 9-74). Label as per institution policy and include the client's name and room number, the name of the medication, the date and time mixed, your initials, and the date and time the infusion was started. In addition, label all intravenous infusion tubing per institution policy.

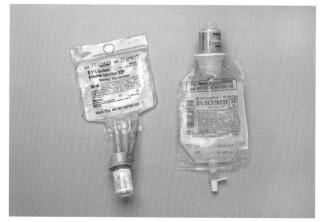

FIG. 9-66 Two types of IVPB medication delivery systems. IVPB medications must be activated before administration to the client.

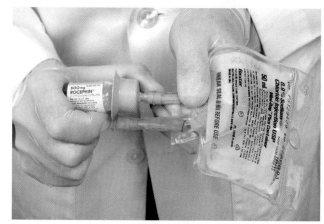

FIG. 9-67 Activating an IVPB infusion bag *(step 1)*.

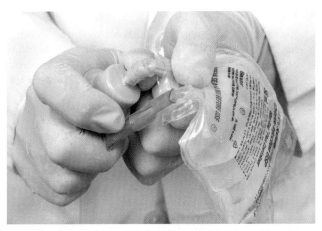

FIG. 9-68 Activating an IVPB infusion bag *(step 2)*.

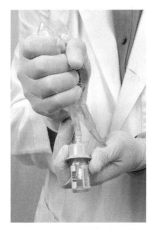

FIG. 9-69 Activating an IVPB infusion bag *(step 3)*.

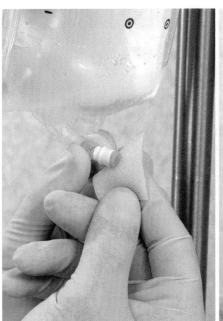
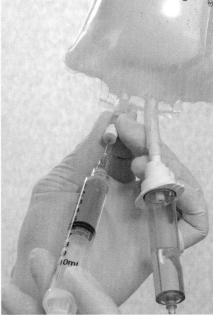
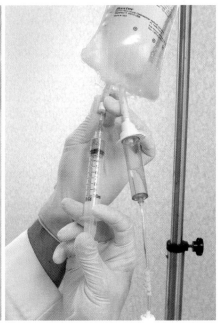

FIGS. 9-70, 9-71, AND 9-72 Adding a medication to an intravenous infusion bag with a needle and syringe.

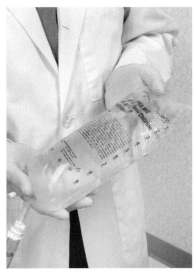

FIG. 9-73 Mix the medication thoroughly before infusing.

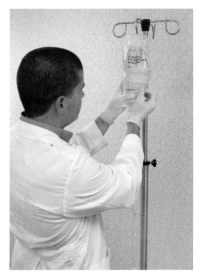

FIG. 9-74 Label the intravenous infusion bag when medication has been added.

Infusions of Intravenous Piggyback Medications

Always begin by washing your hands, and maintain Standard Precautions (see Box 9-1). Gloves should be worn for these procedures.

- Figure 9-75 shows an IVPB medication infusion with a primary gravity infusion. When the IVPB bag is hung higher than the primary intravenous infusion bag, the IVPB medication will infuse until empty, then the primary infusion will take over again.

- When beginning the infusion, attach the IVPB tubing to the upper port on the primary intravenous tubing. A backcheck valve above this port prevents the medication from infusing up into the primary intravenous infusion bag.

- Fully open the clamp of the IVPB tubing and regulate the infusion rate with the roller clamp of the primary infusion tubing. Be sure to note the drip factor of the tubing and calculate the drops per minute to count to set the correct infusion rate for the IVPB.

- Monitor the client during the infusion. Observe for hypersensitivity and for adverse reactions. In addition, observe the intravenous infusion site for infiltration. Have the client report if pain or burning occurs.

- Monitor the rate of infusion during the IVPB administration. Changes in arm position may alter the infusion rate.

- When the infusion is complete, clamp the IVPB tubing and check the primary intravenous infusion rate. If necessary, adjust the clamp to the correct infusion rate.

- Figure 9-76 shows an IVPB medication infusion with a primary infusion that is going through an electronic infusion pump.

- When giving IVPB drugs through an intravenous infusion on a pump, attach the IVPB tubing to the port on the primary intravenous tubing *above* the pump. Open the roller clamp of the IVPB bag. Make sure that the IVPB bag is higher than the primary intravenous infusion bag.

- Following the manufacturer's directions, set the infusion pump to deliver the IVPB medication. Entering the volume of the IVPB bag and the desired time frame of the infusion (such as over 60 minutes) will cause the pump to automatically calculate the IVPB rate. Start the IVPB infusion as instructed by the pump.

- Monitor the client during the infusion, as described earlier.

- When the infusion is complete, the primary intravenous infusion will automatically resume.

- Be sure to document the medication given on the MAR and continue to monitor the client for adverse reactions and therapeutic effects.

- When giving IVPB medications through a saline (heparin) lock, follow the facility's guidelines for flushing protocol before and after the medication is administered.

- Figure 9-77 illustrates a volume-controlled administration set for intravenous medications. The chamber is attached to the infusion between the intravenous infusion bag and the intravenous tubing. Fill the chamber with the desired amount of fluid, and then add the medication via the port above the chamber, as shown in the photo. Be sure to swab the port with an alcohol swab before inserting the needle in the port. Label the chamber with the medication's name, dosage, and time added and your initials. Infuse the drug at the prescribed rate.

- Patient-controlled analgesia (PCA) uses a specialized pump to allow clients to self-administer pain medications, usually opiates (Figure 9-78). These pumps allow the client to self-administer only as much medication as needed to control the pain by pushing a button for intravenous bolus doses. Safety features of the pump prevent accidental overdoses. A client on PCA pump infusions should be monitored closely for his or her response to the drug, excessive sedation, hypotension, and changes in mental and respiratory status. Follow the facility's guidelines for setup and use.

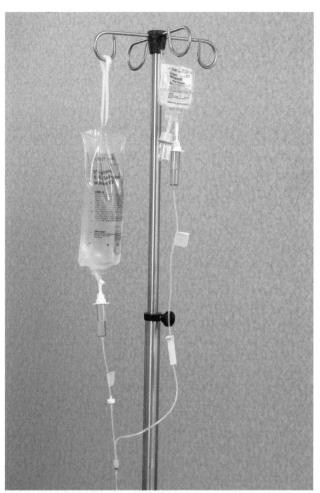

FIG. 9-75 Infusing an IVPB medication with a gravity primary intravenous infusion.

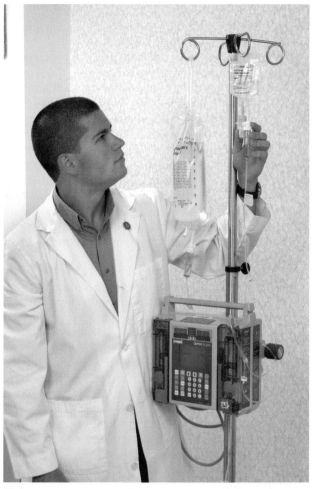

FIG. 9-76 Infusing an IVPB medication with the primary intravenous infusion on an electronic infusion pump.

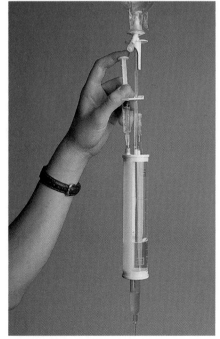

FIG. 9-77 The nurse adds a medication to a volume-controlled administration set.

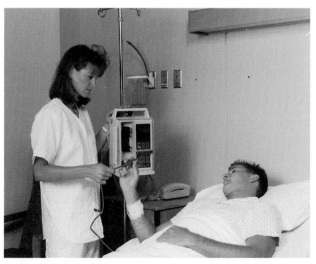

FIG. 9-78 The nurse instructs the client on the use of a patient-controlled analgesia (PCA) pump.

IV Push Medications

Always begin by washing your hands, and maintain Standard Precautions (see Box 9-1).

When administering intravenous push (or bolus) medications, keep in mind the following points:

- Usually the only members of the nursing staff who can give IV push medications are registered nurses, and they may do so only under specified conditions.
- Intravenous push injections allow for rapid intravenous administration of a drug. The term *bolus* refers to a dose given all at once. Intravenous push injections may be given through an existing intravenous line, through an intravenous (saline or heparin) lock, or directly into a vein.
- Because the medication may have an immediate effect, monitor the client closely for adverse reactions, as well as for therapeutic effects.
- Follow the manufacturer's guidelines carefully when preparing an intravenous push medication. Some drugs require careful dilution. Consult a pharmacist if unsure about dilution procedure. Improper dilution may cause an increased risk of phlebitis and other complications.
- Most drugs given by intravenous push injection should be given over a period of 1 to 5 minutes to reduce local or systemic side effects. Always time the dosage with your watch because it is difficult to estimate the time accurately. However, adenosine (Adenocard) must be given rapidly, within 2 to 3 seconds, for optimal action.

Intravenous Push Medications Through an Intravenous Lock

- Prepare two syringes of 0.9 percent normal saline (NS); one should contain 3 mL and the other 5 mL. Prepare medication for injection. (Facilities may differ in protocol for intravenous lock flushes—follow institutional policies.)
- Follow the guidelines for a needleless system, if used.
- Cleanse the injection port of the intravenous lock with an antiseptic swab after removing the cap, if present (Figure 9-79).
- Insert the syringe of 3 mL NS to the injection port (needleless system shown) (Figure 9-80). Open the clamp of the intravenous lock tubing, if present.

- Gently aspirate and observe for blood return. Absence of blood return does not mean that the intravenous line is occluded; further assessment may be required.
- Flush gently with saline while assessing for resistance. If resistance is felt, do not apply force. Stop and reassess the intravenous lock.
- Observe for signs of infiltration while injecting saline.
- Reclamp the tubing (if clamp present) and remove the NS syringe. Repeat cleansing of the port and attach the medication syringe. Open clamp again.
- Inject the medication over the prescribed length of time. Measure time with a watch or clock (Figure 9-81).
- When the medication is infused, clamp the intravenous lock tubing (if present) and remove the syringe.
- Repeat cleansing of the port; attach a 5-mL NS syringe and inject it into the intravenous lock slowly.

Intravenous Push Medications Through an Existing Infusion

- Prepare the medication for injection. Follow the guidelines for a needleless system, if used.
- Check compatibility of the intravenous medication with the existing intravenous solution.
- Choose the injection port that is closest to the client.
- Remove the cap, if present, and cleanse the injection port with an antiseptic swab.
- Occlude the intravenous line by pinching the tubing just above the injection port (Figure 9-82). Attach the syringe to the injection port.
- Gently aspirate for blood return.
- While keeping the intravenous tubing clamped, slowly inject the medication according to administration guidelines. Be sure to time the injection with a watch or clock.
- After the injection, release the intravenous tubing, remove the syringe, and check the infusion rate of the intravenous fluid.

After Injecting an Intravenous Push Medication

- Monitor the client closely for adverse effects. Monitor the intravenous infusion site for signs of phlebitis and infiltration.
- Document medication given on the MAR and monitor for therapeutic effects.

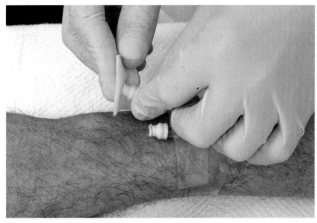

FIG. 9-79 Cleanse the port before attaching the syringe.

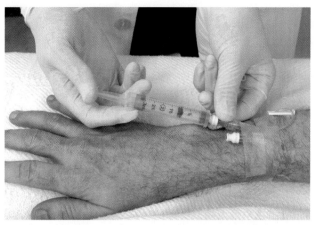

FIG. 9-80 Attaching the syringe to the intravenous lock.

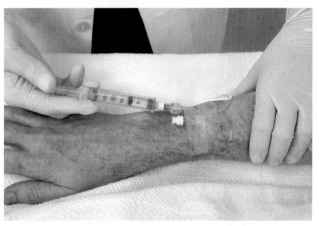

FIG. 9-81 Slowly inject the intravenous push medication through the intravenous lock; use a watch to time the injection.

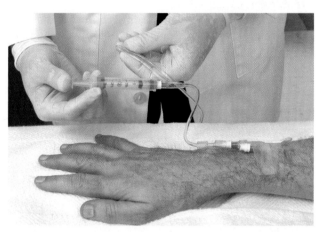

FIG. 9-82 When giving an intravenous push medication through an intravenous line, pinch the tubing just above the injection port.

TOPICAL DRUGS

Administering Optic or Eye Medications

Always begin by washing your hands, and maintain Standard Precautions (see Box 9-1). Gloves should be worn for these procedures. When administering eye preparations, keep in mind the following points:

- Assist the client to a supine or sitting position. The head should be tilted back slightly.
- Remove contact lenses.
- Remove any secretions or drainage with a sterile gauze pad; be sure to wipe from the inner to outer canthus.
- Have the client look up and, with your non-dominant hand, gently pull the lower lid open to expose the conjunctival sac.

Eye Drops

- With your dominant hand resting on the client's forehead, hold the eye medication dropper 1 to 2 cm above the conjunctival sac. Do not touch the tip of the dropper to the eye or with your fingers (Figure 9-83).
- Drop the prescribed number of drops into the conjunctival sac. Never apply eye drops to the cornea.
- If the drops land on the outer lid margins (if the client moved or blinked), repeat the procedure.

Eye Ointment

- Gently squeeze the tube of medication to apply an even strip (about 1 to 2 cm) of medication along the border of the conjunctival sac. Start at the inner canthus and move toward the outer canthus (Fig. 9-84).

After Instilling Eye Medications

- Ask the client to close the eye gently. Squeezing the eye shut may force the medication out of the conjunctival sac. A tissue may be used to blot liquid that runs out of the eye, but the client should be instructed not to wipe the eye.
- You may apply gentle pressure to the client's nasolacrimal duct for 30 to 60 seconds with a gloved finger, wrapped in a tissue. This will help to reduce systemic absorption of the drug through the nasolacrimal duct and may also help to reduce the taste of the medication in the nasopharynx (Figure 9-85).
- Assist the client to a comfortable position.
- Document the medication given on the MAR and check the client for a therapeutic response.

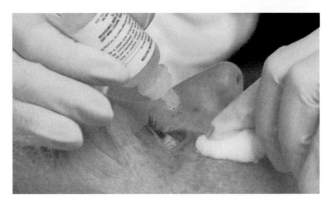

FIG. 9-83 Insert the eye drop into the lower conjunctival sac.

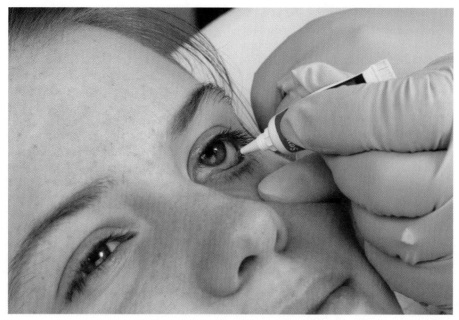

FIG. 9-84 Applying eye ointment.

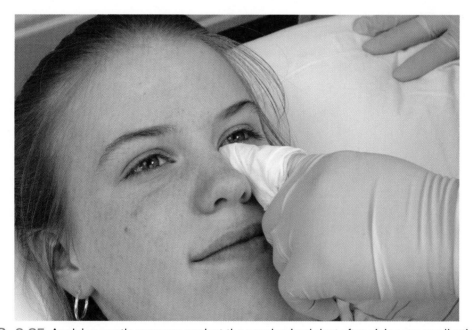

FIG. 9-85 Applying gentle pressure against the nasolacrimal duct after giving eye medications.

Administering Otic or Ear Drops

Always begin by washing your hands, and maintain Standard Precautions (see Box 9-1). Gloves may be worn for these procedures. When administering ear preparations, keep in mind the following points:

- After explaining the procedure to the client, assist the client to a side-lying position with the affected ear facing up. If cerumen (earwax) or drainage is noted in the outer ear canal, remove it carefully without pushing it back into the ear canal.
- Remove excessive amounts of cerumen before instilling medication.
- If refrigerated, the ear medication should be warmed by taking it out of refrigeration for at least 30 minutes before administration. Instillation of cold eardrops can cause nausea, dizziness, and pain.
- For an adult (Figure 9-86) or a child over 3 years of age, the auricle should be pulled upward and outward.
- For an infant or a child under age 3 years of age, the auricle should be pulled down and back (Figure 9-87).
- Administer the prescribed number of drops. Direct the drops along the sides of the ear canal rather than directly onto the eardrum.

- Instruct the client to lie on one side for 5 to 10 minutes. Gently massaging the tragus of the ear with your finger will help to distribute the medication down the ear canal.
- If ordered, a loose cotton pledget, or flat absorbent pad, can be gently inserted into the ear canal to prevent the medication from flowing out. The cotton should still be loose enough to allow any discharge to drain out of the ear canal. To prevent the dry cotton from absorbing the ear drops that were instilled, moisten the cotton with a small amount of medication before inserting the pledget. Cotton that is inserted too deeply may result in increased pressure within the ear canal and on the eardrum.
- Remove the cotton after about 15 minutes.
- If medication is needed in the other ear, wait 5 to 10 minutes after instillation of the first ear drops.
- Document the medication given on the MAR and observe the client for a therapeutic response.

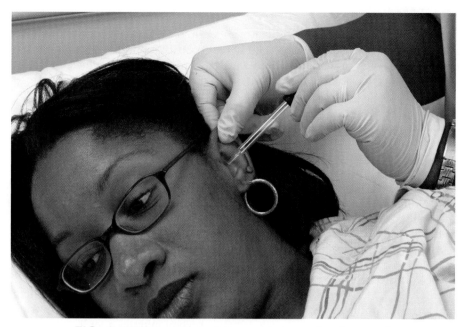

FIG. 9-86 For adults, pull the auricle upward and outward.

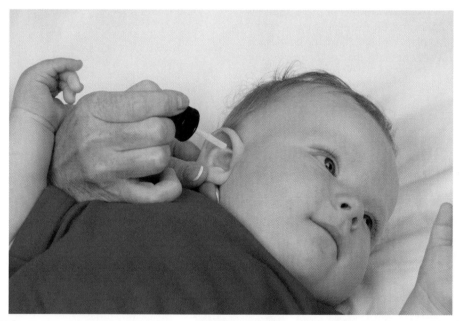

FIG. 9-87 For infants and children under 3 years of age, pull the auricle down and back.

Administering Nasal Medications

Always begin by washing your hands, and maintain Standard Precautions (see Box 9-1). Clients may self-administer some of these drugs, after proper instruction. The nurse should wear gloves for these procedures. When administering nasal medications, keep in mind the following points:

- Before giving nasal medications, explain the procedure to the client and tell him or her that temporary burning or stinging may occur. Instruct the client that it is important to clear the nasal passages by blowing his or her nose, unless contraindicated (increased intracranial pressure [ICP] or nasal surgery), before administering the medication.
- Figure 9-88 illustrates various administration forms of nasal medications: sprays, drops, and dose-measured sprays.
- Position the client in a supine position. Support the client's head as needed.
- If specific areas are targeted for the medication, position as follows:
  - For the posterior pharynx, position the head backward.
  - For the ethmoid or sphenoid sinuses, place the head gently over the top edge of the bed or place a pillow under the shoulders and tilt the head back.
  - For frontal or maxillary sinuses, place the head back and turned toward the side that is to receive the medication.

Nasal Drops

- Hold the nose dropper approximately 1 cm above the nostril. Administer the prescribed number of drops toward the midline of the ethmoid bone (Figure 9-89).
- Repeat the procedure as ordered according to the number of drops per nostril.
- Keep the client in a supine position for 5 minutes.

Nasal Spray

- The client should be sitting upright, with one nostril occluded. After gently shaking the nasal spray container, insert the tip into the nostril. As the client inhales through the open nostril, squeeze the spray bottle into the nostril at the same time (Figure 9-90).
- Repeat the procedure as ordered according to the number of sprays per nostril.

After Administration of Nasal Medicines

- Offer the client tissues for blotting any drainage, but instruct the client to avoid blowing his or her nose for several minutes after instillation of the drops.
- Assist the client to a comfortable position.
- Document the medication administration on the MAR and document drainage, if any. Monitor for adverse reactions and a therapeutic response.

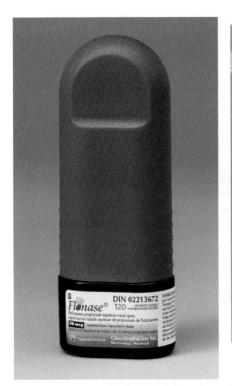
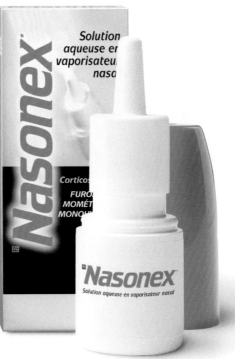

FIG. 9-88 Nasal medications may come in various delivery forms.

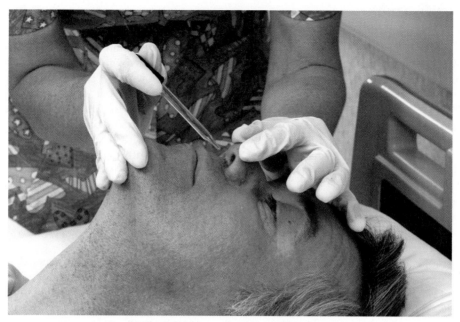

FIG. 9-89 Administering nose drops.

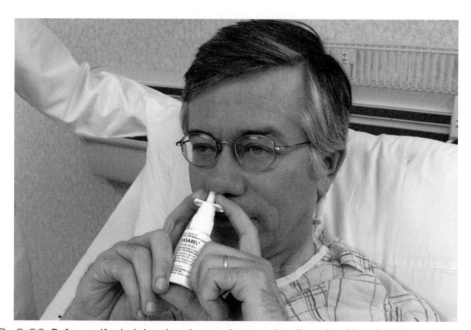

FIG. 9-90 Before self-administering the nasal spray, the client should occlude the other nostril.

Administering Inhaled Drugs

Always begin by washing your hands, and maintain Standard Precautions (see Box 9-1). Gloves may be worn for these procedures. When administering inhaled preparations, keep in mind the following points:

Metered-Dose Inhalers

- There are a variety of metered-dose inhalers (MDIs) available (Figure 9-91). Be sure to check for specific instructions from the manufacturer as needed. Improper use will result in inadequate dosing.
- Shake the MDI gently before using.
- Remove the cap; hold the inhaler upright, and grasp with the thumb and first two fingers.
- Tilt the head back slightly.
- If using the MDI without a spacer:
  1 Have the client open his or her mouth; position the inhaler 3 to 5 cm away from the mouth (Figure 9-92).
  2 Have the client exhale, then press down once on the inhaler to release the medication; have the client breathe in slowly and deeply for 2 to 3 seconds.
  3 Have the client hold his or her breath for approximately 10 seconds, then exhale slowly through pursed lips.
- If using the MDI with a spacer:
  1 Attach the spacer to the mouthpiece of the inhaler after removing the inhaler's cap (Figures 9-93 and 9-94).

  2 Place the mouthpiece of the spacer in the client's mouth.
  3 Have the client exhale.
  4 Press down on the inhaler to release the medication, and have the client inhale deeply and slowly through the spacer. The client should breathe in and out slowly for 2 to 3 seconds, then hold his or her breath for 10 seconds (Figure 9-95).
- If a repeat puff is ordered, wait at least 20 to 30 seconds between puffs.
- If a second type of inhaled medication is ordered, wait 5 to 10 minutes between inhalations, or as prescribed.
- If both a bronchodilator and a steroid inhaled medication are ordered, the bronchodilator should be administered first to allow the passages to be more open for the second medication.
- The client should be instructed to rinse his or her mouth with water after inhaling a steroid medication to prevent the development of an oral fungal infection.
- Document the medication given on the MAR and monitor the client for a therapeutic response, as well as for adverse reactions.
- Teach the client to measure the amount of medication remaining in the MDI canister by immersing it in a large bowl of water. The position of the canister in the water indicates the amount of medication remaining (Figure 9-96).

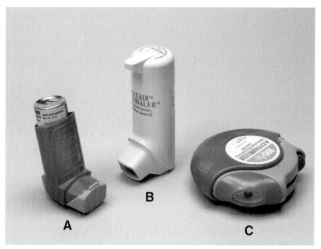

FIG. 9-91 **A,** Metered-dose inhaler (MDI). **B,** Automated MDI. **C,** "Disk-type" MDI that delivers powdered medication.

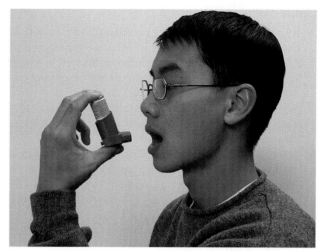

FIG. 9-92 Using an MDI without a spacer.

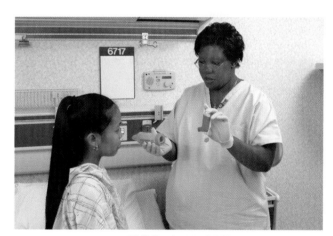

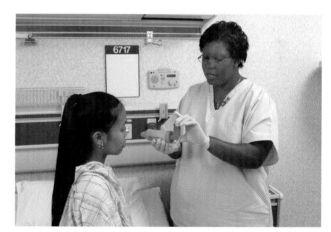

FIGS. 9-93 AND 9-94 Instructing the client on how to use a spacer device.

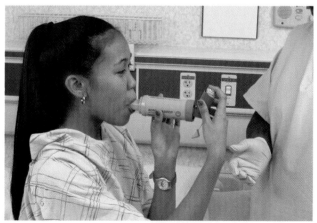

FIG. 9-95 Using a spacer device with an MDI.

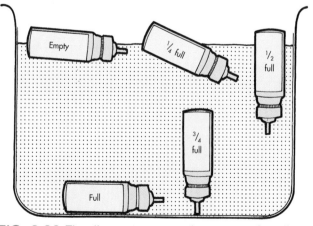

FIG. 9-96 The client can measure the amount of medication remaining in the inhaler canister by immersion in water.

Small-Volume Nebulizers

- In some facilities, the air compressor is located in the wall unit of the room. In other facilities, and at home, a small, portable air compressor will be used. Be sure to follow the manufacturer's recommendations for use.
- Be sure to take the client's baseline heart rate, especially if a beta-adrenergic agent is used. Some drugs may increase the heart rate.
- After gathering the equipment, add the prescribed medication to the nebulizer cup (Figure 9-97). Some medications will require a diluent; others are premixed with a diluent. Be sure to verify before adding a diluent.
- Have the client hold the mouthpiece between his or her lips (Figure 9-98).
- Before starting the nebulizer treatment, the client should take a slow deep breath, hold it briefly, then exhale slowly. Clients who are short of breath should be instructed to hold their breath every fourth or fifth breath.
- Turn on the small-volume nebulizer machine (or turn on the wall unit), and make sure that a sufficient mist is forming.

- Instruct the client to repeat the breathing pattern mentioned previously during the treatment.
- Occasionally tap the nebulizer cup during the treatment and toward the end to move the fluid droplets back to the bottom of the cup.
- Monitor the client's heart rate during and after the treatment.
- If inhaled steroids are given, instruct the client to rinse his or her mouth afterward.
- After the procedure, clean and store the tubing per institutional policy.
- Document the medication given on the MAR and monitor the client for a therapeutic response, as well as for adverse reactions.
- If the client will be using a nebulizer at home, instruct the client to rinse the nebulizer parts after each use with warm, clear water and to air dry. The parts should be washed daily with warm, soapy water and allowed to air dry. Once a week, the nebulizer parts should be soaked in a solution of vinegar and water (four parts water and one part white vinegar) for 30 minutes; rinsed thoroughly with clear, warm water; and air dried. Storing nebulizer parts that are still wet will encourage bacterial and mould growth.

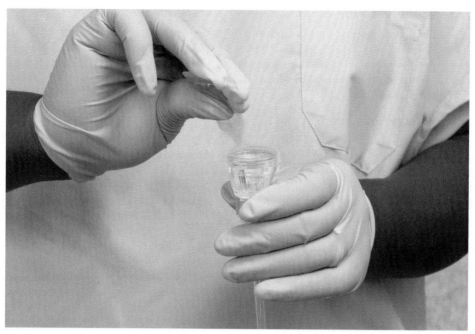

FIG. 9-97 Adding medication to the nebulizer cup.

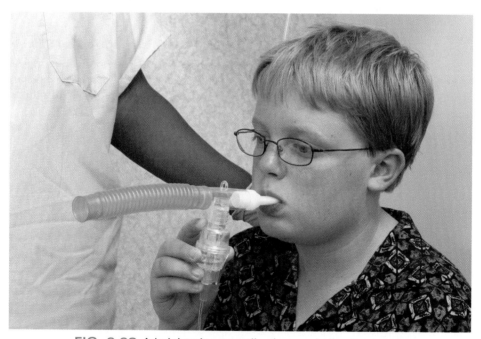

FIG. 9-98 Administering a small-volume nebulizer treatment.

Administering Medications to the Skin

Always begin by washing your hands, and maintain Standard Precautions (see Box 9-1). Gloves should be worn for these procedures. Avoid touching the preparations to your own skin. When administering skin preparations, keep in mind the following points:

Lotions, Creams, Ointments, Powders

- Apply powder to clean, dry skin. Have the client turn his or her head to the other side during application to avoid inhalation of powder particles.
- Apply lotion to clean, dry skin. Remove residue from previous applications with soap and water, if appropriate for the client's condition, and dry the area thoroughly. Also, rotate application sites.
- With lotion, cream, or gel, obtain the correct amount with your gloved hand (Figure 9-99). If the medication is in a jar, remove the dose with a sterile tongue depressor and apply to your gloved hand. Do not contaminate the medication in the jar.
- Apply the preparation with long, smooth, gentle strokes. Avoid excessive pressure (Figure 9-100).
- Some ointments and creams may soil the client's clothes and linens. If ordered, cover the site with gauze over the affected area.
- Nitroglycerin ointment is measured carefully before application (Figure 9-101). Do not massage nitroglycerin ointment into the skin. Apply the measured amount onto a clean, dry site and then secure with plastic wrap and tape. Always remove the old medication before applying a new dose.

Transdermal Patches

- Be sure that the old patch is removed as ordered. Some patches may be removed before the next patch is due—check the order. Cleanse the site of the old patch thoroughly. Observe for signs of skin irritation at the old patch site.
- Give transdermal patches at the same time each day.
- The old patch can be pressed together, then wrapped in a glove as you remove the glove from your hand. Dispose in the proper container according to the facility's policy.
- Select a new site for application and ensure that it is clean and without powder or lotion. The site should be hairless and free from scars, scratches, or irritation. If it is necessary to remove hair, clip the hair instead of shaving to reduce irritation to the skin.
- Remove the backing from the new patch (Figure 9-102). Take care not to touch the medication side of the patch with your fingers.
- Place the patch on the skin site and press firmly (Figure 9-103). Press around the edges of the patch with one or two fingers to ensure that the patch is adequately secured to the skin. Rotate sites of application with each dose.
- Label the patch with the date and time of application.

After Administering Topical Skin Preparations

- Chart the medication given on the MAR and monitor the client for a therapeutic response.
- Provide instruction on self-administration as needed.

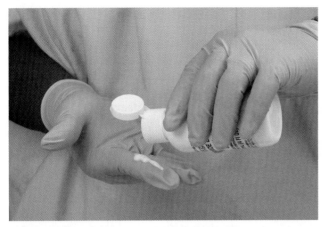

FIG. 9-99 Use gloves to apply topical skin preparations.

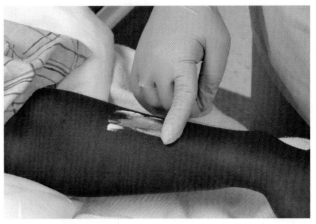

FIG. 9-100 Spread the lotion on the skin with long, smooth, gentle strokes.

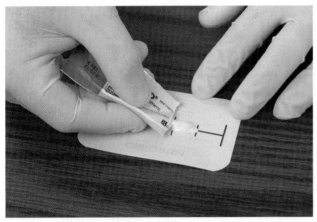

FIG. 9-101 Nitroglycerin ointment is carefully measured before application.

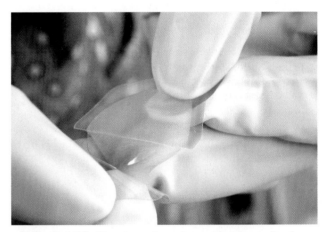

FIG. 9-102 Opening a transdermal patch medication.

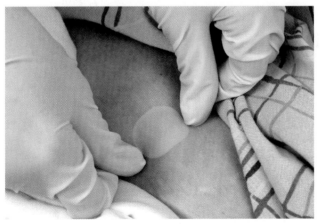

FIG. 9-103 Ensure that the edges of the transdermal patch are secure after applying.

Administering Vaginal Medications

Always begin by washing your hands, and maintain Standard Precautions (see Box 9-1). Gloves should be worn for these procedures. When administering vaginal preparations, keep in mind the following points:

- Vaginal suppositories are larger and more oval than rectal suppositories (Figure 9-104).
- Figure 9-105 shows examples of a vaginal suppository in its applicator and vaginal cream in an applicator.
- Before giving these medications explain the procedure to the client and have her void.
- If possible, administer vaginal preparations at bedtime to allow the medications to remain in place as long as possible.
- Some clients may prefer to self-administer vaginal medications. Provide specific instructions if necessary.
- Position the client in the lithotomy position and elevate the hips with a pillow, if tolerated. Be sure to drape the client to provide privacy.

Creams, Foams, or Gels Applied with an Applicator

- Fit the applicator to the tube of the medication and then gently squeeze the tube to fill the applicator with the correct amount of medication.

- Lubricate the tip of the applicator with water-soluble lubricant.
- Use your non-dominant hand to spread the labia and expose the vagina. Gently insert the applicator as far as possible into the vagina (Figure 9-106).
- Push the plunger to deposit the medication. Remove the applicator and wrap it in a paper towel for cleaning.

Suppositories

- For suppositories, remove the wrapping and lubricate the suppository with a water-soluble lubricant. Be sure that the suppository is at room temperature.
- Using the applicator, insert the suppository into the vagina, then push the plunger to deposit the suppository.
- If no applicator is available, use your dominant index finger to insert the suppository about 5 cm into the vagina (Figure 9-107).
- Have the client remain in a supine position with hips elevated for 5 to 10 minutes to allow the suppository to melt and the medication to spread.
- If the client desires, apply a perineal pad.
- If the applicator is to be reused, wash with soap and water and store in a clean container for the next use.
- Document the medication given and the client's response on the MAR. Monitor for a therapeutic response.

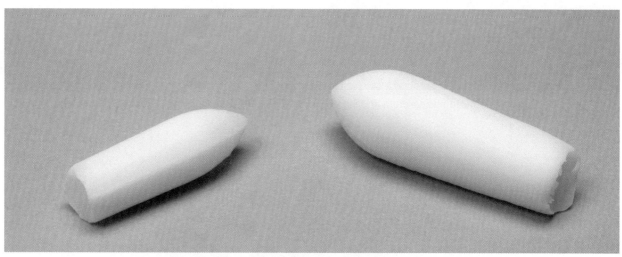

FIG. 9-104 Vaginal suppositories *(right)* are larger and more oval than rectal suppositories *(left)*.

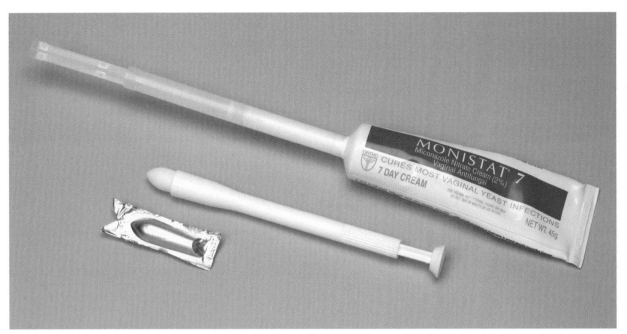

FIG. 9-105 Vaginal cream and suppository, with applicators.

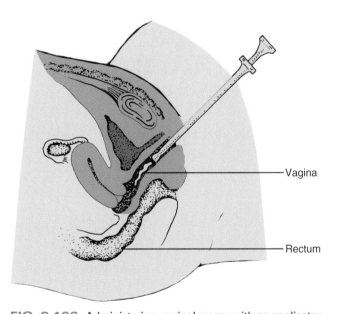

FIG. 9-106 Administering vaginal cream with an applicator.

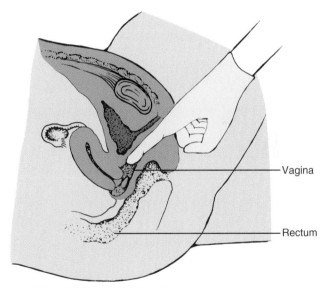

FIG. 9-107 Administering a vaginal suppository.

BIBLIOGRAPHY

Beyea, S., & Nicoll, L. (1996). Back to basics: Administering IM injections the right way. *American Journal of Nursing, 96*(1), 34–35.

Buttaro, M. (1994) Staying on top of transdermal drug patches. *Nursing, 30*(11), 41–44.

Hockenberry, M.J., Wilson, D., Winkelstein, M.L., & Kline, N.E. (2003). *Wong's nursing care of infants and children* (7th ed.). St Louis, MO: Mosby.

James, S., Ashwille, R., & Droske, S.C. (2002). *Nursing care of children* (2nd ed.). Philadelphia: Saunders.

Karch, A., & Karch, F. (2000). Practice errors: A hard pill to swallow. *American Journal of Nursing, 100*(4), 25.

Keen, J. (1995). Drug update: Slow down. *Journal of Emergency Nursing, 21*(4), 323–326.

Lehne, R.A. (2004). *Pharmacology for nursing care* (5th ed.). St Louis, MO: Saunders.

McConnell, E. (1999). Clinical do's and don'ts: Administering a Z-track IM injection. *Nursing, 29*(1), 126.

McConnell, E. (2000). Clinical do's and don'ts: Administering an intradermal injection. *Nursing, 30*(2), 50-52.

McConnell, E. (2002). Clinical do's and don'ts: Administering medications through a gastrostomy tube. *Nursing, 32*(12), 22.

McRoberts, S. (2005). The use of bar code technology in medication administration. *Clinical Nurse Specialist, 19*(2), 55-56.

Miller, D., & Miller, H. (2000). To crush or not to crush? *Nursing, 30*(2), 50–52.

Newton, M., Newton, D., & Fudin, J. (1992). Reviewing the "big three" injection routes. *Nursing, 22*(2), 34–42.

Pullen, R. (2003). Clinical do's and don'ts: Managing IV patient-controlled analgesia. *Nursing, 33*(7), 24.

ILLUSTRATION CREDITS

PART TWO

Drugs Affecting the Central Nervous System: Study Skills Tips

- VOCABULARY
- TEXT NOTATION
- LANGUAGE CONVENTIONS

VOCABULARY

In any subject matter, mastering the vocabulary is essential to mastering the content. But in a complex, technical subject such as nursing pharmacology, if the vocabulary is not mastered, understanding the content will be almost impossible. Most chapters in this text begin with a glossary of unfamiliar terms. As an independent learner, you should spend some time and energy on the vocabulary in the glossary. Do not expect to completely understand and master the terms from the glossary alone. The terms are further defined and explained in the body of the chapter, and it is when you read the chapter that you should expect to fully master the vocabulary. However, the time you spend working on the glossary will pay off when you read the chapter.

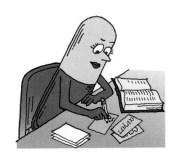

Consider the terms *agonist* and *antagonist* in the Chapter 10 glossary. These terms share a common word part, which means the words are related in meaning. This is an important first step in mastering them. What does *agonist* mean? What is the similarity between *agonist* and *antagonist*? What is the essential difference between the two? Asking these questions as you start to work on Chapter 10 is a valuable technique for beginning to master the language of the content. Do not simply memorize the terms. Learn what they mean, and link relationships between words with common elements. As you practise this technique it will become easier to retain the meaning.

The Chapter 10 glossary has another group of words that should be viewed as a group. The first of these words is *pain*. The definition provided is clear and relatively easy to understand, but your focus should be not just on that single word because there are 14 other words that relate to pain: *acute, cancer, central, chronic, neuropathic, phantom, psychogenic, referred, somatic, superficial, threshold, tolerance, vascular,* and *visceral.* Each of these words defines and categorizes pain in a specific way. As you go about setting up vocabulary cards, look at the opening pages in this chapter. You will find considerable discussion of these terms, which is useful in helping you obtain the fullest understanding of these terms. Do not simply focus on the meaning of each term, but also ask what the similarities and differences are and how these words relate to one another.

TEXT NOTATION

The Study Skills Tips for Part One discussed a method for text underlining. If it is done carefully, this strategy is particularly useful for later review of text material. The object of text underlining is to pick out important terms, ideas, and key information so you can come back to them later for quick review. The three key elements in successful text notation are as follows:

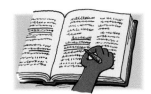

1 You must read the material once before attempting any underlining.

2 You must be acutely aware of the author's language.

3 You must be highly selective. The most common fault in underlining is to mark too much material.

Following are two paragraphs from Chapter 10 that have been underlined. The underlining should be viewed as an example of what can be done. Each reader will mark the text somewhat differently based on his or her background and experience. As you study this example, think not only about what has been underlined but also about *why* that material was chosen.

To fully understand how analgesics work, it is necessary to know what pain is and what its characteristics are. **Pain** is <u>most commonly defined</u> as <u>an unpleasant sensory and emotional experience</u> associated with either actual or potential tissue damage. It is a personal and individual experience. Pain can be defined as whatever a client says it is, and it exists whenever he or she says it does. Although the mechanisms of pain and the nature of pain pathways are becoming better understood, <u>an individual client's perception of pain and appreciation of its meaning are complex processes</u>. Pain involves psychological and emotional processes. Because pain is an individual experience and cannot be quantified, for a caregiver to effectively manage a client suffering from pain, he or she must cultivate a relationship with the client that is built on trust and faith. There is <u>no single approach to effective pain management</u>. Instead pain management has to be individualized and must take into account the cause of the pain, if known; the existence of concurrent medical conditions; the characteristics of the pain; and the client's psychological and ethnocultural characteristics. It also requires ongoing reassessment of the pain and the effectiveness of treatment. Therefore <u>pain</u> is often described as <u>having two elements</u>: a <u>physical element</u> and a <u>psychological element</u>.

The <u>physical element</u> of pain is the <u>client's actual sensation of pain</u>. This involves various nerve pathways and the brain. An important aspect of physical pain is the **pain threshold,** or <u>the level of stimulus needed to produce the perception of pain</u>. This is a <u>measure of the physiological response</u> of the nervous system and is therefore <u>similar for most people</u>. The <u>psychological element</u> represents the <u>client's emotional response</u> to the pain. This response is greatly moulded by the client's age, sex, ethnoculture, previous pain experience, and anxiety level. The <u>psychological element of pain</u> involves **pain tolerance,** <u>or the amount of pain a client can endure without it interfering with normal function</u>. Pain tolerance can vary from client to client because it is a subjective response to pain, not a physiological function. As a result, the client's personality, environment, and ethnocultural background can separately or collectively alter this response. A relatively <u>constant pain threshold exists in all people under normal circumstances</u>. However, pain tolerance, or the point beyond which pain becomes unbearable, varies widely. It can even vary for the same client depending on the circumstances. Table 10-1 lists the <u>various conditions</u> that can alter a person's pain threshold.

LANGUAGE CONVENTIONS

Certain words and phrases are like signal lights at an intersection. They serve to tell the reader that something special, important, or noteworthy is happening. To the attentive, active reader these conventions contribute significantly to understanding what the author is trying to convey. Whether you are highlighting, underlining, writing margin notes, or studying the material using the PURR model, it is important that you become sensitive to these conventions.

The text following the topic heading *Opioid Analgesics: Chemical Structure* contains several examples. The second sentence contains the phrase *classified by.* Whenever an author says that something is being classified it means there are at least two (and perhaps several more) elements of the term or idea that are being classified. This means that you should immediately ask a question about the reading: "What is being classified? How many classifications are there for this?" These questions will help you focus on what to learn and keep your attention firmly fixed on the process of learning.

As you read this chapter, or any other chapter, try to become aware of words and phrases like these that are intended to draw your attention to something the author especially wanted to emphasize. The more aware of language conventions you become, the easier it will be to become a selective reader. Selective readers do not try to remember everything they read but are able to select from the mass of information those concepts and terms that the writers tried to stress.

Analgesic Agents

After reading this chapter, the successful student will be able to do the following:

1 Define analgesia.

2 Describe pharmacological and non-pharmacological approaches to the management and treatment of acute and chronic pain.

3 Discuss the use of non-narcotics, salicylates, non-steroidal anti-inflammatory drugs (NSAIDs), and narcotics in pain management.

4 Identify the various drugs within the analgesic categories listed above.

5 Discuss the difference between opioid agonists, agonist–antagonists, and antagonist agents.

6 Compare the mechanisms of action, drug effects, indications, side effects, adverse effects, cautions, contraindications, and interactions of non-narcotics, salicylates, NSAIDs, narcotic agonists, and agonist–antagonist agents.

7 Discuss "special" pain situations, such as cancer pain, and their management as well as established pain standards for these situations, including those of the World Health Organization (WHO) and consensus guidelines from the Canadian Pain Society.

8 Develop a nursing care plan that includes all phases of the nursing process related to the administration of all classes of analgesics and adjunctive agents for the client experiencing pain.

9 Identify various resources and agencies or professional groups that are involved in establishing standards for the management of all types of pain.

e-LEARNING ACTIVITIES

Student CD-ROM
- Review Questions: see questions 34–48
- Animations
- Medication Administration Checklists
- IV Therapy Checklists

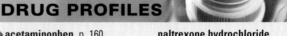 **Web site** (http://evolve.elsevier.com/Lilley/pharmacology/)
- Online Chapter Worksheet • Frequently Asked Questions
- Learning Tips and Content Updates • WebLinks • Online Appendices and Supplements • Mosby/Saunders ePharmacology Update • Access to *Mosby's Drug Consult*

DRUG PROFILES

▸▸ acetaminophen, p. 160
  codeine sulphate, p. 154
  fentanyl, p. 154
  meperidine hydrochloride, p. 157
  methadone hydrochloride, p. 157
▸▸ morphine sulphate, p. 154
▸▸ naloxone hydrochloride, p. 158

naltrexone hydrochloride, p. 158
propoxyphene hydrochloride/napsylate, p. 157
tramadol hydrochloride, p. 158

▸▸ Key drug.

GLOSSARY

Acute pain Pain that is sudden in onset, usually subsides when treated, and typically occurs over a period of less than 3 months.

Addiction Habitual psychological and physiological (physical) dependence on a substance that is beyond normal voluntary control.

Adjuvant analgesic agent A drug that is added as a second drug for combined therapy with a primary drug and may have additive or independent analgesic properties, or both.

Agonist A substance that binds to a receptor and causes a response.

Agonist–antagonist (also known as a *partial agonist)* A substance that binds to a receptor and causes a partial response that is not as strong as that caused by an agonist.

Analgesics Medications that relieve pain without causing loss of consciousness or loss of general sensation (sometimes referred to as *painkillers).*

Antagonist An agent that binds to a receptor and prevents (blocks) a response.

Cancer pain Pain related to a variety of causes as a result of cancer and/or the metastasis of cancer.

Central pain Pain resulting from any disorder that causes central nervous system (CNS) damage.

Chronic pain Persistent or recurring pain that is often difficult to treat. Typically it is pain that lasts longer than 3 months.

Gate theory The most common and well-described theory of pain transmission and pain relief. It uses a gate model to explain how impulses from damaged tissues are sensed in the brain.

Neuropathic pain Pain that results from a disturbance of function or pathological change in a nerve.

Non-opioid analgesics Analgesics that are not classified as opioids.

Non-steroidal anti-inflammatory drugs (NSAIDs) A large, chemically diverse group of drugs that are analgesics and also possess anti-inflammatory and antipyretic activity but are not steroids.

Opioid analgesics Synthetic narcotic agents that bind to the mu, kappa, and delta receptors to relieve pain but are not themselves derived from the opium plant.

Opioid tolerance A physiological result of long-term opioid use in which larger doses of opioids are required to maintain the same level of analgesia.

Opioid withdrawal (opioid abstinence syndrome) The signs and symptoms associated with the abstinence from or withdrawal of opioid analgesics when the body has become physically dependent on the substance.

Pain An unpleasant sensory and emotional experience associated with actual or potential tissue damage. Pain is a subjective and individual experience; it can be defined as whatever the experiencing person says it is and it exists whenever he or she says it does.

Pain threshold The level of stimulus that results in the perception of pain.

Pain tolerance The amount of pain an individual can endure without it interfering with normal function.

Partial agonist A substance that binds to a receptor and causes effects similar to but less pronounced than those of a pure agonist.

Phantom pain Pain experienced in a body part that has been surgically or traumatically removed.

Physical dependence The physical adaptation of the body to the presence of an opioid or other addictive substance.

Psychogenic pain Pain that is psychological in nature but is truly real pain in terms of actual pain impulses that travel through nerve cells.

Psychological dependence (addiction) A pattern of compulsive use of opioids or any other addictive substance characterized by a continuous craving for the substance and the need to use it for effects other than pain relief.

Referred pain Pain occurring in an area away from the organ of origin.

Somatic pain Pain that originates from skeletal muscles, ligaments, or joints.

Superficial pain Pain that originates from the skin or mucous membranes.

Vascular pain Pain that results from a pathology of the vascular or perivascular tissues.

Visceral pain Pain that originates from organs or smooth muscles.

The management of clients experiencing acute or **chronic pain** is an important aspect of nursing care in a variety of settings and across the lifespan. Pain remains one of the more common reasons for clients to seek out the care of a physician, and 80 percent of physician office visits in Canada involve a pain-related component. Surgical and diagnostic procedures often require pain management, and there are many diseases and pathological conditions that also require pain management, such as cancer and AIDS. Pain leads to much suffering and is a tremendous economic burden as a result of loss in productivity and workers' compensation and related health care costs. Because of the personal suffering involved and the prevalence and scope of the problem (e.g., overall 30 percent to 45 percent of cancer clients have pain, and this increases to 75 percent of clients in advanced stages), for nurses to provide quality client care it is critical that they be well informed about pain management, both pharmacological and non-pharmacological (e.g., massage, acupuncture, therapeutic touch, spirituality, relaxation techniques, imagery).

Medications that relieve pain without causing loss of consciousness or loss of general sensation (commonly referred to as *painkillers)* are considered **analgesics.** There are various classes of analgesics. These classes are determined by the chemical structures and mechanisms of action of the agents. This chapter focuses on those agents commonly used to relieve moderate to severe pain—opioid analgesics. The next most common analgesic class consists of **non-steroidal anti-inflammatory drugs (NSAIDs),** which are discussed in Chapter 43.

PHYSIOLOGY AND PSYCHOLOGY OF PAIN

To fully understand how analgesics work, it is necessary to know what pain is and what its characteristics are. **Pain** is most commonly defined as an unpleasant sensory and emotional experience associated with either actual or potential tissue damage. It is a personal and individual experience. Pain can be defined as whatever the client says it is, and it exists whenever he or she says it does. Although the mechanisms of pain and the nature of pain pathways are becoming better understood, an individual client's perception of pain and appreciation of its meaning are complex processes. Pain involves psychological and emotional processes. Because pain is an individual experience and cannot be quantified, for a caregiver to effectively manage a client suffering from pain a relationship with the client must be cultivated that is built on trust and faith. There is no single approach to effective pain management. Instead, pain management has to be individualized and must take into account the cause of the pain, if known; the existence of concurrent medical conditions; the characteristics of the pain; and the client's psychological and ethnocultural characteristics (see the Ethnocultural Implications box). It also requires ongoing reassessment of the pain and the effectiveness of treatment. Therefore pain is often described as having two elements: a physical element and a psychological element.

The physical element of pain is the client's actual sensation of pain. This involves various nerve pathways and the brain. An important aspect of physical pain is the **pain threshold,** or the level of stimulus needed to produce the perception of pain. This is a measure of the physiological response of the nervous system and is therefore similar for most people. The psychological element represents the client's emotional response to the pain. This response is greatly moulded by the client's age, sex, ethnoculture, previous pain experience, and anxiety level. The psychological element of pain involves **pain tolerance,** or the amount of pain a client can endure without it interfering with normal function. Pain tolerance can vary from client to client because it is a subjective response to pain, not a physiological function. As a result, the client's personality, environment, and ethnocultural background can separately or collectively alter this response. A relatively constant pain threshold exists in all people under normal circumstances. However, pain tolerance, or the point beyond which pain becomes unbearable, varies widely. It can even vary for the same client depending on the circumstances. Table 10-1 lists the various conditions that can alter a person's pain threshold.

Pain can also be further classified in terms of its onset and duration as either acute or chronic. Acute and chronic pain differ not only in their onset and duration but also in how they are treated. They are also associated with various diseases or conditions. **Acute pain** is sudden in onset and usually subsides when treated. One example of acute pain is the pain related to the sudden onset of a headache. Chronic pain is persistent or recurring and is often difficult to treat. Table 10-2 lists the characteristics of acute and chronic pain and various diseases and conditions associated with each.

Pain can be further classified according to its source. The two most commonly mentioned sources of pain are somatic and visceral pain. **Somatic pain** originates from skeletal muscles, ligaments, and joints. **Visceral pain** originates from organs and smooth muscles. Sometimes pain originates from the skin and mucous membranes and is called **superficial pain.** Pain treatment may be more appropriately selected when the source of the pain

---

ETHNOCULTURAL IMPLICATIONS

Pain and Pain Management

- Each ethnoculture has its own beliefs, thoughts, and ways of approaching, defining, and managing pain.
- Attitudes, meanings, and perceptions of pain vary with each ethnoculture.
- Many Black and Caribbean Canadians believe in the power of healers who rely strongly on the religious faith of the people and often use prayer and the laying on of hands.
- Many Somali Canadians believe in Quranic readings, the wearing of amulets, and the use of a wide variety of herbs. Illness and healing are often viewed as the will of Allah. The evil eye "al-ayn," spirits called Jinn, or curses may also cause illness. Ritual scarification and fumigation are common, as is cauterization, in which a thin burning stick or heated metal is applied on an affected part.
- Some traditional methods of healing for the Chinese include acupuncture, herbal remedies, yin and yang, and cold treatment. Moxibustion is another form of healing and involves the application of herbal heat to acupoints on the skin. Moxibustion is often used with acupuncture.
- For many Aboriginal Canadians, treatments include massage, the application of heat, sweat baths, herbal remedies, and being in harmony with nature.
- Nurses should be aware of all ethnocultural influences on health-related behaviours, as well as on clients' attitudes toward medication therapy and, ultimately, on its effectiveness. A thorough assessment with questions about the client's ethnocultural background and practices is important to the effective and individualized delivery of nursing care.

TABLE 10-1

CONDITIONS THAT ALTER PAIN THRESHOLD

Pain Threshold	Conditions
Lowered	Anger, anxiety, depression, discomfort, fear, isolation, chronic pain, sleeplessness, tiredness
Raised	Diversion, empathy, rest, sympathy, medications (analgesics, anti-anxiety agents, antidepressants)

TABLE 10-2

ACUTE VERSUS CHRONIC PAIN

Type of Pain	Onset	Duration	Examples
Acute	Sudden (minutes to hours); usually sharp, localized; physiological response (sympathetic nervous system [SNS]: tachycardia, sweating, pallor, increased blood pressure)	Limited (has an end)	Myocardial infarction, appendicitis, dental procedures, kidney stones, surgical procedures
Chronic	Slow (days to months); long duration; dull, persistent aching	Persistent or recurring (endless)	Arthritis, cancer, lower back pain, peripheral neuropathy

SNS, Sympathetic nervous system.

TABLE 10-3

A AND C NERVE FIBRES

Type of Fibre	Myelin Sheath	Fibre Size	Conduction Speed	Type of Pain
A	Yes	Large	Fast	Sharp and well localized
C	No	Small	Slow	Dull and non-localized

is known. For example, visceral and superficial pain usually require opioids for relief, whereas somatic pain usually responds better to **non-opioid analgesics** such as NSAIDs.

Another type of pain is **vascular pain,** which possibly originates from some pathology of the vascular or perivascular tissues and is thought to account for a large percentage of migraine headaches. **Referred pain** happens as a result of visceral nerve fibres synapsing at a level in the spinal cord close to fibres that supply specific subcutaneous tissues in the body. An example is the pain with cholecystitis, which is often referred to the back and scapula areas. **Neuropathic pain** results from injury or damage to peripheral nerve fibres or damage to the central nervous system (CNS) and is often present in the absence of disease or pathological processes. **Phantom pain** occurs in a body part that has been removed—surgically or traumatically—and is characterized as burning, itching, tingling, or stabbing.

Cancer pain, a type of pain that must be taken seriously, has many causes, such as pressure on nerves, organs, or tissues. Other causes of cancer pain include hypoxia; blockage to an organ; metastasis; pathological fractures; muscle spasms; and side effects of radiation, surgery, and chemotherapy. **Psychogenic pain** originates because of psychological factors, not physical conditions or disorders. However, it is still "real" pain in that it results in actual neural pain impulses, as does physical pain. Another type of pain, **central pain,** occurs with tumours, trauma, or inflammation of the brain and may occur with any condition that yields CNS damage, such as cancer, diabetes, stroke, and multiple sclerosis.

Several theories explain pain transmission and pain relief. The most common and well described is the **gate theory.** This theory, proposed by Melzack and Wall in 1965, uses the analogy of a gate to describe how impulses from damaged tissues are sensed in the brain. First, the tissue injury causes the release of several substances, such as bradykinin, histamine, potassium, prostaglandins, and serotonin. Many current pain management strategies are aimed at altering the actions and levels of these substances. Once these substances are released by the damaged tissue, an action potential is initiated. This action potential travels along a sensory nerve fibre and activates a pain receptor. There are two basic types of these nerve fibres: A and C. Table 10-3 summarizes the differences in the size and function of these two types of nerve fibres. The different types of pain experienced are believed to be related to the relative proportions of A and C fibres in a particular area of the body.

These pain fibres, along with other sensory nerve fibres, enter the spinal cord and travel up to the brain. The site where these fibres enter the spinal cord is referred to as the *dorsal (posterior) horn* of the spinal cord. It is here that the so-called *gates* are located. These gates regulate the flow of sensory impulses. If impulses are stopped by a gate at this junction, no impulses are transmitted to the higher centres of the brain. Because it is at these higher centres that impulses are consciously perceived by the client, in this instance there would be no perception of pain. Figure 10-1 depicts the gate theory of pain transmission.

Both the opening and the closing of this gate are influenced by the relative activation of the large-diameter A fibres and the small-diameter C fibres. The closing of the gate seems to be affected by the activation of A fibres. This causes the inhibition of impulse transmission to the brain and thus no perception of pain. Opening of the gate is affected by stimulation of the C fibres. This allows impulses to be transmitted to the brain and pain to be perceived. This gate is also innervated by nerve fibres that originate in the brain. These nerve fibres enable the brain to evaluate, identify, and localize the pain. Thus the brain can control the gate, either keeping the gate closed or allowing it to open so that the brain is stimulated and pain is perceived. The cells that control the gate have a threshold.

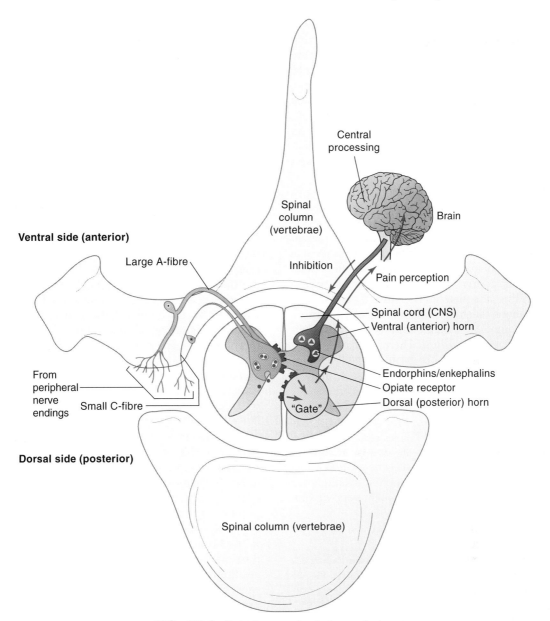

FIG. 10-1 Gate theory of pain transmission.

Impulses that reach these cells must overcome this threshold before an impulse is permitted to travel up to the brain.

The body is equipped with certain endogenous neurotransmitters known as *enkephalins* and *endorphins*. These substances, released whenever the body experiences pain, are considered the body's painkillers. They are capable of binding with opioid receptors and inhibiting the transmission of pain impulses by closing the gate. These endogenous analgesic substances are responsible for the phenomenon of "runner's high." Figure 10-1 depicts this entire process.

The gate theory also explains why massage or applying liniment to the affected area often decreases the pain. Large sensory fibres from peripheral receptors carry impulses to the spinal cord, causing impulse transmission to

be inhibited and the gate to be closed. This in turn reduces the recognition of the pain impulses arriving by means of the small fibres. This is the same pathway that the opioid analgesics use to alleviate pain.

Treatment of Pain in Special Situations

In managing pain associated with malignancies, the main consideration is client comfort and not prevention of drug addiction. Often this means aggressive treatment with large doses of frequently administered narcotic analgesics to relieve the pain and prevent it from recurring. As the disease progresses, the client may develop tolerance and require larger doses and more frequent medication administration using oral, injectable, rectal, transdermal, and/or parenteral routes. However, for long-term use, as with cancer clients, injectable forms are not the first choice, since breaking skin integrity repeatedly can lead to possible infections. Also, if clients are taking long-acting narcotic analgesics, breakthrough pain may require shorter-acting or fast-acting forms on a regular schedule. If a client is requiring larger doses for breakthrough pain, the baseline dose of the narcotic may need to be titrated upward (that is, increased in steps). Other medications, such as antidepressants, may be added. Anti-emetics and laxatives may be used to prevent or relieve the constipation, nausea, and vomiting that are common side effects with narcotic agents.

Sometimes clients may have both chronic pain, as with cancer, but also acute pain from specific disorders or disease complications such as those seen in crises in sickle cell disease, AIDS, and cancer. Acute pain is easier to treat than chronic pain. Although it is difficult to quantify, it is estimated that one of every three Canadians suffers pain, and that pain is poorly understood and often undertreated. Providing adequate pain control in unusual or complex situations, such as with rare diseases, cancer, and AIDS, requires a holistic approach and well-informed healthcare providers. Therapy may include opioid or non-opioid agents (or both), as well as non-pharmacological treatments such as massage, medication, and psychological counselling.

OPIOID ANALGESICS

The analgesics currently known as **opioid analgesics** originated from the opium plant. *Opium* is a Greek word that means "juice." More than 20 different alkaloids are obtained from the unripe seed of the opium poppy plant.

RESEARCH

Pain Management in Nursing Home Clients

A 1999 U.S. study found that nearly 50 000 nursing home residents experienced non-malignant pain daily but that only approximately 26 percent of these clients reported this pain. This same study showed that analgesics were administered less often to clients who were male, over the age of 85 years, cognitively impaired, and of African-American or Hispanic descent. Factors associated with the undertreatment of pain included the belief that discussion and management of pain occurred only if the client was asked if he or she needed pain medication. The study also found that undertreatment resulted from healthcare providers' inadequate knowledge and misinformation about the use and addictive properties of opioids. For example, many believed that pain is a normal process in the aged and should not be treated with opioids due to respiratory depression and the potential for addiction.

From Won, A., Lapane, K., Gambassi, G., Bernabel, R., Mor, V., & Lipsitz, L.A. (1999). Correlates and management of nonmalignant pain in the nursing home. *Journal of the American Geriatrics Society, 47*, 936–942.

The properties of opium and its many alkaloids have been known for centuries. As early as the third century BC, reference to poppy juice is found in the writings of Theophrastus. Arabian physicians were well versed in the uses of opium as well. It was Arabian traders who introduced the drug to East Asia. Opium-smoking immigrants brought opium to Canada, where unrestricted availability of opium prevailed until the early twentieth century.

Chemical Structure

Opioid analgesics are strong pain relievers. They can be classified according to their chemical structure or by their action at specific receptors (see Mechanism of Action and Drug Effects). Of the 20 different alkaloids available from the opium poppy plant, only three are clinically useful: morphine, codeine, and papaverine. Of these three, only morphine and codeine are considered pain relievers; papaverine is a smooth muscle relaxant. Relatively simple chemical modifications of these opium alkaloids have produced the three different chemical classes of opioids: morphine-like drugs, meperidine-like drugs (synthetic), and methadone-like drugs.

Table 10-4 lists the various opioid analgesics and their respective chemical categories.

Mechanism of Action and Drug Effects

Opioid analgesics can also be characterized according to their mechanism of action. They can be agonists, partial agonists, or antagonists. These same concepts also apply to many other pharmacological classes of medications and their respective sites of action (receptor proteins) in the various tissues. In the case of opioid analgesics, an **agonist** binds to an opioid pain receptor in the brain and causes an analgesic response—the reduction of pain sensation. A **partial agonist,** also called an **agonist–antagonist,** binds to a pain receptor and causes only limited actions. The physiological response produced by the binding of a partial agonist is not as pronounced as that produced by an agonist. **Antagonists** are substances that reverse the effects of these agents on pain receptors. Antagonists bind to a pain receptor and exert no response. They may also be referred to as *competitive antagonists* because they compete with

TABLE 10-4
CHEMICAL CLASSIFICATION OF OPIOIDS

Chemical Category	Opioid Agents
meperidine-like agents	Meperidine, fentanyl, remifentanil, sufentanil, alfentanil
methadone-like agents	Methadone, propoxyphene, propoxyphene napsylate
morphine-like agents	Morphine, heroin, hydromorphone, oxymorphone, codeine, hydrocodone, oxycodone

the agonist and antagonist drugs that normally bind to that receptor. The nurse must keep in mind that the body also has its own internal biochemicals that stimulate various receptors. In the case of opioid receptors, these are known as *endorphins,* which stands for "endogenous morphine" because the endorphins are a natural internal mechanism of pain control.

The actual receptors to which opioids bind to relieve pain are listed and their characteristics summarized in Table 10-5. Five types of opioid receptors have been identified to date: mu, kappa, sigma, delta, and epsilon. Mu, kappa, and delta are the primary receptors. Many of the characteristics of a particular opioid, such as its ability to sedate, its potency, and its ability to cause hallucinations, can be attributed to the particular opioid's affinity for these various receptors. Opioid analgesics achieve their beneficial effects by their actions in the CNS. However, they also act outside the CNS, and many of their unwanted effects stem from these actions.

Indications

The main effect of opioids is to alleviate moderate to severe pain. The degree to which pain is relieved or unwanted side effects occur depends on the specific agent, the receptors to which it binds, and its chemical structure. Often drugs from other chemical categories are added to the opioid regimen as **adjuvant analgesic agents** (hereafter referred to as *adjuvants*). These assist the primary agents in relieving pain. Such adjuvant drug therapy may include NSAIDs, antidepressants, anticonvulsants, and corticosteroids, all of which are discussed further in their corresponding chapters. This allows the use of smaller doses of opioids, which accomplishes two important functions. First, it diminishes some of the side effects that are seen with higher doses of opioids, such as respiratory depression, constipation, and urinary retention. Second, it approaches the pain stimulus from another mechanism and has a resulting synergistic beneficial effect in reducing the pain.

Many opioids have an affinity for the CNS. Once there, they suppress the medullary cough centre, which results in cough suppression. The opioid most commonly used for this purpose is codeine. Hydrocodone has also been used in many cough suppressants, either

alone or in combination with other agents. Sometimes the opioid-related cough suppressants have a depressant effect on the CNS and cause sedation. To avoid this problem, dextromethorphan, a non-opioid cough suppressant, is often given instead.

Constipation from decreased gastrointestinal (GI) motility is often an unwanted side effect of opioids related to their anticholinergic effects. Some of the most common opioid-containing antidiarrheal preparations are camphorated opium tincture (paregoric) and diphenoxylate–atropine sulphate.

Strong opioid analgesics such as fentanyl, sufentanil, and alfentanil are commonly used in combination with anaesthetics during surgery. These agents are used not only to relieve pain but also in combination with other drugs to produce *balanced anaesthesia* (see Chapter 11).

Similarly strong opioids such as morphine, meperidine, and oxycodone are often used to control post-operative and other types of pain. All available oxycodone dosage forms are orally administered. The brand name product OxyContin is a sustained-release form of oxycodone that is designed to last up to 12 hours. The "Contin" in the product name stands for "continuous-release," a synonym for any long-acting drug product. There are also immediate-release forms of oxycodone in tablet, capsule, and liquid form. Similarly, the drug product MS Contin is a long-acting or sustained-release form of morphine. The "MS" stands for the salt name morphine sulphate. Morphine is also available in injectable forms. Meperidine is available only in immediate-release dosage forms, both oral and injectable.

Contraindications

Contraindications to the use of opioid analgesics include known drug allergy; severe asthma or other respiratory insufficiency, especially in the absence of resuscitative equipment; conditions involving elevated intracranial pressure; and pregnancy, especially in long-term use or high doses.

Side Effects and Adverse Effects

As previously mentioned, many of the unwanted effects of opioid analgesics are related to their effects on parts of the body other than the CNS. Some of these unwanted effects can be explained by the respective agent's selectivity for the receptors listed in Table 10-5. The various body systems that the opioids affect and their side effects and adverse effects are summarized in Table 10-6.

Opioids that have an affinity for mu receptors and have rapid onset of action produce marked euphoria. These are the opioids that are most likely to be abused and used recreationally. The person taking them to alter his or her mental status will soon become psychologically dependent on them. **Psychological dependence (addiction)** is a pattern of compulsive drug use characterized by a continuous craving for an opioid and the need to use it for effects other than pain relief. In contrast, **physical dependence** occurs when abrupt discontinuation of the

TABLE 10-5

OPIOID RECEPTORS AND THEIR CHARACTERISTICS

Receptor Type	Prototypical Agonist	Effects
Mu	morphine	Supraspinal analgesia, respiratory depression, euphoria, ++sedation
Kappa	butorphanol	Spinal analgesia, ++++sedation, miosis
Delta	enkephalins	Analgesia

PEDIATRIC CONSIDERATIONS

Opioid Administration and Implications

- Assessment of the pediatric client is challenging, and all types of behaviour that may indicate pain, such as muscular rigidity, restlessness, screaming, fear of moving, and withdrawn behaviour, have to be carefully considered.
- Assessment of pain is important in pediatric clients because they are often undermedicated. The nurse should always thoroughly assess the pediatric client and not underestimate the child's complaints.
- When the pediatric client is to receive opioids, the nurse should be careful to recheck dosages against the physician's order and pharmacy references and to double-check the fractions and decimals to prevent errors.
- If suppositories are used, the nurse must be careful to administer the exact dose and not to split, halve, or divide an adult dose into a child's dose because this may result in the administration of an unknown dose.
- The nurse must always monitor pediatric clients closely for any unusual behaviour or signs and symptoms while they are receiving opioids.
- The nurse should report to the physician immediately CNS changes such as dizziness, lightheadedness, drowsiness, hallucinations, changes in the level of consciousness, sluggish pupil reaction and give no further medication until further orders are received from the physician. Drowsiness and changes in level of consciousness are most common and may result in sedating effects.
- The nurse should always monitor and document vital signs before, during, and after the administration of opioid analgesics. Medication is withheld if respirations are <12 breaths/min or if there are any changes in the level of consciousness.
- The nurse should carefully assess respiratory status—respiratory rate, rhythm, character (rate, and difficulty).
- Generally speaking, smaller doses of opioids are indicated for the pediatric client.
- The nurse should maintain frequent client checks and use bed alarms where available.
- Meperidine should be used cautiously in clients younger than 18 years.
- Oral opium derivatives should be given with meals or milk to decrease GI tract distress.
- With opiates, the therapeutic response is a decrease in pain.
- Allergic reactions may include a rash or urticaria.
- Withdrawal symptoms include nausea, vomiting, cramps, faintness, fever, and anorexia.

GERIATRIC CONSIDERATIONS

Opioid Administration and Implications

- The nurse should assess the client carefully before administering opioids because a dose and interval adjustment may be necessary depending on the development of adverse reactions such as confusion, decreased respiration, and excessive CNS depression.
- The nurse should note and record the height and weight of the client before the start of opioid treatment.
- The nurse should carefully monitor and document any changes in geriatric clients who are receiving opioids because they are generally more sensitive to these agents. This includes frequent monitoring of vital signs, respiratory function, and CNS status.
- Smaller doses of opioids are generally indicated for the geriatric client, and idiosyncratic or unexpected reactions may be more likely to occur in clients of this age group.
- Polypharmacy is often a problem in older adults; therefore it is important for the nurse to have a complete list of all medications the client is currently taking and to assess for drug interactions and treatment (drug) duplication.
- The nurse should maintain frequent assessments of clients for their level of consciousness, alertness, and cognitive ability while keeping the environment safe and a call bell or light at the bedside; bed alarms are indicated where available.
- With possible decreased circulation, the absorption of intramuscular (IM) or intravenous (IV) dosage forms will vary and often result in a slower absorption of parenteral forms of opioids.
- The nurse should encourage geriatric clients to ask for medications if needed. They often hesitate to ask for pain medication because they do not want to "bother" the nurse or give in to pain.
- NSAIDs should be used with caution because of renal and GI toxicity. Acetaminophen is the drug of choice for relieving mild to moderate pain but with cautious dosing because of hepatic and renal concerns. The oral route is preferred. The regimen should be as simple as possible to enhance adherence, and the nurse should be sure to note, report, and document any unusual reactions to the opioid agents.

medication results in physical withdrawal symptoms such as rebound pain, tachycardia, elevated blood pressure, and mental agitation. *Tolerance* refers to the need for progressively higher doses to maintain the same analgesic effect. This is obviously a common problem with clients who are addicted to opioids, but it can also result from legitimate control of severe pain in serious illnesses such as cancer. Fear of creating an addiction to opioids may lead well-meaning prescribers to undertreat pain, which is generally considered inhumane and unethical in cases of severe progressive illness. Under these circumstances, control of the client's pain takes ethical and even clinical priority over concerns regarding drug addiction.

All opioids cause some histamine release. It is thought that this histamine release is responsible for many of the unwanted side effects, such as itching or pruritus, rash, and hemodynamic changes. The histamine release causes peripheral arteries and veins to dilate, which leads to flushing

TABLE 10-6
OPIOID-INDUCED SIDE EFFECTS AND ADVERSE EFFECTS BY BODY SYSTEM

Body System	Side Effect or Adverse Effect
Cardiovascular	Hypotension, palpitations, flushing
Central nervous system	Sedation, disorientation, euphoria, light-headedness, dysphoria, lowered seizure threshold, tremors
Gastrointestinal	Nausea, vomiting, constipation, biliary tract spasm
Genitourinary	Urinary retention
Integumentary	Itching, rash, wheal formation
Respiratory	Respiratory depression and aggravation of asthma

and orthostatic hypotension. Morphine-like drugs also blunt the baroreceptor response, which contributes to orthostatic hypotension. The amount of histamine release that an opioid analgesic causes is related to its chemical class. The naturally occurring opiates elicit the most histamine release; the synthetic opioids (e.g., meperidine) elicit the least histamine release. (See Table 10-4 for a list of the various opioids and their respective chemical classes.)

The most serious side effect of opioids is CNS depression, which may lead to respiratory depression. Care should be taken to titrate the dose so that the client's pain is controlled without respiratory function being affected. Individual responses to opioids vary, and clients may occasionally suffer respiratory compromise or the loss of airway reflexes despite careful dose titration. Respiratory depression can be prevented in part by using agents with a short duration of action and no active metabolites. It seems to be more common in clients with a pre-existing condition causing respiratory compromise, such as asthma or chronic obstructive pulmonary disease (COPD). Respiratory depression is strongly related to the degree of sedation. Stimulation of the client may be adequate to reverse mild hypoventilation. If this is unsuccessful, then assisted ventilation by bag and mask or by endotracheal intubation may be needed to support respiration. It may also be necessary to administer naloxone HCl, an opioid reversal agent, to reverse severe respiratory depression. However, the nurse should keep in mind that naloxone will reverse not only the client's respiratory depression but also the pain control. Careful, slow titration of naloxone will prevent over-reversal of the opioid-induced respiratory depression and pain relief. The effects of naloxone are short lived, usually lasting about 1 hour. With long-acting opioids the respiratory depressant effects can reappear after the naloxone has worn off, and redosing may be needed.

GI tract side effects are common in clients receiving opioids. Nausea, vomiting, and constipation are the most common side effects associated with opioid analgesics. Opioids can irritate the GI tract, stimulating the chemoreceptor trigger zone in the CNS, which in turn may cause nausea and vomiting. Opioids slow peristal-

sis and increase water absorption from intestinal contents. These two actions combine to produce constipation. This is more pronounced in a hospitalized client who is non-ambulatory, because lack of daily activity also causes constipation.

Urinary retention, or the inability to void, is another unwanted side effect of opioid analgesics. They cause this by increasing bladder tone. This is sometimes treated with low doses of an opioid **agonist–antagonist** or with an opioid antagonist.

Severe hypersensitivity or anaphylaxis to opioid analgesics is rare. Most clients will experience GI tract or histamine-mediated reactions to opioids and call these "allergic reactions." True anaphylaxis is rare, even with intravenously administered opioids. Some clients may complain of flushing, itching, or weal formation at the injection site, but this is usually local and histamine mediated.

Toxicity and Management of Overdose

Opioid analgesics produce both beneficial effects and toxic or unwanted effects by means of receptors. These receptors and the positive and negative effects they bring about are listed in Table 10-5. The opioid antagonists naloxone and naltrexone bind to and occupy all of these receptor sites (mu, kappa, and sigma). They are competitive antagonists with a strong affinity for these binding sites. In doing so they can reverse the adverse effects induced by the opioid, such as respiratory depression. These agents are used in the management of both opioid overdose and opioid addiction. The commonly used opioid antagonists (reversal agents) are listed in Table 10-7.

For effective management of opioid overdose or toxicity, it is important for the nurse to recognize the signs and symptoms of withdrawal. **Opioid tolerance** may be a physiological result of long-term opioid use; clients with opioid tolerance require larger doses of the opioid agent to maintain the same level of analgesia. The physiological adaptation of the body to the effects of an opioid is referred to as *physical dependence.* Opioid tolerance and physical dependence are expected in clients undergoing long-term opioid treatment and should not be confused with psychological dependence (addiction), manifested by drug abuse behaviour. Confusing these terms in relation to opioid therapy leads to ineffective pain management and contributes to the problem of undertreatment. Physical dependence on opioids is seen when an agent is discontinued abruptly or when an opioid antagonist is administered. This physiological response is referred to as **opioid withdrawal** or **opioid abstinence syndrome** and is manifested by anxiety, irritability, chills and hot flashes, joint pain, lacrimation (tearing), rhinorrhea, diaphoresis, nausea, vomiting, and abdominal cramps and diarrhea.

The timing of the onset of withdrawal symptoms is directly related to the half-life of the opioid analgesic being used. The withdrawal symptoms resulting from the discontinuance or reversal of short-acting opioid therapy (codeine, hydrocodone, morphine, and hydromorphone) will arise within 6 to 12 hours and peak at 24 to 72 hours. The withdrawal symptoms associated with the

TABLE 10-7

OPIOID ANTAGONISTS (REVERSAL AGENTS)

Generic Name	Dosage	Cautions
naloxone (IV)	0.4–2 mg q2–3min (<10 mg); IV infusion: 2 mg in 500 mL (titrate to response)	Raised or lowered blood pressure, dysrhythmias, pulmonary edema, withdrawal
naltrexone (PO)	25–50 mg daily	Nervousness, headache, nausea, vomiting, pulmonary edema, withdrawal

long half-life agents (methadone and transdermal fentanyl) may not appear for 24 hours or more after drug discontinuation and may be milder. The appearance of abstinence syndrome indicates physical dependence on the opioids, which may occur after just 2 weeks of therapy. It does not, however, imply the existence of psychological dependence or addiction. Most clients with cancer take opioid analgesics for more than 2 weeks, and only rarely do they exhibit the drug abuse behaviour and psychological dependence that characterize addiction.

Interactions

Potential drug interactions with opioids are significant. Co-administration of opioids with alcohol, antihistamines, barbiturates, benzodiazepines, phenothiazine, and other CNS depressants can result in additive respiratory depressant effects. The combined use of opioids (such as meperidine) with monoamine oxidase inhibitors (MAOIs) can result in respiratory depression and hypotension.

Laboratory Test Interactions

Opioids can cause an abnormal increase in the serum levels of amylase, alanine aminotransferase, alkaline phosphatase, bilirubin, lipase, creatinine kinase, and lactate dehydrogenase. Other abnormal results include a decrease in urinary 17-keto-steroid level and an increase in urinary alkaloid and glucose concentrations.

Dosages

For the recommended dosages of selected analgesic agents, see the dosages table on p. 155. See Appendix B for some of the common drug brands available in Canada.

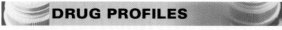

DRUG PROFILES

▶▶ morphine sulphate

Morphine, discussed first because it is the drug prototype for opioids and narcotics, is an alkaloid obtained from opium. Opium is the dried juice of the poppy plant *Papaver somniferum* and is a mixture of opioid and non-opioid alkaloids. As with other narcotics, there is a strong potential for misuse and abuse with morphine. For this reason, morphine is classified as a Narcotic Drug Schedule N in Canada by the Food and Drugs Act (FDA) and the Controlled Drugs and Substances Act (CDSA) and Regulations. However, the nurse's fear of opioids that cause addiction should not result in denying a client adequate pain relief. Gradual withdrawal with chronic use may minimize the development of withdrawal symptoms after long-term use.

Morphine is highly constipating. It is contraindicated in clients showing hypersensitivity to it, and extreme caution is required when administering it to clients with head injuries. It is indicated for treatment of severe pain and may be administered by a variety of routes (oral [PO], intramuscular [IM], sustained-release tablets, intravenous [IV], subcutaneous [SC], rectal, epidural, and intrathecal) depending on the client's condition. Continuous infusions of morphine may also be initiated through a patient-controlled analgesia (PCA) pump. Not usually prescribed for pregnancy. For dosage information, see the table on p. 155.

PHARMACOKINETICS

Half-Life	Onset	Peak	Duration
1.7–4.5 hr	Rapid	IM: 30–60 min	IM: 4–5hr

codeine sulphate

Codeine sulphate (methylmorphine) is the second opioid alkaloid obtained from opium. However, the yield is low, and the high medical consumption of codeine necessitates its synthesis by methylating morphine. Codeine is similar to morphine in terms of its pharmacokinetic and pharmacodynamic properties. However, codeine is less effective as an analgesic and is widely used as an antitussive agent in an array of cough preparations. Fixed combinations using codeine (e.g., with acetaminophen) are classified as Schedule F and are commonly used for control of mild to moderate pain. These combination codeine products have differing controlled substance schedules. Codeine alone is still classified as a Narcotic Drug Schedule N in Canada by the FDA and the CDSA and Regulations, implying a high abuse and addiction potential. For dosage information, see the table on p. 155.

PHARMACOKINETICS

Half-Life	Onset	Peak	Duration
2.5–4 hr	15–30 min	35–45 min	3–4 hr

fentanyl

Fentanyl is a synthetic opioid used to treat moderate to severe pain. It is also used as an adjunct to general anaesthetics. It is available in several dosage forms: transdermal patches, buccal lozenges, and parenteral injections. Fentanyl is a potent analgesic. The potencies of some of the more common opioids as compared with 10 mg of both intramuscular and oral forms of morphine are listed in Table 10-8. Fentanyl at a dose of 0.1 mg given intravenously is equivalent to 10 mg of morphine given intramuscularly.

DOSAGES   Selected Analgesic Agents

Agent	Pharmacological Class	Usual Dosage Range	Indications
OPIOIDS			
codeine sulphate	Opioid; opiate; opium alkaloid	*Pediatric* PO/SC/IM: 2.5 yr, 2.5–5 mg q4–6h—do not exceed 30 mg/day	Antitussive
		Adult/children >12 yr 10–20 mg q4–6h—do not exceed 120 mg/day	Antitussive
		Pediatric 6–11 yr, 5–10 mg q4–6h	Antitussive
		Adult 15–60 mg tid-qid	Opioid analgesic
meperidine HCl	Opioid; synthetic opioid	*Pediatric* PO/IM/SC: 1–1.5 mg/kg q2–3h prn (max 100 mg/dose) IM/SC: 0.5–1 mg/kg 30–90 min before anaesthesia (max 100 mg/day)	Opioid analgesic, pre-op sedation
		Adult PO/IM/SC: 50–150 mg q2–3h prn IM/SC: 50–100 mg IM/SC: 50–100 mg 30–90 min before anaesthesia IV: 50–150 mg q3–4h	Obstetric analgesia, pre-op sedation
methadone HCl	Opioid; synthetic opioid	*Adult* PO for pain 5–10 mg q3–4h; ≥40 mg daily, reduced doses every few days; for addiction 15–30 mg 1×/day up to 120 mg/day	Opioid analgesic, opioid detoxification, opioid addiction maintenance
▸▸morphine sulphate	Opioid; opiate; opium alkaloid	*Pediatric* SC: 0.1–0.2 mg/kg dose—do not exceed a 15-mg single dose	Opioid analgesic
		Adult PO/IM/SC: 5–30 mg q4h Rectal: 10–20 mg q4h IV: 2.5–15 mg IV: 2.5–20 mg q2–6h PO (sustained release: 15 mg q8h to 200 mg q12h)	Opioid analgesic
▸▸naloxone HCl	Opioid antagonist	*Pediatric* IM/IV/SC: 0.01 mg/kg IV followed by 0.1 mg/kg if needed; 0.005–0.01 mg/kg IV—repeat in 2–3 min intervals	Opioid overdose, post-op reversal
		Adult IM/IV/SC: 0.4–2 mg IV—repeat in 2–3 min if needed; 0.1–0.2 mg IV—repeat in 2–3 min intervals	Opioid overdose, post-op reversal
naltrexone HCl	Opioid antagonist	*Adult* PO: 50 mg daily or 100 mg every other day	Maintenance of opioid-free state
Propoxyphene HCl/napsylate	Analgesic	*Adult* PO: 100 mg q4h prn—do not exceed 600 mg/day	Analgesic

OPIOID/ACETAMINOPHEN COMBINATION PRODUCTS
NOTE: There are many others on the market, including combinations with acetylsalicylic acid

acetaminophen/ oxycodone HCl (trade name Percocet) with various strengths of acetaminophen/ oxycodone ratios: 2.5 mg/325 mg; 5 mg/325 mg (Percocet)	Opioid combination	*Pediatric* 6–12 yr: ¼ tab q6h ≥12 yr, 2.5 mg/325 mg: ½ tab q6h *Adult* 2.5 mg/325 mg: 1–2 tabs PO q6h; (not to exceed 4000 mg acetaminophen/24h, assuming normal liver function) 5 mg/325 mg: 1 tab q6h	Combination opioid/ non-opioid analgesic

Continued

DOSAGES **Selected Analgesic Agents—cont'd**

Agent	Pharmacological Class	Usual Dosage Range	Indications
300 mg acetaminophen/ 15 mg caffeine/ 8 mg codeine (Tylenol No.1) 500 mg acetaminophen/ 15 mg caffeine/ 8 mg codeine (Tylenol No.1 Forte)	Opioid combination	1–2 caplets q4h (not to exceed 12 caplets in 24 hrs) 1–2 caplets 3–4× daily (not to exceed 8 caplets in 24 hrs)	analgesic
300 mg acetaminophen/ 15 mg caffeine/ 15 mg codeine (Tylenol No. 2)	Opioid combination	1–2 tablets q4h	analgesic
300 mg acetaminophen/ 15 mg caffeine/ 30 mg codeine (Tylenol No. 3)	Opioid combination	1–2 tablets q4h	analgesic
300 mg acetaminophen/ 15 mg caffeine/ 60 mg codeine (Tylenol No. 4)	Opioid combination	1–2 tablets q4h	analgesic
NON-OPIOID			
▸▸acetaminophen (Tylenol)	Non-opioid	**Pediatric*** PO/PR for: 6–11 mo, 80 mg q4–6h 12–<24 mo, 120 mg q4–6h 2–<4 yr, 160 mg q4–6h 4–<6 yr, 240 mg q4–6h 6–<9 yr, 320 mg q4–6h 9–<11 yr, 400 mg q4–6h 11–<12 yr, 480 mg q4–6h Maximum daily dose not to exceed 65 mg/kg/24 hrs	Mild to moderate pain relief
		Adult PO/PR 325–650 mg q4–6h; do not exceed 4 g/day In alcoholics do not exceed 2 g/day	Mild to moderate pain relief

NOTE: The maximum recommended daily dose of acetaminophen for a typical adult client with *normal* liver function is 4000 mg per 24-hr period. For hepatically compromised clients, this dosage may be 2000 mg or even lower. If in doubt, check with a pharmacist or prescriber regarding a particular client.
*The Canadian Pediatric Association recommends consultation with a physician for infants under 6 months.

Another method of administering fentanyl is the transdermal delivery system, or the Duragesic patch. It has been shown to be highly effective in the treatment of various chronic types of pain syndromes such as cancer-induced pain. It is recommended that clients never before exposed to opioids be started on the lowest strength patch of 25 μg/hr (2.5 mg/10 cm²). However, prior exposure to opioids is common in many clients. In these clients it is necessary to know the appropriate dose (the equipment dose) of transdermal fentanyl to which to convert the client. Table 10-9 is provided to aid in this conversion. The analgesic potency of 10 mg of intramuscular morphine relative to that of 100 μg of intravenous fentanyl was used by the manufacturer to derive the equivalent potency dose of transdermal fentanyl. Thus a 10-mg intramuscular or 60-mg oral dose of morphine given every 4 hours for 24 hours (60 mg daily intramuscularly

or 360 mg daily orally) was considered by the manufacturer to be approximately equivalent to a transdermal fentanyl system that delivered 100 μg/hr. The transdermal fentanyl doses that should be used and the estimated daily equivalent doses of morphine are listed in Table 10-9. (The table was arranged in this manner to avoid the need to prepare a table for every dosage range.) To perform the conversion shown in this table, first the daily (24-hour) opioid requirement of the client should be determined. Second, if the opioid is not morphine, its dose should be converted to the equianalgesic dose of morphine using Table 10-8. Finally, the equipotent transdermal fentanyl dose can be calculated using Table 10-9.

Most clients will experience adequate pain control for 72 hours with this method of fentanyl delivery. A new patch should be applied every 72 hours (see "Nursing Process" on p. 160).

TABLE 10-8
EQUIANALGESIC OPIOID POTENCY

Opioid Analgesic	Equianalgesic Dose (mg)	
	Parenteral	Oral
afentanil	0.4–0.8	Oral not available
codeine	120	200
fentanyl	0.1–0.2	Oral not available
hydromorphone	2	4–6
meperidine	75	300
methadone	10	20
morphine	10	20–30
oxycodone	Injection not available	30
oxymorphone	1.5	Oral not available
propoxyphene	50	100
sufentanil	0.01–0.04	Oral not available

TABLE 10-9
TRANSDERMAL FENTANYL DOSE

Oral 24-Hour Morphine (mg/day)	Intramuscular 24-Hour Morphine (mg/day)	Transdermal Fentanyl (μg/h)
45–134	8–22	25
135–224	23–37	50
225–314	38–52	75
315–404	53–67	100
405–494	68–82	125
495–584	83–97	150
585–674	98–112	175
675–764	113–127	200
765–854	128–142	225
855–944	143–157	250
945–1034	158–172	275
1035–1124	173–187	300

Fentanyl is contraindicated in clients who have shown a hypersensitivity reaction to opioid analgesics and in those with myasthenia gravis. It is available in transdermal doses of 25 μg/hr (2.5 mg/10 cm^2), 50 μg/hr (5 mg/20 cm^2), 75 μg/hr (7.5 mg/30 cm^2), and 100 μg/hr (10 mg/40 cm^2), and as a 50-μg/mL parenteral injection. The commonly recommended transdermal dosages are determined on the basis of a client's prior opioid use. If a client has no such history, the equianalgesic opioid potency table should be used to determine the equivalent transdermal fentanyl dose. This table is conservative in its doses for achieving pain relief, and often supplemental short-acting opioid analgesics should be added as needed. Dosage titration in clients with fentanyl patches should be done as needed every 72 hours. Pregnancy category C.

PHARMACOKINETICS

	Half-Life	Onset	Peak	Duration
IV	1.5–6 hr	Rapid	Minutes	30–60 min
IM	1.5–6 hr	7–15 min	20–30 min	1–2 hr
Transdermal	Delayed	12–24 hr	48–72 hr	13–40 hr

meperidine hydrochloride

Meperidine hydrochloride is a widely used synthetic opioid analgesic. The misuse potential and addiction liability associated with its use are both high. Meperidine should be used with caution, if at all, in geriatric clients and in clients who require chronic analgesia or who have kidney dysfunction. A metabolite, normeperidine, can accumulate and lead to seizures. After 48 hours, meperidine accumulates in the body and is toxic. The drug is contraindicated in clients showing a hypersensitivity to it and in clients currently or recently treated with MAOIs. The concurrent use of MAOIs and meperidine can lead to deep coma and death. Meperidine is available in 50- and 100-mg tablets and several parenteral (injectable) dosage forms. The usual adult dose ranges from 50 to 150 mg every 3 to 4 hours as needed. Pregnancy category D. For dosage information, see the table on p. 155.

PHARMACOKINETICS

Half-Life	Onset	Peak	Duration
3–5 hr	Rapid	30–60 min	2–4 hr

methadone hydrochloride

Methadone hydrochloride is a synthetic opioid analgesic. The potential for misuse and the addiction liability associated with its use are both high. It is the opioid of choice for the detoxification treatment of opioid addicts. The drug has seen widespread use in the methadone maintenance program. The usual dose for methadone maintenance ranges from 40 to 120 mg or higher, given once daily. Concurrent use of agonist–antagonist opioids (e.g., pentazocine) in heroin-addicted or methadone-maintenance clients can induce significant withdrawal symptoms. Methadone is available in 1-, 5-, 10-, and 40-mg tablets and oral solutions, and a parenteral form. Pregnancy category D. For dosage information, see the table on p. 155.

PHARMACOKINETICS

Half-Life	Onset	Peak	Duration
25 hr	30–60 min	1.5–2 hr	24–48 hr

propoxyphene hydrochloride/napsylate

Propoxyphene hydrochloride is an analgesic agent that is structurally related to methadone. Although it is not as potent as methadone, its misuse potential and addiction liability must be considered. It is used for the relief of mild to moderate pain.

Propoxyphene napsylate is more insoluble than propoxyphene hydrochloride, and this makes for more stable dosage formulations. Dextropropoxyphene hydrochloride is available as a 65-mg tablet in Canada and is equivalent to propoxyphene napsylate available as a 100-mg capsule. It is also commonly prescribed as a fixed combination tablet form with acetaminophen (Darvocet). The usual dosage is 65 mg every 3 to 4 hours or 100 mg every 4 hours as needed. Pregnancy category D. For dosage information, see the table on p. 155.

PHARMACOKINETICS

Half-Life	Onset	Peak	Duration
6–12 hr	0.25–1 hr	2–2.5 hr	4–6 hr

OPIOIDS WITH MIXED ACTIONS

Opioids with mixed actions, often also called *partial agonists* or *agonists–antagonists,* bind to the mu receptor and can therefore compete with other substances for these sites. However, they either exert no actions (i.e., they are competitive antagonists) or have only limited actions (i.e., they are partial agonists). The partial agonist opioid analgesics include buprenorphine hydrochloride, butorphanol, and pentazocine. These agents are similar to the agonist opioid agents from the standpoint of their therapeutic indications. They are potent synthetic analgesics, but their misuse potential and addiction liability are both lower than that of the pure agonist opioids. The antagonistic activity of this group can produce withdrawal symptoms in opioid-dependent clients. They are also contraindicated in clients who have shown hypersensitivity reactions to the drugs.

OPIOID ANTAGONISTS

Opioid antagonists are synthetic derivatives of oxymorphone, a potent semi-synthetic opioid. They produce their opioid antagonistic activity by competing with opioids for CNS receptor sites.

▸▸ *naloxone hydrochloride*

Naloxone hydrochloride is a pure opioid antagonist because it possesses no agonist morphine-like properties and works as a blocking agent to the opioid drugs. Accordingly, the drug does not produce analgesia or respiratory depression. Naloxone is the drug of choice for the complete or partial reversal of opioid-induced respiratory depression. It is also indicated in the diagnosis of suspected acute opioid overdose. If its administration does not significantly reverse the opioid overdose, this indicates that the condition may be due to an overdose of non-opioid drugs or the dosing process. Naloxone is available only in injectable dosage forms, including a 0.4-mg/mL and 1-mg/mL form. The usual adult dose for opioid overdose is 0.4 to 2 mg intravenously (for postoperative opioid depression the dose is 0.1 to 0.2 mg), repeated if necessary at 2- to 3-minute intervals. If an intravenous site is not available, then naloxone may be diluted in sterile water for injection. The drug is contraindicated in clients with a history of hypersensitivity to it. Pregnancy category B. For dosage information, see the table on p. 155.

PHARMACOKINETICS

Half-Life	Onset	Peak	Duration
64 min	<2 min	Rapid	Variable depending on dose and route

naltrexone hydrochloride

Naltrexone hydrochloride is an opioid antagonist used as an adjunct for the maintenance of an opioid-free state in former opioid addicts. In the United States it has been identified as a safe and effective adjunct to psychosocial treatments of alcoholism. Naltrexone hydrochloride is contraindicated in clients with hepatitis or liver dysfunction or failure and is also contraindicated in drug hypersensitivity. Nausea and tachycardia are the most common adverse effects and are related to reversal of the opioid effect. Pregnancy category C. For dosage information, see the table on p. 155.

PHARMACOKINETICS

Half-Life	Onset	Peak	Duration
3.9–12.9 hr	Rapid	1 hr	24–72 hr

MISCELLANEOUS ANALGESIC

Tramadol hydrochloride is categorized as a miscellaneous analgesic because of its unique properties.

tramadol hydrochloride

Tramadol hydrochloride is a centrally acting analgesic with a dual mechanism of action. It creates a weak bond to the mu-opioid receptors and inhibits the reuptake of both norepinephrine and serotonin. Although it does have weak opioid receptor activity, tramadol is not currently classified as a controlled substance. Tramadol is indicated for the treatment of moderate to moderately severe pain. The usual dose is 50 to 100 mg every 4 to 6 hours, up to a maximum of 400 mg daily. Tramadol is available in both 50- and 100-mg tablets. A once-daily form of tramadol is in clinical trials. Tramadol is rapidly absorbed and its absorption is unaffected by food. It is metabolized in the liver to an active metabolite (O-dimethyl tramadol) and eliminated via renal excretion. Adverse effects include drowsiness, dizziness, headache, nausea, and constipation. It is contraindicated in clients who have previously demonstrated hypersensitivity to tramadol, another component of this product, or opioids. It is also contraindicated in cases of acute intoxication with alcohol, hypnotics, centrally acting analgesics, opioids, or psychotropic drugs. Seizures have been reported in clients taking tramadol. These seizures have occurred in clients taking normal doses and doses exceeding normal recommended dosages. Clients who may be at risk are those taking tricyclic antidepressants, selective serotonin reuptake inhibitor (SSRI) antidepressants, MAOIs, neuroleptics, or other drugs that reduce the seizure

---

COMMUNITY HEALTH POINTS ▲

Analgesics

- With most opioids the client's mental and physical abilities may be impaired; therefore the nurse should make every effort to instruct the client, family members, and caregivers about the need for safety measures such as not allowing the client to engage in activities requiring mental alertness (e.g., driving a car or operating any type of machinery).
- The nurse should remind clients that to avoid overdose, different opioids should not be mixed in any form or manner unless prescribed by a practitioner familiar with all of the client's medications.
- The nurse should instruct the client and persons caring for the client about careful and accurate pain assessment and the need to keep a journal containing information about the client's pain, precipitating factors, alleviating factors, and the response to pain medication and non-pharmacological measures.

threshold. Pregnancy category C. This drug is currently unavailable in Canada.

PHARMACOKINETICS

Half-Life	Onset	Peak	Duration
5–8 hr	30 min	2 hr	Unknown

NON-OPIOID ANALGESICS (NON-NARCOTICS): FOCUS ON ACETAMINOPHEN

The primary compound considered a non-opioid analgesic is acetaminophen. All drugs in the NSAID class, which includes acetylsalicylic acid, are also non-opioid analgesics, and these agents are discussed in greater depth in Chapter 43. They are commonly used for pain, especially pain associated with inflammatory conditions such as arthritis, because these medications have significant anti-inflammatory effects in addition to their analgesic effects. Acetaminophen is a non-opioid drug that has both analgesic and antipyretic effects but little to no anti-inflammatory effects. It is available in a variety of dosage formulations, both over the counter (OTC) and by prescription. It is also a component of many combination products with opioids.

Mechanism of Action and Drug Effects

The mechanism of action of acetaminophen is similar to that of the salicylates. It is believed to cause pain impulses to be blocked peripherally, in response to the inhibition of prostaglandin synthesis that is produced by acetaminophen. Acetaminophen is believed to lower the body temperature in clients with fever (but rarely in clients with normal body temperatures) by acting on the hypothalamus, the structure in the brain that regulates body temperature. Heat is dissipated as the result of the vasodilation and increased peripheral blood flow that occur.

The drug effects of acetaminophen are limited primarily to its ability to alter the perception of pain (act as an analgesic) and to lower temperature (act as an antipyretic). It has only weak anti-inflammatory effects, in contrast to NSAIDs and is not used when a primary goal is to decrease inflammation (such as with arthritic processes). Also, acetaminophen products do not have any effects on platelets (as compared to acetylsalicylic acid or NSAIDs). Although acetaminophen shares the analgesic and antipyretic effects of the salicylates and NSAIDs, it does not have many of the unwanted effects. Acetaminophen has no drug effects on the cardiovascular or respiratory systems and is not associated with the acetylsalicylate-related acid–base changes, gastric irritation, erosion, prolonged bleeding, or increased excretion of uric acid.

Indications

Acetaminophen is indicated for the treatment of mild to moderate pain and fever. It is an appropriate substitute for acetylsalicylic acid because of its analgesic and antipyretic uses. Acetaminophen is a valuable alternative for clients who cannot tolerate acetylsalicylic acid or in whom acetylsalicylic acid may be contraindicated.

Contraindications

Contraindications to acetaminophen use include known drug allergy, severe liver disease, and the genetic disease known as *glucose-6-phosphate dehydrogenase (G6PD) enzyme deficiency* (discussed in Chapter 2).

Side Effects and Adverse Effects

Acetaminophen is an effective and relatively safe agent. It is therefore available OTC and in many combination prescription drugs. Acetaminophen is generally well tolerated. Side effects may include rash, nausea, and vomiting. Much less common, but more severe, are the adverse effects of blood disorders or dyscrasias (e.g., anemias) and nephrotoxicities, especially if the dosage ranges are not followed per manufacturer guidelines.

Toxicity and Management of Overdose

Many people do not realize that acetaminophen, despite its OTC status, is a potentially lethal drug when overdosed. Depressed clients (especially adolescents) may intentionally overdose on it as an attention-seeking gesture without realizing the grave danger involved.

The ingestion of large amounts of acetaminophen, as in an acute overdose or even chronic unintentional misuse, can cause hepatic necrosis. This is the most serious acute toxic effect. Acute ingestion of acetaminophen doses of 150 mg/kg or more may result in hepatic toxicity.

The standard maximum daily dose of acetaminophen for healthy adults is 4000 mg per day. In most cases, nurses, physicians, and clients should take care to avoid exceeding this dose. Overdosing may occur inadvertently with combination drug products such as tablets that include a fixed ratio of an opioid agent plus acetaminophen.

The long-term ingestion of large doses of acetaminophen is more likely to result in nephropathy. Because the reported or estimated quantity of drug ingested is often inaccurate and not a reliable guide to the therapeutic management of the overdose, a serum acetaminophen concentration should be determined for this purpose no sooner than 4 hours after the ingestion. If a serum acetaminophen level cannot be determined, it should be assumed that the overdose is potentially toxic and treatment should be started with the recommended antidote, acetylcysteine. Acetylcysteine works by preventing the hepatotoxic metabolites of acetaminophen from forming. The treatment regimen consists of an initial loading dose of 140 mg/kg orally, followed by 70 mg/kg every 4 hours for 17 additional doses. If the client vomits within 1 hour of receiving a dose of acetylcysteine, then that dose should be given again immediately. All 17 doses must be given to prevent hepatotoxicity, regardless of the subsequent acetaminophen serum levels.

Interactions

A variety of substances may interact with acetaminophen. Alcohol is potentially the most dangerous. Chronic, heavy alcohol abusers may be at increased risk of liver toxicity from excessive acetaminophen use. The majority of reports involve cases of severe chronic alcoholics exceeding recommended doses, leading to possible overdose. Healthcare professionals should alert clients with regular intake of moderate to large amounts of alcohol not to exceed recommended doses of acetaminophen because of the risk of liver dysfunction and possible liver failure. Other hepatotoxic drugs should also be avoided. Additional potentially interacting drugs include phenytoin, barbiturates, isoniazid, rifampin, beta-blockers, and anticholinergic agents, all of which are discussed in greater detail in later chapters.

Dosages

For dosage information on acetaminophen, see the dosages table on p. 156. See Appendix B for some of the common drug brands available in Canada.

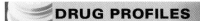

DRUG PROFILES

A variety of drugs could be classified as non-opioid analgesics. Acetaminophen is one of the major drugs in this category and is one of the most widely used non-opioid analgesics. The NSAIDS are discussed in greater detail in Chapter 43.

▶▶ acetaminophen

Acetaminophen is an effective and relatively safe non-opioid analgesic used for mild to moderate pain relief. It is contraindicated in clients with a hypersensitivity to it or an intolerance to tartrazine (yellow dye no. 5), alcohol, sugar, or saccharin. It should be avoided in clients who are anemic or who have renal or hepatic disease. Acetaminophen is available in many oral and rectal dosage formulations. It is available in the form of capsules, solution, suspension, tablets, chewable tablets, film-coated tablets, tablets for solution, and rectal suppositories and in numerous strengths, for use in children or adults. Pregnancy category B. For dosage information, see the table on p. 156.

PHARMACOKINETICS*

Half-Life	Onset	Peak	Duration
1–4 hr	10–30 min	0.5–2 hr	3–4 hr

*For orally administered acetaminophen.

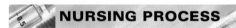

NURSING PROCESS

Clients experiencing pain pose many challenges to the nurse and other healthcare providers. Adequate analgesia, pain relief without complications, and client teaching are all goals of the health care overseen by the nurse. Nurses need to adequately and accurately assess the nature of the client's pain (Box 10-1). Assessment of pain is accepted as a fifth vital sign (along with blood pressure [BP], pulse [P], temperature [T], and respirations [R]). Nurses should also evaluate and monitor the client's response to the analgesic (regardless of whether opioid or non-opioid analgesics are used) to provide safe and effective nursing care. Several organizations and professional groups set standards for pain management. Assessment tools such as the Simple Descriptive Pain Intensity Scale (a 0-to-10 rating scale) and the visual analog scale (VAS) have proved to be valid if the client is capable of answering questions and alert enough to participate in his or her care.

■ Assessment

The management of acute or chronic pain is a common part of clinical practice and a challenging part of nursing and health care. Clients experiencing pain also pose many challenges to significant others or family members. Healthcare providers' goals include adequate analgesia, pain relief without complications, and client teaching. Nurses need to thoroughly assess the nature of the pain and whether it is acute, chronic, or "special."

Before administering an opioid agonist or agonist–antagonist, the nurse should obtain an accurate and thorough medication history to ensure safe use. The nurse should ask and make notes about

- Allergies (to non-opioids [acetaminophen], opioids, partial or mixed agonist–antagonists, pure antagonists)
- Use of other opioids and non-opioid analgesics such as acetaminophen and NSAIDs (the use of other opioids with agonists can lead to toxicity and overdosage; use with agonist–antagonists can lead to an effect antagonistic to the analgesic)
- Use of alcohol
- Pain intensity and character: onset, location, description, intensity, aggravating and relieving factors, previous treatment, and effect of pain on physical and social function
- Severity of pain (e.g., rated on a scale of 1 to 10, with 10 being the worst)
- Type of pain (stabbing, throbbing, dull ache, sharp, diffuse, localized, referred, or knifelike)
- Precipitating and relieving factors
- Home or herbal remedies used and the response to them
- Other pain treatments (both pharmacological and non-pharmacological)

Vital signs (blood pressure, pulse, and respirations) should also be assessed and documented. The nurse should remember that during the acute pain response, stimulation of the sympathetic nervous system (SNS) may result in elevated vital sign values (blood pressure, >120/80 mm Hg, pulse >100 beats/min, respiration >20 breaths/min), and that opioids will depress vital signs. The nurse should always document all findings related to a total-system

BOX 10-1
Assessment of Pain

- Assess factors influencing pain, such as individual reaction; pain tolerance, underlying cause, quality, intensity, duration, type, experience, and threshold; age; physical influences such as sleep and stress; and psychological influences (family roles, spiritual system, meaning of pain, ethnocultural influences, stereotypes, level and stage of growth and development, motivations, personality, fatigue, stress, anxiety, fear). This approach to assessing pain addresses the emotional and psychological components of pain and how they are intertwined with physiological, perceptual, and reflexive components.
- Use a variety of scales to assess pain, such as a numeric rating scale (0 = no pain, 10 = worst possible pain), a VAS, and adjective rating scales (e.g., no pain, little pain, large pain).
- In children under 5 years of age, consider level and stage of growth and development. Pain is often characterized by anger, hostility, and aggressiveness. Use pictures with happy faces (no pain with a scale of "0") and sad faces (pain is "bad" with scale of "5") and tools that the pediatric client can relate to, such as a 15-cm ruler, to show level of pain.
- When assessing geriatric clients, never assume that they do not feel pain as they did when they were younger. Even people with barriers to verbal or nonverbal expression of pain (e.g., dementia, cognitive impairment) experience pain.
- When assessing for chronic pain, consider that pain can occur with or without evident tissue damage and serves

no useful purpose. It is a complex and multifactoral problem that requires a holistic approach, with consideration not only of physical factors but also of psychological factors (insomnia, depression, withdrawal, anxiety, personality changes, and changes in lifestyle). Chronic pain is generally characterized more on the basis of psychological and functional ability changes rather than on physical changes.
- Go the extra mile to assess for chronic pain and then act. Remember that chronic pain is difficult to describe and manage and often not responsive to conventional measures.
- When assessing for cancer pain, remember that this pain should be managed as individually as all other aspects of client care with full belief in the client's pain and suffering. Treatment may include narcotics, possibly in high doses; however, addiction should not be the concern in this situation but rather quality of life for the client.
- Ask the client to keep a daily journal of his or her pain experience, noting precipitating and aggravating factors; measures that alleviate or help the pain; duration and intensity of pain; referred pain; character, onset, and pattern of pain; assessment of his or her meaning of pain; and psychological factors.
- Remember that, in addition to the actual experience of pain, clients with chronic pain and cancer may be suffering from feeling actual or potential loss, including a loss of control.

assessment and continue to monitor (and document) all baseline system-related assessment parameters.

Before administering an opioid, whether a pure agonist or partial agonist, it is essential that the nurse check the route and time of the previous analgesic administration and the client's response. The nurse must always check the client's chart, physician's order, nurses' notes, and medication administration record before administering any additional doses of an analgesic. Clients taking *any* type of analgesic should be reassessed at regular intervals before and during treatment. The 0-to-10 pain rating scale is commonly used.

With regard to the administration of the synthetic agonist–antagonist drugs, it is important for the nurse to determine whether the client is in an addictive state because the administration of an adjunctive opioid may well precipitate withdrawal in such clients. Opioid antagonists such as naloxone hydrochloride and naltrexone have an antagonistic effect on opioid agonists and are used to reverse their effects in the event of toxicity or overdosage from an opioid.

Drug interactions (increased effects) with opioid agonists and agonist–antagonists occur with the following agents: alcohol, other CNS depressants, sedative–hypnotics, muscle relaxants, major tranquilizers, and antipsychotic agents. Opioids are contraindicated in clients with allergies to them, bronchial asthma, opioid addiction, head injuries, and increased intracranial pressure (opioids mask signs and symptoms of possible increasing intracranial pressure from unknown causes or from head injuries). Cautious use, meaning close monitoring of the client's response, reaction, and vital signs during opioid treatment, is called for in clients with any disease or altered state of the liver or kidneys. The nurse should refer to each opioid agonist agent for specific contraindications and cautions.

Contraindications to the use of acetaminophen include intolerance to tartrazine (yellow dye no. 5), alcohol, table sugar, and saccharin. Cautious use is recommended in clients who have anemia, hepatic disease, and chronic alcoholism. The nurse should also monitor liver function studies if long-term therapy is indicated and assess for symptoms of chronic poisoning such as rapid, weak pulse; dyspnea; or cold, clammy extremities. Drug interactions include alcohol, caffeine, colestipol, and cholestyramine.

■ Nursing Diagnoses

Nursing diagnoses appropriate for the client who is taking analgesics include the following:

- Acute pain related to specific pathologies leading to the pain (e.g., chest pain, "fresh" headache, muscle injury)
- Chronic pain related to various pathologies leading to pain (non-cancer pain is usually considered chronic if it occurs for longer than 6 months, e.g., rheumatoid arthritis)
- Risk for injury related to decreased sensorium from opioid agents and associated falls
- Risk for injury related to possible overdosage and severe adverse reactions and/or drug interactions associated with opioids
- Impaired gas exchange related to possible respiratory depression from opioids
- Constipation related to side effects of opioid analgesics
- Risk for infection related to the side effect of urinary retention secondary to the use of opioids and their depressant effects on the CNS
- Deficient knowledge related to unfamiliarity with opioids, their use, and side effects

■ Planning

Goals appropriate to the use of analgesics include the following:

- Client states measures that will enhance the effectiveness of the analgesic.
- Client identifies the rationale and therapeutic and side effects associated with the use of analgesics.
- Client states measures that will decrease the occurrence of commonly associated side effects.

■ *Outcome Criteria*

Outcome criteria related to the use of analgesics are as follows:

- Client demonstrates increased comfort levels as seen by decreased use of analgesics, increased activity, decreased complaints of pain, and decreased rating of pain.
- Client experiences minimal side effects and complications such as nausea, vomiting, and constipation associated with the use of analgesics.
- Client uses non-pharmacological measures such as relaxation therapy, distraction, and music therapy to enhance comfort.
- Client manages side effects associated with analgesics through fluid intake and possible anti-emetic therapy.

■ Implementation

Once the cause of pain has been diagnosed, pain management should begin immediately and aggressively. Pain management is varied, multifaceted, and includes not only pharmacological but also non-pharmacological and alternative approaches to pain relief (see Box 10-2

CASE STUDY

Opioid Administration

Ms. M.B. is 67 years of age and has recently undergone surgery, chemotherapy, and irradiation for breast cancer. She has been in pain after her therapy, for which she has been taking oxycodone/acetaminophen, which has 5 mg of oxycodone and 325 mg of acetaminophen per tablet. Ms. M.B. has been taking two tablets orally (PO) every 4 hours as needed for pain. She has also been taking MS Contin 200 mg SR every 12 hours but remains in pain. Oral thrush has also developed as a result of her chemotherapy and she can no longer tolerate swallowing. The oncology nurse recommends to the physician that Ms. M.B.'s oral medications need to be adjusted or even changed altogether. The physician wants to know her total daily dose of opioids so that the accurate conversion to an equivalent dose of transdermal fentanyl may be made. Answer the following questions using the information provided in the chapter:

- What is the client's total daily dose of oxycodone and morphine?
- What type of side effects and possible complications may occur with the client taking both of these medications, and what information can you share with the client to help decrease these side effects?
- What dose of transdermal fentanyl should this client receive and why?

For answers see http://evolve.elsevier.com/Lilley/pharmacology/.

and the Natural Health Therapies box for feverfew on p. 163). If it is time for the client to receive another dose of an opioid medication, the nurse should administer the opioid, record it in the nurses' notes and medication record, and sign with a full signature. The medication, amount, site, and response should all be documented. When administering opioids, both pure and mixed agents, the nurse must always be sure to medicate clients before the pain becomes severe or when the pain is beginning to return, in order to provide adequate analgesia and pain control. It is often recommended that the oral forms of opioids be taken with food to minimize GI tract upset, specifically nausea. Anti-emetic therapy may be needed if such nausea and vomiting are uncontrollable. Safety measures such as keeping the side rails up (if used in the facility) and placing the bed safety alarm or call bell within the client's reach are crucial to prevent falls stemming from possible confusion, hypotension, and decreased sensorium, especially in the geriatric client.

When administering morphine, meperidine, and similar drugs, the nurse should withhold the dose and contact the physician if there is any decline in the client's condition or if the vital signs are abnormal (see normal values given earlier), especially a respiratory rate of less than 12 breaths/min. When administering an intramuscular injection of an analgesic, the nurse should ensure that the site is adequately and accurately landmarked, skin area

BOX 10-2

Pharmacological and Non-pharmacological Treatment Options for Pain

- Acupressure
- Acupuncture
- Art therapy
- Behavioural therapy
- Comfort measures
- Counselling
- Distraction
- Herbal products
- Hot or cold packs
- Hypnosis
- Imagery
- Massage
- Meditation
- Music therapy
- OTC drugs
- Pet therapy
- Pharmacological cutaneous stimulation
- Prescription drugs
- Reduction of fear
- Relaxation
- Surgery
- Therapeutic baths
- Therapeutic communication
- Therapeutic touch
- Transcutaneous electric nerve stimulation (TENS)
- Yoga

NATURAL HEALTH THERAPIES

FEVERFEW *(Chrysanthemum parthenium)*

Overview
A member of the marigold family known for its anti-inflammatory properties

Common Uses
Treatment of migraine headaches, menstrual problems, arthritis, fever

Adverse Effects
Nausea and vomiting, anorexia, hypersensitivity reactions, muscle stiffness, muscle and joint pain

Potential Drug Interactions
Can increase bleeding with use of acetylsalicylic acid, dipyridamole, and warfarin

Contraindications
Contraindicated in those allergic to ragweed, chrysanthemums, and marigolds, as well as those about to undergo surgery

prepped with an antiseptic (usually a small alcohol swab), and the proper size and gauge needle (usually 22 to 25 gauge, 1½ inch) is used. Analgesics (as well as other parenteral medications) are rarely given intramuscularly, mainly because of the availability of newer dosage forms such as PCA pumps, transdermal patches, and constant subcutaneous or epidural infusions. It is important for the nurse to remember when giving agonists–antagonists that they are effective analgesics when given alone, but when given with other narcotics or given to a client addicted to narcotics they may lead to acute withdrawal and reversal of analgesia. If the client is opioid naïve and not currently taking opioids in any form, partial agents will provide effective analgesia, but reversal will occur with the co-administration of other opioids or narcotics.

There are two basic types of delivery systems for transdermal patch medications such as fentanyl patches. The older reservoir system consists of four layers, beginning with the adhesive layer and ending with the protective backing. Between these two layers are the permeable rate-controlling membrane and the reservoir layer, which holds the drug in a gel or liquid. The newer matrix system consists of two layers: one layer for the active drug with the releasing and adhesive mechanisms within plus the protective impermeable backing layer. The matrix system has several advantages over the reservoir system:

it is slimmer and smaller; it is more comfortable; it is worn for longer (7 days as opposed to 3 to 4 days); and it appears to result in more constant serum drug levels. Additionally, the matrix system is alcohol free; alcohol in the reservoir system often irritates the client's skin. It is important for the nurse to know what type of delivery system is being used in order to follow proper guidelines to enhance the system's effectiveness.

Transdermal patches are to be applied to any clean, non-hairy area and should be changed as ordered and placed on a new site only after the old site has been cleansed. Rotation of sites helps to decrease irritation and enhance drug effects. Transdermal systems are beneficial for many types of medications, especially analgesics, and have the benefit of allowing multi-day therapy with a single application, avoiding first-pass metabolism, improving client adherence, and minimizing frequent dosing. However, the client should be watched carefully for the development of any type of contact dermatitis (the physician or healthcare provider should be contacted immediately if this occurs) and, when at home should maintain a pain journal to inform healthcare professionals and monitor the effectiveness of the medication regimen.

With the intravenous administration of analgesics, the nurse should always follow the insert instructions regarding the diluent and time over which the amount ordered should be delivered. When PCA is used, the amounts and times of dosing should be noted in the appropriate records. When an opioid is used, the nurse should always check and recheck the opioid count and immediately report any errors in counting to the charge nurse, nurse manager, or supervisor. The nurse must never assume that someone else will report or detect the error. The nurse should follow dosage ranges for all non-opioids and opioid drugs, with special consideration given to oxycodone. PCA is an IV infusion controlled by the client and may often be the dosage form of some of the opioids or partial agents when given parenterally (see Chapter 9). However, the nurse is still responsible for monitoring and documenting pain levels, the intravenous needle site, and any side effects or complications. Another point for the nurse to remember when administering analgesics is that each medication, and each route of administration, has a different onset of action, peak, and duration of action. In addition, each client responds differently. See Table 10-10 for opioid administration guidelines. CNS toxicity is always a possibility when administering any type of narcotic or opioid and there is even more risk if the client's renal or liver function is decreased. The nurse must remember to document the client's response to any analgesic, using the 0-to-10 pain scale.

To reverse an opioid overdose or opioid-induced respiratory depression, an opioid antagonist such as naloxone must be administered. If naloxone is the antagonist used, 0.4 to 2 mg should be given either intravenously in its undiluted form and administered over 15 seconds (or as ordered), or the dose should be given as an injection diluted in water, 5 percent dextrose in water, or normal saline solution (see Table 10-7). The guidelines in the package insert should also be followed. Emergency resuscitative equipment should be nearby in the event of respiratory or cardiac arrest.

When administering opioid agonist–antagonist agents such as buprenorphine and nalbuphine, the nurse should remember that they act similarly to the pure opioids when given by themselves; however, when a partial agonist–antagonist is used with a pure opioid, there will be reversal of analgesia, and therefore the same nursing interventions apply. The nurse must be careful to always check the dosages and routes. These drugs, however, have less potential for misuse and addiction than do pure opioids. The nurse should remember that withdrawal symptoms could manifest in individuals who are opioid dependent.

Acetaminophen should be taken as prescribed for all clients, especially pediatric and geriatric clients. Client teaching should emphasize taking the medication as indicated to avoid liver damage and acute toxicity. If a client is taking other OTC medications with acetaminophen, the client should read the labels carefully for other drug–drug interactions. It is important for the nurse to teach the client the signs of acetaminophen overdose. These include bleeding, malaise, fever, sore throat, and easy bruising (due to hepatotoxicity). It is also important for the nurse to inform the client to report fever or pain lasting longer than 3 days, which requires re-evaluation. (Acetylsalicylic acid and NSAIDs are discussed in more depth in Chapter 43.)

To individualize pain management for any type of pain, the nurse should

- At the initiation of pain therapy, review all relevant histories, laboratory values, and diagnostic studies in the client's medical record.
- If there are underlying problems be sure to consider them, but do not forget to treat the client. The nurse

TABLE 10-10

OPIOID ADMINISTRATION GUIDELINES

Narcotic	Nursing Administration
butorphanol	When giving IV, infuse over 3–5 min; always assess respirations. Give IM butorphanol in deep gluteal muscle mass.
codeine	Give PO doses with food to minimize GI tract upset; ceiling effects with oral codeine. Codeine should never be given by direct IV.
fentanyl	IM and IV dosages to be administered slowly and per package insert instructions to prevent muscular rigidity and cardiac arrest; when administered IV or epidurally, should have resuscitative equipment nearby and naloxone at the bedside; patches come in various strengths, so check dosing vs. order very carefully to prevent overdosage; fentanyl will also soon be available in lozenge form for anaesthetic pre-medication in children and adults and an inhalation form is currently in trials for use in breakthrough pain.
hydromorphone	May be given SC, rectally, IV, PO, or IM.
meperidine	Given by a variety of routes; IV, IM, or PO highly protein bound, so watch for interactions and toxicity with PO or IM forms.
methadone	Given PO.
morphine	In a variety of forms: SC, IM, PO, IV, extended and immediate release, and for epidural infusion; morphine sulphate (MS Contin) now available in a 200-mg sustained-release tab.
nalbuphine	IV dosages of 10 mg undiluted over 5 min.
naloxone	Antagonist given for opioid overdose; 0.4 mg usually given IV over 15 seconds or less.
propoxyphene	PO dosing only; high abuse potential.
oxycodone	Often mixed with acetaminophen or acetylsalicylic acid; PO dosage forms. Now available in both immediate and sustained-release tabs.
oxymorphone	IM, IV, and SC dosage forms.
pentazocine	SC, IV, and IM forms; mixed agent; 5 mg IV to be given over 1 min.
sufentanil	Used as adjunct to anaesthesia and so given with oxygen.

must not let the problems overshadow the client's pain.

- Always develop goals for pain management and other aspects of care in conjunction with the client and any family members or significant others.
- Collaborate with other members of the healthcare team to select a regimen that will be easy for the client to follow while in the hospital and, if necessary, at home (e.g., with cancer clients and other chronic pain clients).
- Be aware that most regimens for acute pain include management with short-acting opioids with the addition of other medications such as NSAIDs.
- Be familiar with equianalgesic doses of opioids, because lack of knowledge of equivalencies often leads to inadequate analgesia.
- Use an analgesic appropriate for the situation (e.g., opioids for severe pain secondary to a myocardial infarction, surgery, or kidney stones). For cancer pain, the regimen usually begins with short-acting opioids with eventual conversion to controlled-release formulations and the use of prophylaxis to help avoid side effects. A switch is made to another opioid as soon as possible if the client finds that the medication is intolerable or does not control the pain adequately.

- Consider the option of using adjuvants to analgesia, especially in chronic pain or cancer pain, with the use of other prescribed drugs such as corticosteroids, antidepressants, anticonvulsants, and muscle relaxants.
- Be alert to clients with special needs, such as a client with cancer who is on opioids but needs breakthrough pain management (generally a short-acting version of the long-acting opioid the client is already taking).
- Identify community resources for assistance to the client and any family members or significant others.

Community resources are often located near healthcare facilities. Phone calls to area hospitals may reveal an available pain clinic. Many relevant Web sites can be found by searching using the terms *pain* or *pain clinic.*

Because of the common occurrence of pain in clients of all ages, nurses and other healthcare providers need to think past the basic nursing assessment. A medication history should be taken for all clients, including a list of medications currently used (OTC, prescribed, and

LEGAL and ETHICAL PRINCIPLES

Interventions to Reduce Medication Errors in the Clinical Setting

In the United States more than 600 pharmacists participated in a survey on pharmacy interventions by answering questions about factors facilitating or decreasing pharmacy interventions, types of interventions performed in their pharmacy department, how information was sent out to physicians, and how the information was used. The findings were strongly focused on pharmacy issues, but all healthcare providers can learn from them, especially nurses, who are often the first to assess a client's need for pain medication or intervention.

Assessing the client's health history is an important component of safe care when administering any type of pain medication. For example, the survey revealed a case in which a client who was not diabetic received an oral hypoglycemic agent that so lowered her blood glucose levels that she was admitted to the ICU. Although the client recovered without permanent harm, this is just one concern that healthcare professionals should have when administering medications (especially strong pain medications)—to consider any possible underlying disease processes such as diabetes or liver, kidney, or cardiac disease.

From the Institute for Safe Medication Practices (ISMP). (2002). Pharmacy interventions can reduce clinical errors—Part I of survey findings. *ISMP Medication Safety Alert!*® Newsletter, 7(13), 1–2.

CASE STUDY

Pain Management for Terminal Illness

You are assigned to a client who is in the terminal phases of breast cancer. As a community healthcare nurse, you have many responsibilities; however, you have not cared for many clients who are in the terminal phases of their illness. In fact, most of your clients are post-operative and have only required assessments, dressing changes, and wound care.

Ms. D. is 56 years of age and underwent bilateral mastectomy 4 years ago. She had lymph node involvement at the time of surgery, and recently metastasis to the bone has been diagnosed. She has been taking one 5-mg oxycodone/325-mg acetaminophen tablet q6h at home but is not sleeping through the night and is now complaining of increasing pain to the point that her quality of life has decreased significantly. She wants to stay at home during the terminal phases of her illness but needs to have adequate and safe pain control. Her husband of 28 years is very supportive. They have no children. They are both college graduates.

- Ms. D's recent increase in pain has been attributed to bone metastasis in the area of the lumbar spine. At this time the oxycodone is not beneficial, and you as the community healthcare nurse need to recommend another pain medication to the physician. What medication would you recommend to relieve the bone pain, and what is your rationale for this recommendation? (Provide references from within this chapter for the selection of the specific opioid agent.)
- Identify the client education guidelines for the specific medication you recommended to the physician.
- Outline a comprehensive nursing care plan appropriate to the specific agent used or recommended.

For answers see http://evolve.elsevier.com/Lilley/pharmacology/.

herbal); medication interactions; all medical and psychological pathological disorders; and any medications currently used that have adverse effects that put the client at risk for falls and possible injury, including dizziness, hypotension, postural hypotension, sedation, altered sensorium, and altered level of consciousness. It is important for nurses to assess clients for the potential for falls and to make sure that they take great care to prevent falls, whether by simply checking on a client frequently after he or she has received analgesics, placing a client on a frequent "watch" program, or, in extreme circumstances, getting an order for restraints. If a nurse decides that restraint is necessary to prevent falls, the nurse must follow the facility's policy and procedure regarding orders for and application of restraints and subsequent nursing care. Restraints themselves can cause many injuries; therefore, many facilities never use physical restraints, others have procedures to minimize risks. The nurse should assess, monitor, evaluate, and document the reason for the restraint, as well as document the client's behaviour, type of restraint, and the assessment of the client after the placement of restraints.

For more specific information regarding client teaching, see Client Teaching Tips.

■ Evaluation

During and after the administration of opioid or nonopioid analgesics, it is important for the nurse to monitor the client for both therapeutic and side effects. Therapeutic effects include decreased complaints of pain and increased periods of comfort, with improved activities of daily living (ADL), appetite, and sense of well-being. Side effects vary with each drug (see discussion earlier in this chapter) but often consist of nausea, vomiting, constipation, dizziness, headache, blurred vision, decreased urinary output, drowsiness, lethargy, sedation, palpitations, bradycardia, bradypnea, dyspnea, and hypotension. Should vital signs change, the client's condition decline, or pain continue, the nurse should contact the physician immediately. Respiratory depression may be manifested by a rate of less than 12 breaths/min, dyspnea, diminished breath sounds, and/or shallow breathing.

Positive therapeutic outcomes of acetaminophen use are decreased symptomatology, fever, and pain. Adverse reactions for which the nurse should monitor include anemia and the previously mentioned liver problems with hepatotoxicity. In addition, abdominal pain and vomiting should be reported to the physician.

Although many clients benefit from the administration of prescribed opioids alone, other medications may be needed to help enhance the effects of opioids. During the evaluation process, the nurse should not forget to also evaluate the multimodal approaches to pain management such as relaxation, imagery, art, pet therapy, massage, acupuncture, and music therapy. The nurse should evaluate pain management effectiveness by determining the degree, duration, and nature of pain experienced with drug therapy and by evaluating and reassessing for any new or different complaints of pain.

CLIENT TEACHING TIPS

The nurse should teach the client the following:
▲ To keep a record or journal of his or her pain experience and all methods of treatment, both pharmacological and non-pharmacological.
▲ To follow instructions on the medication vial or bottle regarding the dose, route, and frequency of the medication. Following instructions closely is essential to preventing toxicity or overdose that may result in cardiac or respiratory arrest.
▲ To contact the physician or healthcare provider if emesis occurs while the client is taking an opioid, because nausea and vomiting are common side effects; often medication is needed to alleviate the nausea.
▲ That constipation is a common side effect of opioid use and may be prevented with forced fluids (unless contraindicated) and a high-fibre diet.
▲ To contact the physician should the client show symptoms of allergic reaction such as wheezing or difficulty breathing; itching, rash, or hives; or CNS changes such as weakness, dizziness, or fainting.
▲ The withdrawal symptoms associated with opioids: chills, anxiety, irritability, nausea, vomiting, cramps, fainting spells (syncope), and fever.

▲ To carefully read the directions on all prescription containers as well as on any OTC medications for possible contraindications or drug interactions.
▲ The side effects of analgesics: GI tract upset, constipation, drowsiness, dizziness, headache, sleepiness, tinnitus (ringing of the ears), blurred vision, palpitations, bradycardia, and hypotension.
▲ To change positions slowly to prevent possible orthostatic hypotension.
▲ To inform his or her healthcare providers of the client's use of herbals or homeopathic remedies.
▲ About the risk of dangerous drug interactions if the client does not regularly inform his or her healthcare providers of all medications used. This is important because many prescribed and OTC analgesics may contain the analgesic the client is already taking (e.g., Tylenol PM and cough and cold preparations have varying amounts of acetaminophen, NSAIDs, or even acetylsalicylic acid). Product replication would then be avoided.

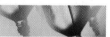

POINTS to REMEMBER

▼ Pain is individualized and involves unpleasant sensations and emotions.

▼ Pain is associated with actual or potential tissue damage and may be worsened (exacerbated) or alleviated depending on the treatment and type of pain.

▼ Pain may be acute or chronic, somatic or superficial.

▼ Analgesics relieve pain without causing loss of consciousness.

▼ Types of analgesics are as follows:
  • Non-opioids include acetaminophen, acetylsalicylic acid, and NSAIDs.
  • Opioids are natural or synthetic agents that either contain or are derived from morphine (opiates)

or have opiate-like effects or activities (opioids). There are pure opioid agonists and partial opioid agonist–antagonist agents.

▼ Nursing considerations include the following:
  • Pain must be managed before it gets uncontrollable.
  • A non-opioid agent is used first in most situations of mild to moderate pain, depending on the pain rating and cause.
  • Stronger analgesics, such as opioids, are used as a next step to pain control (especially moderate to severe pain and special situations such as pain related to cancer). Always document response(s) of the client to the type of pain medication administered.

EXAMINATION REVIEW QUESTIONS

1 A pure narcotic agonist may be used in the treatment of osteoarthritis for the management of which of the following?
  a. Bleeding
  b. Pain
  c. Blood clot formation
  d. Inflammation

2 Which of the following drug classes interact adversely with a pure narcotic agonist?
  a. Acetylsalicylic acid derivatives
  b. CNS depressants
  c. Antihypertensives
  d. Renal toxic drugs

3 Which of the following would be a benefit of using transdermal fentanyl patches in the management of bone pain from the spread of cancer?
  a. More analgesia for longer time periods
  b. Less constipation and minimal dry mouth
  c. Greater CNS stimulation than with oral narcotics
  d. Lower dependency potential and no major side effects

4 You suspect that your client is showing signs of respiratory depression. Which of the following drugs could result in this complication?
  a. Naloxone (Narcan)
  b. Hydromorphone (Dilaudid)
  c. Methamphetamine
  d. Transdermal nicotine patch

5 Which of the following statements best describes the rationale for avoiding the use of narcotics, such as oral meperidine, in cancer clients?
  a. Mood alterations and euphoria are side effects and may be addicting.
  b. Mu receptor stimulation is never indicated and may cause seizure.
  c. It is similar to ultra–long-acting barbiturates and, as such, works well for these clients.
  d. Oral meperidine has a short duration of action and is not available in alternate dosage forms or routes that could be more effective.

For answers see http://evolve.elsevier.com/Lilley/pharmacology/.

CRITICAL THINKING ACTIVITIES

1 What is the purpose of a "drug holiday" with clients who are taking narcotics on a long-term basis?

2 Indicate whether this statement is true or false and explain your answer: Cancer clients should never receive strong narcotics at the beginning of any pain experience because of the fear of addiction.

3 You administer 100 mg meperidine (Demerol) intramuscularly to a client in severe post-operative pain, as ordered. What assessment data should be gathered before and after administering this drug? Explain your answer.

4 Your client complains that the drugs he is receiving for severe pain are really not helping. What would be the most appropriate response to this client?

5 Compare and contrast the effectiveness of oral, intramuscular, and transdermal routes for narcotic administration, considering ease of self-preparation and administration, onset of therapeutic serum concentrations, degree of sedation, side effects, and ease of management in the home setting.

For answers see http://evolve.elsevier.com/Lilley/pharmacology/.

BIBLIOGRAPHY

American Academy of Pain Medicine and American Pain Society: The use of opioids for the treatment of chronic pain, Sept 6, 2001. Retrieved August 1, 2005, from http://www.ampainsoc.org/advocacy/opioids.htm

Anderson, P.O., Knoben, J.E., & Troutman, W.G. (2002). *Handbook of clinical drug data* (10th ed.). New York: McGraw-Hill/Appleton & Lange.

Bral, E.E. (1998). Caring for adults with chronic cancer pain. *American Journal of Nursing, 98* (4), 26.

Canadian Pharmacists Association. (2003). *Therapeutic choices* (4th ed.). Ottawa, ON: Author.

Canadian Pharmacists Association. (2004). *Guide to drugs in Canada.* Toronto, ON: Dorling Kindersley.

Canadian Pharmacists Association. (2005). *Compendium of pharmaceuticals and specialties. The Canadian drug reference for health professionals.* Ottawa, ON: Author. [The subscription-based e-CPS is available at http://www.pharmacists.ca.]

Canadian Consortium on Pain Mechanisms Diagnosis and Management. (2001). The pain experience in Canada. Retrieved July 26, 2005, from http://www.curepain.ca/final3.htm

Elmi A.S. (1999.) *A study on the mental health needs of the Somali community in Toronto.* Toronto, ON: York Community Services Rexdale Community Health Centre. Retrieved August 15, 2005, from http://ceris.metropolis.net/Virtual%20Library/health/elmi1.pdf

Facts and Comparisons. (2004). *Drug facts and comparisons, pocket version* (9th ed.). St Louis, MO: Wolters Kluwer Health.

Gottschalk, A. & Smith, D.S. (2001). New concepts in acute pain therapy: Preemptive analgesia. [Electronic version.] *American Family Physician, 63,* 1979–84, 1985–6.

Hardman, J.G., & Limbird, L.E. (2002). *Goodman and Gilman's the pharmacological basis of therapeutics* (10th ed.). New York: McGraw-Hill.

Health Canada. (2005). Drug product database. Retrieved July 27, 2005, from http://www.hc-sc.gc.ca/hpb/drugs-dpd/

Herman, R.J. (1999). Drug interactions and the statins. *Canadian Medical Association Journal, 161*(10), 1281–1286.

Horgas, A. (2003). Pain management in elderly adults. *Journal of Infusion Nursing, 26*(3), 161–165.

Howard, R.F. (2003). Current status of pain management in children [Special communication]. *The Journal of the American Medical Association, 290*(18), 2464–2469.

Institute for Safe Medication Practices. (2002). Pharmacy interventions can reduce clinical errors—Part 1 of findings from ISMP survey. *ISMP Med Safety Alert,* June 26 issue.

Jovey, R.D., Ennis, J., Gardner-Nix, J., Goldman, B., Hays, H., Lynch., M., et al. (2003). Use of opioid analgesics for the treatment of chronic noncancer pain. A consensus statement and guidelines from the Canadian Pain Society. [Electronic version.] *Pain Research and Management (Supplement), 8,* 3A–14A.

Kasper, D.L., Braunwald, E., Faucey, A., Hauser, S., Longo, D., & Jameson, J.L. (2005). *Harrison's principles of internal medicine* (16th ed.). New York: McGraw-Hill.

Lehne, R.A. (2004). *Pharmacology for nursing care* (5th ed.). St Louis, MO: Saunders.

McCaffery, M., & Pasero, C. (1999). *Pain: clinical manual* (2nd ed.). St Louis, MO: Mosby.

Mosby. (2005). *Mosby's drug consult 2005: The comprehensive reference for generic and brand name drugs* (15th ed.). St Louis, MO: Mosby.

Pasero, C. (1997). Transdermal fentanyl for chronic pain. *American Journal of Nursing, 97*(11), 17.

Skidmore-Roth, L. (2006). *Mosby's 2006 nursing drug reference* (19th ed.). St Louis, MO: Mosby.

Stanik-Hutt, J.A. (2003). Pain management in the critically ill. *Critical Care Nurse, 23*(2), 99.

General and Local Anaesthetics

OBJECTIVES

After reading this chapter, the successful student will be able to do the following:

1 Define anaesthesia.

2 Discuss the differences between and indications for general and local anaesthetics.

3 List the most commonly used general and local anaesthetics with their associated risk factors.

4 Briefly describe the process of anaesthesia, varying levels of consciousness, and nursing considerations appropriate to the various anaesthetics and changes in consciousness.

5 Discuss the differences between depolarizing neuromuscular blocking agents (NMBAs) and non-depolarizing NMBAs.

6 Compare the mechanism of action, indications, side effects, cautions, contraindications, and prioritized nursing implementations for general anaesthesia, local anaesthesia, anaesthesia with depolarizing NMBAs and non-depolarizing NMBAs, and moderate sedation.

7 Develop a nursing care plan that includes pre-anaesthesia and post-anaesthesia care for clients receiving general anaesthesia, local anaesthesia, anaesthesia with NMBAs, and/or moderate sedation.

e-LEARNING ACTIVITIES

Student CD-ROM
- Review Questions: see questions 49–55
- Animations
- Medication Administration Checklists
- IV Therapy Checklists

evolve Web site (http://evolve.elsevier.com/Lilley/pharmacology/)
- Online Chapter Worksheet • Frequently Asked Questions
- Learning Tips and Content Updates • WebLinks • Online Appendices and Supplements • Mosby/Saunders ePharmacology Update • Access to *Mosby's Drug Consult*

DRUG PROFILES

enflurane, p. 173
halothane, p. 173
isoflurane, p. 173
ketamine, p. 173
▸▸lidocaine, p. 176
nitrous oxide, p. 173

pancuronium, p. 180
▸▸propofol, p. 173
▸▸rocuronium bromide, p. 180
sevoflurane, p. 173
▸▸succinylcholine, p. 179

▸▸ Key drug.

GLOSSARY

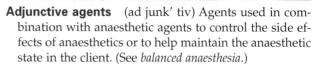

Adjunctive agents (ad junk' tiv) Agents used in combination with anaesthetic agents to control the side effects of anaesthetics or to help maintain the anaesthetic state in the client. (See *balanced anaesthesia*.)

Anaesthesia (an es thee' zhə) A drug-induced state in which the central nervous system (CNS) is altered to produce varying degrees of pain relief, depression of consciousness, skeletal muscle relaxation, and diminished or absent reflexes.

Anaesthetics (an es the' tiks) Agents that depress the CNS to produce depression of consciousness, loss of responsiveness to sensory stimulation, or muscle relaxation.

Balanced anaesthesia The practice of using combinations of drugs rather than a single agent to produce anaesthesia. Common components include sedative–hypnotics, anti-anxiety agents, analgesics, anti-emetics, and anticholinergics.

General anaesthetics Agents that induce a state of global anaesthesia in the whole body, with loss of consciousness.

Local anaesthetics Agents that render a specific portion of the body insensitive to pain without affecting consciousness. Also called *regional anaesthetics.*

Minimum alveolar concentration (MAC) The minimal concentration of the gas in the lungs that is needed to provide anaesthesia in 50% of subjects.

Moderate sedation A form of anaesthesia using combinations of parenteral benzodiazepines and an opiate. It reduces anxiety, sensitivity to pain, and recall of the procedure (also called *conscious sedation*).

Overton-Meyer theory A theory that describes the relationship between the lipid solubility of anaesthetic agents and their potency. It is often used to explain how anaesthetic agents are believed to work.

Parenteral anaesthetics (pə ren′ tər əl) Agents that can be administered directly into the CNS by various spinal injection techniques. In addition, they can be injected adjacent to main nerves to accomplish anaesthesia of the peripheral nervous system.

Rapid Sequence Intubation (RSI) A technique of intubation where a potent sedative or induction agent is administered almost simultaneously with a paralyzing dose of a neuromuscular blocking agent to facilitate rapid tracheal intubation.

Topical anaesthetics A class of local anaesthetics that are applied directly to the skin and mucous membranes. They consist of solutions, ointments, gels, creams, powders, ophthalmic drops, and suppositories.

Anaesthetics are agents that depress the central nervous system (CNS), which in turn produces depression of consciousness, loss of responsiveness to sensory stimulation (including pain), or muscle relaxation. This state of depressed CNS activity is called **anaesthesia.** Anaesthetics accomplish these responses by many mechanisms, but in general they do so by interfering with nerve conduction. They can produce one or all of the actions just mentioned, depending on the agent. Anaesthetics are most commonly classified as either general anaesthetics or local anaesthetics, depending on where in the CNS the particular anaesthetic agent works.

GENERAL ANAESTHETICS

A **general anaesthetic** is an agent that induces a state in which the CNS is altered so that varying degrees of pain relief, depression of consciousness, skeletal muscle relaxation, and reflex reduction are produced. General anaesthesia can be achieved by the use of one drug or a combination of drugs. Often a combination of drugs is used to accomplish general anaesthesia, allowing less of each of the agents to be used and a more balanced, controlled state of anaesthesia to be achieved. General anaesthetic agents are used most commonly to produce deep muscle relaxation and loss of consciousness during surgical procedures. For a historical perspective on general anaesthesia, see Box 11-1.

General anaesthetics are categorized by their routes of administration: mainly inhaled and injectable. Inhaled anaesthetics are volatile liquids or gases that are vaporized in oxygen and inhaled to induce anaesthesia. Injectable anaesthetics are administered intravenously. The different inhaled gases and volatile liquids used as general anaesthetics are listed in Table 11-1.

Intravenously administered anaesthetic agents are used to induce or maintain general anaesthesia, to induce amnesia, and as an adjunct to inhalation-type anaesthetics.

BOX 11-1

General Anaesthesia: An Historical Perspective

Until recently, general anaesthesia was described as having several definitive stages. This was especially true with many of the ether-based inhaled anaesthetic agents. Features of these distinctive stages were easily observable to the trained eye. They included specific physical and physiological changes that progressed gradually and predictably with the depth of the client's anaesthetized state. Gradual changes in pupil size, progression from thoracic to diaphragmatic breathing, vital sign changes, and several other changes all characterized the various stages. However, newer inhalational and IV general anaesthetic drugs often have a much more rapid onset of action and body distribution. As a result, the stages of anaesthesia are no longer sufficiently well defined to be observable. Thus the concept of "stages of anaesthesia" is an outdated one in most modern surgical facilities.

In the United States, registered nurses can pursue advanced training to become a Certified Registered Nurse Anaesthetist (CRNA). This requires a minimum of two years' extensive training and education in the specialty of anaesthesia. A CRNA administers all types of anaesthesia, performs preoperative assessments, and monitors the client in the post-operative period. CRNAs often find this to be a rewarding and interesting area of nursing practice. Some nurses also find that this type of work offers greater flexibility in their work schedule than do other practice areas.

TABLE 11-1

INHALED GENERAL ANAESTHETICS

INHALED GAS
nitrous oxide ("laughing gas")

INHALED VOLATILE LIQUID
desflurane
enflurane
halothane
isoflurane
sevoflurane

TABLE 11-2

INTRAVENOUS ANAESTHETIC AGENTS

Generic Name	Dosage
ketamine	1–4.5 mg/kg IV; 6.5–13 mg/kg IM
propofol†	2–2.5 mg/kg IV (induction); 0.1–0.2 mg/kg/min IV (maintenance)
thiopental	25–250 mg IV as needed

†Dosages for propofol are typically 5–50 mg/kg/min for initiation and maintenance of intensive care unit (ICU) sedation.

These **adjunctive agents** commonly include sedative–hypnotics (barbiturates [e.g., thiopental] and benzodiazepines [e.g., diazepam, midazolam]), narcotics (e.g., morphine sulphate, fentanyl, sufentanil), propofol, and neuromuscular blocking agents (NMBAs) (depolarizing agents [e.g., succinylcholine] and non-depolarizing or competitive agents [e.g., atracurium, mivacurium, pancuronium, rocuronium]). **Balanced anaesthesia** is the use of minimal doses of each anaesthetic agent to achieve the desired level of anaesthesia for the surgical procedure. Such combinations make general anaesthesia possible with smaller amounts of anaesthetic gases, thereby lessening side effects such as dry mouth, bradycardia, nausea, and vomiting. Other than the inhalation drugs, almost all of the agents used in balanced anaesthesia are administered intravenously. The intravenous (IV) anaesthetics, their dosage forms, and the usual doses are listed in Table 11-2. Table 11-3 contains a brief list of the adjunctive agents. These agents are discussed in greater detail in chapters devoted to discussion of the respective classes of agents.

Mechanism of Action and Drug Effects

Many theories have been proposed to explain the actual mechanism of action of general anaesthetics. However, the agents vary widely in their chemical structure and therefore their mechanism of action is not easily explained by a structure–receptor relationship. The concentrations required for different anaesthetics to produce a given state of anaesthesia also differ greatly. The **Overton-Meyer theory** explains some of the properties of anaesthetic agents that may make the mechanism of action of these agents easier to understand. This theory states that there is a relationship between the lipid solubility of an anaesthetic agent and its potency: the greater the solubility of the agent in fat, the greater the effect. Nerve cell membranes have a high lipid content, as does the blood–brain barrier. Anaesthetic agents can therefore easily cross this blood–brain barrier and concentrate in nerve cell membranes. Initially

this produces a loss of the senses of sight, touch, taste, smell, awareness, and hearing, and usually the client becomes unconscious. Even though the heart and lungs (the vital centres responsible for blood pressure and breathing) are controlled by the medulla, they can usually be spared because the medullary centre is depressed last.

Newer data suggest that inhalation anaesthetics activate receptors for gamma-aminobutyric acid (GABA) and cause generalized inhibition of CNS function. GABA is the main inhibitory neurotransmitter in the CNS. It is likely that inhalation anaesthetics activate GABA receptors in two ways. They bind to GABA receptors either at high concentrations, causing direct receptor activation, or at low concentrations, enhancing the effects of GABA (rather than activating receptors directly).

The overall effect of general anaesthetics is an orderly and systematic reduction of sensory and motor CNS functions. They produce a progressive depression of cerebral and spinal cord functions. Therapeutic (anaesthetic) doses cause minimal depression of the medullary centres that govern vital functions. However, an anaesthetic overdose can paralyze the medullary centres, leading to death from circulatory and respiratory failure. The progressive paralysis of nervous system functions produced by general anaesthetics and the level of decreased CNS functioning depends on the anaesthetic used and the dosage and route of administration. The reactions from the CNS to these general anaesthetics are presented in Table 11-4. The previously distinct and identifiable stages of anaesthesia now exist more on a continuum with the newer generation anaesthetics discussed in this chapter. This is especially the case with the now-standardized use of balanced anaesthesia and moderate sedation. Therefore, rather than focusing on the older concept of stages of anaesthesia, the nurse should focus on the agents used and their characteristics, actions, and adverse effects, including any toxic effects.

The **minimum alveolar concentration (MAC)** measures the anaesthetic potency of volatile anaesthetics. This value

TABLE 11-3
ADJUNCTIVE ANAESTHETIC AGENTS

Agent	Pharmacological Class	Usual Dosage Range	Indications
alfentanil fentanyl sufentanil	Opioid analgesic	130–245 µg/kg IV 50–100 µg/kg IV 8–30 µg/kg IV	To induce anaesthesia
diazepam lorazepam midazolam	Benzodiazepine	2–20 mg PO/IV/IM 0.05–0.35 mg/kg IV	To induce amnesia and reduce anxiety
atropine glycopyrrolate scopolamine	Anticholinergic	0.1–0.6 mg IV/IV/SC 0.005 mg/kg IM 0.4–0.6 mg SC/IM	To dry up excessive secretions
meperidine morphine	Opioid analgesic	50–100 mg IM/SC 5–20 mg IM/SC	To prevent and relieve pain
pentobarbital promethazine	Sedative–hypnotic	150–200 mg IM 25–50 mg IM 100 mg PO	To induce amnesia and sedation

IM, intramuscular; *IV*, Intravenous; *PO*, per orally; *SC*, subcutaneous.

TABLE 11-4

EFFECTS OF INHALED AND INTRAVENOUS GENERAL ANAESTHETICS

Organ/System	Reaction
Respiratory	Depressed muscles and patterns of respiration; altered gas exchange and impaired oxygenation; depressed airway protective mechanisms; airway irritation, possible laryngospasms
Cardiovascular	Depressed myocardium; hypotension and tachycardia; bradycardia in response to vagal stimulation
Cerebrovascular	Increased intracranial blood volume and increased intracranial pressure
Gastrointestinal	Reduced hepatic blood flow and so reduced hepatic clearance
Renal	Decreased glomerular filtration
Skeletal muscles	Skeletal muscle relaxation
Cutaneous circulation	Vasodilation
Central nervous system	CNS depression; blurred vision; nystagmus; progression of CNS depression to decreased alertness and sensorium as well as decreased level of consciousness

represents the minimum amount of alveolar air concentration of an inhaled anaesthetic that is required to prevent movement in 50% of the clients in response to pain. By knowing the MAC, the anaesthesiologist will know how much anaesthetic must be in the inspired air to produce anaesthesia. Generally, the alveolar concentration of the gas equals the blood concentration and, a short time later, equals the brain concentration so it can indicate anaesthetic potency. MAC is age-dependent; it is lowest in newborns, peaks in infants, and then decreases progressively with increasing age. MAC values for inhaled anaesthetics are additive; the addition of nitrous oxide (the MAC of nitrous oxide is high) will decrease the MAC of another volatile anaesthetic. The MAC can also be altered following administration of other drugs such as opioids and lithium.

Indications

General anaesthetics are used to produce unconsciousness, skeletal muscular relaxation, and visceral smooth muscle relaxation for surgical procedures.

Contraindications

Contraindications to the various types of anaesthetic agents include known drug allergy and may include pregnancy, narrow angle glaucoma, and known susceptibility to malignant hyperthermia from prior anaesthetic experiences.

Side Effects and Adverse Effects

The adverse effects of general anaesthetics are dose dependent and vary with the individual agents. The heart, peripheral circulation, liver, kidneys, and respiratory tract are the sites primarily affected. Myocardial depression is a common side effect. All of the halogenated anaesthetics are capable of causing hepatotoxicity.

With the development and use of newer agents, many of the unwanted side effects of the older agents (such as hepatotoxicity and myocardial depression) are now a thing of the past. In addition, many of the bothersome side effects such as nausea, vomiting, and confusion have become less common since balanced anaesthesia has become more widely used. This practice prevents many of the unwanted, dose-dependent side effects and toxicity associated with the anaesthetic agents while simultaneously achieving a more balanced general anaesthesia. One medication with a long history of use for prevention or control of post-operative nausea and vomiting is droperidol. Its common dosage range is 0.625 to 1.25 mg intravenously or intramuscularly (IM) every 4 to 6 hours as needed.

Toxicity and Management of Overdose

In large doses all anaesthetics are potentially life threatening, with cardiac and respiratory arrest the ultimate causes of death. However, these agents are almost exclusively administered in a controlled environment by personnel trained in advanced cardiac life support. These agents are also quickly metabolized. In addition, the medullary centre, which governs the vital centres, is the last area of the brain to be affected by anaesthetics and the first to regain function if it is lost. These factors combined make an anaesthetic overdose rare and easily reversible. Symptomatic and supportive therapy, primarily of circulatory and respiratory functions, is usually all that is needed in the event of an anaesthetic overdose.

Malignant hyperthermia is a rare autosomal dominant disorder that can cause a potentially fatal reaction to general anaesthetics. In response to most inhaled anaesthetics (the exception is nitrous oxide) and to the muscle relaxant succinylcholine, a rapid rise in temperature occurs in clients with this disorder, and abnormal calcium regulation in skeletal muscle cells causes severe muscle contractions.

Interactions

Because general anaesthetics produce both desired and adverse effects on so many body systems, they are associated with a wide array of drug interactions that also vary widely in severity. Some of the more common drug–drug interactions occur with antihypertensives, beta-blockers, and tetracycline. These agents have additive effects when given with general anaesthetics. When given with antihypertensives, general anaesthetics may result in increased hypotensive effects; with beta-blockers, increased myocardial depression; and with tetracycline, increased renal toxicity. No significant laboratory test interactions have been reported.

Dosages

For the recommended dosages of selected general anaesthetic agents, see the dosages table on p. 173. See Appendix B for some of the common brands available in Canada.

DOSAGES Selected General Anaesthetic Agents

Agent	Pharmacological Class	Usual Dosage Range	Indications
enflurane	Inhalation general anaesthetic (halogenated ether)	0.5%–3% concentration	General anaesthesia
halothane	Halogenated inhalation general anaesthetic	0.5%–1.5% concentration	General anaesthesia
isoflurane	Inhalation general anaesthetic (enflurane isomer)	0.1%–2% concentration with appropriate drugs	General anaesthesia
nitrous oxide ("laughing gas")	Inorganic inhalation general anaesthetic	20%–40% with oxygen 70% with 30% oxygen	Analgesia Anaesthesia

DRUG PROFILES

All of the agents used for general anaesthesia are, of course, prescription-only drugs. Desflurane, enflurane, sevoflurane, halothane, and isoflurane are all volatile liquids; nitrous oxide is a gas. The dose of each agent depends on the surgical procedure to be performed and the physical characteristics of the client. All of the general anaesthetics have a rapid onset of activity that is maintained for the duration of the surgical procedure by continuous administration of the agent. Propofol is chemically unrelated to the other intravenous anaesthetic agents. Its favourable pharmacokinetics, quick onset of anaesthesia, and quick offset have made it a widely used and attractive agent.

enflurane

Enflurane is a fluorinated ether that produces good muscular relaxation and minimal cardiac sensitivity to catecholamines. The drug can produce seizures in clients who develop hypocapnia (low blood carbon dioxide levels) during anaesthesia and therefore should not be used in clients with convulsive disorders. Dosage information is given in the table above.

halothane

Halothane is a halogenated hydrocarbon (containing three atoms of fluorine and one each of chlorine and bromine) that is commonly used with nitrous oxide. It was a mainstay of general anaesthesia for many years and is still on the Canadian market. However, it causes considerable cardiac sensitivity to catecholamines, it produces poor muscular relaxation when used alone, and its high halogen content can result in significant liver toxicity. Because of these limitations and toxicities, halothane is now less commonly used than the newer, less toxic inhalational anaesthetics. Dosage information is given in the table above.

isoflurane

Isoflurane is similar to enflurane in its chemical structure. However, the differences in its chemical structure give it some favourable characteristics that distinguish it from its chemical relative. Isoflurane has a more rapid onset of action, causes less cardiovascular depression, and overall has been associated with little or no toxicity. Dosage information is given in the table above.

nitrous oxide

Nitrous oxide, also known as "laughing gas," is the only inhaled gas currently used as a general anaesthetic. It is the weakest of the general anaesthetic agents and is primarily used for dental procedures or as a useful supplement to other more potent anaesthetics. Dosage information is given in the table above.

▸▸ propofol

Propofol is an IV sedative–hypnotic agent used for the induction and maintenance of anaesthesia or sedation. Propofol has many favourable characteristics that have led to its widespread use. It produces its effects rapidly, and when it is turned off its effects subside quickly. Propofol also is typically well tolerated, producing few undesirable effects. Propofol can be used to initiate and maintain monitored anaesthesia care sedation during diagnostic procedures in adults. It is also used in intubated, mechanically ventilated adult clients in the intensive care unit (ICU) to provide continuous sedation and control of stress responses. When used in the ICU, typical doses are 5 to 50 mg/kg/min. At higher doses it can be used for induction and maintenance of general anaesthesia. Dosage information is provided in Table 11-2.

sevoflurane

Sevoflurane is another fluorinated ether that is becoming more widely used in Canada following several years of successful use in Japan. Its rapid onset and recovery pharmacokinetics make it especially useful in outpatient surgery settings. It is not irritating to the airway, which greatly facilitates induction of the unconscious state, especially in pediatric clients.

LOCAL ANAESTHETICS

Local anaesthetics are the second class of anaesthetics. They are also called *regional anaesthetics* because they render a specific portion of the body insensitive to pain. They do this by interfering with nerve transmission in specific areas of the body, blocking nerve conduction only in the area where they are applied without causing loss of consciousness. They are most commonly used in clinical settings in which loss of consciousness, whole body mus-

Anaesthesia

- Premature infants, neonates, and pediatric clients are more affected by anaesthesia than young or middle-aged adult clients. Babies' and children's body systems are sensitive to the effects of anaesthesia; therefore the nurse must take all precautions to protect the client and ensure safety during all phases of surgery and all phases of anaesthesia, whether general or regional.
- The pediatric client's hepatic, cardiac, respiratory, and renal systems are either not fully developed or not yet fully functional, which makes these clients more susceptible to problems such as CNS depression, toxicity, atelectasis (lung collapse), pneumonia, and cardiac abnormalities.
- It is important to assess for and document the presence of any disease of the cardiac, renal, hepatic, or respiratory systems because of the attendant increased risk of complications during anaesthesia. Add to this the risk associated with a very young age or with being a newborn or preemie, and the possible complications of surgery and adverse effects of anaesthesia become even more problematic and more likely to occur.
- Neonates are at higher risk of upper airway obstruction or laryngospasms during general anaesthesia because of the airway physical characteristics in this age group.
- A more rapid metabolic rate and small airway diameter also put the neonate at greater risk of complications during general anaesthesia.
- Carefully calculated doses must consider the neonate's weight and/or body surface area (BSA).
- Nitrous oxide is commonly used in pediatric clients because it carries decreased risk of hepatitis.
- Resuscitative equipment should be nearby in any neonatal or pediatric unit.
- Any change in the level of consciousness should be assessed, noted, documented, and reported immediately to a physician, even if it occurs during the postoperative period.

cle relaxation, and loss of responsiveness are either undesirable or unnecessary (e.g., during childbirth). Other uses for local anaesthetics include dental procedures, suturing skin lacerations, spinal anaesthesia, and diagnostic procedures such as lumbar puncture or thoracentesis.

Most local anaesthetics belong to two major groups of organic compounds, esters or amides, and are classified as either topical or parenteral (injectable). **Topical anaesthetics** are applied directly to the skin and mucous membranes. They are available in the form of solutions, ointments, gels, creams, powders, ophthalmic drops, lozenges, and suppositories. These agents, their route of administration, and dosages are listed in Table 11-5. **Parenteral anaesthetics** can be administered directly into the CNS by various spinal injection techniques. Anaesthesia of specific areas of the peripheral nervous system is accomplished either by injecting the agents adjacent to main nerves (to produce a large body area of anaesthesia) or by infiltrating the area with multiple small injections (for a more limited area of anaesthesia). Some of the common types of local anaesthesia are described in Box 11-2. Parenteral anaesthetic agents and their pharmacokinetics are summarized in Table 11-6.

Mechanism of Action and Drug Effects

Local anaesthetics work by interfering with nerve transmission in specific areas of the body, rendering the affected area insensitive to pain. Nerve conduction is blocked only in the area where the anaesthetic is applied, without loss of consciousness. Local anaesthetics block both the generation and conduction of impulses through all nerve fibres (sensory, motor, and autonomic) by blocking the movement of certain ions (sodium, potassium, and calcium) important to this process. They do this by making it more difficult for these ions to move in and out of the nerve fibre. For this reason, some of these agents are also described as membrane stabilizing because they stabilize the cell membrane of the nerve fibre so that it is less permeable to the free movement of ions. The membrane-stabilizing effects occur first in the small fibres, then in the large fibres. In terms of paralysis, usually autonomic activity is affected first, then pain and other sensory functions are lost. Motor activity is the last to be lost. When the effects of the local anaesthetics wear off, they do so in reverse order, as function returns to motor activity, then sensory functions, and last, autonomic activity.

TABLE 11-5

TOPICAL ANAESTHETICS

Agent	Route	Dosage Strength
benzocaine	Topical, aerosol, and spray	0.5%–20% ointment or cream
dibucaine	Injection and topical	0.5%–1% solution, ointment, cream, or suppository
dibucaine	Topical	1% ointment
dyclonine	Topical	0.5%–1% solution
lidocaine	Topical	5% patch, 2% solution, spray
pramoxine	Topical	1% jelly, cream, lotion, or spray
prilocaine/lidocaine	Topical	2.5% prilocaine and 2.5% lidocaine cream
tetracaine	Injection, topical, and ophthalmic	0.5%–2% solution, ointment, or cream

Possible systemic effects of local anaesthetics include effects on circulatory and respiratory function. Such effects are usually unlikely unless large quantities of the drug are injected, which increases the likelihood of significant systemic absorption. Local anaesthetics produce sympathetic blockade, which means that the two neurotransmitters of the sympathetic nervous system (SNS),

norepinephrine and epinephrine, are blocked. The cardiac drug effects of this sympathetic blockade result in decreased stroke volume, cardiac output, and peripheral resistance. The respiratory drug effects can result in reduced respiratory function and altered breathing patterns, though complete paralysis of respiratory function is unlikely because of the large amount of absorbed drug that would be required. Some local anaesthetics, for either infiltration or nerve block anaesthesia, are combined with vasoconstrictors such as epinephrine, phenylephrine, and norepinephrine to help confine the local anaesthetic to the injected area and prevent systemic absorption.

Indications

Local anaesthetics are used for surgical, dental, or diagnostic procedures, as well as for the treatment of certain types of pain. They are administered by two techniques: infiltration anaesthesia and nerve block anaesthesia. Infiltration anaesthesia is commonly used for minor surgical and dental procedures. It involves injecting the local anaesthetic solution intradermally, subcutaneously, or submucosally across the path of nerves supplying the area to be anaesthetized. The local anaesthetic may be administered in a circular pattern around the operative field. Nerve block anaesthesia is used for surgical, dental, and diagnostic procedures and for the therapeutic management of pain. It involves injecting the local anaesthetic directly into or around the nerve trunks or nerve ganglia that supply the area to be numbed.

Contraindications

Contraindications of local anaesthetics include known drug allergy. Only specially designed dosage forms are intended for ophthalmic use.

Side Effects and Adverse Effects

The side effects and adverse effects of the local anaesthetics are, under most circumstances, limited and of little clinical importance. The undesirable effects usually result from high plasma concentrations of the drug, which results from inadvertent intravascular injection, an excessive dose or rate of injection, slow metabolic breakdown, or injection into highly vascularized tissue.

In addition, when a local anaesthetic gets absorbed into the circulation, it can result in adverse reactions similar to those produced by general anaesthetics. When using local anaesthetics containing epinephrine, which has vasocon-

BOX 11-2
Types of Local Anaesthesia

Epidural
The anaesthetic agent is injected via a small catheter into the epidural space, which is just outside the dura mater of the spinal cord. This route is becoming more popular for the administration of opioids for pain management and has longstanding obstetrical use.

Infiltration
Small amounts of anaesthetic solution are injected into the tissue that surrounds the operative site. This approach to anaesthesia is commonly used for such procedures as suturing wounds or dental surgery. Often agents that cause constriction of local blood vessels are also administered to limit the site of action locally (e.g., epinephrine).

Nerve Block
Anaesthetic solution is injected at the site where a nerve innervates a specific area such as a tissue. This allows large amounts of anaesthetic agent to be delivered to a specific area without affecting the whole body. It is often reserved for more difficult to treat pain syndromes such as clients diagnosed with various cancers and chronic orthopedic pain.

Spinal
Anaesthetic solution is injected into the epidural space or the subarachnoid space that surrounds the spinal cord. Different nerves can be anaesthetized depending on the location of the injection. This type of local anaesthesia is commonly used for obstetric procedures.

Topical
The anaesthetic agent is applied directly onto the surface of the skin, eye, or any other mucous membrane to relieve pain or prevent it from being sensed. It is commonly used for diagnostic eye examinations and suturing of skin.

TABLE 11-6
PARENTERAL ANAESTHETIC AGENTS*

Generic Name	Potency†	Onset	Duration	Dose
lidocaine	2nd	Immediate	60–90 min	0.5%–4% injection
mepivacaine	2nd		120–150 min	1%, 2% injection
procaine	3rd	2–5 min	30–60 min	2% injection
tetracaine	1st	5–10 min	90–120 min	0.5% injection

*Other common parenteral anaesthetic agents include bupivacaine, chloroprocaine, and ropivacaine.
†Denotes order of potency from the most (1st) to the least (5th) potent.

strictive properties, care should be taken not to administer into fingers or toes to avoid the possibility of vasospasm.

True allergic reactions to local anaesthetics are rare. However, allergic reactions can occur. They may appear as skin lesions, urticaria, or edema, or they may be acutely anaphylactic. These rare allergic reactions are generally limited to a particular chemical class of anaesthetics called the *ester type*. Box 11-3 separates the local anaesthetic agents into their two chemical families. These two groups have different enzymes that are responsible for their breakdown in the body. Anaesthetics belonging to the ester family are metabolized by cholinesterase in the plasma and liver. They are metabolized to a para-aminobenzoic acid (PABA) compound. This compound is mainly responsible for allergic reactions. The amide type of anaesthetics is metabolized in the liver by other enzymes to active and inactive metabolites. Often when an individual has an undesirable experience after the administration of one of the local anaesthetics, changing from one chemical class to another can prevent these experiences.

Toxicity and Management of Overdose

Local anaesthetics have little opportunity to cause toxicity under most circumstances. However, they can become just as toxic as the general anaesthetics if they are systemically absorbed. To prevent this from occurring, a vasoconstrictor such as epinephrine is co-administered with the local anaesthetic to keep the anaesthetic at its local site of action. Another reason for the lower incidence of toxic effects with local anaesthetics is that doses are on average much smaller than those of general anaesthetics. If for some reason significant amounts of the locally administered anaesthetic get absorbed systemically, cardiovascular and respiratory function may be compromised. Symptomatic and supportive therapy is usually all that is needed to reverse the toxic effects of systemic absorption of the agent, until its eventual metabolism by the body.

Interactions

Few clinically significant drug interactions occur with the local anaesthetics. Some of the more important drug–drug interactions occur with bupivacaine and chloroprocaine. When given with enflurane, halothane, or epinephrine, they can lead to dysrhythmias.

Dosages

For the recommended dosages of a local anaesthetic agent, see the dosages table on p. 177. See Appendix B for some of the common brands available in Canada.

DRUG PROFILES

Besides lidocaine, profiled here, local anaesthetics include bupivacaine, chloroprocaine, mepivacaine, prilocaine, procaine, and tetracaine. There are two major types of local anaesthetics, as determined by their chemical structure: amide and ester. The difference lies

BOX 11-3
Local Anaesthetic Chemical Groups

Ester Type	Amide Type
benzocaine	bupivacaine
chloroprocaine	dibucaine
procaine	lidocaine
tetracaine	mepivacaine
	prilocaine

in the type of linkage between the aromatic ring and the amino group of the agent, two of the structural components that make an anaesthetic an anaesthetic. Lidocaine belongs to the amide type of local anaesthetics. Some clients may report that they have allergic or anaphylactic reactions to "caines," as they may refer to lidocaine and the other amide agents. In these situations it may be wise to try a local anaesthetic of the ester type.

▸▸ *lidocaine*

Lidocaine is one of the most commonly used local anaesthetics. It is available in several strengths, both alone and in different concentrations with epinephrine, and is used for both infiltration and nerve block anaesthesia. It is available as 1-percent and 2-percent parenteral injections and in 1-percent and 2-percent concentrations in combination with epinephrine in a parenteral injection. The epinephrine component reduces blood loss from minor surgical procedures by virtue of its vasoconstrictive properties. Lidocaine is also now available in combination with prilocaine as a 5-percent patch (commonly known as the EMLA patch) for relief from the pain of vaccinations. This patch is administered as a thick layer (2.5 g) covered with an occlusive dressing for at least 1 hr prior to procedure.

Lidocaine is contraindicated in those who have a hypersensitivity to it. Commonly recommended dosages are listed in the table on p. 177.

NEUROMUSCULAR BLOCKING AGENTS (NMBAs)

Neuromuscular blocking agents (NMBAs) prevent nerve transmission in certain muscles, leading to paralysis of the muscle. They are often used with anaesthetics for surgery. Use of NMBAs requires mechanical ventilation because these drugs paralyze respiratory and skeletal muscles, leaving the client unable to breathe independently. The drugs do not cause sedation or relieve pain; therefore the healthcare provider should assume that the paralyzed client is in pain and anxious and should take steps to relieve this with analgesics and anxiolytics.

Snakes and plants played a large role in the discovery of the receptor and the chemical structure of a substance that would cause paralysis. The beginning steps in the identification of the receptor involved study of the seemingly

DOSAGES	Local Anaesthetic Agent		
Agent	**Pharmacological Class**	**Usual Dosage Range**	**Indications**
▸▸lidocaine	Amide local anaesthetic	1%, 2% solution: 5–200 mg	Percutaneous infiltration
		1% solution: 200–300 mg	Caudal obstetric analgesia, thoracic nerve block
		1% solution: 100 mg each side	Paracervical obstetric analgesia
		1% solution: 50–100 mg	Sympathetic lumbar nerve block
		1% solution: 30–50 mg	Paravertebral nerve block
		1% solution: 30 mg	Intercostal nerve block
		1% solution: 50 mg	Sympathetic cervical nerve block
		2% solution: 225–300 mg	Brachial nerve block, caudal surgical anaesthesia
		2% solution: 20–100 mg	Dental procedures
		2% solution: 200–300 mg	Lumbar anaesthesia

irreversible antagonism of neuromuscular transmission by toxins from krait venoms (e.g., *Bungarus multicinctus*) and the venoms of certain varieties of cobra (e.g., *Naja naja*). Once the receptor at which these venoms work was identified, pharmacological agents were studied that would mimic the venoms and produce paralysis.

Curare, a non-depolarizing NMBA, has a long and romantic history. It has been used for centuries by natives of South America along the Amazon and Orinoco rivers and in other parts of that continent for hunting wild animals. Animals shot with arrows soaked in this plant substance would die from paralysis of skeletal muscles. Curare is actually a generic term for various South American arrow poisons. The most potent of all curare alkaloids are the toxiferines, obtained from *Strychnos toxifera*. The seeds of the trees and shrubs of the genus *Erythrina*, widely distributed in tropical and subtropical areas, contain substances with curare-like activity.

NMBAs are traditionally classified as depolarizing or non-depolarizing. Succinylcholine is the only commonly used depolarizing drug. Non-depolarizing NMBAs prevent acetylcholine (ACh) from acting at neuromuscular junctions. Consequently, the nerve cell membrane is not depolarized, the muscle fibres are not stimulated, and skeletal muscle contraction does not occur. Non-depolarizing NMBAs are typically broken down into three groups based on their duration of action: short-, intermediate-, and long-acting agents.

Mechanism of Action and Drug Effects

The prototype drug d-tubocurarine (dTC), the active ingredient of curare, is a naturally occurring plant alkaloid that causes skeletal muscle relaxation or paralysis. dTC is still available in Canada, although rarely used. Most of the newer drugs are synthetic preparations. Succinylcholine works similarly to the neurotransmitter ACh. Initially succinylcholine combines with cholinergic receptors at the motor end plate to produce depolarization and muscle contraction. Repolarization and further muscle contraction are then inhibited as long as an adequate concentration of drug remains at the receptor site. Succinylcholine is metabolized much more slowly than ACh. Because of this slower metabolism, succinylcholine persistently subjects the motor end plate to ongoing depolarizing stimulation and repolarization cannot occur.

As long as sufficient succinylcholine concentrations are present, the muscle loses its ability to contract and a flaccid muscle paralysis results. This muscle paralysis is sometimes preceded by muscle spasms, which may damage muscles. These muscle spasms are termed *muscle fasciculations* and are most pronounced in the muscle groups of the hands, feet, and face. Injury to muscle cells may cause post-operative muscle pain and release potassium into the circulation. Small doses of non-depolarizing NMBAs are sometimes added with succinylcholine to minimize these muscle fasciculations. This reduces the muscle pain caused by depolarizing agents such as succinylcholine. Non-depolarizing NMBAs prevent ACh from acting at neuromuscular junctions. They act as antagonists blocking ACh from binding to the post-synaptic receptors. Consequently, the nerve cell membrane is not depolarized, the muscle fibres are not stimulated, and skeletal muscle contraction does not occur.

If hyperkalemia (excessive potassium in the bloodstream) develops, it is usually mild and insignificant. Rarely cardiac dysrhythmias or even cardiac arrest have occurred. Succinylcholine is normally deactivated by plasma pseudocholinesterase. This enzyme breaks down succinylcholine, freeing up the receptor site and allowing repolarization of the motor end plate. The duration of action of succinylcholine after a single intubating dose is about 5 to 9 minutes as a result of the rapid breakdown of the drug by this enzyme. Some individuals have a pseudocholinesterase deficiency, a rare genetic disorder. Individuals with this disorder are deficient in or have no plasma enzyme pseudocholinesterase, resulting in possible respiratory difficulty if the muscle-relaxing drug succinylcholine is used.

Anticholinesterase drugs, such as neostigmine, pyridostigmine, and edrophonium, are antidotes used to reverse muscle paralysis. They work by preventing the enzyme cholinesterase from breaking down ACh. This causes ACh to build up at the muscle end plate and eventually knocks off the non-depolarizing NMBA, returning the nerve to its original state.

To summarize the drug effects of the NMBAs: The first sensation felt is typically muscle weakness. This is usually followed by a total flaccid paralysis. Small, rapidly moving muscles such as those of the fingers and eyes are typically the first to be paralyzed. The next are those of the limbs, neck, and trunk. Finally the intercostal muscles and the diaphragm are paralyzed. Respirations stop as a result; the client can no longer breathe independently. Recovery of muscles usually occurs in reverse order to that of their paralysis, and thus the diaphragm is ordinarily the first to regain function. Before causing paralysis, depolarizing agents such as succinylcholine evoke transient muscular fasciculations. Muscle soreness may follow the administration of succinylcholine.

CNS effects are usually minimal because of the chemical structure of most of the non-depolarizing agents. They are quaternary ammonium compounds and are not able to penetrate the blood–brain barrier. The effects on the cardiovascular system vary depending on the NMBA used and the individual client. Increases and decreases in blood pressure and heart rate have been seen. Some NMBAs cause a release of histamine, which can result in bronchospasm, hypotension, and excessive bronchial and salivary secretion. The gastrointestinal (GI) tract is seldom affected by NMBAs. When it is affected, decreased tone and motility typically result, which can lead to constipation or even ileus (intestinal blockage).

Indications

The main therapeutic use of NMBAs is to maintain controlled ventilation during surgical procedures. When respiratory muscles are paralyzed by an NMBA, mechanical ventilation is easier because the body's desire to control respirations is eliminated.

NMBAs may also be used for endotracheal intubation and to reduce muscle contraction in an area that needs surgery. Short-acting NMBAs are often used to facilitate intubation with an endotracheal tube. This is commonly done to facilitate a variety of diagnostic procedures such as laryngoscopy, bronchoscopy, and esophagoscopy. When used for this purpose NMBAs are often combined with anxiolytics or anaesthetics. Additional non-surgical applications include reduction of laryngeal or general muscle spasms, reduction of spasticity from tetanus and neurological diseases such as multiple sclerosis, and prevention of bone fractures during electroconvulsive therapy. These drugs are also used as diagnostic agents for myasthenia gravis.

Contraindications

Contraindications to NMBAs include known drug allergy and also may include previous history of malignant hyperthermia, penetrating eye injuries, and narrow-angle glaucoma.

Side Effects and Adverse Effects

The key to limiting side effects and adverse effects with most NMBAs is to use just enough of the agent to block the neuromuscular receptors. Too high a dose increases the risk of affecting other ganglionic receptors, which leads to most of the undesirable effects of NMBAs. The effects of ganglionic blockade in various areas of the body are listed in Table 11-7.

Non-depolarizing NMBAs have relatively few side effects when used appropriately. Their cardiovascular effects include blockade of autonomic ganglia, resulting in hypotension, blockade of muscarinic receptors, resulting in tachycardia, and release of histamine, resulting in hypotension. The depolarizing agent succinylcholine has been associated with hyperkalemia; dysrhythmias; fasciculations; muscle pain; myoglobinuria (the release of muscle contents into the urine); and increased intraocular, intragastric, and intracranial pressure.

Toxicity and Management of Overdose

The primary concern when NMBAs are overdosed is prolonged paralysis requiring prolonged mechanical ventilation. Cardiovascular collapse can also be seen and is thought to be the result of histamine release. Many medical conditions (listed in Box 11-4) can increase sensitivity to NMBAs and prolong their effects, thus predisposing the individual to toxicity.

Some conditions (listed in Box 11-5) make it more difficult for NMBAs to work and therefore require higher doses of NMBAs.

TABLE 11-7

EFFECTS OF GANGLIONIC BLOCKADE BY NEUROMUSCULAR BLOCKING AGENTS

Site	Nervous System Blocked	Physiological Effect
Arterioles	Sympathetic	Vasodilation and hypotension
Veins	Sympathetic	Dilation
Heart	Parasympathetic	Tachycardia
Gastrointestinal	Parasympathetic	Reduced tone and tract motility; constipation
Urinary bladder	Parasympathetic	Urinary retention
Salivary glands	Parasympathetic	Dry mouth

BOX 11-4

Conditions That Predispose Clients to Toxic Effects from Neuromuscular Blocking Agents

Acidosis
Amyotrophic lateral sclerosis
Hypermagnesemia
Hypocalcemia
Hypokalemia
Hypothermia
Myasthenia gravis
Myasthenic syndrome
Neonates
Neurofibromatosis
Paraplegia
Poliomyelitis

Interactions

Many drugs can interact with NMBAs, resulting in either synergistic or opposing effects. Some of the antibiotics when given concomitantly with an NMBA can result in additive effects. The aminoglycoside antibiotics are a common example. They produce neuromuscular blockade by inhibiting ACh release from the preganglionic terminal. The tetracycline antibiotics can also produce neuromuscular blockade, possibly by chelation of calcium, and calcium channel blockers have been shown to enhance neuromuscular blockade. Some of the more notable drugs that interact with NMBAs are listed in Box 11-6.

Dosages

For the recommended dosages of selected neuromuscular blocking agents, see the dosages table on p. 180. See Appendix B for some of the common brands available in Canada.

DRUG PROFILES

NMBAs are one of the most commonly used classes of drugs in the operating room. They are used primarily with general anaesthetics to facilitate endotracheal intubation and to relax skeletal muscles during surgery. In addition to their use in the operating room, NMBAs are commonly used in the ICU to paralyze mechanically ventilated clients. The two basic types of NMBAs are depolarizing and non-depolarizing. The only depolarizing agent is succinylcholine. Non-depolarizing agents can be classified in a variety of ways but are typically classified by their chemical structure or their duration of action. Table 11-8 lists some non-depolarizing agents currently in use.

DEPOLARIZING NEUROMUSCULAR BLOCKING AGENTS

Succinylcholine has a structure similar to the parasympathetic neurotransmitter ACh. It stimulates the same neurons as ACh and produces the same physiological responses initially. Unlike ACh, succinylcholine is metabolized slowly. Because of this slower metabolization, succinylcholine persistently subjects the motor end plate to ongoing depolarizing stimulation. Repolariza-

tion cannot occur. As long as sufficient succinylcholine concentrations are present the muscle loses its ability to contract and flaccid muscle paralysis results. Because of its quick onset, succinylcholine is most commonly used to facilitate endotracheal intubation. It is seldom used over long periods because of the unwanted effects that develop with continuous infusions.

▸▸ *succinylcholine*

Succinylcholine is the only currently available depolarizing NMBA. It is an ultra–short-acting, depolarizing-type skeletal muscle relaxant for intravenous administration. Succinylcholine is indicated as an adjunct to general anaesthesia, to facilitate tracheal intubation, and to provide skeletal muscle relaxation during surgery or mechanical ventilation. It is contraindicated in clients with personal or familial history of malignant hyperthermia, skeletal muscle myopathies, and known hypersensitivity to the drug. It is available as a 20 mg/mL 10-mL solution or 20 mg/mL 5-mL ampoules and 100 mg/mL 5-mL vials. Pregnancy category C. The recommended dosage is given in the table on p. 180.

PHARMACOKINETICS

Half-Life	Onset	Peak	Duration
Seconds	Rapid ≈ 1 min	Rapid	4–6 min

NON-DEPOLARIZING NEUROMUSCULAR BLOCKING AGENTS

Non-depolarizing NMBAs are commonly used to facilitate endotracheal intubation, reduce muscle contraction in an area that needs surgery, and facilitate a variety of diagnostic procedures. They are often combined with anxiolytics or anaesthetics. They may also be used to induce respiratory arrest in clients on mechanical ventilation. Non-depolarizing NMBAs can be classified in a variety of ways but are typically classified by their chemical structure or their duration of action.

BOX 11-5
Conditions That Oppose the Effects of Neuromuscular Blocking Agents

Cirrhosis with ascites (excess fluid in the peritoneal cavity)
Clostridial infections
Hemiplegia
Hypercalcemia
Hyperkalemia
Peripheral nerve transection
Peripheral neuropathies
Thermal burns

BOX 11-6
Drugs That Interact With Neuromuscular Blocking Agents

Additive Effects
aminoglycosides
calcium channel blockers
clindamycin
cyclophosphamide
cyclosporine
dantrolene
furosemide
inhalation anaesthetics
local anaesthetics
magnesium
polymyxin
procainamide
quinidine

Opposing Effects
carbamazepine
corticosteroids
phenytoin

DOSAGES — Selected Neuromuscular Blocking Agents

Agent	Pharmacological Class	Usual Dosage Range	Indications
pancuronium	Non-depolarizing NMBA (long acting)	**Pediatric** IV: 0.02 mg/kg **Adult** IV: 0.04–0.1 mg/kg Continuous infusion: 0.1 mg/kg/hr	Intubation Mechanical ventilation
succinylcholine	Depolarizing NMBA (short acting)	**Pediatric** IV: 1–2 mg/kg IM: 3–4 mg/kg **Adult** IV: 0.3–1.1 mg/kg IM: 3–4 mg/kg	Intubation Mechanical ventilation
▸▸ rocuronium bromide	Non-depolarizing NMBA (intermediate acting)	**Pediatric** IV: 0.6 mg/kg **Adult** IV: 0.6–1.2 mg/kg Continuous infusion: 0.01 to 0.012 mg/kg/min; 0.1 mg/kg/hr	Intubation Mechanical ventilation

pancuronium

Pancuronium is a long-acting non-depolarizing NMBA. It is indicated as an adjunct to general anaesthesia to facilitate tracheal intubation and to provide skeletal muscle relaxation during surgery or mechanical ventilation. It is most commonly used for long surgical procedures that require prolonged muscle paralysis. Pancuronium is contraindicated in clients with known hypersensitivity. It is available as 1 g/mL 10-mL vials and 2 mg/mL 2- and 5-mL ampoules. Pregnancy category C. The recommended dosage is given in the table above.

PHARMACOKINETICS

Half-Life	Onset	Peak	Duration
80–120 min	3–5 min	Rapid	60–100 min

▸▸ rocuronium bromide

Rocuronium bromide, a newer non-depolarizing muscle relaxant (NDMR), is an intermediate-acting non-depolarizing NMBA. It has a rapid to intermediate onset of action, depending on the dosage. It is indicated as an adjunct to general anaesthesia to facilitate both routine tracheal intubation and **rapid sequence intubation (RSI)** and to provide skeletal muscle relaxation during surgery or mechanical ventilation. It is one of the most commonly used NMBAs. Rocuronium bromide is contraindicated in clients with known hypersensitivity. It is available as 10 mg/mL 5 mL vials. Pregnancy category C. The recommended dosage is given in the table above.

PHARMACOKINETICS

Half-Life	Onset	Peak	Duration
14–18 min	1–3 min	2.5 min	25–40 min

TABLE 11-8

CLASSIFICATION OF NEUROMUSCULAR BLOCKING AGENTS

Agent	Structure
SHORT-ACTING AGENT	
mivacurium	Benzylisoquinolinium
INTERMEDIATE-ACTING AGENTS	
atracurium	Benzylisoquinolinium
rocuronium	Steroidal
LONG-ACTING AGENTS	
doxacurium	Benzylisoquinolinium
pancuronium	Steroidal
tubocurarine	Benzylisoquinolinium

MODERATE SEDATION

Many types of procedures, including diagnostic and minor surgical procedures, do not require as great a depth of anaesthesia as do more extensive procedures. A newer trend in anaesthesia is to use an anaesthetic technique known as **moderate sedation** (also known as *conscious sedation*). The client is often given an intravenous combination of both a benzodiazepine (e.g., midazolam) and an opiate analgesic (e.g., meperidine). This combination effectively reduces client anxiety, sensitivity to pain, and recall of the medical procedure, yet it preserves client ability to maintain the airway and respond to verbal commands. In addition, a local anaesthetic (e.g., lidocaine) may be injected or applied topically to the surgical site as needed to further enhance client comfort. This procedure has a more rapid recovery time and greater safety profile than general anaesthesia with its inherent cardiorespiratory risks.

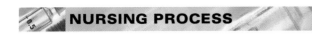

NURSING PROCESS

■ Assessment

One of the most important nursing responsibilities to the client receiving general anaesthesia is to assess the client's status during the various stages of anaesthesia. Each stage of general anaesthesia results in a greater degree of anaesthesia; however, it is also important to assess and document the client's status during the pre-, intra-, and post-operative phases. (Note that it is the anaesthetist's role to assess the level of anaesthesia intra-operatively.) This is assessed by vital signs, pulse (O_2) oximeter, and other appropriate parameters. After the conclusion of the procedure and the termination of any type of general anaesthesia, the nurse's next main concern for the client is summarized by the general rule of ABCs (*a*irway, *b*reathing, and *c*irculation). Once the client is quickly assessed from head to toe and all vital signs are checked, the nurse needs to collect data about the specific anaesthetic used, the procedure done, any allergies, the client's medical history, and any complications during anaesthesia. In addition, the nurse must review the client's current laboratory results and assess the status of any tubes, dressings, intravenous catheters, and equipment. All body systems, including the integumentary system, need to be assessed frequently and thoroughly and the findings documented. It is also important to document intake and output amounts, wound drainage amounts, secretion amounts, level of consciousness, and pain level (rating of 0 [no pain] to 10 [worst pain]). Allergic reactions and either CNS stimulation or depression may occur if the agent has entered the circulation. Frequent assessments will help detect any changes in the client, no matter how small, and prevent further risks of complications.

Intravenously administered general anaesthetic agents usually include various sedative–hypnotics, anti-anxiety agents, opioid and non-opioid analgesics, anti-emetics, and anticholinergics that may decrease some of the undesirable after-effects of excessive doses of the inhaled anaesthetics. Therefore it is particularly important to assess a client on inhaled anaesthetics for any problems with liver, renal, or cardiac functioning. It is important for the nurse to assess and document previous reactions to or problems with general anaesthesia and to inform the appropriate healthcare professionals, such as the anaesthesiologist, nurse anaesthetist, and physician, who are involved with the specific client's care. A baseline assessment is also needed to establish basic parameters, as well as to identify any problems in the client's profile. This includes vital signs, weight, height, electrocardiogram (ECG) and chest X-ray examination (ordered by the physician or anaesthesia personnel), and laboratory values (red blood cell count [RBC], complete blood count [CBC], blood urea nitrogen [BUN], creatinine, alkaline phosphatase, and other liver function studies). Electrolytes and blood glucose levels are also important, even if the client is not having difficulties with these values.

Neurological assessment should include motor and sensory assessments (e.g., reflexes; grasps; strength in lower and upper extremities; ability to follow commands; level of consciousness; alertness and orientation to person, place, and time). Swallowing and gag reflex ability is also important to assess and document. The nurse should question the client about previous responses to general anaesthesia, such as high body temperature or malignant hyperthermia and drug interactions. Drug interactions may occur with any other type of CNS depressants, NMBAs, aminoglycosides, antihypertensives, corticosteroids, anticoagulants, acetylsalicylic acid and acetylsalicylate-containing drugs, and non-steroidal anti-inflammatory drugs (NSAIDs).

Local anaesthesia still carries some potential for causing complications, such as diminished sensation and motor responses and postural hypotension. However, unlike general anaesthesia, the nurse may be the one responsible for administering a topical local anaesthetic in specific situations, such as when assisting a physician in a procedure (e.g., "sewing" up a wound with sutures after a local anaesthetic). In this event, the nurse should be sure to assess whether the client has any pre-existing illnesses and allergies; whether the client uses OTC medications, alcohol, or any prescriptive medications; and whether the client is or has been a smoker. Baseline vital signs are also important to record.

Clients about to undergo anaesthesia with NMBAs need to be assessed head to toe and to have a medical and medication history taken. Great caution is necessary when clients have disorders such as hypothermia, hypokalemia, and hypocalcemia. Conditions that may require higher doses of NMBAs include burns, hyperkalemia, hypercalcemia, and cirrhosis. Drug interactions are common with NMBAs and may involve corticosteroids, carbamazepine, phenytoin, quinidine, magnesium, cyclophosphamide, cyclosporine, furosemide, dantrolene, inhalation anaesthetics, local anaesthetics, aminoglycosides, clindamycin, polymyxin, calcium channel blockers, and procainamide. Some agents, such as succinylcholine, may also cause an increase in intra-ocular and intracranial pressure and should be used cautiously, if at all, in clients with glaucoma or head injuries. In addition, clients receiving NMBAs must have their respiratory system assessed thoroughly because of the paralyzing effect of these drugs. Because NMBAs are often used to induce respiratory arrest (paralysis of respiratory muscles) in clients requiring mechanical ventilation, it is critical to make sure that mechanical ventilation is on hand. In addition, the client needs to be assessed for electrolyte imbalances, especially with potassium and magnesium, because these may lead to increased action of the NMBA. Allergic reactions to NMBAs are characterized by rash, fever, respiratory distress, and pruritus. Drug interactions include, among others, aminoglycosides, clindamycin, lincomycin, quinidine, polymyxin antibiotics, lithium, narcotics, thiazide diuretics, enflurane, isoflurane, magnesium salts, and oxytocin. The physician and/or anaesthesiologist needs to know about these drugs, which will result in increased neuromuscular blockade.

Succinylcholine, a depolarizing NMBA, is contraindicated in clients with personal or familial history of malignant hyperthermia, skeletal muscle myopathies, and known hypersensitivity to the drug. Rocuronium is an intermediate-acting non-depolarizing NMBA and is the most commonly used agent for surgery and for mechanical ventilation. However, long-term use may create difficulty with prolonged paralysis and problems weaning off the mechanical ventilator; therefore it should be used cautiously in these situations. Rocuronium is contraindicated in clients allergic to these types of medications. Pancuronium is a long-acting non-depolarizing NMBA and is most commonly used for long surgical procedures or mechanical ventilation and is contraindicated in clients allergic to the drug. This drug is not contraindicated in pregnancy. It is rated pregnancy category C and, in fact, is often used in newborn infants requiring mechanical ventilation in neonatal ICUs.

To avoid errors and possible death, NMBA medication vials should never be kept on hand in a nursing unit. Because these agents produce apnea, it is important to have the mechanical ventilation and resuscitation equipment in the client's room. The nurse must assess the situation and make sure that the client and family members are prepared adequately and appropriately for the experience of paralysis. Regardless of the level of paralysis, the client will be able to hear and also to sense touch. If possible and appropriate, the nurse should assess baseline hearing.

Assessment of the environment, particularly noise level, is important in any anaesthesia-related scenario because a calm, professional, quiet environment will help to enhance any type of anaesthetic. Always assess for any reversing agent or an antidote because these should always be available instantaneously with the use of many of the general anaesthetics and NMBAs. Peripheral nerve stimulators are used to monitor drug effectiveness with some of the NMBAs and may help avoid overdosage. Depolarizing NMBAs, such as succinylcholine chloride, must be administered carefully by highly qualified individuals, such as a nurse anaesthetist, because too-rapid administration may result in bradycardia and, rarely, in cardiac arrest. The antidote is atropine and neostigmine.

Nursing Diagnoses

Nursing diagnoses appropriate to the client receiving either general or local anaesthesia are as follows:
- Risk for injury related to decreased sensorium resulting from general anaesthesia or related to decreased sensation resulting from local anaesthesia
- Decreased cardiac output related to systemic effects of anaesthesia
- Impaired gas exchange related to CNS depression (respiratory depression) produced by general anaesthesia
- Anxiety related to the use of anaesthesia and the possibility of surgery
- Deficient knowledge related to lack of information regarding and experience with anaesthesia and surgery

Planning

Goals related to the care of the client receiving general or local anaesthesia are as follows:
- Client states the side effects of general or local anaesthesia.
- Client states potential complications of both general and local anaesthesia.
- Client experiences minimal to no injury related to anaesthesia.
- Client describes what to expect during the recovery period of anaesthesia.
- Client adheres with care to decrease the chances of complications after anaesthesia.
- Client follows preoperative instructions regarding his or her care during the post-operative period (see the Community Health Points box on p. 183).
- Client verbalizes anxiety (as needed) regarding surgery and anaesthesia.

Outcome Criteria

Outcome criteria related to the use of general or local anaesthesia are as follows:
- Client experiences minimal to no side effects of general or local anaesthesia, such as myocardial depression, during operative period.
- Client remains free of complications such as injury, falls, and hepatotoxicity during the perioperative period (preoperative, intra-operative, and post-operative).

- Client is free of or experiences minimal anxiety, as evidenced by fewer complaints, better relaxation ability, and decreased post-operative pain.
- Client adheres to all measures and treatments such as turning, coughing, and deep breathing during the perioperative period.

■ Implementation

Regardless of the type of anaesthesia a client is receiving, one of the most important nursing considerations during this time is close and frequent observation of the client and all body systems, with specific attention to the ABCs of nursing care (*a*irway, *b*reathing, and *c*irculation) and vital signs. This should be done as frequently as necessary or per hospital/facility protocol. If any sudden elevation in body temperature (e.g., >40°C) occurs while a client is receiving general anaesthesia, it should be managed immediately because it may indicate the occurrence of malignant hyperthermia. Malignant hyperthermia is a life-threatening emergency and requires prompt medical attention. Other nursing actions include monitoring all aspects of body functions (including the ABCs of care), instituting safety measures, and implementing the physician's orders.

Often, oxygen is administered after a client has received general anaesthesia to compensate for the respiratory depression that occurred during surgery and to elevate oxygen levels in the blood. In addition, hypotension and orthostatic hypotension may occur after anaesthesia because of the vasodilation produced by anaesthetics. When administering pain medication post-operatively, it is important to remember that the dose of any sedative hypnotic, narcotic, other form of analgesic or CNS depressant administered after surgery when the client returns to the room or is in the recovery room is often decreased by one-half to one-fourth to avoid causing or exacerbating CNS depression. For intravenous anaesthesia, any drug antidote and all resuscitative equipment should be kept nearby in case of cardiorespiratory distress or arrest.

Propofol, a newer intravenously administered general anaesthetic, is quick to act and to subside. It is often used to initiate and maintain monitored anaesthesia in adult clients during some diagnostic procedures and is also used in intubated, mechanically ventilated clients (such as those in the ICU) to provide continuous sedation and control over "stress responses." Neurological checks (e.g., reflexes, responses to commands, level of consciousness) and ECG and vital signs monitoring are indicated. The nurse should use critical thinking and clinical judgement to determine how often such checks are needed.

With the use of general anaesthesia, especially combined with succinylcholine, any sudden post-operative elevation in body temperature should be reported to the physician immediately because of the continued risk of malignant hyperthermia. Additional nursing observations during and after general (as well as local and spinal) anaesthesia include the status of breath sounds assessed

COMMUNITY HEALTH POINTS

- Health care in the home plays an important role in the recovery of any client being discharged from the hospital to home. It is a resource for all phases of the rehabilitation and recovery process for clients of any age.
- Community resources are available for clients of all ages during their recovery and rehabilitation at home after surgery. The discharge planning nurse usually evaluates need and then makes the initial contact with healthcare agencies and city-sponsored social service agencies.
- The Meals on Wheels service is often available for the geriatric client, and senior citizen resources and agencies are available through most city governments. Geriatric clients are also encouraged to contact city-sponsored and church-related transportation services.

by auscultation (hypoventilation may be a complication of general anaesthesia); any changes in neurological status (no matter how minute); and any sensation changes in body parts distal to the site of local anaesthesia or distal to where the safety restraints were placed during the surgery. Improper positioning during surgery may lead to the damage of arteries and nerves. When caring for a client who has received either general or local anaesthesia, all body functions should be frequently monitored and safety measures implemented as deemed necessary. Reorienting the client to his or her surroundings and implementing the physician's orders should also be part of the client's care during the post-operative phase.

A client who receives an NMBA should be monitored closely during and after the anaesthesia or induction to mechanical ventilation. Vital signs are constantly monitored during and after the recovery from the administration of NMBAs with measurements of blood pressure, pulse, respirations (rate, depth, pattern, quality), and hand grasp strength (for neuromotor). Intake and output are also monitored every hour. Recovery from the NMBA is manifested by a decrease in paralysis of the face, diaphragm, leg, arm, and remainder of the body. The healthcare provider must reassure the client about his or her condition, because he or she may become frightened if communication is difficult during the recovery process or during intubation.

Any local anaesthetic solution that is cloudy or discoloured or that contains any sort of crystalloids should not be used. Some anaesthesiologists mix the solution with sodium bicarbonate to minimize the local pain during infiltration, but this also causes a more rapid onset of action and a longer duration of sensory analgesia. Resuscitative equipment should be kept nearby. If an anaesthetic ointment or cream is used, the nurse should thoroughly cleanse and dry the area to be anaesthetized before application. If a suppository is used, the nurse should refrigerate it before use, remove the wrapper, moisten the suppository with water or water-soluble lubricant, and then insert it.

If a local anaesthetic is being used in the nose or throat, it is important for the nurse to remember that it may lead to paralysis and/or numbness of the structures of the upper respiratory tract, leading to possible aspiration. Exact amounts of the agent should be used and administered only at the prescribed times. Local anaesthetics are not to be swallowed unless the physician has instructed. If local anaesthetic is swallowed, the nurse needs to closely observe the client, check his or her gag reflex, and withhold food or drink until the client's sensation and/or gag reflex has returned.

Local anaesthesia produces paralysis of certain areas, such as the area below the waist; therefore it is important for the nurse to protect the client from injury resulting from this loss of sensation. Bed side rails should be kept up, and there should be no untoward pressure on the affected skin area because the body's normal sensation and protective mechanisms are diminished. After a spinal anaesthetic, clients must remain flat in bed for up to 12 hours to prevent a spinal headache. They should be well hydrated during this period.

Clients receiving moderate sedation as the method of anaesthesia should receive education about the technique. Generally clients receive this type of anaesthesia for diagnostic and fairly minor surgical procedures. The client is often given a combination of parenteral (specifically intravenous) solutions of a benzodiazepine, such as midazolam, with an opiate analgesic such as meperidine. This combination effectively reduces client anxiety, sensitivity to pain, and recall of the medical procedure, yet it preserves client ability to maintain the airway and respond to verbal commands. In addition, a local anaesthetic (e.g., lidocaine) may be injected or applied topically to the surgical site as needed to further enhance client comfort during the use of moderate sedation. This procedure has a more rapid recovery time and greater safety profile than general anaesthesia with its inherent cardiorespiratory risks.

Teaching tips important for clients receiving either general or local anaesthesia are given in the box below.

■ Evaluation

The therapeutic effects of any general or local anaesthetic include loss of sensation during the procedure (such as loss of sensation in the eye for corneal surgery) or loss of consciousness and other reflexes (such as pain for abdominal or other major procedures). A client who has received general anaesthesia should be constantly monitored for adverse effects, including myocardial depression, convulsions, respiratory depression, allergic rhinitis, and decreased renal or liver function. Clients who have received a local anaesthetic also need to be constantly monitored for adverse effects (mostly stemming from the systemic absorption of the specific agent). These effects include bradycardia, myocardial depression, hypotension, and dysrhythmias. As mentioned earlier, significant overdoses of local agents or direct injection into a blood vessel may result in cardiovascular collapse or cardiac or respiratory depression.

CLIENT TEACHING TIPS

General Anaesthesia

The nurse should do the following:
▲ Obtain a list of all prescription and OTC medications the client is taking so that any possible drug interactions can be averted by discontinuing the medication before surgery. Encourage the client to carry this list at all times.
▲ Educate the client about the procedure and the care required before, during, and after surgery to help alleviate anxiety and promote recovery.
▲ Explain the rationale for the use of preoperative medications as well as the need for the client to be NPO (take nothing by mouth) to prevent aspiration.
▲ Teach the client about turning, coughing, and deep breathing, which are important for recovery and healing whenever general anaesthesia has been used for surgical procedures, especially those requiring an hour or more of anaesthesia.
▲ Teach the client about post-operative pain control methods to alleviate anxiety and promote healing.
▲ Explain the rationale for any other treatments (e.g., the use of drainage tubes, catheters, IV lines).
▲ Discuss with the client the importance of frequent vital sign monitoring to minimize post-operative anxiety and fear.
▲ Instruct the client about the importance of safety features such as calling for assistance to get out of bed. (If the facility is not equipped with bed alarms, keep side rails up. Always have a call light at the bedside.)
▲ Always discuss with the client how the general anaesthesia agents may make him or her feel. For example, with NMBAs used alone, the client may be paralyzed but will be able to hear and feel.

Local Anaesthesia

The nurse should do the following:
▲ Make sure the client understands how local anaesthetics work, their side effects, and why the specific local agent was selected.
▲ Explain that because anaesthetic creams and ointments (such as EMLA cream) require time to take effect, there may be a delay before a procedure can be performed. The EMLA patch is administered as a thick layer (2.5 g) covered with an occlusive dressing at least an hour prior to the procedure.
▲ For clients receiving epidural or spinal anaesthesia, perform vital sign and systems assessments frequently during and after the procedure to monitor for and assess any complications. Inform the client of this to help decrease anxiety.
▲ Remind the client about decreased motor and sensory status so that he or she knows what to expect.

POINTS to REMEMBER

▼ Anaesthesia is a drug-induced state of altered nerve conduction and may be general, local, or moderate sedation.

▼ Anaesthesia allows surgeons to carry out specific and often sophisticated procedures.

▼ The CNS is profoundly altered with general anaesthesia so that pain perception and consciousness are lost; drug effects also include skeletal muscle relaxation and loss of reflexes.

▼ General anaesthetics induce a state of anaesthesia; the effects are global, influencing the entire body.

▼ NMBAs, if given in high doses, may block neuromuscular receptors and other ganglionic receptors, leading to hypotension, tachycardia, decreased GI and genitourinary (GU) tone, and dry mouth.

▼ Moderate sedation often uses a combination of drugs to produce anaesthesia while also maintaining a level of consciousness. It often includes the administration of sedatives, hypnotics, anxiolytics, analgesics, antiemetics, anticholinergics, or an NMBA.

▼ Local anaesthetics are also termed *regional anaesthetics* and render specific portions of the body essentially insensitive to pain without affecting consciousness.

▼ Local anaesthetics may be applied to skin and mucous membranes or injected locally. They are available as parenteral (injectable) solutions, ointments, gels, creams, powders, ophthalmic drops, and suppositories.

▼ Nursing considerations related to the perioperative phase include all nursing actions with a client before (preoperative stage), during (intra-operative stage), and after (post-operative stage) anaesthesia and the surgical process. Each phase demands often complex and specific nursing actions.

▼ NMBAs have many cautions and contraindications and should be used only if mechanical ventilation is being used or is on hand. They should *not* be kept on hand on any nursing unit because of the potential for careless use and the possible induction of apnea.

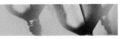

EXAMINATION REVIEW QUESTIONS

1 Your client is in for a lymph node removal from his arm under local anaesthesia. The physician has requested "lidocaine *with* epinephrine." Which of the following provides the most accurate rationale for adding epinephrine?
a. It helps calm the client before the procedure.
b. It helps minimize the risk of an allergic reaction.
c. It enhances the effect of the local lidocaine.
d. It causes vasoconstriction and keeps the anaesthetic local.

2 During your client's surgery, he experiences a sudden elevation in body temperature to about 40.5°C. What is mostly likely occurring with this client?
a. Malignant hyperthermia
b. Spontaneous pneumothorax
c. Severe intra-operative infection
d. Malignant hypermetabolic syndrome

3 Which of the following clients is more prone to complications to general anaesthesia?
a. A 79-year-old female who is about to have her gallbladder removed
b. A 49-year-old male athlete who quit heavy smoking 12 years ago

c. A 30-year-old female who is in perfect health but has never had anaesthesia
d. A 50-year-old female scheduled for outpatient laser surgery for vision correction

4 Which of the following may occur in the client who has been under general anaesthesia for 3 to 4 hours for abdominal–thoracic surgery?
a. Decreased urine output from use of vasopressors as anaesthetics
b. Increased cardiac output related to the effects of general anaesthesia
c. Risk for injury (fall) related to decreased sensorium 2 to 4 days post-operative
d. Decreased gaseous exchange from the CNS depression of general anaesthesia

5 Which of the following should be the nurse's main concern for the client recovering from general anaesthesia during the immediate post-operative period?
a. Airway
b. Pupillary reflexes
c. Return of sensations
d. Level of consciousness

For answers see http://evolve.elsevier.com/Lilley/pharmacology/.

CRITICAL THINKING ACTIVITIES

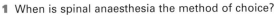

1 When is spinal anaesthesia the method of choice?
2 What is the purpose of adding epinephrine to a local anaesthetic?

3 What are potential complications of local anaesthetics used in dental offices, such as lidocaine with epinephrine, in a client with a variety of cardiac or vessel diseases?

For answers see http://evolve.elsevier.com/Lilley/pharmacology/.

BIBLIOGRAPHY

Albanese, J., & Nutz, P. (2005). *Mosby's 2005 nursing drug cards.* St Louis: MO: Mosby.

Beyea, S.C. (2001). The ideal state for perioperative nursing. *Journal of the American Organization of Registered Nurses, 73,* 5.

Canadian Pharmacists Association. (2003). *Therapeutic choices* (4th ed.). Ottawa, ON: Author.

Canadian Pharmacists Association. (2005). *Compendium of pharmaceuticals and specialties. The Canadian drug reference for health professionals.* Ottawa, ON: Author. [The subscription-based e-CPS is available at http://www.pharmacists.ca.]

Drain, C.B. (2003). *Perianesthesia nursing: A critical care approach* (4th ed.). St Louis, MO: Saunders.

Dripps, R.D., Eckenhoff, J.E., & Vandam, L.D. (Eds.). (1988). *Introduction to anesthesia: The principles of safe practice* (7th ed.). Philadelphia: Saunders.

Facts and Comparisons. (2004). *Drug facts and comparisons, pocket version* (9th ed.). St Louis, MO: Wolters Kluwer Health.

Fetrow, C.W., & Avila, J.R. (2000). *The complete guide to herbal remedies.* Springhouse, PA: Springhouse.

Hardman, J.G., & Limbird, LE. (2002). *Goodman and Gilman's the pharmacological basis of therapeutics* (10th ed.). New York: McGraw-Hill.

Jellin, J.M., Batz, F., & Hitchens, K. (2001). *Natural medicines comprehensive database.* Stockton, CA: Therapeutic Research Faculty.

Johns Hopkins Hospital, Gunn, V.L., & Nechyba, C. (2000). *The Harriet Lane handbook* (16th ed.). St Louis, MO: Mosby.

Katzung, B.G. (2004). *Basic and clinical pharmacology* (9th ed.). New York: McGraw-Hill.

Koda-Kimble, M.A., & Young, L.Y. (2001). *Applied therapeutics: The clinical use of drugs* (7th ed.). Philadelphia: Lippincott Williams & Wilkins.

Lacy, C.F., Armstrong, L.L., Goldman, M.P., & Lance, L.L. (Eds.). (2003). *Drug information handbook* (11th ed.). Hudson, OH: Lexi-Comp.

Lehne, R.A. (2004). *Pharmacology in nursing care* (5th ed.). St Louis, MO: Saunders.

McKenry, L.M., & Salerno, E. (2003). *Mosby's pharmacology in nursing*—revised and updated (21st ed.). St Louis, MO: Mosby.

Mosby. (2005). *Mosby's drug consult 2005: The comprehensive reference for generic and brand name drugs* (15th ed.). St Louis, MO: Mosby.

Skidmore-Roth, L. (2006). *Mosby's 2006 nursing drug reference* (19th ed.). St Louis, MO: Mosby.

Central Nervous System Depressants and Muscle Relaxants

OBJECTIVES

After reading this chapter, the successful student will be able to do the following:

1 Differentiate between a sedative and a hypnotic agent.

2 Describe the differences between benzodiazepines and barbiturates as sedative–hypnotic agents.

3 Identify specific benzodiazepine and barbiturate agents.

4 Discuss the nursing process as it relates to the nursing care of clients receiving sedative–hypnotic agents.

5 Identify mechanisms of action, drug effects, indications, interactions, cautions, contraindications, side and toxic effects, dosage ranges, and routes of administration for sedative–hypnotics and for skeletal muscle relaxants.

6 Understand the importance of always encouraging the use of non-pharmacological approaches to treat sleep disturbances before initiation of pharmacological treatments.

7 Develop education guidelines for clients receiving sedative–hypnotic agents.

8 Discuss the nursing process for clients receiving skeletal muscle relaxants.

e-LEARNING ACTIVITIES

Student CD-ROM
- Review Questions: see questions 56–61
- Animations
- Medication Administration Checklists
- IV Therapy Checklists

evolve Web site (http://evolve.elsevier.com/Lilley/pharmacology/)
- Online Chapter Worksheet • Frequently Asked Questions
- Learning Tips and Content Updates • WebLinks • Online Appendices and Supplements • Mosby/Saunders ePharmacology Update • Access to *Mosby's Drug Consult*

DRUG PROFILES

▶▶baclofen, p. 196
▶▶cyclobenzaprine, p. 197
dantrolene, p. 197
flurazepam, p. 193
lorazepam, p. 193

pentobarbital, p. 191
phenobarbital, p. 191
▶▶temazepam, p. 194
triazolam, p. 194
▶▶zopiclone, p. 194

▶▶ Key drug.

GLOSSARY

Anxiolytic (angk zee o lit′ ik) A medication that relieves anxiety.

Barbiturates (bar bich′ ər əts) A class of drugs that are chemical derivatives of barbituric acid. They can induce sedation and sleep.

Benzodiazepines (ben zo di az′ ə peenz) A chemical category of drugs most frequently prescribed as sedative–hypnotic and anxiolytic agents.

Gamma-aminobutyric acid (GABA) (əmee no bu ter′ ik) An inhibitory neurotransmitter found in the brain.

Hypnotics Drugs that, when given at low to moderate doses, calm or soothe the central nervous system (CNS) without inducing sleep but when given at high doses may cause sleep.

Non–rapid eye movement (non–REM) One of the stages of the sleep cycle. It characteristically has four stages and precedes REM sleep. Most of a normal sleep cycle consists of non-REM sleep.

Rapid eye movement (REM) One of the stages of the sleep cycle. One of the characteristics of REM sleep is the rapid movement of the eyes, vivid dreams, and irregular breathing.

Sedatives Drugs that have an inhibitory effect on the CNS to the degree that they reduce nervousness, excitability, and irritability without causing sleep.

Sedative–hypnotics Drugs that can act in the body either as a sedative or hypnotic.

Sleep A transient, reversible, and periodic state of rest in which there is a decrease in physical activity and consciousness.

Sleep architecture The various steps involved in the sleep cycle, including normal and abnormal patterns of sleep.

Tachyphylaxis (tak ee fə lak′ sis) The rapid appearance of a progressive decrease in response to a drug after repetitive administration of the drug.

Therapeutic index The ratio of the drug's therapeutic dose to its toxic dose.

Drugs that have a calming effect or that depress the central nervous system (CNS) are referred to as *sedatives* and *hypnotics*. A drug is classified as either a sedative or a hypnotic agent depending on the degree to which it inhibits the transmission of nerve impulses to the CNS. **Sedatives** reduce nervousness, excitability, and irritability without causing sleep, but a sedative can become a hypnotic if it is given in large enough doses. **Hypnotics** cause sleep. They have a much more potent effect on the CNS than sedatives do. Many drugs can act in the body as either a sedative or a hypnotic, and for this reason are called *sedative–hypnotics*. Listed in Table 12-1 are some points of interest relating to sedative–hypnotics.

Sedative–hypnotics can be classified chemically into three main groups: barbiturates, benzodiazepines, and miscellaneous agents. Before discussing the sedative–hypnotics in depth, it is important that the physiology of normal sleep be understood because of the significant effects these agents can have on sleep patterns.

SLEEP

Sleep is defined as a transient, reversible, and periodic state of rest in which there is a decrease in physical activity and consciousness. Normal sleep is cyclic and repetitive, and a person's responses to stimuli are markedly reduced during sleep. During waking hours the body is bombarded with stimuli that provoke the senses of sight, hearing, touch, smell, and taste. These stimuli elicit voluntary and involuntary movements or functions. During sleep a person is no longer aware of the sensory stimuli within his or her immediate environment.

Sleep research involves studying the patterns of sleep, or what is sometimes referred to as **sleep architecture.** The architecture of sleep consists of two basic stages that occur cyclically: **rapid eye movement (REM)** sleep and **non–rapid eye movement (non–REM)** sleep. The normal cyclic progression of the stages of sleep is summarized in Table 12-2. Various sedative–hypnotics affect different stages of the normal sleep pattern. If usage is prolonged, emotional and psychological changes can occur. An appreciation of this will help prevent the inappropriate use of long-term sleeping agents.

BARBITURATES

Barbiturates were first introduced into clinical use in 1903 and were the standard agents for treating insomnia and producing sedation. Chemically they are derivatives of barbituric acid. Although there are close to 35 different barbiturates approved for clinical use in Canada, only a handful are in common clinical use today. This is in part due to the favourable safety profile and proven efficacy of the class of drugs commonly referred to as *benzodiazepines*. Barbiturates can produce many unwanted side effects. They are habit-forming and have a narrow **therapeutic index** (the dosage range within which the drug is effective but above which it is rapidly toxic). Barbiturates can be classified into four groups based on their onset and duration of action. Table 12-3 lists the agents within each category and summarizes their pharmacokinetic characteristics.

TABLE 12-1

SEDATIVE–HYPNOTIC AGENTS: POINTS OF INTEREST

Agent	Point
flurazepam	Causes less REM rebound than other benzodiazepines; cautious use in geriatric clients; give 15–30 min before bedtime.
pentobarbital	Short acting; can be given PO, by rectal suppository, or IM; IM injection given deep in large muscle mass; as with any of these agents, clients should avoid caffeine intake 4 hr around the time of dosing because of the decreased effectiveness that results.
phenobarbital	Long acting (up to 16 hr duration); in the body longer and thus can react with other medications such as alcohol and other CNS depressants; because of long duration, use cautiously in the geriatric client who has decreased liver and renal function.
temazepam	Induces sleep within 20–40 min; give 20–30 min before bedtime.
triazolam	Short-term use only; try other medications in this category, as ordered by a physician; cautious use with geriatric clients—causes confusion so protect from injury.

PO, per orally; *IM,* intramuscular(ly); *CNS,* central nervous system.

Mechanism of Action and Drug Effects

Barbiturates are CNS depressants that act primarily on the brainstem in an area called the *reticular formation.* Their sedative and hypnotic effects are dose related, and they act by reducing the nerve impulses travelling to the area in the brain called the *cerebral cortex.* Their ability to inhibit nerve impulse transmission is in part due to their ability to potentiate an inhibitory amino acid known as **gamma-aminobutyric acid (GABA),** which is found in high concentrations in the CNS. Barbiturates are capable of raising the convulsive or seizure threshold and are therefore also effective in treating status epilepticus and tetanus- or drug-induced convulsions. In addition, selected barbiturates are used as prophylaxis for epileptic seizures.

In low doses, barbiturates act as sedatives. Increasing the dose produces a hypnotic effect, but this also decreases the respiratory rate. In normal doses they have little effect on the circulation. Barbiturates as a class are notorious enzyme inducers. They stimulate the enzymes in the liver that are responsible for the metabolism or breakdown of many drugs. By stimulating these enzymes they cause many drugs to be metabolized more quickly, which usually shortens their duration of action.

Warfarin, theophylline, and phenytoin are three such drugs. They are commonly prescribed and potentially dangerous drugs.

Indications

All barbiturates have the same sedative–hypnotic efficacy but differ in their potency, onset, and duration of action. They are used as hypnotics, sedatives, and anticonvulsants and also for anaesthesia during surgical procedures. They are used for the following therapeutic reasons:

Ultra-short: Anaesthetic for short surgical procedures, anaesthesia induction, control of convulsions, narco-analysis (a form of psychotherapy), and reduction in intracranial pressure in neurosurgical clients.

Short: Sedative–hypnotic and control of convulsive conditions.

Intermediate: Sedative–hypnotic and control of convulsive conditions.

Long: Sedative–hypnotic, epileptic seizure prophylaxis, and treatment of neonatal hyperbilirubinemia.

Contraindications

Contraindications to barbiturates include known drug allergy, pregnancy, significant respiratory difficulties, and severe liver disease.

Side Effects and Adverse Effects

The main side effects of barbiturates affect the CNS and include drowsiness, lethargy, dizziness, hangover, and paradoxical restlessness or excitement. Their chronic effects on normal sleep architecture can be detrimental. Sleep research has shown that adequate rest from the sleep process is obtained only when there are proper amounts of REM sleep, which is sometimes referred to as *dreaming sleep.* Barbiturates deprive people of REM sleep, which can result in agitation and an inability to deal with normal stress. When the barbiturate is stopped and REM sleep once again occurs, a rebound phenomenon can occur. During this rebound the proportion of REM sleep is increased, the client's dream time constitutes a larger percentage of the total sleep pattern, and the dreams are often nightmares. The adverse effects of barbiturates relative to the body systems affected are listed in Table 12-4.

TABLE 12-2
STAGES OF SLEEP

Stage	Characteristics	Average Percentage of Time in Each Stage (For Young Adult)
NON–REM SLEEP		
1	Dozing or feelings of drifting off to sleep; person can be easily awakened; insomniacs have longer stage 1 periods than normal.	2%–5%
2	Person is relaxed but can be easily awakened; has occasional REMs and also slight eye movements.	50%
3	Deep sleep; difficult to wake person; respiratory rates, pulse, and blood pressure may decrease.	5%
4	Sleepwalking or bedwetting may occur; difficult to wake person; may be groggy if awakened; dreaming, especially about daily events.	10%–15%
REM SLEEP		
	REMs occur; vivid dreams occur; breathing may be irregular.	25%–33%

Modified from McKenry, L.M., & Salerno, E. 2003. *Mosby's pharmacology in nursing—revised and updated,* 21st ed. St Louis, MO: Mosby.

TABLE 12-3
BARBITURATES: ONSET AND DURATION

Category	Pharmacokinetics		Barbiturates
	Onset	Duration	
Short	IV: <15 min PO: 10–15 min	IV: 10–30 min PO: 2–4 hr	thiopental pentobarbital
Intermediate	PO: 45–60 min	6–8 hr	amobarbital
Long	PO: 60 min	PO: 10–12 hr	phenobarbital

IV, Intravenous; *PO,* oral.

TABLE 12-4

BARBITURATES: ADVERSE EFFECTS

Body System	Side/Adverse Effects
Cardiovascular	Vasodilation and hypotension, especially if given too rapidly
Gastrointestinal	Nausea, vomiting, diarrhea, constipation
Hematological	Agranulocytosis, thrombocytopenia, megaloblastic anemia
Nervous	Drowsiness; lethargy; vertigo; headache; mental depression; and myalgic, neuralgic, arthralgic pain
Respiratory	Respiratory depression, apnea, laryngospasm, bronchospasm, coughing
Other	Hypersensitivity reactions: urticaria, angioedema, rash, fever, serum sickness, Stevens-Johnson syndrome

Toxicity and Management of Overdose

Overdose frequently results in respiratory depression, leading to respiratory arrest. Often this is done therapeutically to induce anaesthesia. In this situation, however, the client is ventilated mechanically and respiration is controlled or assisted mechanically. Another situation in which intentional overdoses are given for therapeutic reasons is the management of uncontrollable seizures. Such clients are sometimes put into what is called a *phenobarbital coma*. Because of the inhibitory effects of barbiturates on nerve transmission in the brain (possibly GABA mediated), the uncontrollable seizures can be stopped until appropriate drug levels of anticonvulsant drugs are achieved.

An overdose of barbiturates produces CNS depression ranging from sleep to profound coma and death. Respiratory depression progresses to Cheyne-Stokes respiration (periodic shallow breathing or apnea), hypoventilation, and cyanosis (bluish skin). Affected clients often have cold, clammy skin or are hypothermic, and later they can exhibit fever, areflexia, tachycardia, and hypotension. Pupils are usually slightly constricted but may be dilated in the event of severe drug toxicity.

Treatment of an overdose is mainly symptomatic and supportive. The mainstays of therapy should consist of maintenance of an adequate airway, assisted respiration, and oxygen administration if needed, along with fluid and pressor support as indicated. The multiple-dose (every 4 hours) nasogastric administration of activated charcoal is highly effective in removing barbiturates from the stomach and the circulation. Barbiturates are highly metabolized by the liver, and they increase enzyme activity there. In an overdose, however, the amount of barbiturate may overwhelm the liver's ability to metabolize it. This is where activated charcoal may be helpful. Activated charcoal helps pull the drug from the circulation and eliminate it by means of the gastrointestinal (GI) system. Some of the barbiturates (e.g., phenobarbital) can be eliminated more quickly by the kidneys when the urine is alkalized. This keeps the drug in the urine and prevents it from being resorbed back into the circulation. Alkalization, along with forced diuresis, can hasten elimination of the barbiturate.

Interactions

The potential drug interactions with barbiturates are considerable in their intensity and often dramatic. The risk encountered in the co-administration of barbiturates with alcohol, antihistamines, benzodiazepines, opioids, and tranquilizers is additive CNS depression. Most of the drug–drug interactions involving barbiturates are secondary to their effects on the hepatic enzyme system. As mentioned previously, barbiturates increase the activity of hepatic microsomal enzymes. This is called *enzyme induction*. Induction of this enzyme system results in increased drug metabolism and breakdown. However, if the two drugs are competing for the same enzyme system for metabolism, this can lead to inhibited drug metabolism or breakdown. Two examples are co-administration of monoamine oxidase inhibitors (MAOIs) or anticoagulants with barbiturates. Co-administration of MAOIs with barbiturates can result in prolonged barbiturate effects. Co-administration of anticoagulants with barbiturates can result in decreased anticoagulation response and possible clot formation. In addition, co-administration of barbiturates with oral contraceptives can result in accelerated metabolism of the contraceptive agent and possible unintended pregnancy. Women taking both types of medication concurrently should be advised to consider an additional method of contraception as a backup.

Laboratory Test Interactions

Barbiturates can also interact with body substances and affect the results of various laboratory tests. Barbiturates can cause an increase in the serum levels of bilirubin, serum glutamate pyruvate transaminase (ALT), serum glutamic-oxaloacetic transaminase (AST), and alkaline phosphatase.

Dosages

As previously mentioned, barbiturates can act as either sedatives or hypnotics depending on their dosage. The various barbiturates and their recommended sedative and hypnotic dosages are listed in the dosages table on p. 191. See Appendix B for some of the common brands available in Canada.

DRUG PROFILES

Barbiturates are available in a variety of dosage forms, including tablets, capsules, elixirs, injections, and suppositories. Studies link certain sedative–hypnotic drug use with birth defects and behavioural abnormalities in babies and so these drugs are not recommended for use during pregnancy. All barbiturates are considered prescription-only drugs because of the potential for misuse and the severe effects that result if they are not

DOSAGES Selected Barbiturates

Agent	Onset and Duration	Usual Dosage Range	Indications
pentobarbital	Short-acting	**Pediatric** IM/IV/PO: 2–6 mg/kg; Rectal: 2 mo–1 yr, 30 mg; 1–4 yr, 30–60 mg; 5–12 yr, 60 mg; 12–14 yr, 60–120 mg HS	Anticonvulsant, pre-op sedative, sedative
		Adult PO: 100–200 mg HS	Hypnotic
		IM: 150–200 mg; Rectal: 120–200 mg HS; IV: 100 mg	Anticonvulsant, pre-op sedative, hypnotic
phenobarbital	Long-acting	**Neonatal** PO: 5–10 mg/kg/day	Hyperbilirubinemia
		Pediatric PO: 1–6 mg/kg in 3 equally divided doses	Sedative
		IM/IV: 1–3 mg/kg	Pre-op sedative
		Adult PO: 60–250 mg/day single or divided	Sedative
		100–320 mg HS	Hypnotic
		IM/IV: 130–200 mg 60–90 min before surgery	Pre-op sedative

HS, at bedtime; *IM*, intramuscular; *IV*, intravenous; *PO*, per orally.

used appropriately. The majority of barbiturates and other sedative–hypnotics are defined as controlled substances, governed by Schedule G of Canada's Food and Drugs Act; the rest are governed by Schedule F. Drugs listed in Schedule F are legally available only with a physician's prescription. Additional restrictions apply to drugs listed in Schedule G. As discussed in Chapter 4, controlled substances are medications that the Controlled Drugs and Substances Act identifies as drugs that have an abuse potential; they are categorized into eight schedules depending on how easily they can be manufactured illegally. Barbiturates are listed under Schedule IV. Provincial laws may place further restrictions on the way these drugs are dispensed; therefore healthcare providers must be careful to comply with both federal and provincial laws. Barbiturates are contraindicated in clients with known hypersensitivity reactions to them, latent porphyria, significant liver dysfunction, and known previous addiction.

pentobarbital

Formerly used as a sedative–hypnotic for insomnia, pentobarbital is now principally used preoperatively to relieve anxiety and provide sedation. In addition, it is used occasionally to control status epilepticus or acute seizure episodes resulting from meningitis, poisons, eclampsia, alcohol withdrawal, tetanus, and chorea. Pentobarbital may also be used to treat withdrawal symptoms in clients who are physically dependent on barbiturates or non-barbiturate hypnotics. Pregnancy category D. The sedative and hypnotic dosages are given in the dosages table above.

PHARMACOKINETICS

	Half-Life	Onset	Peak	Duration
PO:	15–48 hr	10–15 min	30–60 min	3–4 hr
IV:	15–48 hr	<1 min	<30 min	15 min

phenobarbital

Phenobarbital is the most commonly prescribed barbiturate, either alone or in combination with other drugs.

It is considered the prototypical barbiturate and is classified as a long-acting agent. Phenobarbital is used for the prevention of grand mal seizures and fever-induced convulsions. In addition, it has been useful in the treatment of hyperbilirubinemia in neonates. It has also been used for the treatment of Gilbert syndrome. It is only rarely used today as a sedative–hypnotic agent. Pregnancy category D. See the table above for dosages.

PHARMACOKINETICS

	Half-Life	Onset	Peak	Duration
PO:	80–120 hr	60 min	8–12 hr	10–12 hr
IV:	80–120 hr	5 min	30 min	4–10 hr

BENZODIAZEPINES

Benzodiazepines are the most commonly prescribed sedative–hypnotic agents and one of the most commonly prescribed classes of drugs because of their favourable side effect profiles, efficacy, and safety. Even when a drug in this class is taken as the sole agent in an overdose (e.g., not with alcohol), it is relatively benign, resulting in little more than sedation. Benzodiazepines are classified as either anxiolytics or sedative–hypnotics depending on their primary usage. An **anxiolytic** relieves anxiety. The benzodiazepines discussed in Chapter 15 are the ones that work primarily to produce sedation or sleep. There are five such agents commonly used as sedative–hypnotics. They are listed in Table 12-5 and can be further classified on the basis of their duration of action as either long-acting or short-acting.

Mechanism of Action and Drug Effects

As mentioned previously, the sedative and hypnotic action of benzodiazepines is related to their ability to depress activity in the CNS. The specific areas they affect in the CNS appear to be the hypothalamic, thalamic, and

TABLE 12-5

SEDATIVE–HYPNOTIC BENZODIAZEPINES AVAILABLE IN CANADA

LONG-ACTING
chlordiazepoxide
clorazepate
flurazepam

INTERMEDIATE-ACTING
alprazolam
bromazepam
clobazam
clonazepam
lorazepam
nitrazepam
oxazepam
temazepam

SHORT-ACTING*
midazolam (IV only)
triazolam

*Zaleplon and zolpidem share many characteristics with the benzodiazepines but are classified as non-benzodiazepine hypnotic agents and are not available in Canada.

Note: The benzodiazepines discussed in Chapter 15 and those discussed here all have similar pharmacological properties. They all act as anxiolytics and sedative–hypnotics. Different benzodiazepines are just more effective at one or the other pharmacological effect.

limbic systems of the brain. Recent research has indicated that there are specific receptors in the brain for benzodiazepines. These receptors are thought to be the same as those of the CNS inhibitory transmitter GABA. If they are not the same, then they are adjacent to the GABA receptors. Their depressant action on the CNS appears to be related to their ability to inhibit stimulation of the brain. They have many favourable effects compared with the barbiturates. They do not suppress REM sleep to the same extent as barbiturates. They also do not induce hepatic microsomal enzyme activity and are therefore safe to administer to clients who are taking medications that are metabolized by this enzyme system.

In terms of client experience, benzodiazepines have a calming effect on the CNS. This causes the inhibition of hyperexcitable nerves in the CNS that might be responsible for causing seizure activity. Similarly, this calming effect on the CNS makes benzodiazepines useful in controlling agitation and anxiety. It also reduces excessive sensory stimulation and induces sleep. In addition, benzodiazepines have been shown to induce skeletal muscle relaxation. Their receptors in the CNS are in the same area as those that play a role in alcohol addiction. Therefore they are used in the treatment and prevention of the symptoms of alcohol withdrawal (see Chapter 15).

Indications

Benzodiazepines have a variety of therapeutic applications. They are most commonly used for sedation, sleep induction, skeletal muscle relaxation, and anxiety relief. They have also been used in the treatment of alcohol withdrawal, agitation, depression, and epilepsy. They are often combined with anaesthetics, analgesics, and neuromuscular blocking agents (NMBAs) in what is called *balanced anaesthesia*. Their use in this setting is mostly for their amnesiac properties because most people undergoing surgery would rather not remember the events of their procedure.

Contraindications

Contraindications to the use of benzodiazepines include known drug allergy, narrow-angle glaucoma, and pregnancy.

Side Effects and Adverse Effects

As a class, benzodiazepines have a relatively safe side effect profile. The side effects and adverse effects associated with their use are usually mild and they primarily involve the CNS. The more commonly reported undesirable effects are headache, drowsiness, paradoxical excitement or nervousness, dizziness or vertigo, cognitive impairment, and lethargy. However, they can create a significant fall hazard in frail geriatric clients and should be avoided when possible in this population. To help avoid side effects, the lowest effective doses are recommended for all clients, especially geriatric. Because of the benzodiazepines' effect on the normal sleep cycle, a hangover effect is sometimes reported. Other less common side effects and adverse effects are palpitations, dry mouth, nausea, vomiting, hypokinesia, and occasional nightmares.

Toxicity and Management of Overdose

An overdose of benzodiazepines may result in somnolence, confusion, coma, and/or diminished reflexes. An overdose of just benzodiazepines rarely results in hypotension and respiratory depression. These are more commonly seen when benzodiazepines are taken with other CNS depressants such as alcohol or barbiturates. The same holds true for their lethal effects. In the absence of the concurrent ingestion of alcohol or other CNS depressants, benzodiazepine overdose rarely results in death.

The treatment of benzodiazepine intoxication is generally symptomatic and supportive. If ingestion is recent, decontamination of the GI system is indicated. As a rule of thumb, agents that have been orally ingested may be absorbed by activated charcoal. Activated charcoal is beneficial if it can be administered within 2 to 4 hours of ingestion and if the risk of aspiration is minimal. Hemodialysis is not useful in the treatment of benzodiazepine overdose. Flumazenil can be used to acutely reverse the sedative effects of benzodiazepines, though this is normally done only in cases of excessive overdose or sedation. Flumazenil antagonizes the action of benzodiazepines on the CNS by directly competing with benzodiazepines for binding at the benzodiazepine receptor in the CNS. However, it has a stronger affinity for the receptor and knocks the benzodiazepine off the receptor, reversing the sedative action of the benzodiazepine. The dosage regimen to be followed for the reversal of conscious sedation or general

TABLE 12-6
FLUMAZENIL TREATMENT REGIMEN

Indication	Recommended Regimen	Duration
Reversal of conscious sedation or general anaesthesia	0.2 mg (mL) given IV over 15 sec, then give 0.1 mg if consciousness does not occur; may be repeated at 60-sec intervals prn up to 8 additional times (maximum total dose, 1 mg; usual dose is 0.3–0.6 mg)	1–4 hr
Management of suspected benzodiazepine overdose	0.3 mg (3 mL) given IV over 30 sec; wait 30 sec, then give 0.3 mg (3 mL) over 30 sec if consciousness does not occur; further doses of 0.5 mg (5 mL) can be given over 30 sec at intervals of 1 min up to a cumulative dose of 2 mg	1–4 hr

Important note: Flumazenil has a relatively short half-life and duration of effect of 1–4 hr; therefore if using flumazenil to reverse the effects of a long-acting benzodiazepine, the dose of the reversal agent may wear off and the client may become sedated again, requiring more flumazenil.

anaesthesia induced by benzodiazepines and the management of suspected benzodiazepine overdose are summarized in Table 12-6.

Interactions

The potential drug interactions with the benzodiazepines are significant in their intensity, particularly when they are taken in combination with other CNS depressants and MAOIs. The risks associated with the co-administration of other agents are listed and described in Table 12-7.

Laboratory Test Interactions

There are no laboratory test interactions that occur with the five benzodiazepines that are typically used as either sedatives or hypnotics.

Dosages

The benzodiazepines discussed in this chapter are those that are commonly used to treat insomnia. Therefore the dosage recommendations given in the table on p. 194 are those for achieving hypnotic effects. The dosage should be individualized and titrated to achieve the lowest effective dose. All agents used for the treatment of insomnia should be limited to no more than 2 to 4 weeks. With long-term usage, rebound insomnia and severe withdrawal can develop. Geriatric clients should also be started on lower doses because they generally experience a more pronounced effect from benzodiazepines. See Appendix B for some of the common brands available in Canada.

DRUG PROFILES

Benzodiazepines are all prescription-only drugs, and they are designated as Schedule IV controlled substances. All benzodiazepines discussed here have active metabolites, which can accumulate during long-term use, especially in clients who have altered metabolic function (hepatic dysfunction) or altered excretion capabilities (renal dysfunction). There are several other benzodiazepines, but they are more commonly used to treat anxiety or agitation, to produce amnesia, and to relax skeletal muscles. These other

TABLE 12-7
BENZODIAZEPINES: DRUG INTERACTIONS

Drug	Mechanism	Result
cimetidine	Decreased benzodiazepine metabolism	Prolonged benzodiazepine action
Alcohol and other CNS depressants	Additive effects	Increased CNS depression
monoamine oxidase inhibitors (MAOIs)	Decreased metabolism	Increased benzodiazepine effects
Protease inhibitors	Decreased metabolism	Increased benzodiazepine effects

benzodiazepines are discussed in detail in the appropriate chapters.

flurazepam

Flurazepam is available in 15- and 30-mg capsules. It is considered a long-acting hypnotic agent and is indicated for the short-term treatment of insomnia for periods of up to 4 weeks. Flurazepam has two active metabolites that account for its hypnotic effects. These active metabolites have also been shown to be responsible for inducing a hangover effect, causing lethargy or grogginess the morning after the medication has been taken. Because of its rapid onset and its long action, flurazepam is often used for clients who have difficulty not only in falling asleep but also in maintaining sleep. Not recommended for use during pregnancy (pregnancy category X). The recommended dosages for adult and geriatric clients are given in the table on p. 194.

PHARMACOKINETICS

Half-Life	Onset	Peak	Duration
100 hr	15–45 min	30–60 min	7–8 hr

lorazepam

Lorazepam is available in 0.5-, 1-, and 2-mg tablets. It is considered an intermediate-acting hypnotic agent and is indicated for the short-term treatment of insomnia for periods of up to 4 weeks. Because of its short duration, morning drowsiness is not a problem. Pregnancy category X. The recommended dosages for adult and geriatric clients are given in the table below.

PHARMACOKINETICS

Half-Life	Onset	Peak	Duration
10–20 hr	30–60 min	2–4 hr	up to 8 hr

▶▶ temazepam

Temazepam is available in 15- and 30-mg capsules. It is contraindicated in clients who have narrow-angle glaucoma because it can exacerbate the glaucoma. It is indicated for the short-term treatment of insomnia. Pregnancy category X. The common dosages are given in the table below.

PHARMACOKINETICS

Half-Life	Onset	Peak	Duration
10–20 hr	30–60 min	2–3 hr	7–8 hr

triazolam

Triazolam is available in 0.125- and 0.25-mg tablets and is indicated for the short-term treatment of insomnia.

The best approach with this drug is for the nurse to give the smallest effective dose for the shortest possible duration. Pregnancy category X. The common dosages for adult and geriatric clients are given in the table below.

PHARMACOKINETICS

Half-Life	Onset	Peak	Duration
1.5–5 hr	15–30 min	1–2 hr	6–7 hr

▶▶ zopiclone

Zopiclone is a short-acting non-benzodiazepine hypnotic agent. It is indicated for the short-term treatment of insomnia and, as with all benzodiazepines, should be limited to 7 to 10 days of treatment. Zopiclone belongs to a novel chemical class of hypnotics that is structurally unrelated to existing benzodiazepines. However, the pharmacological profile of zopiclone is similar to that of the benzodiazepines. It is available in 5- and 7.5-mg tablets. Pregnancy category B. The recommended dosage is given in the table below.

PHARMACOKINETICS

Half-Life	Onset	Peak	Duration
3.8–6.5 hr	30 min	90 min	4–6 hr

DOSAGES Benzodiazepines: Selected Hypnotic Agents

Agent	Onset and Duration	Usual Dosage Range	Indications
flurazepam	Long-acting	**Adult** PO: 15–30 mg at bedtime	
lorazepam	Intermediate-acting	**Adult** PO: 0.5–1 mg at bedtime	
nitrazepam	Intermediate-acting	**Adult** PO: 5–10 mg at bedtime	
oxazepam	Short-acting	**Adult** PO: 15 mg	
▶▶ temazepam	Intermediate-acting	**Adult** PO: 15 mg at bedtime **Geriatric** PO: 7.5 mg at bedtime	Hypnotic
triazolam	Short-acting	**Adult** PO: 0.125–0.25 mg at bedtime **Geriatric** PO: 0.125–0.25 mg at bedtime	
zolpidem*	Short-acting	**Adult** PO: 10 mg at bedtime **Geriatric** PO: 5 mg at bedtime	
▶▶ zopiclone	Short-acting	**Adult:** PO: 5–7.5 mg at bedtime **Geriatric:** PO: 3.75 mg starting and may be increased up to 7.5 mg at bedtime	

*Zolpidem is classified as a non-benzodiazepine hypnotic agent. It is listed under the Canadian *Benzodiazepines and Other Targeted Substances Regulations* (Targeted Substances Regulations) but is not currently marketed for sale in Canada.

Benzodiazepine Use Among Older Adults

Benzodiazepines are a commonly prescribed drug, especially for older adults, frequently for prolonged periods. Older women are more likely to receive benzodiazepines than older men. Generally benzodiazepines are not recommended to be used for longer than 4 weeks because their long-term efficacy remains unproven. Yet because insomnia is a chronic problem with the older adult, benzodiazepines are frequently prescribed for longer periods of time. As a result, there is an increased risk of dependence. High use of these drugs also leads to memory impairment, daytime drowsiness, accidental falls resulting in hip fractures, motor vehicle crashes, accidental poisonings, hospitalization for depression and other psychiatric problems, as well as attempted and completed suicides. Older adults are more sensitive to the CNS depressant effects of benzodiazepines as aging increases the half-life of the drugs. As a result, the drugs can cause confusion, night wandering, amnesia, loss of balance, hangover effects, and "pseudodementia" (often attributed to Alzheimer's disease). Benzodiazepines without active metabolites (e.g., oxazepam, temazepam) are tolerated better by older adults than those drugs with slowly eliminated metabolites (e.g., chlordiazepoxide, nitrazepam).

MUSCLE RELAXANTS

A variety of conditions such as trauma, inflammation, anxiety, and pain can be associated with acute muscle spasms. Although there is no completely satisfactory form of therapy available for relief of skeletal muscle spasticity, muscle relaxants are capable of providing some relief. The muscle relaxants are a group of compounds that act predominantly within the CNS to relieve pain associated with skeletal muscle spasms. The majority of muscle relaxants are called *central-acting skeletal muscle relaxants* because they have as their site of action the CNS. Central-acting skeletal muscle relaxants are similar in structure and action to other CNS depressants such as diazepam and therefore act within the CNS. It is believed that the muscle relaxant effects of these agents are related to this CNS depressant activity. Only one of these compounds, dantrolene, acts directly on skeletal muscle. It belongs to a group of relaxants known as direct-acting skeletal muscle relaxants. It closely resembles GABA.

These agents are most effective when used in conjunction with rest and physical therapy. When muscle relaxants are taken with alcohol, other CNS depressants, or opioid analgesics, enhanced CNS depressant effects are seen. Close monitoring and dosage reduction of one or both drugs should be considered.

Mechanism of Action and Drug Effects

The majority of the muscle relaxants work within the CNS. Their beneficial effects are believed to come from their sedative effects rather than from direct muscle relaxation. Aside from dantrolene, muscle relaxants have no direct effects on muscles, nerve conduction, or muscle–nerve junctions. One of the more effective agents in this class of drugs, baclofen, is a derivative of GABA. It is believed to work by depressing nerve transmission in the spinal cord. The other agents in this class of drugs are not derivatives of GABA but act by enhancing GABA's central inhibitory effects at the level of the spinal cord. These agents are generally less effective than baclofen. The only agent in the class to act directly on skeletal muscle is dantrolene. Dantrolene acts directly on the excitation–contraction coupling of muscle fibres and not at the level of the CNS. It appears to do this by decreasing the amount of calcium released from storage sites in the sarcoplasmic reticulum.

As noted earlier, muscle relaxants have a depressant effect on the CNS. Their effects are the result of CNS depression in the brain primarily at the level of the brainstem, thalamus, and basal ganglia but also at the spinal cord. Dantrolene has the additive effect of directly affecting skeletal muscles by decreasing the response of the muscle to stimuli. The effects of muscle relaxants are relaxation of striated muscles, mild weakness of skeletal muscles, decreased force of muscle contraction, and muscle stiffness. Other drug effects that may be experienced are generalized CNS depression seen as sedation, somnolence, ataxia (clumsy, unsteady movements), and respiratory and cardiovascular depression.

Indications

Muscle relaxants are primarily used for the relief of painful musculoskeletal conditions such as muscle spasms. They are most effective when used in conjunction with physical therapy. They may also be used in the management of spasticity associated with severe chronic disorders such as multiple sclerosis and other types of cerebral lesions, cerebral palsy, or rheumatic disorders. Some relaxants are used to reduce choreiform (jerky, involuntary) movement in clients with Huntington's chorea, to reduce rigidity in clients with parkinsonian syndrome, or in the relief of pain associated with trigeminal neuralgia. Intravenous dantrolene is used for the management of "full-blown" hypermetabolism of skeletal muscle that is characteristic of a malignant hyperthermia crisis. Another muscle relaxant, baclofen, has been shown to be effective in relieving hiccups.

Contraindications

The only usual contraindication to the use of muscle relaxants is known drug allergy but contraindications may also include severe renal impairment.

Side Effects and Adverse Effects

The primary side effects of muscle relaxants are an extension of their effects on the CNS and skeletal muscles. Euphoria, lightheadedness, dizziness, drowsiness, fatigue, and muscle weakness are often experienced early in treatment. These side effects are generally short lived, with clients growing tolerant to them over time. Less common side effects seen with muscle relaxants include diarrhea, GI upset, headache, slurred speech, muscle stiffness, constipation, sexual difficulties in males, hypotension, tachycardia, and weight gain. Dantrolene has a serious potential to cause hepatotoxicity. However, this is rare, occurring in 0.1 to 0.2 percent of clients treated with the drug for more than 60 days.

Toxicity and Management of Overdose

The toxicities and consequences of an overdose of muscle relaxants primarily involve the CNS. There is no specific antidote or reversal agent for muscle relaxant overdoses. They are best treated with conservative supportive measures. More aggressive therapies are generally needed when muscle relaxants are taken along with other CNS depressant drugs as an overdose. Gastric lavage and close observation of the client are recommended. An adequate airway should be maintained and artificial respiration should be readily available. Electrocardiogram (ECG) monitoring and large quantities of intravenous fluids to avoid crystalluria should be instituted.

Interactions

When muscle relaxants are administered concomitantly with other depressant drugs such as alcohol and benzodiazepines, caution should be used to avoid overdosage. The combination of propoxyphene and orphenadrine has resulted in additive CNS effects. Mental confusion, anxiety, tremors, and additive hypoglycemic activity have been reported as well with this combination. A dosage reduction and/or discontinuance of one or both drugs is recommended.

Laboratory Test Interactions

A reducing substance in the urine of clients receiving methocarbonal may produce false-positive results for glucose determination using cupric sulphate (Benedict's solution, Clinitest, Fehling's solution) but does not interfere with glucose tests using glucose oxidase (Clinistix, Diastix, TesTape). Although these types of testing are somewhat outdated, they are still used in some client care scenarios.

Dosages

For an overview of dosages for the more commonly used muscle relaxants see the table below. See Appendix B for some of the common brands available in Canada.

DRUG PROFILES

Muscle relaxants are all prescription-only drugs and are all (except for one) centrally acting relaxants because of their site of action in the CNS. These include baclofen, chlorzoxazone, cyclobenzaprine, methocarbamol and orphenadrine. Only dantrolene works directly on skeletal muscle and is referred to as a direct-acting relaxant. Muscle relaxants have not been proven safe in pregnancy. They are all contraindicated in clients who have shown a hypersensitivity reaction to them or who have compromised pulmonary function, active hepatic disease, or impaired myocardial function.

▸▸ baclofen

Baclofen is available in 10- and 20-mg tablets and as a 0.5- and a 2-mg/mL concentration for injection. The usual oral (PO) dosage is 5 mg 3 times a day for 3 days. It is then recommended to increase the dose by 5 mg every 3 days until a maximum of 20 mg 3 times/day is reached, titrating to the desired response. The total

DOSAGES — Selected Muscle Relaxants

Agent	Pharmacological Class	Usual Dosage Range	Indications
baclofen	Central-acting	**Adult** PO: 5 mg tid 3 days, then 10 mg tid 3 days, then 15 mg tid, then titrated to response. Intrathecal: 120–1500 μg/day	Spasticity
cyclobenzaprine	Central-acting	**Adult** PO: 10–20 mg tid	Spasticity
dantrolene	Direct-acting	**Pediatric** PO: 0.5 mg/kg/day up to 3 mg/kg/day given in divided doses bid-qid **Adult** PO: 25 mg/day; may increase to 25–100 mg bid–qid **Pediatric and adult** IV: 1 mg/kg, may repeat to total dose of 10 mg/kg	Spasticity and malignant hyperthermia Malignant hyperthermia
tizanidine	Central-acting	**Adult** PO: 2 mg increased by 2–4 mg to optimum effect up to 36 mg/day divided tid	Spasticity

daily dose should not be greater than 80 mg. When given via the intrathecal route a compatible pump must be implanted. With this administration route a test dose should be administered initially to test for a positive response. The injection is diluted before infusion. Pregnancy category C.

PHARMACOKINETICS

Half-Life	Onset	Peak	Duration
2–4 hr	0.5–1 hr	2 hr	>8 hr

▸▸ *cyclobenzaprine*

Cyclobenzaprine is available in a 10-mg dose. It is a central-acting muscle relaxant that is structurally and pharmacologically related to the tricyclic antidepressants. The usual oral dosage is 10 mg 3 times a day for 1 week. It can be increased to a maximum of 60 mg daily. It is recommended for use for short periods (2 to 3 weeks). Pregnancy category B.

PHARMACOKINETICS

Half-Life	Onset	Peak	Duration
1–3 days	1 hr	3–8 hr	12–24 hr

dantrolene

Dantrolene is available in 25- and 100-mg capsules and as a 20-mg parenteral injection. It is a direct-acting muscle relaxant that is pharmacologically different from the central-acting relaxants in that it can work directly on the skeletal muscles. Dantrolene can be administered orally to children at a dosage of 1 mg/kg/day in two to three divided doses or to an adult at a dosage of 25 mg/day. In adults dantrolene can be increased to 25 to 100 mg 2 to 4 times/day when given orally. Dantrolene is also indicated for the acute management of malignant hyperthermia. This serious condition can occur on its own or as a complication of general anaesthesia. When dantrolene is given for malignant hyperthermia it is administered intravenously at a dosage of 1 mg/kg and may be repeated until a total dose of 10 mg/kg has been given. Pregnancy category C.

PHARMACOKINETICS

	Half-Life	Onset	Peak	Duration
PO:	8 hr	0.5–1 hr	5 hr	12–24 hr

MISCELLANEOUS AGENTS

There are several other miscellaneous medications that do not fall into the barbiturate or benzodiazepine drug class. These agents include chloral hydrate, etchlorvynol, tizanidine, and paraldehyde. These are all prescription-only drugs. Of these four sedative–hypnotic agents, chloral hydrate and tizanidine are the ones most commonly prescribed because the other two are associated with severe side effects and are extremely toxic if taken inappropriately or in an overdose.

Chloral hydrate is one of the oldest non-barbiturate, miscellaneous-categorized sedative–hypnotic agents. It

has the favourable characteristic of not suppressing REM sleep at the usual therapeutic doses, and the incidence of hangover effects associated with its use is low because of its relatively short duration of action. One potential disadvantage is that tachyphylaxis can develop rather quickly. **Tachyphylaxis** is the rapid appearance of a progressive decrease in response to a pharmacologically or physiologically active substance after its repetitive administration. This makes chloral hydrate useful only for short-term therapy. High doses lead to dependence and cause GI tract irritation. The combination of alcohol and chloral hydrate, commonly referred to as a "Mickey Finn," leads to rapid loss of consciousness.

Tizanidine is a short-acting, centrally-active alpha-adrenergic receptor agonist similar to clonidine. Tizanidine has been shown to decrease increased muscle tone and the frequency of daytime muscle spasms and nighttime awakenings caused by spasms. It is indicated for increased muscle tone associated with spasticity. It has been used in Europe and Japan for over a decade and was approved for use in Canada in 1999. It is most commonly used in clients with multiple sclerosis or spinal cord injury. The typical starting dose is 2 mg. It is then slowly titrated by 2- to 4-mg steps to optimum effect, not to exceed 36 mg/day. Clients are less likely to suffer from hypotension and bradycardia when it is slowly titrated.

Non-prescription sleeping aids often contain antihistamines, and some may also contain analgesics such as acetylsalicylic acid or acetaminophen. The most common antihistamines contained in over-the-counter (OTC) sleeping aids are doxylamine, diphenhydramine, and pyrilamine. Besides having antihistaminic effects, these agents are heavily sedating. They have a depressant effect on the CNS. Analgesics are sometimes added to offer some pain relief if that is a component of the sleep disturbance or insomnia. As with other CNS depressants, such as barbiturates and benzodiazepines, clients should avoid consuming alcohol when taking them. The combination may result in respiratory depression and death.

NURSING PROCESS

■ Assessment

Before administering any hypnotic or sedative agent, be it a barbiturate, benzodiazepine, or muscle relaxant, the nurse needs to determine whether the client has or has had any of the following conditions or disorders:
- Addictive disorders
- Allergies
- Anxiety
- CNS disorders
- Depression
- Diabetes

- Mental disorders
- Personality disorders
- Sleep disorders (and the previous treatments for these)
- Suicidal thoughts or tendencies
- Thyroid conditions
  The nurse also needs to find out:
- Whether the client consumes alcohol
- Whether the client takes any other CNS depressants or other OTC medications
- Client's renal and liver function status
- Client's age (because of the increased effects of these agents in older adults and young children)
- Nature of the client's sleep patterns
- Client's stress level
- Client's respiratory and cardiac status

Interactions with muscle relaxants include other CNS depressing agents. It is a known fact that sedative–hypnotic agents, when combined with other drugs affecting the CNS, such as anticonvulsants, neuroleptics, and analgesics, have a 90 percent chance of causing adverse drug reactions.

Clients taking sedative–hypnotics should be assessed for allergic reactions to benzodiazepines. Cautious use is indicated in clients who are anemic, are suicidal, have a history of alcohol or other substance abuse, are older, are under the age of 18 years, are pregnant, or are lactating. Caution is also indicated in clients who have seizure disorders, liver or renal disease, chronic obstructive pulmonary disease (COPD), depression, respiratory disease, or sleep apnea.

Before initiating therapy with sedative–hypnotics, the physician may order blood studies (hematocrit [Hct], hemoglobin [Hgb], red blood cell [RBC]) or renal or liver function studies to rule out any problems that might be exacerbated by the drug. The client's mental status (mood, affect, level of consciousness, memory) should be assessed and documented, and a journal of the client's sleep problems should be kept.

In addition, it is important for the nurse to assess the client's vital signs, including supine and erect blood pressures, especially if the intravenous use of any of these agents is planned. For instance, if diazepam is to be administered, the nurse should hold the drug if the systolic blood pressure drops 20 mm Hg or more or if the pulse or respiratory rate declines. Also, the nurse should survey the laboratory data, such as the complete blood count (CBC) and the results of hepatic studies (lactate dehydrogenase, creatine kinase, and bilirubin) and renal studies (blood urea nitrogen [BUN] and creatinine).

■ Nursing Diagnoses

Nursing diagnoses appropriate to the client taking sedative–hypnotic agents include the following:
- Risk for injury, falls, related to decreased sensorium
- Disturbed sleep pattern related to the drug's interference with REM sleep
- Risk for injury related to possible drug overdose, or adverse reactions related to the combined use of the agent with alcohol or other medications such as tranquilizers and analgesics
- Risk for injury, addiction, related to physical or psychological dependency
- Impaired gas exchange related to side effects of respiratory depression with CNS depressants
- Deficient knowledge related to inadequate information about CNS depressants

■ Planning

Goals related to the administration of sedative–hypnotic agents are as follows:
- Client remains free of self-injury and falls related to decreased sensorium.
- Client remains free of further sleep deprivation.
- Client experiences little or no rebound insomnia.
- Client remains free of or experiences minimal side effects and toxic effects from sedative–hypnotic agents or muscle relaxants.
- Client remains free of drug interaction effects.
- Client experiences no problems with addiction.
- Client remains free of respiratory depression.
- Client adheres with drug therapy and keeps follow-up appointments with the physician or other healthcare professional.

■ *Outcome Criteria*

Outcome criteria related to the administration of sedative–hypnotic agents are as follows:
- Client states ways to minimize self-injury and falls related to decreased sensorium, such as changing positions slowly.
- Client states pharmacological and non-pharmacological (relaxation therapy, massage) measures to enhance sleep patterns or enhance relaxation.
- Client states risk for REM interference from sedative–hypnotic agents with associated sleep hangovers and uses non-pharmacological measures as appropriate.
- Client states the common side effects, toxic effects, and symptoms related to sedative–hypnotic agents to be reported to the physician, such as drowsiness, confusion, and respiratory depression.
- Client states the common side effects related to muscle relaxants such as euphoria, dizziness, drowsiness, and fatigue.
- Client minimizes side effects and toxic effects by taking medications as prescribed.
- Client states the common drug interactions with alcohol and other medications (e.g., tranquilizers and analgesics) that may be life-threatening.
- Client states the importance of taking measures to minimize problems with addiction, such as taking medication only as needed.
- Client, family, or significant other states the need to contact physician about possible complications, such as respiratory depression.
- Client demonstrates increased knowledge about pharmacological and non-pharmacological treatment and regimen for sleeping disturbance.

Sedative Hypnotics

An article by Pasero and McCaffery (2002) presents important information about sedation and the nurse's monitoring of this altered level of consciousness. The authors note that benzodiazepines help to relieve pain associated with muscle spasms by relieving muscle contractions. There is also an increased risk of respiratory depression; therefore these agents should be used cautiously. It is important to use basic assessment and monitoring parameters in clients who are taking any type of agent that is mind altering and results in a decreased level of consciousness (e.g., sedative–hypnotics, muscle relaxants, opioid narcotics). It is recommended that sedation scales not include assessment of other conditions. Instead, sedation scales should focus on the necessary characteristics for assessing opioid-induced sedation. Sedation scales can also be used effectively in clients receiving sedative–hypnotics.

The following recommended sedation scale can be used as an important baseline monitoring scale for anyone who is receiving sedative–hypnotics and for anyone who is sedated.

S = Sleep, easy to arouse (acceptable; no action necessary)

1 = Awake and alert (acceptable; no action necessary)

2 = Slightly drowsy, easily aroused (acceptable; no action necessary)

3 = Frequently drowsy, arousable, drifts off to sleep during conversation (unacceptable; actions needed and if on opioids the dose should be decreased up to 25 to 50 percent, add opioid-sparing analgesic such as ketorolac [non-steroidal anti-inflammatory drug (NSAID)] and monitor client's level of sedation and respiratory status)

4 = Somnolent, minimal or no response to physical stimulation (unacceptable; for opioids, stop drug and consider administering a narcotic antagonist such as naloxone)

From Pasero, C., & McCaffery, M. (2002). Monitoring sedation. *American Journal of Nursing* 102(3), 67–68.

■ Implementation

Clients using benzodiazepines may become sedated and sleepy. They should be safely monitored with bed alarm systems on and/or side rails up (as indicated by policy or physician's order) and provided with assistance with ambulation. Clients should be instructed that dependence is possible with long-term use. While taking these agents, clients should avoid driving or doing other activities that require mental alertness. These agents should be taken on an empty stomach for a faster onset; however, this often results in GI upset. To decrease GI upset, clients are then encouraged to take these agents with meals.

Benzodiazepines have an onset of action of about 30 minutes up to 6 hours, depending on the drug (see the pharmacokinetics information for respective agents). Therefore they must be given at the appropriate time before bedtime to maximize their effectiveness in inducing sleep. Most of the benzodiazepines interfere with REM sleep and produce REM rebound (though note that REM rebound is slight with flurazepam). Clients should be informed that rebound insomnia may occur for a few nights after a 3- to 4-week regimen has been discontinued.

Hangover effects are less common with benzodiazepines than with barbiturates, but they still may occur, especially in older adults.

Benzodiazepines should be used with caution in all sleep disorders, particularly with geriatric clients. They should be used for only a short-term period (3 to 4 weeks), and weaning is recommended. They are highly protein bound and may therefore have many drug interactions and increased risk of toxicity. It may take several nights before the full benefits of these agents are noticed. Benzodiazepines and other sedative–hypnotics should be used only after non-pharmacological approaches have been tried, such as relaxation, music, and massage therapies. See the Natural Health Therapies boxes for kava and valerian (see p. 200), herbal agents commonly used to promote sleep and relaxation.

Barbiturates differ in their onset of action, duration, and potency. Short-acting barbiturates (e.g., secobarbital) should be given 15 to 30 minutes before bedtime, as should some of the intermediate-acting agents (e.g., amobarbital). The longer-acting agents such as phenobarbital have an onset of action of 60 minutes. When administering any of these agents by intramuscular (IM) injection, the injection should be given deep into a large muscle mass to prevent tissue sloughing.

Toxicities associated with muscle relaxants are usually treated with supportive measures; therefore early identification of toxicity is critical to prompt treatment and to prevent respiratory depression and related CNS depression. Most of the agents previously discussed are given orally for spasticity, with dantrolene indicated intravenously (1 mg/kg; may repeat to total dose of 10 mg/kg) for malignant hyperthermia. Close monitoring of all vital parameters and level of consciousness is needed with all CNS depressants. Level of sedation and consciousness should be monitored frequently, as indicated by the client's condition and varying levels of sedation or consciousness.

Regardless of the agent given, for the safety of the client and the prevention of injury stemming from decreased sensorium, it is crucial to always protect the client from falls or self-injury resulting from having a decreased sensorium. In years past, it has always been the "standard of care" to keep bedside rails up and some facilities may still use this safety measure; however, most acute and long-term healthcare facilities are using bed alarms that are set off when the client attempts to get out of bed. If the client needs to have side rails up—either one or both sides—the reasons should

KAVA (Piper methysticum)

Overview
Kava rhizome consists of the dried rhizomes of *Piper methysticum*. The drug contains kavapyrones (kawain). Extended continuous intake can cause a temporary yellow discoloration of skin, hair, and nails.

Common Uses
Anxiety, stress, restlessness; promote sleep

Adverse Effects*
Skin discoloration, possible accommodative disturbances such as enlargement of the pupils, scaly skin (with long-term use).

Potential Drug Interactions
Alcohol, barbiturates, psychoactive agents

Contraindications
Contraindicated in clients with Parkinson's disease, liver disease, and alcoholism; those operating heavy machinery; pregnant and breastfeeding clients

*In January 2002, Health Canada issued a consumer warning describing at least 24 case reports including one reported death in other countries involving serious liver toxicity possibly related to the use of kava-containing supplements. Five clients, including one in the United States, even required liver transplantation. As a result of these case reports, health authorities in the United States and several European countries took steps ranging from posting consumer warnings to removing kava-containing products from the market. At the time of this writing, Health Canada continues to investigate a possible relationship between kava and liver disease. It is recommended that clients with known liver disease not use kava-containing products. Other clients who choose to use such products should be advised to report immediately to their healthcare provider any symptoms of liver disease (yellow skin, yellowing of the whites of eyes, brown urine). More non-specific symptoms that should also be considered include nausea, vomiting, light-coloured stools, unusual tiredness or weakness, abdominal pain, and loss of appetite.

Medication Administration Errors

A client erroneously received a diluent with a prescribed drug IV in a post-anaesthesia care unit. When mixing the solution, the nurse intended to mix the medication with a vial of normal saline. Instead, she pulled out a vial in a nearby drug bin of succinylcholine, which is an NMBA. This agent requires that clients be on mechanical ventilation because of the relaxation of the diaphragm. The client was not assisted by mechanical ventilation and went into respiratory arrest. According to the court of law, death was caused by an error in the course of the process of medication administration. Many issues are raised here, especially the issue of proper storage of such potent medications that are hazardous to clients and cause respiratory arrest if the client is not on mechanical ventilation. Another issue is that of checking the medication three times for the "5 Rights" of medication administration, a point that can never be emphasized enough when it comes to safety in medication administration.

VALERIAN (Valeriana officinalis)

Overview
Valerian root, consisting of fresh underground plant parts, contains essential oil with monoterpenes and sesquiterpenes (valerenic acids).

Common Uses
Anxiety, restlessness, sleeping disorders

Adverse Effects
CNS depression, hepatotoxicity, nausea, vomiting, anorexia, headache, restlessness, insomnia

Potential Drug Interactions
CNS depressants, MAOIs, phenytoin, warfarin; may have enhanced relative and adverse effects when taken with other drugs (including other herbal products) that have known sedative properties (including alcohol)

Contraindications
Contraindicated in clients with cardiac disease or when operating heavy machinery

be documented. The rationale for using bed alarms rather than having both side rails up is to prevent injury in those clients who are demented, under the influence of any sort of mind- or conscience-altering drug, or even just sleepy or groggy and try to climb out of the bed and over the side rails, creating the possibility of even greater injury. (The use of bed alarms is mentioned throughout this text, but full explanation of the rationale is only briefly mentioned from this chapter forward.) Also, clients who are taking these agents need to be informed that they should not smoke in bed (especially in the home setting, because most facilities have "no smoking" regulations) and that they should have assistance for any ambulation while under the drug's influence. The call bell or call light should be kept close to the client's side, especially with geriatric clients.

It is important for the nurse to document the dose, route, time of administration, safety measures taken, and response to the drug. Client teaching tips for benzodiazepines and barbiturates are listed below.

■ Evaluation

Some of the criteria by which to determine a client's therapeutic response to a sedative–hypnotic drug include the following: an increased ability to sleep at night, fewer awakenings, shorter sleep induction time, few side effects such as hangover effects, and an improved sense of well-being because of improved sleep. Therapeutic effects related to muscle relaxants include decreased spasticity, reduction of choreiform movements in clients with Huntington's chorea, decreased rigidity of parkinsonian syndrome, and relief of pain from trigeminal neuralgia. The nurse must constantly watch for and document the occurrence of any of the side effects of benzodiazepines, barbiturates, and muscle relaxants. The side effects of benzodiazepines include lethargy, confusion, drowsiness, dizziness, lightheadedness, headache, a hangover effect, sedation during the day, nausea, and vomiting. The side effects of barbiturates include paradoxical excitement in children and older adults, lethargy, confusion, headache, drowsiness, a hangover effect, rash, nausea, vomiting, Stevens-Johnson syndrome (with agents such as phenobarbital), and respiratory depression. Side effects related to muscle relaxants range from short-term euphoria, dizziness, and drowsiness to less common side effects such as slurred speech, GI upset, hypotension, and tachycardia.

CLIENT TEACHING TIPS

The nurse should instruct the client as follows:
▲ Take medication only as prescribed. If one dose does not work, you should not take a double dose. Follow the physician's orders with regard to the dosing of the medication. Overdosage, with muscle relaxants in particular, is usually treated by supportive measures, especially for respiratory function.
▲ Keep a journal of your sleep habits and response to both drug and non-drug therapy.
▲ Avoid driving or operating heavy machinery or equipment and avoid activities requiring mental alertness while on this medication.
▲ Avoid any other type of CNS-altering medications, especially CNS depressants such as tranquilizers, opioids, and alcohol.
▲ Always try measures other than medications to help you sleep because of the REM rebound they cause, which results in your feeling more tired and not rested or in "hangover" effects the morning after. This hangover effect is more common in geriatric clients and is less common with barbiturates.
▲ Keep all medications away from children.
▲ Because of the different characteristics of the benzodiazepines, such as flurazepam, it may take a night or two before you notice an improvement in your sleep patterns.

▲ Always check with your physician first or with the pharmacist before taking any OTC medications because of the many drug interactions associated with sedative–hypnotic agents.
▲ All sedative–hypnotics have the potential to interfere with sleep.
▲ Review sleep patterns and try some of the following interventions, which can be very effective: establish a set sleep pattern; avoid exercise before bedtime, avoid heavy meals late in the evening; drink a warm decaffeinated beverage, such as warm milk, 30 minutes to 1 hour before bedtime.
▲ It often takes 2 to 3 weeks for the therapeutic effects (improved sleep) of the oral forms of barbiturates to occur.
▲ Never stop taking these medications abruptly, especially the barbiturates, because of their highly addictive potential and because of the rebound insomnia you may experience.
▲ If possible, don't use these agents every night or for more than a few days at a time because of their potential to cause side effects, their interference with REM sleep, and their addicting properties.

POINTS to REMEMBER

▼ Sedative agents are commonly used in the hospital setting. They reduce nervousness, excitability, and irritability by producing a calming effect without causing sleep. This information needs to be shared with the client and/or caregivers.
▼ Sedatives may become hypnotic if given in large enough doses, and the effect on the client is generally a greater depression of the CNS with decreased level of consciousness.
▼ Administration of hypnotic agents in clients results in a calming or soothing effect (and CNS depression) to the point of sleep.
▼ Benzodiazepines have fewer addictive properties than barbiturates but can still induce physical dependence.

For clients with a history of alcohol addiction there is an increased risk for cross-addiction.
▼ Muscle relaxants are often used for treatment of muscle spasms, spasticity, and rigidity. They result in varying levels of decreased sensorium and CNS depression depending on the specific drug, dosage, and route of administration.
▼ Anxiolytics are drugs that relieve anxiety (increased nerve stimulation to the brain) and help to calm the CNS. Some of the sedative agents discussed in this chapter also function as anxiolytics.

EXAMINATION REVIEW QUESTIONS

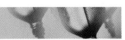

1 Which of the following is an important nursing action for the administration of a benzodiazepine as a sedative–hypnotic agent?
   a. Use IM dosage forms for longer duration.
   b. Administer safely with other CNS depressants for insomnia.
   c. Monitor geriatric clients for the common occurrence of paradoxical reactions.
   d. Evaluate for physical dependence that occurs within 48 hours of beginning the drug.

2 Pediatric and geriatric clients often react with more sensitivity to CNS depressants. This type of sensitivity manifests itself in the development of which type of reaction?
   a. Idiopathic
   b. Teratogenic
   c. Paradoxical
   d. Psychogenic

3 Your client has a history of epilepsy and has been taking barbiturates for a few weeks because of difficulty sleeping. Your main concern for the client, who has stopped taking the barbiturate, would be the occurrence of which of the following?
   a. Seizures
   b. Euphoria

   c. Delirium tremens
   d. Excessive sedation

4 Which of the following is the most common adverse effect related to the use of barbiturates for sleep?
   a. Tachycardia
   b. Hypertension
   c. Polyuria with a protein diuresis
   d. Altered REM sleep with a hangover effect

5 Which of the following is an appropriate nursing intervention for clients who are receiving CNS depressants?
   a. Prevent any activity within the hospital setting while on oral muscle relaxants.
   b. Make sure that the client knows that sedation should be minimal with these agents.
   c. Cardiovascular stimulation, a common side effect, would lead to hypertension.
   d. Make sure the client's call bell/light is close by in case of the need for assistance with activities.

For answers see http://evolve.elsevier.com/Lilley/pharmacology/.

CRITICAL THINKING ACTIVITIES

1 Mrs. L. is a 65-year-old woman who underwent total hip replacement 6 days earlier. She is suffering from a lack of sleep and has tried all of the non-drug therapy techniques. The physician has now ordered chloral hydrate, 250 mg at bedtime prn, for sleep.
   a. What are some of the home health care tips pertinent to the administration of sedative–hypnotic agents in a geriatric client?
   b. Why would chloral hydrate be preferred in this client over the other classes of sedative–hypnotic agents?

2 What instructions should be given to a 31-year-old registered nurse who was found unresponsive after drinking beer all day at a rock concert and who has a 6-year history of grand mal seizures that have been adequately controlled with phenytoin and diazepam?

3 Explain the need for monitoring the following studies when clients are taking long-term barbiturates: hepatic studies—AST, ALT, bilirubin, and lactate dehydrogenase (LDH); laboratory studies—CBC, Hct, Hgb, platelet studies, BUN, and creatine.

4 One of your clients has been told to discontinue flurazepam, which she has been taking for about 1 year. The healthcare provider gave no other instructions. As her home health nurse, does this cause you concern? Why or why not?

5 IV diazepam may be used without any concern. True or false? Explain your answer.

For answers see http://evolve.elsevier.com/Lilley/pharmacology/.

BIBLIOGRAPHY

Aging in Canada. (2004). Benzodiazepine use among seniors. Retrieved November 10, 2005, from http://www.agingin-canada.ca/benzodiazepine_use_among_seniors.htm

Albanese, J., & Nutz, P. (2005). *Mosby's 2005 nursing drug cards.* St Louis, MO: Mosby.

Anderson, P.O., Knoben, J.E., & Troutman, W.G. (2002). *Handbook of clinical drug data* (10th ed.). New York: McGraw-Hill/Appleton & Lange.

Baillargeon, L., Landreville, P., Verreault, R., Beauchemin, J.P., Grégoire, J.P., & Morin, C.M. (2003). Discontinuation of benzodiazepines among older insomniac adults treated with cognitive-behavioural therapy combined with gradual tapering: A randomized trial. *Canadian Medical Association Journal, 169*(10), 1015–1020.

Canadian Pharmacists Association. (2003). *Therapeutic choices* (4th ed.). Ottawa, ON: Author.

Canadian Pharmacists Association. (2004). *Guide to drugs in Canada.* Toronto, ON: Dorling Kindersley.

Canadian Pharmacists Association. (2005). *Compendium of pharmaceuticals and specialties. The Canadian drug reference for health professionals*. Ottawa, ON: Author. [The subscription-based e-CPS is available at http://www.pharmacists.ca.]

Facts and Comparisons. (2004). *Drug facts and comparisons pocket version* (9th ed.). St Louis, MO: Wolters Kluwer Health.

Hardman, J.G., & Limbird, L.E. (2002). *Goodman and Gilman's the pharmacological basis of therapeutics* (10th ed.). New York: McGraw-Hill.

Health Canada. (2002). Advisory. Health Canada is warning consumers not to use any products containing kava. Retrieved July 28, 2005, from http://www.hc-sc.gc.ca/ahc-asc/media/advisories/avis2002/2002_02e.htm

Jellin, J.M., Batz, F., & Hitchens, K. (2003). *Natural medicines comprehensive database*. Stockton, CA: Therapeutic Research Faculty.

Johns Hopkins Hospital, Gunn, V.L., & Nechyba, C. (2002). *The Harriet Lane handbook* (16th ed.). St Louis, MO: Mosby.

Lacy, C.F., Armstrong, L.L., Goldman, M.P., & Lance, L.L. (2003). *Drug information handbook* (11th ed.). Hudson, OH: Lexi-Comp.

Lammon, C.A., & Adams, A.H. (1993). Recognizing benzodiazepine overdose. *Nursing, 23*(1), 33.

Lehne, R.A. (2004). *Pharmacology for nursing care* (5th ed.). St Louis, MO: Saunders.

Mosby: *Mosby's drug consult 2005: The comprehensive reference for generic and brand name drugs* (15th ed.). St Louis, MO: Mosby.

Pasero, C., & McCaffery, M. Monitoring sedation. *American Journal of Nursing, 102*(3), 67–68.

Skidmore-Roth L. (2006). *Mosby's 2006 nursing drug reference* (19th ed.). St Louis, MO: Mosby.

13 Anti-Epileptic Agents

OBJECTIVES

After reading this chapter, the successful student will be able to do the following:

1 Discuss the rationale for the use of the various agents in treating the various forms of epilepsy.

2 List the anti-epileptic drugs according to their classification as well as their indications.

3 Identify the mechanisms of action, cautions, contraindications, dosages, routes of administration, side effects, toxic effects, and various indications for the different classifications of anti-epileptic drugs.

4 Discuss the importance of client education and of adherence in the control of seizure activity.

5 Develop a nursing care plan that includes all phases of the nursing process for clients receiving anti-epileptic drugs.

e-LEARNING ACTIVITIES

Student CD-ROM
- Review Questions: see questions 62–71
- Animations
- Medication Administration Checklists
- IV Therapy Checklists

evolve Web site (http://evolve.elsevier.com/Lilley/pharmacology/)
- Online Chapter Worksheet • Frequently Asked Questions
- Learning Tips and Content Updates • WebLinks • Online Appendices and Supplements • Mosby/Saunders ePharmacology Update • Access to *Mosby's Drug Consult*

DRUG PROFILES

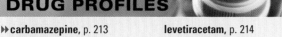

▸▸ **carbamazepine**, p. 213
  clonazepam, p. 211
  clorazepate dipotassium, p. 212
  ethosuximide, p. 212
▸▸ **gabapentin**, p. 213
  lamotrigine, p. 214

  levetiracetam, p. 214
  oxcarbazepine p. 213
▸▸ **phenobarbital**, p. 212
▸▸ **phenytoin**, p. 212
  topiramate, p. 214
▸▸ **valproic acid**, p. 213

▸▸ Key drug.

GLOSSARY

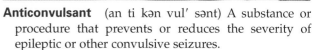

Anticonvulsant (an ti kən vul′ sənt) A substance or procedure that prevents or reduces the severity of epileptic or other convulsive seizures.

Anti-epileptic drug (AED) A substance used that prevents or reduces the severity of epilepsy and different types of epileptic seizures, not just convulsive seizures.

Autoinduction (aw to in dik′ shən) A metabolic process that occurs when a drug increases its own metabolism over time, leading to lower than expected drug concentrations.

Convulsion (kən vul′ shən) A type of seizure involving excessive stimulation of neurons in the brain and characterized by the spasmodic contraction of voluntary muscles. (See also *seizure*.)

Epilepsy (e′ pə lep see) General term for any of a group of neurological disorders characterized by recurrent episodes of convulsive seizures, sensory disturbances, abnormal behaviour, loss of consciousness, or any combination of these.

International Classification of Seizures The most extensively used system of classifying seizures. Both the symptoms and characteristics of the various types of seizures are described.

Narrow therapeutic index (NTI) drugs Drugs that are characterized by a narrow difference between their therapeutic and toxic doses.

Primary or idiopathic epilepsy (id ee o path′ ik) Epilepsy that develops without an apparent cause. More than 50 percent of cases of epilepsy are of unknown origin.

Secondary epilepsy Epilepsy that has a distinct cause (e.g., trauma).

Seizure (see′ zhər) Excessive stimulation of neurons in the brain leading to a sudden burst of abnormal neuron activity that results in temporary changes in brain function.

Status epilepticus (sta′ təs e pə lep′ ti kəs) A common seizure disorder characterized by generalized tonic–clonic convulsions that occur in succession.

Tonic–clonic seizure Formerly called grand mal seizure, this type of epilepsy is characterized by a series of generalized movements of tonic (stiffening) and clonic (rapid, synchronized jerking) muscular contraction.

Unclassified seizures Seizures that are not described by any of the seizure classifications.

EPILEPSY

A seizure disorder, or what is more commonly referred to as *epilepsy,* is not as specific a disease as, say, cancer or diabetes. It is a broad syndrome of central nervous system (CNS) dysfunction that can manifest in many ways, from momentary sensory disturbances to convulsive seizures. Most likely it involves the generation of excessive electrical discharges from nerves located in the area of the brain known as the *cerebral cortex.*

The terms **convulsion, seizure,** and **epilepsy** are often used interchangeably, but they do not have the same meaning. Whereas all convulsions may be called seizures, not all seizures are convulsions. A seizure is a brief episode of abnormal electrical activity in the nerve cells of the brain. A convulsion is characterized by involuntary spasmodic contractions of any or all voluntary muscles throughout the body, including skeletal and facial muscles. Epilepsy is a chronic, recurrent pattern of seizures. These excessive electrical discharges can often be detected by an electroencephalogram (EEG), which is commonly obtained to help diagnose epilepsy. Other helpful diagnostic aids are computerized tomography (CT) and magnetic resonance imaging (MRI). The information yielded by these diagnostic aids in conjunction with the common symptoms of the particular seizure disorder help establish the diagnosis. In particularly severe cases, clients may be observed in a hospital setting or sleep study laboratory with continuous EEG and video monitoring to determine detailed patterns of seizure activity in hopes of tailoring an effective treatment. Commonly reported symptoms are abnormal motor function, loss of consciousness, altered sensory awareness, and psychic changes.

The cause of more than 50 percent of the cases of epilepsy is unknown. The type of epilepsy for which a cause cannot be identified is termed **primary or idiopathic epilepsy.** Other types of epilepsy have a distinct cause such as trauma, infection, cerebrovascular disorder, or other illness. These types of epilepsy are termed **sec-**ondary epilepsy. The chief causes of secondary epilepsy in children and infants are developmental defects, metabolic disease, or injury at birth. Acquired brain disorder is the major cause of secondary epilepsy in adults. Some examples are head injury, disease or infection of the brain and spinal cord, brain attack, metabolic disorder, a primary or metastatic brain tumour, or some other recognizable neurological disease.

The accurate diagnosis of a seizure disorder requires careful client observation, a reliable client history, and an EEG. CT and MRI (which are superior to the clinical examination), EEG, and routine skull radiographs may reveal structural lesions of the CNS as the cause of the seizure disorder. MRI is more sensitive than CT and is now preferred in the evaluation of a client with seizures.

Seizures can be classified into distinct categories based on their characteristics. Traditionally seizures were categorized as grand mal seizures **(tonic–clonic seizures),** petit mal seizures, jacksonian epilepsy, and psychomotor attacks. The newer **International Classification of Seizures** breaks down seizures into two main types: partial seizures and generalized seizures. This system is more extensively used because it more adequately describes the symptoms and characteristics of the various types of seizures. The various types of partial and generalized seizures are listed in Box 13-1. Under this new nomenclature, two other classifications of seizures exist: **unclassified seizures** and status epilepticus. **Status epilepticus** seizures start out as either partial or generalized seizures and become status epilepticus when there is no recovery between attacks.

ANTI-EPILEPTICS

Anti-epileptic drugs (or anti-epileptics) are also called anticonvulsants. The term **anti-epileptic drugs** (or AEDs) is a more appropriate term because many of these medications are indicated for the management of all types of epilepsy, not just convulsions. **Anticonvulsants,** on the other hand, are medications that are used to prevent the seizures typically associated with epilepsy. In practice, however, there is significant overlap between these two terms and both are often used interchangeably.

The combined goal of AED therapy is to control or prevent seizures while maintaining a reasonable quality of life. Many AEDs have side effects, and balancing seizure control with side effects is often a difficult task. In most cases the therapeutic goal is not to eliminate seizure activity but rather to reduce the incidence of seizures as much as possible while minimizing drug-induced toxicity. Many clients must take AEDs for their entire lives. Treatment may eventually be stopped in some, but others will suffer repeated seizures if constant levels of AEDs are not maintained in their blood. In both children and adults there is only a 40 percent chance of recurrence after the first partial or generalized seizure; therefore many physicians choose not to initiate treatment after the first seizure. However, the consensus is that AED therapy should be implemented in clients who have had two or more seizures.

BOX 13-1

International Classification of Seizures

Partial Seizures

Description

Short alterations in consciousness, repetitive unusual movements (chewing or swallowing movements), psychological changes, and confusion.

Simple Partial Seizures

- Symptoms determined by the brain region involved
- No impaired consciousness
- Discrete motor symptoms (most commonly face, arm, or leg)
- Hallucinations of sight, hearing, or taste along with somatosensory changes (tingling)
- Autonomic nervous system responses such as nausea, flushing, salivation, or urinary incontinence
- Personality changes
- Seizures last for 20 to 60 seconds

Complex Partial Seizures

- Impaired consciousness, lack of responsiveness
- Memory impairment
- Behavioural effects such as random walking, mumbling, head turning, or pulling at clothing

- Repetitive, purposeless behaviours (lip smacking, hand wringing) called automatisms
- Aura, chewing and swallowing movements, unreal feelings, bizarre behaviour
- Tonic, clonic, or tonic–clonic seizures
- Seizures last 45 to 90 seconds

Generalized Seizures

Description

Most often seen in children and commonly characterized by temporary lapses in consciousness lasting a few seconds. Staring off into space, daydreaming, and inattentive look are common symptoms. Clients may exhibit rhythmic movements of their eyes, head, or hands but do not convulse. May have several attacks per day.

- Both cerebral hemispheres involved
- Absence, myoclonic, atonic, or tonic–clonic seizures and infantile spasms possible
- Brief loss of consciousness for a few seconds with no confusion
- Head drop or falling-down symptoms

There are several AEDs available. Sometimes a combination of agents must be used to control the disorder. However, most seizure disorders can be controlled. Generally, single-drug therapy must fail before two-drug and then multiple-drug therapy are implemented. A client should always be started on a single AED and the dosage slowly increased until the seizures are controlled or until clinical toxicity occurs. If the first AED does not work, the drug should be tapered slowly while a second AED is introduced. AEDs should never be stopped abruptly unless a severe adverse effect occurs. It is sometimes difficult to control a client's seizures using a single AED, but monotherapy is likely to result in higher serum drug concentrations, fewer adverse effects, and better control.

Serum drug concentrations are useful guidelines in assessing the effectiveness of therapy. They should, however, be only guidelines. Maintaining serum drug levels within therapeutic ranges helps not only to control seizures but also to reduce side effects. There are established normal therapeutic ranges for many AEDs, but these are useful only as guidelines. Each client should be monitored individually and the dosages adjusted based on the individual case. Many clients are maintained successfully below or above the usual therapeutic range. The goal should be to slowly titrate to the lowest effective serum drug level that controls the seizure disorder. This decreases the risk of medication-induced adverse effects and interactions. The serum concentrations of phenytoin, phenobarbital, carbamazepine, and primidone correlate better with seizure control and toxicity than do those of valproic acid, ethosuximide, and clonazepam. Emphasis should be placed primarily on the clinical symptoms and the client's history rather than on strict adherence to established drug concentration ranges.

There are six traditional classes of AEDs, and many new agents have been marketed. These newer agents were developed with the goal of eliminating many of the drug interactions and side effects associated with the older agents. Successful control of a seizure disorder hinges on selecting the appropriate drug class and drug dosage, on ensuring adherence with the treatment regimen, and on limiting toxicity.

The underlying cause of most cases of epilepsy is an excessive electrical discharge from abnormally functioning nerve cells (neurons) within the CNS. Therefore the object of AED therapy is to prevent the generation and spread of these excessive discharges while simultaneously protecting surrounding normal cells.

Mechanism of Action and Drug Effects

Like many classes of drugs, the exact mechanism of action of the AEDs is not known with certainty. However, strong evidence shows that they alter the movement of sodium, potassium, calcium, and magnesium ions. The changes in the movement of these ions induced by AEDs result in stabilized and less responsive cell membranes. This ion theory may explain how AEDs decrease the excitability and responsiveness of brain neurons (nerve cells).

Theoretically the primary pharmacological effects of AEDs are threefold. First, they increase the threshold of activity in the area of the brain called the motor cortex. In other words, they make it more difficult for a nerve to be excited or they reduce the nerve's response to incoming electrical or chemical stimulation. Second, they act to depress or limit the spread of a seizure discharge from its origin. They do this by suppressing the transmission of impulses from one nerve to the next. Third, they can decrease the speed of nerve impulse conduction within a given

TABLE 13-1
ANTI-EPILEPTIC DRUGS OF CHOICE

Partial Seizures		Generalized Seizures					
Simple	Complex	GTC	Absence	Myoclonic	Clonic	Tonic	Atonic
FIRST CHOICE							
CBZ	CBZ	CBZ	ESX	VPA	VPA	VPA	VPA
CBZ	CBZ	CBZ	ESX	VPA	VPA	VPA	VPA
PHB	PHB	PHB	PHB				
PHT	PHT	PHT	VPA				
PMD	PMD	PMD					
VPA	VPA	VPA					
SECOND CHOICE							
CNZ	CNZ	CNZ	AZM	CNZ	CNZ	CBZ	CNZ
CRZ	CRZ	CZP	CNZ			CNZ	
						PHT	

GTC, Generalized tonic–clonic; *CBZ*, carbamazepine; *ESX*, ethosuximide; *VPA*, valproic acid; *PHB*, phenobarbital; *PHT*, phenytoin; *PMD*, primidone; *CNZ*, clonazepam; *AZM*, acetazolamide; *CRZ*, clorazepate.

TABLE 13-2
ANTI-EPILEPTIC DRUGS USED FOR TREATMENT OF STATUS EPILEPTICUS

Drug	Dose (mg/kg)	Onset	Duration	Half-Life	Adverse Effects
diazepam	0.3–0.5 (<30 mg)	3–10 min	Minutes	35 hr	Apnea, hypotension, somnolence
fosphenytoin	15–20 phenytoin equivalents (1.5 mg fosphenytoin = 1 mg phenytoin)	15–30 min	12–24 hr	10–60 hr	Comparable to phenytoin (see below)
lorazepam*	0.05–0.1	1–20 min	Hours	15 hr	Apnea, hypotension, somnolence
phenobarbital	15–20	10–30 min	4–10 hr	53–140 hr	Apnea, hypotension, somnolence
phenytoin	15–20	5–30 min	12–24 hr	10–60 hr	Cardiac dysrhythmias, hypotension

*Off-label use (non–FDA approved indication), but still sometimes used for this purpose.

neuron. AEDs may also have effects outside the neuron, indirectly affecting the area in the brain responsible for the problem by altering, for instance, the blood supply to that area. However, the overall effect is that AEDs stabilize neurons and keep them from becoming hyperexcited and generating excessive nerve impulses to adjacent neurons.

Indications

The major therapeutic indication for AEDs is the prevention or control of seizure activity. They are especially useful for maintenance therapy in clients with the chronic recurring type of seizures that are commonly associated with epilepsy. As evidenced by the wide range of seizure disorders listed in Box 13-1, epilepsy is a diverse disorder. As a result, no one drug can control all types of epilepsy. Although our understanding of epilepsy is still growing, we have a good idea of the primary causes of many of the various seizure disorders. Each involves a distinct area of dysfunction and has certain characteristics that make particular drugs more effective than others in treating it. Therefore particular drugs are indicated for the control of specific seizures. Some of the AEDs and the seizure disorders they are used to treat are listed in Table 13-1.

AEDs are chiefly used for the long-term maintenance treatment of epilepsy. However, AEDs are also useful for the acute treatment of convulsions and status epilepticus. Status epilepticus is a common seizure disorder that

is a life-threatening emergency; it is characterized by generalized tonic–clonic convulsions that occur in succession. Affected clients typically do not regain consciousness between the many convulsions. Hypotension, hypoxia, and cardiac dysrhythmias complicate the disorder, and brain damage and death quickly ensue if prompt, appropriate therapy is not started. Therapy is typically diazepam or lorazepam, considered first-line anticonvulsant medications by the Canadian Pediatric Society. The Canadian Pediatric Society also recommends the use of longer-acting phenytoin for children in status epilepticus who will require long-term anticonvulsant therapy, but are not already on it. Other agents useful for the treatment of status epilepticus are listed in Table 13-2.

Once status epilepticus is controlled, long-term drug therapy is begun with other agents for the prevention of future seizures. Clients who undergo brain surgery or who have suffered severe head injuries may receive prophylactic AED therapy. These clients are at high risk for acquiring a seizure disorder, and often severe complications will arise if seizures are not controlled.

Contraindications

The only usual contraindication to AEDs is known drug allergy. Pregnancy is also a common contraindication, but the prescriber must consider the risks to mother and infant of untreated maternal epilepsy and the increased risks of seizure activity.

Side Effects and Adverse Effects

AEDs are plagued by many side effects, which often limit their usefulness. Agents must be discontinued for many clients because of some of these effects. Each AED is associated with its own diverse set of side effects, which makes it difficult to categorize all of the classes of AEDs according to their common side effects. The various AEDs and their most common side effects are listed in Table 13-3.

Interactions

The drug interactions that can occur with the AEDs are many and varied, and these are summarized in Table 13-4. Significant drug interactions for selected agents are also listed in Table 13-4.

Dosages

Certain AEDs are **narrow therapeutic index (NTI) drugs**; that is, their therapeutic and toxic levels are very close. Table 13-5 lists AEDs that require monitoring of therapeutic plasma levels and their corresponding therapeutic levels. For an overview of dosages, see the dosages table on p. 210. See Appendix B for common brands available in Canada.

It is important for the nurse to understand the nursing process in relation to each of the major classes of drugs used to manage seizure disorders. This discussion focuses on the different groups of the barbiturates, benzodiazepines, and hydantoins. Some of these AEDs, such as the barbiturates and benzodiazepines, are also discussed with the sedative–hypnotic agents (see Chapter 12).

DRUG PROFILES

All AEDs are prescription-only drugs, and should never be taken without the supervision of a qualified medical specialist. They are available in many oral, injectable, and rectal formulations. The U.S. Food and Drug Administration (FDA) uses a pregnancy risk classification of AEDs, summarized in Table 13.6. As Canada has no comparable list, the U.S. FDA classifications are also used as a reference guide.

In most children and adults, epilepsy can be controlled with a first-line AED such as carbamazepine, ethosuximide, phenobarbital, primidone, phenytoin, or valproic acid. For clients who do not respond to the first-line AEDs, a number of second-line AEDs are used occasionally, such as clonazepam, clorazepate, methsuximide, and acetazolamide. These are considered second-line agents because of less favourable efficacy or adverse effect profiles.

Until the 1990s no major new drugs for the treatment of epilepsy had been introduced in Canada since 1978, when valproic acid was introduced. In recent years many investigational AEDs have undergone clinical testing. A few of these have already been recommended for approval by Health Canada, and others have recently been approved and are being marketed. These new drugs show promise, offering possibly better efficacy and toxicity profiles than the older agents.

Gabapentin and lamotrigine have received Therapeutic Products Directorate (TPD) approval at Health Canada. Gabapentin has been available in Canada since 1994. Gabapentin and lamotrigine are primarily used as add-on drugs in adults who have partial seizures alone or with secondary generalized seizures. The most recently approved AEDs are levetiracetam and topiramate. These agents fall under the miscellaneous

TABLE 13-3

ANTI-EPILEPTIC DRUG SIDE EFFECTS

Drug or Drug Class	Side Effects	Drug or Drug Class
Barbiturates	CNS:	Drowsiness, dizziness, lethargy, paradoxical restlessness, excitement
	GI:	Nausea, vomiting
	Other:	Rash, Stevens-Johnson syndrome, urticaria
carbamazepine	Hematological:	Bone marrow suppression (aplastic anemia, agranulocytosis, thrombocytopenia)
	Integumentary:	Exfoliative dermatitis, erythema multiforme, Stevens-Johnson syndrome
	Heart:	Dysrhythmias, heart failure
	Other:	Thrombophlebitis, vision and hearing disturbances, acute urinary retention, dyspnea, pneumonitis, pneumonia
divalproex (valproic acid)	Other:	Pancreatitis, irregular menses, secondary amenorrhea, galactorrhea, rare breast enlargement, weight gain
	Hematological:	Thrombocytopenia
	Pediatric:	Fever, purpura, nervousness, somnolence
Hydantoins	Heart:	Dysrhythmias
	Integumentary:	Exfoliative dermatitis, lupus erythematosus, Stevens-Johnson syndrome
	Hematological:	Bone marrow suppression (agranulocytosis, thrombocytopenia, megaloblastic anemia)
	Other:	Neuropathies, gingival hyperplasia
Succinimides	Hematological:	Agranulocytosis, aplastic anemia, leukopenia, vaginal bleeding
	Integumentary:	Stevens-Johnson syndrome, lupus erythematosus
	Other:	Drowsiness, headache, swollen tongue, gingival hyperplasia

CNS, *Central nervous system;* GI, *gastrointestinal.*

category of AEDs and have greatly expanded the options currently available to clients with seizure disorders. Topiramate is a structurally unique agent chemically related to fructose. It is presently approved as an add-on AED for partial seizures. Topiramate has teratogenic effects in animals and should be avoided during pregnancy if possible. It offers another add-on option for the large number of clients with partial seizures not controlled on first-line AEDs, but cognitive impairment may be troublesome. It has been shown to cause mental slowing (difficulty in word finding, impaired concentration) and fatigue or somnolence.

Carbamazepine, phenytoin, and valproate remain the first-line drugs for treatment of partial seizures. A ready-mixed solution of phenytoin sodium in a vehicle containing 40 percent propylene glycol and 10 percent alcohol in water is available for injection, adjusted to pH 12 with sodium hydroxide. It is irritating to veins when injected. Parenteral phenytoin should be injected slowly (20–30 mg/min not exceeding 50 mg/min in adults), directly into a large vein through a large-gauge needle (preferably >20 gauge) or intravenous (IV) catheter. It should be administered with a 0.22 micron filter and dedicated tubing because of the common problem of precipitation. Each injection of intravenous phenytoin should be followed by an injection of sterile saline through the same needle or intravenous catheter to avoid local venous irritation caused by the alkalinity of the solution. Continuous infusion should be avoided.

Soft tissue irritation and inflammation has occurred at the site of injection with and without extravasation of intravenous phenytoin. Soft tissue irritation may vary from slight tenderness to extensive necrosis, sloughing, and in rare instances amputation. Improper administration, including subcutaneous (SC) or perivascular injection, should be avoided to help prevent the possibility of these occurrences. Local irritation, inflammation, tenderness, necrosis, and sloughing have been reported with or without extravasation of intravenous phenytoin.

Fosphenytoin was developed in an attempt to overcome some of the physical shortcomings of phenytoin sodium. Fosphenytoin is a water-soluble, phosphorylated phenytoin derivative that can be given intramuscularly or intravenously without causing the pain associated with the present product. The physical characteristics of phenytoin sodium were changed to help reduce the tissue irritation and inflammation commonly associated with its intravenous administration (Table 13-7).

New formulations of already available AEDs have also been marketed. An intravenous formulation of valproate has also been released. A new controlled-release system, called the osmotically released oral system (OROS), is now available for carbamazepine, another effective first-line AED. This system offers long-duration and steady carbamazepine serum levels while increasing the likelihood of client adherence due to fewer scheduled daily doses.

TABLE 13-4
ANTI-EPILEPTIC AGENTS: DRUG INTERACTIONS

Drug or Drug Class	Mechanism	Results
CARBAMAZEPINE		
Bone marrow depressants	Additive effect	Increased bone marrow toxicity
doxycycline, phenytoin, theophylline, warfarin	Alters metabolism	Significant decrease in half-life
DIVALPROEX (VALPROIC ACID)		
Barbiturates	Additive effect	Increased CNS depression
clonazepam	Not determined	May produce absence status
phenytoin	Not determined	May produce breakthrough seizures
HYDANTOINS		
disulfiram, isoniazid, valproic acid	Inhibits hepatic enzymes	Increased hydantoin levels
Tricyclic antidepressants	Not determined	Possible seizures
SUCCINIMIDES		
Bone marrow depressants	Additive effects	Increased bone marrow toxicity

TABLE 13-5
THERAPEUTIC PLASMA LEVELS OF NTI ANTI-EPILEPTIC DRUGS

Anti-epileptic Drug	Therapeutic Plasma Level
carbamazepine	17–50 μmol/L
clonazepam	40–230 μmol/mL
divalproex	350–690 μmol/mL
ethosuximide	280–710 μmol/mL
phenobarbital	65–170 μmol/mL
phenytoin	40–80 μmol/L
primidone	23–55 μmol/L
valproic acid	350–700 μmol/mL

NTI, Narrow therapeutic index.

TABLE 13-6
ANTI-EPILEPTIC AGENTS: FDA RISK CLASSIFICATION

Pregnancy Category	Anticonvulsant
C	acetazolamide, ethosuximide, gabapentin, lamotrigine, levetiracetam, oxcarbazepine, topiramate
D	Barbiturates (e.g., phenobarbital), carbamazepine, clonazepam, diazepam, divalproex, phenytoin, primidone, valproic acid

FDA, U.S. Food and Drug Administration.

DOSAGES | Selected Anti-epileptic Agents

Agent	Pharmacological Class	Usual Dosage Range	Indications
▸▸carbamazepine	Iminostilbene	*Pediatric* PO: <9 yr, 10–20 mg/kg/day PO: 6–12 yr, 200–1000 mg/day *Pediatric/adult* PO: >12 yr, 400–1200 mg/day	Partial seizures with complex symptoms; tonic–clonic, mixed seizures; trigeminal—glossopharyngeal neuralgia
clonazepam	Benzodiazepine	*Pediatric* PO: ≤10 yr or 30 kg, 0.1–0.2 mg/kg/day divided tid *Adult* PO: 4–20 mg/day	Lennox-Gastaut; absence, akinetic, and myoclonic seizures
clorazepate dipotassium	Benzodiazepine	*Adult/pediatric >12 yr* PO: 7.5–15 mg bid–qid or single dose of 15–22.5 mg at bedtime *Pediatric 9–11 yr* PO: 7.5 mg bid (max 60 mg/day) *Adult/pediatric >12 yr* PO: 7.5 bid–tid, increase by 7.5 mg/wk (max 90 mg/day)	Anxiety Partial seizures
ethosuximide	Succinimide	*Pediatric* PO: 3–6 yr, 250 mg/day then adjust; >6 yr, 500 mg/day then adjust *Adult* PO: 500 mg/day then adjust	Absence seizures
▸▸gabapentin	GABA analogue	*Pediatric* PO: Children >12, 900–1200 mg/day *Adult* PO: >18 yr, 1800–6400 mg/day	Add-on therapy for partial seizures and neuropathic pain
lamotrigine	Phenyltriazine	*Pediatric (2–12 yr)* PO: 5–15 mg/kg/day depending on other AEDs used *Adult* PO: 75–800 mg/day	Partial seizures, Lennox-Gastaut syndrome, West's syndrome
levetiracetam	Miscellaneous	*Adults only* PO: 500 mg bid–3000 mg/day	Partial seizures
oxcarbazepine	Iminostilbene	*Pediatric (6–16 yr)* PO: 8–10 mg/kg/day divided bid; max 600 mg/day *Adult* 300–600 mg bid	Partial seizures
▸▸phenobarbital	Barbiturate	*Pediatric* PO: 3–5 mg/kg/day IM/IV: 10–20 mg/kg load, may repeat 5 mg/kg every 15–30 min until seizure is controlled or total dose of 40 mg/kg is reached *Adult* PO: 100–300 mg/day IM/IV: 200–800 mg followed by 120–240 mg dose every 20 min until seizure is controlled or a total dose of 1–2 g is reached *Pediatric* PO: 3–6 mg/kg/day	Partial, tonic-clonic seizures Convulsions Partial, tonic–clonic seizures Convulsions Prophylaxis for febrile convulsions

PO, per orally; *AED,* anti-epileptic drug; *IM,* intramuscular; *IV,* intravenous.

DOSAGES Selected Anti-epileptic Agents—*cont'd*

Agent	Pharmacologic Class	Usual Dosage Range	Indications
▶▶phenytoin	Hydantoin	*Pediatric* PO: 4–8 mg/kg/day IV: 15–20 mg/kg *Adult* PO: 300–600 mg/day IV: 15–20 mg/kg	Tonic–clonic; psychomotor seizures Convulsions Tonic–clonic; psychomotor seizures Convulsions
primidone	Barbiturate	*Pediatric* PO: <8 yr, 125–500 mg/tid Dosage for pediatric <8 yr is initially 50–125 mg at bedtime, slowly titrated up to 125–250 mg tid; >8 yr is initially 125–250 mg at bedtime, slowly titrated up to 250 mg; max 2 g/day *Adult/pediatric* PO: >8 yr, 250 mg 4–6 times/day; max 2 g/day	Partial seizures Tonic–clonic seizures
topiramate	Miscellaneous	*Pediatric (2–16 yr)* PO: 1–9 mg/kg/day *Adult (>17 yr)* PO: 25–1600 mg/day	Partial seizures
▶▶valproic acid	Miscellaneous	*Adult/pediatric* PO: 15–60 mg/kg/day divided bid–tid	Multiple seizures

BENZODIAZEPINES

Benzodiazepines are used as first-line agents in the treatment of status epilepticus and generally as second-line agents in the treatment of epilepsy. The prototypical benzodiazepine for the treatment of status epilepticus is diazepam, although lorazepam has also been used for this purpose. (See Table 13-2 for a list of all agents that are commonly used in the treatment of status epilepticus and their important pharmacodynamic and pharmacokinetic properties.) Diazepam remains the drug of choice for the treatment of status epilepticus because of its quick onset. Diazepam can be administered via a variety of routes—intramuscular (IM), intravenous, and a new rectal gel (Diastat). The intravenous and rectal gel routes provide for quick onset of action. Oral tablets and solutions are available as well. Diazepam has a longer biological half-life than lorazepam, approximately 20 to 80 hours, and therefore has a longer duration of action. It is more lipophilic and stays in the CNS longer.

clonazepam

The two benzodiazepines primarily used as second-line AEDs are clonazepam and clorazepate (see next section). Clonazepam is used to treat a variety of seizure disorders. Its greatest value is in the treatment of generalized seizures, but it is also effective in reducing the

TABLE 13-7

PHENYTOIN SODIUM VERSUS FOSPHENYTOIN SODIUM

	phenytoin sodium IV	fosphenytoin sodium IM/IV
pH	12	8.6–9
Maximum infusion rate	50 mg/min	150 mg PE*/min
Admixtures	0.9% saline	0.9% saline or 5% dextrose

*150 mg fosphenytoin sodium = 100 mg phenytoin sodium.
PE, phenytoin sodium equivalents.

frequency of absence, generalized tonic–clonic, and myoclonic seizures. A major factor limiting its use is the high frequency of toxicity. The three most common adverse effects are drowsiness, ataxia, and behavioural and personality changes. The behavioural disturbances can be marked and include hyperactivity, irritability, moodiness, and aggressive behaviour. Many of these can be reduced or prevented by using the lowest effective dose. A tolerance to clonazepam develops in approximately one-third of the clients who initially respond to it, and their seizures recur, usually within

1 to 6 months of starting therapy. Some of these clients respond to an increased dose, but others no longer respond to clonazepam at any dose. Clonazepam is available in 0.25-, 0.5-, 1-, and 2-mg tablets. There is no oral (PO) liquid preparation. It is a prescription-only drug. Studies show a risk to the fetus during pregnancy. Recommended dosages are given in the dosages table on p. 210.

PHARMACOKINETICS

Half-Life	Onset	Peak	Duration
20–80 hr	20–60 min	1–2 hr	6–12 hr

clorazepate dipotassium

Clorazepate dipotassium is a long-acting benzodiazepine anxiolytic used primarily as an add-on drug for clients whose seizures continue despite maximum efforts at treating with a single agent. Clorazepate is a pro-drug that is converted to the active drug N-desmethyldiazepam in the liver. It has been shown to be more effective in the treatment of generalized seizures than in the treatment of other types of seizures. It is available as 3.75-, 7.5-, and 15-mg capsules. It is a prescription-only drug. Pregnancy category C. Recommended dosages are given in the dosages table on p. 210.

PHARMACOKINETICS

Half-Life	Onset	Peak	Duration
100 hr	15 min	0.5–2 hr	4–6 hr

SUCCINIMIDES

ethosuximide

Ethosuximide is a safe and effective first-line AED that is used primarily for the treatment of absence seizures, which occur primarily in childhood. It is also occasionally used as an add-on for adults when valproate is ineffective in controlling primary generalized epilepsy involving seizure types other than absence attacks. Its common side effects are nausea and abdominal discomfort, drowsiness, anorexia, and headache. In rare cases, behavioural changes may be seen, including psychosis. Ethosuximide is available in syrup (250 mg/5 mL) and capsule (250 mg) form. It is a prescription-only drug. Pregnancy category C. Recommended dosages are given in the dosages table on p. 210.

PHARMACOKINETICS

Half-Life	Onset	Peak	Duration
20–60 hr	Reaches steady state in 4–7 days	1–7 hr	12–24 hr

BARBITURATES

▶▶ phenobarbital

Two of the most commonly used AEDs are the barbiturates phenobarbital and primidone. Primidone is metabolized in the liver to phenobarbital and phenylethylmalonamide, both of which have anticonvulsant properties. Phenobarbital has been used since 1912, principally for controlling tonic–clonic and partial seizures. Phenobarbital is also a first-line agent for the management of status epilepticus and is an effective prophylactic drug for the control of febrile seizures. By far the most common adverse effect is sedation, but tolerance to this effect usually develops with continued therapy. In pediatric clients the most common adverse effects are irritability, hyperactivity, depression, sleep disorders, and cognitive abnormalities. Therapeutic effects are generally seen at serum drug levels of 15 to 40 μg/mL. It interacts with many drugs because it is a major "inducer" of hepatic enzymes, causing more rapid clearance of some drugs. Its major advantage is that it has the longest half-life of all the standard AEDs, which allows for once-a-day dosing. This can be a substantial advantage for clients who have a hard time remembering to take their medication or for those who have erratic schedules. A client may take a dose 12 or even 24 hours too late and may still have therapeutic blood levels at that time. In addition, phenobarbital is the most inexpensive AED, costing only pennies a day compared with several dollars a day for other AEDs. It is available for oral administration as capsules (16 mg), tablets (8, 15, 16, 30, 32, 60, 65, 100 mg), and an elixir (15 and 20 mg/5 mL). It is also available as an intravenous injection (30, 60, 65, and 130 mg/mL). It is a prescription-only drug. Pregnancy category D. Recommended dosages are given in the dosages table on p. 210.

PHARMACOKINETICS

	Half-Life	Onset	Peak	Duration
PO:	80–120 hr	60 min	8–12 hr	10–12 hr

HYDANTOINS

▶▶ phenytoin

Phenytoin has been used as a first-line AED for many years. It is primarily indicated for the management of tonic–clonic and partial seizures. The most common side effects are lethargy, abnormal movements, mental confusion, and cognitive changes. Therapeutic drug levels are 40–80 μmol/L. At toxic levels, phenytoin can cause nystagmus (rapid eyeball rolling), ataxia (unsteady and clumsy movements), dysarthria (poorly articulated speech), and encephalopathy (brain disorders). Long-term phenytoin therapy can cause gingival hyperplasia, acne, hirsutism (excess hair growth), and hypertrophy of subcutaneous facial tissue resulting in an appearance known as "Dilantin facies." Scrupulous dental care can help prevent gingival hypertrophy. Another long-term consequence of phenytoin therapy is osteoporosis. Vitamin D therapy may be necessary to prevent this, particularly in women. Phenytoin can interact with other medications for two main reasons. First, it is highly bound to plasma proteins and competes with other highly protein-bound medications for binding sites. Second, it induces hepatic microsomal enzymes, mainly the cytochrome P-450 system, thereby increasing the metabolism of other drugs and decreasing their levels.

Exaggerated phenytoin effects can be seen in clients with low serum albumin concentrations, usually seen with malnutrition or chronic renal failure. With lower levels of albumin in a client's body, more free, unbound, pharmacologically active phenytoin will be present. In these clients it may be necessary to maintain phenytoin levels well below 80 μmol/L. Phenytoin has many advantages from the standpoint of long-term therapy. It is usually well tolerated, highly effective, and relatively inexpensive. It can also be given intravenously if needed. Phenytoin's long half-life allows it to be given only twice a day, and in some cases once a day. As stressed earlier, adherence with AED treatment is important to seizure control. If a client has to remember to take medication only once or twice a day, his or her adherence will be increased and therefore the likelihood of therapeutic drug levels being reached is increased, leading to better seizure control. Phenytoin is available in both oral and intravenous forms. Orally administered phenytoin is available as a suspension (30 and 125 mg/5 mL), chewable "infatablets" (50 mg), regular-release tablets (30 and 100 mg), and capsules (30 and 100 mg). It also is available as a 50-mg/mL injection. Pregnancy category D. Recommended dosages are given in the dosages table on p. 211.

PHARMACOKINETICS

	Onset	Peak	Duration
7–42 hr	2–24 hr	3–12 hr	6–12 hr

▸▸ valproic acid

Valproic acid is used primarily in the treatment of generalized seizures (absence, myoclonic, and tonic–clonic). It has also been shown to be effective for controlling partial seizures. The main side effects are drowsiness; nausea, vomiting, and other gastrointestinal (GI) disturbances; tremor; weight gain; and transient hair loss. The most serious side effects can be fatal: hepatotoxicity and pancreatitis. Valproic acid can interact with many medications. The main reasons for these interactions are protein binding and liver metabolism. It is highly bound to plasma proteins and competes with other highly protein-bound medications for binding sites. It is also highly metabolized by hepatic microsomal enzymes and competes for metabolism. It is available as valproate sodium syrup (250 mg/5 mL), divalproex sodium capsules with sprinkle particles (250 mg), gelatin capsules (250 and 500 mg), liquid-filled capsules (250 and 500 mg), enteric-coated capsules (250 and 500 mg), extended-release divalproex sodium tablets (250 and 500 mg), and valproate sodium injection (100 mg/mL). It is a prescription-only drug. Pregnancy category D. Recommended dosages are given in the dosages table on p. 211.

PHARMACOKINETICS

Half-Life	Onset	Peak	Duration
6–16 hr	15–30 min	3–4 hr	4–6 hr

IMINOSTILBENES

▸▸ carbamazepine

Carbamazepine is the second most commonly prescribed AED in Canada, after phenytoin. It was marketed in the late 1960s for the treatment of epilepsy in adults after its efficacy and safety for the treatment of trigeminal neuralgia were proved. It was granted approval for use in pediatric clients in 1976. It is chemically related to the tricyclic antidepressants and is considered a first-line AED for the treatment of simple partial, complex partial, and generalized tonic–clonic seizures. It is contraindicated in clients with absence and myoclonic seizures and those who have shown a hypersensitivity reaction to it in the past. Carbamazepine is available as an oral suspension (100 mg/5 mL), a 200-mg tablet, and a 100-mg chewable tablet. There are also extended-release tablets available in 100, 200, and 400 mg. The typical therapeutic serum carbamazepine drug level is 4 to 10 μg/mL, but as with all AEDs, the therapeutic concentrations should be used only as a guideline. Carbamazepine is metabolized to carbamazepine epoxide, which has both anticonvulsant and toxic effects. Carbamazepine undergoes **autoinduction**, the process whereby a drug increases its own metabolism over time, leading to lower than expected drug concentrations. With carbamazepine this process usually occurs within the first 2 months after the start of therapy. It is a prescription-only drug. Pregnancy category D. Recommended dosages are given in the dosages table on p. 210.

PHARMACOKINETICS

Half-Life	Onset	Peak	Duration
14–16 hr	Slow	2–24 hr	12–24 hr

oxcarbazepine

Oxcarbazepine is a keto analog of carbamazepine. Its precise mechanism of action is unknown, though it is known to block voltage-sensitive sodium channels, which aids in stabilizing excited neuronal membranes. It is indicated for partial seizures. In adults it may be used as either monotherapy or adjunct therapy with other AED(s). In children it is only recommended as adjunct therapy. In April 2005, Health Canada issued a safety alert about the association of oxcarbazepine with life-threatening dermatological reactions and multiorgan hypersensitivity. It is available in tablet form in 150, 300, and 600 mg, and also in a 60-mg/mL oral suspension. Pregnancy category C. Recommended dosages are given in the dosages table on p. 210.

PHARMACOKINETICS

Half-Life	Onset	Peak	Duration
2–9 hr	2–4 hr	2–3 days	Unknown

MISCELLANEOUS AGENTS

▸▸ gabapentin

Gabapentin is an add-on agent for the treatment of partial seizures and partial seizures with secondary generalization in adults. It is also commonly used to treat neuropathic pain. The exact mechanism of action of gabapentin is unknown. Many believe that it works by increasing the synthesis and accumulation between neurons of the inhibitory neurotransmitter GABA, hence the drug name. It may also work by binding to an as yet undefined receptor site in the brain to produce anticonvulsant activity. Abrupt discontinuation of gabapentin can lead to withdrawal seizures. Its only usual contraindication is known drug allergy. Gabapentin is available as a capsule in 100-, 300-, 400-mg strengths, 600- and 800-mg tablets, and in a 50-mg/mL oral solution. Pregnancy category C. Recommended dosages are given in the dosages table on p. 210.

PHARMACOKINETICS

Half-Life	Onset	Peak	Duration
5–7 hr	Unknown	Unknown	Unknown

lamotrigine

Lamotrigine is indicated for partial seizures in adults and for generalized seizures related to Lennox-Gastaut syndrome in both children and adult clients. It stabilizes neuronal cell membranes by blocking voltage-sensitive sodium channels though its precise antiepileptic mechanism of action is unknown. It has no known contraindications other than drug allergy. Its pharmacokinetic parameters can vary widely when taken concurrently with other AEDs. Lamotrigine is available in 2- and 5-mg chewable tablets, and in 25-, 100-, and 150-mg regular tablets. Pregnancy category C. Recommended dosages are given in the dosages table on p. 210.

PHARMACOKINETICS

Half-Life	Onset	Peak	Duration
25–32 hr	Variable	1.7–2.2 hr	Unknown

levetiracetam

Levetiracetam is indicated as add-on therapy for partial seizures in adults. Its mechanism of action is unknown. However, it is generally well tolerated, with the most common side effects being somnolence, asthenia (loss of strength), and dizziness. Levetiracetam is available in 250-, 500-, and 750-mg tablets. Pregnancy category C. Recommended dosages are given in the dosages table on p. 210.

PHARMACOKINETICS

Half-Life	Onset	Peak	Duration
6–8 hr	Rapid	1 hr	Unknown

topiramate

Topiramate is indicated as add-on therapy for partial seizures in adults and children 2 years of age and older. Its exact mechanism of action is unknown. However, it is believed to work by blocking sodium channels in neurons, blocking glutamate activity, and enhancing GABA activity. Topiramate is available in 15- and 25-mg granular capsules and in 25-, 100-, and 200-mg tablets. Pregnancy category C. Recommended dosages are given in the dosages table on p. 211.

PHARMACOKINETICS

Half-Life	Onset	Peak	Duration
21 hr	Rapid; unaffected by food	2–4 hr	Unknown

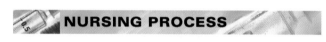

NURSING PROCESS

■ Assessment

When any class of AEDs is to be administered, the nurse should first obtain a thorough health history so that any possible drug interactions (see Table 13-4), drug allergies, and previous unusual or untoward reactions to any of these medications can be known in advance. The nurse needs to gather any information regarding cardiac, respiratory tract, renal, liver, or CNS disorders because of the precautions that may be called for in the use of AEDs. In addition to the traditional AED, it is important to assess liver function studies and CBC laboratory values with the newer agents gabapentin and lamotrigine because of the adverse effects of aplastic anemia and altered liver function. Fosphenytoin and phenytoin are contraindicated in clients with heart problems such as sinus bradycardia, sinoatrial block, second- and third-degree atrioventricular block, and Adams-Stokes syndrome.

Topiramate is contraindicated in clients with hypersensitivity to the drugs themselves. This agent should be used cautiously in clients with renal or liver disease, children under 12 years of age, geriatric clients, and clients who are pregnant or lactating. The client's mental status, sensorium, and level of consciousness also need to be assessed and documented before and during therapy. Topiramate is also to be used cautiously in clients with cardiac disease. Drug interactions for topiramate include digoxin; oral contraceptives; CNS depressants; alcohol (increased effects); and decreased levels of topiramate with phenytoin, carbamazepine, and valproic acid. Renal and liver studies and CBC levels should also be done before initiation of therapy. The newer miscellaneous agents such as topiramate are indicated for use in partial seizures; therefore documentation of this type of seizure activity is important to initiation of drug treatment. Oxcarbazepine is used only as an adjunct with pediatric clients and with clients with partial seizures. It is administered orally; therefore before beginning therapy it is important to assess the status of the GI tract and (as with any CNS depressant) to assess for any type of drug interactions.

■ Nursing Diagnoses

Nursing diagnoses appropriate to the use of anti-epileptic agents include, but are not limited to, the following:

- Risk for injury related to decreased sensorium stemming from drug effects
- Deficient knowledge related to lack of familiarity with and information concerning the use of AEDs
- Non-adherence (to therapeutic regimen) related to client's misuse of drugs or lack of understanding about the seizure disorder and its treatment

■ Planning

The goals of nursing care in a client taking AEDs are as follows:

- Client experiences few or no adverse effects associated with non-adherence and/or with overtreatment or undertreatment.
- Client can identify therapeutic effects of AEDs.
- Client remains adherent with therapy and without major harm to self during AED treatment.

■ *Outcome Criteria*

Outcome criteria related to the use of AEDs include the following:

- Client will state the therapeutic drug effects and side effects of the AED (e.g., sedation, confusion, CNS depression).
- Client (or family members) will state the importance of taking the medication exactly the way it has been prescribed, such as the same time every day.
- Client will state the dangers associated with sudden withdrawal of the medication, such as rebound convulsions.
- Client will maintain a protective environment at home and at work to minimize self-injury.

■ Implementation

Oral AEDs should be taken regularly at the same time of day at the recommended dose and with meals to diminish the GI upset often associated with these agents. Oral suspensions should be shaken thoroughly, and capsules should not be crushed, opened, or chewed. Because there are both extended-release and immediate-release forms of oral hydantoins, it is important for the nurse to be sure which agent is being prescribed. Extended-release agents are usually taken once a day. If there are any questions about the medication order or the medication prescribed, the physician should be contacted immediately for clarification.

When administered intramuscularly, parenteral agents should be given deep in muscles, usually in the gluteal muscles, with rotation of the sites when more than one injection is being given. A 23-gauge, $1\frac{1}{2}$-inch needle (as used for most intramuscular injections) is recommended, but the nurse should follow the manufacturer's recom-

PEDIATRIC CONSIDERATIONS

Anti-epileptic Agent Therapy

- When a skin rash develops in a child or infant taking phenytoin, the drug should be discontinued immediately and the physician notified.
- Chewable dosage forms should not be used for once-a-day administration.
- IM injections of phenytoin should be avoided.
- Family members, parents, significant others, or caregivers should be encouraged to keep a record of signs and symptoms, response to therapy, and any adverse reactions.
- Clients should be encouraged to wear a medical alert bracelet or necklace; medical alert information should be provided to family members, parents, significant others, or caregivers.
- Suspension forms should always be shaken thoroughly before use and an exact graduated device or oral syringe used for more accurate dosing.
- Pediatric clients are much more sensitive to barbiturates and may respond to lower than expected doses; show more profound CNS depressive effects; or exhibit depression, confusion, or excitement (a paradoxical reaction).
- Safe response of neonates to benzodiazepines has not been established. Prolonged CNS depression has been associated with use of these agents in pediatric clients.
- Oral forms of valproic acid should not be given with milk because this may cause them to dissolve early and irritate local mucosa.
- Excessive sedation, confusion, lethargy, or decreased movement should be reported in pediatric clients taking any AED.

mendations and make decisions on the basis of each client's situation.

Parenterally administered AEDs should be given with caution to prevent accidental arterial access and possible cardiac or respiratory arrest. If subcutaneous tissue access does occur as a result of infiltration of the drug at the intravenous infusion site, ischemia and sloughing may occur because of the high alkalinity of some of these agents, specifically the hydantoins. Any of the intravenously administered AEDs, but especially the hydantoins, specifically phenytoin, should be delivered slowly while watching closely for any changes in the vital signs—usually a decrease in pulse (60 beats/min), blood pressure (120/80 mm Hg), and respiratory rate (12 breaths/min). The intravenous infusion site should also be checked for any redness or irritation. When administering phenytoin, the nurse should always check package inserts or drug handbooks for the number of milligrams per seconds or minutes. Phenytoin should not be mixed with any other solution because of the attendant risk of precipitate

NURSING CARE PLAN | Epilepsy

A 68-year-old male client has developed generalized grand mal seizures after experiencing left-sided brain attack 2 months ago. The physician has placed him on phenytoin, 300 mg/day of the extended-release preparation. His caregiver needs discharge instructions about the medication because the client has never taken any type of anti-epileptic medication. The client is aphasic and paralyzed on the right side. He has no major cognitive impairment and has slowed motor activity. His appetite has decreased and his lethargy has increased over the past 2 weeks.

ASSESSMENT	*Subjective Data*	• Client unable to communicate verbally because of left-sided brain attack
	Objective Data	• Client is post-left-sided brain attack
		• Anti-epileptic drug therapy 2 months with increased dose 2 weeks ago
		• Resides in an adult alternative healthcare facility
		• Caregiver eager for instructions
		• Phenytoin ordered for client
		• Problems for 2 weeks with lethargy and decreased appetite

NURSING DIAGNOSIS

Imbalanced nutrition, less than body requirements, related to side effects of medication therapy

PLANNING

Goals
Client will maintain drug therapy with anti-epileptic medications and recommended therapy while at home and before return appointment in 1 month.

Outcome Criteria
Client will show adherence to medication regimen as evidenced by the following:
• Seizure control while at home
• Decreased side effects from taking medication properly
• Lack of complications

IMPLEMENTATION

Client and caregiver instructed on the following:
• Purchase an ID card or medical alert bracelet stating name, diagnosis, drugs being prescribed, phone number, and allergies.
• Client may be drowsy and somewhat sedated when first placed on phenytoin but will gradually develop a resistance to these adverse effects.
• Drug interactions include alcohol, alcohol-containing products (e.g., OTC cough elixirs), and other CNS depressants such as opioids and sedative–hypnotic agents.
• Caregiver should be aware that this medication must be taken as prescribed and not omitted or discontinued abruptly; weaning is recommended after long-term use should client need to discontinue medication.
• Medication may turn client's urine pink, red, or brown; this is a normal reaction.
• Antacids should not be taken at the same time but need to be spaced within 2–3 hr of taking phenytoin.
• Gingival hyperplasia is a side effect so the client needs proper and frequent oral hygiene and regularly scheduled dental appointments.
• Nausea, vomiting, and constipation may occur with this medication.
• Monitor for nausea and vomiting as a side effect of medication; taking medication with meals may be helpful.
• If appetite decreases or nausea and vomiting increase, the client's healthcare provider should be contacted as soon as possible.

EVALUATION

Positive therapeutic outcomes include the following:
• Decreased to no seizure activity
• Tolerance to sedating properties
• Therapeutic blood levels of medication
• No toxicity
• Client should be monitored for common side effects of drowsiness, dizziness, hypotension, nausea and vomiting, gingival hyperplasia, and blood dyscrasias.

formation. Only normal saline solutions are to be used with phenytoin.

With the advent of fosphenytoin and its use to overcome some of the physical shortcomings of phenytoin sodium, the nurse needs to be aware of its dosing in phenytoin sodium equivalents (PE). For example, 375 mg of fosphenytoin is equivalent to 250 mg of phenytoin sodium; 375 mg of fosphenytoin would be labelled as fosphenytoin 250 mg PE. Fosphenytoin should not be administered at a rate exceeding 150 mg PE/min. Hypotension and cardiovascular collapse may occur with a too-rapid intravenous infusion of fosphenytoin, and hypotension and ventricular fibrillation may occur with a too rapid intravenous infusion of phenytoin.

Topiramate should be taken whole and not crushed, broken in half, or chewed. It is often better tolerated with food because of its associated bad taste. These newer medications, as with any AED, should not be discontinued abruptly. Clients taking topiramate are prone to sedation and should have assistance with ambulation and activities of daily living (ADLs). Clients taking topiramate are encouraged to keep a journal of their response to the agent, seizure description, and any side effects. As with any of the other AEDs, clients should avoid driving or other activities that require alertness until the medication levels become stable. Oral forms of oxcarbazepine should be administered as ordered and consistently at the same time every day.

Medical alert tags or identifications (IDs) should be worn or carried by clients taking any AED and by clients with seizure disorders. Clients must be told that therapy may last several years or may be lifelong. Support groups may be an option for the client and caregiver. Client teaching tips are presented in the box below.

■ **Evaluation**

A therapeutic response to AEDs does not mean the client has been cured of the seizures but only that seizure activity is decreased or absent. Any response to the medication should be documented in the nurses' notes. In addition, when monitoring and evaluating the effects of AEDs, the nurse needs to constantly assess the client for mental status, mood and mood changes, sensorium, behavioural changes or changes in the level of consciousness, affect, eye problems or visual disorders, sore throat, and fever (blood dyscrasia is a side effect of the hydantoins). The occurrence of vomiting, diplopia (double vision), cardiovascular collapse, and Stevens-Johnson syndrome indicates toxicity of the bone marrow. If these effects occur, the physician should be contacted immediately and no further doses given.

CLIENT TEACHING TIPS

The client needs to fully understand his or her seizure disorder and the importance of consistent treatment. The nurse should instruct the client as follows:
▲ Report omissions and any problems with dosing to the physician immediately!
▲ Carry an ID card or wear at all times a medical alert bracelet or necklace naming the diagnosis, the medications taken, and any other pertinent facts.

▲ When taking any anticonvulsants, avoid driving or engaging in other activities that require alertness.
▲ Keep a log or journal recording all seizure activity.
▲ Do not take anticonvulsants with alcohol or other medications without checking with your healthcare providers.

POINTS to REMEMBER

▼ The terms *epilepsy*, *seizure*, and *convulsion* have different meanings and should not be used interchangeably:
 • *Epilepsy:* Disorder of the brain manifested as a chronic, recurrent pattern of seizures
 • *Seizure:* Abnormal electrical activity in the brain
 • *Convulsion:* A type of seizure (spasmodic contractions of involuntary muscles)
▼ Specific drugs are indicated for the different classifications of seizure disorders. The more common classifications are as follows:
 • *Partial:* Short alterations in consciousness, repetitive unusual movements, psychological changes, and confusion
 • *Generalized:* Most common in childhood; temporary lapses in consciousness (seconds); rhythmic movement of eyes, head, or hands; does not convulse; and may have several a day
 • *Status epilepticus:* A common seizure disorder—a life-threatening emergency that is characterized by tonic–clonic convulsions and may result in brain damage and death if not treated immediately
▼ Nursing considerations include the following:
 • Nurse must distinguish between focal, primary, secondary, status, tonic–clonic, grand mal, and petit mal seizures.
 • Documentation of any seizure activity and the specific characteristics of the client's movements is important to a diagnosis and to adequate treatment. Non-adherence is the most notable factor leading to treatment failure.

EXAMINATION REVIEW QUESTIONS

1 Which of the following reflects the most appropriate nursing action related to IV fosphenytoin?
   a. Administer IV push at more than 170 mg/mL.
   b. Rectal suppositories are an alternative to the IV form.
   c. Always administer in only 10 percent D5W.
   d. Give IV fosphenytoin at no more than 150 mg (100 mg phenytoin) per minute.

2 A female client who is planning a pregnancy has been taking phenytoin for her AED therapy. Which of the following concerns would dictate that the drug should be changed to another agent? The drug
   a. has teratogenic effects.
   b. often results in pre-eclampsia if taken while pregnant.
   c. may cause maternal tachycardia.
   d. increases fetal weight significantly.

3 Which of the following would you expect in a client with a phenytoin level of 60 μmol/L?
   a. Ataxia
   b. Polyuria
   c. Seizures
   d. Hypertension

4 Which of the following is the most appropriate and effective method of giving an AED?
   a. Administer every 8 hours.
   b. Give one dose IV followed by PO doses every 2 hours.
   c. Maintain a drug regimen based on the half-life of the AED, client response, and as ordered by the physician.
   d. Make sure that PO, IM, and IV routes of any AED are alternated during the first few weeks of therapy.

5 During assessment of a client with a history of epilepsy, which of the following questions would be most important to pose to the client about the disease and its treatment?
   a. "Do you take the capsule or tablet form?"
   b. "Do your seizures interfere with your appetite?"
   c. "Do you have severe migraines with the seizure?"
   d. "Do you experience any unusual sensations or perceptions before the seizure occurs?"

For answers see http://evolve.elsevier.com/Lilley/pharmacology/.

CRITICAL THINKING ACTIVITIES

1 What specific nursing intervention may help minimize the ataxia and other side effects associated with the rapid absorption of some of the AEDs?

2 Why is it critical to effective treatment to assess clients to help determine the most appropriate AED?

3 Why is it so important to be aware of concurrent medication administration, including OTC agents, with clients taking AEDs?

4 What would be the difference between an allergic reaction and a toxic reaction in a client taking phenytoin? What nursing action should you take if either of these occurs in your client?

5 M.M. is a 21-year-old woman who was brought to the emergency room in status epilepticus. The physician has decided to treat the woman with intravenous diazepam and phenytoin. He asks you to give a loading dose of 1.5 g at a rate of 50 mg/min. What rate should you set the pump for (in millilitres per hour)?

For answers see http://evolve.elsevier.com/Lilley/pharmacology/.

BIBLIOGRAPHY

Albanese, J., & Nutz, P. (2004). *Mosby's 2004 nursing drug cards.* St Louis: Mosby.

Blume, W.T. (2003). Diagnosis and management of epilepsy. [Electronic version]. *Canadian Medical Association Journal, 168*(4).

Canadian Pediatric Society. (1996, reaffirmed 2002). Management of the paediatric patient with generalized convulsive status epilepticus in the emergency department. [Electronic version]. *Paediatrics and Child Health, 1* (2), 151-155. Retrieved July 29, 2005, from http://www.cps.ca/english/statements/EP/ep95-01.htm

Canadian Pharmacists Association. (2003). *Therapeutic choices* (4th ed.). Ottawa, ON: Author.

Canadian Pharmacists Association. (2004). *Guide to drugs in Canada.* Toronto, ON: Dorling Kindersley.

Canadian Pharmacists Association. (2005). *Compendium of pharmaceuticals and specialties. The Canadian drug reference for health professionals.* Ottawa, ON: Author. [The subscription-based e-CPS is available at http://www.pharmacists.ca.]

Facts and Comparisons. (2004). *Drug facts and comparisons, pocket version* (9th ed.). St Louis, MO: Wolters Kluwer Health.

Hardman, J.G., & Limbird, L.E. (2002). *Goodman and Gilman's the pharmacological basis of therapeutics* (10th ed.). New York: McGraw-Hill.

Health Canada. (2005). Drug product database (DPD). Retrieved July 30, 2005, from http://www.hc-sc.gc.ca/hpb/drugs-dpd/

Health Canada. (2005). Health Canada endorsed important safety information on TRILEPTAL (oxcarbazepine). Retrieved July 29, 2005, from http://www.hc-sc.gc.ca/dhp-mps/medeff/advisories-avis/prof/trileptal_hpc-cps_e.html

Lehne, R.A. (2004). *Pharmacology for nursing care* (5th ed.). St Louis, MO: Saunders. Manufacturer's package inserts for Gabitril, Keppra, Lamictal, and Neurontin.

Mejia, A.B. (2003). Pediatric epilepsy. What's new? [Electronic version]. *Pharmacy Practice.* Retrieved July 29, 2005, from http://www.apotex.ca/En/ProfessionalAffairs/PracticeTools/PracticeCEFiles/CE200309_prac.pdf

Mosby. (2005). *Mosby's drug consult 2005: The comprehensive reference for generic and brand name drugs* (15th ed.). St Louis, MO: Mosby.

Skidmore-Roth, L. (2006). *Mosby's 2006 nursing drug reference* (19th ed.). St Louis, MO: Mosby.

CHAPTER

14 Antiparkinsonian Agents

OBJECTIVES

After reading this chapter, the successful student will be able to do the following:

1 Briefly discuss the pathophysiology related to Parkinson's disease (PD).

2 Identify the different classes of medications used as antiparkinsonian agents.

3 Discuss the mechanisms of action, dosages, indications, contraindications, cautions, side effects, and toxic effects associated with the use of antiparkinsonian agents.

4 Develop a nursing care plan that includes all phases of the nursing process related to the administration of all classes of antiparkinsonian agents.

e-LEARNING ACTIVITIES

Student CD-ROM
- Review Questions: see questions 72–76
- Animations
- Medication Administration Checklists
- IV Therapy Checklists

evolve Web site (http://evolve.elsevier.com/Lilley/pharmacology/)
- Online Chapter Worksheet • Frequently Asked Questions
- Learning Tips and Content Updates • WebLinks • Online Appendices and Supplements • Mosby/Saunders ePharmacology Update • Access to *Mosby's Drug Consult*

DRUG PROFILES

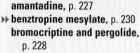

amantadine, p. 227
▸▸ benztropine mesylate, p. 230
bromocriptine and pergolide,
    p. 228
entacapone, p. 228

levodopa, p. 227
▸▸ levodopa-carbidopa, p. 227
▸▸ ropinirole, p. 228
▸▸ selegiline, p. 224
trihexyphenidyl, p. 230

▸▸ Key drug.

GLOSSARY

Akinesia (a ki nee' zhuh) Reduction or lack of psychomotor activity of voluntary muscles.

Anticholinergic agents Drugs that block or impede the activity of the neurotransmitter acetylcholine (ACh) at cholinergic receptors in the brain.

Catechol *O*-methyltransferase (COMT) inhibitors A class of indirect-acting dopaminergic agents that work by inhibiting the enzyme COMT, which catalyzes the breakdown of dopamine.

Chorea (kor ee' uh) A condition characterized by involuntary, purposeless, rapid motions such as flexing and extending the fingers, raising and lowering the shoulders, or grimacing. In some forms the person is also irritable, emotionally unstable, weak, restless, and fretful.

Dopaminergic agents Drugs used to replace the deficiency of dopamine at dopamine receptors in the nerve endings, especially in the brain when treating Parkinson's disease (PD) (can be direct- or indirect-acting or replacement drugs).

Dyskinesia (dis kə nee' zhuh) An impaired ability to execute voluntary movements. Tardive dyskinesia is one type and is caused by brain injury or by prolonged use of certain medications, such as phenothiazine in geriatric clients.

Dystonia (dis to' nee uh) Any impairment of muscle tone. The condition commonly involves the head, neck, and tongue and often occurs as an adverse effect of a medication.

Endogenous Describes any substance produced by the body's own natural biochemistry (e.g., hormones, neurotransmitters).

Exogenous Describes any substance produced outside of the body that may be taken into the body (e.g., a medication, food, or even an environmental toxin). Exogenous substances may be used to replace endogenous substances that are not being produced by the body (or not being produced in sufficient quantities) due to disease. Two examples of medications used in this way are insulin to treat diabetes mellitus and levodopa to treat PD, which is the focus of this chapter.

Parkinson's disease (PD) A slowly progressive, degenerative neurological disorder characterized by resting tremor, pill-rolling of the fingers, a mask-like facies, shuffling gait, forward flexion of the trunk, loss of postural reflexes, and muscle rigidity and weakness. It is usually an idiopathic (of no known cause) disease in people over 60 years of age, although it may occur in younger people, especially after acute encephalitis or carbon monoxide or metallic poisoning.

Presynaptic drugs Drugs that exert their antiparkinson effects before the nerve synapse.

PARKINSON'S DISEASE

Parkinson's disease (PD) is a chronic, progressive, degenerative disorder affecting the dopamine-producing neurons in the brain. Other chronic central nervous system (CNS) neuromuscular disorders are myasthenia gravis (characterized by progressive fatigue and weakness of the skeletal muscles), dementia, and Alzheimer's disease. PD was initially recognized in 1817, at which time it was called "shaking palsy." The symptoms of both the early and advanced stages of the disease, along with the treatment options, were first described by James Parkinson. It was not until the 1960s, however, that the underlying pathological defect was discovered. It was postulated then that a dopamine deficit in the area of the brain called the *substantia nigra* was the cause of the disorder.

PD afflicts approximately 100 000 Canadians. It is primarily a disease of older adults, rarely developing in people under 40 years of age. However, the number of clients with PD will only continue to increase as our geriatric population grows. There is a 2 percent chance of PD developing in a person during his or her lifetime. In most clients the disease becomes apparent between 45 and 65 years of age, with a mean age of onset of 56 years. Men and women are equally affected. Family history does not seem to be a contributing factor. PD is also a prominent cause of disability because of the common accompanying motor complications.

The primary cause of PD is an imbalance in two neurotransmitters—dopamine (DA) and acetylcholine (ACh)—in the area of the brain called the *basal ganglia*. This imbalance is caused by failure of the nerve terminals in the substantia nigra to produce the essential neurotransmitter dopamine. This neurotransmitter acts in the basal ganglia to control movements. Destruction of the substantia nigra leads to dopamine depletion. Dopamine is an inhibitory neurotransmitter, and ACh is an excitatory neurotransmitter in this area of the brain. A correct balance between these two neurotransmitters is needed for the proper regulation of posture, muscle tone, and voluntary movement. Clients who suffer from PD have an imbalance in these neurotransmitters, usually a defi-

ciency of dopamine in the substantia nigra areas of the brain, as mentioned previously. This dopamine deficiency can also lead to ACh (cholinergic) activity due to the lack of a normal dopaminergic balancing effect. Figure 14-1 illustrates the difference in neurotransmitter concentrations in persons with normal balance and in clients with PD.

A significant advance in our understanding of the etiology and pathogenesis of PD came in 1983 with the discovery of the potent neurotoxin 1-methyl-4-phenyl-1,2,3,6-tetrahydropyridine (MPTP) and its metabolic breakdown product 1-methyl-4-phenylpyridine (MPP). This illegal substance has been produced in home laboratories and used for recreational purposes. MPTP and MPP selectively destroy the substantia nigra, or that area of the brain that is dysfunctional in PD. It has been shown that a parkinsonian syndrome almost identical to idiopathic PD develops in laboratory animals injected with this neurotoxin. Others theorize that PD is the result of an earlier head injury or of excess iron in the substantia nigra, which

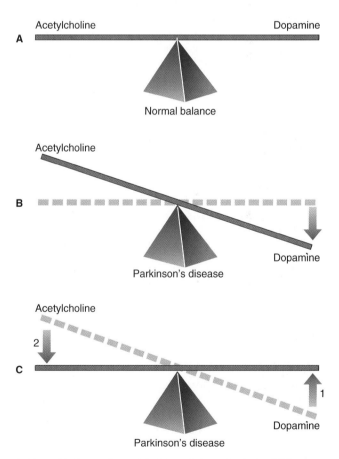

A, Normal balance of acetylcholine and dopamine in the CNS.
B, In Parkinson's disease, a decrease in dopamine results in an imbalance.
C, Drug therapy in Parkinson's disease is aimed at correcting the imbalance between acetylcholine and dopamine. This can be accomplished by either
  1. increasing the supply of dopamine or
  2. blocking or lowering acetylcholine levels.

FIG. 14-1 The neurotransmitter abnormality of Parkinson's disease.

TABLE 14-1
CLASSIC PARKINSONIAN SYMPTOMS

Symptom	Description
Bradykinesia	Slowness of movement
Rigidity	Resistance to passive movement; "cogwheel rigidity," so called because the passively moved joint seems to catch repeatedly
Tremor	Pill rolling: tremor of the thumb against the forefinger, seen mostly at rest, is less severe during voluntary activity; starts usually on one side then progresses to the other; is the presenting sign in 70% of cases
Postural instability	Danger of falling, hesitation in gait as client starts or stops walking

TABLE 14-2
ANTIPARKINSONIAN AGENTS

Drug Category	Agents
Anticholinergic agents	benztropine, biperiden, procyclidine, trihexyphenidyl
Antihistamines (used for their anti-cholinergic effects)	diphenhydramine, orphenadrine
Dopamine receptor agonists (direct-acting)	bromocriptine, levodopa, levodopa-carbidopa, pergolide, pramipexole, ropinirole, selegiline

INDIRECT-ACTING DOPAMINE RECEPTOR AGONISTS

MAO-B inhibitor	selegiline
COMT inhibitor	entacapone
Miscellaneous agents	amantadine

MAO, Monoamine oxidase; *COMT,* catechol *O*-methyltransferase.

undergoes oxidation and causes the generation of toxic free radicals. Still another theory holds that because endogenous dopamine levels naturally decrease with age, PD represents a premature aging of the nigrostriatal cells resulting from environmental or intrinsic biochemical factors, or both. PD is generally believed to result from an interaction of environmental and genetic factors.

No readily available laboratory tests can detect or confirm PD. Results of computerized tomography (CT), magnetic resonance imaging (MRI), cerebrospinal fluid analysis, and electroencephalography are usually normal and of little diagnostic value. A positron emission tomography (PET) scan may offer some additional information. This new type of scanning involves intravenous (IV) injections of deoxyglucose with radioactive fluorine. The various shades of colours that show up indicate areas of abnormalities and assist in the diagnosis of neurological disorders, including PD. CT, MRI, and PET may be useful tools for ruling out other possible diseases as causes of the symptoms. The diagnosis of PD is usually made on the basis of the classic symptoms and physical findings. The classic symptoms of PD are listed in Table 14-1.

Symptoms of PD do not appear until approximately 80 percent of the dopamine store in the substantia nigra of the basal ganglia has been depleted. This means that by the time PD is diagnosed, only approximately 20 percent of the client's original nigral dopaminergic terminals are functioning normally.

Nerve terminals can take up substances, store them, and release them for use when needed. It is this factor that forms the basis for antiparkinsonian treatment. As long as there are functioning nerve terminals that can take up dopamine, the symptoms of PD can be at least partially controlled. The blood–brain barrier does not allow exogenously supplied dopamine to enter the brain; however, it does allow levodopa, a naturally occurring dopamine precursor, to do so. After levodopa has been taken up by the dopaminergic terminal, it is converted into dopamine and then released as needed. Levodopa therapy can thus correct the neurotransmitter imbalance in clients with early PD who still have functioning nerve terminals.

Unfortunately, PD is a progressive condition. With time, the number of surviving dopaminergic terminals that can take up exogenously administered levodopa and convert it into dopamine decreases. Rapid swings in the response to levodopa (known as the *on–off phenomenon*) also occur.

The result is worsening PD when too little dopamine is present or dyskinesia when too much is present. **Dyskinesia** is difficulty in performing voluntary movements. The two dyskinesias most commonly associated with antiparkinsonian therapy are **chorea** (irregular, spasmodic, involuntary movements of the limbs or facial muscles) and **dystonia** (abnormal muscle tone in any tissue).

The first step in the treatment of PD is a full explanation of the disease to the client and his or her family members or significant others. Physical therapy and speech therapy are almost always needed when the client is in the later stages of the disease. As previously discussed, drug therapy is aimed at increasing the levels of dopamine as long as there are functioning nerve terminals. It is also aimed at antagonizing or blocking the effects of ACh and slowing the progression of the disease. The agents available for the treatment of PD and their respective categories are listed in Table 14-2.

See the Geriatric Considerations box for antiparkinsonian agents on p. 223.

SELECTIVE MONOAMINE OXIDASE INHIBITOR THERAPY

In recent years there has been an increasing focus on developing treatment strategies to slow the progression of PD. There are two subclasses of monoamine oxidase (MAO) in the body: MAO-A and MAO-B. However, these treatment strategies' lack of selectivity for MAO type B results in a higher frequency of side effects. Selegiline is a newer, potent, irreversible MAO inhibitor

Antiparkinsonian Agents

- Geriatric clients taking anticholinergics often used for PD are at risk for the development of health problems associated with the side effects of these medications, such as dry mouth, constipation, impaired thought processes, and urinary retention (the latter especially in men with benign prostatic hypertrophy).
- Anticholinergics are contraindicated in clients with narrow-angle glaucoma or with a history of urinary retention.
- Some geriatric clients taking anticholinergic agents experience paradoxical reactions, such as excitement, confusion, or irritability.
- Overheating is a problem in clients taking anticholinergics; therefore geriatric clients should especially avoid excessive exercise during the warm weather and avoid excessive heat exposure.
- Levodopa should be used cautiously, with close monitoring of geriatric clients, especially if there is a history of cardiac, renal, hepatic, endocrine, pulmonary, ulcer, or psychiatric disease.
- The geriatric client taking levodopa is at an increased risk of side effects, especially confusion.
- Levodopa-carbidopa is often started at a low dose because of the increased sensitivity of the older client to these medications.

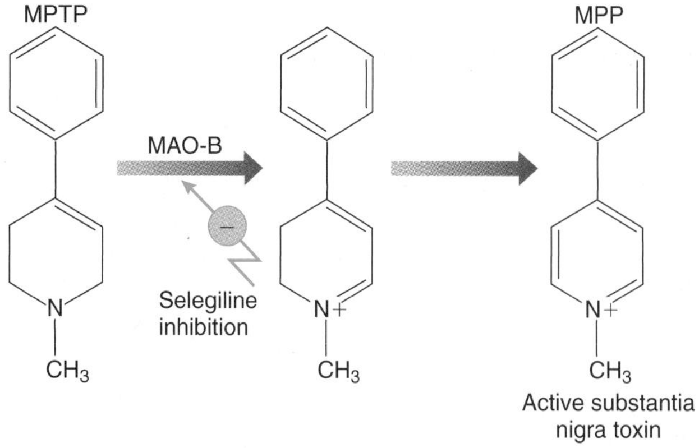

FIG. 14-2 Mechanism of action of selegiline. *MAO-B,* Monoamine oxidase type B; *MPP,* 1-methyl-4-phenylpyridine; *MPTP,* 1-methyl-4-phenyl-1,2,3,6-tetrahydropyridine.

(MAOI) that selectively inhibits MAO-B. It is derived from amphetamine.

As early as 1965, non-selective MAOIs, which inhibit both MAO-A and MAO-B, were being used to improve the therapeutic effect of levodopa in clients with PD. They were also among the first medications used to treat depression and are still used occasionally today for this purpose (see Chapter 15). However, a major adverse effect of these non-selective MAOIs has been that they interact with tyramine-containing foods (cheese, red wine, beer, and yogourt) because of their inhibitory activity against MAO-A. This has been termed the "cheese effect," and one hazardous result can be severe hypertension. This has considerably restricted the therapeutic use of MAOIs. In 1974 selegiline was introduced as an investigational option for PD. As a selective MAO-B inhibitor, selegiline does not elicit the classic cheese effect at doses of 10 mg or less daily. In the years that followed, many investigational studies were conducted, and in October 1989 selegiline received approval from Health Canada's Therapeutic Product Directorate for use in conjunction with levodopa therapy in the treatment of PD. There was earlier speculation by researchers that selegiline, as well as possibly vitamins E (tocopherol) and C (ascorbic acid), might have antiparkinsonian effects due to "neuroprotective" activity at the neuronal (nerve cell) level. The results of some animal studies suggested this as a possibility. However, no human or animal studies to date have con-

clusively demonstrated this to be the case for any of these three substances.

Mechanism of Action and Drug Effects

MAO is one of the two major pathways by which dopamine is degraded. MAO-B accounts for about 70 percent of all MAO activity in the brain. One of the current theories advanced to explain the etiology of PD is that the neurotoxicity that causes the destruction of the cells of the substantia nigra is accomplished by MPP, the enzymatically active toxic metabolite of MPTP. The enzymatic conversion of MPTP to MPP is catalyzed by the enzyme MAO-B. By blocking this enzyme with the MAO-B inhibitor selegiline, MPP is prevented from being produced and the cells of the substantia nigra are spared. Figure 14-2 illustrates this enzymatic inhibition process.

MAOs are widely distributed throughout the body, with higher concentration in the liver, kidney, stomach, intestinal wall, and brain. Most MAO-B is in the CNS, primarily in the brain. The primary role of MAOs is the catabolism or breakdown of catecholamines such as dopamine, norepinephrine, and epinephrine, as well as the breakdown of serotonin. Therefore an MAO-B inhibitor such as selegiline causes an increase in the levels of dopaminergic stimulation in the CNS. This helps to counter the dopaminergic deficiency that arises from the PD pathology.

Indications

Selegiline is currently approved for use in combination with levodopa or levodopa-carbidopa. It is an adjunctive agent used when a client's response to levodopa is fluctuating. It allows the dose of levodopa to be decreased. Improvement in functional ability and decreased severity of symptoms are common after selegiline is added. However, only approximately 50 to 60 percent of clients show a positive response.

Selegiline may be somewhat beneficial as a prophylactic agent. Selegiline administration before exposure to the neurotoxin MPTP has been shown to prevent the onset of a PD-like syndrome in laboratory animals, indicating a possible neuroprotective effect. However, more recent studies in humans have not definitively shown such an effect at the cellular level. Several studies have shown that clients treated with selegiline required levodopa therapy 1.8 times later than control clients. As PD disease progresses, it becomes more and more difficult to control it with levodopa. Ultimately levodopa no longer controls the PD, and the client is seriously debilitated. This generally occurs between 5 and 10 years after the start of levodopa therapy. Prophylactic selegiline use may delay the development of serious debilitating PD for 9 to 18 years. Because the average age of clients at the onset of PD is between 55 and 65 years, such a delay would mean most clients will die of another cause before the functional disability occurs.

Contraindications

Selegiline is normally contraindicated in cases of known drug allergy. Concurrent use of the opioid agent meperidine is contraindicated because of the likelihood of introducing a dangerous condition known as *serotonin syndrome* (see Chapter 15).

Side Effects and Adverse Effects

The most common adverse effects associated with selegiline use are mild and consist of nausea, lightheadedness, dizziness, abdominal pain, insomnia, confusion, and dry mouth (see Table 14-3). Reactions seen when the dosage exceeds 10 mg/day include a hypertensive crisis with the consumption of tyramine-containing food, memory loss, muscular twitches and jerks, and grinding of the teeth.

Interactions

The number of drugs with which selegiline interacts is relatively small, and the degree of interaction is dose dependent. At recommended doses of 10 mg/day, the drug maintains its selective MAO-B inhibition. However, at doses that exceed 10 mg/day, selegiline becomes a non-selective MAOI, contributing to the development of the cheese effect. Meperidine is contraindicated in clients receiving non-selective MAOIs because this combination has been associated with fatal hypertensive episodes. It is suggested that meperidine, as well as other opioids, be avoided in clients taking more than 10 mg/day of selegiline. For the same reasons, selegiline should not be combined with dextroamphetamine, methylphenidate, dextromethorphan, sibutramine, or serotonin-selective reuptake inhibitors (SSRIs) (see Chapter 15).

Dosage

For the recommended dosage of selegiline see the table on p. 225. See Appendix B for some of the common brands available in Canada.

TABLE 14-3

SELEGILINE: ADVERSE EFFECTS

Body System	Side/Adverse Effects
Cardiovascular	Hypotension, dysrhythmia, tachycardia, palpitations, angina, edema
Central nervous	Altered sensation, pain, dizziness, drowsiness, irritability, anxiety, extrapyramidal side effects
Gastrointestinal	Nausea, vomiting, constipation, diarrhea, anorexia
Respiratory	Asthma, shortness of breath

DRUG PROFILES

▸▸ *selegiline*

Selegiline is an MAO-B inhibitor used as an adjunctive agent along with levodopa to decrease the amount of levodopa needed. It has also been shown to exert a neuroprotective effect when started early in therapy. It is a prescription-only drug that is available only in oral (PO) form as a 5-mg tablet and a 5-mg capsule. Selegiline has three active metabolites whose half-lives are listed in the pharmacokinetics table. Pregnancy category C. Recommended dosages are given in the table on p. 225.

PHARMACOKINETICS

Half-Life*	Onset	Peak	Duration
2 hr	1 hr	0.5–2 hr	1–3 days

*Selegiline has three active metabolites with long half-lives of 18–21 hours.

DOPAMINERGIC THERAPY

Because in PD little or no **endogenous** dopamine is produced, ACh is left as the predominant neurotransmitter in the brain, creating a state of imbalance. **Dopaminergic agents** are used to provide **exogenous** replacement of the lost dopamine or enhance the function of the few neurons that are still producing their own dopamine. Dopaminergic agents can be broken down into three categories based on their underlying mechanisms of action: those that release dopamine from remaining functional dopamine vesicles in presynaptic fibres of neurons or that inhibit dopamine-metabolizing enzymes (indirect-acting); those that increase brain levels of dopamine by providing exogenous dopamine in tablet form (replacement); and dopaminergic agonists that act as dopamine substitutes and stimulate dopamine receptors directly in place of dopamine (direct-acting). The ultimate goal is to increase the levels of dopamine in the brain. By doing so and creating a balance with ACh, akinesias, the most detrimental complications of PD, can be reversed. **Akinesias** are symptoms such as a mask-like facial expression and impaired postural reflexes. The course of the disease is progressive; eventually the client's independence is affected.

DOSAGES   Selegiline and Selected Dopaminergic Agents

Agent	Pharmacological Class	Usual Dosage Range	Indications
amantadine	Indirect-acting	**Adult** PO: 100–300 mg/day divided q12h	Triggers release of dopamine
bromocriptine and pergolide	Direct-acting	**Adult** PO: 2.5–40 mg/day divided doses with meals	Dopamine agonists
entacapone	Indirect-acting	**Adult** PO: 200 mg concomitant with levodopa/carbidopa or levodopa/benserazide (max 1600 mg/day)	Adjunct to levodopa and DDC inhibitor–COMT inhibitor
levodopa	Direct-acting	**Adult** PO: 400–8000 mg/day divided bid–qid	Dopamine agonist
▸▸levodopa-carbidopa	Replacement	**Adult** PO: 100/10, 1 tab 3–8 ×/day; 100/25, 1 tab 3–6×/day; 250/25, 1 tab tid–qid CR levodopa 200 mg/carbidopa 50 mg, 1 tab bid; up to 2–8 tabs at 4–12 hr intervals; CR 100/25 to facilitate titration	Replaces dopamine
pergolide	Direct-acting	**Adult** PO: Up to 5 mg/day in combination with levodopa-carbidopa	Dopamine agonist
pramipexole	Direct-acting	**Adult** PO: 1.5–4.5 mg/day divided tid	Dopamine agonist
▸▸ropinirole	Direct-acting	**Adult** PO: 0.25 mg tid slowly titrating to max dose of 24 mg/day	Dopamine agonist
▸▸selegiline	Indirect dopaminergic agent/MAOI	**Adult** PO: 5 mg bid with breakfast and lunch in combination with levodopa-carbidopa, or 10 mg every morning	Parkinson's disease

CR, Controlled release; *DDC*, dopa decarboxylase

Mechanism of Action and Drug Effects

Levodopa and the combination products levodopa-carbidopa and levodopa-benserazide HCl provide exogenous sources of dopamine that directly replace the deficient neurotransmitter dopamine in the substantia nigra. They are considered the cornerstone of the treatment of PD. Levodopa is the biological precursor of dopamine required by the brain for dopamine synthesis. These drugs are also referred to as **presynaptic drugs** or *replacement drugs*. This is because they work presynaptically and attempt to increase brain levels of dopamine. Dopamine must be administered in this form because, as mentioned previously, exogenously administered dopamine cannot pass through the blood–brain barrier, whereas levodopa can. Once it does, it is converted directly into dopamine by the enzyme dopa-decarboxylase. Traditionally, large doses of levodopa had to be administered to get enough dopamine to the brain because much of the levodopa administered was broken down outside the CNS by this same enzyme. These large doses resulted in high peripheral levels of dopamine and many unwanted side effects such as confusion, involuntary movements, gastrointestinal (GI) distress, and hypotension. Levodopa has even been known to cause dysrhythmias. These problems are avoided when levodopa is given with carbidopa or

benserazide, peripheral dopa decarboxylase (DDC) inhibitors that do not cross the blood–brain barrier. Therefore carbidopa and benserazide prevent levodopa breakdown in the periphery, allowing the levodopa to reach and cross the blood–brain barrier without crossing it itself. Once in the brain, the levodopa is converted to dopamine, which can then exert its therapeutic antiparkinsonian effects by offsetting the dopamine–ACh imbalance.

Originally developed and used for the prophylaxis and treatment of viral disorders, amantadine has proved to be a valuable adjunct to the traditional antiparkinsonian drugs. Amantadine appears to exert its antiparkinsonian effect by causing the release of dopamine and other catecholamines from their storage sites in the ends of nerve cells that are still intact and have not yet been destroyed by the disease process. Amantadine also blocks the reuptake of dopamine into the nerve endings, which allows more dopamine to accumulate both centrally and peripherally. Therefore its dopaminergic effects are the result of its indirect actions on the nerve because amantadine does not directly stimulate dopamine receptors as do certain other types of PD drugs. Amantadine also has some anticholinergic properties. This may further help by controlling symptoms of dyskinesias.

Bromocriptine and pergolide are dopaminergic agonists that directly stimulate the dopamine receptors. Chemically, bromocriptine is an ergot alkaloid similar to ergotamine in its chemical structure. Its antiparkinsonian effects are due to its ability to activate dopamine receptors and stimulate the production of more dopamine. This helps correct the imbalance between ACh and dopamine in the CNS. Pergolide, on the other hand, while also an ergot alkaloid, has no effect on dopamine synthesis or dopamine storage sites. It stimulates dopamine receptors in the substantia nigra of the brain, the area believed to be defective in clients with PD. Bromocriptine is a D2 dopamine agonist, whereas pergolide stimulates D1-3 receptors. Another difference between these two postsynaptic drugs is that pergolide is 20 times more potent than bromocriptine and has a half-life three times longer than that of bromocriptine. Pramipexole and ropinirole are two new highly specific D2-3 dopamine agonists released in 1997. They are both non-ergot drugs that are effective in early and late stages of PD.

Entacapone belongs to a totally new class of antiparkinsonian agents, the **catechol *O*-methyltransferase (COMT) inhibitors.** COMT inhibitors help clients with PD by inhibiting COMT, the enzyme responsible for the breakdown of levodopa, the dopamine precursor. In this way, COMT inhibitors are also indirect-acting dopaminergic drugs. Entacapone cannot cross the blood–brain barrier and therefore can act only peripherally. The main positive effect of entacapone is that it prolongs the duration of levodopa benefit. It is administered with levodopa as well as a dopa decarboxylase inhibitor (carbidopa or benserazide) to achieve sustained plasma levels of levodopa. Clients have less "wearing off" and experience prolonged benefits. Along with amantadine, COMT inhibitors are also considered to be indirect-acting agents and work as presynaptic agents.

Indications

The therapeutic effects of the replacement drugs levodopa and levodopa-carbidopa are identical. The only difference is that, as already explained, the combination product is more efficient in increasing the dopamine level in the brain.

The therapeutic effects of the indirect-acting dopaminergic agent amantadine are its antidyskinetic effects (its ability to promote voluntary movements) and its antiviral properties (both prevention and treatment). The direct-acting dopaminergic agents bromocriptine and pergolide also have antidyskinetic effects. In addition they can inhibit lactation, suppress growth hormone production, and inhibit prolactin production. This is because dopamine plays an important role in the regulation of hypothalamic–pituitary function. Dopamine has a direct effect on the adenohypophysis, which is responsible for secretion of growth hormone, prolactin, and other hormones. COMT inhibitors, as mentioned previously, indirectly promote dopamine activity by inhibiting enzymatic breakdown of dopamine. This also helps to control PD symptoms by reducing the dyskinetic effects of the disease.

Contraindications

Contraindications to dopaminergic agents include known drug allergy, history of melanoma or any undiagnosed skin condition, and narrow-angle glaucoma. In addition, these agents should also not be used until at least 14 days after MAOI therapy (except selegiline) is stopped.

Side Effects and Adverse Effects

There are many potential side effects and adverse effects associated with the dopaminergic agents. The most common of these are listed in Table 14-4.

Interactions

The drug interactions involving dopaminergic drugs can cause significant adverse reactions, including a decrease in the efficacy of the dopaminergic drug, a hypertensive crisis, and reversal of the dopaminergic drug's effect. Hydantoins, when given with levodopa, increase the metabolism of levodopa, decreasing its effects. Haloperidol and phenothiazines, when given with levodopa, block dopamine receptors in the brain, resulting in decreased

TABLE 14-4

DOPAMINERGIC AGENTS: ADVERSE EFFECTS

Body System	Side/Adverse Effects
AMANTADINE	
Central nervous	Impaired concentration, dizziness, increased irritability, nervousness, blurred vision
Gastrointestinal	Anorexia, nausea, constipation, vomiting
Other	Purple–red skin spots; dryness of mouth, nose, and throat; increased weakness
ENTACAPONE	
Central nervous	Involuntary movements (dyskinesias)
Gastrointestinal	Nausea, abdominal pain, diarrhea, decreased appetite
Other	Urine discoloration (brownish orange)
LEVODOPA-CARBIDOPA	
Hematological	Hemolytic anemia, agranulocytosis
Cardiovascular	Palpitations, orthostatic hypotension
Central nervous	Agitation; anxiety; psychotic and suicidal episodes; choreiform, dystonic, and other involuntary movements; headache and blurred vision
ROPINIROLE	
Cardiovascular	Syncope sometimes associated with bradycardia, symptomatic orthostatic hypotension
Central nervous	Hallucinations; somnolence; uncontrolled movement of body, face, tongue, arms, hands, and head
Gastrointestinal	Nausea

levodopa levels. Non-selective MAOIs taken concomitantly with dopaminergic drugs can result in inhibited metabolism, leading to a possible hypertensive crisis. Pyridoxine (vitamin B₆) promotes levodopa breakdown and may reverse levodopa effects. Carbidopa may help prevent this adverse outcome. The selective MAO-B inhibitor selegiline may be safely taken concurrently with COMT inhibitors.

Dosages

For the recommended dosages of the dopaminergic agents, see the table on p. 225. See Appendix B for some of the common brands available in Canada.

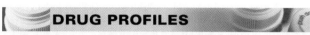

DRUG PROFILES

levodopa

As described earlier, the treatment of PD centres around attempts to replace the dopamine deficiency. Dopamine does not cross the blood–brain barrier, whereas levodopa, a precursor of dopamine, does. However, levodopa is also converted into dopamine in the rest of the body outside the brain. This can cause many unwanted side effects, including cardiac dysrhythmias, hypotension, chorea, muscle cramps, and GI distress.

Levodopa is contraindicated in clients who have shown a hypersensitivity reaction to it, those with narrow-angle glaucoma or a history of melanoma, and those concurrently taking MAOIs. Levodopa is available only in oral form as 50-, 100-, and 200-mg capsules and tablets. Pregnancy category C. Recommended dosages are given in the table on p. 225.

PHARMACOKINETICS

Half-Life	Onset	Peak	Duration
1.5 hr	2–3 wk for therapeutic effect	1–3 hr	<5 hr

▸▸ levodopa-carbidopa

The peripheral decarboxylase inhibitor carbidopa does not cross the blood–brain barrier. However, it does prevent metabolism of levodopa to dopamine in the periphery (i.e., outside the CNS). This, in turn, limits peripheral dopamine-induced side effects such as those described earlier. Instead the levodopa can reach its site of action in the brain without being broken down. As a result, much lower daily doses of levodopa are needed. Levodopa-carbidopa has become the cornerstone in the treatment of PD and is used much more commonly than levodopa alone. It also appears to limit the on–off phenomenon experienced by some clients taking levodopa long term. Such clients may experience periods when they have good control ("on" time) and periods when they have bad control or breakthrough PD ("off" time). A variety of studies have shown that levodopa-carbidopa CR increases on time and decreases off time. When converting clients from conventional levodopa-carbidopa preparations, the dosage of levodopa-carbidopa CR should include 10 to 30 percent more levodopa per day. The interval

between dosages of levodopa-carbidopa CR should be 4 to 8 hours during the waking day. Levodopa-carbidopa CR should not be crushed.

Levodopa-carbidopa is contraindicated in clients who have shown a hypersensitivity reaction to it, those with narrow-angle glaucoma or a history of melanoma, and those concurrently taking MAOIs. This combination agent is available only in oral form as tablets with the following proportions of levodopa to carbidopa, respectively: 100 mg to 10 mg, 100 mg to 25 mg, and 250 mg to 25 mg. There are also controlled-release formulations of this combination product consisting of 100 mg of levodopa and 25 mg of carbidopa or 200 mg of levodopa and 50 mg of carbidopa. Pregnancy category C. Recommended dosages are given in the table on p. 225.

PHARMACOKINETICS

Half-Life	Onset	Peak	Duration
1–3 hr	2–3 wk for therapeutic effect	1–3 hr	<5 h

amantadine

Amantadine is believed to work in the CNS by eliciting the release of dopamine from nerve endings, causing higher concentrations of dopamine in the CNS. It is most effective in the earlier stages of PD when there are still significant numbers of nerves to act on and dopamine to be released. As the disease progresses, however, the population of functioning nerves diminishes, and so does amantadine's effect. Amantadine is usually effective for only 6 to 12 months. After amantadine fails to relieve the hypokinesia and rigidity, a dopamine agonist such as bromocriptine or pergolide is usually tried next.

Amantadine is contraindicated in clients who have shown a hypersensitivity reaction to it, women who are lactating, and children younger than 1 year of age (amantadine is also an antiviral agent). Amantadine is available only in oral form as 100-mg capsules and in an oral solution that provides 50 mg/5 mL of syrup. Pregnancy category C. Recommended dosages are given in the table on p. 225.

PHARMACOKINETICS

Half-Life	Onset	Peak	Duration
15 hr	48 hr	4 hr	6–12 wk

DOPAMINE AGONISTS

The traditional role of dopamine agonists (bromocriptine, pergolide, pramipexole, ropinirole, and cabergoline) has been as adjuncts to levodopa for management of motor fluctuations only. These agents differ from levodopa in that they do not replace dopamine itself but act by stimulation of dopaminergic receptors in the brain. The agents have been evaluated as initial monotherapy and as combination therapy with low-dose levodopa in an attempt to delay levodopa therapy or reduce total exposure to the drug and associated motor complications. The newer agents pramipexole, ropinirole, and cabergoline are more specific for the receptors associated with parkinsonian symptoms, the D2 family (D2, D3, and D4). This in turn may have more specific antiparkinsonian effects with fewer adverse effects associated with generalized dopaminergic stimulation. These newer dopamine agonists have a promising role in the early treatment of PD. They appear to delay the start of levodopa therapy. Another benefit is that they have less ergot-like effects and dyskinesias. Both bromocriptine and pergolide are structurally similar to ergot derivatives and have some of their unwanted effects. These newer agents have also shown efficacy in clients with advanced PD.

bromocriptine and pergolide

Once amantadine becomes ineffective, a dopamine agonist such as pergolide or bromocriptine may be prescribed in its place. Bromocriptine differs from pergolide in that it only stimulates the dopamine 2 (D2) receptors and antagonizes or blocks the dopamine 1 (D1) receptors. Pergolide stimulates or acts as an agonist at both types of receptors. Eventually levodopa-carbidopa is needed to control the client's symptoms, but using amantadine until it fails then a dopamine agonist until it fails may postpone the need for levodopa therapy for up to 3 years. These two agents may also be given with levodopa-carbidopa so that lower doses of the levodopa are needed. This often results in prolonging the on periods, when PD is controlled, and decreasing the off periods, when PD is not controlled.

Bromocriptine is contraindicated in clients who have shown a hypersensitivity reaction to any of the ergot alkaloids, clients with severe ischemic disease, and those with severe peripheral vascular disease. This is primarily because of bromocriptine's ability to stimulate dopamine receptors. Bromocriptine is available only in oral form as 5-mg capsules and as 2.5-mg tablets. Pregnancy category D. Recommended dosages are given in the table on p. 225.

PHARMACOKINETICS: BROMOCRIPTINE

Half-Life	Onset	Peak	Duration
3–5 hr	0.5–1.5 hr	1–3 hr	4–8 hr

Pergolide is contraindicated in clients who have shown a hypersensitivity reaction to it or to other ergot alkaloids. It is available only in oral form as 0.05-, 0.25-, and 1-mg tablets. Pregnancy category B. Recommended dosages are given in the table on p. 225.

PHARMACOKINETICS: PERGOLIDE

Half-Life	Onset	Peak	Duration
27 hr	15–30 min	1–3 hr	1–2 days

▸▸ ropinirole

Ropinirole is a new non-ergot dopamine agonist indicated for monotherapy for PD and adjunctive therapy with levodopa. It is highly selective for the D2 family of dopamine receptors. It is contraindicated in clients who have shown a hypersensitivity reaction to it. Ropinirole is available as 0.05-, 0.25-, and 1-mg tablets. Pregnancy

category C. Recommended dosages are given in the table on p. 225.

PHARMACOKINETICS

Half-Life	Onset	Peak	Duration
3–5 hr	30 min	1–2 hr	6–10 hr

COMT INHIBITORS

A new strategy for prolonging the duration of action of levodopa is to inhibit the naturally occurring enzyme in the body, known as COMT, that breaks down dopamine molecules. One reversible COMT inhibitor is available: entacapone. Entacapone cannot cross the blood–brain barrier and therefore can act only peripherally. Clients have less wearing off and experience prolonged benefits of levodopa. Along with amantadine, this COMT inhibitor is considered to be an indirect-acting agent and works as a presynaptic agent.

entacapone

Entacapone is a new potent COMT inhibitor indicated for the adjunctive treatment of PD. The most recent safety information indicates that entacapone does not appear to be hepatotoxic. Entacapone is taken with levodopa and should be effective from the first dose. A client with PD can feel the benefit of entacapone within a day or two. Entacapone is particularly effective in clients who are experiencing wearing off fluctuations. Entacapone, used with levodopa, can reduce the daily off and increase the daily on time. The levodopa dose and dosing frequency can also be reduced in many cases. It is available in oral form as 200-mg film-coated tablets. It is contraindicated in clients who have shown a hypersensitivity reaction to it. Pregnancy category C. Recommended dosages are given in the table on p. 225.

PHARMACOKINETICS

Half-Life	Onset	Peak	Duration
1.5–3.5 hr	1 hr	0.5–1.5 hr	6 hr

ANTICHOLINERGIC THERAPY

Anticholinergics, or drugs that block the effects of ACh, are sometimes useful in treating the muscle tremors and muscle rigidity associated with PD. These two symptoms are caused by excessive cholinergic activity, which occurs because of lack of the normal dopamine balance. Anticholinergics do little, however, to relieve the bradykinesia (extremely slow movements) associated with PD. The rationale for the use of anticholinergics is to reduce excessive cholinergic activity in the brain. The first agents in this category to be used were the belladonna alkaloids, atropine and scopolamine. However the anticholinergic side effects—dry mouth, urinary retention, blurred vision—can be excessive; therefore new synthetic anticholinergics and antihistamines with better side effect profiles (e.g., benztropine and trihexyphenidyl) were developed.

DOSAGES   Selected Anticholinergic Agents

Agent	Pharmacological Class	Usual Dosage Range	Indications
▸ benztropine mesylate	Anticholinergic	*Adult* PO: 0.5–6 mg/day 1–4 mg bid	Parkinson's disease; drug-induced ex- trapyramidal symptoms
trihexyphenidyl	Anticholinergic	*Adult* PO: 6–10 mg/day 5–15 mg/day	Parkinson's disease; drug-induced ex- trapyramidal symptoms

Mechanism of Action and Drug Effects

All anticholinergics work in some way to block ACh (central cholinergic excitatory pathways). Because of the reduced number of dopamine-producing nerves associated with PD, the ACh-producing nerves are left unchecked and ACh accumulates. This causes an overstimulation of the cholinergic excitatory pathways, resulting in muscle tremors and muscle rigidity. This is sometimes described as *cogwheel rigidity*, because on passive movement, the joint appears to catch repeatedly, as if it were moving over cogs on a wheel. The muscle tremors are usually worse while the client is at rest and consist of a pill-rolling movement and bobbing of the head. Anticholinergic drugs either have the opposite effect or oppose the effects of the neurotransmitter ACh, which is responsible for causing increased *s*alivation, *l*acrimation (tearing of the eyes), *u*rination, *d*iarrhea, increased *G*I motility, and possibly *e*mesis (vomiting). The acronym SLUDGE is often used to describe these cholinergic-induced effects. The effects of anticholinergics are the opposite of the SLUDGE symptoms: antisecretory effects (dry mouth or decreased salivation), urinary retention, decreased GI motility (constipation), dilated pupils (mydriasis), and smooth muscle relaxation.

Indications

Anticholinergic agents decrease salivation and relax smooth muscles. They readily cross the blood–brain barrier and therefore can get right to the site of the imbalance in the CNS—the substantia nigra. It is because of their ability to directly relax smooth muscles that the muscle rigidity and akinesia (little or no movement) are reduced. Besides their use as antidyskinetic agents in PD, anticholinergics are also used for the treatment of drug-induced extrapyramidal reactions such as those related to selected antipsychotic agents (see Chapter 15). The extrapyramidal system is the part of the nervous system that controls muscle reflexes; extrapyramidal symptoms may include tremor, slurred speech, restlessness, and dystonia, as well as anxiety and distress.

Contraindications

Contraindications to anticholinergic agents include known drug allergy, any type of GI or bladder outlet obstruction, and myasthenia gravis.

TABLE 14-5
ANTICHOLINERGIC AGENTS: ADVERSE EFFECTS

Body System	Side/Adverse Effects
Central nervous	Drowsiness, confusion, disorientation, hallucinations
Gastrointestinal	Constipation, nausea, vomiting
Genitourinary	Urinary retention, pain on urination
Other	Blurred vision, dilated pupils (mydriasis), photophobia, dry skin

Side Effects and Adverse Effects

The side effects and adverse effects associated with anticholinergic drug use are many; the most common ones are listed in Table 14-5. They occur more commonly when the agents are given in high doses. Anticholinergic-induced adverse effects are also more common in geriatric clients. However, wise and judicious use of such drugs can lead to effective treatment free of the unwanted side effects.

Interactions

The interactions between anticholinergic drugs and other drugs and drug classes can be damaging. Alcohol, CNS depressants, amantadine, phenothiazines, tricyclic antidepressants, and antihistamines can have an additive effect with anticholinergic drugs, resulting in increased CNS depressant effects. Antacids alter gastric pH and reduce the absorption and therefore the therapeutic effects of anticholinergic drugs.

Dosages

For information on the dosages of benztropine and trihexyphenidyl in the treatment of PD, see the dosage table above. See Appendix B for some of the common brands available in Canada.

DRUG PROFILES

Anticholinergics are helpful in alleviating the muscle tremors and rigidity seen in clients with PD. They are not, however, as effective as the other drug classes used in the treatment of PD in correcting the underlying problem. They are effective for the relief of minimal symptoms and with clients who cannot tolerate or do not respond to dopamine replacement drugs such as levodopa or the dopaminergics such as amantadine and bromocriptine. Anticholinergics are also useful as adjuncts to these primary drugs. Treatment is usually started with small doses, which are gradually increased until the benefits or side effects appear. Some of the more commonly used agents are trihexyphenidyl, ethopropazine diphenhydramine and benztropine mesylate. They must be used cautiously in older adults because significant side effects can develop, such as confusion, urinary retention, visual blurring, palpitations, and increased intraocular pressure. The most commonly used agents are the synthetic anticholinergics, which are associated with fewer of the side effects commonly seen with the belladonna alkaloid derivatives such as atropine and scopolamine.

▶▶ *benztropine mesylate*

Benztropine is a synthetic anticholinergic agent that resembles both atropine and diphenhydramine in its chemical structure. Biperiden is also a synthetic anticholinergic agent used in the treatment of PD. Both benztropine and biperiden have anticholinergic, antihistaminic, and local anaesthetic properties and are primarily used as adjuncts in the treatment of all forms of PD. They are also useful in the treatment of phenothiazine-induced extrapyramidal reactions. Benztropine is available only with a prescription and comes in oral form as 0.5-, 1-, and 2-mg tablets and as an intravenous injection delivering 1 mg/mL. Its use is contraindicated in clients who have shown a hypersensitivity reaction to it; in those who have narrow-angle glaucoma, myasthenia gravis, urinary retention, a history of peptic ulcer disease, megacolon (dilation of the colon), or prostate hypertrophy; and in children under 3 years of age. Pregnancy category C. Recommended dosages are given in the dosages table on p. 229.

PHARMACOKINETICS

Half-Life	Onset	Peak	Duration
4–8 hr	1–2 hrs	2–4 hr	6–10 hr

trihexyphenidyl

Trihexyphenidyl is a synthetic anticholinergic that is used as an adjunctive agent in the treatment of PD. It has weak peripheral anticholinergic effects. It is contraindicated in clients who have shown a hypersensitivity reaction to it and in clients with any of the conditions listed as contraindications to benztropine treatment. Trihexyphenidyl is available only in oral form as a 2-mg/5 mL elixir and 2- and 5-mg tablets. Pregnancy category C. Recommended dosages are given in the dosages table on p. 229.

PHARMACOKINETICS

Half-Life	Onset	Peak	Duration
3–4 hr	<1 hr	2–3 hr	6–12 hr

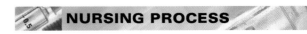

NURSING PROCESS

■ Assessment

Soon after being confronted with the diagnosis of PD, a client learns how the disease can affect every movement and alter activities of daily living (ADLs). Before administering medication, the nurse must perform a thorough assessment and take a thorough nursing history, documenting symptoms and effects on ADLs and identifying any contraindications and cautions. The thorough nursing history should include questions about the following activities and body systems:

• Central nervous system (CNS): ADLs, gait, balance, tremors, weakness, lethargy, and level of consciousness
• Gastrointestinal (GI) and genitourinary (GU): appetite, bladder, and bowel patterns
• Psychological and emotional: mood, affect, depression, and personality changes

Additional signs and symptoms of PD to assess include mask-like expression; speech problems; dysphagia (difficulty swallowing); and rigidity of arms, legs, and neck.

When an anticholinergic agent such as benztropine or trihexyphenidyl is prescribed, the nurse should assess the client carefully for contraindications: a history of urinary retention, bladder difficulties or obstruction, myasthenia gravis, or acute narrow-angle glaucoma (mydriasis leads to an increase in intraocular pressure). Age is a significant factor as well because the physiological changes associated with aging increase the likelihood of side effects or toxicity. Other conditions that these agents can exacerbate include tachycardia, benign prostatic hypertrophy (BPH), and peptic ulcer disease; therefore a client with any of these conditions should be monitored closely. Drugs that interact with these agents include antihistamines, disopyramide, phenothiazines, and tricyclic antidepressants (TCAs) (increase effects). Cholinergic agents decrease the effects of anticholinergics. SSRIs (see Chapter 15) should be avoided when a client is taking antiparkinson agents.

When dopaminergic agents such as levodopa, amantadine, or levodopa-carbidopa are prescribed, the client should be asked whether he or she has a seizure disorder; hypotension; peptic ulcer disease; a renal or hepatic disorder; asthma; a history of myocardial infarction (MI), BPH, or an anemia; or suffers from psychosis or some other affective disorder. These are all contraindications to the use of dopaminergic agents. Drugs that can interact with these agents include MAOIs and furazolidone. Given in combination with the dopaminergic medications, these drugs may result in a hypertensive crisis. Other drug interactions include TCAs, anticholinergics, alcohol, vitamin B$_6$, and antipsychotic agents.

With the newer agent ropinirole, a client with a history of renal or cardiac disease needs to take the drug with caution. Cautious use is also recommended in any client with psychoses, affective disorders, or dysrhythmias. The client needs to be further assessed for involuntary movements seen in parkinsonism such as akinesia, tremors, staggering gait, rigidity, and drooling. Vital signs should be assessed during treatment, with special attention to blood pressure because of the side effects of hypotension and hypertension. Entacapone is contraindicated in clients with hypersensitivity to the drug. Entacapone may be taken safely by clients with a liver disorder. Newer dopamine agonists, such as pramipexole, ropinirole, and cabergoline, are contraindicated in clients with sensitivity to these groups of medications.

Nursing Diagnoses

Nursing diagnoses appropriate to the client with PD taking antiparkinsonian agents include the following:
- Impaired physical mobility related to the disease process and side effects of the medications.
- Disturbed body image related to changes in appearance and mobility due to the disease process.
- Urinary retention with incomplete emptying, related to the effects of the disease on the bladder.
- Constipation with decreased peristalsis, related to the disease process.
- Risk for injury related to the physical limitations produced by the disease process.
- Imbalanced nutrition, less than body requirements, related to pharmacotherapy and associated side effects.
- Deficient knowledge related to lack of exposure to treatment regimen.

Planning

Goals of nursing care related to the administration of antiparkinsonian agents include the following:
- Client remains free of self-injury.
- Client states the purpose of the specific medications prescribed for the disease.
- Client states the side effects and toxic effects of medications.
- Client regains bowel and bladder elimination patterns that are as normal as possible.
- Client maintains adequate nutritional status.
- Client remains as independent as possible.
- Client is less anxious and fearful.
- Client regains a positive self-concept.
- Client remains adherent to therapy.

Outcome Criteria

Outcome criteria related to the administration of antiparkinsonian agents include the following:
- Client (and significant others) states ways of preventing self-injury such as the use of assistive devices.
- Client states purposes, side effects, and toxic effects associated with the specific antiparkinsonian medications such as emesis, nausea, instability, and palpitations.
- Client states ways to prevent some of the side effects and toxic effects of antiparkinsonian medications such as frequent mouth care and increased fluids.
- Client discusses ways to minimize problems associated with drug-induced alterations in bowel and bladder elimination patterns through changes in diet and fluid intake.
- Client discusses measures to ensure an adequate nutritional status with possible anti-emetic therapy.
- Client begins to perform ADLs more independently.
- Client openly verbalizes fears, anxieties, and changes in self-image with members of the healthcare team and support staff.

Implementation

Nursing actions related to the administration of the various antiparkinsonian agents focus primarily on safe drug administration and client education. Oral doses of anticholinergic agents should be taken after meals; a single daily dose should be administered at bedtime. Fluid intake and frequent mouth care should be encouraged because of the dryness of the mouth. Any intravenously administered medications, such as benztropine mesylate, should be given slowly, with the client remaining in bed for 1 hour afterward. The client should be informed not to take any other medications without the physician's consent because of many adverse drug interactions with prescription and over-the-counter (OTC) medications.

During the start of dopaminergic agent therapy, the client should be assisted when walking because of the dizziness caused by these agents. Oral doses should be given with food to help minimize GI upset. It is also important for the nurse to remember that pyridoxine (vitamin B$_6$) in doses greater than 10 mg will reverse the effects of levodopa. Foods high in vitamin B$_6$ should therefore also be avoided. The client should be encouraged to take in extra fluids, unless contraindicated, drinking at least 2000 mL/day, and to consume an adequate amount of food high in fibre. A hypertensive crisis may result if levodopa preparations are taken with MAOIs; therefore these drugs are generally not administered concurrently. At least 2 weeks should be allowed to elapse between the use of these medications. It is also important for the nurse to remember that dopaminergic agents are generally titrated to the client's response. Levodopa-carbidopa CR oral form should not be crushed.

It is important to tell the client to take antiparkinsonian agents as prescribed. The nurse should make sure the client understands the onset of therapeutic benefits. For example, entacapone, a potent COMT inhibitor generally taken with levodopa, should be effective beginning with the first dose. Unlike older agents, which can take weeks, clients normally experience the benefit of entacapone within 1 or 2 days. The newer non-ergot dopamine agonists have been shown to have more efficacy in clients with advanced forms of PD; therefore an important part of client care is teaching about their effects. The client should also be informed that they cause fewer dyskinesia side effects. Entacapone is helpful for clients who are experiencing problems with wearing off fluctuations. This medication comes in film-coated tablets and should not be crushed. To avoid alarm, it is important to tell the client that entacapone turns the urine a brownish orange. Clients taking the newer dopamine agonists pramipexole and ropinirole should be educated about the "sleep attacks" that may occur without warning.

Client teaching tips for dopaminergic agents are presented below.

■ Evaluation

Monitoring the client's response to any of the antiparkinsonian medications is crucial to documenting treatment success or failure. Therapeutic responses to the antiparkinsonian agents include an improved sense of well-being; improved mental status; increase in appetite; ability to perform ADLs, to concentrate, and to think clearly; and less intense parkinsonism manifestations such as tremor, shuffling of gait, muscle rigidity, and involuntary movements. In addition to monitoring for therapeutic responses, the nurse must also watch for the occurrence of side effects, such as confusion, anxiety, irritability, depression, paranoia, headache, weakness, lethargy, nausea, vomiting, anorexia, palpitations, postural hypotension, tachycardia, dry mouth, constipation, urinary retention, blurred vision, dark urine, difficulty swallowing, and nightmares. Therapeutic effects of COMT inhibitors such as entacapone may be noticed within a few days, whereas with other agents it may take weeks. With COMT inhibitors, nurses should monitor for the side effects mentioned previously, although fewer dyskinesias are associated with COMT inhibitors than with dopamine agonists.

CLIENT TEACHING TIPS

The nurse should instruct the client as follows:
▲ Change positions slowly because of the postural hypotension (drop in blood pressure with position changes) that can occur. Take your time changing positions from lying to sitting and then gradually standing. Report excessive twitching, drooling, or eye spasms to your physician (may indicate an overdose).
▲ Always take your antiparkinson medication exactly as prescribed and do not omit or double a dose. If you accidentally skip a dose or make an error, notify the physician immediately.
▲ Do not suddenly stop taking your medication.
▲ If you are taking a levodopa preparation, don't worry if your urine and sweat become darker.
▲ Do not take Vitamin B$_6$ supplements because it enhances metabolism of levodopa, reducing the amount available at sites of action in the brain. (The risk is lower, however, in combination levodopa-carbidopa agents.)
▲ Follow the list you have been given of specific foods to avoid (e.g., bananas, egg yolks, lima beans, meats, peanuts, and whole grain cereals contain large amounts of pyridoxine). The amount of protein in the diet, as well as the time at which high-protein foods (meats, poultry, fish, dairy products, nuts, seeds, and legumes) are eaten may reduce or significantly slow the absorption of levodopa, thereby decreasing its therapeutic effect.
▲ Keep a journal of your progress with treatment and any problems.
▲ If you are taking a controlled-release form, do not crush the tablet.
▲ Take anticholinergics with meals or after meals to minimize stomach upset. Unless your physician has told you to limit fluids, drink at least 2000 mL/day.
▲ Avoid taking any OTC medications while taking any of these drugs unless your healthcare provider approves.
▲ Avoid operating heavy machinery or driving if you feel sedated or drowsy from any of these medications.
▲ If you are prescribed a COMT inhibitor, this is a newer drug that provides a more substantial level of levodopa in the brain and can give you more "good" days. You may improve in a few days. This drug does not replace your levodopa and/or carbidopa, but goes along with it.

POINTS to REMEMBER

▼ The neurotransmitting abnormalities with PD include a chronic, progressive, degenerative disorder of dopamine-producing neurons in the brain, and clients with PD have elevated ACh levels and lowered dopamine levels.
▼ Drug therapy lowers the ACh level and raises the dopamine level.

▼ Signs and symptoms of PD include bradykinesia (slow movements), rigidity (cogwheel), tremor (pill-rolling), and postural instability.
▼ Characteristics of PD include dyskinesias (difficulty performing voluntary movements), chorea (irregular, spasmodic, involuntary movements of limbs or facial muscles), and dystonias (abnormal muscle tone in any tissue).

▼ Drug therapy for PD includes the following mechanisms: MAO inhibition, dopaminergic, and anticholinergic.

▼ Specific antiparkinson drugs include the following:
  • Selegiline, an MAOI, which is specific for MAO-B.
  • Ropinirole and pramipexole, new non-ergot dopamine agonists indicated for monotherapy for PD and for adjunctive therapy with levodopa.
  • Entacapone, a newer COMT inhibitor with a longer duration of action and a quicker onset (1–2 days). The COMT inhibitor is also associated with fewer "wearing off" effects and prolonged therapeutic benefits.

▼ Dopaminergic drugs are classed as indirect-acting, direct-acting, or replacement.
  • *Indirect* agents reduce neuronal reuptake of dopamine from synaptic cleft, or inhibit metabolic breakdown of dopamine
  • *Direct* agents stimulate dopamine receptors (agonists)
  • *Replacement* agents exogenously administer dopamine or a dopamine precursor (levodopa)

▼ Levodopa and levodopa-carbidopa replace deficient dopamine in the brain; levodopa is the biological precursor of dopamine and can pass through the blood–brain barrier to get to the site of action in the brain; dopamine (itself) cannot.

▼ Carbidopa is a peripheral decarboxylase inhibitor, does not cross the blood–brain barrier, and prevents levodopa breakdown in periphery.

▼ Client considerations include long-term care because of the progressive and debilitating nature of this illness.

▼ Client care also requires much support and education about the disease process and the drugs indicated.

▼ "Sleep attacks" may occur with the newer dopamine agonists (pramipexole and ropinirole), and brownish orange discoloration of the urine occurs with entacapone.

EXAMINATION REVIEW QUESTIONS
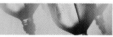

1 Which of the following should alert the nurse to a potential caution or contraindication with use of an anticholinergic agent for treatment of mild PD?
 a. Diarrhea
 b. Drooling
 c. Glaucoma
 d. Irritable bowel syndrome

2 The physician has ordered amantadine for your client. The client is also taking hydrochlorothiazide (HCTZ). Which of the following would be your most appropriate action in this scenario?
 a. Do not be concerned because even though there is a drug interaction; the increased effect of the antiparkinsonian agent by the diuretic is a desirable action.
 b. Contact the healthcare provider about the potential drug interaction with HCTZ leading to toxic effects of amantadine because of its decreased renal excretion.
 c. Encourage the use of both of these agents simultaneously because they are synergistic and result in mood improvement and a decrease in gait abnormalities.
 d. Encourage the client to refuse the medication because research has shown that the use of amantadine with diuretics increases the risk of memory impairment.

3 Client teaching for antiparkinson agents should include which of the following statements?
 a. Twitch and eye spasms indicate adequate dosing.
 b. Changing of positions may be per usual and without concern for dizziness.

 c. There should be concern about antiparkinsonian drug use and brain cancer.
 d. Antiparkinsonian drug use and the occurrence of hypotension may result in postural changes in blood pressure, so change positions slowly.

4 If levodopa therapy is not relieving the symptoms of PD, which of the following antiparkinsonian agents (with corresponding rationale) may the healthcare provider consider switching the client to?
 a. haloperidol with a mechanism of action of dopamine agonism
 b. methyldopa with a mechanism of action of antidopaminergism
 c. amantadine with its exclusive mechanism of action of antiviral effects
 d. levodopa-carbidopa with its exclusive mechanism of action of inhibition of the decarboxylation of peripheral levodopa

5 Which of the following statements should be emphasized and explained during client teaching about the use of levodopa?
 a. "There are few, if any, drug interactions with levodopa."
 b. "Therapeutic effects may take up to several weeks to a few months."
 c. "Make sure that you take a laxative 4 times daily with at least 6000 mL of fluids each 8 to 12 hours."
 d. "Levodopa should be taken as preventive medication to the occurrence of Parkinson's disease."

For answers see http://evolve.elsevier.com/Lilley/pharmacology/.

CRITICAL THINKING ACTIVITIES

1 Mr. P. has been diagnosed with PD and is taking levodopa-carbidopa. He also has Alzheimer's disease and is taking donepezil. What do you think about the use of these two medications together?

2 You discover that your client who has PD and is taking levodopa-carbidopa is also being given some of his wife's phenothiazine medication to make him "feel even better." Why is this combination unsafe and not rational?

3 Your client has been placed on a dopaminergic for the management of PD. She also relates to you during the nursing history that she has a diet high in meats, poultry,

and whole grain cereals. What would be a concern you may have with this client's diet and why?

4 How does levodopa help improve the function of the client diagnosed with PD?

5 After long-term treatment, clients with PD are often placed on a "drug holiday." Explain the rationale for this approach to treatment.

6 Explain the physiology behind the "on-again/off-again" appearance of symptoms that occurs with long-term levodopa treatment.

For answers see http://evolve.elsevier.com/Lilley/pharmacology/.

BIBLIOGRAPHY

Albanese, J., & Nutz, P. (2005). *Mosby's 2005 nursing drug cards.* St Louis, MO: Mosby.

Anderson, P.O., Knoben, J.E., & Troutman, W.G. (2002). *Handbook of clinical drug data* (10th ed.). New York: McGraw-Hill/Appleton & Lange.

Canadian Pharmacists Association. (2003). *Therapeutic choices* (4th ed.). Ottawa, ON: Author.

Canadian Pharmacists Association. (2004). *Guide to drugs in Canada.* Toronto, ON: Dorling Kindersley.

Canadian Pharmacists Association. (2005). *Compendium of pharmaceuticals and specialties. The Canadian drug reference for health professionals.* Ottawa, ON: Author. [The subscription-based e-CPS is available at http://www.pharmacists.ca.]

Facts and Comparisons. (2004). *Drug facts and comparisons pocket version* (9th ed.). St Louis, MO: Wolters Kluwer Health.

Guttman, M., Kish, S.J., & Furukama, Y. (2003). Current concepts in the diagnosis and management of Parkinson's disease. [Electronic version]. *Canadian Medical Association Journal, 168*(3).

Hardman, J.G., & Limbird, L.E. (2002). *Goodman and Gilman's the pharmacological basis of therapeutics* (10th ed.). New York: McGraw-Hill.

Health Canada. (2001). Antiparkinsonian drugs and "sleep attacks." *Canadian Adverse Reaction Newsletter, 11*(2). Retrieved July 30, 2005, from http://www.hc-sc.gc.ca/dph-mps/prodpharma/index_e.html

Health Canada. (2005). Drug product database (DPD). Retrieved July 30, 2005, from http://www.hc-sc.gc.ca/hpb/drugs-dpd/

Katzung, B.G. (2004). *Basic and clinical pharmacology* (9th ed.). New York: McGraw-Hill.

Koda-Kimble, M.A., & Young, L.Y. (2001). *Applied therapeutics: the clinical use of drugs* (7th ed.). Philadelphia: Lippincott Williams & Wilkins.

Lehne, R.A. (2004). *Pharmacology for nursing care* (5th ed.). St Louis, MO: Saunders.

Mosby. (2005). *Mosby's drug consult 2005: The comprehensive reference for generic and brand name drugs* (15th ed.). St Louis, MO: Mosby.

Skidmore-Roth, L. (2006). *Mosby's 2006 nursing drug reference* (19th ed.). St Louis, MO: Mosby.

Psychotherapeutic Agents

After reading this chapter, the successful student will be able to do the following:

1 Identify the various psychotherapeutic drugs, such as anti-anxiety agents, antidepressants, antimanic agents, and antipsychotics.

2 Discuss the mechanisms of action, indications, therapeutic effects, side effects, toxic effects, drug interactions, contraindications, and cautions associated with the various psychotherapeutic agents.

3 Develop a nursing care plan that includes all phases of the nursing process related to the administration of the various psychotherapeutic agents.

4 Develop client education guidelines for clients receiving psychotherapeutic drugs.

𝑒-LEARNING ACTIVITIES

Student CD-ROM
- Review Questions: see questions 77–88
- Animations
- Medication Administration Checklists
- IV Therapy Checklists

evolve Web site (http://evolve.elsevier.com/Lilley/pharmacology/)
- Online Chapter Worksheet • Frequently Asked Questions
- Learning Tips and Content Updates • WebLinks • Online Appendices and Supplements • Mosby/Saunders ePharmacology Update • Access to *Mosby's Drug Consult*

DRUG PROFILES

GLOSSARY

Adjunct therapy Combination drug therapy used when a client's condition does not respond adequately to a single drug (monotherapy), or used when a given combination of medications is known to have therapeutic advantages over a single agent. (See *monotherapy*.)

Affective disorders (a feck' tiv) Emotional disorders that are characterized by changes in mood.

Agoraphobia (a' gə rə fo' bee uh) Fear of leaving the familiar setting of home.

Akathisia Motor restlessness—a distressing experience of uncontrollable muscular movements that can occur as a side effect of many psychotropic medications.

Antihistamine (an tee his' tə meen) Any substance capable of reducing the physiological and pharmacological effects of histamine, including a wide variety of drugs that block histamine receptors.

Antipsychotic (an tee sigh cot' ik) Of or pertaining to a medication that counteracts or diminishes symptoms of psychosis. (See *psychosis*.) An older term for such medications is *neuroleptic*.

Anxiety The unpleasant state of mind in which real or imagined dangers are anticipated and/or exaggerated.

Anxiolytic Capable of reducing anxiety; usually said of a medication.

Benzodiazepine (ben zo die a' zə peen) The most common group of psychotropic agents currently prescribed to alleviate anxiety.

Biogenic amine hypothesis (BAH) Theory suggesting that depression and mania are due to alterations in neuronal and synaptic amine concentrations, primarily the catecholamines dopamine and norepinephrine, as well as the indolamines serotonin and histamine.

Bipolar disorder (BPD)   A major psychological disorder characterized by episodes of mania or hypomania, cycling with depression.

Depression   An abnormal emotional state characterized by exaggerated feelings of sadness, melancholy, dejection, worthlessness, emptiness, and hopelessness that are inappropriate and out of proportion to reality.

Dopamine hypothesis   The view that dopamine dysregulation in certain parts of the brain is one of the primary contributing factors to the development of psychotic disorders (psychoses).

Dysregulation hypothesis   The view that depression and affective disorders as not simply decreased or increased catecholamine and serotonin activity but failures of the regulation of these systems.

Dysthymic disorder or dysthymia   An affective disorder with many of the same symptoms as major depression, except that they are less severe. Dysthymic disorder lasts for at least two years, with only brief interludes of normal mood.

Gamma-aminobutyric acid (GABA)   An inhibitory amino acid in the brain that functions to inhibit nerve transmission in the central nervous system (CNS).

Mania   (may' nee uh) A state characterized by an expansive emotional state; extreme excitement; excessive elation; hyperactivity; agitation; overtalkativeness; flight of ideas; increased psychomotor activity; fleeting attention; and sometimes violent, destructive, and self-destructive behaviour.

Monoamine oxidase inhibitor (MAOI)   (mon o a' meen ok' si dase) Any of a heterogeneous group of drugs used primarily in the treatment of depression.

Monotherapy   Pharmacological therapy involving a single medication for a specific condition. (See *adjunct therapy*.)

Neurotransmitter   Endogenous chemical in the body that serves to conduct nerve impulses between nerve cells (neurons). This type of neurotransmission occurs in both the CNS and the peripheral nervous system. However, the proposed mechanisms of both the pathology of and drug therapy for mental illness centre around neurotransmitter function between neurons in various regions of the brain.

Permissive hypothesis   Implicates reduced concentrations of serotonin (5-HT) as the predisposing factor in individuals with affective disorders.

Psychosis   (sigh ko' sis) (Plural: psychoses) A type of serious mental illness that can take several different forms and is associated with being truly out of touch with reality; that is, unable to distinguish imaginary from real circumstances and events. Psychosis often results in significant disability.

Psychotherapeutics   (sigh ko ther ə pyoo' tiks) Refers to the therapy of emotional and mental disorders. It may involve drug therapy (pharmacotherapy), a variety of counselling techniques, recreational therapy, and in extreme cases electroconvulsive therapy (ECT).

Psychotropic   Capable of affecting mental processes; usually said of a medication.

Seasonal affective disorder   A recurrent episode of depressive illness that occurs most often during the winter months.

Serotonin-selective reuptake inhibitor (SSRI)   Also called *selective serotonin reuptake inhibitors*. Any of a heterogeneous group of newer medications used to treat depression and certain other mental illnesses. They work by selectively reducing post-synaptic reuptake of the neurotransmitter serotonin in the brain.

Stigma   Widespread negative perceptions of and prejudice toward a specific group of people such as those with mental illness.

Tricyclic antidepressants (TCAs)   (try sik' lik) A chemical class of antidepressant agents that block reuptake of the amine neurotransmitters serotonin and norepinephrine. They are so named because their chemical structures include a distinctive three-ring segment.

The treatment of emotional and mental disorders is called **psychotherapeutics.** When a person's ability to cope with his or her environment—to carry out the activities of daily living (ADLs) and to interact with others—is seriously impaired, a **psychotropic** drug may be a treatment option. These drugs are among the most commonly prescribed drugs in Canada today. Because of the inherent subjectivity in the description and reporting of symptoms of mental illness, the effects of these drugs are less easily quantified than for many other types of medications. For example, it is usually not known with certainty how long a given psychotropic drug works in the body (duration of action). Thus the effectiveness of psychotropic drug therapy is often measured by verbal reports from clients regarding the level of improvement (if any) in their social and occupational functioning. There are also several established tools that attempt to quantify client response to psychotropic drug therapy, such as the Hamilton Depression Rating Scale (HAM-D). Of even newer interest is the rapidly expanding area of study known as *pharmacogenomics.* One objective of this field is to

ETHNOCULTURAL IMPLICATIONS

Psychotherapeutic Agents

Many racial and ethnic groups respond to drugs differently. For example, Asians have a lower activity of drug metabolism compared with Caucasians as a result of various enzyme deficiencies. Asians often require lower doses of benzodiazepines and tricyclic antidepressants (TCAs) because they have lower levels of metabolizing enzymes (e.g., CYP2D6) and are therefore more sensitive to these agents. Beta-blockers, specifically propranolol, are also problematic for Asians.

Ethnocultural implications with regard to psychotherapeutic agents involve how a specific ethnic group feels about and deals with mental disorders in general. The nurse must assess family support systems, beliefs about mental illnesses, and the willingness to take or continue with psychotherapeutic drug therapy. Ethnocultural beliefs can lead to treatment failure.

map genetic factors (genetic polymorphisms) that contribute to different patterns of activity of drug-metabolizing enzymes across different ethnic groups. To better understand the nature and goals of this treatment, the types and definitions of various mental disorders are presented first.

OVERVIEW OF MENTAL ILLNESS

Most people experience emotions such as anxiety, depression, and grief. They are normal human emotions. However, the effect of these emotions on a person's ability to engage in normal daily activities and to interact with others can vary considerably. The duration and intensity of these emotions can range from occasional sadness or anxiety to a state of constant emotional distress that interferes with a person's ability to carry on normal ADLs.

There is often considerable overlap among the symptoms of the many different psychiatric disorders, which can make accurate diagnosis difficult. Complicating this issue further is the inherent subjectivity with which different clients experience their symptoms. Often a client will have ongoing symptoms that meet several criteria for more than one, or even several, mental disorders. Such clients may be said to have a spectrum disorder. For example, research shows that more than half of chronically depressed adults also have a co-occurring personality disorder, and one-third have a co-occurring anxiety disorder and/or a substance use problem. Mentally ill people may also be more susceptible to various physical health problems than the general population. For example, obesity is significantly more common in clients with mental disorders. Because of the variety of economic, educational, and psychosocial issues that may preclude a mentally ill person from seeking psychiatric health care, many clients will self-medicate with alcohol, tobacco, and other substances. This generally worsens the problem.

Despite newer, more effective treatments for mental illness, a long-held societal **stigma** continues to be an obstacle for diagnosed clients. The Canadian Alliance on Mental Illness and Mental Health (CAMIMH) is made up of five national organizations with representation from consumers of mental health services, families, core professional service providers, and community organizations. CAMIMH's mission is to advocate for a national mental health strategy. CAMIMH seeks to promote consumer well-being and autonomy through research funding, legislative advocacy, and public education and awareness to reduce stigma. Ideal mental health care usually involves many factors, including a carefully detailed client interview (to help ensure accurate and complete diagnosis); carefully chosen and regularly monitored drug therapy (if indicated); and significant emotional support, which may range from formal psychotherapy to informal support groups, social and family support systems, and spiritual support systems that the client values.

There are three main emotional and mental disorders: psychoses, affective disorders, and anxiety. A **psychosis** is a severe emotional disorder that often impairs mental function to the point of significant disability regarding ADLs. A hallmark of psychosis is a loss of contact with reality. Psychotic disorders primarily include schizophrenia and depressive and drug-induced psychoses.

Affective disorders, also called *mood disorders*, are characterized by changes in mood and range from **mania** (abnormally pronounced emotions) to **depression** (abnormally reduced emotions). Some clients may exhibit both mania and depression, experiencing periodic swings in emotions, from extremely negative emotions to intense, hyperactive emotions. This is referred to as a **bipolar disorder (BPD)**.

Depression is reported to currently have prevalence rates of approximately 6 to 8 percent among Canadians 18 years and older. Major depressive disorders (MDDs) are expected to become the second leading cause of disability by the year 2020. In addition to often drastic reductions in quality of life and occupational and psychosocial functioning, up to 80 percent of clients with depression have major sleep disturbances. Some sleep researchers report that an 1½-hour loss of sleep on any given night may reduce alertness on the following day by 33 percent; therefore insomnia associated with depression has even more far-reaching adverse effects on the client. This loss in the client's state of alertness may then be associated with accidents. Depression also puts the client at risk of suicide. Despite recent advances in pharmacotherapy for depression it remains undertreated in many cases and, in fact, two current and significant epidemiological studies conducted in the United States have demonstrated that clients seeking treatment for depressive symptoms were not even offered antidepressant treatment in 52 percent to 75 percent of cases. It is interesting to note however that the class of psychotherapeutics is the second most prescribed drug in Canada. Effexor XR is the most common drug prescribed.

Dysthymic disorder, also called dysthymia, is a chronic state of low mood (lasting at least two years) with symptoms similar to major depression but less severe. Some people have dysthymia interspersed with episodes of major depression, a condition sometimes called *double depression*. **Seasonal affective disorder (SAD)** is a subtype of depression that affects approximately 2 to 4 percent of the Canadian population. SAD is characterized by recurrent episodes of depressive illness that occur at the same time of year (often late fall or winter) over a period of years and during at least two consecutive years. Most people with SAD have unipolar depression, but as many as 20 percent may have or go on to develop a bipolar or manic-depressive disorder.

Anxiety is the unpleasant state of mind chiefly characterized by a sense of dread and fear. It may be based on actual anticipated or past experiences such as scheduled surgery or prior abuse. It may also stem from exaggerated responses to imaginary negative situations or to common everyday experiences that are only mildly disturbing to a mentally healthy person. Persistent anxiety is divided clinically into several distinct disorders that have been classified by the American Psychiatric Association. This classification is published in the fourth edition of the

Diagnostic and Statistical Manual for Mental Disorders (DSM-IV). This reference delineates the demographic features and diagnostic criteria for the major psychiatric disorders and has categorized anxiety into the following six major disorders:

1 Obsessive–compulsive disorder (OCD)
2 Post-traumatic stress disorder (PTSD)
3 Generalized anxiety disorder (GAD)
4 Panic disorder
5 Social phobia
6 Simple phobia

Anxiety is a normal physiological emotion, but the results of epidemiological studies show that 5 percent of adults suffer from a GAD; 1 to 3.5 percent from a panic disorder; and 2.9 percent to 5 percent from agoraphobia. **Agoraphobia** is defined as *anxiety about being in places or situations from which escape may be difficult (or embarrassing) or in which help might not be readily available in the event of an unexpected or situationally predisposed panic attack.* People with agoraphobia fear being in situations that include being outside the home alone, being in a crowd, being on a bridge, or being on a bus, car, or train. Obsessive-compulsive disorder (OCD) was thought to be rare but is now observed to be twice as common as schizophrenia or panic disorder in the general population. Anxiety may occur as a result of a wide range of medical illnesses, such as cardiovascular or pulmonary disease, hypothyroidism, hyperthyroidism, hypoglycemia, or pheochromocytoma. Many of the anxiety disorders are situational. They arise because of a specific event and subside with time. The treatment of these disorders should be limited to psychotherapy, and possibly short-term drug therapy. However, when the anxiety disorder markedly affects a person's quality of life and relationships or interferes with the ability to function normally over a prolonged period (at least several months), longer-term pharmacotherapy in conjunction with psychotherapy is usually recommended.

The exact causes of mental disorders are not fully understood. Many theories have been advanced in an attempt to explain the causes and pathophysiology of mental dysfunction. In the biochemical imbalance concept, mental disorders are thought to arise as the result of abnormal levels of endogenous chemicals in the brain known as **neurotransmitters.** There is strong evidence indicating that the brain levels of catecholamines (especially dopamine and norepinephrine) and indolamines (serotonin and histamine) play an important role in maintaining mental health. Other biochemicals that seem necessary for the maintenance of normal mental function are **gamma-aminobutyric acid (GABA);** acetylcholine (ACh); and various inorganic ions such as sodium, potassium, and magnesium. Knowledge of these various etiologies, especially the biochemical imbalance theory, can aid in understanding psychotherapeutic drug action because many of the agents used to treat psychoses, affective disorders, and anxiety work by blocking or stimulating the release of these endogenous neurotransmitters.

ANTI-ANXIETY AGENTS

Medications are only one therapeutic option for people afflicted with the various anxiety disorders. Other therapeutic options include the non-pharmacological treatment modalities of psychotherapy, exercise, and meditation. Although benzodiazepines are generally the first-line drug treatment for anxiety disorders, other classes of drugs are also effective. The efficacy of certain classes of medications in the treatment of certain anxiety disorders and their superiority over other drug classes has been documented. These various drug classes are listed in Table 15-1 according to the anxiety disorders they effectively treat.

Mechanism of Action and Drug Effects

Of the several drug classes shown to be effective in the treatment of anxiety disorders, all reduce anxiety by reducing overactivity in the central nervous system (CNS). There are, however, differences among the various drug classes.

Benzodiazepines seem to exert their **anxiolytic** effects by depressing activity in the areas of the brain called the *brainstem* and the *limbic system.* Benzodiazepines are believed to accomplish this by increasing the action of GABA, a neurotransmitter in the brain that inhibits nerve transmission in the CNS. Benzodiazepines have specific receptor proteins (also known as *specific receptor binding sites*) in the same areas of the brain that govern the release of GABA. The binding of benzodiazepines with these sites/receptors produces anxiolytic effects, as well as the effects of sedation and muscle relaxation.

There are a few other drug classes used for the treatment of anxiety disorders. Barbiturates and carbamates are probably the oldest such drug classes. Their anxiolytic properties are related to their ability to depress CNS activity and cause

TABLE 15-1					
VARIOUS ANXIETY DISORDERS: DRUGS OF CHOICE					
Disorder	**TCAs**	**Benzodiazepines**	**MAOIs**	**Buspirone**	**SSRIs**
Panic disorder	+++	++++	+++	0	++++
Generalized anxiety disorder	+	++++	?++	+++	
Obsessive–compulsive disorder	+++	?+	?+	0	++++
Post-traumatic stress disorder	+	?+	+	?+	
Simple phobia	0	+	0	0	
Social phobia	+	+	+	0	

TCA, Tricyclic and tetracyclic antidepressants; *MAOI,* monoamine oxidase inhibitor; *SSRI,* serotonin-selective reuptake inhibitor; 0, no efficacy or use; ?, has shown some efficacy but limited use; + limited use and efficacy; ++, some use and efficacy; +++, frequent use, good efficacy; ++++, most frequent use, best efficacy.

sedation. These agents have many undesirable side effects that make them poor drugs for the long-term treatment of anxiety. They are heavily sedating, they interact with many other drugs, and they interfere with normal sleep patterns (they suppress rapid eye movement [REM] sleep). Meprobamate was one of the more commonly prescribed carbamates used to relieve anxiety. However, its use, and that of the barbiturates, has largely been superseded in anxiety treatment by the newer benzodiazepine agents, which are markedly less hazardous in overdose situations.

Antihistamines have also been used as anxiolytics because of their ability to depress the CNS by sedating the client. The antihistamine most commonly used for the relief of anxiety is hydroxyzine. Its significant sedative effects are related to its antihistaminic properties. This can be advantageous for clients with co-occurring insomnia, often associated with both depression and antidepressant therapy. However, sedative effects of any medication can also be hazardous, and clients should be warned to use caution when driving or operating dangerous machinery. The salt form of hydroxyzine, hydroxyzine hydrochloride, is an effective anxiolytic. However, benzodiazepines, antidepressants, and buspirone (described later in this chapter) have emerged as the mainstays for treatment of ongoing anxiety disorders.

Miscellaneous anxiolytic agents are the third class of anxiolytics and include the single drug buspirone. It has the advantage of being both non-sedating and non–habit-forming. It is described in more detail later in this chapter.

Besides their anxiolytic effects just mentioned, anti-anxiety agents produce several other effects throughout the body, including sedative, hypnotic, appetite stimulating, analgesic, and anticonvulsant effects.

Indications

As stated earlier, both carbamates and barbiturates were used for many years to treat anxiety, but this is now unusual since the introduction of newer agents. Some antihistamines are used to treat anxiety because of their sedative side effects, but their primary pharmacological effect is to block the actions of histamine released during exacerbations of allergic conditions.

Benzodiazepines are the largest and most commonly prescribed anxiolytic drug class because they offer several advantages over the other drug classes used to treat anxiety. At therapeutic doses they have little effect on con-

sciousness, they are safe from the standpoint of their side effect profile, and they do not interact with many other drugs. Six commonly prescribed anxiolytic benzodiazepines are diazepam, lorazepam, alprazolam, clonazepam, chlordiazepoxide, and midazolam. In addition to treating anxiety these drugs are used for sedation, to produce muscle relaxation, to control seizures, to treat alcohol withdrawal, and as adjuvant drug therapy for depression. It should be noted that midazolam is available only in injectable form and is limited to use as a sedative and anaesthetic during invasive medical or surgical procedures. Used for *moderate sedation* (see Chapter 11), it reduces anxiety during painful medical procedures that do not require general anaesthesia; it also reduces the client's memory of the procedure. Midazolam is also used to provide sedation and to control acute anxiety and agitation in intensive care unit (ICU) clients when excessive movement might be harmful (e.g., spinal cord injury in a confused client or a client requiring mechanical ventilation). Benzodiazepines commonly used as sedative–hypnotics, as opposed to anxiolytics per se, are discussed with other CNS depressants and have slightly different therapeutic actions and pharmacokinetics from those of the benzodiazepines used to treat anxiety. Because of their wide range of effects, anxiolytic agents are sometimes used for certain other indications in addition to anxiety, such as seizure disorders, insomnia, agitation, and pain control. The commonly used anxiolytic benzodiazepines and their approved indications are listed in Table 15-2.

Contraindications

Contraindications to anxiolytic agents include known drug allergy, narrow-angle glaucoma, and pregnancy.

Side Effects and Adverse Effects

The most common undesirable effect of the anxiolytic drugs is an overexpression of their therapeutic effects. All of these classes of drugs decrease CNS activity, and many of the unwanted effects of these agents are related directly to this action. The most common side effects and adverse effects of benzodiazepines are listed in Table 15-3. It should also be noted that all benzodiazepines are potentially habit-forming and addictive. Although they can provide significant symptom relief, they should be used judiciously and at the lowest dosages and frequencies effective for symptom control.

ETHNOCULTURAL IMPLICATIONS

Diazepam and Chinese and Japanese Clients

The commonly used anti-anxiety agent diazepam undergoes different metabolic pathways in the Chinese and Japanese population. These two groups are found to be poor "mephenytoin pathway" metabolizers. Approximately 20 percent of these individuals metabolize mephenytoin poorly, resulting in rapid drug accumulation. To prevent possible toxicity, lower doses are generally required. Nurses may need to watch these individuals more closely for sedation, overdosage, and other adverse reactions to diazepam.

TABLE 15-2
BENZODIAZEPINES: APPROVED INDICATIONS

Approved Indications	Benzodiazepines
Alcohol withdrawal	chlordiazepoxide, diazepam, lorazepam, oxazepam
Anxiety	alprazolam, chlordiazepoxide, clorazepate, diazepam, lorazepam, oxazepam
Depression (adjunct)	alprazolam, oxazepam
Muscle spasm	diazepam
Preoperative sedation	chlordiazepoxide, diazepam, lorazepam
Seizure disorders	clorazepate, diazepam

TABLE 15-3

BENZODIAZEPINES: COMMON ADVERSE EFFECTS

Body System	Side/Adverse Effects
Central nervous	Drowsiness, sedation, loss of coordination, dizziness, blurred vision, headaches, paradoxical reactions (insomnia, increased excitability, hallucinations)
Gastrointestinal	Nausea, vomiting, constipation, dry mouth, abdominal cramping
Integumentary	Pruritis, skin rash

Toxicity and Management of Overdose

Overdose of antihistamines is usually not severe but may be associated with excessive sedation, hypotension, and seizures. There is no specific antidote, but in extreme cases a cholinergic drug (see Chapter 19) may be used to treat anticholinergic side effects associated with antihistamines.

When taken alone in normal doses in otherwise healthy clients, benzodiazepines are safe, effective anxiolytics. When taken with other sedating medications or with alcohol, life-threatening respiratory depression or arrest can occur. This serious consequence can also occur in clients whose metabolism or elimination capabilities are impaired because of liver or kidney dysfunction. In such cases, benzodiazepines can accumulate and not be eliminated. This further accentuates their therapeutic and toxic actions. An overdose of benzodiazepines may result in somnolence, confusion, coma, respiratory depression, or a combination of these symptoms. However, coma and respiratory depression are much less likely with benzodiazepines alone than with barbiturates or meprobamate.

The treatment for benzodiazepine intoxication is generally symptomatic and supportive. If ingestion is recent (within 4 hours), activated charcoal and a cathartic may be administered. Hemodialysis is usually not needed or useful in the treatment of benzodiazepine overdose but may be used in more extreme cases, especially those involving multiple types of drugs. A more likely treatment in such severe cases may also be the use of the benzodiazepine-specific antidote flumazenil. This drug is a benzodiazepine receptor blocker (antagonist) that is used to reverse the effects of benzodiazepine overdose. It opposes the actions of benzodiazepines by directly competing with benzodiazepines for binding at the benzodiazepine receptors in the CNS. It has a stronger affinity for these receptors and thus chemically forces the benzodiazepine drug molecules off the receptor, reversing their CNS depressant effects. Caution is recommended when using flumazenil in cases of multiple drug overdose because the associated toxic effects (cardiac arrhythmias and/or convulsions) of the other drugs, especially tricyclic antidepressants, may increase as the effects of the benzodiazepines subside. The treatment regimen for the reversal of benzodiazepine overdose is summarized in Box 15-1.

Interactions

A few notable drug interactions occur with anxiolytics, particularly benzodiazepines. As mentioned earlier, alcohol and CNS depressants, when co-administered with benzodiazepines, can result in additive CNS depression, and

BOX 15-1

Flumazenil Treatment Regimen for Benzodiazepine Overdose

Recommended Regimen
0.3 mg (3 mL) of flumazenil intravenously over 30 seconds by a physician with experience in anaesthesiology, followed by a series of 0.3 mg injections, each administered over a 30-second period, at 60-second intervals, for a total dose of 2 mg.

Duration of Action
Usually 1 hour. If reversing the effects of a long-acting benzodiazepine, may need to readminister flumazenil as it wears off and the effects (e.g., sedation) reappear.

even death. Cimetidine, **monoamine oxidase inhibitors (MAOIs),** and tobacco all can decrease the metabolism of benzodiazepines and result in increased CNS depression.

Dosages

For the recommended dosages of selected anti-anxiety agents, see the dosages table on p. 241. See Appendix B for some of the common brands available in Canada.

DRUG PROFILES

BENZODIAZEPINES

Benzodiazepines are contraindicated in clients who have shown a hypersensitivity reaction to them and in clients who have narrow-angle glaucoma. Benzodiazepines are all considered targeted substances under the Controlled Drugs and Substances Act.

▸▸ alprazolam

Alprazolam is most commonly used as an anxiolytic and as an adjunct for the treatment of depression. It is available only for oral (PO) administration as 0.25-, 0.5-, 1-, and 2-mg tablets. The 0.25-mg tablet is the dose recommended for the geriatric client. Pregnancy category D. The commonly recommended dosages are given in the table on p. 241.

PHARMACOKINETICS

Half-Life	Onset	Peak	Duration
11–16 hr	<1 hr	1–2 hr	6–12 hr

▸▸ chlordiazepoxide

Chlordiazepoxide is used for many indications but is most commonly used for the treatment of alcohol withdrawal, for the relief of anxiety, and as a preoperative sedative agent. Chlordiazepoxide alone is available for oral administration as 5-, 10-, and 25-mg capsules. A combination of chlordiazepoxide and clidinium, an anticholinergic drug, is available as an adjunctive treatment for peptic ulcer and irritable bowel syndrome when associated with excessive anxiety and tension. Pregnancy category D. The commonly recommended dosages are given in the table on p. 241.

PHARMACOKINETICS

Half-Life	Onset	Peak	Duration
9–34 hr	30–60 min	0.5–4 hr	12–24 hr

DOSAGES   Selected Anti-anxiety Agents

Agent	Pharmacological Class	Usual Dosage Range	Indications
▸▸ alprazolam	Benzodiazepine	**Adult** PO: 0.25–0.5 mg tid **Geriatric** PO: 0.25 mg bid–tid	Anxiolytic Anxiolytic
buspirone HCL	Miscellaneous	**Adult only** PO: 15–45 mg/day in 2–3 divided doses	Anxiolytic
▸▸ chlordiazepoxide HCL	Benzodiazepine	**Pediatric** PO: >6 yr, 5 mg bid–qid **Adult** PO: 5–25 mg tid–qid IM/IV: 50–100 mg, then 25 mg tid–qid for severe anxiety IM/IV: 50–100 mg q2–4h for alcoholism IM: 50–100 mg before surgery **Pediatric** PO: >6 mo: 1.25 mg tid–qid **Adult** PO: 2–10 mg bid–qid **Geriatric** PO: 2–2.5 mg once to twice daily **Pediatric** IM/IV: >30 days, 1–2 mg repeated in 3–4 hr prn IM/IV: ≥5 yr: 5–10 mg repeated in 3–4 hr prn IM/IV: >30 days: 0.2–0.5 mg q2–5 min to a max of 5 mg **Adult** IM/IV: 2–10 mg repeated in 3–4 hr prn IM/IV: 10 mg followed by 5–10 mg in 3–4 hr prn IV: 5–10 mg within 5–20 min before procedure IM: 10 mg before surgery PO/IM/IV: 5–10 mg repeated in 3–4 hr prn IM/IV: 5–10 mg repeated at 10– to 15-min intervals to a max of 30 mg, repeat in 3–4 hr prn	Anxiolytic Anxiolytic Anxiolytic, pre-op sedation Anxiety, alcoholism, muscle spasm, convulsive disorders Tetanus Tetanus Status epilepticus Anxiety Alcoholism Cardioversion Pre-op sedation Muscle spasm Status epilepticus
hydroxyzine HCL	Antihistamine	**Pediatric** PO: 30–50 mg/day divided ≥6 yr: PO: 50–100 mg/day divided ≥6 yr: PO: 0.6 mg/kg ≥6 yr: IM: 1.1 mg/kg **Adult** PO: 50–100 mg qid IM: 50–100 mg q4–6h PO: 25 mg tid–qid PO: 50–100 mg IM: 25–100 mg	Anxiolytic/pruritus Pre- and post-op sedation Nausea/vomiting Anxiolytic Anxiolytic Pruritus Pre- and post-partum sedation Nausea/vomiting
▸▸ lorazepam	Benzodiazepine	**Adult** PO: 2–6 mg/day divided PO: 0.5–1 mg at bedtime IM: 0.05 mg/kg to a max of 4 mg IV: 2–4 mg	Anxiolytic Pre-op sedation Pre-op sedation

▸▸ diazepam

Diazepam is one of the most commonly prescribed benzodiazepines. It is indicated for the relief of anxiety, alcohol withdrawal, and seizure disorders (e.g., status epilepticus); for sedation; and as an adjunct for the relief of skeletal muscle spasms. Diazepam has active metabolites that can accumulate in clients who have hepatic dysfunction because it is metabolized primarily in the liver. This can result in additive, cumulative effects that may be manifested as prolonged sedation, respiratory depression, or coma. It is available in oral form as 2-, 5-, and 10-mg tablets and as a 1-mg/mL solution; as a rectal gel (Diastat) in 5-mg/mL amounts; and in intravenous form (Diazemuls) as a 5-mg/mL injection. Pregnancy category D.

PHARMACOKINETICS

Half-Life	Onset	Peak	Duration
20–80 hr	30–60 min	1–2 hr	12–24 hr

▶▶ *lorazepam*

Lorazepam is a widely used benzodiazepine. It is currently approved for use in the management of anxiety disorders, for the short-term relief of acute anxiety, and as a preoperative medication to provide sedation and light anaesthesia and to diminish client recall (amnesia). It has also shown efficacy in the prevention and treatment of chemotherapy-related nausea and vomiting and the symptoms of acute alcohol withdrawal. It is available in oral form as 0.5-, 1-, and 2-mg tablets and as a 4-mg/mL intravenous injection. It may also be administered sublingually (SL) and is available as 0.5-, 1-, and 2-mg tablets. When administered in this fashion, its onset of action is similar to that associated with intravenous administration but without the inconveniences. Pregnancy category D. The commonly recommended dosages are given in the table on p. 241.

PHARMACOKINETICS

Half-Life	Onset	Peak	Duration
IV: 12–16 hr	IV: Rapid	IV: 15–20 min	IV: 4 hr
PO: 12–16 hr	PO: 15–45 min	PO: 2 hr	PO: 12–24 hr

MISCELLANEOUS AGENTS

Several categories of drugs can be used in the treatment of anxiety disorders. Although benzodiazepines are by far the most widely prescribed anxiolytics, often drugs in other categories may be prescribed because of certain advantages they offer. Some of the more commonly used drugs are described in this section. Carbamates, with meprobamate the prototype, have been shown to be effective in treating anxiety disorders. The antihistamine hydroxyzine and the non-benzodiazepine anxiolytic buspirone are also effective anti-anxiety agents.

hydroxyzine HCL

Hydroxyzine is available in hydrochloride salt form (hydroxyzine HCL) and is used to treat anxiety disorders. Hydroxyzine HCL is an antihistamine that suppresses activity in the CNS, which makes it useful as both an anxiolytic and anti-emetic agent. It is available in oral form as a 2- and 10-mg/5 mL solution and in 10-, 25-, and 50-mg capsules. It is also available as 50-mg/mL intramuscular (IM) injections. Pregnancy category C. The commonly recommended dosages are given in the table on p. 241.

PHARMACOKINETICS

Half-Life	Onset	Peak	Duration
3–7 hr	15–30 min	15–30 min	4–6 hr

buspirone HCL

Buspirone HCL is an anxiolytic agent that is distinctly different both chemically and pharmacologically from the benzodiazepines. Its precise mechanism of action is unknown, but it appears to have agonist activity at a subset of both serotonin and dopamine receptors. It is indicated for treatment of anxiety and is always taken on a scheduled (not prn) basis. Its only reported contraindication is drug allergy. The advantages of buspirone HCL over benzodiazepines include its lack of

sedative properties and dependency potential. It does not prevent or treat benzodiazepine withdrawal symptoms, so although it may be used concurrently with benzodiazepines, they still need to be withdrawn gradually if they are to be discontinued. An additional advantage of buspirone HCL is that it does not require dose adjustment for geriatric clients because age has not been shown to affect the pharmacokinetics of the drug in the body. However, the drug is not currently approved for pediatric use. Potential drug interactions include a risk of serotonin syndrome (see the Antidepressants section later in this chapter) when buspirone HCL is used concurrently with any antidepressant with serotonergic activity, such as serotonin-selective reuptake inhibitors (SSRIs), tricyclic antidepressants (TCAs), trazodone, and venlafaxine. Clients receiving both types of medications together should be monitored carefully. It is recommended that MAOIs not be used concurrently with buspirone because of a risk of hypertension. A washout period of at least 14 days after discontinuation of MAOI therapy should occur before starting buspirone. Buspirone HCL is available only in tablet form in 5- and 10-mg strengths. Pregnancy category B. The recommended dosage is given in the table on p. 241.

PHARMACOKINETICS

Half-Life	Onset	Peak	Duration
2–3 hr	Up to 2–3 wk	40–60 min	Unknown

DRUGS USED TO TREAT AFFECTIVE DISORDERS

Several classes of drugs are used in the treatment of affective disorders. The two main drug categories are antimanic agents and antidepressant agents.

ANTIMANIC AGENTS

Clinical evidence indicates that the catecholamines (dopamine and norepinephrine) play an important pathophysiological role in the development of mania. Serotonin also appears to be involved. Lithium salts, the first drug found to effectively alleviate the major symptoms of mania, is still widely used. Lithium also continues to be shown effective in maintenance treatment of BPD. One theory on its effectiveness is that it potentiates serotonergic neurotransmission. A variety of medications may be used in conjunction with lithium to regulate mood or stabilize manic clients. Some of these adjunctive medications are benzodiazepines, carbamazepine, clozapine, dopamine receptor agonists, L-tryptophan, and calcium channel blockers (CCBs). More recently approved medications for acute manic episodes include the anticonvulsant valproic acid (see Chapter 13) and the antipsychotic agent olanzapine (see the Atypical Antipsychotics section later in this chapter).

Antidepressants are often needed as well to control the depressive side of bipolar disorder. A pharmacological challenge is to choose antidepressants that are less likely to evoke manic responses secondary to the expected stimulating effects of the antidepressant medication. Several of the newer third-generation anticonvulsants (see Chapter 13) are also currently under investigation for possible roles in treating BPD. These include lamotrigine and gabapentin. Preliminary studies demonstrate varying degrees of efficacy in treating both acute and long-term depressive and rapid-cycling bipolar symptoms, but not mania. The anticonvulsant topiramate has shown encouraging results in both depressed and manic clients. Further studies are underway to better establish these preliminary findings. Other recent studies have shown the antipsychotic agent risperidone to be effective for acute mania, but more data are needed to firmly establish this finding.

DRUG PROFILES

▶▶ *lithium*

The antimanic effect of lithium is not fully understood. Results of studies indicate that lithium ions alter sodium ion transport in nerve cells, resulting in a shift in catecholamine metabolism. The therapeutic levels of lithium that are required are close to the toxic levels, but there is increasingly greater tolerance to these toxic levels during acute manic phases. For the management of acute mania, a lithium serum level of 0.8 to 1.2 mmol/L is usually required. Desirable long-term maintenance levels range between 0.6 and 0.8 mmol/L. A level of 0.4 to 0.6 mmol/L is desirable for maintenance in the elderly.

Lithium carbonate and lithium citrate are the two currently available salts of lithium. There are no absolute contraindications to lithium therapy, and the side effects and adverse effects are dependent on the serum levels. Levels exceeding 1.5 to 2.0 mmol/L may produce mild to moderate toxicity, while levels exceeding 2.0 to 2.5 mmol/L produce moderate to severe toxicity. The most serious adverse effect is cardiac dysrhythmia. Other effects include drowsiness, slurred speech, epileptic-type seizures, choreoathetotic movements (involuntary wavelike movements of extremities), and hypotension. Long-term treatment may cause hypothyroidism.

The concurrent use of thiazides, angiotensin converting enzyme (ACE) inhibitors, and CCBs can increase lithium toxicity. Lithium is available as 150-, 300-, and 600-mg capsules; a 300-mg tablet; 300- and 450-mg sustained-release tablets; and a 300-mg/5 mL syrup. Pregnancy category D. Lithium's recommended dosage is 450–1200 mg/day in adults and 15–20 mg/kg/day to a maximum of 60 mg/kg/day in children.

PHARMACOKINETICS

Half-Life	Onset	Peak	Duration
18–24 hr	7–14 days*	0.5–2 hr	2–24 hr

*Therapeutic benefit for controlling mania.

ANTIDEPRESSANT AGENTS

Antidepressants are the pharmacological treatment of choice for major depressive disorders (see Research box below). Not only are they effective in treating depression,

they are also useful for treating other disorders, such as dysthymia, schizophrenia (as an adjunct), eating disorders, and personality disorders. Some of these agents are also commonly used in the treatment of various medical conditions, including migraine headaches, chronic pain syndromes, and sleep disorders.

Many of the drugs currently used to treat affective disorders increase the levels of monoamine neurotransmitter concentrations in the CNS. Monoamine neurotransmitters include serotonin (also known as 5-hydroxytryptamine, or 5-HT), dopamine, and norepinephrine. This treatment is based on the belief that alterations in the levels of these types of neurotransmitters in the CNS are responsible for causing depression. One of the most widely held hypotheses advanced to explain depression in these terms is the **biogenic amine hypothesis (BAH).** Specifically, it postulates that depression results from a deficiency of neuronal and synaptic catecholamines (primarily norepinephrine) and mania from an excess of amines at the adrenergic receptor sites in the brain. This hypothesis is illustrated in Fig. 15-1.

RESEARCH

Detecting Depression Among Primary Care Clients

Approximately 3 million Canadians over the age of 18 years have been found to suffer from major depression. In fact, suicide (closely linked to depression) is the second leading cause of death in 10- to 24-year-olds. If untreated, depression can worsen, have a negative impact on one's physical and emotional well-being, and lead to years of suffering and possible suicide. Mental health issues and the use of psychotropic drugs require efficient diagnosing, and with early diagnosis there comes more promise for effective treatment of various mental health illnesses, whether anxiety, mood disorders, depression, bipolar disorders, or schizophrenia. The Mood Disorders Society of Canada as well as the Centre for Addiction and Mental Health (CAMH) publishes information about mental health issues and the need for detecting, in particular, depression. Recently, the Canadian Task Force on Preventive Health Care revised their 1994 position to screen adults for depression and found sufficient evidence to encourage primary care clinicians to formally screen adult clients for depression. This makes the process of identifying depression much easier. This Task Force also called for systems to achieve more accurate diagnoses, effective treatment and management, and adequate follow-up care. Many screening tools are available for depression but there is little evidence that one is more effective than another. Healthcare providers usually choose tools most appropriate for their clients in their healthcare setting. The depression recommendations by the Task Force are available online. In addition, fact sheets and related materials are available from CAMH (http://www.camh.net/) and the Mood Disorders Society of Canada (http://www.mooddisorderscanada.ca/).

From *Screening for depression in primary care: Updated recommendations from the Canadian Task Force on Preventive Health Care.* Retrieved July 31, 2005, from http://www.ctfphc.org/Full_Text/CTF_Depression_TR_2004_final.pdf

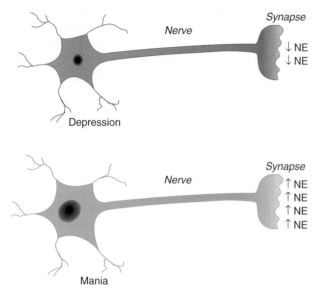

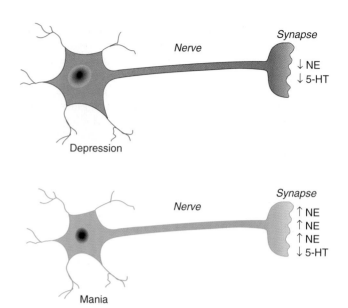

FIG. 15-1 Biogenic amine hypothesis. *NE*, Norepinephrine.

FIG. 15-2 Permissive hypothesis. *NE*, Norepinephrine; *5-HT*, serotonin.

Another explanation, the **permissive hypothesis**, implicates reduced concentrations of serotonin as the predisposing factor for affective disorders. Depression results from decreases in both the serotonin and catecholamine levels, whereas mania results from increased catecholamine but decreased serotonin levels. The permissive hypothesis is illustrated in Fig. 15-2.

A new leading theory, the **dysregulation hypothesis**, is essentially a reformulation of the BAH. It views depression and affective disorders not simply in terms of decreased or increased catecholamine activity but as a failure of the regulation of these systems.

Recent research data indicate that early and aggressive antidepressant treatment increases the chances for full remission. The first 6 to 8 weeks of therapy constitute the acute phase. The primary goals during this time are to obtain a response to drug therapy and improve the client's symptoms. It is currently recommended that antidepressant drug therapy be maintained at the effective dose for an additional 8 to 14 months after remission of depressive symptoms. In choosing an antidepressant for a given client, the client's previous psychotropic drug response history (if any) should be considered. Information regarding any family history of depression with known drug responses may also be helpful. Therapeutic response is measured primarily by subjective client feedback. In addition, a few measurement tools attempt to quantify response to drug therapy, such as the Hamilton Depression Rating Scale (HAM-D) and the Symptom Checklist-90 (SCL-90) anxiety factor score. A therapeutic non-response to antidepressant drug therapy is defined as failure to respond to adequate doses of at least 6 weeks of therapy. Twenty to thirty percent of clients who do not respond to the usual dose of a given antidepressant agent will respond to higher doses. Therefore dose optimization, involving careful upward titration of medication dose for several weeks, is recommended before conclud-

ing that a given drug is ineffective for a particular client. Research indicates that 40 to 60 percent of clients who do not respond to the first drug class attempted will respond to the second drug class attempted.

Non-response to at least two trials, including at least two different classes of antidepressants, is classified as treatment-resistant depression (TRD). Such cases can be treated by switching to a different drug from the same or a different class or augmenting the initial drug therapy by adding a second drug. There is currently limited controlled research data regarding drug combination augmentation strategies, but more research is anticipated on this topic. In the meantime clinicians choosing drug combinations rely on trial and error, clinical experience, and considerations of specific client factors (e.g., co-occurring anxiety). Antipsychotic drugs (discussed in detail later in this chapter) may also be used concurrently with antidepressants in treating some cases of TRD. This practice is currently well established for cases of MDD that also involve psychotic symptoms. Two issues currently under research include the use of antipsychotic drugs as **monotherapy** for psychotic forms of MDD, and the potential use of antipsychotic drugs as **adjunct therapy** for non-psychotic TRD. The most severe cases of TRD may warrant a treatment attempt with electroconvulsive therapy (ECT). Current ECT techniques are greatly refined from similar treatments in past decades and are usually carried out in a post-anaesthesia care unit (PACU) or recovery room setting under general anaesthesia. Seizure activity is induced in the anaesthetized client via externally applied electric shocks to the brain.

Treatment failure in cases of depression may be due to a misdiagnosis or failure to treat co-occurring mental illness (e.g., anxiety disorder, substance abuse) and/or co-occurring non-psychiatric illness (e.g., hypothyroidism). It may also be due to nonadherence to drug therapy, which is the cause in an estimated 20 percent of TRD cases. Careful choice of drug therapy to minimize side effects may improve adherence with treatment and therapeutic outcome. Another reason for treatment failure may be the discouragement associated with depression itself. This alone may cause clients to give up prematurely on their drug therapy, especially because antidepressants often take several weeks to reach their full effect. Effective psychotherapy and support groups can help encourage clients to be consistent with prescribed psychotropic drug therapy.

The drug categories most commonly used in the treatment of affective disorders are the **serotonin-selective reuptake inhibitors (SSRIs)** and the second- and third-generation antidepressants. Less commonly used are the classes informally known as "first-generation" antidepressants. These include the TCAs and MAOIs.

SEROTONIN-SELECTIVE REUPTAKE INHIBITORS AND SECOND- AND THIRD-GENERATION ANTIDEPRESSANTS

These three drug classes can be described together as newer-generation antidepressants (NGAs) and are generally considered superior to TCAs and MAOIs in terms of their side effect profiles. Because of this, they largely replaced TCAs and MAOIs as first-line drug therapy for depression in the 1980s following the introduction of the first SSRI, fluoxetine. The SSRIs include fluoxetine, paroxetine, sertraline, fluvoxamine maleate, citalopram HBr, and escitalopram. Second-generation antidepressants include trazodone and bupropion. Third-generation antidepressants include venlafaxine and mirtazapine. Mirtazapine, a third-generation agent, along with the much less commonly used second-generation agent maprotiline, are also known as *tetracyclic drugs* because of the four connected rings that form the basis of their chemical structure; thus the tetracyclic agents actually span more than one "generation" of antidepressants. In contrast, the TCAs are all solely first-generation drugs. For this reason, the terms *second-* and *third-generation* are more precise and less ambiguous when speaking of the tetracyclic antidepressants. Because maprotiline is rarely used, only mirtazapine is discussed in detail in this chapter.

These newer antidepressants offer several attractive advantages over the traditional TCAs and MAOIs. They are associated with significantly fewer and less severe systemic side effects and adverse effects, especially those to which older adults have little tolerance—anticholinergic and cardiovascular side effects. They are considered safe in adults over the age of 18 years and have few drug–drug or drug–food interactions. However, as with the TCAs and MAOIs, they typically take 4 to 6 weeks to reach maximum clinical effectiveness. In 2004, Health Canada issued a strong warning about SSRIs and other newer antidepressants suggesting that use of these drugs in clients under the age of 18 years may be associated with behavioural and emotional changes, including an increased risk of suicidal ideation and behaviour. It appears these antidepressants, not indicated for use

in children and adolescents, are being prescribed "off-label." However, there is still controversy over whether clear scientific data supports the hypothesis. In 2005, Health Canada issued a warning that the use of paroxetine in the first trimester of pregnancy may have a small increased risk of birth defects compared with other antidepressants.

SSRIs were developed to slow or inhibit the reuptake of serotonin into presynaptic terminals (nerve endings) and thus to increase the levels of serotonin for neurotransmission at the post-synaptic nerve endings. Sertraline is the most selective of the three agents in inhibiting serotonin as opposed to norepinephrine reuptake, and fluoxetine is the least selective. Fluoxetine is the only one that has an active metabolite. Fluoxetine, along with its active metabolite, has an elimination half-life of 2 to 4 days as opposed to a 1-day half-life for sertraline and paroxetine. A newer agent under development in its own unique category is reboxetine. It is a norepinephrine-selective reuptake inhibitor (NSRI). At the time of this writing reboxetine is still being researched for its antidepressant qualities and is only available through Special Access Programme conditions in Canada for clients with refractory depressive disorders.

Mechanism of Action and Drug Effects

The inhibition of serotonin reuptake seems to be the primary clinically significant mechanism of action for the SSRIs, though they may also have weak effects on norepinephrine and dopamine reuptake. Second- and third-generation agents are less selective and have activity at brain serotonin as well as norepinephrine and/or dopamine receptors. They are also referred to as *multimodal* or *multireceptor agents* and have greater receptor specificity than first-generation drugs and a generally improved side effect profile. The second- and third-generation agents have chemical structures different from the SSRIs, and there is significant overlap between the pharmacological activities of these two generations of medications. Trazodone is primarily a serotonin-reuptake inhibitor but also has a smaller inhibitory effect on norepinephrine reuptake. Mirtazapine has both noradrenergic (norepinephrine) and serotonergic (serotonin) effects but works by promoting presynaptic release of these two neurotransmitters and does not inhibit either their pre- or post-synaptic reuptake. The antidepressant activities of bupropion and venlafaxine are believed to affect all three major neurotransmitters: serotonin, norepinephrine, and—to a lesser degree—dopamine. The latest research is starting to suggest that these newer-generation multireceptor agents may offer significant improvement outcomes in depression treatment over even the highly acclaimed SSRI agents. Larger clinical studies are anticipated with these newer drugs, either alone or in combination with SSRI therapy.

The increase in serotonin, norepinephrine, or dopamine reuptake causes increased concentrations of these various neurotransmitters at nerve endings in the CNS, resulting in numerous functional changes associated with enhanced amine neurotransmission. This increased neurotransmitter concentration in the CNS also seems to lead to a decrease in REM sleep. In addition, it has a potentiating effect when given with opioid analgesics in that the increased serotonin concentration at nerve endings appears to work synergistically with the opioid analgesic in relieving pain.

A primary advantage of SSRIs over TCAs and MAOIs, as well as the second- and third-generation antidepressants, is that SSRIs have little or no effect on the cardiovascular system, apparently because they have no substantial anticholinergic activity, alpha$_1$-adrenergic blocking activity, catecholamine-potentiating effects, or quinidine-like cardiotoxic effects. They also seem to have little if any effect on the cardiac conduction system. Although all NGAs are associated with varying degrees of weight gain or loss, SSRIs are more commonly associated with anorectic activity and weight loss. This appetite-inhibiting action may result from the blocking of serotonin reuptake and the attendant increase in the serotonin concentration at the nerve endings. For this reason, SSRIs are sometimes used to treat eating disorders, such as bulimia nervosa, that involve compulsive overeating.

Indications

All three classes of NGAs have been used to treat many affective disorders. Depression, BPD, obesity, eating disorders, OCD, panic attacks or disorders, social anxiety disorder, PTSD, premenstrual dysphoric disorder, and the neurological disorder myoclonus are only some of the many disorders that this highly effective drug class can be used to treat. This list is expanding with continued research. These newer antidepressant classes have also shown some beneficial effects in the treatment of various substance abuse problems such as alcohol dependence.

Contraindications

Contraindications to NGA use include known drug allergy, use sooner than 14 days after stopping MAOI therapy, and therapy with certain antipsychotic drugs such as thioridazine or mesoridazine. Bupropion is also contraindicated in cases of eating disorder and also seizure disorder because it can lower the seizure threshold.

Side Effects and Adverse Effects

NGAs generally are much safer than TCAs and MAOIs and have fewer side effects and adverse effects. However, some side effects can be bothersome enough to cause clients to discontinue their antidepressant drug therapy. Up to two-thirds of all depressed clients may discontinue therapy because of drug side effects. Some of the most common and bothersome side effects include insomnia, weight gain, and sexual dysfunction. Bupropion and mirtazapine are associated with a reduced incidence of sexual side effects. One potentially hazardous adverse effect of any drug or combination of drugs that have serotonergic activity is known as *serotonin syndrome*. It usually includes involuntary muscle twitches, **akathisia**, tremor, and, in the most severe cases, seizures and coma. Fortunately it is usually self-limiting on discontinuation of the drugs. The various side effects and adverse effects that can occur in clients taking second-generation antidepressants are listed in Table 15-4.

Interactions

NGAs are highly bound to plasma proteins such as albumin. When given with other drugs that are also highly bound to protein (warfarin and phenytoin), both compete for binding sites on the surface of albumin. This results in more free, unbound drug and therefore a greater, more pronounced drug effect.

NGAs also may inhibit cytochrome P-450, an enzyme in the liver that is responsible for the metabolism of

TABLE 15-4

NEWER GENERATION ANTIDEPRESSANTS: ADVERSE EFFECTS

Body System	Side/Adverse Effect
Central nervous	Headache, dizziness, tremor, nervousness, insomnia, fatigue
Gastrointestinal	Nausea, diarrhea, constipation, dry mouth, weight loss/gain
Other	Sweating, sexual dysfunction

TABLE 15-5

NEWER GENERATION ANTIDEPRESSANTS: DRUG INTERACTIONS

Drug	Mechanism	Result
carbamazepine	Decreases carbamazepine metabolism	Increased carbamazepine levels, carbamazepine toxicity, ocular changes, vertigo, tremor
MAOIs	Enhances serotonin activity	Hyperthermia, diaphoresis, shivering, tremor, seizures, ataxia, autonomic instability
TCAs	Increases TCA toxicity	Sedation, decreased energy, lightheadedness, dry mouth, constipation, elevated TCA levels
warfarin	Warfarin displaced from protein binding sites	Increased warfarin effects

several drugs. This finding is controversial, however; many studies have shown minimal or no inhibition. Inhibition of cytochrome P-450 results in higher levels of drugs because they accumulate rather than break down to their inactive metabolites. This also prolongs the action of drugs metabolized by the cytochrome P-450 system. The SSRIs fluoxetine and paroxetine seem to be more potent inhibitors of this enzyme system than sertraline. The most common and significant drug interactions are listed in Table 15-5.

To prevent the potentially fatal pharmacodynamic interactions that can occur between NGAs and MAOIs, a 2- to 5-week washout period is recommended between uses of the two classes of medications. NGAs that have a longer half-life, such as fluoxetine, require the longer washout period.

Dosages

For dosage information for selected NGAs, see the dosages table below. See Appendix B for some of the common brands available in Canada.

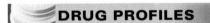

DRUG PROFILES

The 1980s and 1990s were decades of much development in psychotropic pharmacotherapy. Several new classes of antidepressants alone were introduced during this period. TCAs and MAOIs may be thought of as first-generation antidepressants. Two drugs introduced in the 1980s, now classified as second-generation antidepressants, are trazodone and bupropion. Both are still commonly used. There are six currently available

SSRIs, five introduced during the 1980s and 1990s and one more recently in 2004. In chronological order they are fluoxetine, sertraline, paroxetine, fluvoxamine, citalopram, and escitalopram. The 1990s saw the introduction of another major class of antidepressants: the third-generation antidepressants. These are venlafaxine and mirtazapine. Both of these newer drugs have proved to be valuable additions to the antidepressant armamentarium. They are highly effective as antidepressants and are associated with few serious side effects and adverse effects, especially when compared with first-generation antidepressants. They are now considered first-line agents in the treatment of depression, especially for clients with concurrent symptoms of anxiety, clients with depression with suicidal ideations, and clients unable to tolerate adverse reactions to other agents. One notable hazard of the first-generation agents, especially the TCAs, is their tendency to cause fatal cardiac dysrhythmias following overdose. Because depressed clients are generally at greater risk for suicide attempt, the newer generations of antidepressant agents usually provide a safer drug choice.

trazodone

Trazodone was the first of the second-generation antidepressants that could selectively inhibit serotonin reuptake but that negligibly affected norepinephrine reuptake. Thus, unlike the TCAs, it has minimal adverse effect on the cardiovascular system. It is, however, sedating. This can be severe and can impair cognitive function in older adults. However, the sedating effect of trazodone is often advantageous in promoting effective sleep for depressed clients, who commonly have co-occurring anxiety and/or insomnia. Trazodone has rarely

DOSAGES | Selected NGAs

Agent	Pharmacological Class	Usual Dosage Range*	Indications
trazodone	Second generation	PO: 150–600 mg/day, with larger doses divided	Depression
▸▸ bupropion	Second generation	PO: 100–300 mg/day, divided	Depression, smoking cessation
▸▸ fluoxetine	SSRI	PO: 20–80 mg/day, once or twice a day	Depression, OCD, bulimia nervosa
sertraline	SSRI	PO: 25–200 mg, taken daily	Depression, OCD, panic disorder
paroxetine	SSRI	PO: 10–50 mg/day, taken daily	Depression, OCD, panic disorder, social anxiety disorder, GAD, PTSD
venlafaxine	Third generation	PO: 75–375 mg/day, taken daily	Depression; GAD
fluvoxamine	SSRI	50–300 mg/day, with larger doses divided bid	Depression, OCD
▸▸ mirtazapine	Third generation	15–45 mg/day at bedtime	Depression
▸▸ citalopram	SSRI	20–40 mg/day taken daily—qam or qpm	Depression
escitalopram	SSRI	10–20 mg/day	Depression, GAD

*All dosages reflect usual adult dosage ranges. Pediatric doses may be more variable and should be specified by a pediatric practitioner.
OCD, obsessive–compulsive disorder; *GAD*, generalized anxiety disorder; *PTSD*, post-traumatic stress disorder.

been associated with transient non-sexual priapism. This is reportedly the result of alpha-adrenergic blockade. When trazodone is combined with certain drugs (ketoconazole [an antifungal agent], ritonavir and indinavir [protease inhibitors used in the treatment of HIV], or carbamazepine [an anti-epileptic therapy]) clients may experience nausea, low blood pressure, temporary loss of consciousness (increased trazodone levels), or decreased trazodone levels.

Trazodone's use is contraindicated in clients who have shown a hypersensitivity reaction to it. It is available only in oral form as 50-, 68.25-, 100-, and 150-mg tablets. Pregnancy category C. The commonly recommended dosages are given in the table on p. 247.

PHARMACOKINETICS

Half-Life	Onset	Peak	Duration
6–9 hr	1–2 wk*	2–4 wk*	Weeks*

*Therapeutic effects.

▶▶ bupropion

Bupropion, a second-generation antidepressant, is a unique antidepressant in terms of both its structure and mechanism of action. It has no appreciable effect either on the uptake of serotonin or norepinephrine or on the activity of MAO. It does, however, have a modest effect on the blockade of dopamine reuptake. A new sustained-release form of bupropion, Zyban, has recently been approved as first-line therapy in smoking cessation treatment. Zyban is the first nicotine-free prescription medicine to treat nicotine dependence.

Bupropion is contraindicated in clients who have shown a hypersensitivity reaction to it, those with a seizure disorder (bupropion can lower the seizure threshold) or who currently or in the past have suffered from anorexia nervosa or bulimia, and those currently on MAOI treatment. It is available as 100- and 150-mg sustained-release tablets. Pregnancy category B. The commonly recommended dosages are given in the table on p. 247.

PHARMACOKINETICS

Half-Life	Onset	Peak	Duration
1–14 hr	Up to 4 wk*	3 hr	Weeks to months

*Therapeutic effects.

▶▶ fluoxetine

Fluoxetine was the first SSRI marketed for the treatment of depression in 1988. It is contraindicated in clients who have shown a hypersensitivity reaction to it and in those taking MAOIs.

Fluoxetine is available in oral form as 10-, 20-, and 40-mg capsules and a 20-mg/5 mL solution. Pregnancy category B. The commonly recommended dosages are given in the table on p. 247.

PHARMACOKINETICS

Half-Life	Onset	Peak	Duration
1–3 days	1–4 wk*	6–8 hr	2–4 wk

*Therapeutic effects.

sertraline

Sertraline, another SSRI, is the most selective of the three discussed here in inhibiting serotonin reuptake and has little effect on the inhibition of the cytochrome P-450 enzyme system in the liver. This allows it to be used in renally impaired clients. Sertraline is often used successfully to treat depression in even frail geriatric clients with or without renal compromise. It has no metabolites with clinically significant activity. It is contraindicated in clients who have shown a hypersensitivity to it and those taking MAOIs or pimozide. Sertraline is available in oral form as 25-, 50-, and 100-mg capsules. Pregnancy category B. The commonly recommended dosages are given in the table on p. 247.

PHARMACOKINETICS

Half-Life	Onset	Peak	Duration
24 hr	1–8 wk*	6–8 hr	Unknown

*Therapeutic effects.

paroxetine

Paroxetine, another SSRI, is contraindicated in clients who have shown a hypersensitivity reaction to it and those taking MAOIs. Paroxetine is available in oral form as 10-, 20-, and 40-mg tablets and 12.5- and 25-mg sustained-release tablets. Pregnancy category B. The commonly recommended dosages are given in the table on p. 247.

PHARMACOKINETICS

Half-Life	Onset	Peak	Duration
14 hr	1–4 wk*	5–8 hr	Unknown

*Therapeutic effects.

fluvoxamine

Fluvoxamine, an SSRI, can have antidepressant activity like the other SSRIs, but it also has potent anti-obsessional activity. For this reason it is more commonly used to treat OCD, one of the anxiety disorders mentioned earlier, rather than depression. However, because clients with all types of anxiety disorders often have co-occurring depressive symptoms, OCD clients may also benefit from the antidepressant effects of the drug. Fluvoxamine does inhibit certain of the cytochrome P-450 enzyme systems in the liver and thus has the potential for interactions with many other classes of drugs. In particular, any medications with serotonergic effects (e.g., other SSRIs, buspirone, meperidine) may interact with fluvoxamine to cause serotonin syndrome. Such combinations should either be avoided or the client monitored carefully with concurrent use. Fluvoxamine is contraindicated in cases of drug allergy and in clients taking MAOIs. Fluvoxamine is available only in oral form as 50- and 100-mg tablets. Pregnancy category C. Dosage information is provided in the table on p. 247.

PHARMACOKINETICS

Half-Life	Onset	Peak	Duration
13–15 hr	1–4 wk*	3–8 hr	Unknown

*Therapeutic effects.

▸▸ *citalopram*

Citalopram is one of the newest of the SSRIs currently indicated for treatment of depression only. However, research is underway to evaluate its effectiveness for nicotine and alcohol addiction, senile dementia, OCD, and even kidney failure associated with diabetes. This drug has significant effects on various cytochrome P-450 enzyme systems, increasing the likelihood of interactions with other drugs that are metabolized by these systems. Citalopram is contraindicated in cases of drug allergy and is not recommended in clients who have had difficulty tolerating other SSRI agents. It is also contraindicated with concurrent MAOI use; a 14-day washout period is recommended when discontinuing either drug before starting the other. Citalopram is available in oral form as tablets of 20 and 40 mg. Citalopram is being replaced in practice by a newer agent, escitalopram, which is simply one (of two) chemical enantiomers of citalopram and can have similar efficacy with lower dosages. Pregnancy category C. Dosage information is provided in the table on p. 247.

PHARMACOKINETICS

Half-Life	Onset	Peak	Duration
24–48 hr	1–4 wk*	1–6 hr	Unknown

*Therapeutic effects.

venlafaxine

Venlafaxine, a third-generation antidepressant, is unique in that it is chemically unrelated to all other available antidepressants and that it has a trimodal mechanism of action on the activity of three major brain neurotransmitters. Specifically, it has potent inhibitory effects on both serotonin and norepinephrine reuptake and weaker, though still significant, inhibitory effects on dopamine reuptake. Given this multi-neurotransmitter activity, it is not surprising that venlafaxine, along with many other newer antidepressants, is often associated with activating side effects such as nervousness and insomnia. However, clients often report rapid improvement in depressive symptoms. Venlafaxine does have significant metabolic effects on various cytochrome P-450 enzyme systems and is contraindicated in cases of drug allergy and in combination with MAOIs. Concurrent use with other serotonergic drugs carries the risk of serotonin syndrome and is generally not recommended. Venlafaxine is available in oral form in immediate and extended-release (XR) capsules in 37.5, 75, and 150 mg strengths. Pregnancy category C. The commonly recommended dosages are given in the table on p. 247.

PHARMACOKINETICS

Half-Life	Onset	Peak	Duration
3–11 hr	1–7 days	1–2 hr	Unknown

▸▸ *mirtazapine*

Mirtazapine, the newest of the third-generation antidepressants, is unique in that it promotes the presynaptic release in the brain of both serotonin and norepinephrine because of its antagonist activity in the presynaptic alpha$_2$-adrenergic receptors (see Chapter 17) but does not inhibit the reuptake of either of these neurotransmitters. It is strongly associated with sedation in over 50 percent of clients because of its histamine (H$_1$) receptor activity and so is usually dosed once daily at bedtime. However, it has demonstrated significant improvement of symptoms in depressed clients, including frail geriatric clients in the nursing home setting. Furthermore, although clearance of the drug may be somewhat reduced in geriatric clients, no dosage adjustment is currently recommended. Mirtazapine is contraindicated in cases of drug allergy and concurrent use of MAOIs. It is available in both regular and disintegrating tablets (which dissolve in the mouth) in strengths of 15, 30, and 45 mg. Pregnancy category C. The commonly recommended dosages are given in the table on p. 247.

PHARMACOKINETICS

Half-Life	Onset	Peak	Duration
20–40 hr	1–3 wk	2 hr	Unknown

TRICYCLIC ANTIDEPRESSANTS

Among the original, first-generation antidepressants, **tricyclic antidepressants** (TCAs) have largely been superseded as first-line antidepressant drug therapy following the introduction of the SSRIs in the 1980s, beginning with fluoxetine. At this point TCAs are generally considered second-line drug therapy for clients who fail NGAs or as adjunct therapy with NGAs.

Mechanism of Action and Drug Effects

TCAs are believed to work by correcting the imbalance in the neurotransmitter concentrations of serotonin and norepinephrine at the nerve endings in the CNS (the biogenic amine hypothesis). This is accomplished by blocking the reuptake of the neurotransmitters and thus causing these neurotransmitters to accumulate at the nerve endings. Some also believe that these agents may help regulate malfunctioning nerves (the dysregulation hypothesis).

TCAs have several advantageous therapeutic effects, but their use is also associated with many adverse effects. Both the advantageous and adverse effects can be explained by the functions of the various receptors these agents affect. As previously mentioned, the therapeutic effects of TCAs result from their ability to inhibit the reuptake of norepinephrine and serotonin at the nerve endings, but they also block muscarinic, histaminergic, adrenergic, dopaminergic, and serotonergic receptors. This non-selective antagonism of multiple receptor types contributes to their adverse effects. The therapeutic and undesirable effects as they relate to the receptors affected are presented in Table 15-6.

Indications

TCAs are used to treat depression. They have been available for more than 40 years. Overall they have demonstrated a remarkable efficacy, and their side effect profiles are well established. They are also considerably less expensive than most of the newer agents, with many of them available in generic formulations. Some of the TCAs have additional specific indications besides depression. For example, imipramine is used as an adjunct in the treatment of childhood enuresis (bedwetting), and clomipramine is useful in the treatment of OCD. Besides their beneficial antidepressant effects, TCAs are useful as adjunctive analgesics. TCAs have also been used in the treatment of trigeminal neuralgia.

Contraindications

Contraindications for TCAs include known drug allergy, use sooner than 14 days after stopping MAOI therapy, and pregnancy. They are also not recommended in clients with any acute or chronic cardiac problems because of their ability to cause disturbances in cardiac conduction. It is this effect that usually results in death when these medications are overdosed by a suicidal client.

Side Effects and Adverse Effects

The most common undesirable effects of TCAs are due to their effects on various receptors, mostly the muscarinic receptors. Blockade of these receptors by TCAs results in many undesirable anticholinergic side effects and adverse effects, the most common being sedation, erectile dysfunction, and orthostatic hypotension. Geriatric clients have a tendency to suffer more from dizziness, postural hypotension, constipation, delayed micturition, edema, and muscle tremors. The various undesirable effects as they relate to body systems are listed in Table 15-7.

Toxicity and Management of Overdose

TCA overdoses are notoriously lethal. It is estimated that 70 to 80 percent of clients who die of TCA overdose do so before reaching the hospital. The primary organ systems affected are the CNS and cardiovascular system, and death usually results from either seizures or dysrhythmias. There is no specific antidote for TCA poisoning. Consultation with a Poison Control Centre is recommended. Treatment is symptomatic and supportive. Management efforts are aimed at decreasing drug absorption through the administration of multiple doses of activated charcoal. Administration of an alkaline agent such as sodium bicarbonate speeds up elimination of the TCA by alkalinizing the urine to a pH of greater than 7.55. CNS damage may also be minimized through the administration of diazepam, and cardiovascular events may be minimized by giving antidysrhythmics to control cardiac dysrhythmias. Other care includes basic life support in an intensive care setting to maintain vital organ functions. These processes must continue until enough of the TCA is eliminated to permit restoration of normal organ function.

Interactions

Adrenergics, when taken with TCAs, may result in increased sympathetic stimulation. Anticholinergics and phenothiazines taken with TCAs may result in increased anticholinergic effects. CNS depressants, when taken with TCAs, will have additive CNS depressant effects. MAOIs, when taken with TCAs, may result in increased therapeutic and toxic effects. TCAs can inhibit the metabolism of warfarin, resulting in increased anticoagulation effects.

Dosages

For the recommended dosages for selected TCA agents, see the dosages table on p. 251. See Appendix B for some of the common brands available in Canada.

TABLE 15-6
TRICYCLIC ANTIDEPRESSANTS: THERAPEUTIC AND UNDESIRABLE DRUG EFFECTS BY RECEPTOR SITE

Blockade of	Drug Effect*
Adrenergic receptors	Orthostatic hypotension, antihypertensive effects
Dopaminergic receptors	Extrapyramidal and endocrine side effects
Histaminergic receptors	Sedation, weight gain
Muscarinic receptors	Dry mouth, constipation, blurred vision, tachycardia, urinary retention, confusion
Norepinephrine reuptake	*Antidepressant*, tremors, tachycardia, additive pressor effects with sympathomimetic drugs
Serotonergic receptors	Alleviation of rhinitis, hypotension
Serotonin reuptake	*Antidepressant*, nausea, headache, anxiety, sexual dysfunction

*Italicized effects are the therapeutic ones.

TABLE 15-7
TRICYCLIC ANTIDEPRESSANTS: ADVERSE EFFECTS

Body System	Side/Adverse Effects
Cardiovascular	Tremors, tachycardia, orthostatic hypotension, dysrhythmias
Central nervous	Anxiety, confusion, extrapyramidal effects, sedation
Gastrointestinal	Nausea, constipation, dry mouth
Other	Blurred vision, urinary retention, weight gain, erectile dysfunction

DRUG PROFILES

TCAs are effective agents in the treatment of various affective disorders, but they are also associated with serious side effects. Therefore clients taking them need to be monitored closely. For this reason, all antidepressants are available only with a prescription, with the exception of some herbal products such as St. John's wort (see the Natural Health Therapies box at right). Many drugs in this class are rated as pregnancy category D agents, making their use by pregnant women relatively more hazardous than most of the NGAs.

There are many drugs in the TCA drug class, including the tertiary-amine and secondary-amine TCAs. The secondary-amine TCAs have a stronger noradrenergic (norepinephrine) receptor effect and may have a structural advantage over the tertiary-amine TCAs in augmenting drug therapy with SSRIs in TRD. Box 15-2 lists the various cyclic antidepressants according to their respective categories.

▸▸ amitriptyline

Amitriptyline is one of the oldest and most widely used of all the TCAs. It is the prototypical tertiary-amine TCA and is also used in the treatment of various pain disorders such as trigeminal neuralgia. It has potent anticholinergic properties, which can lead to many adverse effects such as dry mouth, constipation, blurred vision, urinary retention, and dysrhythmias. There is one combination product that contains amitriptyline: Etrafon, which also contains perphenazine. Amitriptyline is available in oral form as 10-, 25-, 50-, and 75-mg tablets. The commonly recommended dosages are given in the table below.

PHARMACOKINETICS

Half-Life	Onset	Peak	Duration
10–50 hr	7–21 days*	2–12 hr	6–12 hr

*Therapeutic antidepressant effect.

nortriptyline

Nortriptyline is one of the prototypical secondary-amine TCAs. It is available only in oral form as 10- and 25-mg capsules. Pregnancy category D. The commonly recommended dosages are given in the table below.

PHARMACOKINETICS

Half-Life	Onset	Peak	Duration
18–90 hr	1–2 hr	7–8.5 hr	Variable

NATURAL HEALTH THERAPIES

ST. JOHN'S WORT (Hypericum perforatum)

Overview
St. John's wort consists of the dried, above-ground parts of the plant species *Hypericum perforatum* gathered during flowering season. It is available over the counter in numerous oral dosage forms. St. John's wort is sometimes referred to as the "herbal Prozac."

Common Uses
Depression, anxiety, sleep disorders, nervousness

Adverse Effects
GI upset, allergic reactions, fatigue, dizziness, confusion, dry mouth, possible photosensitization (especially in fair-skinned individuals)

Potential Drug Interactions
MAOIs, SSRIs, sympathomimetic amines, piroxicam, tetracycline, tyramine-containing foods

Contraindications
Contraindicated in clients with BPD, schizophrenia, Alzheimer's disease, or dementia

DOSAGES   Selected Tricyclic Antidepressants

Agent	Usual Dosage Range	Indications
▸▸ amitriptyline	**Adult** PO: 15–200 mg/day divided **Geriatric** PO: 100–150 mg/day divided	Depression
nortriptyline	**Pediatric** PO: 6–12 yr, 10–20 mg/day divided **Adolescent** PO: 30–150 mg/day divided **Adult** PO: 25–100 mg/day divided **Geriatric** PO: 10–75 mg/day at bedtime	Depression

BOX 15-2
Cyclic Antidepressant Categories

Tertiary Amine TCAs
amitriptyline
doxepin
imipramine
trimipramine

Secondary Amine TCAs
desipramine
nortriptyline

Tetracyclic Antidepressants
maprotiline
mirtazapine

MONOAMINE OXIDASE INHIBITORS

MAOIs, along with TCAs, represent the first generation of antidepressant drug therapy. Although MAOIs are potent drugs, they are now considered to be second- or third-line agents for the treatment of TRD: depression that is not responsive to other pharmacological therapies such as the SSRIs or TCAs. The adverse effects of MAOIs are listed in Table 15-8. A serious disadvantage of MAOIs is their potential to cause a hypertensive crisis when taken with a substance containing tyramine, which is found in many common foods and beverages (see Table 15-9). Note that tyramine, which comes from exogenous food and beverage sources, is not to be confused with tyrosine, an amino acid that is a biochemical precursor of dopamine.

Two available MAOI antidepressants, phenelzine and tranylcypromine, are non-selective inhibitors of both types A and B MAO. Both types of MAO are widely distributed throughout the body, including the brain. MAO-A preferentially metabolizes serotonin, norepinephrine, and tyramine. MAO-B preferentially metabolizes dopamine. Inhibiting the MAO enzyme system means that amines such as dopamine, serotonin, and norepinephrine are not broken down and therefore higher levels occur. This in turn alleviates the symptoms of depression. However, higher levels of tyramine can also result in the hazardous drug–food interaction associated with MAOIs. This interaction is described in the following section on MAOI toxicity. There is also an MAO type B-selective inhibitor called selegiline (see Chapter 14). This medication is used solely for treating Parkinson's disease (PD) and is not used for depression. Dosage information for selected MAOIs appears in the table on p. 253.

Toxicity and Management of Overdose

Clinical symptoms of MAOI overdose generally do not appear until about 12 hours after ingestion. The primary signs and symptoms are cardiovascular and neurological in nature. The most serious cardiovascular effects are tachycardia and circulatory collapse, and the neurological symptoms of major concern are seizures and coma. Hyperthermia and miosis are also generally present in overdose. Consultation with a Poison Control Centre is recommended. Treatment is symptomatic and supportive. The recommended treatment is aimed at eliminating the ingested toxin with the use of activated charcoal and protecting the organs at greatest risk for damage—the brain and heart. MAOIs are one of the few drug classes that are capable of interacting with food, leading to a severe reaction. In this case food containing the amino acid tyramine is the primary culprit, and a hypertensive crisis is the reaction. It is essential for both the client and the nurse to know the various foods and drinks that should be avoided; these are listed in Table 15-9. Treatment of hypertensive crisis resulting from consumption of tyramine-containing foods or beverages may require intravenous administration of hypotensive agents along with careful monitoring in an intensive care setting.

Interactions

A wide variety of drug interactions can occur with MAOIs. Sympathomimetic agents can also interact with the MAOIs and together cause a hypertensive crisis. MAOIs can markedly potentiate the effects of meperidine and therefore concurrent use is contraindicated. In addition, concurrent use of MAOIs with SSRIs carries the risk of serotonin syndrome. A washout period of at least 2 weeks after discontinuation of fluoxetine, sertraline, paroxetine, or citalopram should occur before initiation

TABLE 15-8

MAOIs: ADVERSE EFFECTS

Body System	Side/Adverse Effects
Cardiovascular	Orthostatic hypotension, tachycardia, palpitations, edema
Central nervous	Dizziness, drowsiness, restlessness, insomnia, headache
Gastrointestinal	Anorexia, abdominal cramps, nausea
Other	Blurred vision, impotence, skin rashes

TABLE 15-9

FOOD AND DRINK TO AVOID WHEN TAKING MAOIs

Food/Drink	Examples
HIGH TYRAMINE CONTENT—NOT PERMITTED	
Aged mature cheeses	Cheddar, blue, Swiss
Smoked/pickled meats, fish, or poultry	Herring, sausage, corned beef, salami, pepperoni
Aged/fermented meats, fish, or poultry	Chicken or beef liver pate, game
Yeast extracts	Brewer's yeast
Red wines	Chianti, burgundy, sherry, vermouth
Italian broad beans	Fava beans
MODERATE TYRAMINE CONTENT— LIMITED AMOUNTS ALLOWED	
Meat extracts	Bouillon, consommé
Pasteurized light and pale beer	
Ripe avocado	
LOW TYRAMINE CONTENT—PERMISSIBLE	
Distilled spirits (in moderation)	Vodka, gin, rye, scotch
American and mozzarella cheeses	Cottage cheese, cream cheese
Chocolate and caffeinated beverages	
Fruit	Figs, raisins, grapes, pineapple, oranges
Soy sauce	
Yogourt, sour cream	

of MAOI therapy. A 5-week washout period is necessary if switching to MAOIs from fluoxetine.

Dosages

For recommended dosages for selected MAOI agents, see the table below. See Appendix B for some of the common brands available in Canada.

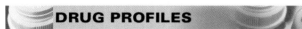

DRUG PROFILES

MAOIs are contraindicated in clients with the following conditions: cerebrovascular or cardiovascular disorders, pheochromocytoma, a known hypersensitivity reaction to MAOIs, and liver or renal dysfunction. MAOIs should also not be used in combination with adrenergic agents, tyramine-rich foods, NGAs, or meperidine. All MAOIs are classified as pregnancy category C agents. Of the agents prescribed for the treatment of depression, phenelzine tends to be more commonly prescribed and tranylcypromine may be more activating (perhaps because of its structural similarity to amphetamine). They are equally effective, although most physicians lean toward a favourite.

Occasionally a TCA is combined with an MAOI in the treatment of depression refractory to treatment with a TCA alone or with some other agent. Typically this is done by giving an MAOI to a client already taking a TCA, or the two may be started together at 50 percent of the usual dose of each. If a client's depression is stabilized on an MAOI but the physician wishes to switch to a TCA, then there must be at least a 2-week washout period before the start of TCA treatment. Without this washout period, the client might experience hyperthermia, delirium, convulsions, and coma.

phenelzine

Phenelzine is an MAOI that has been used for the treatment of affective disorders such as depression. In investigational studies it has also shown some effectiveness in the treatment of panic disorders. It is generally indicated for those clients who do not respond to other antidepressants. It is available only in oral form as a 15-mg tablet. Pregnancy category C. The commonly recommended dosages are given in the table below.

PHARMACOKINETICS

Half-Life	Onset	Peak	Duration
Variable	2 wk*	≤6 wk	2 wk*

*Therapeutic effects.

tranylcypromine

Tranylcypromine is an MAOI used for the treatment of depression. It is structurally similar to amphetamine. It is available only in oral form as a 10-mg tablet. Pregnancy category C. The commonly recommended dosages are given in the table below.

PHARMACOKINETICS

Half-Life	Onset	Peak	Duration
2–3 hr	<2 hr	1.5–3 hr	3–10 days

ANTIPSYCHOTIC AGENTS

Antipsychotic agents are used to treat serious mental illness such as depressive and drug-induced psychoses and schizophrenia. Antipsychotics are also used to treat extreme mania (as an adjunct to lithium), BPD, certain movement disorders (e.g., Tourette's syndrome), and certain other medical conditions (e.g., nausea, intractable hiccups). Antipsychotics have also been referred to as *tranquilizers* or *neuroleptics* because they produce a state of tranquility and work on abnormally functioning nerves. However, these are both older terms that are now less commonly used.

Constituting about two-thirds of all antipsychotics, phenothiazines are the largest group of antipsychotic drugs. Like many other drugs, phenothiazines were discovered by chance, in this case during research for new antihistamines. In 1951 chlorpromazine was the first phenothiazine to be discovered in this way. Although phenothiazines can provide much relief to the mentally ill client, they can also cause many undesirable side effects. These agents are associated with a high incidence of anticholinergic side effects because they are so closely related to antihistamines. Therefore since the early 1950s researchers have been working on developing phenothiazines with fewer side effects.

Phenothiazines can be divided into three groups based on structural differences: aliphatic, piperidine, and piperazine. Besides the phenothiazine antipsychotics, four other categories of drugs are commonly used to treat mental illness: thioxanthenes, butyrophenones, dihydroindolones, and dibenzoxazepines. Many of the therapeutic and toxic effects of the antipsychotics are the consequence of their chemical structures.

DOSAGES	Selected MAOIs		
Agent	**Usual Dosage Range**		**Indications**
phenelzine	PO: Initial dose 15–90 mg/day divided tid, followed by dose reduction to minimal effective dose after therapeutic effect achieved		Atypical depression
tranylcypromine	20–30 mg/day divided bid		Depression phase of bipolar disorder

TABLE 15-10

MAJOR DOPAMINE SYSTEMS IN THE BRAIN

DA System	DA-Related Function	Effects of DA Receptor Blockade
Hypothalamic–pituitary	Regulates prolactin secretion, temperature, appetite, emesis	Increased prolactin levels resulting in galactorrhea, amenorrhea, and decreased libido; loss of temperature regulation, increased appetite, and anti-emetic effects
Mesocortical	Regulates behaviour	Therapeutic antipsychotic effects
Mesolimbic	Regulates stereotypical and other behaviours	Therapeutic antipsychotic effects
Nigrostriatal	Mediates function of the extrapyramidal motor system (EPS movement)	*Reversible:* Dystonia, pseudoparkinsonism, akathisia *Irreversible:* Tardive dyskinesia (must catch early to reverse!)

DA, Dopamine; *EPS,* extrapyramidal symptoms

There is little difference between traditional antipsychotics in their mechanisms of action; therefore selection of an antipsychotic is based primarily on the least undesirable drug side effect and the client's type of psychosis. Of the currently available antipsychotic agents, no single drug stands out as either more or less effective in the treatment of the symptoms of psychosis. It should also be stressed that antipsychotic drug therapy does not provide a cure for mental illness but is only a way of chemically controlling the symptoms of the illness. These agents represent a significant advance in our treatment of mental illnesses; before the 1950s, the treatment of mental illness consisted largely of such extreme measures as isolation, physical restraint, shock therapy, and even lobotomy.

Over the last 6 or 7 years a new class of antipsychotic medications has evolved. They are referred to as *atypical antipsychotics (AAPs)* or *second-generation antipsychotics,* and they differ from first-generation agents in both their mechanisms of action and their side effect profiles. Some of these newer AAPs include clozapine, risperidone, olanzapine, and quetiapine. Ziprasidone is currently in clinical trials in Canada. Newer antipsychotics gaining approval and showing great promise include sertindole and zotepine.

Mechanism of Action and Drug Effects

One thing that all antipsychotics have in common is some degree of blockage of dopamine receptors in the brain, thus decreasing the dopamine concentration in the CNS. Specifically, the older phenothiazines block the receptors to which dopamine normally binds post-synaptically in certain areas of the CNS, such as the limbic system and the basal ganglia. These are the areas associated with emotions, cognitive function, and motor function. This results in a tranquilizing effect in psychotic clients. Both the therapeutic and toxic effects of these agents are the direct result of the dopamine blockade in these areas.

The newer AAPs block specific dopamine receptors called *dopamine 2 [D2] receptors,* as well as specific serotonin receptors in the brain called *serotonin 2 [5-HT2] receptors.* The different mechanisms of action of the AAPs are responsible for their improved efficacy and improved safety profiles.

Antipsychotics have many effects throughout the body. Besides blocking the dopamine receptors in the CNS, they also block alpha receptors, which can result in hypotension and other cardiovascular effects. Many of the adverse effects of these drugs stem from their ability to block histamine receptors (anticholinergic effects). They also block serotonin receptors. This, in combination with their ability to block dopamine receptors in the chemoreceptor trigger zone and peripherally and with their ability to inhibit neurotransmission in the vagus nerve in the GI tract, accounts for the ability of certain antipsychotics to function as anti-emetics. Additional blocking of dopamine receptors in the brainstem reticular system also allows AAPs to have anti-anxiety effects. The older first-generation agents such as phenothiazines and haloperidol can also augment prolactin release, which can result in swelling of the breasts and milk secretion in women taking these agents. Gynecomastia can also be a distressing side effect in male clients.

Indications

The major therapeutic effect of antipsychotic agents is the result of blockade of dopamine receptors in certain areas of the CNS. These are the areas where regulation of dopamine activity tends to be dysfunctional in psychotic clients. The extent to which such antidopaminergic drug therapy has been shown to control psychotic symptoms is one of the major factors supporting the **dopamine hypothesis** regarding the origins of the various psychotic disorders. Note that this type of drug therapy is in direct contrast to that for PD treatment, where dopaminergic activity needs to be enhanced instead of reduced. The various areas within the CNS where antipsychotics have a major effect are listed in Table 15-10.

Contraindications

Contraindications to the use of antipsychotic agents include known drug allergy; comatose state; and possibly significant CNS depression, brain damage, liver or kidney disease, blood dyscrasias, and uncontrolled epilepsy.

Side Effects and Adverse Effects

The side effects of the individual antipsychotic drugs are many and are important to remember. The goal is to choose a drug with the least bothersome side effect

TABLE 15-11
ANTIPSYCHOTICS: RECEPTOR-RELATED SIDE EFFECTS

Receptor	Side/Adverse Effect	Drug Category
Alpha-adrenergic	Postural hypotension, lightheadedness, reflex tachycardia	Low-potency drugs
Dopamine	Extrapyramidal movement disorders, dystonia, pseudoparkinsonism, akathisia, tardive dyskinesia	High-potency drugs
Endocrine	Prolactin secretion (galactorrhea, gynecomastia), menstrual changes, sexual dysfunction	Low-potency drugs
Histamine	Sedation, drowsiness, hypotension, weight gain	Low-potency drugs
Muscarinic (cholinergic)	Blurred vision, worsening of narrow-angle glaucoma, dry mouth, tachycardia, constipation, urinary retention, decreased sweating	Low-potency drugs

profile for a given client. Individual clients may vary widely in their response to, and tolerance of, a given medication. These individual variances are usually not predictable, and so often the medication(s) that best help a given client are discovered through a trial and error process. The common side effects caused by blockade of the dopamine, muscarinic (synonymous with cholinergic), histamine, and alpha-adrenergic receptors are listed in Table 15-11. These undesirable effects can also be classified according to the body system affected. Severe hematological effects may include agranulocytosis and hemolytic anemia. Integumentary effects may include exfoliative dermatitis. CNS effects include drowsiness, neuroleptic malignant syndrome (NMS), extrapyramidal symptoms (EPS), and tardive dyskinesia (TD). NMS is a potentially life-threatening adverse effect that may include high fever, unstable blood pressure (BP), and myoglobinemia. EPS involves involuntary motor symptoms similar to those associated with PD (pseudoparkinsonism), akathisia (distressing motor restlessness), and acute dystonia (painful muscle spasms). Tardive is a word that means "late-appearing." TD involves involuntary contractions of oral and facial muscles (e.g., involuntary tongue-thrusting) and choreoathetosis (wavelike movements of extremities) that usually appear only after continuous long-term antipsychotic therapy. Ocular adverse effects include blurred vision, corneal lens changes, epithelial keratopathy, and pigmentary retinopathy. Cardiovascular effects include postural hypotension. Additionally, electrocardiogram (ECG) changes, notably prolonged QT interval, are associated to varying degrees with all classes of antipsychotic agents. Baseline and periodic ECGs, as well as serum potassium and magnesium levels, can help determine if a client is at risk for such effects or diagnose newly acquired cardiac dysrhythmias. In such cases, another drug choice may still control symptoms without causing cardiac effects.

The common side effects and adverse effects caused by antipsychotic drugs are listed in Table 15-12.

Low-potency antipsychotic agents generally have a low incidence of EPS and a high incidence of sedation, anticholinergic side effects, and cardiovascular side effects. The opposite is true for high-potency antipsychotic agents. They have a high incidence of EPS and a low incidence of sedation, anticholinergic side effects, and cardiovascular side effects.

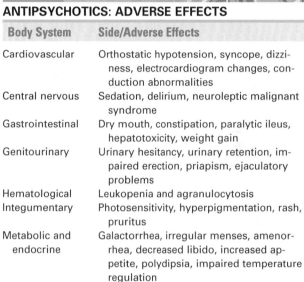

TABLE 15-12
ANTIPSYCHOTICS: ADVERSE EFFECTS

Body System	Side/Adverse Effects
Cardiovascular	Orthostatic hypotension, syncope, dizziness, electrocardiogram changes, conduction abnormalities
Central nervous	Sedation, delirium, neuroleptic malignant syndrome
Gastrointestinal	Dry mouth, constipation, paralytic ileus, hepatotoxicity, weight gain
Genitourinary	Urinary hesitancy, urinary retention, impaired erection, priapism, ejaculatory problems
Hematological	Leukopenia and agranulocytosis
Integumentary	Photosensitivity, hyperpigmentation, rash, pruritus
Metabolic and endocrine	Galactorrhea, irregular menses, amenorrhea, decreased libido, increased appetite, polydipsia, impaired temperature regulation

Interactions

Antacids can decrease antipsychotic absorption. Antihypertensives may have additive hypotensive effects and CNS depressants may have additive CNS-depressant effects when taken with antipsychotics.

Dosages

For recommended dosages for selected antipsychotic agents, see the table on p. 256. See Appendix B for some of the common brands available in Canada.

DRUG PROFILES

Antipsychotics are prescription-only medications that are indicated for the treatment of various psychotic disorders. Of the currently available agents, no single drug has stood out as being either more or less effective in the treatment of the symptoms of psychosis. Some of the factors that should be considered before selecting an antipsychotic agent are the client's history of response to an agent and the desired side effect profile. It is also important to start with the lowest possible dose of an orally administered drug.

DOSAGES Selected First-Generation Antipsychotic Agents

Agent	Pharmacological Class	Usual Dosage Range	Indications
chlorpromazine	Alipathic phenothiazine	**Adult** PO, IM: 25–400 mg/day with larger doses divided; IM is usually for acute care only **Pediatric >6 months** PO, IM, IV: 0.5–1 mg/kg/dose q6–8 h	Psychotic disorders, mania
fluphenazine	Piperidine phenothiazine	**Adult only** PO: 2.5–20 mg/day with larger doses divided tid–qid IM: 1.25–10 mg/day with larger doses divided tid–qid	
haloperidol	Butyrophenone phenyl-butylpiperidine	**Adult** PO, IM: 1.5–20 mg bid–tid **Pediatric 3–12 years** PO: 0.25–1.5 mg/kg/day bid–tid IM (acute care only): 2–5 mg q1h to maximum of 20 mg prn Depot: 10–15 × normal oral dose, q4weeks	Psychotic disorders
loxapine	Dibenzoxazepine dipenzepine	**Adult only** PO: 10 mg bid up to 100 mg/day divided bid–qid IM: 12.5–50 mg q4–6h	
thiothixene	Thioxanthenes	**Adult** 5 mg tid to 60 mg/day divided tid	

PHENOTHIAZINES

chlorpromazine

Chlorpromazine has strong anticholinergic and sedative effects and is a strong anti-emetic. It is considered a low-potency neuroleptic agent and therefore the associated incidence of EPS is low. The incidence of sedative, anticholinergic, and cardiovascular side effects is high, however. It is indicated for the symptomatic relief of nausea, vomiting, hiccups, and porphyria; for preoperative sedation; and for the treatment of psychotic disorders.

Chlorpromazine is contraindicated in clients who have shown a hypersensitivity reaction to phenothiazines and in those suffering from circulatory collapse, liver dysfunction, blood dyscrasias, comatose state, bone marrow depression, or alcohol or barbiturate withdrawal. It is available in oral, rectal, and intravenous dosage formulations. In the oral form it is available as 10-, 25-, 50-, 100-, and 200-mg tablets; a 44.5-mg/mL syrup; and 25- and 100-mg/mL concentrated solutions. In its rectal formulation it is available as 100-mg suppositories. The intravenous and intramuscular forms of chlorpromazine are available as a 25-mg/mL injection. Pregnancy category C. The commonly recommended dosages are given in the table above.

PHARMACOKINETICS

Half-Life	Onset	Peak	Duration
PO: 6 hr	PO: 30–60 min	PO: Unknown	PO: 4–6 hr
PR: 6 hr	PR: 1–2 hr	PR: Unknown	PR: 3–4 hr
IM: 6 hr	IM: Unknown	IM: Unknown	IM: 4–8 hr
IV: 6 hr	IV: Rapid	IV: Unknown	IV: Unknown

PR, Per rectum (suppository).

fluphenazine

Fluphenazine is available in three different salt forms, which give it varying degrees of antipsychotic potency. The decanoate and enanthate (latter not available in Canada) salt forms have the longest durations of action, and the hydrochloride salt form is fairly short in duration. Fluphenazine has the greatest potency of all the phenothiazines: 1 mg of the drug has the antipsychotic potency of 200 mg of chlorphenazine. It is primarily used to treat psychotic disorders and schizophrenia. It is considered a high-potency antipsychotic and is therefore associated with a high incidence of EPS; however, the associated incidence of sedative, anticholinergic, and cardiovascular effects is low. It is contraindicated in clients who have shown a hypersensitivity reaction to phenothiazines and in those suffering from circulatory collapse, liver dysfunction, blood dyscrasias, comatose state, bone marrow depression, or alcohol or barbiturate withdrawal. Fluphenazine decanoate is available as 25- and 100-mg/mL intramuscular/subcutaneous injections. The hydrochloride salt form is available in oral form as a 0.5-mg/mL elixir; 1-, 2-, 2.5-, and 5-mg tablets; and 15- and 30-mg capsules. It is also available as a 2.5-mg/mL intramuscular injection. Pregnancy category C. The commonly recommended dosages are given in the table above.

PHARMACOKINETICS

Half-Life	Onset	Peak	Duration
PO: 15–16 hr*	PO (HCI): 1 hr	PO (HCI): 1.5–2 hr	PO (HCI): 6–8 hr
IM: Up to 2 wk†	IM (HCI): 1 hr	IM (HCI): 1.5–2 hr	IM (HCI): 6–8 hr
	IM (decanoate): 24–72 hr	IM (decanoate): Unknown	IM (decanoate): ≥4 wk

*Following single dose.
†Following multiple intramuscular injections.

DOSAGES Selected Anti-anxiety Agents			
Agent	**Pharmacological Class**	**Usual Dosage Range***	**Indications**
clozapine	Dibenzodiazepine dibenzepine	12.5–50 bid initially increased to achieve 300–900 mg/day with larger doses divided tid	Treatment-resistant schizophrenia
▸▸ risperidone	Benzisoxazole	1–10 mg/day–bid	Schizophrenia and related disorders
▸▸ olanzapine	Thienobenzodiazepine dibenzepine	5–20 mg/day	Schizophrenia, bipolar mania
quetiapine	Dibenzothiazepine dibenzepine	25–800 mg/day with larger doses divided bid–tid	Schizophrenia

*All dosages reflect usual adult dosage ranges. Pediatric doses may be more variable and should be specified by a pediatric practitioner.

THIOXANTHENES

thiothixene

Thiothixene is a high-potency antipsychotic agent. Its use is associated with a high incidence of EPS but a low incidence of sedative, anticholinergic, and cardiovascular side effects. Thiothixene is primarily used for the treatment of psychotic disorders, schizophrenia, and acute agitation. It is contraindicated in clients who have shown a hypersensitivity reaction to it and in those suffering from circulatory collapse, liver dysfunction, blood dyscrasias, bone marrow depression, comatose state, narrow-angle glaucoma, or alcoholism. Thiothixene is available in oral form as 2-, 5-, and 10-mg capsules. Pregnancy category C. The commonly recommended dosages are given in the table on p. 256.

PHARMACOKINETICS

Half-Life	**Onset**	**Peak**	**Duration**
PO: 34 hr	PO: Days to weeks	PO: Unknown	PO: Unknown

BUTYROPHENONES

haloperidol

Haloperidol is structurally different from the thioxanthenes and the phenothiazines but has similar antipsychotic properties. It is a high-potency neuroleptic agent that has a favourable cardiovascular, anticholinergic, and sedative side effect profile but can often cause EPS. Haloperidol is available in three salt forms: base, decanoate, and lactate (not available in Canada). Haloperidol decanoate has an extremely long duration of effect. It is used primarily for the long-term treatment of psychosis and is especially useful in clients who show non-adherence with their drug treatment. It is contraindicated in clients who have shown a hypersensitivity reaction to it, those in a comatose state, those taking large amounts of CNS depressants, and those with PD. The base form is available in oral form as 0.5-, 1-, 2-, 5-, 10-, and 20-mg tablets and as a 2-mg/mL oral solution. The long-acting decanoate salt comes as 50- and 100-mg/mL injections for intramuscular use; the other shorter-acting haloperidol comes as a 5-mg/mL injection. Pregnancy category C. The commonly recommended dosages are given in the table on p. 256.

PHARMACOKINETICS

Half-Life	**Onset**	**Peak**	**Duration**
PO/IM: 13–35 hr	PO: 2 hr	PO: 2–6 hr	PO: 8–12 hr
	IM (lactate): 20–30 min	IM (lactate): 30–45 min	IM (lactate): 4–8 hr
	IM (decanoate): 3–9 days	IM (decanoate): Unknown	IM (decanoate): 1 mo

ATYPICAL ANTIPSYCHOTICS

There are a number of antipsychotics on the market. All show some efficacy for the positive symptoms of schizophrenia, and over time the improvement may even increase. These so-called *positive symptoms* are hallucinations, delusions, and conceptual disorganization. Unfortunately, first-generation antipsychotics are much less effective for *negative symptoms*: apathy, social withdrawal, blunted affect, poverty of speech, and catatonia. It is these negative symptoms that account for most of the social and vocational disability caused by schizophrenia. Another drawback to first-generation antipsychotics is that they all cause EPS, including rigidity, tremor, bradykinesia (slow movement), and bradyphrenia (slow thought). To summarize, first-generation antipsychotics such as haloperidol are effective for controlling symptoms, but not all symptoms, not in all clients, and not without serious side effects.

Between 1975 and 1990 there was not a single new antipsychotic drug approved in Canada. Then in 1991 came the approval of clozapine, the first of the AAPs. Clozapine was followed in the late 1990s in quick succession by risperidone, olanzapine, and quetiapine. The *atypical antipsychotics* (AAPs) show less effect on prolactin levels than older agents and improvement in the negative symptoms associated with schizophrenia. Though they are still fairly new compared with their first-generation counterparts, they also show a lower risk of NMS, EPS, and TD. These new agents—plus several more in clinical trials—are in the process of revolutionizing the treatment of psychosis and schizophrenia. For these reasons, AAPs are also referred to as *second-generation antipsychotic agents*. All four of the currently available AAPs have several pharmacological properties in common.

Antagonist activity at the dopamine D_1 receptor is believed to be the mechanism of antimanic activity. Serotonergic (serotonin agonist) activity at various serotonin (5-HT) receptor subtypes and alpha$_2$-adrenergic (agonist) activity are both associated with antidepressant activity. Alpha$_1$-adrenergic receptor antagonist activity is associated with orthostatic effects, and histamine H_1 receptor antagonist activity is associated with both sedative and appetite stimulating effects. This last effect accounts for a common side effect of weight gain that is associated to various degrees with AAP agents. This can cause or worsen obesity and even bring about diabetes. Clozapine and olanzapine are associated with the most weight gain, and risperidone and quetiapine with less. Sedative effects may diminish over time and can actually be helpful for clients with insomnia. Although these drugs all have similar pharmacological properties, they vary in the degree of affinity that each may have for the various types of receptors. These subtle pharmacological differences, along with often unknown and unpredictable physiological client differences, help to explain why some clients respond better to one medication than to another.

clozapine

Clozapine is a unique antipsychotic agent. It is similar to loxapine in its chemical structure in that it is a piperazine-substituted tricyclic antipsychotic; however, pharmacologically it is different from all other currently available antipsychotics in terms of its mechanism of action. It also more selectively blocks the dopaminergic receptors in the mesolimbic system. Other antipsychotic agents block dopamine receptors in an area of the brain called the *neostriatum,* but blockade in this area of the brain is believed to give rise to the unwanted EPS. Because clozapine has weak dopamine-blocking abilities in this area, it is associated with minor or no EPS. In fact, clozapine is currently the AAP with the lowest reported incidence of such effects. This often makes clozapine the drug of choice for psychotic disorders in clients with co-occurring PD because it will not worsen motor symptoms. However, clozapine is associated with hematological adverse effects, and newer AAPs may be better tolerated.

Clozapine has been extremely useful for the treatment of clients who have failed treatment with other antipsychotic agents, especially those with schizophrenia. Clients taking clozapine must be monitored closely for the development of agranulocytosis, a dangerous lack of white blood cell (WBC) production that is drug induced. The risk of agranulocytosis developing as the result of clozapine therapy is 1 to 2 percent after the first year; this compares with a risk of 0.1 percent to 1 percent for phenothiazines. For this reason, clients beginning clozapine therapy require weekly monitoring of WBC count for the first 6 months of therapy. If the count falls below 3×10^9/L, the drug should be withheld until the count rises above this value. Weekly WBC counts are also recommended for 4 weeks after discontinuation of the drug. Clozapine is available only in oral form

as 25- and 100-mg tablets. Its use is contraindicated in clients who have shown a hypersensitivity reaction to it and in those with myeloproliferative disorders, severe granulocytopenia, CNS depression, or narrow-angle glaucoma or those who are in a comatose state. Pregnancy category B. The commonly recommended dosages are given in the table on p. 257.

PHARMACOKINETICS

Half-Life	Onset	Peak	Duration
12 hr	1–6 hr	Weeks	4–12 hr

▶▶ risperidone

Risperidone was the second atypical antipsychotic to receive Health Canada approval. It is even more active than clozapine at the serotonin (5-HT 2A and 2C) receptors. It also has high affinity for alpha$_1$- and alpha$_2$-adrenergic receptors and histamine H_1 receptors. It has lower affinity for the serotonin 5-HT 1A, 1C, and 1D receptors and the dopamine D1 receptor. It is effective for refractory schizophrenia, including negative symptoms, and causes minimal EPS at therapeutic dosages (1 to 6 mg/day). It also is not associated with the hematological hazards and need for frequent WBC count monitoring that is necessary with clozapine. However, it can cause mild to moderate elevation of serum prolactin levels. It is available as 0.25-, 0.5-, 1-, 2-, 3-, and 4-mg oral tablets; 0.5-mg disintegrating tablet; 1-mm/mL oral solution; and as Risperdal Consta, a 25-, 37.5- and 50-mg/mL solution. The use of risperidone is contraindicated in clients who have shown a hypersensitivity reaction to it. Pregnancy category C. The commonly recommended dosages are given in the table on p. 257.

PHARMACOKINETICS

Half-Life	Onset	Peak	Duration
20–30 hr	1–2 wk*	Unknown	7 days

*Therapeutic effects.

▶▶ olanzapine

Olanzapine is the third of the AAPs to receive Health Canada approval. It interacts with dopamine D1-4 and serotonin 5-HT2A and 2C receptors. Like clozapine, it has blocking action on a variety of other receptors such as other serotonin receptors, alpha$_1$-adrenergic receptors, and histamine receptors. Olanzapine is a thienobenzodiazepine derivative. It was designated *1S* (new molecular entity) by the Notice of Compliance to Health Canada and approved to speed its availability for clients with schizophrenia. Many previously disabled clients experienced dramatic improvement in their level of day-to-day functioning. Olanzapine has only minor effects on the hepatic cytochrome P-450 enzyme systems, greatly reducing the likelihood of significant drug interactions. It also lacks the requirement for frequent monitoring of WBC count that is necessary with clozapine. However, it is associated with both weight gain and sedation. Its only absolute contraindication is drug allergy. Olanzapine is available as an orally disintegrating tablet in 5, 10, and 15 mg. It is also available in regular tablet form in 2.5-, 5-, 7.5-, 10-, and 15-mg strengths and as an intramuscular form of 10 mg/5 mL. In 2004 Health Canada issued safety information warning about the use of olanzapine in elderly clients with dementia. In clinical trials, the use of olanzapine is associated with increased incidence of cerebrovascular adverse events (brain attack and transient ischemic attacks) including fatalities. Pregnancy category C. The commonly recommended dosages are given in the table on p. 257.

PHARMACOKINETICS

Half-Life	Onset	Peak	Duration
21–54 hrs	>1 wk	6 hr	Unknown

quetiapine

A fourth AAP is quetiapine. It is a dibenzothiazepine antipsychotic similar in structure to clozapine but seems to be much safer, especially from a hematological standpoint. Quetiapine has affinity for dopamine D_2 and D_1 receptors; serotonin 5-HT1A, 2A, and 2C receptors; muscarinic (cholinergic) M_1 receptors; histamine H_1 receptors; and alpha$_1$- and alpha$_2$-adrenergic receptors. It also has minor effects on hepatic cytochrome P-450 enzyme systems, thus reducing the likelihood of serious drug interactions. The drug also blocks histamine and alpha-adrenergic receptors. This medication can cause ocular cataracts and clients should have eye examinations every 6 months. Quetiapine is available in oral form as 25-, 100-, 150-, 200-, and 300-mg tablets. Pregnancy category C. The commonly recommended dosages are given in the table on p. 257.

PHARMACOKINETICS

Half-Life	Onset	Peak	Duration
6 hr	2 days	1–2 hr	Unknown

Antipsychotic Agents Summary

All of these agents have a place in the treatment of schizophrenia. The lack of traditional neurological side effects is a tremendous benefit of the newer-generation atypical agents. This encourages the early use of antipsychotics when therapy is most beneficial. Physicians have been reluctant in the past to prescribe drugs early in therapy. With the evolution of the AAPs, early therapy is not only possible but safe and well tolerated.

▨ NURSING PROCESS

▮ Assessment

Both the physical and emotional status of clients taking psychotherapeutic drugs need to be thoroughly assessed before, during, and after initiation of therapy. The potential for drug interactions, drug toxicity, and other adverse effects associated with these drugs is great. If the more potent psychotherapeutic drugs and older agents are taken incorrectly, the risk for toxicity and overdosage are high. Suicidal tendencies must be assessed thoroughly because many of these drugs may be used by themselves or in combination with other agents for the purpose of committing suicide. Also, many of the clients needing these medications are so mentally distressed that their physical needs go unmet, resulting in a complexity of other problems such as insomnia, poor health status, and weight loss or gain. It is critical to client safety that physical parameters be assessed before therapy is initiated with any of the psychotherapeutic agents. Baseline BP, pulse rate, and body temperature must be obtained and documented not only before treatment is initiated but also during therapy. Postural (lying and standing) BP readings are particularly important with the use of some of the more potent psychotherapeutics so that the degree of a drop in BP caused by medication effects may be identified quickly and dealt with appropriately by healthcare personnel. Many of the older psychotherapeutic drugs, such as the MAOIs and TCAs, are known for their postural hypotensive effects.

The client's level of consciousness, mental alertness, and level of motor and cognitive functioning must be assessed and documented as well. The Mini-Mental Status Examination (MMSE) is one tool that may be used to assess the cognitive impairment found with so many mental illnesses. The MMSE is simple and cost efficient and can be completed in about 20 minutes by the nurse clinician. The MMSE is included in most psychiatric–mental health nursing textbooks. It includes an assessment with scoring of points in four major areas: level of orientation, attention and calculation ability, recall testing, and language skills. The MMSE is a commonly used assessment tool, but there are others, such as those for dementia (e.g., the six-item Blessed Orientation-Memory-Concentration Test, Clock Drawing Tasks, Functional Activities Questionnaire). There are additional assessment tools for other disease processes and associated mental functioning, such as the Alzheimer's Disease Assessment Scale, the Mattis Dementia Rating Scale, and the Severe Impairment Battery.

It is also important to have laboratory studies performed before, during, and after psychotropic drug therapy. These are especially important in clients on long-term therapy so that complications and potential toxicity can be prevented or identified early. Some of these tests may include a complete blood cell count (CBC), erythrocyte sedimentation rate, serum electrolytes, glucose levels, blood urea nitrogen (BUN), liver function studies, serum vitamin B_{12}, and thyroid studies. If the client is experiencing forms of dementia, other types of testing may be needed, such as genetic studies, computed tomography (CT) scan, or magnetic resonance imaging (MRI).

With any of the psychotherapeutic agents, the nurse should always check the client's mouth to make sure the client has swallowed the entire oral dosage. This helps to prevent hoarding of medications, a form of non-adherence that may lead to drug toxicity or overdose. Use of liquid preparations when available may minimize such problems. Appetite, sleeping patterns, addictive behaviours, elimination difficulties, hypersensitivity, and other conditions and complaints also need to be watched for and documented.

Specific contraindications and cautions apply to *anti-anxiety agents*. Contraindications include hypersensitivity to the drug, chemical abuse, pregnancy, and narrow-angle and open-angle glaucoma. In addition, the anti-anxiety drugs should not be used in clients under 12 years of age (see Pediatric Considerations box on p. 261). These drugs are also contraindicated, or should be used cautiously, in clients with liver or renal dysfunction, in geriatric clients, or in anyone in a debilitated state (see Geriatric Considerations box on p. 261). If these clients have to take these drugs, they need to be closely monitored and observed for oversedation and CNS depression for the duration of the therapy. Any time there is concern for the client's safety and risk of adverse effects or toxicity, it is critical for the nurse to document these findings and make safety a top priority. Before the start of an anti-anxiety (anxiolytic) medication, serum laboratory studies should be performed, including CBC, lactate dehydrogenase (LDH), creatinine, alkaline phosphatase, and BUN. If systolic BP drops by 20 mm Hg or more, the physician must be informed immediately. Verapamil, lithium, and parenteral solution incompatibilities are also common with the benzodiazepines.

Eye problems may occur with the *benzodiazepines*. Individuals taking these drugs long term should have baseline visual functioning determined not only with basic Snellen chart examinations but also by an ophthalmologist. Allergic reactions to clonazepam are characterized by a red, raised rash and may result in a significant reduction in bone marrow functioning with resulting blood dyscrasias, fever, sore throat, bruising, and jaundice. Midazolam has the same contraindications and cautions as the other benzodiazepines but has additional cautions for use in those clients with chronic obstructive pulmonary disease (COPD) and heart failure. Also, if an obese client is receiving midazolam as a part of operative sedation he or she needs to be closely monitored for drug toxicity because of the possibility of an increased half-life.

Some of the benzodiazepines have names that sound or look like other drug names. To avoid medication errors, it is especially important to check the drug order for the right drug. For example

- clonazepam may be confused with clonidine
- diazepam may be confused with ditropan
- lorazepam may be confused with alprazolam

The following are more assessment-related parameters for benzodiazepines:

- Lorazepam should be given cautiously (under close supervision) if the client is suicidal because it is often used in suicide attempts.

- Alprazolam should be administered only after assessment of mental status, anxiety, mood, sensorium, sleep patterns, and dizziness. The nurse should assess the client's knowledge of this drug and educate the client as needed about the potential for physical dependency with possible withdrawal symptoms of anxiety, panic attacks, convulsions, nausea, and vomiting. (Note: These withdrawal symptoms may occur with any of the benzodiazepines.)
- Chlordiazepoxide requires monitoring for any blood dyscrasias (altered blood counts) and assessing gait for any evidence of ataxia.
- Clonazepam is commonly associated with blood dyscrasias; therefore blood studies such as red blood cell (RBC) count, hematocrit (Hct), hemoglobin (Hgb), and reticulocytes should be performed every week for the first 4 weeks and then monthly. In addition, the therapeutic blood level, which is 20 to 80 μg/L, should be monitored. The usual eye, hepatic, and renal cautions apply with this drug.

With benzodiazepines, it is important for the nurse to monitor and assess BP readings. In general, systolic BP drops of 20 mm Hg have been reported; therefore clients need to have their BP taken and documented in some sort of journal or graphing document. Hepatic and renal studies should be performed, including aspartate aminotransferase (AST), alanine aminotransferase (ALT), bilirubin, creatinine, LDH, and alkaline phosphatase. For pregnant clients, a careful assessment is always needed of the safety of any of these drugs. Older adults have many age-related difficulties with metabolizing drugs and therefore physicians often order shorter-acting drugs that have no metabolites, such as lorazepam, oxazepam, and alprazolam, so that there is less risk of serum drug accumulation and toxicity. Drug interactions include phenytoin, digitalis drugs, alcohol, MAOIs (increased drug levels), cimetidine, and antacids (decreased absorption of drug). Clonazepam also interacts, in particular, with herbal product kava, and may result in an increased CNS depressant effect. Buspirone interacts with grapefruit juice, resulting in increased blood levels of buspirone. Other drugs that interact with benzodiazepines include other CNS depressants (including prescription, OTC, and herbal agents), opiates, and barbiturates. Cautious use of benzodiazepines and other anti-anxiety agents is recommended in clients with a history of benign prostatic hypertrophy, urinary retention, anemia, seizure disorder, psychosis, suicidal thoughts, narrow-angle and open-angle glaucoma, liver or renal dysfunction, thyroid disease, and cardiac disease; in geriatric clients; and in clients under 12 years of age.

Antimanic drugs, specifically lithium, are contraindicated in clients who have shown a hypersensitivity reaction to these drugs; in those with renal disease, liver disease, organic brain syndrome, brain trauma, schizophrenia, severe dehydration, or cardiac disease; in pregnant or lactating women; and in chil-

PEDIATRIC CONSIDERATIONS

Psychotherapeutic Agents

- Pediatric clients are more likely to experience side effects from psychotropic agents, especially EPS. Always closely monitor pediatric clients taking psychotropic agents!
- The incidence of Reye's syndrome and other adverse reactions is greater in pediatric clients taking psychotropic agents who have had chickenpox, CNS infections, measles, acute illnesses, or dehydration.
- Lithium may lead to decreased bone density or bone formation in children; therefore children receiving it should be closely monitored for signs and symptoms of lithium toxicity and bone disorders.
- TCAs are generally not prescribed for clients under 12 years of age. However, some antidepressants are used in children with enuresis, attention deficit disorders, and major depressive disorders and may be associated with adverse reactions such as changes in the ECG, nervousness, sleep disorder, fatigue, elevated BP, and GI upset. Pediatric clients are generally more sensitive to the effects of most drugs, and this group of agents is no exception. Be aware of the toxicity risk, which can be fatal. Should confusion, lethargy, visual disturbances, insomnia, tremors, palpitations, constipation, or eye pain occur, report this to the physician immediately.

GERIATRIC CONSIDERATIONS

Psychotherapeutic Agents

- Geriatric clients have higher serum levels of psychotherapeutic agents because of changes in the drug distribution and metabolism processes, less serum albumin, decreased lean body mass, less water in tissues, and increased body fat. Because of these changes, geriatric clients generally require lower doses of antipsychotic and antidepressant agents.
- Orthostatic hypotension, anticholinergic side effects, sedation, and EPS are more common in geriatric clients taking psychotherapeutic agents. Careful evaluation and documentation of baseline values and neurological findings are therefore important to the safe use of these agents.
- Increased anxiety is often associated with the use of TCAs. Clients with a history of cardiac disease may be at greater risk for dysrhythmias, tachycardia, stroke, myocardial infarction, or heart failure.
- Lithium is more toxic in geriatric clients and lower doses are often necessary. Close monitoring is important to its safe use in this age group. CNS toxicity, lithium-induced goitre, and hypothyroidism are more common in the geriatric client.

dren younger than 12 years of age. Cautious use is recommended in geriatric clients, clients with endocrine disorders such as diabetes mellitus and thyroid disorders, and those with a seizure disorder or urinary retention. Baseline urine laboratory studies should include measurement of the albumin, uric acid, and glucose levels and of the specific gravity. Baseline assessment of sodium intake and skin turgor is important because decreased sodium and fluid intake may lead to lithium toxicity, whereas increased sodium and fluid intake may lead to lithium loss. Baseline assessments of consciousness, gait and mobility levels, and neuromotor functioning are also important because poor coordination, tremors, and weakness that arise after the start of therapy can be symptoms of toxicity.

Lithium must be taken for approximately 3 weeks before therapeutic blood levels are reached, and clients should be closely monitored during this time and given supportive care. Contraindications include hypersensitivity to lithium (as with any drug) and use of the following: antithyroid agents, potassium iodide (increased hypothyroid effects), haloperidol and thioridazine (neurotoxicity), indomethacin, diuretics, NSAIDs (increased lithium toxicity), theopyllines, and urea and urine alkalizers (decreased effects of lithium). Other drug interactions to assess for with the use of lithium include thiazides, ACE inhibitors, and CCBs; the effect with these drugs is increased lithium toxicity. Irreversible brain damage is also

possible when lithium is used with haloperidol. Before administering lithium the nurse should document the client's weight so that the nurse can assess for edema, which is associated with lithium use.

Antidepressants include a wide variety of newer agents, as well as many older drugs:

- MAOIs, including phenelzine, tranylcypromine, fluvoxamine, and citalopram
- TCAs, including amitriptyline and nortriptyline
- SSRIs, including fluoxetine, paroxetine, and sertraline
- Second-generation agents, including trazodone and bupropion
- Third-generation agents, including mirtazapine and venlafaxine

There are many cautions, contraindications, and interactions, and other assessment parameters associated with antidepressant use. These are discussed by grouping or classification of drugs. Contraindications for all antidepressants include hypersensitivity to the drug.

Serotonin syndrome may occur with the use of any serotonergic medication, especially when combining two or more such drugs. Any of the following agents can cause this hazardous adverse effect: SSRIs; MAOIs; tryptophan; and the herbal products ephedra, ginseng, and St. John's wort. Signs and symptoms of this syndrome include mental status changes, restlessness, agitation, myoclonus (involuntary jerky motions), hyper-reflexia (overactive reflexes), diaphoresis (excessive sweating), shivering, tremor, diarrhea, nausea, headaches, and ataxia (lack of coordination).

Because the newer antidepressants are associated with fewer and less potent side effects, only a few *MAOIs* are used today in psychiatric mental health settings. Clients receiving MAOIs who have a history of suicide attempts or suicidal ideations, or who have seizure disorders, hyperactivity, diabetes, or psychosis need to be closely monitored for hoarding because of the suicide potential of these drugs. Cautious use is also recommended in clients with severe depression. These clients should be under the care of a healthcare professional (such as a psychiatrist, physician, or nurse practitioner) so that they may be closely monitored for destructive behaviors.

MAOIs are also known for their potentiation of hypertensive crisis when used with SSRIs, meperidine, or TCAs. Other drugs that should be avoided while taking MAOIs are anticholinergics, anaesthetics, haloperidol, lithium, warfarin, phenytoin, diazepam, CNS depressants, sympathomimetics, cyclic antidepressants, and the newer antidepressants. Another significant drug interaction is that between MAOIs and fluoxetine, an SSRI. It is recommended that the fluoxetine be discontinued for a period of 5 weeks before MAOI therapy is begun.

MAOIs have significant contraindications, cautions, drug–drug interactions, and drug–food interactions. Foods that contain tyramine (see Table 15-9) interact adversely with the MAOIs.

Because MAOIs can cause postural hypotension, it is important for the nurse to take BPs, both supine and standing. If the client is hospitalized it is recommended that the nurse assess supine and standing or sitting BPs *at least* 4 times a day. The nurse should wait 1 to 2 minutes after taking supine BP before taking standing or sitting BP. Pulse rate and laboratory values such as those indicative of hepatic functioning (ALT, AST, bilirubin) and CBCs are needed to rule out any further contraindications or cautions resulting from the side effect of blood dyscrasias.

Contraindications to the use of *TCAs* such as amitriptyline and nortriptyline are hypersensitivity, narrow-angle glaucoma, pregnancy, and recovery from myocardial infarction. Cautious use is indicated in children under the age of 12 and in clients with suicidal ideation; convulsive disorders; benign prostatic enlargement; severe depression; increased intraocular pressure (IOP); urinary retention; and cardiac, renal, or hepatic disease. Geriatric clients should also be carefully monitored if taking TCAs. The parameters of BP, pulse, CBCs, hepatic and renal studies, daily weights, and weekly weights are needed so that the nurse can assess for some of the adverse effects of these drugs. The parkinsonism-like syndrome or side effects are especially common in older adults and result in symptoms that are often seen in PD, such as tremors, inability to

carry out ADLs, and progressive deterioration of motor activities. Drug interactions with TCAs include cimetidine, fluoxetine, phenothiazines, oral contraceptives, antidepressants (increased effects of the TCA), clonidine and other antihypertensives, and ephedrine (decreased effects of TCAs). A hyperpyretic crisis (dangerously high fever) may occur if TCAs are used with MAOIs and clonidine or with clients exhibiting high fever, convulsions, or a hypertensive crisis. The herbal product kava may cause increased CNS depression if used with TCAs.

Often the *SSRIs* and the second- and third-generation antidepressants are discussed together. Because assessment as related to the SSRIs has been discussed, the other agents are presented here. Second-generation antidepressants include trazodone and bupropion. Third-generation antidepressants include venlafaxine and mirtazapine. Mirtazapine is also called a *tetracyclic drug,* as is the drug maprotiline, a rarely used second-generation antidepressant.

With *second-generation antidepressants,* cautious use with close monitoring is recommended in clients who are pregnant or lactating, in geriatric clients, and in clients who have diabetes. Trazodone, a second-generation TCA, is associated with fewer cardiac side effects and has minimal anticholinergic effects and so is often preferred over other TCAs. However, the male client needs to be assessed for his level of knowledge and understanding about this drug because one of the more common side effects, priapism (prolonged penile erection), occurs in younger men taking higher doses of this drug. Male clients must be informed to discontinue the drug immediately and seek medical advice if this side effect occurs.

Bupropion, a second-generation SSRI agent, may be preferred over other antidepressants because it has fewer anticholinergic, antiadrenergic, and cardiotoxic effects. However, the therapeutic effect of bupropion may not be reached for up to 4 weeks; therefore it is critical for the nurse to assess the client for suicidal tendencies and support systems to ensure client safety. (This applies to any drug with a delayed onset of therapeutic effects.) Those clients with seizure disorders should be informed about the risks of seizures associated with bupropion and should not take this drug. All second-generation antidepressants should be used cautiously in children. Drug interactions associated with the second-generation antidepressants include MAOIs, any highly protein-bound drugs, lithium, carbamazepine, alcohol, benzodiazepines, and SSRIs such as sertraline, cimetidine, diazepam, tolbutamide, and warfarin. It is important to client safety that the client understand that overdosage with bupropion may result in grand mal seizures, hallucinations, tachycardia, and neurotoxicity. Bupropion should not be given to anyone who is suffering from anorexia nervosa or bulimia or who is taking MAOIs, and should not be given to anyone with a seizure disorder.

Third-generation antidepressants have several advantages over the older antidepressants, but they still have contraindications, cautions, and drug interactions. Venlafaxine lacks many of the histamine-, cholinergic-, and adrenergic-related side effects associated with other antidepressants, such as TCAs; however, hypersensitivity to the drug would be a contraindication. Cautious use is needed with venlafaxine in the presence of GI disorders, loss of appetite, and hypertension. Venlafaxine should also be given with great caution to geriatric clients and to those with renal, hepatic, or cardiac disease. Mirtazapine is contraindicated with hypersensitivity to the drug and with MAOIs. Geriatric clients who have decreased renal functioning should not take this or any other third-generation drug. Drug interactions are few with the third-generation agents because they are not as highly protein bound as older agents. However, interactions do occur with MAOIs, other beta-blockers, haloperidol, and lorazepam. Also, concurrent use of third-generation antidepressants with any of the serotonergic drugs carries the risk of serotonin syndrome.

Haloperidol is similar to other high-potency *neuroleptics* in that its sedating effects are low but the incidence of EPS is high. These include tremors and muscle twitching and result from the blockade of the dopamine receptors, which has an inhibitory effect on specific movements in the musculoskeletal system. Extrapyramidal movement disorders are manifested as parkinsonism-like motor disturbances and are irritating and uncomfortable for the person experiencing them. Drug interactions for phenothiazines include antacids, antihypertensives, alcohol, and CNS depressants. Contraindications to these agents generally include hypersensitivity to the agent, liver dysfunction, blood dyscrasias, bone marrow suppression, and alcohol or barbiturate withdrawal. For community health points, see the box below. Haloperidol, as a butyrophenone, is also contraindicated in clients who take large doses of CNS depressants and in clients with PD, angina, urinary retention, or narrow-angle glaucoma.

Phenothiazines are one of the major groups of antipsychotics and include chlorpromazine and promazine. These agents are rarely used because of the high degree of sedation and severe orthostatic hypotension associated with them, as well as moderate degrees of EPS. If any of the phenothiazine drugs are used it is crucial to client safety for the nurse to know about their contraindications and cautions. Contraindications include use in geriatric clients and in pregnancy (some studies have shown that weeks 4 through 10 are dangerous times for taking antipsychotics). Drug interactions to the phenothiazine antipsychotics are many and include amphetamines, antacids, antidysrhythmics, anticholinergics, antihistamines, antihypertensives, anticonvulsants, barbiturates, beta-blockers, alcohol, lithium, haloperidol, antiparkinson drugs, narcotics, nicotine, SSRIs, MAOIs, and TCAs.

Quetiapine, an atypical agent used for the treatment of psychosis, is much like clozapine. Contraindications include hypersensitivity. Cautious use with close monitoring is recommended with children and geriatric clients; during pregnancy and lactation; and with clients with seizure disorders, breast cancer, or hepatic disease. Drug interactions include cimetidine, phenytoin, barbiturates, thioridazine, glucocorticoids, levodopa, and lorazepam. A thorough mental status examination should be performed and documented in the nurse's notes before initiation of the drug. An assessment of musculoskeletal functioning and monitoring for any EPS reactions is also important. Laboratory studies to be assessed before and during treatment include bilirubin and other liver function studies, CBC, and urinalysis. BPs, supine and standing, should also be assessed and documented. A drop of 20 mm Hg or more should be reported to the physician immediately. In addition, with geriatric clients the healthcare provider may order reduced doses, and antiparkinsonian agents may be indicated for prevention or treatment of EPS reactions.

Other atypical antipsychotic drugs carry the same assessment concerns. In addition, they should be used cautiously in overweight clients because weight gain may occur with these drugs. These drugs are also associated with a high degree of sedation and therefore should be used cautiously not only in geriatric clients but in any client who may be at risk for personal injury or harm. Clozapine is contraindicated in clients with a hypersensitivity reaction to it and in clients with blood dyscrasias, CNS depression, coma, or narrow-angle glaucoma.

COMMUNITY HEALTH POINTS

Phenothiazines

- Inform clients taking phenothiazines to tell the physician if they experience dizziness, lightheadedness, or palpitations. These symptoms may be indicative of postural hypotension and may be prevented by changing positions slowly, especially from lying to sitting or standing. Encourage clients to sit on the side of the bed for a few minutes before standing.
- Teach clients about the need to protect themselves from sun exposure and avoid tanning beds. Sunscreen should be used whenever there is a possibility of sun exposure, such as when going for a walk outdoors or working in the yard. This is to prevent solar erythema due to photosensitivity.
- Encourage clients to regularly schedule dental care to prevent infections and oral candidiasis related to drug-induced dry mouth.
- Teach clients about the need to avoid temperature extremes (e.g., sitting in hot tubs or saunas, spending time outside in high temperatures) because of the increased risk of hyperthermia leading to heat prostration.
- Encourage follow-up medical visits, therapy sessions, and follow-up laboratory studies to monitor therapeutic drug levels.

Because of the significance of leukopenia and platelet disorders, the nurse needs to assess for the risk for infections as well as clotting problems (e.g., easy bruising and increased bleeding potential). Grapefruit juice and nicotine alter clozapine levels.

Other *atypical antipsychotics,* like risperidone, are contraindicated in those clients with hypersensitivity to them. Orthostatic hypotension may occur with risperidone, so it should be used cautiously in geriatric clients and those who have unstable BPs. Olanzapine is associated with fewer problems with orthostasis and may not be as much of a culprit for orthostatic hypotension, but it does have a high degree of sedation and should be used cautiously with geriatric clients.

Loxapine and thiothixene (non-phenothiazine antipsychotic agents) are miscellaneous antipsychotic agents. Each is associated with contraindications, cautions, and drug interactions. These drugs should not be given to clients with hypersensitivity to them. Other contraindications for loxapine and similar drugs include blood disorders (such as different types of anemias), brain damage, bone marrow depression, or alcohol or barbiturate withdrawal. These drugs are contraindicated for use in children. They should be used cautiously in pregnant or lactating women; clients with cardiac, seizure, or liver disorders; men with benign prostatic hypertrophy; and clients younger than 16 years of age. Thiothixene is contraindicated in clients with blood dyscrasias or bone marrow depression. It should be used with caution in clients showing adverse reactions; in women who are pregnant or lactating; and in clients with seizure disorders, high BP, or hepatic or cardiac disease. These clients should be closely monitored, so the nurse should assess the client's history carefully with regard to cardiac disease because orthostatic hypotension and tachycardia are possible adverse effects of these agents. Thiothixene may lead to more profound side effects in the geriatric client because of their exaggerated response. The client's medication history and current medication list should be carefully noted because of possible drug interactions.

Antipsychotic drugs in general interact with several drugs and drug classes, including oral contraceptives, MAOIs, TCAs, SSRIs, erythromycin, quinolone antibiotics, the antibiotic ciprofloxacin, and nicotine. They can also interact with foods grilled over charcoal. Using these drugs with alcohol, antihistamines, anti-anxiety agents, barbiturates, meperidine, and morphine may result in additive antipsychotic effects and cause further CNS depressive effects.

Antipsychotic drugs are potent agents that deserve close monitoring and attention. Nurses knowledgeable about these agents are able to assess clients more thoroughly and to help these clients have more therapeutic responses and fewer side effects.

In summary, all healthcare professionals who prescribe or administer psychotherapeutic drugs must remain informed and cautious. Safety is a major concern for any client, and the concern is even greater when the drug being administered has significant adverse effects, contraindications, cautions, and drug interactions. The nurse must always take the time to assess the client thoroughly before administering any psychotherapeutic (or other) drug.

Nursing Diagnoses

Nursing diagnoses appropriate to the nursing care of clients receiving any of the psychotherapeutic agents include the following:
- Risk for injury related to disease state and possible side effects of medications.
- Disturbed thought processes related to impaired mental state.
- Impaired social interaction related to disease state and isolation from others.
- Imbalanced nutrition, less than body requirements, related to influence of mental disorder.
- Disturbed sleep patterns related to the mental illness or to drug therapy.
- Situational low self-esteem related to disease process or to side effects of medication.
- Urinary retention related to side effects of psychotherapeutic agents.
- Deficient knowledge related to lack of information about the specific psychotherapeutic drugs and their side effects.

Planning

Goals related to the administration of psychotherapeutic medications include the following:
- Client does not sustain injury while on medication.
- Client experiences no further deterioration in thought processes.
- Client exhibits improved nutritional status.
- Client regains normal sleep patterns.
- Client exhibits (overtly and covertly) a more positive self-image.
- Client remains free of any alterations in urinary elimination patterns.
- Client remains adherent with therapy.
- Client is free of complications associated with the drug and with food and drug interactions.

Outcome Criteria

Outcome criteria related to the aforementioned goals include the following:
- Client is free from falls, dizziness, and fainting attributable to side effects.
- Client demonstrates improved or no deterioration in thought processes and is less hostile, withdrawn, and delusional once medication has reached steady state.
- Client demonstrates more open and appropriate behaviour and communication with healthcare team and significant others.

- Client shows healthy nutrition habits with appropriate weight gain (if needed) and a diet that includes foods from Canada's Food Guide.
- Client reports improved sleep patterns and feeling more rested.
- Client openly discusses feelings of poor self-image and self-concept with staff.
- Client reports any problems with urinary retention.
- Client states the importance of taking medications exactly as prescribed at the same time every day and without omissions.
- Client states the importance of appointments with the physician or other healthcare providers to follow improvement and monitor therapy.
- Client states the common side effects of the medication and those adverse effects (e.g., confusion and changes in level of consciousness) to be reported to the physician.
- Client lists those medications and foods to be avoided while taking any psychotherapeutic medication.

Implementation

Regardless of the psychotherapeutic agent prescribed, several general nursing actions are important to the safe administration of the agent. First and foremost is a firm (unless the client is confrontational or aggressive) but patient attitude. Simple explanations should be given about the drug and its effects and the length of time before therapeutic effects can be expected. Vital signs should be monitored during therapy, especially in geriatric clients and in clients with a history of cardiac disease. The name of the drug, the dosage and route of administration, and more specifically the client's response should all be documented. Abrupt withdrawal of any of these medications should be avoided.

More specific nursing actions in clients taking *anti-anxiety agents* include frequent checks of vital signs because of the orthostatic hypotension that can occur. Clients may be told to wear elastic compression stockings if orthostatic hypotension is problematic. The nurse should advise clients to change positions slowly, especially from a sitting or reclining position, and to avoid operating heavy equipment or machinery or driving should sedation or drowsiness occur. It is important to tell clients that they will develop tolerance to the sedating properties of the *benzodiazepines.* If clients are allergic to one benzodiazepine agent they will most likely be allergic to the other benzodiazepines. The nurse should educate clients that many OTC drugs interact with the anti-anxiety drugs and therefore clients should always check with their healthcare provider before using any OTC drugs. Taking anti-anxiety agents during pregnancy or lactation is discouraged because of possible adverse effects to the fetus or baby. Clients should also be reminded to keep these drugs and other medications out of the reach of children because of the potential for severe effects and possibly death. In some clients only small amounts of medications may be dispensed at any one time to minimize the risk of

suicide attempt. When administering hydroxyzine intramuscularly, the nurse should use the Z-track method to prevent tissue injury at the site of injection. Lorazepam is often administered intravenously as an adjunct to anaesthesia; in this setting it should be administered with the proper diluent in equal amounts and infused at a rate of 2 mg or less over 1 minute. Lorazepam given intramuscularly should be given deep into a large muscle mass. Clients should always be advised to take the medication as directed and never to abruptly withdraw it.

The *antimanic drug* lithium is used mainly for clients who are in a manic state, but its exact mechanism of action is unknown. Crucial to its safe use, however, is keeping the client adequately hydrated and in a state of electrolyte balance because its excretion is decreased (therefore leading to increased serum levels) under conditions of hyponatremia. If fluids are not restricted, clients should be encouraged to consume plenty to reduce thirst and to maintain normal fluid balances. High levels of sodium increase the excretion of lithium and may decrease blood levels of the drug. Clients who are dehydrated may also experience lithium toxicity. Lithium should be taken on a regular basis at the same time every day; if a dose is forgotten the client should contact his or her healthcare provider. With initial treatment the side effects of fine hand tremors, increased thirst and urination, nausea, diarrhea, and anorexia may occur and will be transient. Side effects to report to the healthcare provider immediately include extreme hand tremors, sedation, muscle weakness, vomiting, and vertigo.

Antidepressants must be administered carefully per the physician's order, and it is important for clients to realize that it often takes 1 to 3 or even 4 weeks before the therapeutic effects are evident. The nurse must make sure that the client understands this and continues to take the medication as prescribed. Careful monitoring of the client and providing supportive care and therapy are important during this time. Taking these drugs with food often helps to decrease GI upset. Taking them with 4 to 6 ounces of water or other fluid also helps. The more potent and often older drugs, such as the *MAOIs* and *TCAs,* are associated with more side effects. If the sedation that may occur with some of the antidepressants continues after a period of 2 to 3 weeks, the physician should be notified. When administering an antidepressant for the first time, especially to geriatric or weakened clients, the nurse should assist them with ambulation and other activities during which falls may occur as a result of drowsiness or postural hypotension. Clients should be encouraged to consume at least 6 to 8 glasses of water a day to help with hydration and decrease the side effects of dry mouth and constipation. An increase in fibre intake may also help to counteract constipation. Sucking on hard candy (diet forms available), chewing gum, and using OTC saliva drops may be helpful in relieving the discomfort of dry mouth that may occur with some of these drugs.

SSRIs, a safer group of antidepressants with a lower potential for overdosage, are often preferred for the treatment of depression. Clients on long-term therapy with SSRIs, such as 4 to 6 months, need to be closely monitored for the therapeutic effects of the drug and they also need information about possible problems with GI upset, sexual dysfunction, and weight gain. It is important for nurses to know that the SSRI "discontinuation syndrome" will be diminished if the client has his or her SSRI tapered while coming off the drug. Tapering should take place over a minimum of 1 to 2 months. Brief periods of forgetting to take the medication may result in the client experiencing discontinuation syndrome, with symptoms of dizziness, diarrhea, movement disorders, insomnia, irritability, visual disturbance, lethargy, anorexia, and lowered mood. As mentioned previously, serotonin syndrome may occur when the SSRI is taken along with MAOIs, St. John's wort (herbal product), or tryptophan (a serotonin precursor). Signs and symptoms of this syndrome include diarrhea, nausea, abdominal cramping, mental status changes, restlessness, diaphoresis, shivering, tremors, ataxia, headaches, and hyper-reflexia. These symptoms need to be immediately reported to the prescribing physician or, if necessary, to any other healthcare professional. Sexual dysfunction may be managed by taking the following measures:

1 Waiting to see if the side effect goes away as a result of tolerance to the drug.

2 Reducing the current dose of the drug (the healthcare professional—not the client!).

3 The physician inducing a "drug holiday" where the client is monitored closely—sometimes in a hospital setting—while the drug is discontinued.

4 Substituting medication and using agents such as sildenafil citrate, bethanechol, and yohimbine to reverse anorgasmia.

It is important for the nurse to inform the client that the initial sedation with the SSRI demands extra safety measures when participating in activities; it may be wise to avoid driving for a brief period. The nurse should discourage the use of OTC products when the client has a cold or the flu and encourage the client to contact his or her healthcare provider for an acceptable prescription for the symptoms. This is important because many OTC preparations and cough preparations interact adversely with the SSRIs and may precipitate serotonin syndrome.

MAOIs are potent antidepressants and are reserved for those clients who do not respond to TCAs or other modes of therapy. Both the MAOIs and TCAs may be replaced therapeutically with the SSRIs. The side effects of these agents are often severe, and include orthostatic hypotension, dysrhythmias, ataxia, hallucinations, seizures, tremors, dry mouth, and erectile dysfunction. Clients should be told to contact their physician if any of these side effects occur. In addition, tachycardia, seizures, respiratory depression, mental confusion, and restlessness may occur as a result of overdose and can persist for several weeks. The onset of any of these symptoms should be immediately reported to and discussed with the physician. The desired antidepressant effects of MAOIs do not usually occur until 1 to 4 weeks after the start of therapy. Clients should be weaned carefully from these medications a few weeks before any surgical procedure.

If a client who has been taking *TCAs* is scheduled to undergo a surgical procedure, it is important to wean him or her off the medication a few days beforehand so that an interaction with the anaesthetic agents does not occur; however, this is only done with a physician's order. During TCA treatment, it is important for the nurse to recognize and document the occurrence of blurred vision, excessive drowsiness or sleepiness, urinary retention, or constipation and to consult and discuss this with the physician. It is also important to emphasize the need for the client on long-term therapy to wear a medical alert bracelet or tag naming the agent being taken.

Second- and *third-generation antidepressants* have fewer systemic and less severe side effects than the MAOIs and TCAs, and geriatric clients seem to tolerate them fairly well. As a result they are more commonly used. However, it is important for the nurse to inform clients that maximum clinical effectiveness may take up to 6 weeks to reach with these drugs. Clients should know if their agent causes sedation (e.g., trazodone) and should be told that a tolerance to this side effect will develop. It is important to educate male clients taking trazodone about the potential for priapism (prolonged penile erection), which occurs more often in younger men who are on high dosages but can also occur with recommended dosages. Should this side effect occur, the client should stop the medication immediately and seek medical advice. Emergency or surgical intervention may be needed in a small percentage of cases.

Bupropion and venlafaxine both come in sustained-release formulations and therefore a convenient once- or twice-a-day dosing is allowed. In addition to its use for treatment of depression, bupropion may be used as an antidote for SSRI-induced sexual dysfunction. Mirtazapine is effective with depression and may also be used for its anxiolytic properties. As with the other newer-generation antidepressants, mirtazapine may also be used as an antidote for SSRI-induced sexual dysfunction. It is better tolerated than other antidepressants in clients who are medically ill and/or taking multiple medications.

Haloperidol, along with its use for treating psychotic disorders, is also indicated and used to treat Tourette's syndrome and is used in pediatric psychiatry. Its use in children is mainly because it has fewer anticholinergic side effects and milder hypotensive effects. Clients need to be aware that when taking haloperidol they need to take it exactly as prescribed and to be adherent (often difficult with the clients it is used with, such as those with schizophrenia) because it is associated with a narrow "therapeutic window," meaning that serum levels below 4 μg/L and above 22 μg/L may result in either lack of therapeutic effects (with the lower level) or toxicity (with the higher level). Therefore haloperidol is not necessarily the best agent to use because of the risk for under- or overmedicating.

Antipsychotic agents come in a variety of "packages." Atypical agents—such as clozapine, risperidone, olanzapine, and quetiapine—are used because of the minimal risk for TD, lower incidence of EPS, and an increase in cognition. The older, more traditional drugs, such as chlorpromazine, are more highly protein-bound and therefore have many drug interactions. They are also associated with more side effects, which may be severe, such as anticholinergic effects (photophobia, dry mouth, mydriasis with increased intraocular pressure [IOP], sedation, constipation, urinary retention); antiadrenergic effects (hypotension); and the risk of dysrhythmias, decreased cardiac output, and tachycardia. EPS occur in up to 90 percent of the clients taking these older, more traditional antipsychotics, and up to 50 percent have side effects such as dystonias, TD, neuroleptic malignant syndromes, and many others as presented earlier in this chapter. Thus it is easy to understand why they may not be commonly used in certain clients. When using these traditional, older agents, clients should be taught to avoid the following:

1 Hot baths and saunas (precipitates further drop in BP)
2 Abrupt withdrawal of the drug (induces withdrawal psychosis)
3 Sun exposure (because of photosensitivity)
4 Ignoring signs and symptoms of sore throat, malaise, fever, and bleeding
5 Hot climates (to prevent further drops in BPs and hyperthermia)

In general the phenothiazine antipsychotics should be taken as prescribed: often a once-a-day dosing at the same time each day; without street drugs, alcohol, or OTCs (unless approved by the healthcare provider); and for the entire duration—often lifelong.

With any of the antipsychotic drugs, it is important for the nurse to monitor the drug therapy and determine whether the client is adherent. If not, then it is important to get the client switched to a parenteral dosage form such as depot (longer releasing preparation) intramuscular injections. Antipsychotic drugs available for injection include chlorpromazine, fluphenazine, haloperidol, loxapine, perphenazine, thiothixene, and trifluoperazine.

Because all antipsychotic agents are quite potent, the nurse must be sure that any oral dosage form has been swallowed and not tucked in the side of the mouth or under the tongue. Oral forms of the antipsychotics are generally well absorbed and will cause less GI upset if taken with food or a full glass of water. Hard candy or gum may be used to relieve dry mouth. Perspiration may be

increased; therefore clients should be warned about engaging in excessive activity or being exposed to hot or humid climates. Excessive sweating could lead to dehydration and then drug toxicity.

With the newer antipsychotic agent, quetiapine, the nurse should assist clients with ambulation until they have been stabilized on the medication. Clients should be taught to change positions slowly to avoid fainting caused by postural hypotension. Increasing fluids may help decrease constipation, and sips of water, candy, and gum may help with dry mouth. Some of the other atypical antipsychotic agents have the characteristics of fewer EPS, increased cognition, and reduction of TD and therefore may be used more commonly. The newer drugs (dibenzodiazepine [clozapine], benzisoxazole [risperidone], thienobenzodiazepine [olanzapine], or dibenzothiazepine [quetiapine]) may be used more commonly. It is important for the nurse to remember that although these drugs have different qualities and fewer of the most serious side effects, there are still side effects and concerns associated with their use. These newer drugs do appear to be more efficient for those individuals who are treatment resistant or who are exhibiting many adverse effects. However, lethal blood dyscrasias (the nurse should monitor CBCs more frequently) and EPS, anticholinergic, antiadrenergic, and antihistamine adverse effects may occur with the use of clozapine, limiting its use.

Client education and adherence are the keys to successful treatment. Often it is the mental disorder itself that causes clients to not adhere to treatment. Clients must be taught that overdoses can occur when these drugs are mixed with alcohol and other CNS depressants, leading to respiratory and/or cardiovascular collapse, which are often fatal.

In summary, with all of the psychotropic medications, clients need to know how to properly self-medicate and when to contact the physician. Drug interactions and factors to avoid (e.g., hot climates, saunas, certain foods) need to be reinforced, as well as the need for follow-up appointments and repeat laboratory studies to assess blood levels of the drug, electrolyte levels, and even possible side effects. Also, clients need to be involved in some form of professional counselling with a mental healthcare provider (psychiatrist or nurse practitioner) and/or a licensed clinical worker so that they are always monitored. Group therapy sessions are also available for the client and significant others. Client teaching tips for these agents are presented on p. 269.

■ Evaluation

Both the therapeutic effects of psychotropic medications and the client's progress within the treatment regimen must be monitored. Mental alertness, cognition, affect, mood, the ability to carry out ADLs, appetite, and sleep patterns need to be closely monitored and documented.

In addition to drug therapy, the client must work and seek consultation to acquire effective coping skills. Psychotherapy, relaxation therapy, and an increase in exercise can all help in this regard. Before evaluation of the specific psychotherapeutic drugs is discussed it is important to mention that blood levels are often drawn with these drugs so that therapeutic levels are maintained and toxic levels and/or undermanagement are prevented.

The therapeutic effects of *anti-anxiety agents* are evidenced by improved mental alertness, cognition, and mood; fewer anxiety and panic attacks; improved sleep patterns and appetite; more interest in self and others; less tension and irritability; and fewer feelings of fear, impending doom, and stress. Adverse effects to watch for in clients taking anti-anxiety agents include hypotension, lethargy, fatigue, drowsiness, confusion, constipation, dry mouth, blood dyscrasias, lightheadedness, and insomnia.

Adverse reactions to *antidepressants* in general consist of drowsiness, dry mouth, constipation, dizziness, postural hypotension, sedation, blood dyscrasias, and tremors. Overdose is evidenced by irritability, agitation, CNS irritability, seizures, and then progression to CNS depression with respiratory or cardiac depression.

Lithium's therapeutic effects are characterized by less mania, and it is during the manic phase that lithium is better tolerated by the client. Therapeutic levels of lithium range from 1.0 to 1.5 mmol/L and should be determined frequently, every few days initially and then at least every few months while the client is on the drug. The nurse should also monitor the client's mood, affect, and emotional stability. Adverse reactions to lithium include dysrhythmias, hypotension, sedation, slurred speech, slowed motor abilities, and weight gain. GI symptoms such as diarrhea and vomiting, drowsiness, weakness, and unsteady gait are indicative of overdose. The physician should be consulted immediately if these occur. Clients taking clozapine should exhibit improvement in their schizophrenic state. When evaluating for adverse effects such as development of agranulocytosis, it is important for the nurse to remember that it is associated with minor to no EPS.

As antidepressants, *SSRIs* may take up to 8 weeks to reach a full therapeutic effect. They are also associated with the therapeutic effects of improved mood/mental status; improved ability to carry out ADLs; and less insomnia without an overproduction of the side effects of weight gain, sedation, headache, insomnia, GI upset and complaints, dizziness, agitation, and sexual dysfunction. Serotonin syndrome is characterized by tachycardia, confusion, malaise, manic-like states, hyperthermia, profuse sweating, NMS, and eventually cardiovascular collapse.

Other therapeutic effects of the SSRIs and other antidepressants are improved sleep patterns and nutrition, increased feelings of self-esteem, decreased feelings of hopelessness, and an increased interest in self and appearance.

MAOIs are potent antidepressants, but therapeutic effects do not occur for up to 4 weeks after the start of therapy. The effects are similar to those produced by *TCAs*. Adverse effects include sedation, dry mouth, constipation, postural hypotension, blurred vision, seizures, and tremors. Toxic reactions are manifested by confusion or hypotension and possibly by respiratory or cardiac distress. The potential for drug–food interactions cannot be overemphasized because of the violent hypertension that can result when these agents are taken with foods and beverages high in tyramine.

The therapeutic effects of *haloperidol*, another antipsychotic agent, are similar to those of the other agents, but the nurse should monitor the client for adverse reactions particular to haloperidol. These include sedation; tic-like, trembling movements of the hands, face, neck, and head; hypotension; and dry mouth. Overdose is manifested by severe sedation, hypotension, respiratory depression, and coma. It takes approximately 3 weeks for the therapeutic effects of haloperidol to appear, but it is still important for the nurse to watch the client for possible dyskinesia and trembling during this early period. Should these occur, the nurse should consult the physician immediately to discuss possible actions.

The therapeutic effects of *antipsychotic drugs* (e.g., phenothiazines, non-phenothiazines, and quetiapine; AAPs) should include improvement in mood and affect and alleviation of the psychotic symptoms and episodes. Emotional instability, hallucinations, paranoia, delusions, garbled speech, and inability to cope should begin to abate once the client has been on the medication for several weeks. It is critical that the nurse carefully monitor a client's potential to injure himself or herself or others during the delay between the start of therapy and symptomatic improvement. It is also important that the nurse watch the client for the development of adverse reactions to phenothiazines. These include dizziness and syncope stemming from orthostatic hypotension, tachycardia, confusion, drowsiness, insomnia, hyperglycemia, blood dyscrasias, and dry mouth. Overdose is manifested by excessive CNS depression, severe hypotension, and EPS such as dyskinesias and tremors. These symptoms should be reported immediately to the physician. Other side effects to monitor for with the AAPs include the anticholinergic-, antiadrenergic-, antihistaminic-, and prolactin-related side effects, as well as the risk for extrapyramidal side effects.

CLIENT TEACHING TIPS

The nurse should teach the following to clients, as appropriate:

▲ It might take 2 to 4 weeks to notice the full therapeutic effects of antidepressants. These drugs remain in the body long after they have been discontinued. Close monitoring during this lag time is crucial to your safety. (Note: A short-term drug may be used for a brief period to help with symptoms while the client is waiting for the main drug to have its onset of action.)

▲ Take medications as prescribed and do not discontinue them abruptly. If the doctor decides to stop this medication, you will probably be "weaned off": that is, your dose will be gradually reduced.

▲ Do not skip or omit any doses and do not double up on the medication. If you remember you have not taken your medication and it is within 1 or 2 hours of the time you would have taken it, then go ahead and take the dose. If it is more than 2 hours after this time, skip that dose and take the medication at the next scheduled time.

▲ Keep medications out of the reach of children.

▲ Change positions slowly to avoid fainting or dizziness. Call your physician immediately should you experience any fainting episodes while taking these medications.

▲ If you experience drowsiness and sedating effects, do not operate heavy equipment or machinery.

▲ Avoid consuming alcohol and taking other CNS depressants.

▲ Do not take OTC medications or any other medications without checking with your physician first.

▲ Report palpitations, confusion, fatigue, mania, and high fever to your healthcare provider immediately. (Note: Serotonin syndrome may occur when SSRIs are taken with MAOIs, tryptophan, and St. John's wort or when any of these agents is used alone.)

▲ Report any sexual dysfunction as well, because of the possible interventions that may help.

▲ You may experience more drowsiness during the beginning of treatment. With the TCAs this should decrease after the first few weeks of therapy.

▲ Contact your physician if you experience sores in the mouth, fever, sore throat, hallucinations, confusion, disorientation, shortness of breath, difficulty in breathing, yellow discoloration of the skin or eyes, or irritability.

▲ Consumption of caffeine and caffeinated beverages such as cola, tea, and coffee, as well as nicotine, decrease the effectiveness of your medication.

▲ Keep all appointments and follow-up visits with your physician and other healthcare providers.

▲ Always carry or wear a medical alert tag naming the medication you are taking.

▲ The therapeutic effects of MAOIs may not occur for up to 4 weeks. Therefore do not alter your dosing if you are not feeling better before this time.

▲ With MAOIs, remember that a hypertensive crisis may occur if you consume foods and beverages high in tyramine, such as cheese, beer, wine, avocados, bananas, and liver. Avoid caffeinated beverages as well. Remember that the drug will remain in the body for up to 2 weeks after discontinuing the medication. Contact your physician should you experience chest pain, a severe throbbing headache, rapid pulse, or nausea.

▲ Avoid abrupt withdrawal of MAOIs.

▲ Take all antipsychotic medications exactly as prescribed; do not double, omit, or skip doses. Remember, it may be several weeks before an improvement is experienced.

▲ Phenothiazines may cause drowsiness, dizziness, or fainting; therefore change positions slowly.

▲ Wear sunscreen when taking phenothiazines because of photosensitivity. Avoid taking antacids or antidiarrheal preparations within 1 hour of a phenothiazine dose. Notify your physician immediately should you note fever, sore throat, yellow discoloration of the skin, or uncontrollable movements of the tongue while taking a phenothiazine.

▲ Do not take phenothiazines or haloperidol with alcohol or with any other CNS depressant.

▲ Long-term haloperidol therapy may result in tremors, nausea, vomiting, or uncontrollable shaking of small muscle groups, and any of these symptoms should be reported to your physician. Avoid abrupt withdrawal with this drug.

▲ Lithium is to be taken exactly as prescribed; do not double, skip, or omit doses; do not discontinue abruptly. It may take several weeks before any improvement related to the drug therapy is noted.

▲ With lithium, fluid volume status is important. If you become ill with vomiting or diarrhea or are unable to eat or drink, it is important that you notify your physician of this immediately. Dehydration of any type, even as the result of excessive sweating, may result in lithium toxicity.

▲ Many of the side effects of lithium will disappear with time; however, you should contact your physician if you experience any excessive vomiting, tremors, weakness, or any involuntary movements.

▲ Make sure to keep your appointments while taking lithium, especially when blood is to be drawn to determine the serum lithium levels. Always carry or wear a medical alert tag with medications identified. Do not discontinue this drug abruptly.

POINTS to REMEMBER

▼ Psychosis is a major emotional disorder that impairs mental function. A person suffering from psychosis cannot participate in everyday life and shows the hallmark symptom of loss of contact with reality.

▼ Affective disorders are emotional disorders characterized by changes in mood and range from mania (abnormally elevated emotions) to depression (abnormally reduced emotions).

▼ Anxiety, a normal physiological emotion, may be a healthy reaction but becomes pathological when it becomes life altering.

▼ There are six main types of anxiety disorder: OCD, PTSD, GAD, panic disorder, social phobia, and simple phobia.

▼ Situational anxiety arises with specific life events.

▼ Anxiety, if life altering, may be treated with psychotherapy and drugs. This is indicated when the anxiety markedly affects quality of life, relationships, or normal functioning.

▼ Benzodiazepines remain the drug of choice for treatment of anxiety, are most often prescribed, are considered to be fairly safe, and do not interact with many other drugs.

▼ Flumazenil, a benzodiazepine antagonist, blocks the benzodiazepine receptor; it directly opposes the actions of the benzodiazepines and is used to reverse the sedative effects of benzodiazepines.

▼ SSRIs are fairly new and are considered second-generation antidepressants.

▼ SSRIs are often prescribed because of their superiority to TCAs and MAOIs in terms of side effect and safety profiles.

▼ SSRIs specifically and potently inhibit presynaptic serotonin reuptake.

▼ *Antipsychotics* and *neuroleptics* are terms that refer to the drugs commonly used to treat serious mental illnesses. They are used to treat BPD, psychoses, schizophrenia, and autism.

▼ In the past antipsychotics were called *tranquilizers* because they produce a state of tranquility.

▼ *Neuroleptics* are thus termed because they work on abnormally functioning nerves.

▼ Nursing considerations related to psychotherapeutic agents include astute assessment of medication and drug history and medical past and present history.

▼ Nursing actions focus on adequate use of the nursing process with all types of psychotherapeutic medications and informing clients that their medications must be taken exactly as prescribed and that they need to avoid alcohol and other CNS depressants (as well as many other medications) to maintain client safety. Frequent blood studies are needed to monitor therapeutic levels of the drugs.

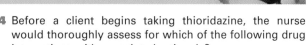

EXAMINATION REVIEW QUESTIONS

1 One of your clients has been diagnosed with delusional thoughts and depression and has been placed on thioridazine 25 mg tid. The physician wants to see how the client responds to the medication. When assessing the client for side effects of this medication, what would the nurse most likely expect to see?
   a. Polyuria with gross proteinuria
   b. Hypertension with severe emesis
   c. Various anemias accompanied by bradydysrhythmias
   d. GI complaints accompanied by possible photosensitivity

2 TCAs are sometimes ordered for depression. Client teaching with these agents would include which of the following points?
   a. Therapeutic effects may take up to 2 to 3 weeks.
   b. Alcohol is permitted with these agents, unlike with other groups of antidepressants.
   c. The medication may be withdrawn without regard to a weaning period.
   d. If a dose is missed, it is important for the client to double up on the doses to maintain adequate blood levels.

3 Depression is a complex disorder that is manifested by other symptoms besides a change in mood. TCAs, used to treat depression, may also help decrease which of the other manifestations of depression?
   a. Hepatitis
   b. Nephritis
   c. Anorexia
   d. Akathisia

4 Before a client begins taking thioridazine, the nurse would thoroughly assess for which of the following drug interactions with associated rationale?
   a. Acetaminophen, because it enhances thioridazine's constriction on vessels
   b. Alcohol, because it vasoconstricts and would increase thioridazine's side effect of hypertension
   c. Beta-blockers, because they will exacerbate the orthostatic hypotension associated with thioridazine
   d. Sodium warfarin, because it potentiates thioridazine's common side effect of hemorrhage

5 Which of the following, when administered with lithium, increases the risk of toxicity?
   a. Diuretics
   b. Lomefloxacin
   c. Calcium iodide
   d. Sodium bicarbonate

For answers see http://evolve.elsevier.com/Lilley/pharmacology/.

CRITICAL THINKING ACTIVITIES

1 What conditions would be responsible for decreasing the excretion of lithium from the body? Explain the impact of this decrease on the client.

2 Mrs. B. has inadvertently been given too much lorazepam and is experiencing respiratory arrest. The benzodiazepine reversal agent flumazenil has been ordered. The dose called for is 0.2 mg delivered over 15 seconds, then another 0.2 mg if consciousness does not occur after 45 seconds. This is to be repeated at 60-second intervals as needed up to four additional times for a maximum total dose of 1 mg. Flumazenil is available as a 0.1-mg/mL vial. What dose should you draw up into the needle to deliver 0.2 mg each time?

3 Mr. H. has a psychotic disorder that has been controlled on chlorpromazine therapy (50 mg q4h) until recently, when severe anticholinergic side effects from chlorpromazine, a low-potency antipsychotic, have necessitated

his being switched to haloperidol, a high-potency antipsychotic. The physician would like to know what the equivalent daily dose of haloperidol would be. What is the equivalent daily dose of haloperidol?

4 A 51-year-old client arrives at the doctor's office for his annual physical. As the intake nurse, you do a brief assessment and take a short drug history. He states that he has started taking St. John's wort for depression and wants to know what the doctor thinks. You document this in the chart and research this information because you are not that familiar with herbal products. What is St. John's wort? Is it safe for clients to use for depressive symptoms? What information is important to remember about this herbal product? What information is really crucial to share with clients in the future if they state that they are taking this supplement?

For answers see http://evolve.elsevier.com/Lilley/pharmacology/.

BIBLIOGRAPHY

Albanese, J., & Nutz, P. (2005). *Mosby's 2005 nursing drug cards.* St Louis, MO: Mosby.

Anderson, I. (2001). Meta-analytical studies on new antidepressants. *British Medical Bulletin, 57,* 161–178.

Aquila, R. (2002). Management of weight gain in patients with schizophrenia. *Journal of Clinical Psychiatry, 63*(Suppl 4), 33–36.

Bakish, D. (2001). New standard of depression treatment: Remission and full recovery. *Journal of Clinical Psychiatry, 62*(Suppl 26), 5–8.

Bowden, C. (2001). Clinical correlates of therapeutic response in bipolar disorder. *Journal of Affective Disorders, 67*(1–3), 257–265.

Brady, K., & Kaltsounis-Puckett, J. (2002). Major depressive disorder with anxiety symptoms or sleep disturbance. *Journal of Clinical Psychiatry, 63*(Suppl 1), 5–7.

Buckley, P. (2001). Broad therapeutic uses of atypical antipsychotic medications. *Biological Psychiatry, 50*(11), 912–924.

Calabrese, J, Shelton M, Rapport, D. J., & Kimmel, S. E. (2002). Bipolar disorders and the effectiveness of novel anticonvulsants. *Journal of Clinical Psychiatry, 63*(Suppl 3), 5–9.

Canadian Pharmacists Association. (2003). *Therapeutic choices* (4th ed.). Ottawa, ON: Author.

Canadian Pharmacists Association. (2004). *Guide to drugs in Canada.* Toronto, ON: Dorling Kindersley.

Canadian Pharmacists Association. (2005). *Compendium of pharmaceuticals and specialties. The Canadian drug reference for health professionals.* Ottawa, ON: Author. [The subscription-based e-CPS is available at http://www.pharmacists.ca.]

Enns, M.W., Swenson, J.R., McIntyre, R.S., Swinson, R.P., & Kennedy, S.H. (2001). Clinical guidelines for the treatment of depressive disorders. VII. Comorbidity. *Canadian Journal of Psychiatry, 46*(Suppl 1), 77–90S.

Facts and Comparisons. (2004). *Drug facts and comparisons pocket version* (9th ed.). St Louis, MO: Wolters Kluwer Health.

Fortinash, K.M. & Holoday Worret, P.A. (2004). *Psychiatric mental health nursing* (3rd ed.). St. Louis, MO: Mosby.

Garland, E.J. (2004). Facing the evidence: Antidepressant treatment in children and adolescents. *Canadian Medical Association Journal, 170*(4), 489–491.

Glassman, A. (2002). Clinical management of cardiovascular risks during treatment with psychotropic drugs. *Journal of Clinical Psychiatry, 63*(Suppl 9), 12–17.

Hardman, J.G., & Limbird, L.E. (2002). *Goodman and Gilman's the pharmacological basis of therapeutics* (10th ed.). New York: McGraw-Hill.

Health Canada. (2004). Health Canada advises Canadians of stronger warnings for SSRIs and other newer anti-depressants. Retrieved July 31, 2005, from http://www.hc-sc.gc.ca/ ahc-asc/ media/advisories-avis/2004/2004_31_e.htm

Health Canada. (2004). Health Canada is advising Canadians that antidepressant trazodone may interact with certain medications. Retrieved July 31, 2005, from http://www.hc-sc. gc.ca/ahc-asc/media/advisories-avis/2004/2004_38_e.htm

Health Canada. (2005). Public Advisory. Health Canada endorsed important safety information on Paxil (paroxetine). Retrieved November 11, 2005 from http://www.hc-sc.gc.ca/dhp-mps/ medeff/advisories-avis/public/paxil_3_pa-ap_e.html

Health Canada. (2005). Drug product database (DPD). Retrieved August 1, 2005, from http://www.hc-sc.gc.ca/hpb/drugs-dpd/

IMS Health. (2005). In Canada, depression ranks as fast-growing diagnosis. Retrieved August 1, 2005, from http://www.imshealth.com/ims/portal/front/articleC/ 0,2777,6599_41382706_57069115,00.html

Johns Hopkins Hospital, Gunn, V.L., & Nechyba, C. (2002). *The Harriet Lane handbook* (16th ed.). St Louis, MO: Mosby.

Keck, P., & McElroy, S. (2002). Clinical pharmacodynamics and pharmacokinetics of antimanic and mood-stabilizing medications. *Journal of Clinical Psychiatry, 63*(Suppl 4), 3–10.

Keltner, N.L., & Folks, D.G. (2003). *Psychotropic drugs* (3rd ed.). St Louis, MO: Mosby.

Kennedy, S., Eisfeld, B., & Cooke, R. (2001). Quality of life: An important dimension in assessing the treatment of depression? *Journal of Psychiatry & Neuroscience, 26*(Suppl), S23–28.

Kennedy, S.H., Lam, R.W., Cohen, N.L., & Ravindran, A.V. (2001). Clinical guidelines for the treatment of depressive disorders. IV. Medications and other biological treatments. *Canadian Journal of Psychiatry, 46*(Suppl 1), 38–58S.

Kullar, A., & McIntyre, R.S. (2004). An approach to managing depression. [Electronic version]. *Canadian Family Physician.* Retrieved August 1, 2005, from http://www.cfpc.ca/cfp/2004/Oct/vol50-oct-cme-1.asp

Lacy, C.F., Armstrong, L.L., Goldman, M.P., & Lance, L.L. (2003). *Drug information handbook* (11th ed.). Hudson, OH: Lexi-Comp.

Lin, K., & Smith, M. (2001). Culture and psychopharmacology. *Psychiatric Clinics of North America, 24*(3), 523–538.

Malhotra, S., & McElroy, S. (2002). Medical management of obesity associated with mental disorders. *Journal of Clinical Psychiatry, 63*(Suppl 4), 24–30.

Mitchell, P., & Malhi, G. (2002). The expanding pharmacopoeia for bipolar disorders. *Annual Review of Medicine, 53,* 173–188.

Mosby (2005). *Mosby's drug consult 2005: The comprehensive reference for generic and brand name drugs* (15th ed.). St Louis, MO: Mosby.

Naber, D., &, Karow, A. (2001). Good tolerability equals good results: The patient's perspective. *European Neuropsychopharmacology, 11*(Suppl 4), S391–396.

MacMillan, H.L., Patterson, C.J.S., Wathen, C.N., & the Canadian Task Force on Preventive Health Care. (2005). Screening for depression in primary care: Recommendation from the Canadian Task Force on Preventive Health Care. [Electronic version]. *Canadian Medical Association Journal, 172*(1). Retrieved July 31, 2005, from http://www.cmaj.ca/cgi/data/172/1/33/DC1/1

Milin, R., Walker, S., & Chow, J. (2003). Major depressive disorder in adolescence: A brief review of the recent treatment literature. [Electronic version]. *Canadian Journal of Psychiatry, 48.*

Olver, J., Burrows, G., & Norman, T. (2001). Third-generation antidepressants: Do they offer advantages over the SSRIs? *CNS Drugs, 15*(12), 941–954.

Parikh, S.V., & Lam, R.W. (2001). Clinical guidelines for the treatment of depressive disorders. I. Definitions, prevalence, and health burden. *Canadian Journal of Psychiatry, 46*(Suppl 1), 13–20S.

Piepho, R. (2001). Cardiovascular effects of antipsychotics used in bipolar illness. *Journal of Clinical Psychiatry, 63*(Suppl 4), 20–23.

Reesal, R.T., & Lam R.W. (2001). Clinical guidelines for the treatment of depressive disorders. II. Principles of management. *Canadian Journal of Psychiatry, 46*(Suppl 1), 21–28S.

Segal, Z.V., Kennedy, S.H., & Cohen, N.L. (2001). Clinical guidelines for the treatment of depressive disorders. V. Combining psychotherapy and pharmacotherapy. *Canadian Journal of Psychiatry, 46*(Suppl 1), 59–62S.

Segal, Z.V., Whitney, D.K., & Lam, R.W. (2001). Clinical guidelines for the treatment of depressive disorders. III. Psychotherapy. Canadian Journal of Psychiatry, 46(Suppl 1), 29–37S.

Shriqui, C.L. (2002). Atypical antipsychotics. *The Canadian Journal of CME 65.* Retrieved August 1, 2005, from http://www.stacommunications.com/journals/pdfs/cme/julycme/g.pdf

Shulman, K. (2002). A review of mood stabilizers in old age: Focus on bipolar disorders. *Journal of Geriatric Care, 1*(3), 275–283.

Skidmore-Roth, L. (2006). *Mosby's 2006 nursing drug reference* (19th ed.). St Louis, MO: Mosby.

Strakowski, S., DelBello, M., & Adler, C. (2001). Comparative efficacy and tolerability of drug treatments for bipolar disorder. *CNS Drugs, 15*(9), 701–718.

Thase, M. (2002). What role do atypical antipsychotic drugs have in treatment-resistant depression? *Journal of Clinical Psychiatry, 63*(2), 95–103.

Thorpe, L., Whitney, D.K., Kutcher, S.P., & Kennedy, S.H. (2001). Clinical guidelines for the treatment of depressive disorders. VI. Special populations. *Canadian Journal of Psychiatry, 46*(Suppl 1), 63–76S.

Van Ameringen, M., & Mancini, C. (2001). Pharmacotherapy of social anxiety disorder at the turn of the millennium. *Psychiatric Clinics of North America, 24*(4), 783–803.

Whiskey, E., Werneke, U., &Taylor, D. (2001). A systematic review and meta-analysis of *Hypericum perforatum* in depression: A comprehensive clinical review. *International Clinical Psychopharmacology, 16*(5), 239–252.

Yatham, L. (2002). The role of novel antipsychotics in bipolar disorders. *Journal of Clinical Psychiatry, 63*(Suppl 3), 10–14.

Central Nervous System Stimulant Agents

OBJECTIVES

After reading this chapter, the successful student will be able to do the following:

1 Identify the various central nervous system (CNS) stimulants with indications and contraindications.

2 Discuss the effects associated with the use of CNS stimulants.

3 Define *analeptic, anorexiant, hyperactivity, attention-deficit disorder,* and *attention-deficit/hyperactivity disorder.*

4 Discuss the mechanisms of action, indications, contraindications, cautions, side effects, and toxic effects of the various CNS stimulants.

5 Identify the various conditions and disorders treated with CNS stimulants.

6 Develop a nursing care plan as related to the nursing process and drugs that stimulate the CNS.

e-LEARNING ACTIVITIES

Student CD-ROM
- Review Questions: see questions 89–93
- Animations
- Medication Administration Checklists
- IV Therapy Checklists

evolve Web site (http://evolve.elsevier.com/Lilley/pharmacology/)
- Online Chapter Worksheet • Frequently Asked Questions
- Learning Tips and Content Updates • WebLinks • Online Appendices and Supplements • Mosby/Saunders ePharmacology Update • Access to *Mosby's Drug Consult*

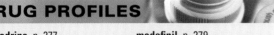

DRUG PROFILES

▶▶**dexedrine**, p. 277
▶▶**caffeine**, p. 276
▶▶**methylphenidate hydrochloride**, p. 279

modafinil, p. 279
orlistat, p. 277
▶▶**sibutramine**, p. 277
▶▶**sumatriptan**, p. 280

▶▶Key drug.

GLOSSARY

Amphetamines (am fet' ə meenz) Central nervous system (CNS) stimulants that produce mood elevation or euphoria, increase mental alertness and capacity to work, decrease fatigue and drowsiness, and prolong wakefulness.

Analeptics (an ə lep' tiks) CNS stimulants that have generalized effects on the brainstem and spinal cord, which in turn produces an increase in responsiveness to external stimuli and stimulates respiration.

Anorexiants (an ə rek' see ənts) Drugs used to control or suppress appetite. These also stimulate the CNS.

Attention-deficit/hyperactivity disorder (ADHD) Syndrome affecting children, adolescents, and adults. It is characterized by a persistent pattern of inattention, hyperactivity–impulsivity, or both that may contribute to learning difficulties and behavioural problems.

Central nervous system (CNS) stimulants Drugs that stimulate a specific area of the brain or spinal cord.

Narcolepsy (nar' ko lep see) Syndrome characterized by sudden sleep attacks, cataplexy, sleep paralysis, and visual or auditory hallucinations at the onset of sleep.

Serotonin agonists (ser ə toe' nin ag' ə nists) A new class of CNS stimulants used to treat migraines; they work by stimulating 5-HT1 receptors in the brain and are sometimes referred to as selective serotonin receptor agonists (SSRAs) or triptans.

Sympathomimetic agents (sim' pə tho mi met' ik) Another name for CNS stimulants.

CENTRAL NERVOUS SYSTEM STIMULANTS

Central nervous system (CNS) stimulants are drugs that stimulate a specific area of the brain or spinal cord. Many of the actions mimic those of the sympathetic nervous system (SNS) neurotransmitters norepinephrine and epinephrine. For this reason they are sometimes referred to as **sympathomimetic agents.** CNS stimulants elevate mood, produce a sense of increased energy and alertness, decrease appetite, and enhance the performance of tasks impaired by fatigue or boredom. Two of the oldest known stimulants are cocaine and amphetamine. These are also the prototypical agents. Cocaine is a natural alkaloid that was first extracted from the plant *Erythroxylon coca* in the mid-nineteenth century but had been used by natives of the Andes for its stimulant effects for centuries before. Caffeine, which is contained in coffee and tea, is another plant-derived CNS stimulant.

CNS activity is regulated by a checks-and-balances system, which consists of both excitatory and inhibitory systems. CNS stimulation can result from either excessive stimulation of the excitatory neurons or blockade of the inhibitory neurons; however, most CNS stimulants act by stimulating the excitatory neurons in the brain. There are many such drugs, but only a few have therapeutic properties.

There are two ways to classify these therapeutic CNS stimulants. The first is according to their location of action in the CNS, and hence the site where they produce their therapeutic effects (Table 16-1). CNS stimulants may also be classified on the basis of structural similarities (Table 16-2). However CNS stimulants are classified, their therapeutic applications are limited to five areas. They can be used as analeptics (CNS stimulants); as appetite suppressants; and for the treatment of **attention-deficit/hyperactivity disorder (ADHD),** narcolepsy, and migraine headache.

Amphetamines produce mood elevation or euphoria, increase mental alertness and the capacity for work, decrease fatigue and drowsiness, and prolong wakefulness. They are used to treat narcolepsy and ADHD. Amphetamines produce tolerance and psychological dependence. They are associated with a high abuse potential and are therefore classified as Schedule G of Canada's Food and Drugs Regulations (FDR) and Schedule III of the Controlled Drugs and Substances Act (CDSA) and are legally available only by prescription. Because of this high abuse potential, this class of CNS stimulants is used more commonly for non-medical (recreational) purposes than for therapeutic ones.

Analeptics were used primarily to stimulate respiration when the natural reflex was lost. However, their use has waned as effective modern techniques of mechanical respiratory therapy have become available. In addition, respiratory paralysis caused by overdoses of opioids, alcohol, barbiturates, and general anaesthetics can now be appropriately treated with reversal agents or by more reliable and effective methods of mechanical assistance.

Anorexiants suppress appetite and are used in the treatment of exogenous obesity. According to Statistics Canada, 23 percent of adult Canadians are 20 percent or more overweight. At any given time, 70 percent of overweight women and 48 percent of overweight men are trying to lose weight. An estimated 5.5 million Canadians are overweight. Eight percent of children aged 2 to 17 (approximately 500 000) are considered obese. Aboriginal people, children, and immigrant groups have higher rates of obesity in Canada. Obesity increases the risk for hypertension, coronary artery disease, type 2 diabetes mellitus, gallbladder disease, sleep apnea, gout, and certain types of cancer. One in 10 deaths each year (9.3 percent) is attributed to obesity, making it a leading cause of preventable deaths in Canada. The cost to society is around $1.8 billion annually, yet most people who attempt weight loss do so for cosmetic reasons, not for health reasons. Even healthcare professionals may have a prejudice against overweight people, often believing that the obese do not deserve medical treatment for their condition and insisting that the client lose weight before receiving treatment for other medical conditions (e.g., hypertension).

In June 2001 the Therapeutic Products Program of Health Canada took steps to remove a sympathomimetic anorexiant, phenylpropanolamine (PPA), from the market, alone or in combination with other products. This action followed the lead of the U.S. Food and Drug Administration's Non-prescription Drug Advisory Committee, based on a Yale University study (Kernan et al., 2000), among other data. The conclusion was that the use of PPA is associated with increased incidence of hemorrhagic stroke. Most of these cases involved women but men could also be at risk.

TABLE 16-1
CNS STIMULANTS: SITE OF ACTION

Site of Action	CNS Stimulant
Brainstem	Serotonin agonist
Cerebral cortex	Amphetamines
Hypothalamic and limbic regions	Anorexiants
Medulla and brainstem	Analeptics

TABLE 16-2
STRUCTURALLY RELATED CNS STIMULANTS

Chemical Category	CNS Stimulant
Amphetamines	dextroamphetamine, methylphenidate
Serotonin agonists	naratriptan, rizatriptan, sumatriptan, zolmitriptan
Sympathomimetics	phentermine
Xanthines	caffeine, theophylline

Serotonin agonists, also referred to as selective serotonin receptor agonists (SSRAs), have made dramatic improvements in the treatment of migraine headaches. They have quickly become a standard for the initial choice of therapy for an acute migraine attack. Migraines are a common type of chronic headache and affect about 7 out of 100 people. Migraines most commonly occur in women and usually begin between 12 and 46 years of age, with women between the ages of 25 and 54 years more severely affected. In some cases migraines appear to be hereditary.

Often tension headaches are confused for migraine. Tension headaches are caused by the contraction of the muscles surrounding the skull, decreasing blood flow to the brain. Rarer than migraine, and more painful, are cluster headaches, which usually attack men. The cause of clusters is somewhat of a mystery. Research, however, is providing clues that cluster headaches may be related to the sinuses, the nervous system, and serotonin.

Mechanism of Action and Drug Effects

CNS stimulants have varying mechanisms of action and many effects on the CNS. Analeptics (aminophylline, theophylline, and caffeine) have generalized effects on the brainstem and spinal cord and, as previously stated, tend to stimulate respiration. Methylxanthine analeptics (caffeine, aminophylline, and theophylline) work by inhibiting the enzyme phosphodiesterase. This enzyme breaks down a substance called *cyclic adenosine monophosphate* (cAMP). When the breakdown of cAMP is blocked, cAMP accumulates. This results in relaxation of smooth muscle in the respiratory tract, dilation of pulmonary arterioles, and stimulation of the CNS. Caffeine can stimulate the CNS at almost any level depending on the dose. Its ability to stimulate areas in the CNS is greater than that of the other two methylxanthines.

Anorexiants are believed to work by suppressing appetite control centres in the brain, although this has yet to be proved scientifically. There are some minor differences between these agents in terms of their individual actions. Mazindol resembles the amphetamines from the standpoint of their activity in the CNS, but diethylpropion has little effect on the cardiovascular system. Orlistat works by irreversibly inhibiting the enzyme lipase. This results in decreased amounts of ingested dietary fat absorption and increased fecal fat excretion. Sibutramine works by centrally inhibiting the reuptake of serotonin (enhancing satiety) and norepinephrine (raising metabolic rate). Phentermine has little effect on mood but does cause some cardiovascular stimulation.

As previously mentioned, amphetamines are used to treat ADHD and narcolepsy. These agents are potent stimulators of the CNS, and therefore the potential for problematic use is high. Amphetamines increase the amount and the duration of effect of catecholamine neurotransmitters in the CNS responsible for stimulation, mainly norepinephrine and dopamine. The drugs used to treat ADHD and narcolepsy cause an increase in the release of these neurotransmitters and block their reuptake. As a result of this blockade, norepinephrine and dopamine are in contact with their receptors longer, and therefore their duration of action and effectiveness are prolonged. A novel new agent for the treatment of narcolepsy is modafinil. It is a non-amphetamine stimulant that works by decreasing gamma-aminobutyric acid (GABA)-mediated neurotransmission in the brain.

Many of the effects of CNS stimulants are dose related. Their pharmacological actions are similar to the actions of the SNS in that the CNS and the respiratory system are the primary body systems affected. The CNS effects most commonly noted are increased motor activity and mental alertness, diminished sense of fatigue, emotional or mood elevation, and mild euphoria. The respiratory effects most commonly seen are relaxation of bronchial smooth muscle, increased respiration, and dilation of pulmonary arteries. Other body systems can also be affected by CNS stimulants, including the cardiovascular, gastrointestinal (GI), genitourinary (GU), and endocrine systems. Often stimulation of these other body systems results in the unwanted effects discussed later in this chapter.

Indications

The therapeutic effects of CNS stimulants are varied and best discussed from the standpoint of the individual drug category. The therapeutic effects of analeptics are limited to the relaxation of smooth muscle in the respiratory tract; dilation of pulmonary arterioles; and stimulation of areas within the CNS that control respiration, mainly the medulla and spinal cord.

Anorexiants primarily work by broadly stimulating the CNS. As mentioned previously, it is believed that their action specifically targets the appetite control centres in the brain, but this has yet to be proved. Some evidence points toward increased fat mobilization, decreased absorption of dietary fat, and increased cellular glucose uptake as other possible therapeutic effects.

The agents used to treat ADHD stimulate the areas of the brain responsible for mental alertness and attentiveness—the cerebral cortex and subcortical structures such as the thalamus. This results in increased motor activity and mental alertness and a diminished sense of fatigue.

Narcolepsy is a condition in which clients unexpectedly fall asleep in the middle of normal activity. An agent that can increase mental alertness would be most beneficial in treating a condition such as this, and that is what the amphetamines, the primary agents used to treat narcolepsy, do. The amphetamines' main sites of action in the CNS appear to be the cerebral cortex and possibly the reticular activating system. Stimulation of these areas also results in increased motor activity and a diminished sense of fatigue.

Other therapeutic effects are seen with CNS stimulants such as caffeine. Caffeine may induce diuresis and is a helpful agent in the treatment of migraines when co-administered with other drugs. It does this by increasing blood flow to the kidneys and decreasing the resorption of sodium and water. The constriction of the cerebral blood vessels that caffeine may induce also potentiates the action of the other agents given in combination with it. The constriction of cerebral blood vessels by SSRAs accounts for their beneficial effects in the treatment of migraines as well. However, the mechanism by which SSRAs do this is much different than that of caffeine.

Contraindications

Contraindications to the use of CNS stimulants include known drug allergy, marked anxiety or agitation, glaucoma, Tourette's syndrome, tic disorders, and use of any monoamine oxidase inhibitor (MAOI) within the preceding 14 days.

Side Effects and Adverse Effects

CNS stimulants have a wide range of adverse effects that most often arise at doses higher than the therapeutic doses. These drugs tend to "speed up" body systems. For

example, effects on the cardiovascular system include increased heart rate and blood pressure. The most common undesirable effects associated with the administration of CNS stimulants are listed in Table 16-3 according to the body system affected.

Interactions

The drug interactions associated with CNS stimulants vary greatly from class to class. The drug interactions that occur with analeptics and anorexiants differ from those seen with amphetamines. Those drug interactions most commonly encountered for the three classes of CNS stimulants are listed in Table 16-4.

Dosages

The recommended dosages for selected CNS stimulants are given in the table on p. 278. See Appendix B for some of the brands available in Canada.

DRUG PROFILES

ANALEPTICS

Most analeptic CNS stimulants are highly toxic and have a high potential for problematic use and are therefore only available by prescription. Caffeine is the exception. The profiles for aminophylline and theophylline can be found in Part Six on respiratory system drugs.

▶▶ caffeine

Caffeine is a CNS stimulant that can be found in over-the-counter (OTC) drugs and combination prescription drugs. It is also contained in many beverages and foods. Just a few of the many foods and drugs that contain caffeine are listed in Table 16-5. Caffeine is contraindicated in clients with a known hypersensitivity to it and should be used with caution in clients who have a history of peptic ulcers or cardiac dysrhythmias or who have recently had a myocardial infarction (MI). Caffeine is available in oral (PO) form as 100-mg regular-release tablets. Pregnancy category B. For the recommended

TABLE 16-3
CNS STIMULANTS: COMMON ADVERSE EFFECTS

Body System	Side/Adverse Effects
Cardiovascular	Palpitations, tachycardia, hypertension, angina, dysrhythmias
Central nervous	Nervousness, restlessness, jitteriness, anxiety, insomnia, headache, tremor, blurred vision
Endocrine*	Hypoglycemia, hyperglycemia, increased metabolic rate
Gastrointestinal	Nausea, vomiting, diarrhea, abdominal pain, dry mouth
Genitourinary	Increased urinary frequency, diuresis

*Effects apply only to methylxanthines, such as theophylline.

TABLE 16-4
CNS STIMULANTS: COMMON DRUG INTERACTIONS

Drug	Mechanism	Result
AMPHETAMINES		
Beta-blockers	Increase alpha-adrenergic effects	Hypertension, bradycardia, dysrhythmias, heart block
CNS stimulants	Additive toxicities	Cardiovascular adverse effects, nervousness, insomnia, convulsions
Digoxin	Additive toxicity	Increased risk of dysrhythmias
MAOIs	Increase release of catecholamines	Headaches, dysrhythmias, severe hypertension
TCAs	Additive toxicities	Cardiovascular adverse effects (dysrhythmias, tachycardia, hypertension)
ANOREXIANTS AND ANALEPTICS		
CNS stimulants	Additive toxicities	Nervousness, irritability, insomnia, dysrhythmias, seizures
MAOIs	Increase release of catecholamines	Headaches, dysrhythmias, severe hypertension
Quinolones	Interfere with metabolism	Reduce clearance of caffeine and prolong caffeine's effect
Serotonergic agents	Additive toxicity	Cardiovascular adverse effects, nervousness, insomnia, convulsions

MAOI, monoamine oxidase inhibitor; *TCA*, tricyclic antidepressant.

TABLE 16-5
CAFFEINE-CONTAINING FOODS AND DRUGS

Medications	Amount of Caffeine
NON-PRESCRIPTION MEDICATIONS	
Analgesics	
Anacin; Anacin Extra-Strength	32 mg/tab
Excedrin Extra-Strength	65 mg/tab
Stimulants	
Wake-Up Tablets	100 mg/tab
Acetaminophen compound caplets with codeine	15 mg/caplet
PRESCRIPTION MEDICATIONS (FOR MIGRAINES)	
Fiorinal	40 mg/tab
Cafergot	100 mg/tab
	100 mg/suppository

Beverages	Amount of Caffeine
Coffee (brewed)	80–150 mg/150 mL
Coffee (instant)	80–150 mg/150 mL
Coffee (decaffeinated)	2–4 mg/150 mL
Tea (brewed)	30–75 mg/150 mL
Soft drinks	35–60 mg/360 mL
Cocoa	5–40 mg/150 mL

adult and neonate dosages, refer to the table on p. 278.

PHARMACOKINETICS

Half-Life	Onset	Peak	Duration
3–4 hr	15–45 min	50–75 min	<6 hr

ANOREXIANTS

The majority of anorexiants are CNS stimulants. Diethylpropion and sibutramine suppress appetite control centres in the brain by elevating levels of neurotransmitters such as norepinephrine, serotonin, and dopamine. Until recently the anorexiants were all closely related in chemical structure and mechanism of action. Orlistat, however, is an anorexiant that works by altering fat metabolism. Sibutramine and orlistat are the newest anorexiant agents and appear to offer advantages over older agents with respect to safety and tolerability.

orlistat

Orlistat, one of the newer anorexiants, is unrelated to any of the other anorexiants. It works by blocking the absorption of fat from the GI tract rather than suppressing appetite. Orlistat binds to gastric and pancreatic enzymes called *lipases*. This binding results in inactivation of the enzyme, which prevents absorption of about 30 percent of dietary fat. Restricting dietary intake of fat to less than 30 percent of total calories can help reduce some of the GI side effects. Flatulence with discharge, oily spotting, and fecal urgency can occur in 20 to 40 percent of clients. Decreases in serum concentrations of vitamins A, D, and E and beta-carotene are seen as a result of the blocking of fat absorption. Supplementation with fat-soluble vitamins corrects this deficiency. Orlistat is available in 120-mg capsules. It is

contraindicated in cases of known drug allergy, malabsorption syndrome, or paralysis of the bile tract. Pregnancy category B. Recommended dosages are given in the table on p. 278.

PHARMACOKINETICS

Half-Life	Onset	Peak	Duration
1–2 hr	3 mo*	6–8 hr	Unknown

*Therapeutic effects.

▶▶ sibutramine

Sibutramine is one of the newest anorexiants and is structurally related to amphetamine. It is approved for treatment of obesity and is classified as a Schedule F of the Food and Drug Regulations and requires a prescription. Sibutramine works by inhibiting primarily the reuptake of norepinephrine and serotonin. These neurotransmitters, along with dopamine, are elevated in the brain, resulting in decreased appetite.

The most common side effects are dry mouth, headache, insomnia, and constipation. As with the other amphetamines, some concerns exist over increases in blood pressure (BP) and heart rate. However, to date no heart valve abnormalities have occurred like those that led to the removal of fenfluramine and dexfenfluramine from the market. Another benefit is that clients taking sibutramine have not developed primary pulmonary hypertension, which occurred rarely with some of the other anorexiants.

Sibutramine should not be used with other drugs that elevate serotonin, such as the serotonin-selective reuptake inhibitors (SSRIs) used for depression, SSRAs used for migraines, lithium, meperidine, fentanyl, dextromethorphan, or pentazocine, or within 2 weeks of using an MAOI. It is contraindicated in clients who have shown a hypersensitivity reaction to it or in clients receiving MAOIs, clients who have anorexia nervosa, or clients taking other centrally acting appetite-suppressant drugs. Sibutramine is available as 10- and 15-mg capsules. Pregnancy category C. Recommended dosages are listed in the table on p. 278.

PHARMACOKINETICS

Half-Life	Onset	Peak	Duration
14–16 hr	8 wk	6 mo*	12 mo*

*Therapeutic effects.

AMPHETAMINES

Amphetamines treat ADHD and narcolepsy by increasing the amount and duration of effect of the catecholamine neurotransmitters. The overall response is global CNS excitement and stimulation, with improved mental alertness and attentiveness as the therapeutic effects.

▶▶ dexedrine

Dextroamphetamine is the prototypical CNS stimulant used to treat ADHD and narcolepsy in Canada. When used in the treatment of these conditions it is only as an adjunct to psychological, educational, and social therapies. Its use is associated with a wide array of CNS effects, many of which are undesirable or unintended. It is for these reasons that many of the other drugs used

DOSAGES Selected CNS Stimulants

Agent	Pharmacological Class	Usual Dosage Range	Indications
almotriptan	Serotonin receptor agonist	**Adult only** PO: 6.25–12.5 mg 1 dose; may repeat in 2 hr for a max of 12.5 mg/24 hr	Acute migraine
dextroamphetamine	CNS stimulant	**Pediatric 6–12 yr** PO: 2.5–5 mg daily qid and increased 5 mg weekly until desired effect to a daily max of 40 mg **Adult >12 yr** PO: 10 mg bid or tid; increased 10 mg weekly until desired effect to a daily max of 60 mg	ADHD Adjunctive for narcolepsy
caffeine	Xanthine cerebral stimulant	**Adult** PO: 100–200 mg prn	Aids in staying awake
eletriptan	Serotonin receptor agonist	**Adult only** PO: 20–40 mg × 1 dose; may repeat in 2 hr for a max of 40 mg/24 hr	Acute migraine
methylphenidate (extended-release)	CNS stimulant	**Pediatric and adult** 18–54 mg/day in a single dose	ADHD
methylphenidate	CNS stimulant	**Pediatric ≥6 yr** PO: 5 mg bid before breakfast and lunch and increased weekly until desired effect to a daily max of 60 mg **Adult** PO: 20–60 mg/day divided bid–tid 30–45 min ac	ADHD Narcolepsy
methylphenidate (slow-release)	CNS stimulant	**Pediatric and adult** 20–60 mg/day in a single dose	ADHD
modafinil	CNS stimulant	**Adult** PO: 200 mg/day, up to 400 mg/day	Narcolepsy
orlistat	Lipase inhibitor	**Adult** PO: 120 mg tid with each meal containing fat	Decreases fat absorption
sibutramine	CNS stimulant (anorexiant)	**Adult** PO: 10 mg/day, up to max of 15 mg/day	Appetite control in obesity
sumatriptan	Serotonin agonist	**Adult** PO: 25, 50, or 100 mg, can repeat after 2 hr (max 200 mg/day) SC: 6 mg, can repeat in 1 hr (max 2 injections/day) Nasal spray: 5 or 20 mg, can repeat after 2 hr (max 40 mg/day)	Migraines

to treat narcolepsy and ADHD were developed. Dextroamphetamine is contraindicated in clients who have shown a hypersensitivity reaction to it, as well as in those with the contraindications that apply to the other CNS stimulants. It is available in oral form as 5-mg tablets and 10- and 15-mg slow-release spansules. The latter release an immediate therapeutic dose followed by the remaining dose released gradually to sustain the effects of the drug for 10 to 12 hours. A mixture of amphetamine salts (dextroamphetamine sulphate, dextroamphetamine saccharate, amphetamine sulphate, and amphetamine aspartate) is known as Adderall. In 2005 dextroamphetamine was briefly suspended and removed from the Canadian market because of sudden deaths, heart-related deaths, and strokes in children and adults taking usual recommended doses of dextroamphetamine. Although none of the reported deaths occurred in Canada, 14 deaths occurred in children and 2 in adults internationally. In August 2005, the drug was reinstated with revisions to the labelling warning against using dextroamphetamine XR in clients with structural heart abnormalities. Another warning will advise about the dangers of misusing amphetamines. Dextroamphetamine is a Schedule G drug of the FDR, CDSA Schedule III controlled substance. Pregnancy category C. For recommended dosages, refer to the table on p. 278.

PHARMACOKINETICS

Half-Life	Onset	Peak	Duration
7–14 hr*	30–60 min	<2 hr	10 hr

*pH <6.6

▸▸ methylphenidate hydrochloride

Methylphenidate has become the drug of choice for the treatment of ADHD and narcolepsy. Much attention has been focused on this CNS stimulant because of its dramatic effect in the treatment of ADHD, a condition that may affect adults as well as children. However, this heightened interest may have more to do with the better diagnosis and a growing awareness of the disorder than with the drug's particular attributes. There is some controversy regarding its use, especially among concerned and apprehensive parents. However, proper diagnosis of the disorder, proper dosing of the drug, and regular medical monitoring of the client can significantly help many children in terms of school performance and social skills. Psychosocial problems within a child's family should be ruled out or addressed if they are contributing to the child's problems, regardless of whether the medication is prescribed. Adults affected by significant attention-deficit problems can similarly benefit from use of this medication. Like the other CNS stimulants, its use should be considered adjunctive to psychological, educational, social, and other remedial measures in the treatment of ADHD and narcolepsy. The side effect profile of methylphenidate is more favourable than that of many other CNS stimulants. It can therefore be used in more clients without as much concern with regard to some of the more severe toxicities seen with other CNS stimulants. Overstimulation of the CNS may still occur, with severe cardiovascular and nervous system complications; however, this

is less common. Methylphenidate is contraindicated in clients with a history of marked anxiety, tension, and agitation. It is also contraindicated in clients with glaucoma and in those with a known hypersensitivity to it. It is available in oral form as 10- and 20-mg tablets and 18-, 20-, 36-, and 54-mg extended-release tablets. Pregnancy category C. For recommended dosages, refer to the table on p. 278.

PHARMACOKINETICS

Half-Life	Onset	Peak	Duration
1–3 hr	30–60 min	2–5 hr	4–6 hr

modafinil

Modafinil is indicated to improve wakefulness in clients with excessive daytime sleepiness associated with narcolepsy. It is pharmacologically unrelated to methylphenidate or dextroamphetamine, and has less potential for problematic use. Modafinil appears to work indirectly by decreasing GABA-mediated neurotransmission. Some of the most common side effects

OTC Drug for Migraines

In 1999 in the United States, the FDA expanded the indications for Excedrin Migraine, an OTC drug produced by Bristol-Myers Squibb. This product contains 250 mg of acetaminophen, 250 mg of acetylsalicylic acid, and 65 mg of caffeine and has an indication of "treats migraines." The label states that the drug is "for the temporary relief of mild to moderate pain associated with migraine headache." The entire range of symptoms often accompanying migraines is also listed, including severe pain, nausea, and sensitivity to light. Excedrin Migraine is the first FDA-approved OTC drug for migraine and its accompanying symptoms. In three separate clinical trials, researchers found that Excedrin Migraine was highly effective in treating all levels of migraine pain and the associated symptoms. Even clients with severe migraine attacks stated that they experienced a noticeable reduction in their pain within 30 minutes and that they noticed major improvements in their ability to take part in ADLs. According to the experts who tested Excedrin Migraine, this pain reliever has an excellent safety profile and is tolerated well. However, it is not approved for use in Canada.

It is important to keep clients well informed of the various non-prescription drugs and natural health products available to treat migraines. Following are some resources that may be helpful to clients who suffer from migraines:

Online Resources and Newsletters
http://www.clusterheadaches.ca
http://www.sleepnet.com/

Professional/Consumer Associations
American Academy of Neurology (AAN)
   http://www.aan.com/
American Council for Headache Education (ACHE)
   http://www.achenet.org/
American Headache Society (AHS)
   http://www.ahsnet.org/
American Institute of Stress
   http://www.stress.org/
Canadian Health Network
   http://www.canadian-health-network.ca
College of Family Physicians of Canada
   http://www.cfpc.ca/
Mind-Body Medical Institute
   http://www.mbmi.org/
National Headache Foundation
   http://www.headaches.org/
National Sleep Foundation
   http://www.sleepfoundation.org/
Society for Light Treatment and Biological Rhythms (SLTBR)
   http://www.websciences.org/sltbr/
Women's Health Matters
   http://www.womenshealthmatters.ca/
World Headache Alliance
   http://www.w-h-a.org/wha2/index.asp

Data from the Excedrin Headache Resource Center at http://www.excedrin.com/.

are headache, nausea, nervousness, anxiety, and insomnia. It is available as 100-mg tablets. Modafinil is listed under Schedule F of the FDR and Schedule III of the CDSA and is contraindicated in cases of known drug allergy. Pregnancy category C. Recommended dosages are given in the table on p. 278.

PHARMACOKINETICS

Half-Life	Onset	Peak	Duration
10 hr	1–2 mo*	2–4 hr	Unknown

*Therapeutic effects.

SEROTONIN AGONISTS

The serotonin agonists are a new class of CNS stimulants used to treat migraine headache. They can often produce relief from moderate to severe migraines within 2 hours in 70 to 80 percent of clients. They work by stimulating 5-HT$_1$ receptors in the brain and are sometimes referred to as SSRAs or triptans. This stimulation results in constriction of dilated blood vessels in the brain and decreased release of inflammatory neuropeptides. They are available in a variety of formulations including subcutaneous (SC) self-injections, oral formulations, and nasal sprays. Self-injection and nasal sprays are useful options because many people with migraines experience nausea and vomiting and cannot tolerate oral medications. Sprays and injections are also typically quicker in onset, producing relief in some clients in 10 to 15 minutes, compared with 1 to 2 hours with tablets.

Currently six SSRAs are available: zolmitriptan, naratriptan, rizatriptan, sumatriptan, eletriptan hydrobromide, and almotriptan malate. Sumatriptan was the original prototype drug for this class, and the rest of these agents represent newer generations of triptans with slight differences. Sumatriptan, as the oldest drug in this class, has a greater body of clinical experience and more available dosage forms: subcutaneous injection, tablets, and nasal spray. Of the available oral SSRAs, zolmitriptan and rizatriptan have the most rapid onset of action. Rizatriptan is also available as a wafer that dissolves on the tongue. This may be advantageous both for speed of onset and for clients who cannot take tablets because of nausea, vomiting, and disabling pain or cannot absorb them well because of decreased GI motility. Naratriptan has the longest half-life and therefore may have the longest protection against recurrence of migraines.

▶▶ *sumatriptan*

Sumatriptan is indicated in the acute treatment of migraines. Sumatriptan is contraindicated in clients with ischemic heart disease, signs and symptoms consistent with ischemic heart disease, or Prinzmetal's angina (unstable angina caused by coronary artery spasm). It is possible to experience a slight increase in BP after administration; therefore it is also contraindicated in clients with uncontrolled or severe hypertension. It should not be given to clients who have a history, symptoms, or signs of ischemic cardiac, cerebrovascular, or peripheral vascular syndromes or underlying cardiovascular disease (atherosclerosis, congenital heart disease). It is also contraindicated in clients who have severe liver impairment or are hypersensitive to sumatriptan or any of its active ingredients.

Sumatriptan has some important drug interactions. It should not be taken concurrently with an MAOI or within 2 weeks of discontinuing one. It should not be taken within 24 hours of an ergotamine-containing or ergot-like compound such as dihydroergotamine (DHE) or methysergide. Clients should not take other triptans for 24 hours after taking sumatriptan. Sumatriptan is available as 25-, 50-, and 100-mg tablets, a 6-mg/0.5 mL injection, and a 5- and 20-mg nasal spray. Pregnancy category C. Recommended dosages are given in the table on p. 278.

PHARMACOKINETICS

Half-Life*	Onset	Peak	Duration
2 hr	30 min	2 hr	4 hr

*For orally administered sumatriptan.

NURSING PROCESS

■ Assessment

CNS stimulants are most often used for the treatment of drug-induced or post-anaesthetic respiratory depression. These agents are also used for the treatment of ADHD, narcolepsy, and exogenous obesity. Before administering these agents, the nurse must carefully assess the client and gather data from the nursing history regarding potential contraindications, cautions, and drug interactions. Clients need to be questioned about other medications they are taking, specifically whether they are taking MAOIs or vasopressors, antihypertensive agents, oral anticoagulants, tricyclic antidepressants (TCAs), or anticonvulsants. The nurse should also ask about the use of any

natural health or OTC products that contain ephedra or ginseng. These agents also stimulate the CNS, and many complications may occur, such as seizures, palpitations, and abnormal cardiac rhythms. The Natural Health Therapies box below lists selected herbal products used for nervous system stimulation.

Contraindications to the use of these medications include a hypersensitivity to them, seizure disorders, and liver dysfunction. Vital signs, especially BP in clients with a history of cardiac disease, should be assessed and the findings recorded for baseline purposes. For clients with ADHD it is particularly important to assess thoroughly their vital signs, BP, and pulse rate and rhythm. Typical behaviour, attention span, and history of social problems or problems in school are also important to assess and document. Because these agents may retard growth, the height and weight of children who are taking methylphenidate should be measured and recorded before therapy is initiated, and their growth rate should be plotted during therapy.

Sibutramine, a newer anorexiant similar to amphetamines, should not be used with other drugs that elevate serotonin, such as the SSRIs (used to treat depression) or SSRAs (used for migraines). It is also contraindicated with the use of lithium, meperidine, fentanyl, and dextromethorphan. Sibutramine should be avoided within 2 weeks of using an MAOI. Sibutramine is also contraindicated in clients who have shown an allergic reaction to MAOIs, have anorexia nervosa, or are taking any other centrally-acting appetite suppressant.

Orlistat is another anorexiant used to treat obesity. It is the first drug in a new class of non-systemically acting anti-obesity agents to be used in clients with a body mass index (BMI) of 30 or more, or in clients with a BMI of 27 who are also hypertensive or have high cholesterol or diabetes. (A client who is 175 cm tall and weighs 82 kg

NATURAL HEALTH THERAPIES

SELECTED HERBAL COMPOUNDS USED FOR NERVOUS SYSTEM STIMULATION*

Common Name(s)	Uses	Possible Drug Interactions (Avoid Concurrent Use)
Ephedra,[†] ma huang	Nervous system stimulation, appetite suppression	MAOIs, ephedrine, beta-blockers, phenothiazines, pseudoephedrine, theophylline
Ginkgo biloba, ginkgo	To treat dementia, poor memory; to enhance mental alertness	Warfarin, acetylsalicylic acid
Ginseng	To treat impaired mental function and concentration	Drugs for diabetes that lower blood sugar (e.g., insulin, oral hypoglycemic agents), MAOIs
Guarana	Nervous system stimulation, appetite suppression	Adenosine, disulfiram, quinolones, oral contraceptives, beta-blockers, iron, lithium, phenylephrine (e.g., nasal spray), cimetidine, theophylline, tobacco

Data from Fetrow, C.W., & Avila, J.R. (2000). *The complete guide to herbal remedies.* Springhouse, PA: Springhouse.
*The information in this box does not imply author or publisher endorsement of these products. Though individual consumers often experience satisfying results with various herbal products, there is often little, if any, rigorously controlled research to demonstrate their efficacy at treating particular condition(s). Clients should always be advised to communicate regularly with their healthcare practitioner(s) about all medications used, including herbal remedies, to decrease the likelihood of possibly hazardous drug interactions.
†In January 2002 Health Canada restricted the amount of ephedra available for sale. Maximum allowable dosages for *Ephedra*/ephedrine in products are 8 mg ephedrine/single dose or 32 mg ephedrine/day. Health Canada also issued a warning not to use ephedra products for weight loss. In the United States the use of dietary supplements containing ephedra is banned because of significant cardiovascular health risks.

has a BMI of about 30.) Nutritional assessments and a physician's order are needed. The nurse should keep in mind that this medication may lead to a reduction of some fat-soluble vitamins (A, D, E, K) and beta-carotene. Orlistat has become a popular agent for obesity because most anorexiant agents are systemic and increase the risk for addiction, pulmonary hypertension, valvular heart disease, and hypertension. However, this newer drug acts directly at the site of the lumen of the stomach and small intestine, affecting fat absorption and decreasing the incidence of systemic-related adverse effects seen with the CNS stimulants.

The serotonin agonists are a newer class of CNS stimulants and are commonly used in the treatment of migraines, but not without concern for possible adverse reactions or for contraindications and drug interactions. Most of these agents are contraindicated in clients with a history of ischemic heart disease or in those with symptoms consistent with ischemic heart, cerebrovascular, or peripheral vascular syndromes, or Prinzmetal's angina. Because a (usually slight) elevation in BP may occur, these agents should not be used in clients with uncontrolled hypertension. Clients with CAD should not receive serotonin agonists unless they have had a thorough cardiac evaluation and their use is approved. They should not be administered to anyone with severe liver impairment. Serotonin agonists should not be administered within 2 weeks of MAOI use or within 24 hours of use of ergotamine-containing products or even DHE or methysergide. Other triptans should not be taken within 24 hours of taking sumatriptan.

Nursing Diagnoses

Nursing diagnoses appropriate to clients taking CNS stimulants include the following:
- Imbalanced nutrition, less than body requirements, related to side effects of the medication.
- Disturbed sleep pattern (decreased sleep) related to drug effects.
- Decreased cardiac output related to side effects of palpitations and tachycardia.
- Situational low self-esteem related to the impact of possible altered growth in children.
- Anxiety related to drug effects.
- Deficient knowledge related to lack of information about drug regimen.

Planning

Goals associated with the use of CNS stimulants include the following:
- Client maintains normal body weight and height.
- Client continues normal growth and development while on medications.
- Client experiences minimal sleep deprivation.
- Client is free of cardiac symptoms and associated complications of drug therapy.
- Client maintains positive self-esteem.
- Client appears less anxious.

- Client remains adherent to drug therapy.
- Client remains free of complications related to antimigraine treatment.

Outcome Criteria

Outcome criteria related to the nursing care of clients receiving CNS stimulants include the following:
- Client maintains normal body weight and height (if pediatric client, continues normal growth and development patterns with weight and height falling within normal limits on growth chart) while taking CNS stimulants.
- Client shows improved sensorium and level of consciousness with increased attentiveness.
- Client experiences more restful sleep using non-pharmacological measures.
- Client's vital signs, specifically BP and pulse, are within normal limits.
- Client communicates openly any feelings of anxiety or anger and any problems with self-image or self-esteem.
- Client states symptoms (e.g., palpitations, chest pain) to report to the physician immediately.
- Client reports a decrease in headaches.

Implementation

Methylphenidate should be administered at least 6 hours before bedtime to diminish the insomnia it may cause, and it is recommended that it be given approximately 45 minutes before meals. There is now a longer-acting product (Concerta) leading to more stimulant in the blood for a longer period. Because dry mouth is an expected side effect, the client should perform frequent mouth care; sucking on hard candy or frequently sipping fluids may provide some relief. If the client is taking the CNS stimulant for the treatment of obesity, a holistic approach should be used that includes exercise and dietary teaching, all under the supervision of a physician. Use of a journal to record responses to the drug therapy at home, play, and school is important for charting the effectiveness of the drug for the child. In addition, counselling is generally a part of the treatment, with the family involved in goal setting for the treatment regimen. Use of a journal to record any side effects—such as weight loss, hypertension, and changes in sensorium or affect—is also important to the progress of the client.

Phentermine and other cerebral stimulants used for control of appetite should be given at least 6 hours before bedtime (often recommendations are 10 to 14 hours before retiring) to avoid problems with insomnia. Most of these agents are usually given 30 minutes before meals, but the physician's orders should be followed. Gum, hard candy, and frequent sips of water may help decrease dry mouth. Clients should be encouraged to have follow-up visits with their physician because some of the newer agents (anorexiants) are recommended to be taken on a short-term basis.

When taking sibutramine, clients should be informed that the therapeutic effects may take up to

8 weeks to occur and peak effects occur at about 6 months. Strict dietary instructions should be given to clients taking any anorexiant, and the need for exercise with any weight-control program should be emphasized. Clients may need approval from their physician before beginning exercise, especially if they are not used to a regular exercise program. As sibutramine elevates blood pressure and heart rate in some clients, blood pressure should be monitored regularly (every 2 weeks is recommended) in the first 3 months of treatment, then at 1- to 3-month intervals. With orlistat, clients need to be careful of dietary fat intake; restricting the intake of fat to less than 30 percent of total caloric intake may help to decrease the occurrence of the GI side effects. However, orlistat is to be taken with meals that contain fat. Supplementation with fat-soluble vitamins may be indicated.

Serotonin agonists come in a variety of dosage forms. Rizatriptan comes in a wafer that dissolves on the tongue, leading to rapid absorption even if the client is experiencing nausea and vomiting. The nasal spray or self-injectable forms of the serotonin agonists are desirable especially in clients experiencing the nausea and vomiting that often occurs with migraine headache. Oral forms are well tolerated but only if nausea and vomiting are not occurring. Self-injectable forms and nasal sprays also have the benefit of an onset of action of about 10 to 15 minutes as compared with 1 to 2 hours with tablet forms. Client teaching should include instructions about the dosing. The subcutaneous injection for adults is not to exceed 12 mg/24 hr; the oral form is a maximum of 100 mg; and the nasal spray is one dose in one nostril with repeating of the dose in 2 hours at 40 mg/24 hr. Also, foods containing tyramine should be avoided because tyramine is known to precipitate severe headaches. Tyramine-containing foods include beer, wine, aged cheese, food additives, preservatives, artificial sweeteners, chocolate, and caffeine. The client will often complain of pain at the injection site, along with a tingling, hot sensation, and burning at the site. A journal of headaches, precipitating factors, and response to drug therapy is also encouraged to properly follow the client's progress.

Client teaching tips for CNS stimulants are presented on p. 284.

■ Evaluation

Therapeutic responses to agents used in the management of hyperkinesia include decreased hyperactivity, increased attention span and concentration, and improved behaviour. The therapeutic response to agents used for the management of narcolepsy is the ability to remain awake. Anorexiants should cause the client's appetite to decrease and weight loss to occur. The nurse needs to monitor the client for the development of adverse effects to these medications; these include mental status changes and changes in sensorium, mood, affect, and sleep patterns; physical dependency; irritability; and withdrawal symptoms such as headache, nausea, and vomiting.

Therapeutic effects of sibutramine include appetite control and weight loss for the treatment of obesity. Adverse effects of sibutramine include dry mouth, headache, insomnia, and constipation. Concerns also exist for increases in BP and heart rate because of the similarity of structure to amphetamines or CNS stimulation. However, less concern exists about heart valve abnormalities, and the same concern does not exist about pulmonary hypertension as with previous anorexiants that were removed from the market (fenfluramine and dexfenfluramine). Therapeutic effects of orlistat (an anorexiant that is a lipase inhibitor instead of a CNS stimulant) include appetite control in obesity. Adverse effects mainly caused by the drug's action of inhibiting lipase include flatulence with discharge of an oily type, spotting, and fecal urgency. The client also needs to be closely evaluated for decreases in fat-soluble vitamins (A, D, E, and beta-carotene) because these vitamins are affected by the decrease in absorption of fats.

Therapeutic responses to modafinil include a decrease in sleepiness associated with narcolepsy. Clients taking modafinil should be monitored for adverse effects including headache, nausea, nervousness, and anxiety.

Therapeutic responses to the serotonin agonists include a decrease in the frequency, duration, and severity of migraine headaches with improved daily functioning and performance because of the decrease in headaches. Adverse effects for which to monitor include pain at the injection site (temporary); flushing; chest tightness or pressure; weakness; sedation; dizziness; sweating; increase in BP and pulse; and bad taste with the nasal spray formulation, which may precipitate nausea.

CLIENT TEACHING TIPS

The nurse should instruct the client as follows:

▲ Avoid other sources of CNS stimulants such as caffeine, which is found in coffee, tea, cola products, and chocolate.

▲ Take your medication exactly as prescribed by your physician, including taking the medication at the same time every day. Do not skip, omit, or double up on doses.

▲ Do not take OTC preparations unless they are approved by your physician. Avoid herbal products such as ephedra and ginseng.

▲ Do not drink alcohol or consume any products that contain alcohol. Be aware that there is alcohol in some OTC cold products such as cough syrups.

▲ Keep a log of your daily activities and record how the drug is working and any side effects.

▲ Do not stop taking this medication abruptly.

▲ Take your medication at least 6 hours before bedtime to decrease insomnia.

▲ If taking medication for treatment of obesity, take it 30 to 45 minutes before meals.

▲ To minimize dry mouth, suck on hard candy, chew gum, or sip fluids.

▲ If you are taking a serotonin agonist, or any other CNS stimulant, avoid tyramine-containing foods.

▲ To ensure safe use of any serotonin agonist, take the exact dose you have been prescribed, at the prescribed frequency.

▲ Use a journal to record headaches, treatment, and results.

▲ With appetite suppressants, decrease caffeine consumption to avoid excessive CNS stimulation. Foods and beverages high in caffeine include chocolate, tea, coffee, and cola.

▲ To avoid serious drug interactions with appetite suppressants, avoid OTC preparations unless your physician is contacted and approves.

▲ If you are going to stop taking this medication, you may need to taper off rather than abruptly discontinuing, because this medication can cause physical dependency. Don't make any changes in your medication without checking with your physician first.

POINTS to REMEMBER

▼ CNS stimulants are drugs that stimulate the brain or spinal cord (e.g., cocaine and caffeine).

▼ Actions of these stimulants mimic those of the SNS neurotransmitters norepinephrine and epinephrine.

▼ CNS stimulants are also called *sympathomimetic agents* because they mimic the SNS neurotransmitters.

▼ Included in the family of CNS stimulants are the amphetamines, analeptics, and anorexiants, with therapeutic uses for appetite control, ADHD, and narcolepsy.

▼ Amphetamines elevate mood or produce euphoria, increase mental alertness and capacity for work, decrease fatigue and drowsiness, and prolong wakefulness.

▼ The analeptics have generalized effects on the brainstem and spinal cord, increase responsiveness to external stimuli, and stimulate respiration.

▼ Because the analeptics stimulate respiration, they may be used to treat respiratory paralysis caused by overdose of opioids, alcohol, barbiturates, and general anaesthetic agents.

▼ Anorexiants control or suppress appetite. They may also be used to stimulate the CNS and work by suppressing appetite control centres in the brain.

▼ Contraindications to the use of anorexiants, as well as any CNS stimulant, include hypersensitivity, seizure activity, convulsive disorders, and liver dysfunction.

▼ The serotonin agonists are a newer class of CNS stimulants generally used to treat migraine headaches. They are to be avoided by clients who have ischemic cardiac, cerebrovascular, or peripheral vascular syndromes, cardiovascular disease (atherosclerosis, congenital heart disease), and Prinzmetal's (spastic) angina.

▼ Nursing considerations for children who take methylphenidate include recording baseline height and weight before initiating drug therapy and continuing to plot height and weight in a journal during therapy.

▼ Therapeutic responses to agents used in the treatment of hyperkinesia include decreased hyperactivity, increased attention span and concentration, and improved behaviour patterns.

▼ Side effects to monitor for in individuals taking CNS stimulants include changes in mental status or sensorium, mood, affect, and sleep patterns; physical dependency; and irritability.

▼ Serotonin agonists may be administered subcutaneously, as a nasal spray, and as oral tablets.

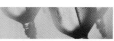

EXAMINATION REVIEW QUESTIONS

1 A client with narcolepsy and obesity will probably be prescribed a CNS stimulant. Which of the following side effects is this client likely to encounter?
a. Bradycardia
b. Nervousness
c. Mental clouding
d. Drowsiness at night

2 One of your clients is to begin treatment with an anorexiant. Which side effect may be anticipated with this drug?
a. Polyuria
b. Irritability
c. Bradycardia
d. Drowsiness at all times

3 Clients being treated with anorexiants are most likely being treated for which of the following nursing diagnoses?
a. Deficient fluid volume
b. Excess fluid volume

c. Imbalanced nutrition, less than body requirements
d. Imbalanced nutrition, more than body requirements

4 Which of the following drugs cannot be administered with an amphetamine drug?
a. Caffeine
b. Estrogen
c. Morphine
d. Meperidine

5 Which of the following would alert the nurse to a possible contraindication or caution to the use of an anorexiant?
a. Fatigue
b. Overweight
c. Questionable alcohol abuse
d. Headaches 1 to 2 times per year

For answers see http://evolve.elsevier.com/Lilley/pharmacology/.

CRITICAL THINKING ACTIVITIES

1 Narcolepsy has been diagnosed in Ms. P., a 68-year-old retired nurse, and she has been on a CNS stimulant for the past 6 months. Formulate a list of questions to ask her caregiver that will help to determine the effectiveness of her drug therapy.

2 Why would you, as a nurse practitioner, recommend or not recommend appetite suppressants for an adult who is obese?

For answers see http://evolve.elsevier.com/Lilley/pharmacology/.

BIBLIOGRAPHY

Albanese, J., & Nutz, P. (2005). *Mosby's 2005 nursing drug cards.* St Louis, MO: Mosby.

Canadian Institutes of Health Research. (2004). Obesity. Retrieved August 2, 2005, from http://www.cihr-irsc.gc.ca/e/24942.html

Canadian Pharmacists Association. (2003). *Therapeutic choices* (4th ed.). Ottawa, ON: Author.

Canadian Pharmacists Association. (2004). *Guide to drugs in Canada.* Toronto, ON: Dorling Kindersley.

Canadian Pharmacists Association. (2005). *Compendium of pharmaceuticals and specialties. The Canadian drug reference for health professionals.* Ottawa, ON: Author. [The subscription-based e-CPS is available at http://www.pharmacists.ca.]

Cheng, A., Williams, B.A., & Sivarajan, B.V. (Eds.). *The HSC handbook of pediatrics* (10th ed.). Toronto, ON: Elsevier.

DG News. (2002). Canada approves Xenical (Orlistat) for treatment of excess weight/obesity in type 2 diabetes. Retrieved August 17, 2005, from http://www.docguide.com/news/content.nsf/news/8525697700573E1885256C2100531249

Evans, C., Blackburn, D., Butt, P., & Dattani, D. (2004). Use and abuse of methylphenidate in attention deficit/hyperactivity disorder. [Electronic version]. *Canadian Pharmacy Journal, 137*(6).

Facts and Comparisons. (2004). *Drug facts and comparisons pocket version* (9th ed.). St Louis, MO: Wolters Kluwer Health.

Fetrow, C.W., & Avila, J.R. (2000). *The complete guide to herbal remedies.* Springhouse, PA: Springhouse.

Health Canada. (2001). Health Canada withdraws drug products containing phenylpropanolamine (PPA) from the market. Retrieved August 2, 2005, from http://www.hc-sc.gc.ca/ahc-asc/media/advisories-avis/2001/2001_61e.htm

Health Canada. (2005). Advisory: Health Canada suspends the market authorization of ADDERALL XR®, a drug prescribed for Attention Deficit Hyperactivity Disorder (ADHD) in children. Retrieved August 2, 2005, from http://www.hc-sc.gc.ca/ahc-asc/media/advisories-avis/2005/2005_01.html

Health Canada. (2005) Drug product database (DPD). Retrieved August 2, 2005, from http://www.hc-sc.gc.ca/hpb/drugs-dpd/

Health Canada. (2005). News release. Health Canada allows Adderall XR® back on the Canadian Market. Retrieved November 11, 2005 from http://www.hc-sc.gc.ca/ahc-asc/media/nr-cp/2005/2005_92_e.html

Kernan, W.N., Viscoli, C.M., Brass, L.M., Broderick, J.P., Brott, T., & Feldmann, E., (2000). Phenylpropanolamine and the risk of hemorrhagic stroke. *New England Journal of Medicine, 343*(25), 1826–1832.

Lacy, C.F., Armstrong, L.L., Goldman, M.P., & Lance, L.L. (2003). *Drug information handbook* (11th ed.). Hudson, OH: Lexi-Comp.

Martin, S. (2001). Prevalence of migraine headache in Canada. *Canadian Medical Association News Pulse, 164*(10), 1481.

Mosby. (2005). *Mosby's drug consult 2005: The comprehensive reference for generic and brand name drugs* (15th ed.). St Louis, MO: Mosby.

Skidmore-Roth, L. (2006). *Mosby's 2006 nursing drug reference* (19th ed.). St Louis, MO: Mosby.

Statistics Canada. (2005). Canadian Community Health Survey: Obesity among children and adults. Retrieved August 2, 2005, from http://www.statcan.ca/Daily/English/050706/d050706a.htm

PART THREE

Drugs Affecting the Autonomic Nervous System: Study Skills Tips

- PURR APPLICATION

PURR APPLICATION

Planning for the Part

The basic explanation provided for the PURR model in the Study Skills Tips for Part One demonstrates the application process as it relates to individual chapters. Another useful application of the PURR model encourages the learner to take a broader view of the assignment. In the case of this text, you have noticed that the chapters are grouped together into multiple chapter blocks called *parts*. Part organization is not some random process applied by the authors to further complicate the subject. Part organization is a carefully thought-out process to put content together in a logical and meaningful fashion. Since the authors have spent considerable time trying to link the chapters together in the most logical pattern, it is to your advantage as a student to learn to take advantage of the work already done for you.

Part Title

Begin the process of part planning by looking at the Part Three title, "Drugs Affecting the Autonomic Nervous System." Then look at the part structure. Part Three contains four chapters. All these chapters must be concerned with the autonomic nervous system. Even before you have done any reading in any chapter, you are beginning to look for the links that will establish relationships among ideas in individual chapters. You are also looking for the broader link that connects the four chapters in this part with each other and with the ideas that have come in earlier parts and will follow in later parts.

There is a clear example in this part of the way in which parts relate to one another. Look back at Part Two, "Drugs Affecting the Central Nervous System." Clearly

that part deals with some aspect of the nervous system, as does this part. One learning objective you should establish for yourself is to grasp the relationship between these two parts. You must be able to define and explain *central nervous system* and *autonomic nervous system.* However, stopping there limits the learning you can achieve. Ask yourself some additional questions that will help you establish a connection between these parts. "What is the difference in functions of the central and the autonomic nervous systems?" "Are there pharmacological agents that have application in both the central and autonomic nervous systems?" The principle is to keep stressing the links that must exist throughout all the parts and chapters you are studying. Most students focus on the individual chapters, but to fully understand the subject it is essential to encompass the broader scope of chapter and part.

Part Chapters

After considering the part title and looking for relationships between the new part and past parts studied, the next step in applying the Plan step of PURR to a part is to spend a few minutes studying the chapter titles and looking for the relationships that must exist. Part Three has four chapters, and there is a clear pattern in these chapters. Chapters 17 and 18 both contain the term *adrenergic*. Clearly the two chapters are dealing with the same broad topic. However, Chapter 17 covers adrenergic agents and Chapter 18 covers adrenergic-blocking agents. Apply questioning strategies at this point. "What does adrenergic mean?" "What is an adrenergic agent?" These two questions are essential in mastering the content of Chapter 17, and you should ask them almost without thinking. However, the next step, while easily overlooked, can greatly enhance your understanding when you start to read the material. Notice that Chapter 17 deals with agents and Chapter 18 deals with blocking agents. There must be a difference between an agent and a blocking agent. Focus now with a few questions that will keep you aware that the content in Chapter 17 has a direct relationship to the content in Chapter 18. "What is the difference between an agent and a blocking agent? When is the pharmacological application of an agent appropriate? Under what conditions should a blocking agent be chosen?" Then ask a question to help maintain the focus on the concept of the entire part. "What aspects of the autonomic nervous system are related to the adrenergic agents and blocking agents?"

Chapters 19 and 20

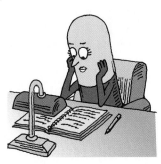

Once you begin to focus on the relationship of chapters within a part, certain things will begin to become apparent. Chapters 19 and 20, too, cover agents and blocking agents. These two chapters develop the concept as related to cholinergics, rather than adrenergics. But the same questions you used as a focus for Chapters 17 and 18 can be recycled in setting up the study of Chapters 19 and 20. Simply replace the term adrenergic with cholinergic and you are ready to begin reading these two chapters with a clear personal learning objective.

Active Questioning

This is the key concept to master in working through the process of planning your learning for an entire part rather than for single chapters. The idea is to view the part as a whole rather than seeing only the content of individual chapters. In the preceding discussion we have provided a number of sample questions to help you begin the process. These are not the only questions you should ask, but rather samples to help you develop a questioning process.

Some of the questions will prove to be useful when reading the chapters. Others may have little or no application as you read and understand the content of an individual chapter. Do not worry about the quality of the questions when planning on the part level. Questions can (and sometimes should) be revised or discarded when the details of the chapter become clearer. The important point is that you begin the part with some questions to help you focus your own reading and learning. Also, you will find that the more you apply active questioning as a part of your learning strategy, the better your questions will become.

Adrenergic Agents

OBJECTIVES

After reading this chapter, the successful student will be able to do the following:

1 Briefly discuss the sympathetic nervous system (SNS) as related to drug therapy—specifically, the affects of adrenergic stimulation or sympathomimetic effects.

2 List the various adrenergic agonists with associated indications.

3 Discuss the mechanisms of action of adrenergic agonists, as well as their therapeutic effects, indications, adverse and toxic effects, cautions, contraindications, interactions, and any available antidotes to overdosage.

4 Discuss the nursing process related to the administration of adrenergic agents, including specific teaching points for clients and caregivers.

e-LEARNING ACTIVITIES

Student CD-ROM
- Review Questions: see questions 94–100
- Animations
- Medication Administration Checklists
- IV Therapy Checklists

evolve **Web site** (http://evolve.elsevier.com/Lilley/pharmacology/)
- Online Chapter Worksheet • Frequently Asked Questions
- Learning Tips and Content Updates • WebLinks • Online Appendices and Supplements • Mosby/Saunders ePharmacology Update • Access to *Mosby's Drug Consult*

DRUG PROFILES

▶▶dobutamine, p. 298
▶▶dopamine, p. 299
▶▶epinephrine, p. 295, 299
   isoproterenol, p. 299
   isoproterenol hydrochloride, p. 295
   midodrine, p. 299

▶▶norepinephrine, p. 299
   phenylephrine, p. 299
▶▶pseudoephedrine hydrochloride, p. 297
▶▶salmeterol, p. 296
▶▶salbutamol, p. 295
   tetrahydrozoline, p. 297

▶▶ Key drug.

GLOSSARY

Adrenergic receptors Receptor sites for the sympathetic neurotransmitters norepinephrine and epinephrine.

Adrenergics (ad' rən er' jiks) Drugs that stimulate the sympathetic nervous system (SNS). They are also referred to as *adrenergic agonists* or *sympathomimetics* because they mimic the effects of the sympathetic neurotransmitters norepinephrine and epinephrine.

Alpha-adrenergic receptors Adrenergic receptors that are further divided into alpha$_1$- and alpha$_2$-adrenergic receptors and are differentiated by their location on nerves.

Autonomic functions Bodily functions that are involuntary and result from physiological activity of the autonomic nervous system. The functions often occur in pairs of opposing actions between the sympathetic and parasympathetic divisions of this nervous system. Adrenergic stimulation mimics the sympathetic division of the autonomic nervous system and includes end results such as dilation of bronchioles (SNS or adrenergic effects) or constriction of the bronchioles (parasympathetic nervous system [PSNS] or adrenergic blocking effects), cardiac acceleration with increased pulse rate (SNS or adrenergic agonists) or cardiac deceleration with decreased pulse rate (PSNS or adrenergic blockers), and peristaltic contractions of intestinal smooth muscle (parasympathetic activity) vs. decreased motility of the same intestinal smooth muscle (sympathetic activity).

Autonomic nervous system (ANS) Controls autonomic bodily functions, as described previously. Consists of the SNS and PSNS.

Beta-adrenergic receptors Located on post-synaptic effector cells—the cells, muscles, and organs that the nerves stimulate. Beta$_1$-adrenergic receptors differ from beta$_2$-adrenergic receptors in that they are primarily in the heart; beta$_2$-adrenergic receptors are located in the smooth muscle of the bronchioles and arterioles and in visceral organs.

Catecholamines (kat' ə kol' ə meenz) Substances that can produce a sympathomimetic response. They are either endogenous catecholamines (such as epinephrine, norepinephrine, and dopamine) or synthetic catecholamines (such as isoproterenol and dobutamine).

Dopaminergic receptors (do' pə mən er' jik) Adrenergic receptors that, when stimulated by dopamine, cause the renal, mesenteric, coronary, and cerebral arteries to dilate and the flow of blood to increase.

Mydriasis Pupillary dilation, whether natural (physiological) or drug-induced.

Ophthalmics (off thal' miks) Topically applied eye medications.

Positive chronotropic effect (kron' o trop' ik) An increased heart rate.

Positive dromotropic effect (drom' o trop' ik) An increase in conduction through the atrioventricular node.

Positive inotropic effect (in' o trop' ik) An increased force of contraction of the heart muscle (myocardium).

Synaptic cleft (si nap' tik) The space between the nerve ending and the effector organ.

Adrenergics are a large group of both exogenous (synthetic) and endogenous (naturally occurring) substances. They have a wide variety of therapeutic uses depending on their site of action and their effect on receptors. Adrenergics stimulate the sympathetic nervous system (SNS) and are also called *adrenergic agonists,* or *sympathomimetics,* because they mimic the effects of the SNS neurotransmitters norepinephrine and epinephrine, which are referred to chemically as **catecholamines.** When describing the adrenergic class of medications, it is helpful to understand how the SNS operates in relation to the rest of the nervous system.

SYMPATHETIC NERVOUS SYSTEM

Figure 17-1 depicts the divisions of the nervous system, showing the relationship of the SNS to the entire nervous system. The SNS is the counterpart to the parasympathetic nervous system (PSNS); together they make up the **autonomic nervous system (ANS).** They provide a checks-and-balances system for maintaining the normal homeostasis of the **autonomic functions** of the human body.

Throughout the body there are receptor sites for the catecholamines (norepinephrine and epinephrine). These are referred to as **adrenergic receptors,** and these are the sites where adrenergic drugs bind and produce their effects. Adrenergic receptors are located at many anatomic sites, and many physiological responses are produced when they are stimulated or blocked. Adrenergic receptors are further divided into **alpha-adrenergic** and **beta-adrenergic receptors,** depending on the specific physiological responses caused by their stimulation. Both types of adrenergic receptors have subtypes, designated 1 and 2, providing a further means of checks and balances that control stimulation and blockade, constriction and dilation, and the increased and decreased production of a substance.

Alpha$_1$- and alpha$_2$-adrenergic receptors are differentiated by their location on nerves. Alpha$_1$-adrenergic receptors are located on post-synaptic effector cells (the cell, muscle, or organ that the nerve stimulates). Alpha$_2$-adrenergic receptors are located on the presynaptic nerve terminals. They control the release of neurotransmitters. The predominant alpha-adrenergic agonist response is vasoconstriction and central nervous system (CNS) stimulation.

Beta-adrenergic receptors are all located on post-synaptic effector cells. Beta$_1$-adrenergic receptors are primarily located in the heart; beta$_2$-adrenergic receptors are located in the smooth muscle of the bronchioles, arterioles, and visceral organs. A beta-adrenergic agonist response results in bronchial, gastrointestinal (GI), and uterine smooth muscle relaxation; glycogenolysis; and cardiac stimulation. Table 17-1 contains a more detailed listing of the adrenergic receptors and the responses elicited when they are stimulated by a neurotransmitter or a drug that acts like a neurotransmitter (see also Figure 17-2).

Another type of adrenergic receptor is the **dopaminergic receptor.** When stimulated by dopamine, these receptors cause the vessels of the renal, mesenteric, coronary, and cerebral arteries to dilate, increasing blood flow to these tissues. Dopamine is the only substance that can stimulate these receptors.

Catecholamines are produced by the SNS and are stored in vesicles or granules located in the ends of nerves. Here the transmitter waits until the nerve is stimulated, whereupon the vesicles move to the nerve ending and release their contents into the space between the nerve ending and the effector organ, called the **synaptic cleft.** The released contents of the vesicle (catecholamines) then have the opportunity to bind to the receptor sites located all along the effector organ. Once the neurotransmitter binds to the receptors, the effector organ responds. Depending on the function of the particular organ, this elicits smooth muscle contraction, an increased heart rate, the increased production of a substance, or contraction of a blood vessel. This process is stopped by the action of enzymes and by reuptake of the neurotransmitter. Catecholamines are specifically metabolized by two enzymes, monoamine oxidase (MAO) and catechol O-methyltransferase (COMT). Each enzyme breaks down catecholamines but is responsible for doing it in a different area. MAO breaks down the catecholamines that are in the nerve ending, and COMT breaks down the catecholamines that are outside the nerve ending at the synaptic cleft. The neurotransmitter is also actively taken back up into the nerve ending by a

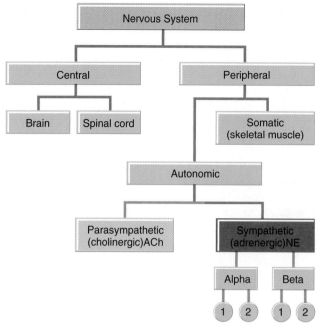

FIG. 17-1   The sympathetic nervous system in relation to the entire nervous system.

TABLE 17-1

ADRENERGIC RECEPTOR RESPONSES TO STIMULATION

Location	Receptor	Response
CARDIOVASCULAR		
Blood vessels	Alpha$_1$/beta$_2$	Constriction/dilation
Cardiac muscle	Beta$_1$	Increased contractility
Atrioventricular node	Beta$_1$	Increased heart rate
Sinoatrial node	Beta$_1$	Increased heart rate
ENDOCRINE		
Pancreas release	Beta$_1$	Decreased insulin
Liver	Beta$_2$	Glycogenolysis
Kidney	Beta$_2$	Increased renin secretion
GASTROINTESTINAL		
Muscle	Beta$_2$	Decreased motility
Sphincters	Alpha$_1$	Constriction
GENITOURINARY		
Bladder sphincter	Alpha$_1$	Constriction
Bladder (detrusor muscle)	Beta$_2$	Relaxation
Penis	Alpha$_1$	Ejaculation
Uterus	Alpha$_1$/Beta$_2$	Contraction/relaxation
RESPIRATORY		
Bronchial muscles	Beta$_2$	Dilation

pump. This restores the catecholamine to the vesicle and provides another means of maintaining an adequate supply of the substance. This process is illustrated in Figure 17-2.

ADRENERGIC DRUGS

Drugs that have effects similar to or that mimic the effects of the SNS neurotransmitters norepinephrine, epinephrine, and dopamine are referred to as adrenergics. As mentioned previously, these neurotransmitters are referred to as *catecholamines*. This term also refers specifically to an adrenergic drug that has a basic chemical structure similar to that of norepinephrine, epinephrine, or dopamine. Catecholamines produce a sympathomimetic response and are either endogenous substances such as epinephrine, norepinephrine, and dopamine, or synthetic substances such as isoproterenol, dobutamine, and phenylephrine.

Catecholamines used therapeutically produce the same result as the endogenous ones but without the need to stimulate the nerve to release the neurotransmitter. Instead, when epinephrine, dobutamine, or any of the adrenergic drugs are given, they bathe the area between the nerve and the effector organ (synaptic cleft). Once there, they have the opportunity to induce a response. This can be accomplished in one of three ways: direct stimulation, indirect stimulation, or a combination of the two.

A direct-acting sympathomimetic binds directly to the receptor and causes a physiological response (Figure 17-3). Epinephrine is an example of such an agent. An indirect-acting sympathomimetic is an adrenergic drug that causes the release of the catecholamine from the storage sites

(vesicles) in the nerve endings, which then binds to the receptors and causes a physiological response (Figure 17-4). Amphetamine and other related anorexiants are examples of such agents. A mixed-acting sympathomimetic both directly stimulates the receptor by binding to it and indirectly stimulates the receptor by causing the release of the neurotransmitter stored in vesicles at the nerve endings (Figure 17-5). Ephedrine is an example of a mixed-adrenergic drug.

There are also non-catecholamine adrenergic drugs such as phenylephrine, orciprenaline, and salbutamol. These are structurally dissimilar to the endogenous catecholamines and generally have a longer duration of action than either the endogenous or synthetic catecholamines.

Catecholamines and non-catecholamines can act to varying degrees at different types of adrenergic receptors depending on the amount of drug administered. Examples of a few of the catecholamines and the dose-specific selectivity of these agents for various adrenergic receptors are given in Table 17-2. Non-catecholamine agents show comparable patterns of activity. Although adrenergics work primarily at post-ganglionic receptors (the receptors that immediately innervate the effector organ, gland, muscle, and so on), they may also work more centrally in the nervous system at the preganglionic sympathetic nerve trunks. The ability to do so depends on the potency of the specific drug and the dose used.

Although adrenergic agents are most technically classified by their specific receptor activities, they may also be thought of in terms of their clinical effects. For

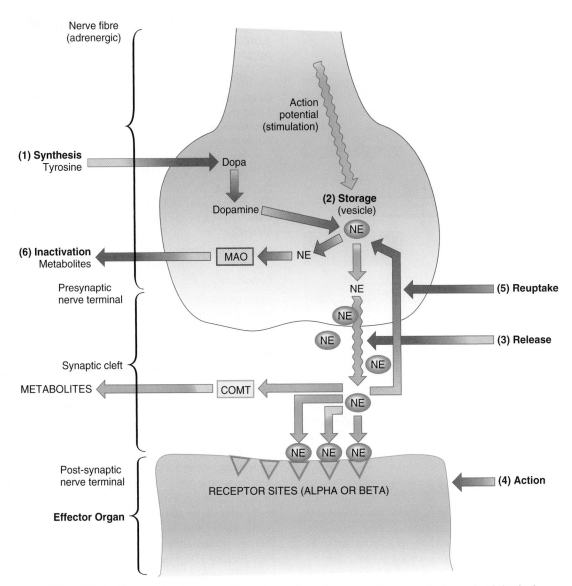

FIG. 17-2 The mechanism by which stimulation of a nerve fibre results in a physiological process; adrenergic drugs mimic this same process. *NE*, norepinephrine.

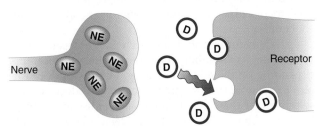

FIG. 17-3 Mechanism of physiological response by **direct-acting** sympathomimetics. *D*, Drug; *NE*, norepinephrine.

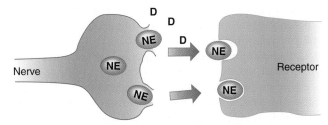

FIG. 17-4 Mechanism of physiological response by **indirect-acting** sympathomimetics. *D*, Drug; *NE*, norepinephrine.

example, phenylephrine might be thought of in practice as an alpha$_1$-agonist and salbutamol thought of as a bronchodilator. Both methods are correct for most clinical purposes. However, it may sometimes be necessary to carefully choose an adrenergic agent with greater se-

lectivity for a particular receptor type to avoid undesired clinical effects. In such a situation, detailed knowledge of the comparative type and degree of receptor selectivity between different drugs may become more important.

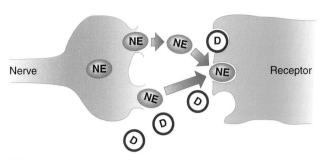

FIG. 17-5 Mechanism of physiological response by **mixed-acting** sympathomimetics. *D,* Drug; *NE,* norepinephrine.

TABLE 17-2

CATECHOLAMINES AND THEIR DOSE-RESPONSE RELATIONSHIP

Drug	Dosage	Receptor
dobutamine	Maintenance: 2–15 μg/kg/min High: 40 μg/kg/min	Beta$_1$>>beta$_2$>alpha$_1$
dopamine	Low: 0.5–2 μg/kg/min	Dopaminergic
	Moderate: 2–4 or <10 μg/kg/min	Beta$_1$
	High: 20–30 μg/kg/min	Alpha$_1$
epinephrine	Low: 1–4 μg/min	Beta$_1$>beta$_2$>>alpha$_1$
	High: 4–40 μg/min	Alpha$_1$ $\geq$ beta$_1$

Mechanism of Action and Drug Effects

To fully understand the mechanism of action of adrenergics it is necessary to have a working knowledge of normal adrenergic transmission, which takes place at the junction between the nerve (post-ganglionic sympathetic neuron) and the innervated organ (effector organ or receptor site). The process of SNS stimulation is illustrated in Fig. 17-2 and discussed earlier in this chapter. When adrenergic drugs stimulate alpha$_1$-adrenergic receptor sites located on smooth muscles, vasoconstriction most commonly occurs. Many areas of the body are covered by smooth muscles with alpha-adrenergic receptors on them. The binding of adrenergic drugs to these alpha$_1$-adrenergic receptors on the smooth muscle of blood vessels, for instance, causes vasoconstriction; at other sites, it causes the relaxation of GI smooth muscle; contraction of the uterus and bladder; male ejaculation; decreased insulin release; and contraction of the ciliary muscles of the eye, causing the pupils to dilate (see Table 17-1). Stimulation of alpha$_2$-adrenergic receptors actually tends to reverse sympathetic activity but is not of great significance either physiologically or pharmacologically speaking.

There are beta$_1$-adrenergic receptors on the myocardium and in the conduction system of the heart, the sinoatrial (SA) node, and the AV node. Stimulating these beta$_1$-adrenergic receptors by an adrenergic drug results in an increased force of contraction **(positive inotropic effect),** an increased heart rate **(positive chronotropic effect),** and an increase in conduction through the AV node **(positive dromotropic effect).** Activation of beta$_2$-adrenergic receptors produces relaxation of the bronchi (bronchodilation) and uterus. Beta$_2$-adrenergic receptors also cause stimulation in the liver with glycogenolysis and an increase in renin secretion in the kidneys (see Table 17-1).

Indications

Adrenergics, or sympathomimetics, are employed in the treatment of a wide variety of illnesses and conditions. Their selectivity for either alpha- or beta-adrenergic receptors and their affinity for certain tissues or organs determine the settings in which they are most commonly used. Some adrenergics are used as adjuncts to diet in the short-term treatment of obesity. These drugs are discussed in greater detail in Chapter 16.

Respiratory Indications

Certain adrenergic drugs have an affinity for the adrenergic receptors located in the respiratory system and are classified as bronchodilators. They tend to preferentially stimulate the beta$_2$-adrenergic receptors rather than the alpha-adrenergic receptors and cause bronchodilation. Of the two subtypes of beta-adrenergic receptors, these adrenergic agents are predominantly more attracted to the beta$_2$-adrenergic receptors on the bronchial, uterine, and vascular smooth muscles rather than the beta$_1$-adrenergic receptors on the heart. These drugs are helpful in treating conditions such as asthma and bronchitis. Some common bronchodilators that are classified as predominantly beta$_2$-selective adrenergic agents include formoterol, isoproterenol, orciprenaline, salbutamol, salmeterol, and terbutaline.

Indications as Topical Nasal Decongestants

The intranasal application of certain adrenergics can cause the constriction of dilated arterioles and a reduction in nasal blood flow, thus decreasing congestion. These adrenergic drugs work by stimulating alpha$_1$-adrenergic receptors and have little or no effect on beta-adrenergic receptors. These nasal decongestants include epinephrine, ephedrine, oxymetazoline, and phenylephrine.

Ophthalmic Indications

In another topical application, some adrenergics can be applied to the surface of the eye. These are called **ophthalmics** and work much the same way as nasal decongestants, except that they affect the vasculature of the eye. When administered they stimulate alpha-adrenergic receptors located on small arterioles in the eye and temporarily relieve conjunctival congestion. The ophthalmic adrenergics include epinephrine, naphazoline, phenylephrine, and tetrahydrozoline.

Adrenergics can also be used to reduce intraocular pressure (IOP) and dilate pupils (mydriasis), properties that make them useful in the treatment of open-angle glaucoma. They accomplish these tasks by stimulating alpha- or beta$_2$-adrenergic receptors, or both. The adrenergics used for this purpose are epinephrine, apraclonidine, and dipivefrin.

Vasoactive Indications

The final group of adrenergics is sometimes referred to as vasoactive sympathomimetics, pressors, inotropes, or cardioselective sympathomimetics because they are used to support the cardiovascular system during cardiac failure or shock. These agents have a variety of effects on the various alpha- and beta-adrenergic receptors, and these effects can also be related to the specific dose of the adrenergic agent. Common vasoactive adrenergic agents include dobutamine, dopamine, ephedrine, epinephrine, isoproterenol, norepinephrine, orciprenaline, and phenylephrine.

Contraindications

The usual contraindications to adrenergic agents are known drug allergy and severe hypertension.

Side Effects and Adverse Effects

Some of the most common unwanted CNS effects of the alpha-adrenergic agents are headache, restlessness, excitement, insomnia, and euphoria. Possible cardiovascular side effects of the alpha-adrenergics include vasoconstriction, hypertension, tachycardia, and palpitations or dysrhythmias. Effects on other body systems include anorexia, or loss of appetite; dry mouth; nausea; vomiting; and, rarely, taste changes.

Beta-adrenergic agents can adversely stimulate the CNS, causing mild tremors, headache, nervousness, and dizziness. Beta-adrenergic agents can also have unwanted effects on the cardiovascular system, including increased heart rate (positive chronotrope), palpitations (dysrhythmias), and fluctuations in blood pressure (BP). Other significant effects include sweating, nausea, vomiting, and muscle cramps. See the Pediatric and Geriatric Considerations boxes below for additional information.

PEDIATRIC CONSIDERATIONS

Administration of Beta-Adrenergic Agonists

- Children are usually more sensitive to most medications; therefore watch children closely for excessive cardiac or CNS stimulations with palpitations, tachycardia, irritability, and chest pain.
- Terbutaline is generally not used in children ≤12 years of age.
- Other medications, including OTC medications, should not be used unless physician has been notified and approves concurrent use.

Toxicity and Management of Overdose

The toxic effects of adrenergic drugs are mainly an extension of their common adverse effects (e.g., seizures, hypotension or hypertension, dysrhythmias, palpitation, nervousness, dizziness, fatigue, malaise, insomnia, headache, tremor, dry mouth, and nausea). The two most life-threatening toxic effects involve the CNS and cardiovascular system. In the acute setting, seizures can be effectively managed with diazepam. Intracranial bleeding can also occur, often as the result of an extreme elevation in BP. Such elevated BP poses the risk of hemorrhage not only in the brain but elsewhere in the body as well. The best and most effective treatment in this situation is lowering the BP using a rapid-acting alpha-adrenergic–blocking drug. This can directly reverse the adrenergic-induced state.

Many adrenergic drugs are either synthetic analogues of the naturally occurring neurotransmitters (norepinephrine, epinephrine, and dopamine) or are the actual endogenous adrenergic compound. Therefore when these drugs are taken in an overdose or signs and symptoms of toxicity develop, reversing these effects takes a relatively short time. The majority of these compounds have short half-lives, and therefore their effects are relatively short lived. Stopping the drug should quickly cause the toxic symptoms to subside. The recommended treatment of overdoses often involves treating the symptoms and supporting the client. If death occurs, it is usually the result of either respiratory failure or cardiac arrest. The treatment of an overdose should be aimed at the support of these two body systems.

Interactions

The potential drug interactions that can occur with adrenergic agents are significant. Although many of the interactions result only in a diminished adrenergic effect

GERIATRIC CONSIDERATIONS

Administration of Beta-Adrenergic Agonists

- Older people are more sensitive to medications so monitor for excessive cardiac and CNS stimulation.
- Because of the possible presence of other medical conditions such as hypertension, peripheral vascular disease, and cardiovascular disease, geriatric clients need to be monitored carefully before, during, and after the use of these medications.
- Immediately report any chest pain, palpitations, blurred vision, headache, seizures, or hallucinations to the physician.
- Cautious use is recommended with OTC and other medications. Contact the physician for further instructions.
- Monitor vital signs, especially BP and pulse rate, with these medications because of their cardiovascular effects.
- Geriatric clients often have poor manual dexterity; therefore special instructions are needed to help with proper inhaler technique.

because of direct antagonism at and competition for receptor sites, some reactions can be life threatening. Alpha- and beta-adrenergic agents, when given with adrenergic antagonists, directly antagonize each other, resulting in reduced therapeutic effects. Adrenergics, when given with anaesthetic agents, can cause increased risk of cardiac dysrhythmias. Tricyclic antidepressants (TCAs), when given with adrenergics, can cause increased vasopressor effects, acute hypertensive crisis, and possibly respiratory depression. Adrenergic agents, when given with MAO inhibitors (MAOIs), can cause a possibly life-threatening hypertensive crisis. Antihistamines and thyroid preparations can increase the adrenergic effects of this class of drugs. Antihypertensives and adrenergics may directly antagonize each other's therapeutic effects.

Laboratory Test Interactions

Alpha-adrenergic agents can cause the serum levels of corticosteroids to be increased and the glucose levels to be increased. Therefore interpretations of these laboratory results should be done with caution in clients taking these medications. Alpha-adrenergic agents can cause the plasma cortisol and corticotropin concentrations to be elevated.

Dosages

For the recommended dosages of various adrenergic agents, see the dosages tables on pp. 296–298. See Appendix B for some of the common brands available in Canada.

DRUG PROFILES

Adrenergics are used in the treatment of a variety of illnesses, and there are many indications for their use. Their selectivity for either alpha- or beta-adrenergic receptors and their affinity for various tissues or organs define the settings in which they are most commonly used. Four commonly used therapeutic classes of adrenergic agents are the bronchodilators (see Chapter 36), ophthalmic agents (Chapter 56), nasal decongestants (Chapter 35), and vasoactive agents, which are emphasized in this chapter and in Chapter 23.

BRONCHODILATORS

The bronchodilating adrenergic agents act primarily to stimulate beta$_2$-adrenergic receptors. They are effective as anti-asthmatic agents and are used in the treatment of acute attacks because of their rapid onset of action and efficacy. Ephedrine and epinephrine also possess alpha-adrenergic activity. These agents are prescription-only drugs.

Activation of beta$_2$-adrenergic receptors causes the bronchi to dilate. The selective beta$_2$-adrenergics are the preferred bronchodilators because they produce fewer cardiac-related side effects (e.g., tachycardia) than the non-selective beta agents. These drugs are available primarily in oral (PO) and aerosol forms, with one available for intravenous use. Common dosage information for selected bronchodilators appears in the table on p. 296.

▸▸ salbutamol sulphate

Salbutamol is a selective beta$_2$-adrenergic bronchodilator. It is contraindicated in clients with a known hypersensitivity to it. It can be administered orally and by inhalation. The dosage should be individualized. According to Canadian guidelines, if salbutamol is required more than three times a week (excluding its use for exercise-induced asthma), anti-inflammatory therapy should be added as part of the asthma regimen. Increasing use usually indicates worsening asthma. It is available in a metered-dose inhaler (MDI), oral syrup, inhalation solution, inhalation capsules, intramuscular injection, and intravenous infusion. Pregnancy category C. See the table on p. 296 for the most common dosage information.

PHARMACOKINETICS

Half-Life	Onset	Peak	Duration
PO: 4 hr	PO: 30 min	PO: 2.5 hr	PO: 6–8 hr
Inhaler: 4 hr	Inhaler: 5–15 min	Inhaler: 1–1.5 hr	Inhaler: 3–6 hr

▸▸ epinephrine

Epinephrine is a naturally occurring catecholamine produced by the adrenal medulla. It is a potent mixed alpha- and beta-adrenergic agent that produces vasoconstriction, increased BP, cardiac stimulation, and dilation of the bronchioles. Its primary use is for the relief of respiratory distress due to bronchospasm and for the treatment of anaphylaxis. In addition, epinephrine is used to treat open-angle glaucoma; to restore cardiac rhythm in cardiac arrest; for symptomatic relief of serum sickness, urticaria, and angioneurotic edema; and to control bleeding in surgical procedures. It is also used to relax uterine muscles and to inhibit uterine contractions. Furthermore, it is used as an ophthalmic agent and a nasal decongestant and to prolong the activity of infiltrated local anaesthetics. Its use is contraindicated in several conditions, including hypersensitivity, narrow-angle glaucoma, shock due to trauma, halogenated general anaesthetics, coronary insufficiency, and labour. In addition, its use with local anaesthetics administered in the toes or fingers is not recommended because distal circulation may be decreased due to its vasoconstricting properties. For those OTC products that contain epinephrine, such as Primatene Mist, cautious (if any) use is recommended because of the potential CNS stimulation and subsequent adverse effects. Pregnancy category C. See the table on p. 296 for selected dosage information.

PHARMACOKINETICS

Half-Life	Onset	Peak	Duration
Variable (min)	SC: 5–10 min	SC: 20 min	SC: 4 hr
	PO inhalation, IV: 1 min	PO inhalation, IV: <30 min	

isoproterenol hydrochloride

Isoproterenol is a non-selective beta-sympathomimetic (beta$_1$-beta$_2$) anti-asthmatic agent. The beta$_1$-adrenergic activity results in a positive inotropic and chronotropic cardiac effect with a corresponding increase in the stroke volume and oxygen consumption of the myocardium. Beta$_2$-adrenergic activation produces bronchial, GI tract, and uterine smooth muscle relaxation. Isoproterenol is indicated for the treatment of acute and chronic forms of asthma, bronchitis, emphysema, and other chronic forms of bronchopulmonary disorders where bronchospasm is a complication. Other indications include cardiac arrest, carotid sinus hypersensitivity, Adams-Stokes syndrome, ventricular dysrhythmias resulting from atrioventricular (AV) block, laryngobronchospasm during anaesthesia, and as adjunctive therapy during shock. Isoproterenol is contraindicated in clients with a known hypersensitivity to it and in those suffering from digitalis-induced tachycardia or with pre-existing cardiac dysrhythmias. Pregnancy category C. See the table below for selected dosage information.

PHARMACOKINETICS

Half-Life	Onset	Peak	Duration
IV: 2 min	IV: Immediate	IV: <15 min	IV: <1 hr

▸▸ *salmeterol*

Salmeterol is a new beta$_2$-agonist indicated for long-term maintenance treatment of asthma, prevention of bronchospasm, and prevention of exercise-induced bronchospasm. It is not indicated for acute exacerbations of asthma or bronchospasms. It is contraindicated in clients with known hypersensitivity to salmeterol. In 2005, Health Canada updated its safety information to reflect the results

| DOSAGES | Selected Bronchodilator Agents |

Agent	Pharmacological Class	Usual Dosage Range	Indications
▸▸ salbutamol	Beta-adrenergic agonist (beta$_2$-predominant)	***Adult/pediatric >4 yr*** MDI (aka inhalation aerosol): 1–2 puffs q4–6h (adults not to exceed 8 puffs/day; children >4 yr not to exceed 4 puffs/day) ***Pediatric 2–6 yr*** PO syrup: 0.1 mg/kg tid–qid ***Pediatric 6–12 yr*** PO syrup: 2 mg tid–qid ***Adult/pediatric >12 yr*** PO syrup: 2–4 mg tid–qid ***Adult*** IM: 8 μg/kg q4h prn, max 2000 μg/day IV: 5 μg/min, increased to 10 μg/min & 20 μg/min q15–30 min intervals prn ***Adult*** Ventodisk blisters/Diskhaler: 200–400 μg tid–qid, max 1600 μg ***Pediatric >6 yr*** Ventodisk blisters/Diskhaler: 200 μg tid–qid, max 800 μg ***Adult/pediatric ≥12 yr*** Inhalation solution/nebules (via nebulizer device): 2.5–5 mg qid diluted in 2.5–5 mL sterile NS ***Pediatric 5–12 yr*** Inhalation solution (via nebulizer device): 1.25–2.5 mg qid diluted in 2–5 mL sterile NS	Bronchodilation
▸▸ epinephrine	Adrenergic agonist (alpha$_1$, beta$_1$, beta$_2$)	***Adult*** IM/SC: 0.2–1 mg (1:1000 solution); repeated at 20-min to 4-hr intervals based on response ***Pediatric*** SC: 0.01 mg/kg (1:1000 solution) to max of 0.5 mg; repeat at 20-min to 4-hr intervals based on response	
formoterol	Beta-adrenergic agonist (beta$_2$-predominant)	***Adult/pediatric ≥6 yr*** Inhalation capsule: 12–24 μg bid, max 48 μg	
isoproterenol	Beta-adrenergic agonist (beta$_2$-predominant)	***Adult only*** IV: 10–20 μg of a diluted solution	
▸▸ salmeterol	Beta-adrenergic agonist (beta$_2$-predominant); long-acting	***Adult/pediatric ≥4 yr*** Inhalation aerosol: 2 inhalations q12h Inhalation powder: 1 inhalation q12h	
terbutaline	Beta-adrenergic agonist (beta$_2$-predominant)	***Adult/pediatric ≥6 yr*** MDI Inhalation powder: 1–2 inhalation with 5 min between inhalations prn, max 6 inhalations/day	

MDI, Metered-dose inhaler; *NS,* normal saline.

of the United States Salmeterol Multi-Center Asthma Research Trial (SMART) (Health Canada, 2005). Salmeterol is to be used *as alternative additional therapy for those clients with asthma who have unsatisfactory symptom control despite an optimal dose of inhaled corticosteroids (ICS)*. The SMART study showed an *increased risk of asthma-related death and other serious respiratory-related outcomes in clients who used salmeterol* in addition to their regular asthma therapy. The use of concurrent ICS appears to have a protective effect; however, this protective effect was to a lesser degree for Blacks. It is available as a 25-μg/dose aerosol inhaler and a 50-μg/dose powder inhalation device. Pregnancy category C. Recommended dosages are given in the table on p. 296.

PHARMACOKINETICS

Half-Life	Onset	Peak	Duration
5.5 hr	10–20 min	3 hr	12 hr

NASAL DECONGESTANTS

The sympathomimetic agents used as nasal decongestants consist of both alpha- and alpha-beta-adrenergic agents. The alpha-adrenergic activity of these agents is responsible for causing vasoconstriction in the nasal mucosa. This produces shrinkage of the mucosa, which promotes easier nasal breathing and reduces nasal secretions. However, excessive use of nasal decongestants can lead to greater congestion because of a rebound phenomenon that occurs when use of the product is stopped. This is not seen with the oral agents. The decongestants are administered topically with nasal drops or sprays, which are instilled into each nostril. The ephedrine salts, phenylephrine hydrochloride, and pseudoephedrine can produce nasal decongestion when taken either as single therapy or in multiple therapy such as in combination with allergy, cold, cough, and sinus relief preparations. Phenylephrine is usually administered via intranasal spray for this purpose, whereas pseudoephedrine is taken orally.

Relative contraindications to the use of the nasal decongestants are the same for all of the agents and include hypersensitivity, diabetes, hypertension, thyroid disorders, and enlargement of the prostate gland. With routine use, side effects due to systemic absorption of nasally administered decongestants are usually minimal. However, all practitioners should be aware of the possibility of systemic side effects and educate clients accordingly if they are prescribed these agents.

▸▸ pseudoephedrine hydrochloride

Pseudoephedrine is a natural plant alkaloid that is obtained from the ephedra plant. It is a stereoisomer of ephedrine and is a widely used, orally administered decongestant. It is available in infant oral drops, oral solution, and tablet form. Some dosage forms are available without prescription. Because ephedra is also a component of certain OTC herbal dietary supplements, it may be unsafe for clients to use these supplements concurrently with pseudoephedrine. Pregnancy category C. See the table below for recommended dosages.

PHARMACOKINETICS

Half-Life	Onset	Peak	Duration
Variable (min)	15–30 min	30–60 min	4–6 hr
			SR: 8–12 hr

OPHTHALMIC DECONGESTANTS

Ophthalmic decongestants are adrenergics that are applied topically to the eye. When instilled into the eye, they stimulate alpha-adrenergic receptors located on the small arterioles in the eye. This results in arteriolar vasoconstriction, which reduces conjunctival congestion, thus decreasing redness in the eye. Although epinephrine, phenylephrine, and naphazoline are all used as ophthalmic decongestants, tetrahydrozoline is the one most widely used.

tetrahydrozoline

Tetrahydrozoline is applied topically to the eye to temporarily relieve congestion, itching, and minor irritation in clients with red and irritated eyes. It causes constriction of the blood vessels of the eye and is sometimes also used during some diagnostic eye procedures. It is the active ingredient in such OTC products as Visine and Visine Clear eye drops. It is contraindicated in clients with a hypersensitivity reaction to it and in those with narrow-angle glaucoma. Pregnancy category C. The recommended dosages are given in the table below.

PHARMACOKINETICS

Half-Life	Onset	Peak	Duration
Variable (min)	<3 min	Short (min)	4–8 hr

DOSAGES Selected Nasal and Ophthalmic Decongestant Adrenergics

Agent	Pharmacological Class	Usual Dosage Range	Indications
▸▸ pseudoephedrine	Alpha-beta-adrenergic	**Adult** PO tabs: 60 mg q4–6h, max 240 mg/day **Pediatric 6–12 yr** PO tabs: 30 mg q4–6h, max 120 mg/day **Pediatric 2–5 yr** PO tabs: 15 mg q4–6h, max 60 mg/day	Nasal decongestant
tetrahydrozoline	Alpha-adrenergic	1–2 drops into eye(s) up to qid	Ophthalmic decongestant

VASOACTIVE ADRENERGICS

Adrenergics that have primarily cardioselective effects are referred to as vasoactive adrenergics. They are used to support a failing heart or to treat shock. They may also be used to treat individuals with orthostatic hypotension. These agents have a wide range of effects on alpha- and beta-adrenergic receptors, depending on the dose. The vasoactive adrenergics are potent, quick-acting, injectable drugs. Although dosage recommendations are given in the table below, all of these drugs are titrated to the desired physiological response. All of the vasoactive adrenergics (with the exception of midodrine) are rapid in onset, and their effects quickly cease when they are stopped. Therefore careful titration and monitoring of vital signs and electrocardiogram (ECG) are required in clients receiving them.

▸▸ dobutamine

Dobutamine is a beta$_1$-selective vasoactive adrenergic drug that is structurally similar to the naturally occurring catecholamine dopamine. By stimulating the beta$_1$ receptors on the heart (myocardium), it increases cardiac output by increasing contractility (positive inotropy), which increases the stroke volume, especially

DOSAGES Selected Vasoactive Adrenergics			
Agent	**Pharmacological Class**	**Usual Dosage Range**	**Indications**
▸▸ dobutamine	Beta$_1$-adrenergic	**Pediatric** IV infusion: 2.5–15 μg/kg/min **Adult** IV infusion: 2.5–40 μg/kg/min	Cardiac decompensation
▸▸ dopamine	Beta$_1$-adrenergic	**Adult/pediatric** IV infusion: 1–50 μg/kg/min	Shock syndrome, cardiopulmonary resuscitation
▸▸ epinephrine	Alpha-beta-adrenergic	**Pediatric** SC: 10 μg/kg repeated q15min × 2 then q4h prn **Adult** SC: 0.1–0.5 mg repeated q10–15min if required **Neonatal** IV: 10–30 μg/kg q3–5min if required **Pediatric** IV: 10 μg/kg q3–5min if required **Adult** IV: 0.5–1 mg q3–5min if required	Anaphylaxis, cardiopulmonary resuscitation
isoproterenol	Beta-adrenergic	**Adult only** IV infusion: 0.5–20 μg/min IM: 0.2 mg, subsequently 0.02–1 mg SC: 0.2 mg, subsequently 0.15–0.2 mg IV bolus: 0.02–0.06 mg, subsequently 0.01–0.2 mg Intracardiac: 0.02 mg	Heart block/dysrhythmias
midodrine	Alpha$_1$-adrenergic	**Adult only** PO: 2.5–10 mg tid–qid max 30 mg/day	Orthostatic hypotension
▸▸ norepinephrine	Alpha-beta-adrenergic	**Adult** IV infusion: 2–4 μg/min	Hypotensive states
phenylephrine	Alpha-adrenergic	**Pediatric** (for hypotension during spinal anaesthesia) SC or IM: 0.1 mg/kg/dose **Adult** IV infusion: 10 mg/250 or 500 mL IV solution, start at 100–180 μg/min and titrate down to 40–60 μg/min IM/SC: 2–5 mg IV: 0.1–0.5 mg	Hypotension, paroxysmal supraventricular tachycardia

in clients with heart failure. Dobutamine is available only as an intravenous (IV) injectable drug. Pregnancy category B. The recommended dosages are listed in the table on p. 298.

PHARMACOKINETICS

Half-Life	Onset	Peak	Duration
2–5 min	<2 min	<10 min	<10 min

▸▸ dopamine

Dopamine is a naturally occurring catecholamine neurotransmitter in the SNS. It has potent dopaminergic and beta$_1$- and alpha$_1$-adrenergic receptor activity, depending on the dose. Dopamine, when used at low doses, can dilate blood vessels in the brain, heart, kidneys, and mesentery, which increases blood flow to these areas (dopaminergic receptor activity). At higher infusion rates dopamine can improve cardiac contractility and output (beta$_1$-adrenergic receptor activity). The drug is contraindicated in clients who have a catecholamine-secreting tumour of the adrenal gland known as a *pheochromocytoma*. It is available only as an intravenous injectable drug. Pregnancy category C. The recommended vasoactive dosages are given in the table on p. 298.

PHARMACOKINETICS

Half-Life	Onset	Peak	Duration
<2 min	2–5 min	Rapid	10 min

▸▸ epinephrine

Epinephrine is also an endogenous vasoactive catecholamine. It acts directly on both the alpha- and beta-adrenergic receptors of tissues innervated by the SNS. It is used in emergency situations and is one of the primary vasoactive drugs used in many advanced cardiac life support (ACLS) protocols. The physiological response it elicits is dose related. At low dosages it stimulates mostly beta$_1$-adrenergic receptors, increasing the force of contraction and heart rate. It is also used for anaphylactic shock at these doses because it has significant bronchodilatory effects via the beta$_2$-adrenergic receptors in the lungs. At high dosages it stimulates mostly alpha-adrenergic receptors, causing vasoconstriction, which elevates the BP. Pregnancy category C. The dosages recommended for the treatment of various disorders are given in the table on p. 298.

PHARMACOKINETICS

Half-Life	Onset	Peak	Duration
<5 min	<2 min	Rapid	5–30 min

isoproterenol

Isoproterenol acts directly on the beta-adrenergic receptors. In normal doses it has little or no effect on alpha-adrenergic receptors. The main effects of therapeutic doses of isoproterenol are cardiac stimulation via beta$_1$ receptor activity. It also causes relaxation of the smooth muscle of the bronchial tree, GI tract, uterus, and peripheral blood vessels by stimulating the beta$_2$-adrenergic receptors. In addition, isoproterenol inhibits the anaphylaxis-induced release of histamine and may be used to treat clients experiencing an anaphylactic reaction. Pregnancy category C. Common dosages are given in the table on p. 298.

PHARMACOKINETICS

Half-Life	Onset	Peak	Duration
<2 min	Immediate	<15 min	8–50 min

midodrine

Midodrine is a pro-drug converted to its active form, desglymidodrine, in the liver. It is this active metabolite that accounts for the primary pharmacological action of midodrine, which is alpha$_1$-adrenergic receptor stimulation. Alpha$_1$ stimulation causes constriction of both arterioles and veins, resulting in peripheral vasoconstriction. Midodrine is primarily indicated for the treatment of symptomatic orthostatic hypotension. Midodrine is available as 2.5- and 5-mg tablets. Pregnancy category C. Common dosages are given in the table on p. 298.

PHARMACOKINETICS

Half-Life	Onset	Peak	Duration
3–4 hr	45–90 min	1 hr	6–8 hr

▸▸ norepinephrine

Norepinephrine acts predominantly by directly stimulating alpha-adrenergic receptors. It also has some direct-stimulating beta-adrenergic effects on the heart (beta$_1$-adrenergic receptors) but none on the lung (beta$_2$-adrenergic receptors). The most evident effects, however, are those on the alpha-adrenergic receptors, which lead to vasoconstriction. Norepinephrine is directly metabolized to dopamine and is primarily used in the treatment of hypotension and shock. Pregnancy category D. Common dosages are given in the table on p. 298.

PHARMACOKINETICS

Half-Life	Onset	Peak	Duration
<5 min	Immediate	1–2 min	1–2 min

phenylephrine

Phenylephrine works almost exclusively on the alpha-adrenergic receptors. It is primarily used as a short-term agent to augment BP in clients in shock, to control some dysrhythmias (supraventricular tachycardias), and to produce vasoconstriction with regional anaesthesia. It is also administered topically as an ophthalmic agent and as a nasal decongestant. Common vasoactive dosages are listed in the table on p. 298.

PHARMACOKINETICS*

Half-Life	Onset	Peak	Duration
<5 min	Immediate	Rapid	15–20 min

*Intravenous use.

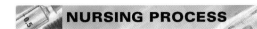
NURSING PROCESS

■ Assessment

Adrenergic drugs have a variety of effects depending on the receptors they stimulate. Stimulation of the alpha-adrenergic receptors results in vasoconstriction, stimulation of beta$_1$-adrenergic receptors produces cardiac stimulation, and stimulation of the beta$_2$-adrenergic receptors results in bronchodilation. Because of these properties, the use of adrenergics requires careful client assessment to minimize the possible side effects and maximize the therapeutic effects.

In a thorough assessment the nurse first gathers information about the client's allergies and past and present medical conditions. A system overview and a thorough medication history should also be part of this assessment. Pertinent questions for the nurse to ask the client are as follows:

- Are you allergic to any medication, food, topical products, environmental products, and so on?
- Are you asthmatic? If so, how frequent and severe are the attacks?
- What are their manifestations and precipitating factors?
- What previous treatment have you received for the asthma? Has it been successful or has it failed?
- Do you have a history of hypertension, cardiac dysrhythmias, or any other cardiovascular disease?

Assessment of renal and hepatic functioning is also important before initiating treatment. Adrenergic drugs may precipitate tachycardia, hypertension, myocardial infarction (MI), or heart failure. Therefore the drugs should be given cautiously in any clients receiving them who are at risk of exacerbation of disease states and/or side effects, such as geriatric clients and those individuals with cardiac disease. Baseline vital signs and assessment of peripheral pulses, skin colour, temperature, and capillary refill should be obtained and documented. In particular for midodrine, postural BPs (supine, sitting, and standing—as ordered) and pulse rates should be documented before and during drug administration. This should be done for both short- and long-term management. Clients requiring midodrine are often those who are having difficulty with postural hypotensive episodes with dizziness, lightheadedness, and even syncope. They already have problems with their BP and therefore will need close assessment before, during, and after the drug has been given. Assessments of the client's symptoms and his or her perception of either disease progression or a decrease in symptoms are important for effective and successful treatment; therefore it is important for the client to have basic knowledge of the disease and its treatment. The nurse should assess and document lung sounds and any abnormalities, mainly for baseline and comparative purposes.

In particular with salmeterol, contraindications include hypersensitivity to it or to adrenergic amines. It is also not to be used for clients during an acute asthmatic attack because of its prolonged effect. Cautious use is recommended with clients who have a history of cerebrovascular disease, dysrhythmias, tachycardia, CNS disorders such as seizures, or diabetes; during pregnancy and lactation; and in geriatric clients. Drug interactions include MAOIs (salmeterol must not be used within 2 weeks after the discontinuation of MAOIs), TCAs, and beta-blockers.

■ Nursing Diagnoses

Nursing diagnoses associated with the use of adrenergic agonists include, but are not limited to, the following:
- Acute pain related to side effects of tachycardia and palpitations
- Deficient knowledge regarding therapeutic regimen, side effects, drug interactions, and precautions related to use of adrenergic agents
- Risk for injury related to possible side effects (nervousness, vertigo, hypertension, or tremors) or from potential drug interactions
- Disturbed sleep pattern related to CNS stimulation caused by adrenergic agents
- Non-adherence with drug therapy related to lack of information about the importance of taking the medication as ordered

■ Planning

Goals for the client receiving sympathomimetics include the following:
- Client takes drugs as ordered and follows directions explicitly.
- Client's symptoms are relieved.
- Client remains adherent with the drug therapy.
- Client demonstrates an adequate knowledge about the use of the specific medications.

■ *Outcome Criteria*

Outcome criteria related to the administration of adrenergic agonists include the following:
- Client states the importance of pharmacological and non-pharmacological treatment of the respiratory or other disorder that is present, such as asthma.
- Client states the importance of adherence with the therapy and the risks and complications associated with overuse of the medication, such as excessive CNS stimulation, insomnia, and tachycardia.
- Client states conditions and side effects that should be reported to the physician, such as chest pain, restlessness, and insomnia.
- Client states the importance of scheduling and keeping follow-up appointments with the physician to monitor the effectiveness of drug therapy.
- Client's condition improves once on the medication regimen with decreased signs and symptoms, such as decreased coughing or wheezing.

■ Implementation

There are several nursing interventions that can maximize the therapeutic effects of adrenergic agents and minimize the side effects. The nurse should always check the package inserts concerning dilutional agents and recommended dilutional amount. For the subcutaneous (SC) administration of the adrenergic agonists for asthma, a tuberculin syringe should be used so that accurate, small doses are administered into the subcutaneous space as indicated. When an inhaler or nebulizer is ordered, the nurse should teach the client how to correctly administer the agent and how to properly use and clean the equipment. A spacer may be ordered for more effective inhaled doses of the drug, and client education must be thorough (see the Client Teaching Tips on p. 302). The nurse must be careful not to administer two adrenergic agents at the same time because of the high risk of precipitating severe side effects such as tachycardia and hypertension. At least 4 hours should elapse between doses of these medications to prevent the occurrence of serious cardiac dysrhythmias. The nurse must emphasize to clients that they must be sure to use these medications exactly as prescribed with regard to amount, timing, and spacing of doses. Often these medications (especially asthmatics) are used in combination with other agents because of their synergistic effects; therefore client education about the possible interactions and exacerbation of side effects is important.

When administering intravenous infusions of these agents for shock-related symptoms (hypotension), the nurse should check the intravenous site frequently for patency and rule out infiltration every hour because of the potential for tissue necrosis from excessive vascular vasoconstriction. Phentolamine is often used for the treatment of infiltration (see Chapter 18, p. 308). Also, with intravenous infusions the nurse must make sure to use only clear solutions, mix in 5 percent dextrose in water (D5W), and administer with an infusion device such as an intravenous pump (all vasoactive substances should be administered via intravenous pump) in conjunction with cardiac monitoring. The agent must be infused slowly to avoid precipitating drastic and possibly dangerous cardiovascular changes in the client's BP and/or pulse rate.

If the ophthalmic form of these agents is given, the nurse must make sure that the medication has not expired. The eye dropper must not be allowed to touch the eye. This helps to prevent possible contamination of the remaining solution. With ophthalmic administration, the nurse must always make sure to use a currently dated and clear solution and apply the drops into the conjunctival sac—not directly onto the eye itself.

Clients with chronic lung disease receiving an adrenergic agent should avoid any of the factors that may exacerbate their condition (e.g., allergens, foods, cigarette smoking) and try to diminish the risk of respiratory infection. This may include avoiding those who are ill with colds and flu, avoiding crowded areas, and remaining well-nourished and rested. In addition, fluid intake of up to 3000 mL/day should be encouraged to ensure adequate hydration, unless contraindicated. Clients should also be encouraged to keep a journal of their symptoms and any improvement or worsening in their condition while on medication. Midodrine, which is given orally in clients with orthostatic intolerance (postural hypotension), should be taken as prescribed. Medications are often to be taken before the client gets out of bed in the morning. Doses are also often "front loaded," or ordered to be taken before 2 pm, when the client may be most symptomatic and most active. Clients should avoid taking these drugs after 6 pm to prevent insomnia and possible supine hypertension.

Salmeterol is indicated for asthma and prevention of bronchospasms in clients over 12 years of age who may need long-term maintenance. It is not to be used for relief of acute symptoms, and education about its dosing is important. Dosing of salmeterol is usually 2 puffs twice daily 12 hours apart for maintenance effects. For prevention of exercise-induced asthma, it is recommended that clients take 2 puffs ½ hour to 1 hour before exercise and no additional doses for 12 hours. If another type of inhalant is used, such as a steroid, the bronchodilator should be used first, with a 5-minute waiting period afterward. All equipment should be rinsed, and the client should be encouraged to perform mouth care after the use of any inhalant forms of medication.

Client teaching tips for the adrenergic agents are listed in the box on p. 302.

Evaluation

Clients receiving adrenergic agents for the treatment of hypotension, shock, or cardiac arrest should be monitored for therapeutic effects including a decrease in edema, increased urinary output, return to normal vital signs (BP $\geq$120/80 mm Hg or increase in BP with each reading, pulse >60 but <120 beats/min, respiratory rate >12 but <20 breaths/min), improved skin colour (pallor to pink) and temperature (cool to warm), and increased level of consciousness. Improvement in the condition of clients with bronchial asthma would be evidenced by return to a normal respiratory rate (>12 but <20 breaths/min); improved breath sounds throughout the lung field with less rales; increased air exchange, including that in the lung bases; decreased to no cough; less dyspnea; improved gas levels; and increased tolerance of activity. If these agents are used for nasal congestion, the client should report less congestion and a better ability to breathe. Therapeutic effects of midodrine include improved level of functioning and activities of daily living (ADLs), fewer episodes of postural intolerance (dizziness, lightheadedness, and possibly syncopal episodes), and more energy.

Clients should be aware of side effects including (but not limited to) cardiac dysrhythmias, hypertension, tachycardia, nervousness, anxiety, tremors, insomnia, and restlessness. Rebound nasal congestion, rhinitis, and nasal mucosa ulcerations are possible adverse effects of the nasal decongestants. Side effects related to the use of midodrine include "goose bumps," itchy scalp, and possible hypertension and even supine hypertension, which may worsen during sleep.

Therapeutic response to salmeterol (and other adrenergics used for asthma) includes an improvement in asthma with improved lung sounds, less wheezing, less respiratory distress, and an overall improved respiratory status. Side effects include CNS stimulation with headache, nervousness, hyperactivity, dizziness, GI upset, tremors, tachycardia, elevated BP, and palpitations.

CLIENT TEACHING TIPS

The nurse should instruct the client as follows:

▲ Always take medications as prescribed; excessive dosing may overstimulate your heart and nervous system, causing problems such as palpitations and a faster heartbeat.

▲ When taking inhaled forms of medication for metered-dose administration, shake the container thoroughly, exhale through the nose, and administer the medication by aerosol while inhaling or breathing in deeply through the mouthpiece of the inhaler. Hold your breath for a few seconds and exhale slowly. When using the inhaler for more than one breath application, wait 2 minutes between inhalations and take only the amount ordered. If you are using a spacer or aerochamber, attach it to the mouthpiece of the inhaler itself. Make sure you understand how to do this. Place the mouthpiece in your mouth, then press down on the inhaler to release the medication with one puff while inhaling slowly. Then breathe slowly for 2 to 3 seconds and then hold your breath for about 10 seconds. If you are supposed to take more than one puff, wait one minute between puffs.

▲ If you have a history of diabetes mellitus, hypertension, hyperthyroidism, dysrhythmias (irregular heartbeat), chest pain, or seizures, make sure your physician knows of these conditions and of any other medications you may be taking for these conditions. (Note: Because of the CNS and cardiovascular stimulation produced by adrenergic agents, these medical conditions need to be closely monitored and the agents must be carefully used to prevent worsening of the pre-existing disorder.)

▲ Do not take any other medications (including OTC medications and natural health supplements) without your physician's approval.

▲ If your respiratory difficulties increase with use of these medications, contact your physician immediately.

▲ If you have a sublingual (SL) form of this medication, hold it under your tongue and don't swallow until it is completely dissolved. Rinse out your mouth afterward to prevent dental problems such as tooth decay.

▲ If you are using an adrenergic agent to treat nasal congestion, there may be a "rebound phenomenon"—that is, it is possible that your congestion will get worse. If this happens, stopping the drug will eventually stop the rebound congestion.

▲ If you carry an EpiPen, you should be aware that it has a recommended 16-month shelf life.

POINTS to REMEMBER

▼ Dopaminergic receptors have a predominant vasodilation response when stimulated and the receptors are located on post-synaptic effector cells, blood vessels, and organs.

▼ Drugs that stimulate the SNS are also called *adrenergic agonists* or *sympathomimetics* and they mimic the effects of the CNS neurotransmitters norepinephrine and epinephrine.

▼ Catecholamines are substances that produce a sympathomimetic response (stimulate the SNS). Naturally occurring or endogenous catecholamines include epinephrine, norepinephrine, and dopamine. Dobutamine is a synthetic or exogenous catecholamine.

▼ Nursing considerations with adrenergic agonists used for respiratory disorders include telling clients to avoid respiratory irritants and to stay away from people with infections. Clients should also avoid OTCs or prescribed medications because of possible drug interactions with adrenergic agonists.

▼ With nasal preparations, rebound nasal congestion or ulcerations of the nasal mucosa may occur if drugs are overused; therefore clients need to be educated to use these products only as directed.

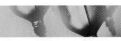

EXAMINATION REVIEW QUESTIONS

1 Which of the following actions of beta-agonist drug therapy describes its cardiac effect? Increased
  a. contractility and pulse rates
  b. conduction, but only through the Bundle of His.
  c. nodal firing and ectopic foci firing.
  d. conduction, but it decreases contractility.

2 Which of the following would be expected in a client who is on daily doses of pseudoephedrine?
  a. Bradycardia
  b. Polyuria
  c. Hypertension
  d. Dysphagia

3 Which of the following would be expected in the client who has postural hypotension and is taking 10 mg of oral midodrine?
  a. More normal ranges of blood pressure
  b. Cardiac arrest
  c. Acute diabetes
  d. "Shocky" signs and symptoms

4 A client is receiving dobutamine for a worsening of her heart failure secondary to the stress of surgery 2 days ago.

Vital signs upon return to the unit post-operatively were as follows: BP 150/88, P 110, R 16. Vital signs now are as follows: BP 170/94, P 110, R 20. She is also complaining of "chest tightness." Which of the following is most appropriately related to the presentation of symptoms?
  a. The changes in vital signs are reflective of a therapeutic response to the drug.
  b. She most likely needs a dose of a beta-agonist to elevate the heart rate and help with the heart failure.
  c. Dobutamine should not be used with heart failure, which explains the symptoms and changes in vital signs.
  d. The new complaint of chest tightness and changes in vital signs need to be re-evaluated immediately by the nurse and physician.

5 Which of the following would occur with use of a positive inotropic drug?
  a. Improved SA nodal firing
  b. Bronchodilation
  c. Sinus bradycardia
  d. Enhanced myocardial contractility

For answers see http://evolve.elsevier.com/Lilley/pharmacology/.

CRITICAL THINKING ACTIVITIES

1 Why is it important to carefully assess the geriatric client for the presence of medical conditions before administering any beta-adrenergic agonist agents?

2 Discuss the rationale for careful titration and monitoring of clients receiving vasoactive adrenergic agents.

For answers see http://evolve.elsevier.com/Lilley/pharmacology/.

BIBLIOGRAPHY

Albanese, J., & Nutz, P. (2005). *Mosby's 2005 nursing drug cards.* St Louis, MO: Mosby.

Anderson, P.O., Knoben, J.E., & Troutman, W.G. (2002). *Handbook of clinical drug data* (10th ed.). New York: McGraw-Hill/ Appleton & Lange.

Canadian Pharmacists Association. (2003). *Therapeutic choices* (4th ed.). Ottawa, ON: Author.

Canadian Pharmacists Association. (2004). *Guide to drugs in Canada.* Toronto, ON: Dorling Kindersley.

Canadian Pharmacists Association. (2005). *Compendium of pharmaceuticals and specialties. The Canadian drug reference for health professionals.* Ottawa, ON: Author. [The subscription-based e-CPS is available at http://www.pharmacists.ca.]

Cheng, A., Williams, B.A., & Sivarajan, B.V. (Eds.). *The HSC handbook of pediatrics* (10th ed.). Toronto, ON: Elsevier.

Facts and Comparisons. (2004). *Drug facts and comparisons pocket version* (9th ed.). St Louis, MO: Wolters Kluwer Health.

Hardman, J.G., & Limbird, L.E. (2002). *Goodman and Gilman's the pharmacological basis of therapeutics* (10th ed.). New York: McGraw-Hill.

Health Canada. (2005). Drug product database (DPD). Retrieved August 4, 2005, from http://www.hc-sc.gc.ca/hpb/drugs-dpd/

Health Canada. (2005). Health Canada endorsed important safety information on Serevent. Retrieved November 11, 2005, from http://www.hc-sc.gc.ca/dhp-mps/medeff/advisories-avis/ prof/serevent_2_hpc-cps_e.html

Health Canada. (2005). Safety information about a class of asthma drugs known as long-acting beta-2 agonists. Retrieved February 3, 2006, from http://www.hc-sc.gc.ca/ahc-asc/media/ advisories-avis/2005/2005_107_e.html

Katzung, B.G. (2004). *Basic and clinical pharmacology* (9th ed.). New York: McGraw-Hill.

Lacy, C.F., Armstrong, L.L., Goldman, M.P., & Lance, L.L. (2003). *Drug information handbook* (11th ed.). Hudson, OH: Lexi-Comp.

Lehne, R.A. (2004). *Pharmacology for nursing care* (5th ed.). St Louis, MO: Saunders.

Mosby (2005). *Mosby's drug consult 2005: The comprehensive reference for generic and brand name drugs* (15th ed.). St Louis, MO: Mosby.

Skidmore-Roth, L. (2006). *Mosby's 2006 nursing drug reference* (19th ed.). St Louis, MO: Mosby.

CHAPTER

18 Adrenergic-Blocking Agents

OBJECTIVES

After reading this chapter, the successful student will be able to do the following:

1 Discuss the normal anatomy and physiology of the autonomic nervous system as it pertains to adrenergic-blocking agents or sympatholytics.

2 List examples of the various adrenergic antagonists or adrenergic blockers.

3 Discuss the mechanisms of action, therapeutic effects, indications, and adverse and toxic effects of adrenergic antagonists, as well as cautions, contraindications, dosages and routes of administration.

4 Identify the antidotes used to treat overdose with adrenergic-blocking agents.

5 Develop a nursing care plan that includes all phases of the nursing process as related to the administration of the various adrenergic antagonists.

e-LEARNING ACTIVITIES

Student CD-ROM
- Review Questions: see questions 101–109
- Animations
- Medication Administration Checklists
- IV Therapy Checklists

  evolve Web site (http://evolve.elsevier.com/Lilley/pharmacology/)
- Online Chapter Worksheet • Frequently Asked Questions
- Learning Tips and Content Updates • WebLinks • Online Appendices and Supplements • Mosby/Saunders ePharmacology Update • Access to *Mosby's Drug Consult*

DRUG PROFILES

acebutolol, p. 311
▸▸atenolol, p. 311
carvedilol, p. 311
ergotamine tartrate, p. 307
▸▸esmolol, p. 311
labetalol, p. 311

▸▸metoprolol, p. 311
▸▸phentolamine, p. 307
▸▸prazosin, p. 308
▸▸propranolol, p. 311
sotalol, p. 313

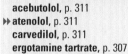 Key drug.

GLOSSARY

Agonists (ag′ ə nists) Drugs with a specific cellular affinity that produces a "mimic" response.

Angina (an jy′ nuh) Paroxysmal chest pain caused by myocardial ischemia.

Antagonists (an tag′ ə nists) Drugs that bind to adrenergic receptors and inhibit or block neurotransmitters.

Cardioprotective The characteristic of beta-blockers to inhibit stimulation of the heart by circulating catecholamines.

Cardioselective beta-blockers Beta-blocking drugs that are selective for beta$_1$-adrenergic receptors. Also called beta$_1$-blocking agents.

Dysrhythmia (dis rith′ mee uh) Irregular heartbeat.

Extravasation (ek′ strav ə say′ shən) Leaking of fluid from the blood vessel into the tissues.

Glycogenolysis (gly′ koe jə nol′ ə sis) The production of glucose from glycogen in the liver, which is reduced by beta-blockers.

Intrinsic sympathomimetic activity (ISA) (in trin′ zik sim′ pə tho mi met′ ik) Action of agents within the beta-blocking class. A drug that mimics the activity of the adrenergic system, such as certain beta-blockers (acebutolol).

Lipophilicity (lip′ o fil is′ ət ee) Attraction to lipid or fat.

Non-selective beta-blockers Beta-blocking drugs that block both beta$_1$- and beta$_2$-adrenergic receptors.

Orthostatic hypotension (or′ tho stat′ ik hy′ poe ten′ shən) Abnormally low blood pressure occurring when a person stands up.

Oxytocics (ok′ si to′ siks) Drugs used to treat postpartum and post-abortion bleeding caused by uterine relaxation and enlargement. They stimulate the smooth muscle of the uterus to contract.

Pheochromocytoma (fee' o kroe' moe sy toe' muh) Vascular tumour that secretes norepinephrine and stimulates the central nervous system (CNS).

Sympatholytics Another name for adrenergic antagonists.

Vaughan Williams classification System of classifying antidysrhythmic agents.

The autonomic nervous system consists of the parasympathetic and sympathetic nervous systems. The class of drugs discussed in this chapter works primarily on the sympathetic nervous system (SNS). As discussed in Chapter 17, the adrenergic agonist drugs stimulate the SNS. These drugs are called **agonists** because they bind to receptors and cause a response. The adrenergic blockers have the opposite effect and are therefore referred to as **antagonists.** They also bind to adrenergic receptors but in doing so inhibit or block stimulation of the SNS. They are also referred to as **sympatholytics** because they "lyse," or inhibit, SNS stimulation.

Throughout the body there are receptor sites for the sympathetic neurotransmitters norepinephrine and epinephrine. These are called the *adrenergic receptors,* and there are two basic types—alpha and beta. There are subtypes of both the alpha- and beta-adrenergic receptors, designated 1 and 2. Alpha$_1$- and alpha$_2$-adrenergic receptors are differentiated by their location on nerves. Alpha$_1$-adrenergic receptors are located on the cell, muscle, or organ that the nerve is stimulating (post-synaptic effector cells). The alpha$_2$-adrenergic receptors are located on the actual nerves that stimulate the presynaptic effector cells. Beta$_1$-adrenergic receptors are located primarily on the heart. Beta$_2$-adrenergic receptors are located primarily on the smooth muscles of the bronchioles and blood vessels. It is at these receptors that adrenergic blockers work, and these agents are classified by the type of adrenergic receptor they block—alpha or beta. Hence they are called *alpha-blockers* and *beta-blockers.*

ALPHA-BLOCKERS

Alpha-adrenergic–blocking agents, or alpha-blockers, interrupt or block the stimulation of the SNS at the alpha-adrenergic receptor. Various physiological responses occur when the stimulation of the alpha-adrenergic receptors is inhibited. Adrenergic blockade at the alpha-adrenergic receptors leads to vasodilation, decreased blood pressure (BP), miosis or constriction of the pupil, or suppressed ejaculation. The ergot alkaloids dihydroergotamine mesylate, ergoloid mesylate, ergotamine tartrate, and ergonovine maleate are alpha-blockers that are used mainly for their vasoconstrictor properties. The alpha-blockers doxazosin, prazosin, and terazosin are used as antihypertensive agents because they cause vasodilation. Each of these two groups of agents blocks alpha-adrenergic receptors, but they have an affinity for different sites in the body and therefore the resultant effects differ. Phentolamine is another alpha-blocker.

Mechanism of Action and Drug Effects

As mentioned earlier, alpha-blockers work by blocking or inhibiting the normal stimulation of the SNS. They do this either by directly competing with the SNS neurotransmitter norepinephrine or by a non-competitive process. Most alpha-blockers are competitive in their actions. They have a higher affinity for the alpha-adrenergic receptor than norepinephrine and occupy the receptor before the neurotransmitter can do so. Once this competitive alpha-blocker binds to the receptor, it causes the receptor to be less responsive. This blockade is reversible. Non-competitive alpha-blockers work in a different fashion. They also bind to the alpha-adrenergic receptors, but this type of bond (a covalent bond) is irreversible. Regardless of which way the blockade is accomplished, the result is a decreased response to stimulation of the SNS. Figure 18-1 illustrates these two mechanisms.

Alpha-blockers have many effects on the normal physiological functions of the body. The effects of each agent can differ depending on the agent's selectivity for particular tissues or cells in the body. Ergot alkaloids, for example, can cause peripheral and cerebral vasoconstriction as well as the constriction of dilated arteries. Certain alpha-blockers can stimulate uterine contractions. Others can block alpha-adrenergic receptors on both vascular and non-vascular smooth muscle. The vascular smooth muscle for which these alpha-blockers have an affinity is that in the bladder and its sphincters, the gastrointestinal (GI) tract and its sphincters, the prostate, and the ureters. The non-vascular smooth muscle for which these agents have an affinity is in the CNS, liver, and kidneys. Unlike ergot alkaloids, some alpha-blockers can induce arterial and venous dilation and thus decrease peripheral vascular resistance and BP. Alpha-blockers can also affect certain concentrations of neurotransmitters, causing a depletion of catecholamines such as norepinephrine and epinephrine. Others can directly block a neurotransmitter such as serotonin (5-hydroxytryptamine) or indirectly cause it to be depleted.

Indications

Alpha-blockers have many therapeutic effects, but these effects differ greatly depending on the particular agent. Ergot alkaloids constrict dilated arterioles in the brain that are often responsible for causing vascular headaches, such as migraines. The vasoconstriction that results from these drugs helps relieve the symptoms associated with vascular migraines due to dilated arteries. They are also used as **oxytocics,** agents used to control post-partum and post-abortion bleeding caused by uterine relaxation and enlargement. These agents increase the intensity of uterine contractions and induce local vasoconstriction.

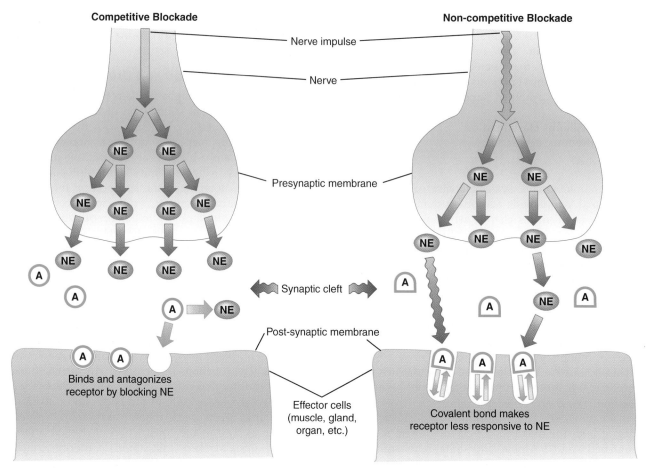

FIG. 18-1 Alpha-blocker mechanisms for alpha-adrenergic competitive and non-competitive blockade. *NE*, norepinephrine; *A*, antagonist.

Alpha-blockers such as doxazosin, prazosin, terazosin, and tamsulosin cause both arterial and venous dilation. This reduces peripheral vascular resistance and BP; thus these agents are used to treat hypertension. Alpha-adrenergic receptors are also present on the prostate and bladder. By blocking stimulation of alpha$_1$-receptors, these agents reduce smooth muscle contraction of the bladder neck and prostatic portion of the urethra. For this reason, alpha-blockers are used in clients with benign prostatic hyperplasia (BPH) to decrease resistance to urinary outflow. This reduces urinary obstruction and relieves some of the effects of BPH. Tamsulosin is used exclusively for treating BPH.

Other alpha-blockers can inhibit excitatory responses to adrenergic stimulation. These agents non-competitively block alpha-adrenergic receptors on smooth muscle and various exocrine glands. Because of this action, these alpha-blockers are useful in controlling or preventing hypertension in clients who have a **pheochromocytoma,** a tumour that forms on the adrenal glands on top of the kidneys and secretes norepinephrine, thus causing SNS stimulation. Alpha-blockers are also useful in the treatment of clients who have increased endogenous alpha-adrenergic agonist activity. Three such conditions are frostbite, Raynaud's disease, and acrocyanosis. Still other alpha-blockers are effec-

tive at antagonizing responses caused by injected catecholamines such as epinephrine and norepinephrine. This causes peripheral vasodilation and decreases peripheral resistance by blocking catecholamine-stimulated vasoconstriction. They can also be used to treat pheochromocytomas. Because of their potent vasodilating properties and their fast onset of action, they are also used to prevent skin necrosis and sloughing after the **extravasation** of vasopressors such as norepinephrine or epinephrine. When these drugs extravasate, or leak out of the blood vessel into the surrounding tissue, this causes vasoconstriction and ultimately tissue death, or necrosis. If the vasoconstriction is not reversed quickly, the whole limb can be lost. Phentolamine, an alpha-blocker, can reverse this potent vasoconstriction and restore blood flow to the ischemic, vasoconstricted area.

Contraindications

Contraindications of alpha-blocking agents include known drug allergy and peripheral vascular disease and may include hepatic and renal disease, coronary artery disease, peptic ulcer, and sepsis.

Side Effects and Adverse Effects

The primary side effects and adverse effects of alpha-blockers are those related to their effects on the vascula-

TABLE 18-1
ALPHA-BLOCKERS: ADVERSE EFFECTS

Body System	Side/Adverse Effects
Cardiovascular	Palpitations, orthostatic hypotension, tachycardia, edema, dysrhythmias, chest pain
Central nervous	Dizziness, headache, drowsiness, anxiety, depression, vertigo, weakness, numbness, fatigue
Gastrointestinal	Nausea, vomiting, diarrhea, constipation, abdominal pain
Other	Incontinence, nose bleeding, tinnitus, dry mouth, pharyngitis, rhinitis

TABLE 18-2
ALPHA-BLOCKERS: COMMON DRUG INTERACTIONS

Drug	Mechanism	Results
Beta-blockers Calcium channel blockers Diuretics	Additive effects	Profound hypotension
Protein-bound drugs	Compete for plasma protein-binding sites	Increased free drug levels in plasma

ture. The alpha-blockers' primary side effects and adverse effects are listed by body system in Table 18-1.

Toxicity and Management of Overdose

In an acute overdose, consultation with a Poison Control Centre is recommended. Activated charcoal can be administered to bind to the drug and remove it from the stomach and the circulation. To hasten elimination of the drug bound to the activated charcoal, the first dose is given with a cathartic such as sorbitol. Symptomatic and supportive measures should be instituted as needed, such as BP support with the administration of fluids, volume expanders, and vasopressor agents and the administration of anticonvulsants such as diazepam for the control of seizures.

Interactions

The most severe of the drug interactions with alpha-blockers are the ones that potentiate the alpha-blockers' effects. Alpha-blockers as a whole are highly protein bound and compete for binding sites with other drugs that are highly protein bound. With limited sites for binding on protein and increased competition for these sites, the result is that more drug is not bound; therefore more drug circulates freely in the bloodstream. Because drug that is not bound to protein is active, the result is a more pronounced drug effect. Some of the common drugs that interact with alpha-blockers and the results of these interactions are listed in Table 18-2.

Dosages

For the recommended dosages of alpha-blockers, see the table on p. 308. See Appendix B for some of the common brands available in Canada.

DRUG PROFILES

Alpha-blockers are prescription-only drugs that are available in many dosage forms. The oral (PO) forms include tablets only. Parenteral formulations include intravenous (IV) and intramuscular (IM) injections. They are also available as rectal suppositories.

Most alpha-blockers are rated as pregnancy category C agents by the U.S. Food and Drug Administration (FDA) and Canada uses these categories as guidelines. Ergot alkaloids, however, are rated as pregnancy category X drugs.

ergotamine tartrate

Ergotamine is an ergot alkaloid. All ergot alkaloids are obtained from a fungus called *Claviceps purpurea* that grows on rye. It causes dilated blood vessels in the brain, the carotid arteries, to constrict. These dilated arteries are responsible for causing vascular headaches such as migraines and cluster headaches. In Canada ergotamine tartrate is available only in combination with other agents. The addition of caffeine to ergotamine facilitates the absorption of ergotamine when taken in the oral or suppository form, which leads to a more effective and rapid onset of vasoconstriction. It is contraindicated in clients with peripheral vascular disease, coronary artery disease, severe hypertension, sepsis, shock, impaired hepatic or renal functions, as well as in pregnant women. It is available as a tablet containing 1 mg of ergotamine and 100 mg of caffeine and as a rectal suppository that contains 2 mg of ergotamine and 100 mg of caffeine. There are also several other combination-drug preparations available in oral tablet form. These combinations vary; some of the other agents combined with ergotamine in these preparations are belladonna alkaloids, phenobarbital, and diphenhydramine. See the table on p. 308 for dosing information.

PHARMACOKINETICS

Half-Life	Onset	Peak	Duration
2.7 hr	30 min–2 hr	2 hr	24–48 hr

▸▸ phentolamine

Phentolamine is an alpha-blocker that reduces peripheral vascular resistance and is also used to treat hypertension. It can be used to help establish the diagnosis of pheochromocytoma and to treat the high BP caused by this catecholamine-secreting tumour. To help establish a diagnosis of pheochromocytoma, a single intravenous dose of phentolamine is given to the hypertensive client who is suspected of having the tumour. If the blood pressure declines rapidly (by more than 35 mm Hg systolic and 25 mm Hg diastolic), it is highly likely that the client has a pheochromocytoma. It is available

DOSAGES **Selected Alpha-Adrenergic Blocking Agents**

Agent	Pharmacological Class	Usual Dosage Range	Indications
ergotamine tartrate-caffeine	Alpha-blocker	**Adult** PO tabs: 2 mg; repeat at ½-hr intervals; do not exceed 6 mg/day or 10 tabs/wk Suppos: 2 mg; repeat at 1 hr intervals; do not exceed 6 mg/day or 5 suppos/wk **Pediatric 6–12 yr** PO tabs: 1 mg; repeat × 2/day (or 1½ supp/day; do not exceed 5 mg/wk Supp: 0.5 mg (½ supp); repeat at 1 hr intervals; do not exceed 1½/day or 2½ supp/wk	Migraine
▶▶phentolamine	Alpha-blocker	**Adult** IV: 2–5 mg 1–2 hr pre-op and repeat if necessary **Pediatric >8 yr** IV: 1 mg 1–2 hr pre-op	Control/prevention of hypertension in clients with pheochromocytoma preoperatively and during surgery
		Adult IM/IV: 5 mg; repeat if necessary	Hypertensive episodes with pheochromocytoma
		Adult 5–10 mg diluted in 10 mL NS injected into extravasation site within 12 hr **Pediatric >8 yr** 1 mg into extravasation site	Treatment of alpha-adrenergic drug extravasation
▶▶prazosin	Alpha₁-blocker	**Adult only** PO: 0.5 mg bid (initial dose HS); maintenance range 1–5 mg/day divided bid–qid; do not exceed 20 mg/day	Hypertension

NS, Normal saline.

only as an intravenous preparation, but this confers some advantages because it can then be used to treat the extravasation of vasoconstricting intravenous drugs such as norepinephrine, epinephrine, and dopamine, which when given intravenously can leak out of the vein, especially if the intravenous tube is not correctly positioned. If the drug is allowed to extravasate into the surrounding tissue, this leads to intense vasoconstriction, decreased blood flow, necrosis, and potential loss of the limb. When phentolamine is injected subcutaneously in a circular fashion around the extravasation site, this causes alpha-adrenergic receptor blockade and vasodilation, which in turn increases blood flow to the ischemic tissue, thus preventing permanent damage. It is contraindicated in clients who have shown a hypersensitivity to it or to sulphites, those who have suffered a myocardial infarction (MI), and those with coronary artery disease or hypotension. The recommended dosages are given in the table above.

PHARMACOKINETICS

Half-Life	Onset	Peak	Duration
19 min	Immediate	2 min	15–30 min

▶▶ *prazosin*

Prazosin is an alpha₁-adrenergic–blocking agent primarily used to treat hypertension and to reduce urinary obstruction in men with BPH. Other drugs that are chemically and pharmacologically related to prazosin are doxazosin, terazosin, and tamsulosin. Its primary antihypertensive effects are related to its selective and competitive inhibition of alpha₁-adrenergic receptors. In men with BPH, prazosin relieves the impaired urinary flow and urinary frequency by relaxing and dilating the vasculature and smooth muscle in the area surrounding the prostate. It also rather dramatically lowers BP. A client's ability to tolerate this drop in BP must be taken into consideration when prescribing alpha-blockers for the treatment of BPH. Often when clients are first started on the drug, they become lightheaded and may even pass out when standing up after sitting or lying down. This is referred to as **orthostatic hypotension.** Although it is a fairly common problem specific to the alpha₁-blockers prazosin, doxazosin, terazosin, and tamsulosin, clients quickly acquire a tolerance to it, most after the first dose. Often clients taking their first dose are told to take it at bedtime to circumvent the problem. Prazosin is contraindicated in clients who have shown hypersensitivity reactions to it. It is available orally in 1-, 2-, and 5-mg capsules. The normally recommended dosages of prazosin are given in the table above.

PHARMACOKINETICS

Half-Life	Onset	Peak	Duration
2–4 hr	2 hr	1–3 hr	6–12 hr

BETA-BLOCKERS

Beta-adrenergic–blocking agents (beta-blockers) block SNS stimulation of the beta-adrenergic receptors by competing with the endogenous catecholamines norepinephrine and epinephrine. Beta-blockers can be either selective or non-selective, depending on the type of beta-adrenergic receptors they antagonize or block. As mentioned earlier, beta$_1$-adrenergic receptors are located primarily on the heart. Beta-blockers selective for these receptors are sometimes called **cardioselective beta-blockers,** or beta$_1$-blocking agents. Other beta-blockers block both beta$_1$- and beta$_2$-adrenergic receptors, the latter located primarily on the smooth muscles of the bronchioles and blood vessels. Beta-blockers that block both types of beta-adrenergic receptors are referred to as **non-selective beta-blockers.** The agents within the beta-blocker class can be further categorized according to whether they have **intrinsic sympathomimetic activity (ISA).** Agents with ISA (acebutolol, pindolol) not only block beta-adrenergic receptors but also partially stimulate them. This was initially believed to be an advantageous characteristic, but clinical use has not borne this out. Some beta-blockers also have alpha-receptor-blocking activity, especially at higher doses; examples of these drugs include carvedilol and labetalol. Box 18-1 lists the currently available beta-blockers.

Mechanism of Action and Drug Effects

Because beta-blockers compete with and block norepinephrine and epinephrine at the beta-adrenergic receptors located throughout the body, the beta-adrenergic receptor sites can then no longer be stimulated by the neurotransmitters and SNS stimulation is blocked. Although beta-adrenergic receptors are located throughout the body, the most important ones in terms of these agents are the ones located on the surface of the heart, the smooth muscle of the bronchi, and the smooth muscle of blood vessels.

Cardioselective beta$_1$-blockers block the beta$_1$-adrenergic receptors on the surface of the heart. This reduces myocardial stimulation, which in turn reduces heart rate, slows conduction through the atrioventricular (AV) node, prolongs sinoatrial (SA) node recovery, and decreases myocardial oxygen demand by decreasing myocardial contractile force (contractility). Non-selective beta-blockers also have this effect on the heart, but they block beta$_2$-adrenergic receptors on the smooth muscle of the bronchioles and blood vessels as well.

Smooth muscle also surrounds the airways in the lungs called *bronchioles.* When beta$_2$-adrenergic receptors are blocked on these, the smooth muscle contracts, causing these airways to narrow. This may lead to shortness of breath. Additionally, the smooth muscle that surrounds blood vessels controls the size of the blood vessels and can cause them to dilate or constrict depending on whether the alpha$_1$- or beta$_2$-adrenergic receptors are stimulated. When beta$_2$-SNS stimulation at these smooth muscles is blocked by a beta-blocker, these muscles are

BOX 18-1

Currently Available Beta-Blockers

Non-selective Beta-Blockers
carvedilol
labetalol*
nadolol
oxprenolol
pindolol
propranolol
sotalol
timolol

Cardioselective Beta-Blockers
acebutolol
atenolol
betaxolol
bisoprolol
esmolol
metoprolol

*Blocks both alpha- and beta-adrenergic receptors.

then stimulated by unopposed SNS activity at the alpha$_1$-adrenergic receptors, which causes them to contract. This in turn increases peripheral vascular resistance. Furthermore, catecholamines promote **glycogenolysis,** the production of glucose from glycogen, and mobilize glucose in response to hypoglycemia. Non-selective beta-blockers impair this process and also impair the secretion of insulin from the pancreas, which causes an elevated blood glucose level.

Finally, beta-blockers can cause the release of free fatty acids from adipose tissue. This may result in moderately elevated blood levels of triglycerides and reduced levels of the "good cholesterol" known as high-density lipoproteins (HDLs).

Indications

The drug effects mentioned in the preceding section vary from beta-blocker to beta-blocker depending on the specific chemical characteristics of the agent. Some beta-blockers are used primarily in the treatment of **angina,** or chest pain. These work by decreasing demand for myocardial energy and oxygen consumption, which helps shift the supply-and-demand ratio to the supply side and allows more oxygen to get to the heart muscle. This in turn helps relieve the pain in the heart muscle caused by the lack of oxygen.

Other beta-blockers are considered **cardioprotective** because they inhibit stimulation by the circulating catecholamines. Catecholamines are released during muscle damage such as that caused by an MI, or heart attack. When a beta-blocker occupies their receptors, the circulating catecholamines cannot then bind to the receptors. Thus the beta-blockers "protect" the heart from being stimulated by these catecholamines, which would only further increase the heart rate and the contractile force, thereby increasing myocardial oxygen demand. As a result, beta-blockers are commonly given to clients after they have suffered an MI to protect the heart from the effects of these released catecholamines.

As mentioned previously, beta-blockers also have a profound effect on the conduction system of the heart. The AV node normally receives impulse stimulation from the SA node and slows it down so that the ventricles have time to fill before they are stimulated to contract. Conduction in the SA node, which spontaneously depolarizes at the most frequent rate, is further slowed by beta-blockers, resulting in a decreased heart rate. They also slow conduction through the AV node. These effects of beta-blockers on the conduction system of the heart make them useful agents in the treatment of various types of irregular heartbeats called **dysrhythmias.** In the **Vaughan Williams classification** of antidysrhythmic drugs (see Chapter 22), all beta-blockers are in the class II category, with the exception of sotalol, which is class III.

Their ability to reduce SNS stimulation of the heart, including heart rate and the force of myocardial contraction, renders beta-blockers useful in treating hypertension. Traditionally beta-blockers were thought to worsen heart failure. However, recent studies have shown benefit when using beta-blockers. Certain beta-blockers such as carvedilol and metoprolol have had the best results to date. The form of heart failure that has a diastolic dysfunction component responds favourably to beta-blockers.

Because of their **lipophilicity** (attraction to lipid or fat), other beta-blockers can easily gain entry into the CNS and brain. These beta-blockers are used to treat migraine headaches. In addition, the topical application of beta-blockers on the eye has been effective in treating ocular disorders such as glaucoma.

TABLE 18-3
BETA-BLOCKERS: COMMON ADVERSE EFFECTS

Body System	Side/Adverse Effects
Cardiovascular	AV block, bradycardia, heart failure, peripheral vascular insufficiency
Central nervous	Dizziness, mental depression, lethargy, hallucinations
Gastrointestinal	Nausea, dry mouth, vomiting, constipation, diarrhea, cramps, ischemic colitis
Hematological	Agranulocytosis, thrombocytopenia
Other	Erectile dysfunction, rash, alopecia, bronchospasms

Contraindications

Contraindications of beta-blockers include known drug allergies and may include uncompensated heart failure, cardiogenic shock, heart block or bradycardia, pregnancy, severe pulmonary disease, and Raynaud's disease.

Side Effects and Adverse Effects

The side effects and adverse effects of beta-blockers are primarily extensions of their pharmacological activity. Most such effects are mild and diminish with time. Some of the most serious undesirable effects can be caused by acute withdrawal of the drug. This may exacerbate the underlying angina they are being used to treat, or it may precipitate an MI. Beta-blockers may also mask the signs and symptoms of hypoglycemia. Beta-blockers may precipitate bronchospasm in clients with asthma and chronic obstructive pulmonary disease (COPD). Beta-blocker–induced side effects and adverse effects are listed by body site in Table 18-3.

Toxicity and Management of Overdose

After the acute ingestion of an overdose of a beta-blocker, consultation with a Poison Control Centre is recommended. Treatment consists primarily of symptomatic and supportive care. Atropine may be given intravenously for the management of bradycardia. If the bradycardia persists despite atropine treatment, isoproterenol may be administered. If the bradycardia still persists, placement of a transvenous cardiac pacemaker should be considered. For the treatment of severe hypotension, vasopressors should be titrated until the desired BP and heart rate are achieved. Intravenously administered diazepam may be useful for the treatment of seizures. Most beta-blockers are dialyzable; therefore hemodialysis may be useful in enhancing elimination in the event of severe overdose.

Interactions

Most of the drug interactions with beta-blockers result from either the additive effects of co-administered medications with similar mechanisms of action, or the antagonistic effects of the agents (see Table 18-4).

Dosages

For information on the recommended dosages for selected beta-blockers, see the table on p. 312. See Appendix B for some of the common brands available in Canada.

TABLE 18-4
BETA-BLOCKERS: DRUG INTERACTIONS

Drug	Mechanism	Result
Antacids (aluminum hydroxide type)	Decrease absorption	Decreased beta-blocker activity
Antimuscarinics/anticholinergics	Antagonism	Reduced beta-blocker effects
Diuretics and cardiovascular drugs	Additive effect	Additive hypotensive effects
Neuromuscular blocking agents	Additive effect	Prolonged neuromuscular blockade
Oral hypoglycemic agents	Antagonism	Decreased hypoglycemic effects

DRUG PROFILES

Beta-blockers are prescription-only drugs that are available in oral preparations as tablets and capsules and in parenteral forms as intermittent injections or continuous intravenous infusions. Topically administered forms are also available. Beta-blocker eye drops are used in the treatment of glaucoma. Most beta-blockers, except acebutolol and sotalol, are rated as pregnancy category C agents. However, acebutolol is a category D agent, and sotalol a category B agent.

acebutolol

Acebutolol is a cardioselective beta$_1$-blocker used for the treatment of hypertension and angina. It is commonly used alone as an antihypertensive agent or in combination, often with a thiazide diuretic for the additive antihypertensive effects. It is one of the few beta-blockers that possess ISA. It is contraindicated in clients who have had a hypersensitivity reaction to it; in those with severe bradycardia, heart block greater than first degree, or malignant hypertension; and in those in cardiogenic shock or cardiac failure. It is available orally in 100-, 200-, and 400-mg capsules. Pregnancy category D. The commonly recommended dosages are given in the table on p. 312.

PHARMACOKINETICS

Half-Life	Onset	Peak	Duration
3–4 hr	1.5–3 hr	2.5–3.5 hr	10–24 hr

▶▶ atenolol

Atenolol is a cardioselective beta-blocker that is commonly used to prevent future MIs in clients who have had an MI. It is also used in the treatment of hypertension and angina. It is available for intravenous use and orally in 25-, 50-, and 100-mg tablets. It is also available in combination with the diuretic chlorthalidone. Pregnancy category C. See the table on p. 312 for the recommended dosages.

PHARMACOKINETICS

Half-Life	Onset	Peak	Duration
6–7 hr	IV: Immediate	IV: <5 min	IV: <12 hr
	PO: <30 min	PO: 2–4 hr	PO: 24 hr

carvedilol

Carvedilol is a newer beta-blocker. It has many actions, including acting as a non-selective beta-blocker, an alpha$_1$-blocker, a calcium channel blocker (CCB), and possibly an antioxidant. It is primarily used in the treatment of heart failure but is also beneficial in hypertension and angina. It has been shown to slow progression of heart failure and decrease the frequency of hospitalization in clients with mild to moderate (Class II or III) heart failure. Carvedilol is most commonly added to digoxin, furosemide, and angiotensin converting enzyme (ACE) inhibitors when used to treat heart failure. It is contraindicated in clients with Class IV decompensated heart failure, asthma, second- or third-degree AV block, cardiogenic shock, and severe bradycardia. It is available as 3.125-, 6.25-, 12.5-, and 25-mg tablets. Pregnancy category C. Recommended dosages are given in the table on p. 312.

PHARMACOKINETICS

Half-Life	Onset	Peak	Duration
7–10 hr	30 min	1–2.3 hr	24 hr

▶▶ esmolol

Esmolol is a potent short-acting beta$_1$-blocker. It is primarily used in emergencies to provide rapid, temporary control of the ventricular rate in clients with supraventricular tachydysrhythmias (SVTs). Because of its short half-life, it is only given as an intravenous infusion, and the serum levels are titrated to control the client's symptoms. It is available in 10-mg/mL concentrate for intravenous injection. Pregnancy category C. Recommended dosages are given in the table on p. 312.

PHARMACOKINETICS

Half-Life	Onset	Peak	Duration
9 min	Immediate	5 min	15–20 min

labetalol

Labetalol is unusual in that it can block both alpha- and beta-adrenergic receptors. It is interesting to note that the action of labetalol is 4 times greater on the beta receptors than the alpha receptors. It is used in the treatment of severe hypertension and hypertensive emergencies to quickly lower the BP before permanent damage is done. It is available both parenterally as a 5-mg/mL intravenous injection and orally as 100- and 200-mg tablets. Pregnancy category C. The normal dosages are given in the table on p. 312.

PHARMACOKINETICS

Half-Life	Onset	Peak	Duration
6–8 hr	IV: 2–5 min	IV: 5–15 min	IV: 2–4 hr
	PO: 20–120 min	PO: 1–4 hr	PO: 8–24 hr

▶▶ metoprolol

Metoprolol is a beta$_1$-blocker that has become popular for use in the post-MI client. Recent studies of metoprolol have shown increased survival in clients given the agent after they have suffered an MI. It is also used in the management of hypertension and angina. It is available as a 1-mg/mL injection or as 25-, 50-, 100-, and 200-mg tablets and 200-mg extended-release tablets. It is also available in combination with the diuretic hydrochlorothiazide (HCT). Pregnancy category C. Commonly recommended dosages are given in the table on p. 312.

PHARMACOKINETICS

Half-Life	Onset	Peak	Duration
3–4 hr	IV: Immediate	IV: 10 min	IV: 5–8 hr
	PO: 10 min	PO: 1.5–5 hr	PO: 24 hr

▶▶ propranolol

Propranolol is the prototypical non-selective beta$_1$- and beta$_2$-blocking agent. It was one of the first beta-blockers to be used. Lengthy experience has yielded many uses for it. Besides the indications mentioned for acebutolol, propranolol has also been used in the treatment of the tachydysrhythmias associated with cardiac glycoside

DOSAGES Selected Beta-Adrenergic Antagonists ("Beta-Blockers")

Agent	Pharmacological Class	Usual Dosage Range	Indications
acebutolol	Beta₁-blocker	**Adult** PO: 400–800 mg/day divided bid 200–600 mg/day divided bid	Hypertension Angina
▸▸atenolol	Beta₁-blocker	**Adult** PO: 50–100 mg/day, taken daily 50–200 mg/day divided once or twice daily	Hypertension Angina
bisoprolol	Beta₁-blocker	**Adult** PO: 5 mg/day; may be titrated every 2 wks up to max 20 mg/day	Mild to moderate hypertension
carvedilol	Alpha₁- and beta-blocker	**Adult** PO: 3.125 mg bid; may double dose every 2 wk to highest tolerated dose, max 50 mg/day	Heart failure
▸▸esmolol	Beta₁-blocker	**Adult** IV: Bolus of 0.5 mg/kg/min over 1 min, followed by 4 min at 0.05 mg/kg/min and evaluate IV: 1.5 mg/kg bolus over 30 sec followed by 0.15–0.3 mg/kg/min infusion	Supraventricular tachydysrhythmias Intra-operative/post-operative tachycardia and hypertension
labetalol	Alpha- and beta-blocker	**Adult** PO: 200–1200 mg/day divided bid IV: 20 mg over 20 min with additional doses of 40 mg at 10-min intervals until desired effect or a total dose of 300 mg is injected; maintenance infusion of 2 mg/min initially and titrate to response	Hypertension Severe hypertension
▸▸metoprolol	Beta₁-blocker	**Adult** PO: 100–400 mg/day divided bid SR tabs: 100–200 mg/day am IV/PO: 3 bolus injections of 5 mg at 2-min intervals followed in 15 min by 50 mg PO q6h for 48 hr; thereafter 100 mg PO bid	Hypertension, late MI, angina Early MI
▸▸propranolol	Beta-blocker	**Adult** PO: maintenance 60–320 mg/day divided bid–qid 180–240 mg divided tid 20–40 mg tid–qid 120–130 mg/day 160–240 mg/day divided 30–60 mg/day divided for 3 days before surgery with an alpha-blocker also IV: 1 mg slow IV push, may repeat every 5 min up to 5 mg	Prophylaxis for angina, hypertension Post-MI Hypertrophic subaortic stenosis Essential tremor Migraine Pheochromocytoma surgery Serious dysrhythmias
sotalol (Betapace)	Beta-blocker	**Adult** PO: 160–320 mg/day divided	Life-threatening ventricular dysrhythmias

MI, Myocardial infarction.

intoxication and for the treatment of hypertrophic subaortic stenosis, pheochromocytoma, thyrotoxicosis (excessive thyroid hormone), migraine headache, and essential tremors, as well as many other conditions. The same contraindications that apply to the cardioselective beta-blockers (cited in the discussion on acebutolol) apply to propranolol as well. In addition, it is contraindicated in clients with bronchial asthma. It is available as a 1-mg/mL intravenous injection; as 60-, 120-, and 160-mg oral long-acting capsules; and as 10-, 20-, 40-, 80-, and 120-mg tablets. Pregnancy category C. The recommended dosages are given in the table above.

PHARMACOKINETICS

Half-Life	Onset	Peak	Duration
4–6 hr	30 min	1–1.5 hr	6–8 hr

sotalol

Sotalol is a non-selective beta-blocker that has potent antidysrhythmic properties. It is commonly used for the management of difficult-to-treat dysrhythmias. Often these dysrhythmias are life-threatening ventricular dysrhythmias such as sustained ventricular tachycardia. It has both Class II and Class III antidysrhythmic properties (see Chapter 22). Because it is a non-selective beta-blocker, it causes some of the unwanted side effects typical of these agents. It is available in oral form in 80-, 160-, and 240-mg tablets. Pregnancy category B. Commonly recommended dosages are given in the table on p. 312.

PHARMACOKINETICS

Half-Life	Onset	Peak	Duration
10–20 hr	<1 hr	2.5–4 hr	8–12 hr

NEWER BETA-BLOCKERS

Many of the newer beta-blockers are cardioselective, and thus do not produce some of the unwanted side effects associated with non-selective beta-blockers, such as bronchiole constriction and increased peripheral vascular resistance. Another advantage is that many need to be taken only once a day, which promotes client adherence, especially among clients taking several other medications to control hypertension and possibly other diseases. Examples of these agents are betaxolol and bisoprolol.

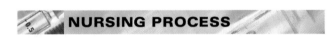 **NURSING PROCESS**

■ Assessment

Adrenergic-blocking agents, or sympatholytics, produce a variety of effects on the client, depending on the type of receptor blocked. Because of their clinical impact on the cardiac and respiratory systems, all these agents require careful client assessment to minimize side effects and maximize therapeutic effects. It is important to remember some basic anatomy and physiology: If an adrenergic-blocking agent is "non-selective," it blocks both alpha- and beta- (beta$_1$- and beta$_2$-) receptors with blocking effects of blood vessels (alpha), heart rate (beta$_1$), and bronchial smooth muscle (beta$_2$). This leads to the following actions:

- Alpha-blocking: a block to the sympathetic effects on blood vessels (vasoconstriction), resulting in vasodilation and thus a decrease in BP.
- Beta$_1$-blocking: a block to the sympathetic effects on the heart rate, contractility, and conduction, resulting in bradycardia, negative inotropic effects (inotropic means contractility, so negative inotropic effects means a decrease in contractility), and a decrease in conduction, helping with several types of dysfunctional irregularities of heart rates.
- Beta$_2$-blocking: a block to the sympathetic effects on bronchial smooth muscle (bronchodilating effects from smooth muscle relaxation), resulting in bronchoconstricting effects in the lungs.

These basic physiological concepts help the nurse better understand all of the aspects of drug administration that alter the SNS (in this chapter, blocking sympathetic effects).

To begin a thorough assessment, information should be gathered about the client's allergies and past and present medical conditions. A system overview and a thorough medication history should be part of this process. The following questions may be posed:

- Are you allergic to any medications or foods?
- Do you have a history of a chronic obstructive pulmonary disease such as emphysema, asthma, or chronic bronchitis?
- Do you have a history of hypotension, cardiac dysrhythmias, bradycardia, heart failure, or any other cardiovascular disease?

These questions are important because alpha-blockers may precipitate hypotension, whereas non-selective beta-blockers may precipitate bradycardia, hypotension, heart block, heart failure, and bronchoconstriction or increased airway resistance; therefore, such pre-existing conditions may be contraindications. Beta$_1$-blocking agents may exacerbate conditions or diseases such as bradycardia, decreased cardiac contractility, and decreased conduction. Beta$_2$-blocking agents, by increasing bronchoconstriction, may exacerbate conditions or diseases involving increased airway resistance. In summary, alpha-blockers may precipitate hypotension and are therefore contraindicated in hypotensive states, myocardial ischemia, peripheral vascular disease, and cardiac disease. Non-selective beta-blockers (which block both beta$_1$ and beta$_2$ receptors) may precipitate bradycardia and hypotension; they are contraindicated in decompensated Class IV heart failure and asthma.

Clients should be asked whether they are taking any drugs that could possibly interact with the adrenergic-blocking agent that has been prescribed for them. These interactions include alpha- and beta-agonists (or stimulators). For more drug interactions, see Table 18-4 on p. 310. Remember that beta$_1$-blockers work mainly on the beta$_1$ receptors in the heart. The blocking of these receptors leads to a decrease in heart rate (negative chronotropic), a decrease in conduction (negative dromotropic), and a decrease in myocardial contraction (negative inotropic). Beta$_2$-blockers block mainly the bronchial smooth muscle and result in bronchoconstriction. Therefore if the client has heart disease and respiratory disease, then a beta$_1$-blocker, or *cardioselective agent,* would be beneficial because it would lack the beta$_2$-constriction or increased airway resistance.

■ Nursing Diagnoses

Nursing diagnoses related to the use of adrenergic antagonists, or sympatholytics, include, but are not limited to, the following:

- Deficient knowledge related to therapeutic regimen, side effects, drug interactions, and precautions to be taken.
- Risk for injury related to possible side effects of the adrenergic blockers (e.g., numbness and tingling of fingers and toes).

- Imbalanced nutrition, less than body requirements, because of nausea and vomiting related to the use of adrenergic blockers.
- Ineffective tissue perfusion, cerebral and cardiovascular, related to side effects of the disease of hypertension and side effects of the drug.
- Disturbed sensory perception related to CNS adverse effects of drug.

■ Planning

Goals for the client receiving sympatholytics include, but are not limited to, the following:
- Client takes medication exactly as prescribed.
- Client experiences relief of the symptoms for which the medication was prescribed.
- Client remains adherent with the drug therapy.
- Client demonstrates an adequate knowledge concerning the use of the specific medications, the side effects, and the appropriate dosing routine to be followed at home.
- Client is free of injury to self as the result of adverse effects of the medications.

■ *Outcome Criteria*

Outcome criteria related to the administration of adrenergic blockers include the following:
- Client states the importance of both the pharmacological and non-pharmacological treatment of his or her migraine headaches, hypertension, or other reason for drug therapy.
- Client states reasons for adherence with the medication therapy and the risks and complications such as syncope, dizziness, and hypotension arising as a result of overuse of the medication.

CASE STUDY ▸◆▸

Nutritional Supplements for Migraine Headaches

Your 47-year-old client has a 20-year history of migraine headaches. She has decided to try to treat her headaches, which have improved over the last 2 years, with nutritional supplementation. She is currently in excellent health. She takes one capsule of Fiorinal #3 every 6 hours as needed for headache pain and one 25-mg tablet of promethazine every 6 hours as needed for nausea and vomiting occurring with the headache. In your client teaching session, you are to inform her of nutritional remedies used to help with migraines.
- After doing research, what type of supplementation would you recommend (if you were able to prescribe) and why?
- What side effects have occurred with the type of supplement that you think is best?
- If nutritional supplementation does not work, what other types of therapeutic modalities could you recommend?

For answers see http://evolve.elsevier.com/Lilley/pharmacology/.

- Client demonstrates the correct method of taking BP with self-taking digital cuff or by using community resources.
- Client identifies community resources for monitoring BP (e.g., rescue squads, fire departments).
- Client taking these medications for the treatment of migraine headaches states the importance of remaining in a quiet and dark room during a headache.
- Client states conditions of which the physician should be informed immediately, such as palpitations, chest pain, insomnia, and excessive agitation.
- Client keeps all follow-up appointments with the physician to maintain safe therapy.
- Client follows instructions regarding the avoidance of sudden withdrawal of hypertensive agents to avoid rebound hypertensive crises and experiences minimal complications.

■ Implementation

Several nursing interventions can maximize the therapeutic effects of adrenergic-blocking agents and minimize the side effects. Thorough client education is a must to ensure good adherence. Clients taking alpha-blockers should be encouraged to change positions slowly to prevent or minimize postural hypotension. Because beta-blockers can cause cardiac depression, clients should be taught how to take their BP and their apical pulse for 1 full minute. They should contact the physician if the systolic blood pressure decreases to less than 100 mm Hg or the pulse decreases to less than 60 beats/min. The physician should also be notified if the BP continues to decrease, even by a few millimetres of mercury. Clients should also know to immediately report weakness; shortness of breath; edema; or weight gain, especially 1 kg or more in a 24-hour period or 2 kg or more within one week. The nurse should make sure that clients are weaned off these medications slowly, if this is indicated, because of the possible rebound hypertension or chest pain that rapid withdrawal can precipitate. Also, the nurse should remember basic anatomy and physiology; it will always help guide nursing actions and considerations related to these agents.

Carvedilol—a beta-blocker and alpha$_1$-blocker with antioxidant properties—is generally given at 3.125 mg twice daily with possible doubling of dosage every 2 weeks until reaching the highest tolerated dose. Therefore client education regarding side effects is important to the safe dosing of this agent. Because carvedilol is often used with digoxin, furosemide, and ACE inhibitors, it is crucial to teach clients to consume potassium, to record pulse rates before doses, and to report adverse effects (e.g., postural hypotension and bradycardia). Clients should be encouraged to keep a journal of their responses to the medication regimen and to record their daily (or more frequent) BPs. Carvedilol should be taken with food to reduce the rate of absorption and hence the orthostatic effects that may occur with titration.

Client teaching tips for all types of adrenergic-blocking agents are listed on p. 316.

■ Evaluation

Therapeutic effects to monitor for in clients receiving adrenergic-blocking agents include, but are not limited to, the following:

- Decrease in BP, pulse rate, and palpitations in clients with a pheochromocytoma
- Return to normal BP and pulse with lowering of the BP toward 120/80 mm Hg or the pulse to within normal limits (60 beats/min)
- Decrease in chest pain in clients with angina

Clients must also be monitored for the occurrence of the side effects of these medications, which include, but are not limited to, the following:

- Bradycardia
- Heart failure

- Depression
- Fatigue
- Heart block
- Hypotension
- Increased airway resistance
- Insomnia
- Lethargy
- Tachycardia (alpha-blockers)
- Vivid nightmares

NURSING CARE PLAN | **Hypertension and Use of Metoprolol**

Ms. K., a 48-year-old professional journalist, is about to be discharged from the cardiac unit. The physician has prescribed metoprolol 100 mg bid. This drug is ordered for a new diagnosis of hypertension, and she has a significant family history for hypertension and stroke. She has also been diagnosed with mitral valve prolapse, moderate degree. Ms. K. is asking many questions about the medication because this is a newly diagnosed condition. She is curious about the drug's mechanism of action and side effects, as well as how she can minimize these side effects. You are about to begin a teaching session related to the administration of metoprolol and you have decided to give her a printed copy to take home because of her strong interest.

ASSESSMENT	Subjective Data	• "What type of medication am I going to be on?" • "Will I have to take this medication forever?" • "What kind of side effects can I expect, and when is it necessary to see a physician?"
	Objective Data	• Recent diagnosis of hypertension and mitral valve prolapse • No major complications related to the disease • Education level: 4 years of university • Readiness level: asking questions about the medication
NURSING DIAGNOSIS		Risk for injury or fall related to possible postural hypotension or bradycardia as a side effect of metoprolol
PLANNING	Goals	Client is free of dysrhythmias and elevated BPs on return to physician's office in 1 mo.
	Outcome Criteria	Client shows adherence to medication therapy as evidenced by the following: • No complaints of palpitations or chest discomfort • Normal ECG on return to physician's office • BP return within normal limits, with projected target systolic pressure of 130 mm Hg and diastolic pressure 85 mm Hg • Decreased side effects because of proper home administration of medications • Lack of complications of drug therapy
IMPLEMENTATION		Inform client of the following information about metoprolol therapy: • There are many drug interactions with metoprolol, including alcohol, nitroglycerin, certain anaesthetics, reserpine, guanethidine, antipsychotics, antimalarials, antifungals, indomethicin, prazosin, H₂-antagonists, oral antidiabetic agents, MAOIs, SSRIs, digitalis, xanthines, antiarrhythmics (quinidine, propafenome), clonidine, rifampin, and verapamil. You should be aware of these interactions to prevent side effects, particularly reoccurrence of dysrhythmias, chest pain, and palpitations. • These interactions may result in decreased effectiveness, more pronounced action, and other problems.

Continued

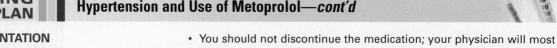

NURSING CARE PLAN | Hypertension and Use of Metoprolol—*cont'd*

IMPLEMENTATION (cont'd)

- You should not discontinue the medication; your physician will most likely taper your dose over a 2-wk period. Stopping this medication abruptly may lead to rebound hypertensive effects and possible stroke and myocardial ischemia.
- Take the medication as ordered.
- To help prevent complications or adverse interactions, do not use OTC products containing alpha-adrenergic stimulants (nasal decongestants, cold preparations).
- Avoid alcohol because it will adversely affect the action of metoprolol.
- We will teach you how to monitor your pulse so that you will know when to contact your physician (i.e., pulse 50 beats/min because bradycardia is a side effect).
- Make sure that you adhere with all aspects of your medication regimen, such as adequate exercise, dietary changes, weight control, and any other changes your healthcare provider has ordered.
- It is suggested that you purchase a medical alert bracelet or tag stating your name, diagnosis, drugs being prescribed, phone number, and allergies.
- Remember that this medication controls symptoms but does not provide a cure.
- Should you experience shortness of breath, coughing at night, swelling of feet, pulse <50 beats/min, dizziness, fever, or depression, it is important to contact your physician.
- Do not skip any doses or double up on this medication and do not stop taking this medication. Always contact the physician or other healthcare providers for assistance with any problems with the medication or with adherence.
- BP may be lowered because of medication and should be monitored.
- Syncope may occur if postural hypotension occurs.
- Change positions slowly to avoid dizziness or syncope.

EVALUATION

- Positive therapeutic outcomes include the following:
  - Absence or decreased occurrence of elevated BPs
  - Absence or decreased occurrence of palpitations and other side effects
  - No chest pain and no postural hypotensive-limiting side effects
- Client is monitored for common side effects of insomnia, fatigue, dizziness, mental changes, constipation, hiccups, depression, nightmares, nausea, and diarrhea.

CLIENT TEACHING TIPS

The nurse should instruct the client as follows:
- ▲ Take your medication exactly as prescribed and never abruptly stop taking the drug. Avoid OTC medications because of risk of drug interactions.
- ▲ Keep alpha-blockers and all other medications out of the reach of children.
- ▲ Notify your physician if you have palpitations, difficulty breathing, nausea, or vomiting.
- ▲ Avoid caffeine and any other CNS stimulant because of excessive irritability.
- ▲ Avoid alcohol.
- ▲ If you are taking a beta-blocker, always take your medication as prescribed, no more and no less, and never abruptly stop taking the medication. If you do, you could suffer rebound hypertension or chest pain. If you become ill and are unable to take the prescribed doses, notify your physician.
- ▲ If you are taking a beta-blocker, report to your healthcare provider any weight gain of 1 kg or more over a 24-hour period or 2 kg or more within a week. Also report any problems with fluid collection or swelling of the feet or ankles, shortness of breath, excessive fatigue or weakness, fainting, or dizziness.
- ▲ If you are taking a beta-blocker, your blood pressure may go too low if you change positions quickly, such as from sitting or lying to standing, which could result in dizziness and/or syncope. This may occur with exercise, exposure to heat (due to more vasodilation and more of a drop in BP), or increased activity.
- ▲ Report constipation or the development of any urinary hesitancy or bladder distention (discomfort over symphysis pubis) to your healthcare provider for further instructions about the drug, its dosage, and these side effects.
- ▲ If you experience confusion, depression, hallucinations, nightmares, palpitations, or dizziness, report this to your physician or other healthcare provider immediately.

POINTS to REMEMBER

▼ Alpha-blockers block the stimulation of the alpha$_1$- and alpha$_2$-adrenergic receptors with a net result of blocking the effects of either norepinephrine or epinephrine. This may create a variety of physiological responses depending on what receptors are blocked.

▼ Some agents may stimulate effects on the alpha-adrenergic receptors at regular doses yet block them at high doses.

▼ With alpha-blockers, the predominant response is vasodilation due to blood vessel relaxation.

▼ Vasodilation of blood vessels with the alpha-blockers results in a drop in BP and a reduction in urinary obstruction that may lead to increased urinary flow rates.

▼ Beta-blockers block the stimulation of beta-adrenergic receptors by blocking the effects of the SNS neurotransmitters norepinephrine, epinephrine, and dopamine.

▼ The predominant response when beta receptors are blocked is blood vessel dilation and cardiac depression. Beta-blockers are classified into two groups: selective and non-selective.

▼ Cardioselective beta-blockers block just beta$_1$-adrenergic receptors on the heart; receptors are located on postsynaptic effector cells (cells, muscles, and organs that nerves stimulate).

▼ Beneficial effects of the cardioselective beta-blockers include decreased heart rate, cardiac conduction, and myocardial contractility.

▼ Non-selective beta-blockers block both beta$_1$- and beta$_2$-adrenergic receptors and affect the heart and smooth muscle.

▼ Nursing considerations for clients on alpha- and/or beta-blockers include teaching clients to avoid sudden changes in position because of possible postural hypotension.

EXAMINATION REVIEW QUESTIONS

1 Atenolol works by which of the following actions?
a. Beta-blocker
b. Alpha-blocker
c. Sympathomimetic
d. Parasympatholytic

2 Which of the following statements is most correct for a client taking beta-blockers?
a. It may be discontinued without any time restraints.
b. Postural hypotension is not a problem with this agent.
c. Weaning off the medication is necessary to prevent rebound hypertension.
d. The client should stop taking the medication at once should he or she gain 1 to 2.5 kg in a week.

3 Beta$_1$-blockers result in which of the following?
a. Tachycardia
b. Tachypnea
c. Bradycardia
d. Bradypnea

4 Clients taking alpha-adrenergic blockers need to be assessed for which of the following conditions and/or disorders due to a possible caution or contraindication?
a. Hypertension
b. Hirsutism
c. Hypotension
d. Hyperplasia

5 The newer "once-a-day" dosing of beta-blockers may result in which of the following?
a. Polyuria
b. Severe anaphylaxis
c. Better adherence
d. Difficulty breathing due to higher risk of toxicity

For answers see http://evolve.elsevier.com/Lilley/pharmacology/.

CRITICAL THINKING ACTIVITIES

1 Develop client teaching plans for the use of the following medications:
a. ergotamine tartrate/caffeine
b. prazosin
c. atenolol

2 One of your clients, a 46-year-old mother of two adolescent children, is now taking propranolol for the control of tachycardia and hypertension. What should you tell her if she says, "Well, if it doesn't work after a month or two, I'll just quit taking it!"?

3 You have just come on your shift and are taking over for a nurse who already has your client's heart rate controlled on an esmolol infusion. It is running at a rate of 54 mL/hour. The physician is making rounds and asks you how many μg/kg/min of esmolol the client is controlled on. The client weighs 90 kg and the normal concentration of esmolol is 10 μg/mL. How many μg/kg/min of esmolol is the client receiving?

For answers see http://evolve.elsevier.com/Lilley/pharmacology/.

BIBLIOGRAPHY

Albanese, J., & Nutz, P. (2005). *Mosby's 2005 nursing drug cards.* St Louis, MO: Mosby.

Canadian Pharmacists Association. (2003). *Therapeutic choices* (4th ed.). Ottawa, ON: Author.

Canadian Pharmacists Association. (2004). *Guide to drugs in Canada.* Toronto, ON: Dorling Kindersley.

Canadian Pharmacists Association. (2005). *Compendium of pharmaceuticals and specialties. The Canadian drug reference for health professionals.* Ottawa, ON: Author. [The subscription-based e-CPS is available at http://www.pharmacists.ca.]

Cheng, A., Williams, B.A., & Sivarajan, B.V. (Eds.). *The HSC handbook of pediatrics* (10th ed.). Toronto, ON: Elsevier.

Health Canada. (2005). Drug product database (DPD). Retrieved August 5, 2005, from http://www.hc-sc.gc.ca/hpb/drugs-dpd/

Mosby (2005). *Mosby's drug consult 2005: The comprehensive reference for generic and brand name drugs* (15th ed.). St Louis, MO: Mosby.

Skidmore-Roth, L. (2006). *Mosby's 2006 nursing drug reference* (19th ed.). St Louis, MO: Mosby.

Cholinergic Agents

After reading this chapter, the successful student will be able to do the following:

1 Briefly discuss the normal anatomy and physiology of the autonomic nervous system (ANS), including the events that occur during synaptic transmission within the parasympathetic divisions.

2 Cite various examples of the cholinergic drugs, including newer drug therapy for treating Alzheimer's disease.

3 Discuss the mechanisms of action, therapeutic effects, indications, adverse effects, and antidotes to overdose of the cholinergic drugs.

4 Develop a nursing care plan that includes all phases of the nursing process related to the administration of the various cholinergic agents.

e-LEARNING ACTIVITIES

Student CD-ROM
- Review Questions: see questions 110–115
- Animations
- Medication Administration Checklists
- IV Therapy Checklists

evolve **Web site** (http://evolve.elsevier.com/Lilley/pharmacology/)
- Online Chapter Worksheet • Frequently Asked Questions
- Learning Tips and Content Updates • WebLinks • Online Appendices and Supplements • Mosby/Saunders ePharmacology Update • Access to *Mosby's Drug Consult*

DRUG PROFILES

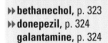

▸▸ **bethanechol,** p. 323   ▸▸ **physostigmine,** p. 325
▸▸ **donepezil,** p. 324   ▸▸ **pyridostigmine,** p. 325
 galantamine, p. 324   rivastigmine, p. 325
 memantine, p. 325

▸▸ Key drug.

GLOSSARY

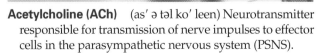

Acetylcholine (ACh)   (as′ ə təl ko′ leen) Neurotransmitter responsible for transmission of nerve impulses to effector cells in the parasympathetic nervous system (PSNS).

Alzheimer's disease   A disease characterized by progressive mental deterioration manifested by confusion, disorientation, loss of memory, loss of ability to calculate, and loss of visual–spatial orientations.

Cholinergic agents   (ko′ lin er′ jik) Drugs that stimulate the parasympathetic nervous system (PSNS).

Cholinesterase   (ko′ lin es′ tər ays) Enzyme responsible for the breakdown of ACh.

Direct-acting cholinergic agonists   Agents that bind to cholinergic receptors to activate them.

Indirect-acting cholinergic agonists   Agents that make more ACh available at the receptor site.

Irreversible cholinesterase inhibitors   Agents that form a permanent covalent bond with cholinesterase.

Miosis   Contraction of the pupil.

Muscarinic receptors   (mus′ kə rin′ ik) Cholinergic receptors located post-synaptically in the smooth muscle, cardiac muscle, and glands of the parasympathetic fibres and in the effector organs of the cholinergic sympathetic fibres; can be stimulated by the alkaloid muscarine.

Nicotinic receptors   (nik′ o tin′ ik) Cholinergic receptors located in the ganglia of both the PSNS and the sympathetic nervous system (SNS); can be stimulated by the alkaloid nicotine.

Parasympathomimetics   Another name for cholinergic agents that mimic the effects of ACh.

Reversible cholinesterase inhibitors Agents that bind to cholinesterase for minutes to hours but do not form a permanent bond.

Cholinergic agents, *cholinergics, cholinergic agonists,* and *parasympathomimetics* are all terms that refer to the class of drugs that stimulate the parasympathetic nervous system (PSNS). To better understand how these agents work, it is helpful to know how the PSNS operates in relation to the rest of the nervous system.

PARASYMPATHETIC NERVOUS SYSTEM

The parasympathetic nervous system (PSNS) is the opposing system to the sympathetic nervous system (SNS) in the autonomic nervous system (ANS) (Figure 19-1). The neurotransmitter responsible for the transmission of nerve impulses to effector cells in the PSNS is **acetylcholine (ACh).** The receptor that binds the ACh and mediates its actions is called a *cholinergic receptor.* There are two types of cholinergic receptor, as determined by their location and their action once stimulated. **Nicotinic receptors** are located in the ganglia of both the PSNS and SNS. They are called *nicotinic* because they can be stimulated by the alkaloid nicotine. The other cholinergic receptors are the **muscarinic receptors.** These receptors are located post-synaptically in the smooth muscle, cardiac muscle, and glands of the parasympathetic fibres and in the effector organs of

the cholinergic sympathetic fibres. They are called *muscarinic* because they are stimulated by the alkaloid muscarine, a substance isolated from mushrooms. Figure 19-2 shows how the nicotinic and muscarinic receptors are arranged in the PSNS.

CHOLINERGIC AGONISTS

Cholinergic agonists mimic the effects of ACh and are therefore sometimes referred to as **parasympathomimetics.** These drugs can stimulate their receptors either directly or indirectly. **Direct-acting cholinergic agonists** bind to cholinergic receptors and activate them. **Indirect-acting cholinergic agonists** act by making more ACh available at the receptor site, thereby allowing the ACh to bind to and stimulate the receptor. They do this by inhibiting **cholinesterase,** the enzyme responsible for breaking down ACh. The indirect-acting cholinergic agents bind to the cholinesterase in one of two ways: reversibly or irreversibly. **Reversible cholinesterase inhibitors** bind to cholinesterase for a period of minutes to hours; **irreversible cholinesterase inhibitors** bind to cholinesterase and form a permanent covalent bond. The body must then generate new enzymes to override the effects of the irreversible agents. Box 19-1 lists the direct- and indirect-acting cholinergics.

These agents are used primarily to reduce intraocular pressure (IOP) in clients with glaucoma or in those undergoing ocular surgery, to treat various gastrointestinal (GI) and bladder disorders, to diagnose and

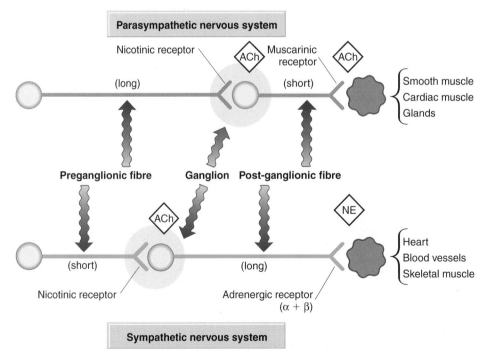

FIG. 19-1 The parasympathetic and sympathetic nervous systems and their relationships to one another. *ACh,* Acetylcholine; *NE,* norepinephrine.

treat myasthenia gravis (chronic progressive muscular weakness due to myoneural conduction defect), to treat **Alzheimer's disease,** and to treat excessive dry mouth (xerostomia) resulting from a disorder known as *Sjögren's syndrome.*

Mechanism of Action and Drug Effects

As described, cholinergic drugs all work by stimulating the PSNS. The direct-acting cholinergics act as an agonist at the receptor, directly binding to the ACh receptors and causing stimulation. Indirect-acting agents protect ACh from being broken down by acetylcholinesterase (AChE), making more of this neurotransmitter available to act directly with the receptor. When ACh directly binds to its receptor, stimulation occurs. Once binding occurs on the effector cells (the cell membranes of the target organs), the permeability of the cells changes and calcium and sodium are permitted to flow into the cells. This depolarizes the cell membrane and stimulates the muscle.

The effects of direct- and indirect-acting cholinergics are those that are generally seen when the PSNS is stimulated. There are many ways to remember these effects. One way is to think of the PSNS as the "rest-and-digest" system. Another way of remembering the effects of cholinergic poisoning is by using the acronym SLUDGE, which stands for *s*alivation, *l*acrimation, *u*rinary incontinence, *d*iarrhea, *G*I cramps, and *e*mesis.

Cholinergic drugs stimulate the intestine and bladder, resulting in increased gastric secretions, GI motility, and increased urinary frequency. They also stimulate the pupil to constrict, causing **miosis.** This helps decrease IOP. In addition, stimulation of the PSNS by the parasympathomimetics causes increased salivation and sweating. The cardiovascular effects are decreased heart rate and vasodilation. These agents also cause the bronchi of the lungs to constrict and the airways to narrow.

ACh is also needed for normal brain function. It is in short supply in clients with Alzheimer disease. At recommended doses, cholinergics primarily affect the muscarinic receptors, but at high doses the nicotinic receptors can also be stimulated. The desired effects come from muscarinic receptor stimulation; many of the undesirable effects are due to nicotinic receptor stimulation. The various beneficial and undesirable effects of the cholinergic agents are listed in Table 19-1 according to the receptors stimulated.

Indications

Most of the direct-acting agents (carbachol and pilocarpine) are used topically to reduce IOP in clients with glaucoma or in those undergoing ocular surgery. They are poorly absorbed orally because they have large quaternary amines in their chemical structure. This is what limits their use to mostly topical application. One exception is the direct-acting cholinergic drug bethanechol, which can be administered orally (PO). It primarily affects the detrusor muscle of the urinary bladder and the smooth muscle of the GI tract. When given, it causes increased bladder and GI tract tone and motility, thereby increasing the movement of contents through these areas. It also causes the sphincters in the bladder and the GI tract to relax, allowing them to empty. It is therefore used to treat atony of the bladder and GI tract, which sometimes occurs after a surgical procedure.

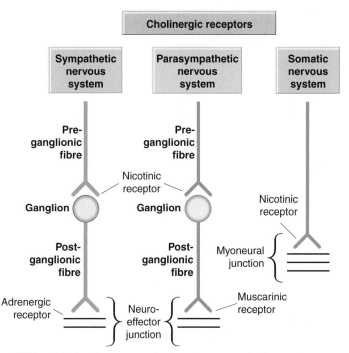

FIG. 19-2 The sympathetic, parasympathetic, and somatic nervous systems. Note the location of the nicotinic and muscarinic receptors within the parasympathetic nervous system.

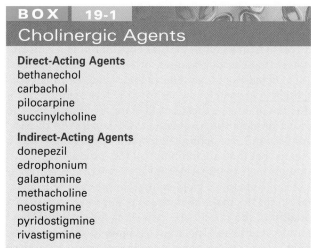

BOX 19-1
Cholinergic Agents

Direct-Acting Agents
bethanechol
carbachol
pilocarpine
succinylcholine

Indirect-Acting Agents
donepezil
edrophonium
galantamine
methacholine
neostigmine
pyridostigmine
rivastigmine

TABLE 19-1

CHOLINERGIC AGENTS: DRUG EFFECTS

Body Tissue	Response to Stimulation	
	Muscarinic	Nicotinic
Bronchi (lung)	Increased secretion, constriction	None
Cardiovascular		
Blood vessels	Dilation	Constriction
Heart rate	Slowed	Increased
Blood pressure	Decreased	Increased
Eye	Pupil constriction, decreased accommodation	Pupil constriction, decreased accommodation
Gastrointestinal		
Tone	Increased	Increased
Motility	Increased	Increased
Sphincters	Relaxed	None
Genitourinary		
Tone	Increased	Increased
Motility	Increased	Increased
Sphincter	Relaxed	Relaxed
Glandular secretions	Increased intestinal, lacrimal, salivary, and sweat gland secretion	—
Skeletal muscle	—	Increased contraction

Indirect-acting agents work by increasing ACh concentrations at the receptor sites stimulating the effector cells. They cause skeletal muscle contraction and are therefore used for the diagnosis and treatment of myasthenia gravis. Their ability to inhibit AChE also makes them useful for the reversal of neuromuscular blockade produced either by neuromuscular blocking agents (NMBAs) or by anticholinergic poisoning. For this reason, physostigmine is considered the antidote for anticholinergic poisoning, as well as poisoning by irreversible cholinesterase inhibitors such as organophosphates and carbonates, the common insecticides. Physostigmine is a restricted drug in Canada and only available through the Special Access Programme.

In the treatment of Alzheimer's disease, cholinergic agents increase concentrations of ACh in the brain, thereby improving cholinergic function. The ability to increase ACh levels in the brain by inhibiting AChE and preventing the degradation of endogenously released ACh increases or maintains memory and learning capabilities. Fortunately, the last decade has seen the introduction of new medications that are specifically used to arrest or slow the progression of Alzheimer's disease. All are indirect-acting anticholinergic agents, which means that they are inhibitors of the enzyme AChE. Although their therapeutic efficacy is often limited, their use can sometimes yield enough improvement in mental status to make a noticeable improvement in the quality of life for clients, as well as for caregivers and family members. The most commonly used of these medications at this time is donepezil, but it should be

RESEARCH

Alzheimer's Disease

The initial results of clinical trials to test the safety and efficacy of a potential vaccine for Alzheimer's disease have shown that the vaccine is well tolerated in humans. Researchers are using animals to test how a vaccine may work to clear the plaques out of the brain in those with Alzheimer's disease. Plaques are a characteristic of this disease and are formed by sticky "protein" substances called *beta-amyloid.* The plaques, along with "neurofibrillary tangles," damage healthy brain cells and cause the brain tissue to shrink. The specific vaccine, AN-1792, had been tested on mice and other animals. Unfortunately, early human trials had to be stopped because some of the subjects developed potentially lethal brain inflammation to the antibodies of the beta amyloid. However, in recent studies in mice, researchers are using newer conjugates of the beta amyloid peptides to develop a novel synthetic vaccine to prevent and treat Alzheimer's disease. Although amyloid plaques are found in the brains of individuals with Alzheimer's disease, it is still not known whether these plaques cause the disease or are a result of the disease process. Other promising areas in Alzheimer research include genetic studies; the use of neurotransmitter receptor measurements in older adults and those with Alzheimer's; and the use of the drug nefiracetam to help improve memory, thinking ability, and daily activities with those diagnosed in the mild to moderate stages of the disease. Other clinical trials, such as with NSAIDs and specifically naproxen (an OTC NSAID), are examining the relationship between the drug and a related slowing down of the progression of mental decline. Alzhemed, currently in clinical development, is in Stage III clinical trials in Canada. Other clinical trials and research studies continue in the hope of learning more about this disease and, ultimately, finding a cure.

From The Alzheimer Society of Canada. (2005). Treatment. Clinical trials and research studies. Retrieved August 6, 2005, from http://www.alzheimer.ca/english/treatment/trials-listing.htm#drugs

kept in mind that client response to these agents, as with most other drug classes, is highly variable. For this reason, a failure to respond to maximally titrated doses of one of these agents should not necessarily rule out the prospect of attempting therapy with another. Dosage information for all of these agents appears in the dosages table on p. 324.

Contraindications

Contraindications to cholinergic agents include known drug allergy, GI or genitourinary (GU) tract obstruction (which may require surgical correction), bradycardia, defects in cardiac impulse conduction, hyperthyroidism, epilepsy, hypotension, chronic obstructive pulmonary disease (COPD), and Parkinson's disease.

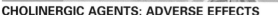

TABLE 19-2

CHOLINERGIC AGENTS: ADVERSE EFFECTS

Body System	Side/Adverse Effects
Cardiovascular	Bradycardia, hypotension, conduction abnormalities (AV block and cardiac arrest)
Central nervous	Headache, dizziness, convulsions
Gastrointestinal	Abdominal cramps, increased secretions, nausea, vomiting
Respiratory	Increased bronchial secretions, bronchospasms
Other	Lacrimation, sweating, salivation, loss of binocular accommodation, miosis

AV, Atrioventricular.

Side Effects and Adverse Effects

The primary side effects and adverse effects of cholinergic agents are the consequence of overstimulation of the PSNS. They are extensions of the cholinergic reactions that affect many body functions. The major effects are listed by body system in Table 19-2.

Interactions

Severe drug interactions can occur with the cholinergics. Anticholinergics (such as atropine), antihistamines, and sympathomimetics may antagonize cholinergic agents, resulting in decreased response to them. Other cholinergic drugs may have additive effects.

Toxicity and Management of Overdose

There is little systemic absorption of the topically administered agents and therefore little systemic toxicity. When administered locally in the eye, they can cause transient but bothersome ocular changes such as blurring and dimming of vision. Systemic toxicity with topically applied cholinergics is seen most commonly when longer-acting agents are given repeatedly over a long period. This can result in overstimulation of the PSNS and in all the attendant responses. Treatment is generally symptomatic and supportive, and the administration of a reversal agent is rarely required.

The likelihood of toxicity is greater for cholinergics given orally or intravenously. The most severe consequence of an overdose is a cholinergic crisis, which may include circulatory collapse, hypotension, bloody diarrhea, shock, and cardiac arrest. Early signs include abdominal cramps, salivation, flushing of the skin, nausea, and vomiting. Transient syncope, transient complete heart block, dyspnea, and orthostatic hypotension may also occur. These can be reversed promptly by the administration of atropine, a cholinergic antagonist. Severe cardiovascular reactions or bronchoconstriction may be alleviated by epinephrine, an adrenergic agonist. Janssen Pharmaceutica, the makers of cisapride, stopped marketing the drug on July 14, 2000. As of May 31, 2000, Health Canada had received at least 44 reports of heart rhythm abnormalities,

including 10 reports of death, associated with the use of cisapride. Most of these events occurred in clients who were taking other medications or suffering from underlying conditions known to increase the risk of cardiac dysrhythmia. Since May 31, 2000, cisapride has been available only through the Special Access Programme.

Dosages

For recommended dosages of the cholinergic agents, see the dosages table on p. 324. See Appendix B for some of the common brands available in Canada.

DRUG PROFILES

Of the direct-acting cholinergic agents, bethanechol is the only one administered orally. Pilocarpine and a drug formulation of acetylcholine itself are applied topically to the eye for the treatment of glaucoma or for a reduction in IOP during ocular surgery. These agents are discussed in greater detail in Chapter 56, as are the indirect-acting cholinergics neostigmine and pyridostigmine, which are used primarily for the treatment of eye disorders or for surgical purposes. The cholinergics are available in oral form as tablets, in topical form as eye drops, and parenterally as intravenous (IV) and subcutaneous injections. The cholinergics are all prescription-only drugs.

▸▸ *bethanechol*

Bethanechol is a direct-acting cholinergic agonist that stimulates the cholinergic receptors located on the smooth muscle of the bladder. This stimulation results in increased bladder tone, increased motility, and relaxation of the sphincter of the bladder. It is used in the treatment of acute post-operative and post-partum non-obstructive urinary retention and for the management of neurogenic atony of the bladder with retention. It has also been used to prevent and treat the side effects of other classes of drugs, such as phenothiazine- and tricyclic antidepressant (TCA)–induced bladder dysfunction. In addition, it is used in the treatment of post-operative GI atony and gastric retention, chronic refractory heartburn, and familial dysautonomia (abnormal functioning of the autonomic nervous system), as well as in the diagnostic test for infantile cystic fibrosis. Intramuscular and intravenous use are contraindicated. Bethanechol is contraindicated in clients with hyperthyroidism, peptic ulcer, active bronchial asthma, pronounced bradycardia or hypotension, cardiac disease or coronary artery disease, epilepsy, and parkinsonism. It should also be avoided in clients with conditions in which the strength or integrity of the GI tract or bladder wall is questionable or with conditions in which increased muscular activity could prove harmful. Bethanechol is available as oral tablets in 10-, 25-, and 50-mg strengths. Pregnancy category C. Commonly recommended dosages are given in the table on p. 324.

PHARMACOKINETICS

Half-Life	Onset	Peak	Duration
Variable	30–90 min	<30 min	1–6 hr

DOSAGES **Selected Cholinergic Agonist Agents**

Agent	Pharmacological Class	Usual Dosage Range	Indications
▸▸bethanechol	Direct-acting muscarinic	**Adult** PO: 10–50 mg tid–qid (usually start with 5–10 mg, repeating hourly until urination, max 50 mg/cycle)	Post-operative and post-partum functional urinary retention
memantine	NMBA-receptor antagonist	**Adult only** PO: Initial dose is 5 mg/day; may titrate by 5 mg per week up to a max daily dose of 20 mg	Moderate to severe Alzheimer Disease
▸▸physostigmine	Anticholinesterase (indirect acting)	**Pediatric** IM/IV: 0.01–0.03 mg/kg repeated at 5–10 min intervals until desired effect or a dose of 2 mg reached **Adult** IM/IV: 0.5–2 mg repeated q20min if needed	Reversal of anticholinergic drug effects and TCA overdose
▸▸pyridostigmine	Anticholinesterase (indirect acting)	**Pediatric** PO: 7 mg/kg/day divided into 5–6 doses **Adult** PO: 60–1500 mg/day divided to provide maximum therapeutic effect SR tabs: 180–540 mg once to twice daily	Myasthenia gravis Myasthenia gravis Reversal of non-depolarizing NMBAs

Currently Available Cholinergic Agonist Agents Specifically for Treating Alzheimer's Disease

Agent	Pharmacological Class	Usual Dosage Range	Indications
▸▸donepezil	Anticholinesterase (indirect acting)	**Adult** PO: 5–10 mg/day as a single dose	Alzheimer's disease
galantamine	Anticholinesterase (indirect acting)	**Adult** PO: 16–32 mg divided bid	Alzheimer's disease
rivastigmine	Anticholinesterase (indirect acting)	**Adult** PO: 3–12 mg divided bid	Alzheimer's disease

NMBA, neuromuscular blocking agent.

▸▸ *donepezil*

Donepezil is an indirect-acting anticholinesterase drug that works centrally in the brain to increase levels of ACh by blocking its breakdown. It is used in the treatment of mild to moderate Alzheimer's disease. Drugs with anticholinergic properties should be avoided in clients on donepezil because they may counteract the effects of donepezil.

Donepezil offers many advantages over tacrine, the first agent of this class of indirect acting anticholinesterase drugs. Introduced in 1997, tacrine has a short half-life that requires 4 doses a day. Because of the dosing schedule and its effect on the liver, it is not available in Canada. Donepezil is taken only once a day. It is specific for AChE in the central nervous system (CNS), which decreases the incidence of drug interactions. Donepezil is available orally in 5- and 10-mg tablets. Pregnancy category C. Recommended dosages are given in the table above.

PHARMACOKINETICS

Half-Life	Onset	Peak	Duration
72–80 hr	3 wk*	3–4 hr	2 wk*

*Therapeutic effects.

galantamine

Galantamine is an indirect-acting cholinergic agent. Its mechanism of action is through inhibition of the enzyme AChE. It is indicated for treating clients with mild to moderate dementia associated with Alzheimer's disease. Its only known contraindication is drug allergy. Reduced dosages are recommended for clients with moderate renal or hepatic impairment. This drug is *not* recommended for clients with severe renal or hepatic impairment. Side effects include nausea, vomiting, dizziness, anorexia, and syncope. This drug, along with others in its class, has been shown in some cases to alter cardiac conduction in clients with and without prior cardiovascular disease. Therefore all clients treated with galantamine, as well as other cholinergic agents, should be considered at risk for cardiac conduction effects. Galantamine is available as 4-, 8-, and 12-mg tablets. Pregnancy category B. The recommended dosage is given in the table on p. 324.

PHARMACOKINETICS

Half-Life	Onset	Peak	Duration
4–10 hr	Variable*	1 hr	Unknown*

*Onset and duration of drug action for this and other cholinergic agents used for Alzheimer dementia are difficult to quantify because both may vary significantly among clients. The practitioner should judge the therapeutic effect of these medications according to the degree of change in the client's mental status.

▸▸ physostigmine

Physostigmine is a synthetic quaternary ammonium compound that is similar in structure to edrophonium. In Canada, physostigmine is available only under the Special Access Programme. It is an indirect-acting cholinergic agent that works to increase ACh by inhibiting the enzyme that breaks down ACh. It has been shown to improve muscle strength and is therefore used in the symptomatic treatment of myasthenia gravis. Neostigmine and pyridostigmine are the standard agents used for the symptomatic treatment of myasthenia gravis. Edrophonium, another indirect-acting cholinergic agent, is commonly used to diagnose this disorder. It is also useful for reversing the effects of non-depolarizing neuromuscular blocking agents (NMBAs) after surgery. It may also be used in the treatment of severe TCA overdose. It is contraindicated in clients who have shown a hypersensitivity or severe cholinergic reaction to it. It should be used in caution in clients with epilepsy, bronchial asthma, bradycardia, recent coronary artery occlusion, hyperthyroidism, cardiac dysrhythmias, or peptic ulcer. Pregnancy category C. Recommended dosages are given in the table on p. 324.

PHARMACOKINETICS

Half-Life	Onset	Peak	Duration
15–40 min	<5 min	5 min	30–60 min

▸▸ pyridostigmine

Pyridostigmine is a synthetic quaternary ammonium compound that is similar structurally to edrophonium and neostigmine. It is an indirect-acting cholinergic agent and is used in the symptomatic treatment of myasthenia gravis. It is also useful for reversing the effects of non-depolarizing NMBAs after surgery. It is contraindicated in clients who have shown a hypersensitivity or severe cholinergic reaction to it. It should be used with caution in clients with epilepsy, bronchial asthma, bradycardia, recent coronary artery occlusion, vagotonia, hyperthyroidism, cardiac dysrhythmias, or peptic ulcer. It is available in oral form as a regular 60-mg tablet and an 180-mg extended-release tablet. Pregnancy category B. Recommended dosages are given in the table on p. 324.

PHARMACOKINETICS

Half-Life	Onset	Peak	Duration
Variable	PO: 20–30 min	PO: 2–5 hr	PO: 6–12 hr

rivastigmine

Rivastigmine is an indirect-acting cholinergic agent. Its mechanism of action is through the inhibition of the enzyme AChE. It is indicated for treating clients with mild to moderate dementia associated with Alzheimer's disease. It is contraindicated in clients with a known drug allergy to rivastigmine or other carbamate compounds. It should be used with caution in clients with epilepsy, bronchial asthma or obstructive pulmonary disease, bradycardia, coronary artery disease or congestive heart failure, and gastrointestinal conditions. It should also be used with caution in clients with serious co-occurring disorders and in those who have known renal and liver impairments. The lowest effective dose should be used with these clients and close monitoring is recommended. Common side effects include dizziness, headache, nausea, vomiting, diarrhea, and anorexia (loss of appetite). Rivastigmine is available in oral form as 1.5-, 3, 4.5-, and 6-mg capsules and as a solution of 2 mg/mL. Pregnancy category B. The recommended dosage is given in the table on p. 324.

PHARMACOKINETICS

Half-Life	Onset	Peak	Duration
1.5 hr	Variable*	1 hr	Unknown*

*Onset and duration of drug action for this and other cholinergic agents used for Alzheimer dementia are difficult to quantify because both may vary significantly between clients. The practitioner should judge the therapeutic effect of these medications according to the degree of change in the client's mental status.

MISCELLANEOUS ALZHEIMER'S DISEASE MEDICATION
memantine

In 2004, Health Canada approved a new medication for treating Alzheimer's disease. Memantine is classified as an NMDA-receptor antagonist because of its inhibitory activity at the N-methyl-D-aspartate receptors in the CNS. Stimulation of these receptors is believed to be part of the Alzheimer disease process. Memantine blocks this stimulation, thereby helping to reduce or arrest the client's degenerative cognitive symptoms. As with all other currently available medications for this debilitating illness, the effects of this drug are likely to be temporary but may still afford some improved quality of life and general functioning for some clients. Its only current contraindication is known drug allergy. It is available in 10-mg tablets. No pregnancy category is currently listed. The recommended dosage is given in the table on p. 324.

NURSING PROCESS

▮ Assessment

Cholinergic drugs, or parasympathomimetics, produce a variety of effects stemming from their ability to stimulate the PSNS and mimic the action of ACh. These agents have the following effects:

* Decreased heart rate
* Increased GI and GU tone through increasing the contractility of the smooth muscle

- Increased contractility and tone of bronchial smooth muscle
- Increased respiratory secretions
- Miosis (papillary constriction)

Clients who are to receive a cholinergic agent need to be assessed to determine whether they suffer from GI or GU obstruction, asthma, peptic ulcer disease, or coronary artery disease because of the potential for these agents to exacerbate these problems. Information about the client's allergies and past and present medical conditions should also be gathered. In addition, a system overview and a thorough medication history should be done to identify any possible drug interactions or contraindications.

Before donepezil is administered for Alzheimer's disease, the client needs to be assessed for allergies to this agent or to any piperidine derivative. Cautious use is indicated in clients with sick sinus syndrome, asthma, GI bleeding, liver disease, ulcer disease, GU obstruction, seizure disorders, or COPD; in pediatric clients; and during pregnancy or lactation. Drug interactions include synergistic effects with cholinesterase inhibitors and succinylcholine. Cholinesterase inhibitors have the potential to interfere with the activity of anticholinergic medications. Before initiation of drug therapy with donepezil, it is important for the nurse to assess and document the client's vital signs, GI and GU history and status, mental status, mood, affect, changes in behaviour, depression, suicidal tendencies, and level of consciousness. Once the client has begun the medication, it is crucial for the nurse to assess the client's response to the drug; if no improvement is noted within a 6-week period, the healthcare provider may find it necessary to adjust the dosing.

Rivastigmine and galantamine, some of the newer agents for Alzheimer's disease–related dementia, are to be used cautiously in clients with renal, hepatic, and cardiac diseases, as well as those with seizure disorders, ulcers, asthma, urinary obstructions, pregnancy, and lactation. Drug interactions for these agents include other cholinesterase inhibitors and cholinomimetics and other specific agents mentioned later in this section. With clients taking galantamine, reduced dosages are recommended for those with renal or hepatic dysfunction, and this drug is not to be given if there is severe impairment of these organs. Cardiac conduction may also be affected by galantamine; therefore this drug should be used cautiously in clients with a history of cardiac symptoms or disease. Also, assess for use of herbal products, such as ginkgo (see Natural Health Therapies box on p. 327) because of its use in organic brain syndrome.

■ Nursing Diagnoses

Nursing diagnoses associated with the use of cholinergics include, but are not limited to, the following:
- Acute pain related to the side effects of abdominal cramping due to drug therapy.
- Deficient knowledge regarding therapeutic regimen, side effects, drug interactions, and precautions related to the use of cholinergic agents.

- Risk for injury related to possible side effects of cholinergic agents (bradycardia and hypotension).
- Decreased cardiac output related to the cardiovascular side effects of dysrhythmias, hypotension, and bradycardia.
- Disturbed sensory perception related to adverse CNS effects of cholinergic drugs.

■ Planning

Goals for the client receiving cholinergic agents include, but are not limited to, the following:
- Client receives or takes medications as prescribed.
- Client experiences relief of the symptoms for which the medication was prescribed.
- Client remains adherent with the drug therapy regimen.
- Client demonstrates an adequate knowledge concerning the use of the specific medication, its side effects, and the appropriate dosing at home.
- Client remains free of self-injury resulting from adverse effects of the medication.

■ *Outcome Criteria*

Outcome criteria related to the administration of cholinergic agents include the following:
- Client states the importance of both the pharmacological and non-pharmacological treatment of GI or GU disorder or glaucoma in achieving good health.
- Client states reasons for adherence with the medication therapy and the risks associated with non-adherence as well as the complications associated with overuse of the medication, such as bronchospasms, increased abdominal cramping, and decreased pulse and BP.
- Client states conditions under which to contact the physician, such as wheezing, bradycardia, and increased abdominal pain.
- Client states the importance of scheduling and keeping follow-up appointments with the physician as related to management of the disorder for which medication has been prescribed.

■ Implementation

Several nursing interventions can maximize the therapeutic effects of cholinergic agents and minimize their side effects. One is to always make sure clients who have undergone surgery ambulate as early as possible as ordered after their procedure to help minimize or prevent gastric and urinary retention. For myasthenia gravis, giving the medication about 30 minutes before meals allows for onset of action and decreased dysphagia. The packaging inserts should always be checked for instructions concerning dilutional agents and the route of administration. Atropine is the antidote to the cholinergics; therefore this medication should be available as necessary and per facility protocol and after a physician's order.

Donepezil is not a cure for Alzheimer disease or dementia. The nurse should be honest with the client and caregivers about the fact that this drug is only for symptomatic improvement. While beginning the medication clients will most likely need continued assistance with ADLs and help with ambulation because the medication may initially increase dizziness and cause gait imbalances. Clients and family members or caregivers also need to understand the importance of taking the medication exactly as ordered. In addition, clients should be instructed not to abruptly stop the medication or increase the dosage without physician approval because of the potential for serious complications or overdosage.

Rivastigmine has severe GI side effects (nausea and vomiting), which may be dose limiting. BPs should be recorded before, during, and after initiation of therapy, as should the client's mental status and level of consciousness. Administering this drug with meals is helpful in decreasing the GI side effects, although absorption may be decreased too. Clients who become dizzy with the therapy should be assisted with ambulation.

For client safety with galantamine, the nurse should take BP and pulse and should have electrocardiogram (ECG) baseline studies available, especially if there is any history of cardiac conduction disorders or cardiac disease. Clients should be encouraged to report to their healthcare provider any new cardiac distress.

Client teaching tips are presented in the box below.

■ Evaluation

Following are some therapeutic effects to monitor for in clients receiving cholinergic agents. In clients with myasthenia gravis, the signs and symptoms of the disease should be alleviated (see the Client Teaching Tips). In clients suffering a decrease in GI peristalsis post-operatively, increased peristalsis should be evident in increased bowel sounds, the passage of flatus, and bowel movements. In clients suffering from a hypotonic bladder with urinary retention, micturition (voiding) should occur within about 60 minutes of the administration of bethanechol.

The nurse must also be alert to side effects, including increased respiratory secretions, bronchospasms, diffi-culty breathing, nausea, vomiting, diarrhea, abdominal cramping, dysrhythmias, hypotension, bradycardia, increased sweating, and an increase in the frequency and urgency of the voiding patterns.

Therapeutic effects of donepezil may not occur for up to 6 weeks but include an improvement of the symptoms of the disease. Adverse effects include hypotension or hypertension, dizziness, insomnia, headache, fatigue, syncope, nausea, vomiting, and anorexia. Therapeutic effects of rivastigmine and galantamine include improved mood and a decrease in confusion. Side effects of these drugs include nausea, vomiting, dizziness, syncope, confusion, tremors, ataxia, depression, hypo- or hypertension, anorexia, liver toxicity, GI bleeding, cough, and urinary incontinence and frequency. Cardiac conductive disorders and hepatic problems are the associated side effects with galantamine.

NATURAL HEALTH THERAPIES

GINKGO *(Ginkgo biloba)*

Overview
The dried leaf of the plant contains flavonoids, terpenoids, and organic acids, which help ginkgo preparations exert their positive effects as an antioxidant and inhibitor of platelet aggregation.

Common Uses
Organic brain syndrome, peripheral arterial occlusive disease, vertigo, tinnitus

Adverse Effects
Stomach or intestinal upset, headache, bleeding, allergic skin reaction

Potential Drug Interactions
Acetylsalicylic acid, NSAIDs, warfarin, heparin, anticonvulsants, ticlopidine, clopidogrel, dipyridamole, TCAs

Contraindications
None

CLIENT TEACHING TIPS

The nurse should instruct the client as follows:
▲ Always take your medication as ordered because an overdose can cause life-threatening problems.
▲ You will get the best effects from your medication if you space doses evenly.
▲ Call your physician or other healthcare provider if you experience increased muscle weakness, abdominal cramps, diarrhea, or difficulty breathing.
▲ If you are taking this medication for the treatment of myasthenia gravis, your symptoms should abate. That

is, you should experience less eyelid drooping (ptosis), less double vision (diplopia), less difficulty swallowing and chewing, and less weakness.
▲ If you have myasthenia gravis, take your medication 30 minutes before meals to help improve swallowing and chewing.
▲ If you have a sustained-release tablet, do not break, crush, or chew it.
▲ It is a good idea to wear a medical alert bracelet or tag in case you need emergency treatment.

POINTS to REMEMBER

▼ *Cholinergics, cholinergic agonists,* and *parasympathomimetics* are all appropriate terms for the class of drugs that stimulate the PSNS (the branch of the ANS that opposes the SNS).

▼ The main neurotransmitter of the PSNS is ACh.

▼ There are two types of cholinergic receptors: nicotinic and muscarinic.

▼ Nicotinic receptors are located on preganglionic nerve fibres in the PSNS, SNS, and adrenal medulla.

▼ Muscarinic receptors are located on post-synaptic cells, muscles, and glands (*not* on nerve).

▼ Cholinesterase is the enzyme responsible for the breakdown of ACh.

▼ Indirect-acting cholinergic agents work by inhibiting cholinesterase so that ACh accumulates at the synapse.

▼ Nursing considerations for cholinergic agents: Give as directed and monitor the client carefully for the occurrence of bradycardia, hypotension, headache, dizziness, respiratory depression, or bronchospasms. If these occur in a client taking cholinergics, the healthcare provider needs to be contacted immediately.

▼ Clients taking cholinergics should always be encouraged to change positions slowly to avoid dizziness and fainting resulting from postural hypotension.

EXAMINATION REVIEW QUESTIONS

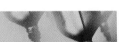

1 Which of the following is the rationale for the use of cholinergic agents with clients who have bladder atony?
   a. Blockage of ACh occurs with increased bladder wall pressure.
   b. The synthetic drugs work predominantly in the muscarinic receptors.
   c. Increased bladder tone and motility occur with increased emptying of the bladder.
   d. Decreased dopamine levels occur with a stimulation of alpha-cholinergic receptors.

2 The geriatric client needs to be more cautious when taking bethanechol because of which of the following side effects?
   a. Dyspnea
   b. Diaphoresis
   c. Hypotension
   d. Hyperthermia

3 Which of the following client education instructions for use of ophthalmic pilocarpine should not be included?
   a. Store medication away from heat, light, and children
   b. Apply pressure to the inner canthus to prevent systemic absorption

   c. Open eyelid and pull lower eyelid away from the eye for administration into the conjunctival sac
   d. Wash your hands, put on sterile gloves, and place the drug in the inner canthus for greater drug distribution

4 Your client is taking oral bethanechol and has been taking it before meals. He has begun to complain of nausea and vomiting. Which of the following statements would not be an appropriate response?
   a. "Take with meals if nausea is problematic."
   b. "Urecholine is best tolerated if all doses are taken at bedtime."
   c. "If you take it with at least 180 mL of fluid you may decrease GI upset."
   d. "If nausea and vomiting are severe, contact your healthcare provider for further instructions."

For answers see http://evolve.elsevier.com/Lilley/pharmacology/.

CRITICAL THINKING ACTIVITIES

1 Your client had a bladder resection 3 days ago and is now experiencing difficulty urinating. The physician orders bethanechol, starting with 10 mg PO tid. What should you do?

2 Discuss the implications for assessment of clients on either a direct- or an indirect-acting parasympathomimetic.

3 Discuss the advantages and disadvantages of the available cholinergic agents that are specifically intended for use in Alzheimer disease.

BIBLIOGRAPHY

Albanese, J., & Nutz, P. (2005). *Mosby's 2005 nursing drug cards*. St Louis, MO: Mosby.

Alzheimer Society of Canada. (2005). Treatment. Clinical trials and research studies. Retrieved August 6, 2005, from http://www.alzheimer.ca/english/treatment/trials-intro.htm

Canadian Pharmacists Association. (2003). *Therapeutic choices* (4th ed.). Ottawa, ON: Author.

Canadian Pharmacists Association. (2004). *Guide to drugs in Canada*. Toronto, ON: Dorling Kindersley.

Canadian Pharmacists Association. (2005). *Compendium of pharmaceuticals and specialties. The Canadian drug reference for health professionals*. Ottawa, ON: Author. [The subscription-based e-CPS is available at http://www.pharmacists.ca.]

Cheng, A., Williams, B.A., & Sivarajan, B.V. (Eds.). (2003). *The HSC handbook of pediatrics* (10th ed.). Toronto, ON: Elsevier.

Facts and Comparisons. (2004). *Drug facts and comparisons pocket version* (9th ed.). St Louis, MO: Wolters Kluwer Health.

Hardman, J.G., & Limbird, L.E. (2002). *Goodman and Gilman's the pharmacological basis of therapeutics* (10th ed.). New York: McGraw-Hill.

Health Canada. (2000). Warning. PREPULSID® to be withdrawn as a result of cardiac complications. Retrieved from http://www.hc-sc.gc.ca/ahc-asc/media/advisories-avis/2000/2000_56_e.html

Health Canada. (2005). Drug product database (DPD). Retrieved August 6, 2005, from http://www.hc-sc.gc.ca/hpb/drugs-dpd/

Health Canada Therapeutic Drugs Directorate. (2004). Conditional approval of Ebixa. Fact sheet. Retrieved August 6, 2005, from http://www.hc-sc.gc.ca/dhp-mps/prodpharma/index_e.html

Katzung, B. G. (2004). *Basic and clinical pharmacology* (9th ed.). New York: McGraw-Hill.

Koda-Kimble, M.A., & Young, L.Y. (2001). *Applied therapeutics: The clinical use of drugs* (7th ed.). Philadelphia: Lippincott Williams & Wilkins.

Lacy, C.F., Armstrong, L.L., Goldman, M.P., & Lance, L.L. (2003). *Drug information handbook* (11th ed.). Hudson, OH: Lexi-Comp.

Lehne, R.A. (2004). *Pharmacology for nursing care* (5th ed.). St Louis, MO: Saunders.

Mosby. (2005). *Mosby's drug consult 2005: The comprehensive reference for generic and brand name drugs* (15th ed.). St Louis, MO: Mosby.

Skidmore-Roth, L. (2006). *Mosby's 2006 nursing drug reference* (19th ed.). St Louis, MO: Mosby.

CHAPTER

20 Cholinergic-Blocking Agents

OBJECTIVES

After reading this chapter, the successful student will be able to do the following:

1 Contrast normal anatomy and physiology of the autonomic nervous system with the events that are blocked with the use of anticholinergic agents.

2 Identify the various anticholinergic drugs with specific information related to their use.

3 Compare the mechanisms of action, therapeutic effects, indications, and adverse and toxic effects of the various anticholinergic drugs and any antidotes.

4 Identify the drug interactions associated with the use of anticholinergics.

5 Evaluate the therapeutic vs. side effects of the different anticholinergic agents.

6 Develop a nursing care plan that includes all phases of the nursing process related to the administration of the various anticholinergic agents.

e-LEARNING ACTIVITIES

Student CD-ROM
- Review Questions: see questions 116–121
- Animations
- Medication Administration Checklists
- IV Therapy Checklists

evolve **Web site** (http://evolve.elsevier.com/Lilley/pharmacology/)
- Online Chapter Worksheet • Frequently Asked Questions
- Learning Tips and Content Updates • WebLinks • Online Appendices and Supplements • Mosby/Saunders ePharmacology Update • Access to *Mosby's Drug Consult*

DRUG PROFILES

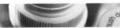

▶▶ atropine, p. 333
▶▶ benztropine (Chapter 14), p. 230
▶▶ dicyclomine, p. 333
  glycopyrrolate, p. 333
  scopolamine, p. 335
▶▶ tolterodine, p. 335
  trihexyphenidyl (Chapter 14), p. 230

▶▶ Key drug.

GLOSSARY

Anticholinergic (an' tee ko' lə ner' jik) Another name for a cholinergic-blocking agent.
Cholinergic-blocking agent Any agent that blocks the action of acetylcholine (ACh) and substances sim-

ilar to ACh at receptor sites in the synapse. Such agents in effect block the action of cholinergic nerves that transmit impulses through the release of ACh at their synapses.
Competitive antagonist A drug or other substance that is an antagonist or that resembles a normal human metabolite and interferes with its function in the body, usually by competing for the metabolite's receptors or enzymes. Also called an *antimetabolite*.
Mydriasis (mi dry' ə sis) Dilation of the pupil of the eye caused by contraction of the dilator muscle of the iris.

Cholinergic blockers, anticholinergics, parasympatholytics, and *antimuscarinic agents* are all terms for the class of drugs that block or inhibit the actions of acetylcholine (ACh) in the parasympathetic nervous system (PSNS). **Cholinergic-blocking agents** block the action of the neurotransmitter ACh at the muscarinic receptors in the PSNS. ACh released from the stimulated nerve fibre is then unable to bind to the receptor site and fails to produce a cholinergic effect. This is why the cholinergic blockers are also referred to as **anticholinergics.** Blocking the parasympathetic nerves allows the sympathetic (adrenergic) nervous system (SNS) to dominate. Because of this, cholinergic blockers have many of the same effects as the adrenergics. Figure 20-1 illustrates the site of action of the cholinergic blockers within the PSNS.

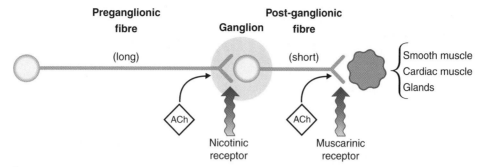

FIG. 20-1 Site of action of cholinergic blockers within the parasympathetic nervous system.

Cholinergic blockers have many important therapeutic uses and are one of the oldest groups of therapeutic agents. Originally they were derived from various plant sources, but today these naturally occurring substances are only part of a larger group of cholinergic blockers that include both synthetic and semi-synthetic agents. Box 20-1 lists the currently available cholinergic blockers grouped according to their chemical class.

Mechanism of Action and Drug Effects

Cholinergic blockers are largely **competitive antagonists.** They compete with ACh for binding at the muscarinic receptors of the PSNS. Once they have bound to the receptor, they inhibit nerve transmission at these receptors. This generally occurs at the neuroeffector junction of smooth muscle, cardiac muscle, and exocrine glands. Cholinergic blockers have little effect at the nicotinic receptors, although at high doses they can have partial blocking effects.

The major sites of action of the anticholinergics are the heart, respiratory tract, gastrointestinal (GI) tract, urinary bladder, eye, and exocrine glands. In general the anticholinergics have effects opposite those of the cholinergics at these sites of action. The blockade of ACh by cholinergic blockers causes the pupils to dilate and increases intraocular pressure (IOP). This can occur because the ciliary muscles and the sphincter muscle of the iris are innervated by cholinergic nerve fibres. Cholinergic blockers can therefore keep the sphincter muscle of the iris from contracting and allow unopposed radial muscle stimulation. This results in a dilated pupil **(mydriasis)** and a relaxed eye (cycloplegia). However, this can be detrimental to clients with glaucoma because it results in increased IOP.

In the GI tract, cholinergic blockers cause a decrease in GI motility, GI secretions, and salivation. In the cardiovascular system these agents cause an increased heart rate. In the genitourinary (GU) system, anticholinergics lead to decreased bladder contraction, which can result in urinary retention. In the skin they reduce sweating, and in the respiratory system they dry mucous membranes and cause bronchial dilation. These effects are listed according to body system in Table 20-1. Many of these cholinergic-blocking agents are available in a variety of forms (intravenous [IV], intramuscular [IM], oral [PO], subcutaneous [SC].

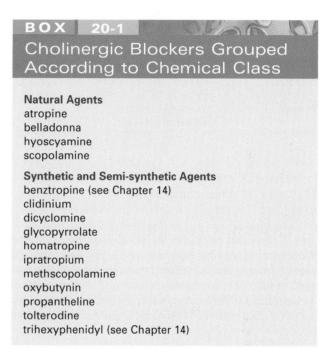

BOX 20-1

Cholinergic Blockers Grouped According to Chemical Class

Natural Agents
atropine
belladonna
hyoscyamine
scopolamine

Synthetic and Semi-synthetic Agents
benztropine (see Chapter 14)
clidinium
dicyclomine
glycopyrrolate
homatropine
ipratropium
methscopolamine
oxybutynin
propantheline
tolterodine
trihexyphenidyl (see Chapter 14)

Indications

The central nervous system (CNS) effects of cholinergic blockers have the therapeutic effect of decreasing muscle rigidity and diminishing tremors. This is of benefit in the treatment of both Parkinson's disease (see Chapter 14) and drug-induced extrapyramidal reactions. The therapeutic cardiovascular effects of anticholinergics are related to their cholinergic-blocking effects on the heart's conduction system. At low doses the anticholinergics slow the heart rate by means of their effects on the cardiac centre in the portion of the brain called the *medulla*. At high doses, cholinergic blockers block the inhibitory vagal effects on the pacemaker cells of the sinoatrial (SA) and atrioventricular (AV) nodes and accelerate the heart rate. Atropine is primarily used for cardiovascular disorders, such as for the diagnosis of sinus node dysfunction, the treatment of clients with symptomatic second-degree AV block, and advanced life support in the treatment of sinus bradycardia that is accompanied by hemodynamic compromise.

TABLE 20-1
CHOLINERGIC BLOCKERS: DRUG EFFECTS

Body System	Cholinergic Blocker Effects
Cardiovascular	*Small doses:* Decrease heart rate
	Large doses: Increase heart rate
Central nervous	*Small doses:* Decrease muscle rigidity and tremors
	Large doses: Drowsiness, disorientation, hallucinations
Eye	Dilate pupils (mydriasis), decrease accommodation by paralyzing ciliary muscles (cycloplegia)
Gastrointestinal	Relax smooth muscle tone of GI tract, decrease intestinal and gastric secretions, decrease motility and peristalsis
Genitourinary	Relax detrusor muscle of bladder, increase constriction of internal sphincter; these two may result in urinary retention
Glandular	Decrease bronchial secretions, salivation, sweating
Respiratory	Decrease bronchial secretions, dilate bronchial airways

TABLE 20-2
CHOLINERGIC BLOCKERS: ADVERSE EFFECTS

Body System	Cholinergic-Blocking Effects
Cardiovascular	Increased heart rate, dysrhythmias
Central nervous	CNS excitation, restlessness, irritability, disorientation, hallucinations, delirium
Eye	Dilated pupils, decreased visual accommodation, increased IOP
Gastrointestinal	Decreased salivation, gastric secretions, motility
Genitourinary	Urinary retention
Glandular	Decreased sweating
Respiratory	Decreased bronchial secretions

When the cholinergic stimulation of the PSNS is blocked by cholinergic blockers, the SNS effects go unopposed. In the respiratory tract this results in decreased secretions from the nose, mouth, pharynx, and bronchi. It also causes relaxation of the smooth muscles in the bronchi and bronchioles, which results in decreased airway resistance and bronchodilation. Because of this, the cholinergic blockers have proved beneficial in treating exercise-induced bronchospasms, chronic bronchitis, asthma, and chronic obstructive pulmonary disease (COPD).

Gastric secretions and the smooth muscle responsible for producing gastric motility are both under the control of the PSNS, which is primarily under the control of muscarinic receptors. Cholinergic blockers antagonize these receptors, causing decreased secretions, relaxation of smooth muscle, and decreased GI motility and peristalsis. For these reasons cholinergic blockers are commonly used in the treatment of irritable bowel disease and GI hypersecretory states.

Although cholinergic blockers were commonly used in the past for treating peptic ulcer disease, their use for this purpose has largely been superseded by newer drug categories such as histamine H_2 receptor antagonists and proton pump inhibitors (PPIs). These agents are covered in Chapter 49.

The effects that anticholinergics have on the bladder have made them useful in the treatment of such GU tract disorders as reflex neurogenic bladder and incontinence. They relax the detrusor muscles of the bladder and increase constriction of the internal sphincter. The cholinergic blockers' ability to decrease glandular secretions also makes them potentially useful agents for reducing gastric and pancreatic secretions in clients with acute pancreatitis.

Contraindications

Contraindications to the use of anticholinergic agents include known drug allergy, narrow-angle glaucoma, acute asthma or other respiratory distress, myasthenia gravis, acute cardiovascular instability, and GI or GU tract obstruction or other acute illness in these areas.

Side Effects and Adverse Effects

Many body systems are affected adversely by cholinergic blockers. This is a function of the cholinergic blockers' site of action. The muscarinic receptors are located in a variety of tissues, organs, glands, and cells throughout the body. Therefore blockade of these receptors by the anticholinergics produces a wide range of effects, some desirable, as described in the previous section, and some not so desirable. The various side effects and adverse effects of cholinergic blockers are listed by body system in Table 20-2.

Other factors contributing to the wide variety of possible adverse effects of cholinergic blockers are the affinity of the muscarinic receptors for specific drugs and the drug dose. Certain client populations are more susceptible to the effects of these drugs. These include infants, older adults, fair-skinned children with Down syndrome, and children with spastic paralysis or brain damage.

Interactions

Significant drug interactions can occur with cholinergic blockers. Knowledge of the broad categories of drugs that should not be co-administered with cholinergic blockers can help prevent potentially serious consequences. Additive cholinergic effects can be seen when antihistamines, phenothiazines, tricyclic antidepressants (TCAs), and monoamine oxidase inhibitors (MAOIs) are given with cholinergic blockers.

Toxicity and Management of Overdose

The dose of cholinergic blockers is particularly important because these drugs have a narrow therapeutic index: that is, there is a relatively small difference between therapeutic and toxic doses. The treatment of cholinergic blocker overdose consists of symptomatic and supportive therapy. Consultation with a Poison Control Centre is recommended. The client should be hospitalized, and close, continuous monitoring should be initiated, including continuous electrocardiogram (ECG) monitoring. Activated charcoal has proven to be effective in removing drug that is already absorbed.

Fluid therapy and other standard measures used for the treatment of shock should be instituted as needed. Delirium, hallucinations, coma, and cardiac dysrhythmias respond favourably to physostigmine treatment. Its routine use as an antidote for cholinergic blocker overdose is controversial, however, and it is available in Canada only under the Special Access Programme. It has the potential for producing severe adverse effects such as seizures and asystole and should therefore be reserved for the treatment of clients showing extreme delirium or agitation who could inflict injury on themselves.

Dosages

For the recommended dosages of selected cholinergic blockers, see the table on p. 334. See Appendix B for some of the common brands available in Canada.

DRUG PROFILES

All cholinergic blockers are prescription-only drugs. They are available in many dosage formulations: oral, topical, and injectable. Most of the cholinergic blockers are classified as pregnancy category C agents; dicyclomine is classified as a pregnancy category B agent.

Among the oldest and best known naturally occurring cholinergic blockers are the belladonna alkaloids. It is the belladonna alkaloid contained in these agents that is responsible for their therapeutic effects. Of these, atropine is the prototypical agent. It has been in use for hundreds of years and continues to be widely used because of its effectiveness. Besides atropine, scopolamine is the other major naturally occurring drug. These drugs come from a variety of plants within the potato family (Solanaceae). Some examples are *Atropa belladonna* (deadly nightshade), *Hyoscyamus niger* (henbane), and *Datura stramonium* (jimsonweed or thorn apple).

Of the semi-synthetic and synthetic cholinergic blockers, there are many therapeutically useful agents. These agents are used in the treatment of a variety of illnesses and conditions ranging from peptic ulcer disease and irritable bowel syndrome to the symptoms of the common cold, as well as preoperatively to dry up secretions. They are the synthetic derivatives of the plant-derived belladonna alkaloids and are generally more specific in binding predominantly with muscarinic receptors. They may also be associated with fewer side effects.

▶▶ atropine

Atropine is a naturally occurring antimuscarinic. It may be prepared synthetically but is usually obtained by extraction from various members of the Solanaceae family of plants (deadly nightshade or jimsonweed). In general, atropine is more potent than scopolamine in its cholinergic-blocking effects on the heart and in its effects on the smooth muscles of the bronchi and intestines. Atropine is effective in the treatment of many of the conditions listed in the Indications section. It is also used preoperatively to reduce salivation and GI secretions, as is glycopyrrolate. It is contraindicated in clients with pyloric stenosis, thyrotoxicosis, narrow-angle glaucoma, certain types of asthma (not cholinergic associated), advanced hepatic and renal dysfunction, intestinal atony, obstructive GI or urinary conditions, and severe ulcerative colitis and toxic megacolon. It is used with caution in clients with coronary artery disease, congestive heart failure, cardiac dysrhythmias, and hypertension. It is available as a parenteral injection in several concentrations and strengths, as well as various ophthalmic preparations (Chapter 56). Pregnancy category C. The recommended dosages are given in the table on p. 334.

PHARMACOKINETICS

Half-Life	Onset	Peak	Duration
IV: 2.5 hr	IV: Immediate	IV: 2–4 min	IV: 4–6 hr

▶▶ benztropine

For a discussion of benztropine, see p. 230 in Chapter 14.

▶▶ dicyclomine

Dicyclomine is a synthetic antispasmodic cholinergic blocker used primarily in the treatment of functional disturbances of GI motility such as irritable bowel syndrome. It has also been used for the treatment of colic and enterocolitis in infants. It is most commonly administered in oral form as either a 10- or 20-mg tablet. It is also available as an orally administered syrup that contains 10 mg/5 mL of the drug. As a parenteral preparation, it is available as a 10-mg/mL intramuscular injection. Intravenous administration is not recommended. It is contraindicated in infants less than 6 months of age, clients who have a known hypersensitivity to anticholinergics, and in those with GI obstruction, myasthenia gravis, paralytic ileus, GI atony, severe ulcerative colitis, reflux esophagitis, glaucoma, or unstable cardiovascular status. Pregnancy category B. The recommended dosages can be found in the table on p. 334.

PHARMACOKINETICS

Half-Life	Onset	Peak	Duration
9–10 hr	1–2 hr	1–1.5 hr	3–4 hr

glycopyrrolate

Glycopyrrolate is a synthetic antimuscarinic agent that blocks receptor sites in the autonomic nervous system that control the production of secretions and the

DOSAGES	Selected Cholinergic Antagonist (Anticholinergic) Agents		
Agent	**Pharmacological Class**	**Usual Dosage Range**	**Indications**
▸ atropine	Anticholinergic	***Pediatric*** 0.01–0.02 mg/kg/dose pre-op and/or q4–6hr	Pre-op (for secretion control), therapeutic anticholinergic effect
		0.01–2 mg/kg, max 1–2 mg (child to adolescent respectively)	Bradycardia
		0.02–0.05 mg/kg initial dose q10–20min until effect, then q1–4hr × 24 hr	Anticholinesterase effect for organophosphate or carbamate poisoning (e.g., insecticides)
		Inhalation: 0.03–0.05 mg/kg/dose in 3–5 mL NS tid–qid; max 2.5 mg/dose	Bronchospasm
		Adult IM: 1 mg	Hypotonic radiography
		IV: 0.5–1 mg every 3–5 min to 0.03–0.04 mg/kg	Bradycardia, CPR
		IV: 1–3 mg/dose, repeat q 5–60 min until signs of atropine intoxication appear (e.g., tachycardia); continue until definite improvement	Anticholinesterase effect for organophosphate or carbamate poisoning (e.g., insecticides)
		Inhalation: 0.025 mg/kg/dose in 3–5 mL NS tid–qid; max 2.5 mg/dose	Bronchospasm
▸ dicyclomine	Anticholinergic	***Pediatric 6 mo–2 yr*** PO: 5–10 mg tid–qid; max 40 mg/day ***Pediatric 2–12 yr*** PO: 10 mg tid–qid ***Adult*** PO: 80–160 mg/day divided tid–qid	Irritable bowel syndrome
glycopyrrolate	Anticholinergic	***Pediatric*** IM/IV: 0.1–0.2mg tid–qid	Control of secretions
		IV (intra-operative): 0.005 mg/kg may repeat q2–3min prn; max 0.1 mg/dose	Control of secretions (intra-operative)
		Adult and pediatric IM/IV: 0.1–0.2 mg tid–qid	Peptic ulcer
		IM: 0.005 mg/kg 30–60 min pre-op	Pre-op for control of secretions
		IV (intra-operative): 0.1 mg, may repeat q2–3min prn	Control of secretions (intra-operative)
		Adult and pediatric 0.2 mg for each 1 mg of neostigmine or 5 mg of pyridostigmine	Reversal of neuromuscular blockade
oxybutynin	Anticholinergic	***Pediatric >5 yr*** PO: 5 mg bid–tid ***Adult*** PO: 5 mg bid–qid ***Adult only*** PO ER tab: 5–30 mg/day as single or divided doses	Antispasmodic for neurogenic bladder (e.g., following spinal cord injury), overactive bladder
scopolamine	Anticholinergic	***Pediatric*** 0.006 μg/kg/dose	Pre-op for control of secretions
		Adult IM, IV, SC: 0.3–0.6 mg; may repeat 3–4/day	Pre-op for control of secretions
		Transdermal patch: 1.5 mg patch behind ear q3days (delivers approx 1 mg scopolamine over 3 days); apply at least 12 hr before transportation	Motion sickness
▸ tolterodine	Anticholinergic	***Adult only*** PO: 1–2 mg bid PO ER cap: 2–4 mg daily	Overactive bladder

CPR, Cardiopulmonary resuscitation; *NS,* normal saline; *ER,* extended release.

concentration of free acids in the stomach. It is most commonly used as a preoperative medication to reduce salivation and excessive secretions in the respiratory and GI tracts and for the management of gastrointestinal disorders when oral medication is not tolerated or rapid effect is required. It is contraindicated in clients who have a hypersensitivity to it and in those with narrow-angle glaucoma, myasthenia gravis, GI or GU obstruction, tachycardia, myocardial ischemia, hepatic disease, paralytic ileus, severe ulcerative colitis, and toxic megacolon, as well as in elderly or debilitated clients with chronic lung disease. Glycopyrrolate is available parenterally as a 0.2-mg/mL intramuscular or intravenous injection. Pregnancy category B. The normal recommended dosages are given in the table on p. 334.

PHARMACOKINETICS

Half-Life	Onset	Peak	Duration
Variable	IV: 1 min	IV: 10–15 min	IV: 4 hr

scopolamine

Scopolamine is another naturally occurring cholinergic blocker and one of the principal belladonna alkaloids. It appears to be the most potent antimuscarinic for the prevention of motion sickness. It seems to accomplish this by correcting the imbalance between ACh and norepinephrine in the higher centres in the brain, particularly in the vomiting centre, responsible for the symptoms of motion sickness. Ipratropium, a derivative of scopolamine, has potent effects on the lungs and is discussed in Chapters 35 and 36. It is available in several different delivery systems that make it useful for various indications. For the prevention of motion sickness it is available in a convenient transdermal delivery system, a patch that can be applied just behind the ear 12 hours before the anti-emetic effect is required. It is also available in two parenteral formulations for injection by various routes: intravenous, intramuscular, and subcutaneous. The transdermal patch is available by prescription. The contraindications that apply to atropine apply to it as well. Pregnancy category C. The recommended dosages for various indications can be found in the table on p. 334.

PHARMACOKINETICS

Half-Life	Onset	Peak	Duration
Variable	IV: 30–60 min	IV: 30–45 min	IV: 4 hr
	Patch: 4–5 hr	Patch: 12 hr	Patch: 72 hr

▸▸ tolterodine

Tolterodine is new muscarinic receptor blocker now being widely promoted for treatment of urinary frequency, urgency, and urge incontinence caused by bladder (detrusor) overactivity. Another drug that is commonly used to treat these conditions is oxybutynin, which is one of the most commonly prescribed. Other agents also used include propantheline, hyoscyamine, flavoxate, and the TCA imipramine. These agents are less commonly used because of their antimuscarinic adverse effects, particularly dry mouth. Tolterodine appears to have a much lower incidence of dry mouth in part because of its specificity for the bladder as opposed to the salivary glands.

Tolterodine should not be used in clients with uncontrolled narrow-angle glaucoma or urinary retention.

Clients with markedly decreased hepatic function or poor metabolizers taking drugs that inhibit CYP3A4, such as erythromycin or ketoconazole, should not receive doses greater than 1 mg twice a day. It is available as 1- and 2-mg tablets. Pregnancy category C. Recommended dosages are given in the table on p. 334.

PHARMACOKINETICS

Half-Life	Onset	Peak	Duration
2–4 hr	1 hr	1–2 hr	5 hr

trihexyphenidyl

For a discussion of trihexyphenidyl, see p. 230 in Chapter 14.

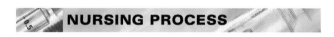

NURSING PROCESS

■ Assessment

Anticholinergic drugs, or parasympatholytics, produce a variety of effects resulting from the blocking of ACh in the PSNS. Because of their various effects at different body sites (e.g., smooth muscle relaxation, decreased glandular secretion, mydriasis) the nurse must perform a thorough medical and medication history and a head-to-toe assessment to reveal any contraindications. These include benign prostatic hypertrophy, glaucoma, tachycardia, myocardial infarction (MI), heart failure, and hiatal hernia. In general the cholinergic blockers should not be used in clients with GI or GU obstruction and in children under 3 years of age. Geriatric clients are also more vulnerable to side effects, particularly confusion, delirium, constipation, blurred vision, and tachycardia, necessitating more careful use in this population. Drug interactions are discussed earlier in this chapter. The head-to-toe assessment will also help document baseline findings related to the disease and to assess drug effectiveness.

Atropine and atropine-like drugs (dicyclomine, glycopyrrolate, and scopolamine) are contraindicated in those with glaucoma, unstable cardiac disease or symptoms, asthma, GI and/or GU tract obstruction, paralytic ileus or intestinal atony, and ulcerative colitis. Cautious use with close monitoring is recommended with debilitated clients and with clients who experience reflux esophagitis, autonomic neuropathies, impaired liver or renal functioning, hypertension, hyperthyroidism, and diarrhea. Drug interactions associated with atropine and atropine-like drugs include antacids, anticholinergics, antihistamines, phenothiazines, and TCAs (such as amitriptyline).

Tolterodine and oxybutynin are anticholinergic agents used to treat urinary incontinence. Tolterodine is a muscarinic-receptor-blocking agent that has been most recently introduced for treatment of a variety of urinary symptoms and problems ranging from frequency and urgency to incontinence. Tolterodine and oxybutynin are the agents most commonly used at this time. Both of these drugs are contraindicated in clients with GI or GU obstruction, GI hemorrhage, glaucoma, urinary retention, cardiac and/or hepatic disease, colitis, and myasthenia gravis, and cautious use is recommended for clients who are pregnant, lactating, geriatric, or under 12 years of age. Clients who have narrow-angle glaucoma or urinary retention should not take tolterodine. For clients with poor renal function or who are taking drugs that inhibit CYP3A4, the enzyme for metabolism (such as erythromycin or ketoconazole), a lower dosage such as 1 mg twice daily may be recommended. Drug interactions for both tolterodine and oxybutynin include many of the antihypertensive agents, sympathomimetics, alcohol, barbiturates, benzodiazepines, atenolol, digoxin, acetaminophen, haloperidol, levodopa, MAOIs, antidepressants, and phenothiazines.

Nursing Diagnoses

Nursing diagnoses associated with the use of cholinergic-blocking agents include, but are not limited to, the following:

- Ineffective tissue perfusion, cardiopulmonary, related to drug-induced tachycardia.
- Risk for injury related to possible excessive CNS stimulation and side effects resulting in tremors, confusion, sedation, and amnesia.
- Constipation related to side effects of the drug.
- Impaired gas exchange related to thickened respiratory secretions from side effects of the drug.
- Urinary retention related to loss of bladder tone as a result of side effects of the drug.
- Risk for injury related to decreased sweating and loss of normal heat-regulating mechanisms (especially in geriatric clients and in those who engage in excessive exercise or who are in high environmental temperatures) and possible heat stroke due to effects of the drug on the temperature-regulating mechanisms.
- Risk for falls related to changes in vision related to the mydriatic (pupil dilation) effects of the medication.
- Deficient knowledge of therapeutic regimen, side effects, drug interactions, and precautions related to the use of anticholinergic agents.

Planning

Goals for the client receiving cholinergic-blockers include, but are not limited to, the following:

- Client self-administers medications as prescribed.
- Client experiences relief of symptoms for which the medication was prescribed.
- Client remains adherent with the drug therapy.
- Client demonstrates an adequate knowledge about the use of the specific medications, side effects, and the appropriate dosing at home.
- Client is free of injury to self resulting from side effects from the medication.

Outcome Criteria

Outcome criteria include the following:

- Client states the rationale for the use of cholinergic blockers in preoperative preparation, such as decreasing the risk of complications associated with anaesthesia.
- Client states the importance of adherence with the medication regimen, such as avoiding complications of Parkinson's disease.

- Client states the importance of taking the medication as prescribed and not suddenly withdrawing the medication, which could increase symptoms.
- Client states those conditions of which the physician should be notified immediately (e.g., palpitations, dysrhythmias, chest pain).
- Client keeps follow-up appointments with the physician to avoid unnecessary adverse effects of complications from treatment or non-adherence.

Implementation

A preventive-type approach as a focus for nursing care is important to the effective use of cholinergic-blocking agents, especially in teaching clients how to possibly decrease their need for these medications. Several nursing interventions may also serve to maximize the therapeutic effects of anticholinergics and minimize the side effects. For example, encouraging clients to take the medications as prescribed; to take the exact dose ordered by the healthcare provider; and, if therapeutic effects are limited or side effects are troubling, to contact their healthcare provider for other treatment or recommendations.

Because atropine is compatible with some of the other commonly used preoperative medications, such as meperidine and morphine, it is often used in combination and mixed in the same syringe for pre-anaesthetic medication. However, whenever mixing several medications together in one syringe, the doses must always be calculated carefully. When administering optical solutions of the cholinergic-blocking medications to produce mydriasis, the nurse must always check the concentration of medication and apply pressure to the inner canthus to prevent more systemic absorption. Atropine, in small doses such as 0.03 mg, is combined with other agents such as hyoscyamine (another cholinergic-blocking agent) for treatment of lower urinary tract discomfort due to hypermotility. Atropine and atropine-like drugs have been used in the treatment of diarrhea and in preoperative formulations and should be given exactly as directed and at the time ordered, whether "on-call" to the operating room (OR) or at a daily specified time. Sedation and dry mouth are just two of the side effects that create concerns for nursing, such as making sure that clients remain safe and free from injury and that they get the needed mouth care to prevent the problems that often arise from the use of these drugs.

When using cholinergic-blocking agents for urinary tract disorders or dysfunction, such as for urinary or bladder instability, clients need to be aware of the importance of dosing as indicated, which may be up to three times a day depending on the drug. For example, oxybutynin is generally taken up to three times a day and tolterodine is administered twice daily. In addition, oxybutynin may need to be decreased in dosage or dosing frequency because it will result in significant renal or hepatic dysfunction when administered along with drugs that are CYP3A4 inhibitors (e.g., erythromycin). Tolterodine should be taken as directed and is usually well tolerated when taken with food. Oxybutynin should be taken as directed with fluids 1 hour before or 2 hours after meals, if tolerated. Dry mouth associated with these drugs may be handled best by performing frequent mouth care, chewing gum, or sucking on hard candy. For cholinergic-blocking agents used for urinary incontinence, constipation and the inability to sweat or perspire should be managed with increased fluids and bulk and avoidance of extremes of heat. Clients taking medications for urinary disorders should also be told to report immediately to their healthcare provider any unresolved constipation, palpitations, alterations in gait, excessive dizziness, or difficulty in urinating.

Client teaching tips are presented in the box below.

■ Evaluation

Therapeutic effects for cholinergic-blocking drugs include the following:

- For Parkinson's disease, clients experience improved ability to do ADLs and fewer problems with tremors, salivation, and drooling.
- For relief of GI symptoms such as hyperacidity, clients report improved comfort and a decrease in symptoms of abdominal pain, nausea, vomiting, and heartburn.
- For urological problems, clients show an improvement in urinary patterns with less hypermotility and increased time between voiding.
- For preoperative situations, clients experience fewer bronchospasms with induction of anaesthesia and fewer problems with secretions because the cholinergic-blockers (anticholinergic agents) dry them out, making them more thick and viscous.

The nurse must evaluate the client for the occurrence of the side effects of these medications, such as constipation, tachycardia, tremors, confusion, hallucinations, CNS depression (which occurs with large doses of atropine), sedation, urinary retention, hot and dry skin, and fever. Toxicity with these drugs includes possible CNS depression with confusion and hallucinations and cardiovascular stimulation with severe tachycardia and palpitations.

CLIENT TEACHING TIPS

The nurse should instruct the client as follows:

▲ Always take your medication as ordered because an overdose can cause life-threatening heart or nervous system problems.

▲ Dry mouth is a common side effect of these medications; therefore if you are taking them on a long-term basis, brush your teeth regularly to avoid cavities. Chew gum or suck on hard candy to relieve dryness— as long as these are not contraindicated. Sugar-free formulations are available.

▲ Be careful when engaging in various activities such as driving a car or operating machinery because of the blurred vision that commonly occurs with these medications.

▲ You may experience sensitivity to light and may therefore want to wear dark glasses or sunglasses.

▲ Always consult with your physician before taking any other medication, including OTC medications.

▲ (For older clients) Since these drugs can put you at risk of heat stroke, avoid strenuous exercise and exposure to high temperatures. Limit physical exertion and always remember the importance of adequate fluid and salt intake, if this is allowed. Use fans, air conditioners, and adequate ventilation to prevent overheating.

▲ Contact your physician if you experience urinary hesitancy and/or retention, constipation, palpitations, tremors, confusion, sedation or amnesia, excessive dry mouth (especially if you have chronic lung infections or other chronic lung disease), or fever.

POINTS to REMEMBER

▼ Cholinergic blockers, anticholinergics, parasympatholytics, and antimuscarinics are all terms used for the drugs that block or inhibit the actions of ACh in the PSNS.

▼ The use of these cholinergic blockers allows the SNS to dominate. Their chemical classifications are natural, semi-synthetic, and synthetic.

▼ Anticholinergics may be competitive antagonists (blockers) and compete with ACh at the muscarinic receptors. In high doses they result in partial blocking actions at nicotinic receptors.

▼ Anticholinergics bind to and block ACh at muscarinic receptors located on the cells that the parasympathetic nerve stimulates.

▼ Contraindications to the use of anticholinergics include a history of benign prostatic hypertrophy, glaucoma, tachycardia, MI, heart failure, and hiatal hernia.

▼ Anticholinergics should be used with caution in clients with GI or GU obstruction or in children under 3 years of age.

▼ Anticholinergics are used commonly in the treatment of urinary instability such as with urinary or bladder hypermotility.

EXAMINATION REVIEW QUESTIONS

1 Which of the following points should the nurse remind geriatric clients of when taking anticholinergics?
   a. Avoid exposure to high temperatures
   b. Take the drug without concern if also taking antiglaucoma medications
   c. Participate in exercises and use a hot tub for relaxation
   d. Don't be alarmed if you have constipation, confusion, and palpations

2 Contraindications to the use of anticholinergics include which of the following?
   a. Preoperative status
   b. Peptic ulcer disease
   c. Irritable bowel syndrome
   d. Benign prostatic hypertrophy (BPH)

3 Side effects associated with the use of cholinergic blockers include which of the following?
   a. Diaphoresis
   b. Dry mouth
   c. Diarrhea
   d. Decreased sensorium

4 Which of the following is an expected effect from a parasympatholytic?
   a. Miosis
   b. Increased muscle rigidity
   c. Increased bronchial secretions
   d. Decreased motility and peristalsis

5 During an assessment of a client about to receive a cholinergic-blocking agent, the nurse should assess for which of the following drug interactions?
   a. Narcotics
   b. Phenothiazines
   c. Meperidine
   d. Bethanechol

For answers see http://evolve.elsevier.com/Lilley/pharmacology/.

CRITICAL THINKING ACTIVITIES

1 You are getting ready to administer preoperative medications to a 75-year-old woman undergoing minor surgery. She has a history of smoking, heart failure, and open-angle glaucoma. What is the rationale for not administering the atropine preoperatively to this client, as ordered? Also, what is your rationale for contacting the physician about this drug interaction and your subsequent action?

2 You are caring for a client who has just arrested in the cardiac care unit. The client is in second-degree heart block, has sinus bradycardia with a heart rate of 30, and has passed out. You recommend that the cholinergic blocker _____ be given to _____ the heart rate.
   a. belladonna; slow
   b. esmolol; slow
   c. atropine; increase
   d. atropine; decrease

3 You are chaperoning a group of 8-year-old children on a deep sea fishing trip. The mother of one of these children is an anaesthesiologist. She has given all the children a medication to prevent seasickness. Three hours into the fishing expedition you notice that the children are disoriented, hallucinating, irritable, and cannot sit still. You realize the children are suffering from _____ side effects from the cholinergic blocker _____.
   a. central nervous system; scopolamine
   b. cardiovascular; belladonna
   c. respiratory; pilocarpine
   d. central nervous system; pilocarpine

4 In the situation described in question 3, you are asked to give 0.5 mg of atropine to your client. The vial concentration is 1 mg/mL. In the haste of this emergency situation, 5 mL of atropine is given. How many milligrams of atropine were given to your client?

5 If the SNS is for mobilizing the organism in times of stress or during emergency situations, what is the importance of the PSNS? Why are clients at risk for hyperthermia when taking drugs such as atropine?

6 Post-operatively, the client receives prochlorperazine IV. Subsequently, the client develops extrapyramidal symptoms for which the physician orders an anticholinergic. What is the rationale for this order?

For answers see http://evolve.elsevier.com/Lilley/pharmacology/.

BIBLIOGRAPHY

Albanese, J., & Nutz, P. (2005). *Mosby's 2005 nursing drug cards.* St Louis, MO: Mosby.

Canadian Pharmacists Association. (2003). *Therapeutic choices* (4th ed.). Ottawa, ON: Author.

Canadian Pharmacists Association. (2004). *Guide to drugs in Canada.* Toronto, ON: Dorling Kindersley.

Canadian Pharmacists Association. (2005). *Compendium of pharmaceuticals and specialties. The Canadian drug reference for health professionals.* Ottawa, ON: Author. [The subscription-based e-CPS is available at http://www.pharmacists.ca.]

Cheng, A., Williams, B.A., & Sivarajan, B.V. (Eds.). (2003). *The HSC handbook of pediatrics* (10th ed.). Toronto, ON: Elsevier.

Facts and Comparisons. (2004). *Drug facts and comparisons: pocket version* (9th ed.). St Louis, MO: Wolters Kluwer Health.

Hardman, J.G., & Limbird, L.E. (2002). *Goodman and Gilman's the pharmacological basis of therapeutics* (10th ed.). New York: McGraw-Hill.

Health Canada. (2005). Drug product database (DPD). Retrieved August 6, 2005, from http://www.hc-sc.gc.ca/hpb/drugs-dpd/

Katzung, B.G. (2004). *Basic and clinical pharmacology* (9th ed.). New York: McGraw-Hill.

Koda-Kimble, M.A., & Young, L.Y. (2001). *Applied therapeutics: the clinical use of drugs* (7th ed.). Philadelphia: Lippincott Williams & Wilkins.

Lacy, C.F., Armstrong, L.L., Goldman, M.P., & Lance, L.L. (2003). *Drug information handbook* (11th ed.). Hudson, OH: Lexi-Comp.

Lehne, R.A. (2004). *Pharmacology for nursing care* (5th ed.). St Louis, MO: Saunders.

Mosby. (2005). *Mosby's drug consult 2005: The comprehensive reference for generic and brand name drugs* (15th ed.). St Louis, MO: Mosby.

Skidmore-Roth, L. (2006). *Mosby's 2006 nursing drug reference* (19th ed.). St Louis, MO: Mosby.

Turkoski, B.B., & Lance, B.R., & Bonfiglio, M.F. (2000). *Drug information handbook for nursing* (2nd ed.). Cleveland, OH: Lexi-Comp.

PART FOUR

Drugs Affecting the Cardiovascular and Renal Systems: Study Skills Tips

- LINKING LEARNING
- TEXT NOTATION

LINKING LEARNING

The Part Three Study Skills Tips stressed the importance of planning for the part as a whole. With that in mind, what is the focus of Part Four? The part title is "Drugs Affecting the Cardiovascular and Renal Systems." What is the first question you think you should ask about this part? You might begin by asking, "What are the cardiovascular and renal systems?" This is an obvious question and might seem to be so basic that it need not be asked, but the next eight chapters will all develop around this part title. Asking the obvious question is sometimes the best way to get started.

Chapter Structure

Just as there is a structure to each part in the text, which is constant from one part to the next, there is also a structure in the chapters. This structure is a repeating model created by the authors to organize the material and present it in the clearest way possible. The chapter structure is a valuable learning asset for those who make use of it.

Chapter Objectives

Each chapter begins with a set of objectives. These are established by the authors and serve to tell you what they expect you will know and be able to do when you have completed the chapter. It is sometimes tempting to ignore the objectives and get right on with the task of reading the chapter. Do not give in to that temptation. Read the objectives and spend some time thinking about what they reveal about the content of the chapter.

Example Based on Chapter 21 Objectives

Objective 1. Define *inotropic, chronotropic,* and *dromotropic.*

What can you learn from this objective? First, there is the vocabulary. This objective makes it clear that you have some terms to learn. This means that you may want to have some blank note cards available to start setting up vocabulary cards for this chapter. Write each of the terms in objective 1 on a separate card and be ready to complete the card as the terms are introduced and explained in the chapter.

The next thing that stands out in this first objective is that the three terms contain a common element, tropic. This should bring active questioning into play. What does the suffix "tropic" mean? Asking this question now is a way of noting that these three terms do have some common meaning. Also it serves to provide an immediate focus for personal learning when you begin to read the chapter.

Objective 2. Briefly discuss the effect of cardiac glycosides and other positive inotropics on the damage resulting from several forms of heart disease.

From this comes the potential for a new question relating to the first objective. What do inotropic, chronotropic, and dromotropic have to do with the heart? Just as it is essential to see the relationship between parts and chapters, it is also essential to see relationships within the chapters. These first two objectives should cause you to consider those relationships and make your own learning much more active.

Chapter Headings

The next chapter structure to consider in this process is the chapter headings. Chapter 21 has the major sections Heart Failure and Cardiac Dysrhythmias, Cardiac

Glycosides, Phosphodiesterase Inhibitors, Miscellaneous Heart Failure Agent, and Nursing Process. What is the importance of this heading structure? It tells you that the authors will focus on the pharmacological aspects first and then explain how this relates to nursing. This does not tell the learner a great deal about what to anticipate in terms of chapter content, but it does make clear a structure that is consistent in most of the chapters in this text.

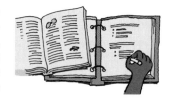

Cardiac Glycosides is broken down into subsections in this chapter. Spend several minutes considering the organization of these subsections. The first subtopic to be treated is "Mechanism of Action and Drug Effects." What is the mechanism of action of cardiac glycosides? How do they act? What effect do they have on the heart? It does not matter that you cannot answer these questions at this point. What is important is that you ask them as a means of fostering an active and participatory learning attitude when you begin to read the chapter. Think, question, anticipate, and then read. This sequence will enhance your learning.

Continue this process of looking at the subtopics and thinking ahead to what will be explained in the chapter. These subsections are the same in every chapter, and this thinking process should quickly become automatic.

Glossary

The next chapter structure has already been stressed in previous Study Skills Tips, and it is essential to learning. The glossary is a mini-dictionary for each chapter. Words that have not been introduced earlier in the text and that are central to the content of this chapter are presented here. The listing is in alphabetical order, which means that the glossary terms will not necessarily occur in the same order in the body of the chapter.

As you read terms as presented in the glossary, be aware of the nature of the definition. A glossary definition is specific and brief. It is a useful place to begin to learn the new terms in the chapter, but the definition presented may not be enough for full understanding. You will find that full understanding will come after reading the chapter and encountering the term within the fuller context of sentences and paragraphs of text that explain not only the term but how it applies in the particular situation.

Glossary and Text Relationship

The term *inotropic agent* is defined in the Chapter 21 glossary. As you read it you understand that inotropic has to do with force or energy of muscle contractions. The glossary states that a positive inotropic agent is a drug that increases myocardial contractility. Some of this information is clear, and some of it is still somewhat hazy. It should become clearer when connected with the chapter text. The first paragraph of the chapter introduces inotropic agents: "Drugs that increase the force of myocardial contraction are called positive **inotropic agents,** and such drugs have a beneficial role in the treatment of a failing heart muscle."

With this sentence you should have a much clearer understanding of what is meant by inotropic agents, as well as knowing that there are positive inotropic drugs. This is what must happen to fully master the content-specific vocabulary. You must see the core definition as presented in the glossary, but you must also read to determine how that core definition is expanded and exemplified in the body of the text.

When preparing vocabulary cards it is not a good idea to simply copy the definition from the glossary and assume that definition will serve your purpose. Wait to fill out the card until after you encounter the same term in the body of the chapter, and then pick and choose the information from the glossary and the body that will provide you with the clearest understanding of the term. Also, when placing information on vocabulary cards, it is always useful to include chapter number and page numbers so that you can locate the source of your definition quickly later.

These chapter structures can provide you with a clear picture of what you are expected to learn and the organizational pattern in which the material will be presented. Being aware of the structures and making use of them in this way will improve your concentration when you begin to read the chapter for understanding and memory. The time spent working with chapter structure is not wasted and does not significantly increase the study time of the chapter. In fact, the time you spend working with the objectives, headings, and glossary will generally save time when you are doing intensive reading and study.

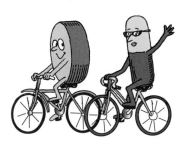

TEXT NOTATION

Highlighting or underlining text materials can be helpful when rehearsing and reviewing materials after the study reading. The problem, as discussed in the *Study Guide*, is that it is often difficult to limit the quantity of material that is marked. Although a good general guideline is to try to limit yourself to marking no more than 20 to 25 percent of the total, this guideline applies to large blocks of material. However, some paragraphs contain essential information and must be marked extensively, while other paragraphs may need only one or two sentences marked. In this Study Skills Tips section, the object is to look at how the author's structure and language can help you to select what should be marked.

Text Notation Application

Reproduced below are the first two paragraphs from Chapter 26 with model underlining completed, followed by a discussion of the reasons for these particular choices. You should not view the underlining shown here as a "perfect" model. The decision as to what to mark is an individual choice based on a number of factors, including prior experience with the subject matter and awareness of personal learning objectives and needs. This example is intended to provide you with a basic model to adapt to your own learning style and needs.

Chapter 26, Paragraphs One and Two

"Fluid and electrolyte management is one of the cornerstones of client care. Most disease processes, tissue injuries, and surgical procedures greatly influence the physiological status of fluids and electrolytes in the body. A prerequisite to understanding fluid and electrolyte management is knowledge of the extent and composition of the various body fluid compartments.

"About 60 percent of the adult human body is water. This is referred to as the *total body water* (TBW), and it is distributed to the three main compartments in the following proportions: **intracellular fluid (ICF), 67 percent, interstitial fluid (ISF), 25 percent, and plasma volume (PV), 8 percent**. This distribution is illustrated in Figure 26-1. Typical fluid volumes are shown in Table 26-1."

Discussion. The first thing you should notice is that the underlining here exceeds the 20 to 25 percent guideline. These are the first paragraphs in the chapter. First paragraphs are usually introductions to the topic and may vary a great deal in the quantity of important information. This selection seemed to contain a number of key points that must be considered. Because the content seems important, more is underlined.

Sentence one was chosen because of the word "cornerstones." This word suggests that fluid management is extremely important in client care and the reader must be sure to keep that focus throughout the chapter. Paying careful attention to the author's word choices plays a major role in selecting materials for text notation.

Paying attention to language led to the third sentence, which begins: "A prerequisite to understanding. . . " That phrase should immediately capture your attention. The phrase says that there is something that must be understood before anything else that follows will make complete sense. The phrase should also serve as an instant cue to generate a question for reading. "What is the prerequisite to understanding fluid and electrolyte management?" This question is answered directly by the sentence containing the phrase. The phrase serves as a language cue that there is something important. This in turn suggests that you probably will want to underline or highlight some information. The question helps you select what should be marked. Everything you do at this point serves as a guide to help you establish clear learning objectives and makes the process of selecting the best information for marking easier.

The next segment was chosen because it stands out from the body of the paragraph. *"Total body water"* is italicized. This is a print convention used as a means of putting emphasis on something that the author believes to be of special importance. The decision to underline words and phrases that are already emphasized is a personal one. You may feel that, since the author has already

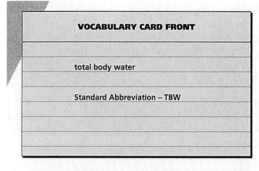

marked it, you have no need to add your own marks. Some students find that their own marking, even of italicized or bold print material, serves as a double reminder of the importance of the information. This is an excellent illustration of the statement that text notation is highly personal. Whether you choose to add your own marking or not there is one aspect of this phrase that is essential. "Total body water" is part of the vocabulary of fluids and electrolytes. That means it is time to add to your vocabulary cards.

This term served as a lead-in to the next key point marked. The next statement is "[TBW] is distributed to the three main compartments. . . " Whenever you see a phrase with a number and a word such as "main," you should be aware that this is potentially important material. This phrase should generate a new question that will aid in your selection of material to mark. "What are the three main compartments?" You see immediately that the rest of this sentence answers that question, and therefore identifies what needs to be marked. This marking also identifies three additional vocabulary items to be added to your cards for this chapter. As you set up your cards, be careful. One fluid is "intra-," and the second is "inter-." It would be easy to confuse the two, but they have different meanings. If you are not sure what the difference is between intra- and inter-, use a dictionary.

Chapter 26, Paragraph Three

" . . .The TBW can be described as being in or out of the blood vessels, or vasculature. If this terminology is used, then the term **intravascular fluid (IVF)** describes fluid inside the blood vessels, and the term **extravascular fluid (EVF)** describes the fluid outside the blood vessels. The term **plasma** is used to describe the fluid that flows through the blood vessels (intravascular). . . **ISF** is the fluid that is in the space between cells, tissues, and organs. Both plasma and ISF make up *extracellular* volume. Both ISF and ICF make up *extravascular volume*. These terms are often confused and misused. Table 26-1 lists these definitions for further clarity and understanding."

Discussion. The language conventions and the print conventions, **bold** and *italics,* are the same that I used to help in the previous paragraph. This paragraph also makes a point about the possibility of confusing and/or misusing the terms introduced. Being told that there is confusing material suggests that it is crucial that you be able to identify, define, and explain each of the terms used, and that it will take some careful thought to do so. There is one additional point in this paragraph that is important. The last sentence points you to a table, Table 26-1. There are many tables in this text. Tables are often used to simplify complex material and to clarify the relationships between the items presented. In these opening paragraphs, with the repeated reference to the confusing nature of the descriptions, Table 26-1 will almost certainly be important to your learning.

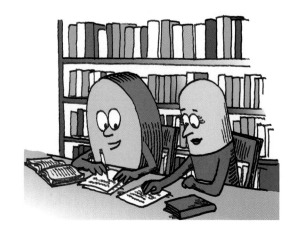

Positive Inotropic Agents

OBJECTIVES

After reading this chapter, the successful student will be able to do the following:

1 Define *inotropic, chronotropic,* and *dromotropic.*

2 Briefly discuss the effect of cardiac glycosides and other positive inotropics on the damage resulting from several forms of heart disease.

3 Compare the mechanisms of action, pharmacokinetics, indications, dosages, dosage forms and routes of administration, cautions, contraindications, side effects, and toxicity of the cardiac glycosides and other positive inotropics.

4 Contrast the different dosages and processes of rapid vs. slow digitalization, including nursing considerations.

5 Identify significant drug, laboratory test, and food interactions associated with the various positive inotropic agents.

6 Explain why specific diseases, conditions, and drugs are considered interactions, cautions, or contraindications to the use of a digoxin and other positive inotropic agents.

7 Discuss the nurse's responsibility to clients experiencing toxicity from digoxin or other designated drugs.

8 Develop a nursing care plan that includes all phases of the nursing process for clients undergoing treatment with positive inotropics.

e-LEARNING ACTIVITIES

Student CD-ROM
- Review Questions: see questions 122–131
- Animations
- Medication Administration Checklists
- IV Therapy Checklists

evolve **Web site** (http://evolve.elsevier.com/Lilley/pharmacology/)
- Online Chapter Worksheet • Frequently Asked Questions
- Learning Tips and Content Updates • WebLinks • Online Appendices and Supplements • Mosby/Saunders ePharmacology Update • Access to *Mosby's Drug Consult*

DRUG PROFILES

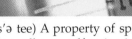

▸▸**digoxin,** p. 349   **milrinone,** p. 352
digoxin immune Fab, p. 350

▸▸ Key drug.

GLOSSARY

Automaticity (aw′ to mə tis′ə tee) A property of specialized excitable tissue that allows self-activation through the spontaneous development of an action potential, as in the pacemaker cells of the heart.

Cardiac glycoside (gly′ kə side) A glycoside is any of several carbohydrates that yield a sugar and a nonsugar as the result of hydrolysis. The plant species *Digitalis purpurea* yields a glycoside used in the treatment of heart disease; these glycosides are called *cardiac glycosides.*

Chronotropic agent (kron′ o trop′ ik) An agent that influences the rate of the heartbeat. A positive chronotropic agent increases the heart rate, whereas a negative chronotropic agent decreases it.

Dromotropic agent (drom′ o trop′ ik) An agent that influences the conduction of electrical impulses. A positive dromotropic agent enhances the conduction of electrical impulses in the heart.

Ejection fraction The proportion of blood that is ejected during each ventricular contraction compared with the total ventricular filling volume. It is an index of left ventricular function, and the normal fraction is 65 percent (0.65).

Heart failure An abnormal condition in which cardiac pumping is impaired as the result of myocardial infarction, ischemic heart disease, or cardiomyopathy. Failure of the ventricle to eject blood efficiently results in volume overload, chamber dilation, and elevated intracardiac pressure. The retrograde transmission of increased hydrostatic pressure from the left ventricle leads to pulmonary congestion; elevated right ventricular pressure leads to systemic venous congestion and peripheral edema.

Inotropic agent (in' o trop' ik) An agent that affects the force or energy of muscular contractions, particularly contraction of the heart muscle. Positive inotropic agents are drugs that increase myocardial contractility.

Left ventricular end-diastolic volume (LVEDV) (ven trik' yə lər dye' ə stol' ik) Ventricular diastole begins with the onset of the second heart sound and ends with the first heart sound. The left ventricular end-diastolic volume is the total amount of blood in the ventricle before it contracts, or the pre-load.

Refractory period The period during which a pulse generator (e.g., the sinoatrial node of the heart) is unresponsive to an input signal of specified amplitude and during which it is impossible for the myocardium to respond. This is the period when the cardiac cell is readjusting its sodium and potassium levels and cannot be depolarized again until completion of the refractory period.

Therapeutic window The drug level range in the blood that is considered beneficial as opposed to toxic.

Recall from Chapter 17 that adrenergic agents (e. g. dopamine, dobutamine) are also inotropic agents. This chapter includes a comprehensive discussion of the inotropic agents. Drugs that increase the force of myocardial contraction are called positive **inotropic agents,** and such drugs have a beneficial role in the treatment of a failing heart muscle. A drug that increases the rate at which the heart beats is called a positive **chronotropic agent.** Drugs may also affect how quickly electrical impulses travel through the conduction system of the heart (the sinoatrial [SA] node, atrioventricular [AV] node, bundle of His, and Purkinje fibres). Drugs that accelerate conduction are referred to as positive **dromotropic agents.** This chapter focuses on two of the main classes of positive inotropic agents: **cardiac glycosides** and phosphodiesterase inhibitors.

It is estimated that over 350 000 Canadians are affected with **heart failure**. It is the number one reason for hospitalization in elderly Canadians and mortality rates range from 25 to 40 percent one year post-diagnosis. Findings yielded by one of the largest and most frequently cited studies involving clients with heart failure, the Framingham study, show that the 5-year survival rate in clients with heart fail-

ure is approximately 50 percent. Therefore any drug that could lengthen survival in affected clients or help the failing heart perform its essential functions would be extremely valuable. The glycosides have generally been viewed as an important tool for this purpose. However, a 1997 study (Digitalis Investigation Group) showed that using digoxin as a first-line treatment for heart failure did not lower mortality rates. Angiotensin converting enzyme (ACE) inhibitors and diuretics were recommended as the mainstays. However, digoxin may still offer benefit in some clients.

HEART FAILURE AND CARDIAC DYSRHYTHMIAS

Heart failure is a pathological state in which the heart is unable to pump blood in sufficient amounts from the ventricles (i.e., cardiac output) to meet the body's metabolic needs. The signs and symptoms typically associated with heart failure constitute the syndrome of heart failure. This syndrome can be limited to the left ventricle (producing pulmonary edema and symptoms of dyspnea or cough) or the right ventricle (producing symptoms such as pedal edema, jugular venous distention, ascites [accumulation of fluid in the peritoneal cavity], and hepatic congestion), or it may affect both ventricles.

In clients with heart failure, the overworked, failing heart cannot meet the demands placed on it and blood is not ejected efficiently from the ventricles. This occurs because of a decrease in the **ejection fraction**—the amount of blood ejected with each contraction compared with the total amount of blood in the ventricle just before contraction (**left ventricular end-diastolic volume**). (Normally the ejection fraction is approximately 65 percent [0.65].) As more blood accumulates in the right and left ventricles, more pressure builds up in the blood vessels leading to the heart. The retrograde transmission of this increased hydrostatic pressure from the left ventricle leads to pulmonary congestion, whereas elevated right ventricular pressure causes systemic venous congestion and peripheral edema.

Because the heart cannot then meet the increased demands placed on it, the blood supply to certain organs is reduced. The organs most dependent on blood supply, the brain and heart, are the last to be deprived of blood. As an organ that is relatively less dependent on blood supply, the kidney has its blood supply shunted away. Therefore the filtration of fluids and removal of waste products is impaired. When these fluids and waste products accumulate, the client experiences such symptoms as pulmonary edema and shortness of breath, resulting from kidney failure.

The physical defects producing heart failure are of two types: (1) a cardiac defect (myocardial deficiency such as myocardial infarction [MI] or valve insufficiency), which leads to inadequate cardiac contractility and filling; and (2) a defect outside the heart (systemic defect such as coronary artery disease, pulmonary hypertension, or diabetes), which results in an overload on an otherwise normal heart. Both of these defects may be present in the same client. Common causes of myocardial deficiency and systemic defects are listed in Box 21-1.

Myocardial Deficiency and Increased Workload: Common Causes

Myocardial Deficiency	Increased Workload
Inadequate Contractility	***Pressure Overload***
Myocardial infarction	Hypertension
Coronary artery disease	Outflow obstruction
Cardiomyopathy	
Infection	***Volume Overload***
	Hypervolemia
Inadequate Filling	Congenital abnormalities
Atrial fibrillation	Anemia
Infection	Thyroid disease
Tamponade	
Ischemia	

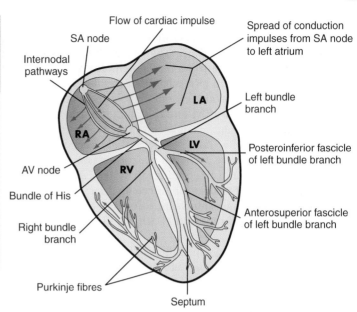

FIG. 21-1   Conduction system of the heart. *AV,* Atrioventricular; *LA,* left atrium; *LV,* left ventricle; *RA,* right atrium; *RV,* right ventricle; *SA,* sinoatrial. (Modified from Kinney, M., et al. (1996). *Comprehensive cardiac care* (8th ed.). St Louis, MO: Mosby; Lewis, S.M., Heitkemper, M.M., & Dirksen, S.R. (2004). *Medical-surgical nursing: Assessment and management of clinical problems* (6th ed.). St Louis, MO: Mosby.)

In clients with supraventricular dysrhythmias, atrial fibrillation, or atrial flutter, the top aspects of the heart (atria) are contracting several hundred times a minute. Not only are the atria contracting frequently, but several areas in the atria besides the SA node are then acting as the pacemaker of the heart. Normally the AV node controls how slowly or quickly impulses arrive in the ventricles, and it also has the ability to receive all of these depolarizations and to allow only a certain number to pass through the ventricles. This keeps the client from going into ventricular fibrillation, which is fatal. It also gives the ventricles time to fill with blood, which is equally important. However, during atrial fibrillation or flutter, clients may show symptoms of heart failure.

All cells in the heart can depolarize spontaneously, a property called **automaticity.** The **refractory period** is the time when the cardiac cells are readjusting their sodium and potassium levels. During this time the cardiac cells cannot depolarize again. It is the sodium–potassium adenosinetriphosphatase (ATPase) pump that is responsible for the movement of potassium ions in and sodium ions out of the cardiac cells after they have depolarized, an action potential has been generated, and the electrical impulse has been generated. In clients with either atrial fibrillation or flutter, the AV node is circumvented and the impulses arrive in the ventricle before the refractory period is over. The resultant slow spread of impulses from the atrium through refractory muscle results in continuous atrial excitation—atrial fibrillation or flutter. Figure 21-1 illustrates the conduction system of the heart. (The cardiac conduction system and the abnormalities responsible for causing dysrhythmias are described in greater detail in Chapter 22.)

CARDIAC GLYCOSIDES

Based on the survival statistics cited earlier, any drug that can lengthen survival in clients with heart failure by helping the failing heart perform its essential functions would be extremely valuable. Glycosides may be able to do this in certain clients. They are one of the oldest and most widely used groups of drugs. Not only do they have beneficial effects in the failing heart but they also help control the ventricular response to atrial fibrillation or flutter. They were originally obtained from either the *Digitalis purpurea* or the *Digitalis lanata* plant, both commonly referred to as *foxglove.* Cardiac glycosides have been the mainstay of therapy for heart failure for more than 200 years, and they continue to be one of the most commonly used positive inotropic agents. Digoxin is the most commonly prescribed digitalis preparation. Critically ill clients can be restored to near-normal states within hours after digitalization. It should be noted, however, that this chapter regarding heart failure focuses on systolic dysfunction or inadequate ventricular action during the pumping action of systole, the ventricular contractions. Less common but still important is diastolic dysfunction. This condition is most commonly associated with left ventricular hypertrophy secondary to chronic hypertension. However, it may also result from cardiomyopathy (e.g., virus-induced), pericardial disease, and diabetes. Inotropic agents (including digoxin) and vasodilators (see Chapter 24) may not be the drugs of choice for diastolic failure. Diuretic agents (see Chapter 25) are often used for both conditions.

Mechanism of Action and Drug Effects

The primary beneficial effect of a cardiac glycoside (e.g., digoxin) is thought to be an increase in myocardial contractility. This occurs secondarily to the inhibition of the sodium pump. By inhibiting this enzyme complex, the cellular sodium concentration and subsequently the calcium concentration increase. The overall result is enhanced myocardial contraction. Digoxin also augments vagal tone, resulting in increased diastolic filling.

Cardiac glycosides also change the electrical conduction properties of the heart, and this markedly affects the conduction system and cardiac automaticity. Glycosides decrease the velocity (rate) of electrical conduction and prolong the refractory period in the conduction system. The particular area of the conduction system where this occurs is between the atria and the ventricles (SA node to AV node through the ventricles). The cardiac cell remains in a state of depolarization and is unable to start another electrical impulse.

Cardiac glycosides, especially digitoxin and digoxin, are almost identical in their ability to treat heart failure and dysrhythmias. The two glycosides vary, however, in terms of their water solubility, half-life, and excretion, and the clinical profile of the client determines which glycoside is selected. All cardiac glycosides produce dramatic inotropic, chronotropic, and dromotropic cardiac effects. (Inotropic refers to the force or energy of muscular contractions; chronotropic refers to the rate of the heartbeat; and dromotropic refers to the conduction of electrical impulses.) These effects include the following:

- A positive inotropic effect resulting in an increase in the force and velocity of myocardial contraction without a corresponding increase in oxygen consumption
- A negative chronotropic effect producing a reduced heart rate
- A negative dromotropic effect that decreases automaticity at the SA node, decreases AV nodal conduction, reduces conductivity at the bundle of His, and prolongs the atrial and ventricular refractory periods
- An increase in stroke volume
- A reduction in heart size during diastole
- A decrease in venous blood pressure (BP) and vein engorgement
- An increase in coronary circulation
- Promotion of diuresis as the result of improved blood circulation
- Palliation of exertional and paroxysmal nocturnal dyspnea, cough, and cyanosis

Indications

Cardiac glycosides are primarily used in the treatment of heart failure and supraventricular dysrhythmias. In heart failure the therapeutic effects of digoxin are secondary to its ability to increase the force of contraction, its positive inotropic action. There are many therapeutic benefits to this action. Increasing the force of contraction increases the ejection fraction compared with the left ventricular end-diastolic volume, or pre-load. As more blood is ejected with each contraction of the heart, there is less blood remaining in the ventricle and thus less pressure. The symptoms of pulmonary edema, pulmonary hypertension, and right-sided ventricular failure subside.

Another benefit of positive inotropic action is that it promotes diuresis by ensuring that adequate blood is supplied to the kidneys. As a result, fluids are filtered and waste products removed, resulting in the relief of shortness of breath and pulmonary edema.

Cardiac glycosides are also effective in the treatment of dysrhythmias such as atrial fibrillation and atrial flutter because of their negative chronotropic (decreased heart rate) and negative dromotropic (slowed conduction velocity) actions. Automaticity, conduction velocity, and the refractory period are all affected. Digoxin can slow the depolarization of the SA node and other areas of the atria that may be acting as pacemakers. Thus glycosides such as digoxin directly slow conduction through the AV node (decreasing the ventricular rate) and increase the vagal action on the heart. In addition, the cardiac glycosides lengthen the refractory period, which allows the correct levels of sodium and potassium ions to be reached before depolarization.

Contraindications

Contraindications to the use of cardiac glycosides include known drug allergy and may include second- or third-degree heart block, concurrent atrial fibrillation, ventricular tachycardia or fibrillation, heart failure resulting from diastolic dysfunction, sick sinus syndrome, and subaortic stenosis (obstruction in the left ventricle below the aortic valve).

Side Effects and Adverse Effects

The side effects and adverse effects associated with cardiac glycoside use can be serious. The primary cardiac glycoside in use today is digoxin, and it is essential to monitor closely clients' clinical response to it and the possible development of toxic symptoms. Digoxin has a narrow **therapeutic window,** meaning there is a small range of the drug level in the blood that is considered therapeutic. After the drug reaches steady state, levels need to be monitored only if there is suspicion of toxicity, nonadherence, or deteriorating renal function. Low potassium levels increase its toxicity; therefore frequent serum electrolyte level checks are also important. It has been estimated that as many as 20 percent of clients taking digoxin exhibit toxic symptoms. The common undesirable effects associated with cardiac glycoside use are listed in Table 21-1.

TABLE 21-1

CARDIAC GLYCOSIDES: COMMON ADVERSE EFFECTS

Body System	Side/Adverse Effect
Cardiovascular	Any type of dysrhythmia including bradycardia or tachycardia
Central nervous	Headache, fatigue, malaise, confusion, convulsions
Eye	Coloured vision (i.e., green, yellow, or purple), halo vision, or flickering lights
Gastrointestinal	Anorexia, nausea, vomiting, diarrhea

Toxicity and Management of Overdose

The treatment strategies for digoxin toxicity depend on the severity of the symptoms. These strategies can range from simply withholding the next dose to instituting aggressive therapies. Consultation with a Poison Control Centre is recommended. The steps usually taken in the management of cardiac glycoside toxicity are listed in Table 21-2.

When significant toxicity develops as a result of cardiac glycoside therapy, digoxin immune Fab may be indicated. Digoxin immune Fab is an antibody that recognizes digoxin as an antigen and forms an antibody–antigen complex, thus inactivating the free digoxin. This therapy is not indicated in every client showing signs of digoxin toxicity. It may be indicated in the following circumstances:

- Hyperkalemia (serum potassium level >5 mmol/L) in a digitalis-toxic client
- Life-threatening cardiac dysrhythmias, sustained ventricular tachycardia or fibrillation, and severe sinus bradycardia or heart block unresponsive to atropine treatment or cardiac pacing
- Life-threatening digoxin or digitoxin overdose: >10 mg of digoxin in adults; >4 mg of digoxin in children

Interactions

A number of significant drug interactions are possible with cardiac glycosides. The common ones are listed in Table 21-3. One food interaction, bran in large amounts, may decrease the absorption of oral digitalis drugs. Other food interactions are mentioned in Table 21-3. The herbal supplement hawthorn, which is used for hypertension and angina, can reduce the effectiveness of cardiac glycosides.

Dosages

For dosage information on the cardiac glycosides, see the table on p. 351. See Appendix B for some of the common brands available in Canada.

DRUG PROFILES

Cardiac glycosides get their name from their chemical structures. Glycosides are complex, steroid-like structures linked to sugar molecules. Because the particular drugs derived from the digitalis plant have potent ac-

tions on the heart, they are referred to as *cardiac glycosides*, with digoxin by far the most commonly prescribed digitalis preparation. Digitoxin is a less commonly prescribed preparation. The widespread and longstanding popularity of cardiac glycosides such as digoxin is the result of their unequalled efficacy in the treatment of heart failure. Cardiac glycosides are prescription-only drugs and are classified as pregnancy category C agents.

▸▸ digoxin

Digoxin is by far the most commonly prescribed digitalis glycoside. It is a highly effective agent for the treatment of both heart failure and atrial fibrillation and flutter. It may also be used clinically to improve myocardial contractility and thus reverse cardiogenic shock or other low cardiac output states. Digoxin is contraindicated in clients who have shown a hypersensitivity to it and in those with ventricular tachycardia and fibrillation, beriberi heart disease, incomplete AV block, or hypersensitive carotid sinus syndrome. It is unwarranted in the treatment of obesity. Normal therapeutic drug levels of digoxin should be between 0.8 and 2 ng/mL. Levels higher than 2 ng/mL are typically desirable for the treatment of atrial fibrillation. (Note that the unit here is a nanogram, one-thousandth of a microgram.) Digoxin is available in oral (PO) form as a 0.05-mg/mL elixir and 0.0625-, 0.125-, and 0.25-mg tablets. It comes in parenteral form as 0.05- and 0.25-mg/mL intravenous (IV) injections. Because of digoxin's fairly long duration of action and half-life, a loading, or "digitalizing," dose is often given to bring serum levels of the drug up to a desirable therapeutic level more quickly. See the table on p. 351 for the recommended digitalizing doses and the daily oral and intravenous adult and pediatric dosages.

PHARMACOKINETICS

Half-Life	Onset	Peak	Duration
1.5–2 days	30–120 min	2–6 hr	2–4 days

TABLE 21-2
DIGOXIN TOXICITY: STEP-BY-STEP MANAGEMENT

Step	Instructions
1	Discontinue drug.
2	Begin continuous electrocardiographic monitoring for cardiac arrhythmias; administer any appropriate antidysrhythmic drugs as ordered.
3	Determine serum digoxin and electrolyte levels.
4	Administer potassium supplements for hypokalemia if indicated, as ordered.
5	Institute supportive therapy for gastrointestinal symptoms (nausea, vomiting, or diarrhea).
6	Administer digoxin antidote (i.e., digoxin immune Fab) if indicated, as ordered.

PEDIATRIC CONSIDERATIONS
Cardiac Glycosides

- Digoxin should be given according to a regular time schedule 1 hour before or 2 hours after the child's or infant's feeding.
- Close monitoring is needed, along with individualized dosing and nursing care. Extra caution is important in calculating doses because a one-decimal-point placement error may result in a tenfold dosage error, which would be fatal. Because digoxin has a narrow margin of error, all medication calculations should be double-checked by another registered nurse or by a pharmacist or physician.
- Toxicity is manifested in children by nausea, vomiting, bradycardia, anorexia, and dysrhythmias.
- The physician should be notified immediately should the following symptoms indicative of heart failure develop: increased fatigue, sudden weight gain (>1 kg in 1 wk), respiratory distress, or profuse scalp sweating.

TABLE 21-3

CARDIAC GLYCOSIDES: DRUG INTERACTIONS

Drug	Mechanism	Result
Adrenergics reserpine succinylcholine	Increase cardiac irritability	Increased digoxin toxicity
Antibiotics	Increase digoxin absorption	Increased digoxin toxicity
amphotericin B chlorthalidone Loop diuretics Laxatives Steroids (adrenal) Thiazide diuretics	Hypokalemia	Increased digoxin toxicity
Antacids Antidiarrheals cholestyramine colestipol	Decrease oral absorption	Reduced therapeutic effect
Anticholinergics	Increase oral absorption	Increased therapeutic effect
Barbiturates	Enzyme inducer	Reduced therapeutic effect
Beta-blockers	Blocks beta$_1$-receptors in heart	Increased bradycardic effect of digoxin
Calcium channel blockers	Blocks calcium channels in myocardium	Enhances bradycardic and negative inotropic effects of digoxin
quinidine verapamil	Decrease clearance	Increased digoxin levels (2×); digoxin dose should be carefully individualized

A digoxin preparation can also interfere with the results of several laboratory tests. It can cause the plasma levels of estrone to be raised and the levels of lactate dehydrogenase and testosterone to be lowered. It can also cause the erythrocyte sodium concentration to be increased and the erythrocyte potassium concentration to be reduced.

In addition to the drug and laboratory test interactions, digoxin can also interact with certain foods. The consumption of excessive amounts of potassium-rich food can decrease its therapeutic effect, whereas the consumption of excessive amounts of licorice can increase digoxin toxicity as the result of the hypokalemia produced.

digoxin immune Fab

Digoxin immune Fab is the antidote for severe digoxin overdose and is indicated for the reversal of such life-threatening cardiotoxic effects as severe bradycardia, advanced heart block, severe ventricular tachycardia or fibrillation, and severe hyperkalemia. It has also been used for life-threatening toxicity due to digitoxin. It has a unique mechanism of action. As previously mentioned, it is believed to work by binding to free (unbound) digoxin, which then blocks or reverses all of the drug effects and symptoms of toxicity. Digoxin immune Fab is contraindicated in clients who have shown a hypersensitivity to it. It is available only in parenteral form as a 38-mg vial. Digoxin immune Fab is dosed either in milligrams or by the number of vials, depending on the dose calculation method or the reference chart used. It is commonly dosed based on the client's serum digoxin level in conjunction with the client's weight. The recommended dosages vary according to the amount of cardiac glycoside ingested. Each vial containing 38 mg of purified digoxin-specific Fab fragments will bind approximately 0.05 mg of digoxin or digitoxin. For recommended dosages the nurse should consult the manufacturer's latest dosage table recommendations. It is important to bear in mind that after digoxin immune Fab is given, all subsequent digoxin serum levels will be elevated for days to weeks because of the presence of both the free (unbound) digoxin (toxic digoxin) and the digoxin that has been bound by the digoxin immune Fab (nontoxic digoxin). Therefore, at this point, the clinical signs and symptoms of digoxin toxicity rather than the digoxin serum levels should be used to monitor the effectiveness of reversal therapy.

PHARMACOKINETICS

Half-Life	Onset	Peak	Duration
15–20 hr	Immediate	Immediate	Days to weeks

PHOSPHODIESTERASE INHIBITORS

As the name implies, phosphodiesterase inhibitors are a group of inotropic agents that work by inhibiting an enzyme called *phosphodiesterase*. The inhibition of this enzyme results in two beneficial effects in an individual with heart failure: a positive inotropic response and vasodilation. For this reason this class of drugs may also be referred to as *inodilators* (inotropes and dilators). These agents were discovered in the search for positive inotropic drugs with a wider therapeutic window than digoxin. There is presently only one agent in this category available in Canada: milrinone. Milrinone shares a similar pharmacological action with methylxanthines such as theophylline. They both inhibit phosphodiesterase, resulting in an increase in intracellular cyclic adenosine monophosphate (cAMP). However, milrinone is more specific for phosphodiesterase type III, which is especially common in the heart and vascular smooth muscles.

DOSAGES   Agents for Heart Failure

Agent	Pharmacological Class	Usual Dosage Range	Indications

▸▸ digoxin	Digitalis cardiac glycoside	**Pediatric**
		Digitalizing dose
		IV: Premature: 0.015–0.025 mg/kg
		      Newborn: 0.020–0.030 mg/kg
		      1 mo–2 yr: 0.030–0.050 mg/kg
		      2–5 yr: 0.025–0.035 mg/kg
		      5–10 yr: 0.015–0.030 mg/kg
		      >10 yr: 0.008–0.012 mg/kg
		PO: Premature: 0.020–0.030 mg/kg
		      Newborn: 0.025–0.035 mg/kg
		      1 mo–2 yr: 0.035–0.060 mg/kg
		      2–5 yr: 0.030–0.040 mg/kg
		      5–10 yr: 0.020–0.035 mg/kg
		      >10 yr: 0.010–0.015 mg/kg
		Usual maintenance dose, 25–35% of
		   digitalizing dose
		Adult
		PO/IV: Usual digitalizing dose, 1–1.5 mg/day;
		   usual maintenance dose, 0.125–0.5 mg/day
			Heart failure, supraventricular dysrhythmias

milrinone	Phosphodiesterase inhibitor	**Adult** IV loading dose: 50 μg/kg IV continuous infusion dose: 0.375–0.75 μg/kg/min	Heart failure Heart failure

Mechanism of Action and Drug Effects

The mechanism of action of a phosphodiesterase inhibitor differs from other inotropic agents such as cardiac glycosides and catecholamines. The beneficial effects of a phosphodiesterase inhibitor come from cAMP, the build-up of a substance that the phosphodiesterase enzyme normally breaks down. Milrinone works by selectively inhibiting phosphodiesterase type III, which is in high concentrations in the heart and vascular smooth muscle. Inhibition of phosphodiesterase results in more calcium being available for the heart to use in muscle contraction. It also results in dilation of blood vessels, which in turn decreases the workload of the heart. The effects on heart muscle result in an increase in the force of contraction (i.e., positive inotropic action). The effects on the smooth muscle that surrounds blood vessels result in relaxation of smooth muscle and therefore cause dilation of blood vessels. The increased calcium present in heart muscle is also taken back up into its storage sites in the sarcoplasmic reticulum at a much faster rate than normal. This results in the heart muscle relaxing more than normal, as well as being more compliant. In summary, phosphodiesterase inhibitors have positive inotropic and lusitropic (relaxing blood vessels) effects. They may also increase heart rate in some instances and therefore may also have positive chronotropic effects.

Indications

Phosphodiesterase inhibitors are primarily used for the short-term management of heart failure. In heart failure the therapeutic benefits of the inodilators are secondary to their ability to increase the force of contraction (inotropic effects) and to relax blood vessels (lusitropic effects). The inodilators have 10 to 100 times greater affinity for smooth muscle surrounding blood vessels than for heart muscle. This suggests that the primary beneficial effects of inodilators are due to their ability to dilate blood vessels. This causes a reduction in afterload, or the force that the heart has to pump against to eject its volume.

Traditionally, phosphodiesterase inhibitors are given to clients who can be closely monitored and who have not responded adequately to digoxin, diuretics, and/or vasodilators. Phosphodiesterase inhibitors do not require a receptor-mediated effect to increase contraction. Other positive inotropic agents, such as beta-agonists (e.g., dobutamine, dopamine), require stimulation of a receptor to increase contraction. The repetitive stimulation of these receptors can cause the body to become less sensitive to stimulation over time. In clients with end-stage heart failure who require positive inotropic support, a continual dosage increase would be needed to maintain positive results. As these drug dosages are increased they produce more unwanted cardiac effects. Because phosphodiesterase inhibitors do not use receptors to increase force of contraction, they do not pose this problem. Many hospitals that treat large numbers of clients with heart failure now treat end-stage heart failure clients with weekly 6-hour infusions of phosphodiesterase inhibitors. This has been shown to increase the quality of life and decrease the number of readmissions to the hospital for exacerbations of heart failure.

Contraindications

Contraindications to the use of phosphodiesterase inhibitors include known drug allergy and may include the presence of severe aortic or pulmonary valvular disease and heart failure resulting from diastolic dysfunction.

Side Effects and Adverse Effects

The primary side effect seen with milrinone therapy is dysrhythmia, mainly ventricular. Ventricular dysrhythmias occur in 12.6 percent of clients treated with milrinone. Other side effects are ventricular ectopic activity (9.0 percent), ventricular tachycardia (3.6 percent), hypotension (3.1 percent), angina (chest pain) (1.4 percent), hypokalemia (0.7 percent), tremor (0.5 percent), headache of mild to moderate severity (2.4 percent), and thrombocytopenia (0.5 percent). Although rare, anaphylactic shock, bronchospasm, and skin reactions such as rash were reported in post-market research. Liver function test abnormalities have been reported but are uncommon.

Toxicity and Management of Overdose

No specific antidote exists for an overdose of milrinone. The primary effects of excessive doses are cardiac arrhythmia and hypotension due to the drug's ability to cause vasodilation. If excessive hypotension occurs, the phosphodiesterase inhibitor should be reduced or discontinued until the client's condition is stabilized. Consultation with a Poison Control Centre and general measures for circulatory support are also recommended.

Interactions

Limited data are available regarding potential drug interactions with phosphodiesterase inhibitors. They are given concurrently with a wide variety of cardiovascular medications in intensive care settings without interactions. The few data that are present indicate safe concurrent administration of phosphodiesterase inhibitors with digoxin, lidocaine, quinidine, hydralazine, prazosin, isosorbide dinitrate, nitroglycerine, chlorthalidone, furosemide, hydrochlorothiazide, spironolactone, captopril, heparin, warfarin, diazepam, insulin, and potassium supplements. Furosemide must not be injected into intravenous lines of milrinone because it will precipitate immediately.

Dosages

For dosage information on the phosphodiesterase inhibitor, see the dosages table on p. 351. See Appendix B for some of the common brands available in Canada. Because of the high incidence of heart failure, an understanding of the nursing implications associated with its medical treatment is critical to the safe and effective care of clients receiving cardiac glycosides as the mainstay of treatment. Owing to the narrow therapeutic index of cardiac glycosides, the nurse needs to constantly assess the client, update the plans of care, intervene appropriately, and evaluate or monitor the therapeutic and adverse effects of the drug.

DRUG PROFILES

milrinone

Milrinone is the only available phosphodiesterase inhibitor. Milrinone is referred to as an inodilator because it exerts both a positive inotropic effect and a vasodilatory effect. This agent is contraindicated in clients who have shown hypersensitivity to it. Milrinone is available only as an intravenous product in 1-mg/mL vials. It is classified as a pregnancy category C agent. Recommended dosages are given in the table on p. 351.

PHARMACOKINETICS

Half-Life	Onset	Peak	Duration
2.3 hr	5–15 min	6–12 hr	8–10 hr

 NURSING PROCESS

■ Assessment

Before the administration of a cardiac glycoside, a thorough assessment of the client is required so that the drug can be used in the safest manner possible. An assessment of the client's medical history, including both diseases and conditions, is crucial and may yield findings that either dictate cautious use of the agent or even contraindicate its use (Table 21-4). Before the nurse initiates digoxin therapy, and even during maintenance therapy, several

TABLE 21-4

CONDITIONS PREDISPOSING TO DIGITALIS TOXICITY

Condition/ Disease	Significance
Cardiac pacemakers	Clients with these devices may exhibit digitalis toxicity at lower-than-usual doses.
Hepatic dysfunction	Decreased hepatic elimination of digitoxin necessitating a reduction of digitoxin.
Hypokalemia	Increases a client's risk of serious dysrhythmias and renders the client more predisposed to digitalis toxicity.
Hypercalcemia	Places the client at higher risk of suffering sinus bradycardia, dysrhythmias, and heart block.
Atrioventricular block	Heart block may worsen with increasing levels of digitalis.
Dysrhythmias	Dysrhythmias may occur that did not exist before digitalis use and thus could be related to digitalis toxicity.
Hypothyroid, respiratory, or renal disease	Clients with these disorders require lower doses because of the resultant delayed drug excretion.
Advanced age	Because of decreased renal function and the resultant diminished drug excretion along with decreased body mass in this client population, a lower-than-usual dose is needed to prevent toxicity. The practice of polypharmacy may also lead to toxicity.
Ventricular fibrillation	Ventricular rate may actually increase with digitalis use.

clinical parameters need to be assessed. These include the following:

- BP
- Apical pulse for 1 full minute (to be documented next to the dose administered with the rate noted as well)
- Heart sounds
- Breath sounds
- Weight
- Intake and output amounts
- Serum laboratory values such as potassium, sodium, magnesium, and calcium
- Electrocardiograms (ECGs)
- Renal function laboratory values (blood urea nitrogen [BUN] and creatinine)
- Liver function values (aspartate aminotransferase [AST], alanine aminotransferase [ALT], creatine phosphokinase, lactate dehydrogenase [LDH], and alkaline phosphatase)

The baseline status of electrolytes is crucial to the safe use of digitalis drugs. Because electrolyte disorders, especially hypokalemia, may precipitate digitalis toxicity, it is crucial that serum potassium levels, as well as other electrolyte levels (e.g., calcium, magnesium, and sodium), are obtained and documented before and during drug therapy. Also, the occurrence of any edema (weight gain of 1 kg a day or 2.5 kg in one week), confusion, nausea, vomiting, anorexia, or diarrhea needs to be documented. The client's dietary habits and medication record or a list of current medications need to be assessed. Medication history must include past and present drug therapies, over-the-counter (OTC), herbal, prescription, and illegal drugs used. Drug allergies must also be assessed for digitalis products and other positive inotropics. In addition, the nurse should always be on the lookout for possible drug interactions because several drugs can interact with digitalis, such as antacids, calcium channel blockers (CCBs), beta-blockers, and thyroid preparations (may result in decreased digoxin levels). In addition, large amounts of bran taken with digoxin will decrease its absorption. The newer agent milrinone is used for the short-term intravenous therapy of heart failure. Before its use clients should be assessed for any allergy to it, and it should be used cautiously with clients with COPD, aortic or pulmonary valvular diseases, ventricular dysrhythmias, atrial fibrillation or flutter, or renal dysfunction. It is also used cautiously in pregnancy. The client's vital signs and ECG should be monitored during infusion of the drug.

Nursing Diagnoses

Nursing diagnoses related to the administration of positive inotropic agents include the following:

- Ineffective tissue perfusion, cardiopulmonary, related to the pathophysiological influence of heart failure.
- Deficient knowledge related to the first-time use of a cardiac glycoside and lack of information on heart failure and its treatment.

- Risk for injury related to the pathological impact of heart failure and the potential side effects of medication therapy.
- Imbalanced nutritional status, less than body requirements, related to GI side effects and potential digoxin toxicity.
- Non-adherence to therapy related to lack of information about the drug effects and adverse effects.

Planning

Goals of care related to the administration of positive inotropic agents include the following:

- Client exhibits improved cardiac output once therapy is initiated.
- Client states use, action, side effects, and toxic effects of therapy.
- Client is free from injury related to medication therapy.
- Client's appetite is improved or client is free of anorexia while on positive inotropic agents.

It is important for the nurse to check the dosage when administering either digoxin or digitoxin because of the difference in the pharmacokinetic properties of these drugs; for example, 80 percent of digoxin is excreted by the kidneys and 90 percent of digitoxin is first metabolized by the liver. These differences, in conjunction with the client's particular medical history, often determine whether the physician prescribes digoxin (preferred in clients with impaired liver function) or digitoxin (preferred in clients with impaired renal function).

Outcome Criteria

Outcome criteria in clients receiving a positive inotropic agent include the following:

- Client has improved to strong peripheral pulses, increased endurance for activity, decreased fatigue, and pink, warm extremities.
- Client has increased urinary output resulting from therapeutic effects of the drug.
- Client has improved heart and lung sounds with decreased dysrhythmias and rales.
- Client loses appropriate weight and has less edema (increased urinary output due to increased cardiac output).
- Client's skin and mucous membranes (colour and temperature) are improved to pink and warm.
- Client maintains appetite while on therapy and reports any anorexia, nausea, or vomiting immediately to physician.
- Client is free of toxicity as evidenced by no bradycardia or complaints of anorexia, nausea, or vomiting.
- Client demonstrates proper technique for taking radial pulse for 1 full minute before taking medication.
- Client is able to cite drug-related problems to report to the physician, such as palpitations, dysrhythmias, chest pain, and pulse less than 60 beats/min.

■ Implementation

Before administering any dose of a cardiac glycoside, the nurse should count the client's apical pulse (auscultate the apical heart rate—found at the point of maximal impulse [PMI] at the fifth left midclavicular intercostal space—for 1 full minute). If the pulse is 60 beats/min or less or greater than 120 beats/min, then the dose should be withheld and the physician notified of the problem. In addition, the physician should be contacted if the client experiences any of the following manifestations of toxicity: anorexia, nausea, vomiting or diarrhea, or visual disturbances such as blurred vision or the perception of green or yellow halos around objects. Most institutions and/or nursing units follow some protocol or policy and procedures with regard to digitalis and its administration, and the nurse must be sure to refer to these instructions as well.

Other nursing interventions include checking the dosage form and amounts and the physician's order carefully to make sure that the specific drug ordered has been dispensed (such as digitoxin vs. digoxin). Digoxin may be administered with meals but not with foods high in fibre because the fibre will bind to the digitalis, which will make less drug available for absorption. If the medication is to be given intravenously, the following interventions are critical: administer undiluted intravenous forms at around 0.25 mg/min or over more than 5 minutes. The administration of intramuscular (IM) forms of cardiac glycosides is extremely painful and is not recommended because tissue necro-

sis and erratic absorption may ensue. Digoxin and digitoxin are incompatible with any other medication in solution or syringe. It is important for the nurse to remember that, regardless of the dosage form, if the client's apical pulse is less than 60 beats/min or more than 120 beats/min, the dose should be withheld, the physician notified of the problem, the vital signs monitored, and all interventions documented. Should toxicity become life threatening, digoxin immune Fab, the antidote to digoxin or digitoxin toxicity, should be administered over 30 minutes or given as an intravenous bolus if cardiac arrest is imminent. See the Community Health Points box below.

The nursing interventions for clients undergoing digitalization need to be considered separately. Although not commonly used in contemporary practice, digitalization may still be done in some areas of practice for the management of heart failure. Rapid digitalization (to get faster action) is generally reserved for clients with heart failure who are in acute distress. Such clients are hospitalized because digitalis toxicities can appear quickly with the high drug concentrations used. Should the client undergoing rapid digitalization exhibit any of the manifestations of toxicity, the physician should be contacted immediately. Such clients should be observed constantly and serum digoxin or digitoxin levels measured frequently. Slow digitalization is generally performed on an outpatient basis in clients with heart failure who are not in such acute distress. Any toxic effects will appear later (depending on the specific drug's half-life) than

---

COMMUNITY HEALTH POINTS

Digoxin

- Clients should be instructed to take radial pulse before each dose of digoxin. For geriatric and physically or mentally challenged clients it is important to have community health care personnel supervise the medication regimen because these individuals are at risk for possible interactions with other medications or for possible toxicity.
- Clients should keep a journal at home to record date, day, time of dose, amount of medication taken, dietary intake, any unusual side effects or changes in conditions, and pulse rate. Below is an example of a chart-type journal, which may help to identify therapeutic and side effects and toxicity.

- Clients should be encouraged to contact the physician or healthcare provider with any unusual complaints or if the pulse is below 60 beats/min or erratic, or if they are experiencing anorexia, nausea, or vomiting. Any changes in visual acuity should also be reported to their healthcare provider or home health care nurse.
- Clients taking digoxin should be encouraged to wear a medical alert bracelet or tag. This should be ordered before discharge from the hospital.
- A weight gain of 0.5 or 1 kg a day or 2.5 kg in 1 wk should be reported to the healthcare provider or to the home health care nurse.

Drug dose	Date and time	Apical pulse rate	Weight	Side effects	Diet intake	Any changes or unusual complaints	Misc.

with rapid digitalization. Slow digitalization is safer and can be done on an outpatient basis and with oral dosage forms. However, it takes longer for the therapeutic effects to occur and the symptoms of toxicity are more gradual, and therefore more insidious, in onset. Intake and output, heart rate, BP, daily weight, respiration, and all other vital signs should be monitored closely during milrinone therapy.

Milrinone should only be infused using an infusion pump. During treatment, the client should be monitored for any discomfort at the intravenous site, numbness, tingling of the extremities, and/or difficulty breathing.

Client teaching tips for these agents are listed on p. 356.

■ Evaluation

Monitoring clients after the administration of positive inotropic agents is crucial for identifying therapeutic effects and side effects. Because positive inotropic agents increase the force of myocardial contractility (positive inotropic effect), alter electrophysiological properties (decrease rate negative chronotropic effect), and decrease AV node conduction (negative dromotropic effect), the therapeutic effects include the following:

- Increased urinary output
- Decreased edema
- Decreased shortness of breath, dyspnea, and rales
- Decreased fatigue
- Resolving of paroxysmal nocturnal dyspnea
- Improved peripheral pulses, skin colour, and temperature

While monitoring for the therapeutic effects, it is essential (because of the low therapeutic index of digitalis preparations) for the nurse to watch for side effects such as anorexia, nausea, vomiting, diarrhea, ventricular dys-

rhythmias, heart block, bradycardia, and confusion. Laboratory values should also be monitored, such as serum creatinine, potassium, calcium, sodium, and chloride levels, as well as levels of digoxin (therapeutic range 0.8–2.0 ng/mL) or digitoxin (therapeutic range 13–25 ng/mL). If a client experiences toxicity on digoxin or digitoxin, and/or as ordered by the physician, the antidote, digoxin immune Fab, may be used. Digoxin immune Fab is available only in parenteral form, dosed by the number of vials, depending on the dose calculation method or the reference chart used. It is commonly dosed based on the client's serum digoxin level in conjunction with the client's weight; the recommended dosages vary according to the amount of cardiac glycoside ingested. Each vial of digoxin immune Fab can neutralize 0.5 mg of digoxin or digitoxin. For recommended dosages consult the manufacturer's latest dosage table recommendations. It is important for the nurse to bear in mind that after digoxin immune Fab is given, all subsequent digoxin serum levels will be elevated for days to weeks because of the presence of both the free (unbound) digoxin (toxic digoxin) and the digoxin that has been bound by the digoxin immune Fab (non-toxic digoxin). Therefore at this point the clinical signs and symptoms of digoxin toxicity rather than the digoxin serum levels should be used to monitor the effectiveness of reversal therapy.

Therapeutic effects of milrinone include an improvement in cardiac function with less severe symptoms of heart failure. Side effects for which to monitor include hypotension, dysrhythmias, headache, ventricular fibrillation, chest pain, and hypokalemia. Clients on milrinone should be evaluated for significant hypotension, and the drug should be discontinued or the infusion rate decreased per the physician's orders.

NURSING CARE PLAN ▌ Heart Failure

Mr. D., a 72-year-old man admitted with heart failure, has been started on digoxin 0.125 mg for maintenance doses. He will be on your nursing unit for the next 1 to 2 days and will require frequent monitoring of the effects of the cardiac glycoside. Vital parameters are as follows on admission to your unit: confused in early pm, UO about 240 cc/shift, P110, RR 33, BP 100/56, 11 pitting pedal edema, SOB, DOE, energy levels, unable to dress self, and skin intact. Lab studies show normal H&H, BUN, urinalysis, but K^1 at 3.4.

ASSESSMENT	**Subjective Data**	• Complaints of SOB, DOE, pedal edema
	Objective Data	• Rales lower bases
		• Weight 1 kg in 5 days
		• RR 32
		• P 102
		• BP 100/60
NURSING DIAGNOSIS		Ineffective tissue perfusion related to tachycardia from heart failure

Continued

NURSING CARE PLAN | Heart Failure—*cont'd*

PLANNING

Goals Client will show improved tissue perfusion within 48 hr of treatment

Outcome Criteria Client will have increased tissue perfusion (cardiopulmonary) within 8 hr as evidenced by the following:
- Urinary output 30 mL/hr
- Decreased weight resulting from fluid loss
- Rales
- P<60<100
- RR 16–20
- Decreased pedal edema

IMPLEMENTATION
- Take client's vital signs q4h and prn, including apical pulse
- I&O q8h
- Daily weights
- Monitor digitalis levels as ordered
- Monitor serum electrolytes
- Take apical pulse for 1 full minute and notify physician if P<60; hold drug until further orders
- Breath sounds q4h and prn
- Elevate head of bed
- Keep feet elevated at all times
- Passive ROM

EVALUATION
Client will show the following therapeutic responses to digitalis treatment:
- Decreased weight
- Ease of breathing
- Increased UO
- Decreased edema
- Decreased SOB/DOE
- Increased ability to perform ADLs
- Vital signs within normal limits

Client will be monitored for (and experience minimal) side effects associated with digitalis therapy such as bradycardia, headache, GI symptoms, blurred vision, anorexia.

UO, Urinary output; *P,* pulse; *RR,* respiratory rate; *BP,* blood pressure; *SOB,* shortness of breath; *DOE,* dyspnea on exertion; *H&H,* hematocrit and hemoglobin; *BUN,* blood urea nitrogen; *K¹,* potassium; *I&O,* intake and output; *ROM,* range of motion; *ADLs,* activities of daily living.

CLIENT TEACHING TIPS

The nurse should instruct clients as follows:
▲ Take your medication at the same time every day and exactly as ordered. Never double up on a dose and never skip a dose unless told to do so by your physician, or unless you have certain problems listed below.
▲ Do not discontinue the drug abruptly.
▲ Use only the dropper supplied with the elixir form to administer the medication. Never guess or estimate dosages of these drugs.
▲ Do not change brands when refilling prescriptions unless specifically prescribed by the physician.
▲ Check with your physician before taking any other medication with the digoxin, whether a prescribed or an over-the-counter (OTC) medication or natural health product.
▲ If your pulse goes below 60 beats/min or above 120 beats/min or if it is erratic, don't take the next dose,

and contact your healthcare provider immediately. The same applies if you experience loss of appetite, nausea, vomiting, diarrhea, or blurred vision, or if you see green or yellow halos around objects. These are early signs of digitalis toxicity.
▲ Inform your physician if you experience a weight gain of 1 kg or more per day or 2.5 kg or more in one week.
▲ Wear a medical alert bracelet or necklace at all times and always carry a written note in your wallet or purse naming the medication or medications you are taking and your cardiac condition. Contact your local emergency medical services department to find out how to post information in your home about your condition and medications.

▲ If you take antacids or eat ice cream, yoghurt, cheese, or other milk products, take your dose 2 hours before or after these medications or foods.

▲ Consume foods high in potassium, especially if you are also taking a potassium-depleting diuretic.

▲ Report any signs and symptoms of weakness, fatigue, or lethargy.

▲ Family members or caregivers must also be taught the side effects and the importance of taking the client's pulse before giving the drug, as well as the signs and symptoms of toxicity.

POINTS to REMEMBER

▼ *Inotropic* is a term that refers to the force of myocardial contraction; therefore positive inotropics (e.g., digoxin) increase the force of contractions and negative inotropics (e.g., beta-blockers, CCBs) decrease myocardial contractility.

▼ Negative inotropic agents decrease force of contraction

▼ *Chronotropic* refers to the rate at which the heart beats (beats/min); positive chronotropic agents (e.g., epinephrine, atropine) increase the heart rate and negative chronotropic agents decrease the heart rate.

▼ *Dromotropic* refers to the conduction of electrical impulses through the heart; positive dromotropic agents increase the speed of the electrical impulse through the heart, whereas negative agents have the opposite effect.

▼ Digitalis drugs, specifically digoxin, are one of the oldest and most effective groups of drugs obtained from a plant source. The digitalis plant, *foxglove*, has been the mainstay of heart failure treatment for over 200 years; however, newer positive inotropics are also helpful in specific heart failure diagnoses.

▼ A client's ejection fraction reflects the contractility of the heart and is at about 65 percent (0.65) in a normal heart. This value decreases as heart failure progresses; therefore clients with heart failure have low ejection fractions because their hearts are failing as effective "pumps."

▼ Contraindications to the use of digoxin include allergy to the digitalis medications, ventricular tachycardia and fibrillations, beriberi heart disease, AV block, and hypersensitive carotid sinus syndrome.

▼ Predisposers to digitalis toxicity include hypokalemia, hypercalcemia, hypothyroid states, renal dysfunction, and advanced age.

▼ Taking an apical pulse for 1 full minute is a standard of care expected when administering digoxin.

▼ A physician should be notified at the first signs of anorexia, nausea, vomiting, and for bradycardia with a pulse below 60 beats/min for a client receiving digoxin; however, policies regarding the management of digitalis-related bradycardia vary from institution to institution and from doctor to doctor.

▼ Hypotension, dysrhythmias, and thrombocytopenia are major adverse effects of milrinone.

EXAMINATION REVIEW QUESTIONS

1 Which of the following statements best describes digoxin toxicity?
a. Digoxin has maximal concentrations without loading doses and may actually cure the individual with heart failure.
b. Digoxin immune Fab is another form of digoxin and is used only in children for prevention of severe hypokalemia, thus improving digoxin toxicity.
c. Monitor digoxin and electrolyte levels with an alert to BUN levels because if lower than normal levels exist, the client may then have more problems with toxicity.
d. Hypokalemia is one of the major causes of digoxin toxicity, and digoxin therapeutic levels should be monitored and be 2 ng/dL.

2 Digoxin immune Fab therapy is indicated in which of the following situations?
a. Severe sinus tachycardia
b. Digoxin level of 1.5 ng/dL
c. Serum potassium level 5 mmol/L
d. Life-threatening cardiac dysrhythmias

3 Which of the following is an added benefit to the positive inotropic action of digoxin? Digoxin promotes
a. increased cardiac output and thus more diuresis and improved heart failure.
b. proteinuria because protein leaves the body resulting in less fluid overload in heart failure.
c. bradycardia leading to a diminished oxygen consumption, demand, and supply.
d. chronotropy with improved conduction, not contractility.

4 Bradycardia, as a side effect of digoxin, is related to which of the following effects?
a. Positive chronotropic
b. Negative chronotropic
c. Positive chromotropic
d. Negative chromotropic

5 Which of the following medication classifications would antagonize the therapeutic effects of digoxin?
a. Calcium channel blockers
b. Antidepressants
c. Benzodiazepines
d. Diuretics

For answers see http://evolve.elsevier.com/Lilley/pharmacology/.

CRITICAL THINKING ACTIVITIES

1 Atrial fibrillation develops in the client for whom you are caring. The client is not currently on any agent to treat this and is becoming quite symptomatic. The physician prescribes digoxin at a dosage of 0.5 mg intravenously stat, followed by 0.25 mg intravenously q6h for two doses. On hand is a vial of digoxin with the strength of 0.25 mg/mL. How much digoxin (in millilitres) is generally recommended each time you administer the drug? Explain your answer.

2 Your client, a 78-year-old-man, has a potassium level of 3.0 mmol/L. He states that he has been nauseous and without an appetite and has experienced some diarrhea. He has been taking digoxin for the past few weeks for the treatment of recently diagnosed heart failure. Discuss the implication of hypokalemia in a client who is on digoxin and any negative consequences.

3 Explain why the geriatric client with hypothyroid disease is at increased risk for digitalis toxicity.

For answers see http://evolve.elsevier.com/Lilley/pharmacology/.

BIBLIOGRAPHY

Albanese, J., & Nutz, P. (2005). *Mosby's 2005 nursing drug cards.* St Louis, MO: Mosby.

Anderson, P.O., Knoben, J.E., & Troutman, W.G. (2002). *Handbook of clinical drug data* (10th ed.). New York: McGraw-Hill/Appleton & Lange.

Berne, R., & Levy, M. (2002). *Principles of physiology* (3rd ed.). St Louis, MO: Mosby.

Boron, W.F., & Boulpaep, E.L. (2003). *Medical physiology.* Philadelphia: Saunders.

Canadian Pharmacists Association. (2003). *Therapeutic choices* (4th ed.). Ottawa, ON: Author.

Canadian Pharmacists Association. (2004). *Guide to drugs in Canada.* Toronto, ON: Dorling Kindersley.

Canadian Pharmacists Association. (2005). *Compendium of pharmaceuticals and specialties. The Canadian drug reference for health professionals.* Ottawa, ON: Author. [The subscription-based e-CPS is available at http://www.pharmacists.ca.]

Clayton, B.D., & Stock, Y.N. (2004). *Basic pharmacology for nurses* (13th ed.). St Louis, MO: Mosby.

Digitalis Investigation Group. (1997). The effect of digoxin on mortality and morbidity in patients with heart failure. *New England Journal of Medicine, 336,* 525.

Ducharme, A., Doyon, O., White, M., Rouleau, J.L., & Brophy, J.M. (2005). Impact of care at a multidisciplinary congestive heart failure clinic: A randomized trial. *Canadian Medical Association Journal, 173*(1), 40–45.

Facts and Comparisons. (2004). *Drug facts and comparisons pocket version* (9th ed.). St Louis, MO: Wolters Kluwer Health.

Health Canada. (2005) Drug product database (DPD). Retrieved August 7, 2005, from http://www.hc-sc.gc.ca/hpb/drugs-dpd/

Heart and Stroke Foundation of Canada. (2003). *The growing burden of heart disease and stroke in Canada 2003.* Ottawa, ON: Author.

Johns Hopkins Hospital, Gunn, V.L., & Nechyba, C. (2002). *The Harriet Lane handbook* (16th ed.). St Louis, MO: Mosby.

Kasper, D.L., Braunwald, D., Faci, A., Hauser, S., Longo, D., & Jameson, J.L. (2005). *Harrison's principles of internal medicine* (16th ed.). New York: McGraw-Hill.

Lacy, C.F., Armstrong, L.L., Goldman, M.P., & Lance, L.L. (Eds.). (2003). *Drug information handbook* (11th ed.). Hudson, OH: Lexi-Comp.

Liu, P., Arnold, J.M., Belenkie, I., Demers, C., Dorian, P., Gianetti, N., et al. (2003). The 2002/3 Canadian Cardiovascular Society consensus guideline update for the diagnosis and management of heart failure. *Canadian Journal of Cardiology, 19*(4), 347–356.

MacAulay, S., & Jorgenson, D. (2003). Beta-blockers for the management of chronic heart failure. A summary of the evidence. *Canadian Pharmacy Journal, 136*(5), 35–41.

Mosby. (2005). *Mosby's drug consult 2005: The comprehensive reference for generic and brand name drugs* (15th ed.). St Louis, MO: Mosby.

Skidmore-Roth, L. (2006). *Mosby's 2006 nursing drug reference* (19th ed.). St Louis, MO: Mosby.

Tierney, L.M., McPhee, S.J., & Papadakis, M.A. (2002). *2002 Current medical diagnosis and treatment: Adult ambulatory and inpatient management.* New York: McGraw-Hill.

Turkoski, B.B. (1999). *Drug information handbook for nursing 1999–2000: Including assessment, administration, monitoring guidelines, and patient education* (2nd ed.). Cleveland, OH: Lexi-Comp.

Tsuyuki, R.T., Shibata, M.C., Nilsson, C., & Hervas-Malo, M. (2003). Contemporary burden of illness of congestive heart failure in Canada. *Canadian Journal of Cardiology, 19*(4), 436–438.

Woods, S.L., Sivarajan Froelocher, E.S., Underhill Motzer, S., & Bridges, E.J. (2005). *Cardiac Nursing* (5th ed.). Philadelphia: Lippincott Williams & Wilkins.

Antidysrhythmic Agents 22

OBJECTIVES

After reading this chapter, the successful student will be able to do the following:

1 Define the term *dysrhythmia*.

2 Compare the various dysrhythmias and their impact on the structures of the heart.

3 Identify the most commonly encountered dysrhythmias and summarize the precipitating factors for each type.

4 Compare the anatomy and physiology of a normal heart, including the electrical system, with that of a heart with abnormal conduction and/or rhythm.

5 Contrast the various classes of antidysrhythmics using specific drug examples in each class, in terms of mechanisms of action, routes of administration, dosing, specific drug protocols and related indications, side effects, cautions, contraindications, drug interactions, and any toxic reactions.

6 Develop a nursing care plan that includes all phases of the nursing process for each class of antidysrhythmics.

e-LEARNING ACTIVITIES

Student CD-ROM
- Review Questions: see questions 132–141
- Animations
- Medication Administration Checklists
- IV Therapy Checklists

evolve **Web site** (http://evolve.elsevier.com/Lilley/pharmacology/)
- Online Chapter Worksheet • Frequently Asked Questions
- Learning Tips and Content Updates • WebLinks • Online Appendixes and Supplements • Mosby/Saunders ePharmacology Update • Access to *Mosby's Drug Consult*

DRUG PROFILES

adenosine, p. 373
▶▶ amiodarone, p. 371
▶▶ atenolol, p. 370
bretylium, p. 372
▶▶ diltiazem, p. 373
disopyramide, p. 365
esmolol, p. 370
flecainide, p. 369
▶▶ lidocaine, p. 369

▶▶ metoprolol, p. 371
mexiletine, p. 369
procainamide, p. 365
propafenone, p. 370
▶▶ propranolol, p. 371
quinidine, p. 366
▶▶ sotalol, p. 371
▶▶ verapamil, p. 373

▶▶ Key drug.

GLOSSARY

Action potential An electrical impulse consisting of a self-propagating series of polarizations and depolarizations that is transmitted across the cell membranes of a nerve fibre during the transmission of a nerve impulse and across the cell membranes of a muscle cell during contraction or other activity of the cell.

Action potential duration (APD) The interval during which a cell is repolarizing to its baseline membrane potential.

Arrhythmia (uh rith' mee uh) In the most literal sense, the absence of a rhythmic pattern. A term also commonly used to refer to any deviation from the normal pattern of the heartbeat (see *dysrhythmia*).

Cardiac Arrhythmia Suppression Trial (CAST) The name of the major research study conducted by the National Heart, Lung, and Blood Institute to investigate the possibility of eliminating sudden cardiac death in clients with asymptomatic, non–life-threatening ectopy that has arisen after a myocardial infarction.

Dysrhythmia (dis rith' me uh) Any disturbance or abnormality in a normal rhythmic pattern.

Effective refractory period (ERP) The period after the firing of an impulse during which a cell may respond to a stimulus but the response will not be passed along or continued.

359

Fast channels, sodium channels Other terms for *fast-response channels*. These cells can rapidly conduct electrical impulses.

Internodal pathways, Bachmann's bundle Special pathways in the atria that carry electrical impulses that are spontaneously generated by the sinoatrial node. These impulses cause the heart to beat.

Relative refractory period (RRP) The time during which a depressed response to a strong stimulus is possible.

Resting membrane potential (RMP) The transmembrane voltage that exists when the heart muscle is at rest.

Sodium–potassium ATPase pump A mechanism for transporting sodium and potassium ions across cell membranes against an opposing concentration gradient. Energy for this transport system is obtained from the hydrolysis of adenosine triphosphate (ATP) by means of an enzyme called adenosine triphosphatase (ATPase).

Sudden cardiac death Unexplained cessation, or death, of cardiac function.

Threshold potential (TP) The spontaneous depolarization of cells after a critical state of electrical tension is reached.

Vaughan Williams classification The most commonly used system used to classify antidysrhythmic drugs.

DYSRHYTHMIAS AND NORMAL CARDIAC ELECTROPHYSIOLOGY

A **dysrhythmia** is any deviation from the normal rhythm of the heart. The term **arrhythmia,** which is also used to refer to these deviations, literally means "no rhythm," which implies asystole, or no heartbeat at all. A person in asystole is dead. Thus the more accurate term for an irregular heart rhythm is *dysrhythmia.* There are many conditions in which dysrhythmias can develop. Some of the more common arise after a myocardial infarction (MI) or

cardiac surgery or as the result of coronary artery disease. These dysrhythmias are usually serious and require treatment with an antidysrhythmic agent, though not all have to be treated.

Disturbances in cardiac rhythm are the result of abnormally functioning cardiac cells. To understand the pathological mechanism responsible for dysrhythmias it is first necessary to review the electrical properties of cardiac cells. Figure 22-1 illustrates the process from the standpoint of a single cardiac cell. Inside a cardiac cell there exists a net negative charge relative to the outside of the cell. This difference in the electronegative charge exists in all types of cardiac cells and is referred to as the **resting membrane potential (RMP).** The RMP results from an uneven distribution of ions (sodium, potassium, and calcium) across the cell membrane. This uneven distribution of ions is maintained by the **sodium–potassium ATPase pump,** an energy-requiring ionic pump. Cardiac cells become excited when there is a change in this distribution of ions across their membrane, and this movement of ions results in the propagation of an electrical impulse and the subsequent contraction of the myocardial muscle. This is called an **action potential** and consists of four phases. Phase 1 of the action potential starts when the fast sodium channel closes and a period of rapid repolarization begins. During phase 2, calcium ion influx occurs through the slow channels. This causes a plateau phase during which the membrane potential changes only slightly. Over time potassium ions flow outward and the cell is repolarized to its baseline level (phase 3). To restore the cell to its original state, the energy-dependent sodium-potassium ATPase pump, or sodium pump, moves sodium ions out of and potassium ions into the cell. Phase 4 is the RMP.

The movement of ions across the cardiac cell's membranes (action potential) varies in speed from one area to another in the heart's conduction system. Figure 22-2 illustrates the action potential in two different types of cells found in the conduction system of the heart. The action

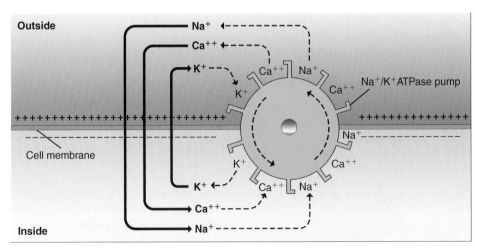

FIG. 22-1 Resting membrane potential of a cardiac cell.

potential of the specialized electrical conducting cells in the sinoatrial (SA) node is shown in Figure 22-2, *A,* and the action potential of a Purkinje cell (fibre) located in the specialized electrical conducting system is depicted in Figure 22-2, *B.* Figure 22-3 also illustrates the movement of sodium, potassium, and calcium ions into and out of a Purkinje cell during the four phases of the action potential. There are several important differences in the action potentials of the SA node and Purkinje cell. The RMP in the Purkinje cell is approximately −80 to −90 mV, compared with −50 to −60 mV in the SA nodal cell. The level of the RMP (phase 4) is an important determinant of the rate of impulse conduction to other cells. The less negative the RMP at the onset of phase 0, the slower the upstroke velocity of phase 0. The slope or rate of rise of phase 0 is directly related to the impulse conduction velocity or speed. If the slope of phase 0 is steep, as it is in the Purkinje cells, electrical conduction through these cells is fast.

The action potential of the Purkinje cells illustrated in Figure 22-2, *B,* has a rapid rate of rise of phase 0 and

therefore electrical impulses are conducted quickly. These cells are referred to as *fast-response cells,* or *fast-channel cells.* During this phase, channels open, permitting a rapid influx of sodium ions into the cell. The terms **fast channels** and **sodium channels** both refer to these fast-response channels. Many antidysrhythmic agents affect the RMP and sodium channels, which in turn affects the rate of impulse conduction.

Because the cells of the SA or atrioventricular (AV) nodes have RMPs of −50 to −60 mV, they have a much slower upstroke velocity, or a slower phase 0. This slow rate of rise in phase 0 of the SA and AV nodes is primarily dependent on the entry of calcium ions through the slow channel. These cells are therefore called *slow-channel tissue,* or *calcium channels,* and conduction in these cells is slower than that in the myocardial or other electrical conduction tissue. Drugs that affect calcium ion movement into or out of these cells tend to have significant effects on the SA and AV nodal conduction rates.

The interval between phase 0 and phase 4 when the cell is repolarizing and returning to its RMP is called the

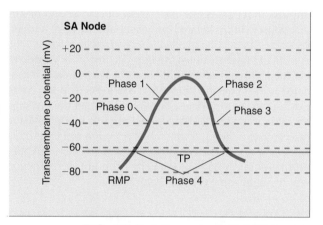
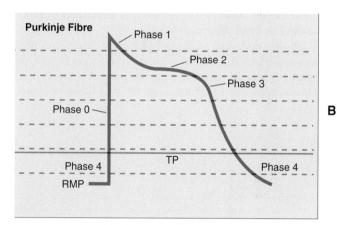

FIG. 22-2 Action potentials. *RMP,* Resting membrane potential; *SA,* sinoatrial; *TP,* threshold potential.

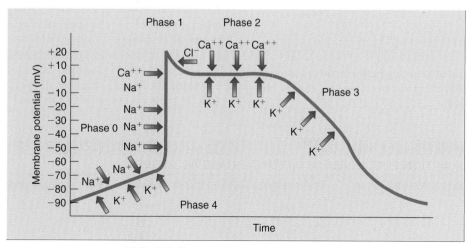

FIG. 22-3 Purkinje fibre action potential.

action potential duration (APD). The period between phase 0 and midway through phase 3 is called the absolute or **effective refractory period (ERP).** During the ERP the cardiac cell cannot be stimulated to depolarize and conduct electricity. During the remainder of phase 3 until the return to the RMP (phase 4), the cardiac cell is vulnerable to depolarization if it receives an impulse. This period is referred to as the **relative refractory period (RRP),** and during it a strong stimulus can initiate a premature depolarization. If a cardiac cell receives a strong enough stimulus during the RRP, it will be when the cell is at a lower membrane potential (less negative), which will result in slow impulse conduction. Figure 22-4 illustrates these various aspects of an action potential.

The RMP of certain cardiac cells gradually and spontaneously decreases (becomes less negative) over time, and this is probably secondary to small changes in the flux of sodium and potassium ions. Depolarization eventually occurs when a certain critical voltage is reached **(threshold potential [TP]).** This process of spontaneous depolarization is referred to as *automaticity,* or *pacemaker activity.* It is normal when it occurs in the SA node, AV node, and His-Purkinje system (see Figure 21-1). When other tissues assume the property of spontaneous depolarization, dysrhythmias occur.

The SA node, AV node, and His-Purkinje cells all possess automaticity, but the SA node is the pacemaker of the heart because it spontaneously depolarizes the fastest. The SA node has an intrinsic rate of 60 to 100 depolariza-tions, or beats per minute (beats/min); that of the AV node is 40 to 60 beats/min; and that of the ventricular Purkinje fibres is 40 or fewer beats/min. The action potentials in different areas of the heart, along with other characteristics of the cells in these different areas, are compared in Table 22-1.

As the natural pacemaker of the heart, the SA node, which is located near the top of the right atrium, generates the electrical impulse needed to produce the heartbeat. This impulse then travels through the atria via specialized pathways called the **internodal pathways** or **Bachmann's bundle.** While the impulse is traveling through these specialized pathways, it is causing the myocardial muscle in the atria to contract. This impulse is then received by the AV node, which is located near the bottom of the right atrium. The AV node slows this fast-moving electrical impulse just long enough to allow the ventricles to accept the blood that the atria have just squeezed into them. If the AV node did not slow the impulse, the ventricles would contract almost at the same time as the atria, resulting in a smaller volume of blood being injected (decreased cardiac output).

Upon stimulation the AV node generates an electrical impulse that passes into the bundle of His, a band of cardiac muscle fibres located between both the right and left ventricles in what is called the *ventricular septum.* The bundle of His distributes the impulse into both ventricles via the right and left bundle branch. Each branch terminates in the Purkinje fibres that are located in the myocardium of the ventricles. The stimulation of the Purkinje fibres causes ventricular contraction and blood to leave the ventricles, going to the lungs from the right ventricle and to the rest of the body from the left ventricle. Any abnormality in cardiac automaticity or impulse conduction will result in some type of dysrhythmia.

ANTIDYSRHYTHMIC AGENTS

Numerous drugs are available to treat dysrhythmias. They are classified on the basis of where and how they affect cardiac cells. The most commonly used system is the **Vaughan Williams classification,** which is based on the effect produced by the particular agent on the action potential. This approach has yielded four major groups of agents. Class I antidysrhythmics are considered membrane-stabilizing agents, but they are further divided into Ia, Ib, and Ic agents, depending on the magnitude of their effects on phase 0, the APD, and the ERP.

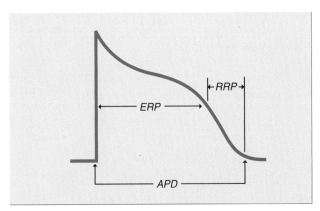

FIG. 22-4 Aspects of an action potential. *APD,* Action potential duration; *ERP,* effective refractory period; *RRP,* relative refractory period.

TABLE 22-1				
COMPARISON OF ACTION POTENTIALS IN DIFFERENT CARDIAC TISSUE				
Tissue	**Action Potential Wave**	**Speed of Response**	**Threshold Potential (mV)**	**Conduction Velocity (m/sec)**
SA node	⌒	Slow	−60	<0.05
Atrium	⋀	Fast	−90	~1
AV node	⌒	Slow	−60	<0.05
His-Purkinje	⋀	Fast	−95	3
Ventricle	⋀	Fast	−90	1

Class II drugs are beta-blockers that depress phase 4 depolarization. Class III drugs primarily prolong repolarization during phase 3. Class IV drugs depress phase 4 depolarization and prolong repolarization during phases 1 and 2. Calcium channel blockers (CCBs) (slow channel blockers) such as verapamil belong to class IV. The various agents in these four classes are listed in Table 22-2. Several antidysrhythmics exert more than one type of effect on the action potential. There is a gradual current trend away from the use of class Ia agents. The formerly available class Ic agent encainide was removed from the market after research indicated that its risk of inducing fatal cardiac dysrhythmias overshadowed its dysrhythmia suppression effects. For similar reasons the other two class Ic agents, flecainide and propafenone, are generally used only in clients intolerant of other agents. Nonetheless, several class I agents of all types remain available on the Canadian market as therapeutic options and so are included in this discussion. The class III agents are currently among the most widely used antidysrhythmics. The class IV agents (CCBs), unlike most of the other classes, have limited usefulness in tachydysrhythmias (dysrhythmias associated with tachycardia). The role of class II agents (beta-blockers) continues to grow in the field of cardiology, including dysrhythmia management. Digoxin, the cardiac glycoside discussed in Chapter 21, retains a role in dysrhythmia management, especially with regard to preventing dangerous ventricular tachydysrhythmias secondary to atrial fibrillation.

Mechanism of Action and Drug Effects

Antidysrhythmic drugs can correct abnormal cardiac electrophysiological function by various mechanisms of action. As the membrane-stabilizing agents, class I drugs exert their actions on the sodium (fast) channels; however, as already noted, there are some slight differences in the actions of the agents within this class, resulting in three subgroups of agents. Class Ia agents (quinidine, procainamide, and disopyramide) block sodium channels by binding to the sodium channel in the open state; more specifically they delay repolarization and increase the APD. Class Ib agents (mexiletine and lidocaine) block the sodium channels in the inactivated state, but unlike class Ia agents, they accelerate repolarization and decrease the APD. Class Ic agents (flecainide and propafenone) have a more pronounced effect on the blockade of sodium channels in the open state but have little effect on repolarization or the APD.

Class II agents are beta-blockers. They work by reducing or blocking sympathetic nervous system stimulation to the heart and, as a result, the transmission of impulses in the heart's conduction system. This results in depression of phase 4 depolarization. These drugs mostly affect slow tissue.

Class III agents (amiodarone, bretylium, and sotalol) increase the APD by prolonging repolarization in phase 3. They affect fast tissue and are most commonly used to manage dysrhythmias that are difficult to treat.

Class IV agents are calcium channel blockers (CCBs). As their name implies, they work by inhibiting the slow-channel pathways, or the calcium-dependent channels. By doing this, they depress phase 4 depolarization. Diltiazem and verapamil are by far the most commonly used CCBs for cardiac rhythm disturbances.

The mechanisms of action of the major classes of antidysrhythmics are summarized in Table 22-3. The effects for the various classes of agents are summarized in Box 22-1.

Indications

Antidysrhythmic agents are effective in treating a variety of cardiac dysrhythmias. The antidysrhythmic drugs and the most common indications for their use are listed in Table 22-4.

Contraindications

Contraindications to the use of antidysrhythmic agents include known drug allergy to a specific product and may include second- or third-degree AV block, bundle branch block, cardiogenic shock, sick sinus syndrome, or any other major electrocardiogram (ECG) changes as rated by expert opinion, preferably that of an experienced cardiologist. The safe prescribing of antidysrhythmic therapy is an area of drug therapy that requires especially strong clinical expertise and careful judgement on a case-by-case basis.

TABLE 22-2

VAUGHAN WILLIAMS CLASSIFICATION OF ANTIDYSRHYTHMIC AGENTS

Functional Class	Drugs
Class Ia: ↑ blockade of sodium channel, delay repolarization, ↑APD	quinidine, disopyramide, procainamide
Class Ib: ↑ blockade of sodium channel, accelerate repolarization, ↓ APD	mexiletine, lidocaine
Class Ic: ↑↑↑ blockade of sodium channel ± on repolarization	flecainide, propafenone
Class II: Beta-blocking agents	All beta-blockers
Class III: Principal effect on cardiac tissue is to ↑ APD	amiodarone, bretylium, sotalol
Class IV: Calcium channel blockers	verapamil, diltiazem
Other: Antidysrhythmic drugs that have the properties of several classes and therefore cannot be placed in one particular class	digoxin, adenosine

APD, Action potential duration; ↑, increase; ↓, decrease; ±, increase or decrease.

TABLE 22-3

ANTIDYSRHYTHMIC AGENTS: MECHANISMS OF ACTION

Vaughan Williams class	I	II	III	IV
Action	Blocks sodium channels, affects phase 0	Decreases spontaneous depolarization, affects phase 4	Prolongs APD	Blocks slow calcium channels
Tissue	Fast	Slow	Fast	Slow
Effect on action potential				

APD, Action potential duration.

BOX 22-1

Drug Effects of Antidysrhythmic Agents

Class Ia (disopyramide, procainamide, quinidine)
• Depression of myocardial excitability
• Prolongation of the ERP
• Elimination or reduction of ectopic foci stimulation
• Decrease in inotropic effect
• Anticholinergic (vagolytic)

Class Ib (lidocaine, mexiletine)
• Decrease in myocardial excitability in the ventricles
• Elimination or reduction of ectopic foci stimulation in the ventricles
• Minimal effect on the SA node and automaticity
• Minimal effect on the AV node and conduction
• Minimal anticholinergic (vagolytic) activity

Class Ic (flecainide, propafenone)
• Dose-related depression of cardiac conduction, especially in the bundle of His–Purkinje system
• Minimal effect on atrial conduction
• Elimination or reduction of ectopic foci stimulation in the ventricles
• Minimal anticholinergic (vagolytic) activity
• Flecainide now reserved for the most serious dysrhythmias

Class II (acebutolol, esmolol, propranolol)
• Block of beta-adrenergic cardiac stimulation
• Reduction in SA node activity
• Elimination or reduction of atrial ectopic foci stimulation
• Reduction in ventricular contraction rate
• Reduction in cardiac output and BP

Class III (amiodarone, bretylium, sotalol)
• Prolongation of the ERP
• Prolongation of myocardial action potential
• Block of both alpha- and beta-adrenergic cardiac stimulation

Class IV (diltiazem, verapamil)
• Prolongation of AV node ERP
• Reduction of AV node conduction
• Reduction of rapid ventricular conduction caused by atrial flutter

AV, Atrioventricular; *SA,* sinoatrial; *ERP,* effective refractory period; *BP,* blood pressure.

Side Effects and Adverse Effects

Side effects and adverse effects common to most antidysrhythmics include hypersensitivity reactions, nausea, vomiting, and diarrhea. Other common effects include dizziness, headache, and blurred vision. In addition, any antidysrhythmic is capable of producing a proarrhythmic (dysrhythmic) effect. This occurs most commonly in association with quinidine, amiodarone, and propafenone therapy.

Toxicity and Management of Overdose

The main toxic effects of the antidysrhythmics involve the heart, circulation, and central nervous system (CNS). Specific antidotes are not available, and the management of an overdose involves maintaining adequate circulation and respiration using general support measures and any required symptomatic treatment (Table 22-5).

Interactions

Antidysrhythmics can interact with many different categories of drugs. The most serious drug interactions are the ones that can result in dysrhythmias, hypotension or hypertension, respiratory distress, or a summation of either the therapeutic or toxic effects. See Table 22-6 for a summary of the drug interactions.

Dosages

For information on the dosages of the various antidysrhythmics see the dosages table on p. 367. See Appendix B for some of the common brands available in Canada.

TABLE 22-4

ANTIDYSRHYTHMIC AGENTS: INDICATIONS

Drug	Indications
CLASS Ia disopyramide procainamide quinidine	Atrial fibrillation, premature atrial contractions, premature ventricular contractions, sustained ventricular tachycardia
CLASS Ib lidocaine mexiletine	Ventricular dysrhythmias only (premature ventricular contractions, ventricular tachycardia, ventricular fibrillation)
CLASS Ic flecainide propafenone	Severe ventricular dysrhythmias only May use in atrial fibrillation/flutter
CLASS II Beta-blockers atenolol esmolol metoprolol propranolol	General myocardial depressants for both supraventricular and ventricular dysrhythmias
CLASS III amiodarone bretylium sotalol	Life-threatening ventricular tachycardia or fibrillation Atrial fibrillation or flutter in acute settings
CLASS IV CCBs diltiazem verapamil	Paroxysmal supraventricular tachycardia; rate control for atrial fibrillation and flutter

CCB, Calcium channel blocker.

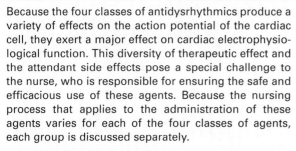

DRUG PROFILES

Because the four classes of antidysrhythmics produce a variety of effects on the action potential of the cardiac cell, they exert a major effect on cardiac electrophysiological function. This diversity of therapeutic effect and the attendant side effects pose a special challenge to the nurse, who is responsible for ensuring the safe and efficacious use of these agents. Because the nursing process that applies to the administration of these agents varies for each of the four classes of agents, each group is discussed separately.

CLASS IA DRUGS

Class Ia drugs are considered membrane-stabilizing drugs because they possess local anaesthetic properties. They stabilize the membrane and have depressant effects on phase 0 of the action potential. All class Ia agents are classified as pregnancy category C agents.

disopyramide

Disopyramide is used primarily for the treatment of documented life-threatening ventricular dysrhythmias. Its therapeutic efficacy is comparable to that of quinidine and procainamide, but it can produce significant side effects, including anticholinergic effects, ventricular dysrhythmias, and particularly cardiovascular depression. For these reasons its use is limited, especially in clients with poor left ventricular (LV) function. Significant adverse reactions from disopyramide are hypotension and widening of the QRS interval on the ECG, as well as those mentioned for quinidine and procainamide. Disopyramide has been known to cause development of a positive antinuclear antibody (ANA) test with or without symptoms of lupus erythematosus-like syndrome; however, this is less than that associated with the use of procainamide. Contraindications to its use are similar to those of quinidine and procainamide. Disopyramide is available only in oral (PO) form as 100- and 150-mg regular-release and 250-mg extended-release capsules. Pregnancy category C. Common dosages are listed in the dosages table on p. 367.

PHARMACOKINETICS

Half-Life	Onset	Peak	Duration
PO: 4–10 hr	PO: 30 min–3.5 hr	PO: 1–2 hr LA: 4.5–6.2 hr	PO: 6–12 hr

procainamide

The electrophysiological effect of procainamide is similar to that of quinidine, but its indirect effect (anticholinergic action) is weaker. Procainamide is useful in the management of atrial and ventricular tachydysrhythmias. It is reported to be more effective in the treatment of ventricular disturbances, especially in suppressing premature ventricular contractions and preventing the recurrence of ventricular tachycardia. The intravenous (IV) form of procainamide is generally preferred over that of quinidine. Procainamide is chemically related to the local anaesthetic procaine. Significant adverse effects of the agent include ventricular dysrhythmias and granulocytopenia. It can cause a positive ANA test with or without symptoms of a drug-induced lupus erythematosus-like syndrome, which occurs in slightly more than 1 percent of clients on long-term therapy. It can also cause gastrointestinal (GI) effects such as nausea, vomiting, and diarrhea, but these are less intense than those of quinidine. Other side effects include fever, thrombocytopenia, maculopapular rash, urticaria, pruritus, eosinophilia, hypergammaglobulinemia, psychosis with hallucinations, and convulsions.

Procainamide is contraindicated in clients who have shown hypersensitivity reactions to it and in those with complete heart block, lupus erythematosus, and second- or third-degree heart block. It should not be administered to clients having "les torsades de pointes" (QT interval prolongation) ventricular arrhythmias. It is available in three different oral forms: 250-mg capsules; 250-, 500-, and 750-mg extended-release film-coated tablets; and 250-, 500-, and 750-mg film-coated tablets. It is also available as a 100-mg/mL injection. Pregnancy category C. Common dosages are listed in the dosages table on p. 368.

PHARMACOKINETICS

Half-Life	Onset	Peak	Duration
IV/IM: 3 hr PO: 3 hr	IV/IM: 10–30 min PO: 0.5–1 hr	IV/IM: 10–60 min PO: 1–2 hr	IV/IM: 3 hr PO: 3 hr*

*8-hr extended release.

TABLE 22-5

ANTIDYSRHYTHMIC AGENTS: MANAGEMENT OF OVERDOSE

Drug	Toxic Effect	Management
acebutolol	Bradycardia	1–3 mg IV atropine divided
	Bronchospasm	Aminophylline or isoproterenol
	Cardiac failure	Digitalization
	Hypotension	Vasopressor
adenosine	Usually self-limiting due to a short half-life	Competitive antagonists caffeine or theophylline
amiodarone	Bradycardia	Temporary pacing
	Hypotension	Positive inotropic agent or vasopressor
bretylium	Hypertension	Nitroprusside
	Hypotension	Dopamine or norepinephrine and fluid therapy
digoxin	Decrease clearance	Lidocaine, quinidine, procainamide, and beta-adrenergic agents; increase digoxin levels
disopyramide	Loss of consciousness, cardiac and respiratory arrest	Neostigmine for anticholinergic effects, activated charcoal, symptomatic treatment, and hemodialysis
esmolol	Same as acebutolol	Same as acebutolol
flecainide	Reduced heart rate	Dopamine, dobutamine, or isoproterenol; acidify very alkaline urine to promote excretion of drug
lidocaine	Convulsions	Diazepam or thiopental
mexiletine	Bradycardia, hypotension	Atropine; acidify urine to promote excretion
procainamide	Severe hypotension, ventricular fibrillation	IV pressor agents and supportive measures
propafenone	Convulsions	Diazepam and mechanical assisted respiration
propranolol	Hypotension, bradycardia, ventricular tachycardia/fibrillation	Temporary pacing, isoproterenol, dopamine
quinidine	Severe hypotension, cardiac dysrhythmias, heart block, heart failure	Sodium bicarbonate reduces toxicity except in alkalosis; dopamine, dobutamine, isoproterenol, norepinephrine, intra-aortic balloon pump
sotalol	Same as acebutolol	Same as acebutolol
verapamil	Bradycardia	Atropine
	Cardiac failure	Dopamine or dobutamine
	Conduction problems	Isoproterenol
	Hypotension	Cardiac pacing
		Vasopressors, calcium gluconate solution

TABLE 22-6

ANTIDYSRHYTHMIC AGENTS: DRUG INTERACTIONS

Drug	Mechanism	Result
Anticoagulants	Anticoagulant displaced from protein-binding sites	More pronounced anticoagulant effects
Antidysrhythmics	Additive	Pro-arrhythmic, may cause dysrhythmias
Sulphonylurea compounds	Sulphonylurea displaced from protein-binding sites	More pronounced sulphonylurea effects

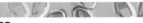

quinidine

Quinidine has both a direct action on the electrical activity of the heart and an indirect (anticholinergic) effect. Its anticholinergic action results in inhibition of the parasympathetic nervous system (PSNS) and allows sympathetic nervous system (SNS) activity to go unopposed. This accelerates the rate of electrical impulse formation and conduction. The most common cardiovascular adverse effect is ventricular tachycardia, primarily torsades de pointes, or ventricular fibrillation. Significant adverse effects include cardiac asystole and ventricular ectopic beats. Like other cinchona alkaloids and the salicylates, quinidine can cause cinchonism, which is a condition caused by an overdose of quinine or its natural source, cinchona bark. Symptoms of mild cinchonism include tinnitus, vertigo, headache, dizziness, loss of hearing, slight blurring of vision, and GI upset. Contraindications to the use of the drug include hypersensitivity to it, thrombocytopenic purpura resulting from previous therapy, AV block, intraventricular conduction defects, and abnormal rhythms (proarrhythmic effects such as torsades de pointes). Quinidine is available both in oral and parenteral forms and in three different salt forms. The oral preparations consist of 200- and 325-mg regular-release and 250-mg extended-release quinidine bisulphate tablets. Parenteral quinidine sulphate is available as a 190-mg/mL injection. Parenteral quinidine gluconate is available through the Special Access Programme. Pregnancy category C. Common dosages are listed in the dosages table above.

PHARMACOKINETICS

Half-Life	Onset	Peak	Duration
PO: 6–7 hr	PO: 1–3 hr	PO: 0.5–6 hr	PO: 6–8 hr*

*12-hr sustained-release.

DOSAGES ▶ Selected Antidysrhythmic Agents

Agent	Pharmacological Class	Usual Dosage Range	Indications
adenosine	Unclassified anti-dysrhythmic	**Adult** IV: 6-mg bolus over 1–2 sec; a second rapid bolus of 12 mg as needed (prn), which may be repeated a second time as needed **Pediatric <50 kg** IV: 0.05–0.1 mg/kg rapid bolus	Supraventricular tachy-cardia, conversion to normal sinus rhythm
▶▶amiodarone	Class III antidys-rhythmic	**Adult** IV: 150 mg over 10 min, then 60 mg/hr for 6 hr, then 30 mg/hr as maintenance dose PO: 800–1600 mg/day for 1–3 wk, reduced to 600–800 mg/day for 5 wk; usual maintenance dose 400 mg/day PO: 200–400 mg/day	Ventricular dysrhythmias Atrial dysrhythmias
▶▶atenolol	Beta$_1$-blocker (class II anti-dysrhythmic)	**Adult** IV: 5 mg over 5 min followed by 5 mg over 10 min followed by 50 mg PO 10 min after last IV injection and another 50 mg PO 12 hr later, then 100 mg/day PO for a further 6–9 days	Acute MI
bretylium	Class III antidys-rhythmic	**Adult** IM/IV: 5–10 mg/kg repeated at 5–30 min intervals as needed to a total dose of 30–35 mg/kg	Ventricular dysrhythmias
▶▶diltiazem	Calcium channel blocker	**Adult** IV: Bolus dose 0.25 mg/kg over 2 min, second dose 0.35 mg/kg over 2 min after 15 min as needed, then 5–10 mg/hr or higher by continu-ous infusion	Supraventricular dysrhythmias
disopyramide	Class Ia antidys-rhythmic	**Adult** PO: 400–800 divided daily; LA: 250 mg bid	Ventricular dysrhythmias
esmolol	Beta$_1$-blocker (class II antidys-rhythmic)	**Adult** IV: Bolus dose of 0.5 mg/kg/min for 1 min followed by 4 min of 0.05 mg/kg/min and evaluate	Supraventricular tachyarrhythmias
flecainide	Class Ic antidys-rhythmic	**Adult** PO: 50 mg q12h can be increased by 50 mg bid q4d until desired effect with a daily max of 300 mg for PSVT 100 mg q12h with increment of 50 mg bid q4d as needed; usual dose 150 mg q12h with daily max of 400 mg	Paroxysmal supraven-tricular tachycardia–paroxysmal atrial flutter/fibrillation Sustained ventricular tachycardia
▶▶lidocaine	Class Ib antidys-rhythmic	**Pediatric** IV: Suggested bolus dose, 1 mg/kg; usual main-tenance infusion rate, 20–50 μg/kg/min **Adult** IV: Bolus dose 50–100 mg; may be repeated in 10 min; do not exceed 200–300 mg over 1 hr; usual maintenance infusion rate 1–2 mg/min	Ventricular dysrhythmias Ventricular dysrhythmias
▶▶metoprolol	Beta$_1$-blocker	**Adult** IV/PO: 3 bolus injections of 5 mg at 2-min inter-vals followed by 50 mg PO q6h for 48 hr, thereafter 100 mg bid PO: 100 mg bid	Early MI Late MI

MI, Myocardial infarction.

Continued

DOSAGES Selected Antidysrhythmic Agents—cont'd

Agent	Pharmacological Class	Usual Dosage Range	Indications
mexiletine	Class Ib antidys-rhythmic	**Adult** PO: Start with 200 mg q8h; a minimum of 2–3 days is required between dosage adjustments, which are 50- or 100-mg increments up or down; for rapid control, 400 mg followed by 200 mg in 8 hr; stabilized clients may be put on a 12–hr schedule with a maximum dose of 450 mg q12h	Ventricular dysrhythmias
procainamide	Class Ia antidys-rhythmic	**Adult** PO: initial dose, 1.25 g; 0.75 g in 1 hr; 0.05–1 g q2h until results or tolerance PO: initial dose 1 g; 50 mg/kg divided q3h until results or tolerance SR (maintenance): 50 mg/kg divided q6h doses IV: 20 mg/min (total 17 mg/kg), then maintenance infusion of 1–4 mg/min	Atrial fibrillation, paroxysmal atrial tachycardia Ventricular tachycardia Rapid dysrhythmia control
propafenone	Class Ic antidys-rhythmic	**Adult** PO: Start with loading dose 300 mg; then 100 mg q6h; may increase to 150–200 mg q6h; usual range, 400–800 mg/day 4 divided doses	Ventricular dysrhythmias
▸▸propranolol	Beta-blocker (class II antidys-rhythmic)	**Adult** IV: 1–3 mg; if needed, repeated in 2 min and additional doses as needed q≥4h; switch to PO as soon as possible PO: 60–320 mg/day divided bid–qid	Serious dysrhythmias Angina
quinidine	Class Ia antidys-rhythmic	**Adult** *Bisulphate Durules (0.25 g/Durule)* Test dose in the A.M.; 2 Durules in P.M.; then A.M. 2–3 Durules q12 hr; maintenance 0.5–1.25 g bid *Sulphate* PO: 200 mg q2–3h up to 8 doses with daily increases until sinus rhythm is restored or toxic effects occur 300–400 mg q6h to max 3–4 g IV: 200–300 mg q6–8h or loading dose 12 mg/kg with maintenance dose of 6 mg/kg q4–6h PO: 400–600 mg q 2–3h until effect	Ventricular and supraventrical dysrhythmias Atrial fibrillation or flutter Conversion of atrial fibrillation Premature atrial and ventrical contractions Paroxysmal supraventrical tachycardia
▸▸sotalol	Class II antidys-rhythmic	**Adult** PO: 160–320 mg/day divided into 2 doses	Life-threatening dysrhythmias
▸▸verapamil	Calcium channel blocker (class IV antidysrhythmic)	**Pediatric** IV: ≤1 yr: 0.1–0.2 mg/kg bolus over 2 min; repeat dose after 30 min IV: 1–15 yr: 0.1–0.3 mg/kg bolus over 2 min; do not exceed 5-mg dose; repeat dose not exceeding 10 mg may be given after 30 min **Adult** PO: Start with 80 mg tid–qid; daily range 240–480 mg IV: 5–10 mg bolus over 2 min; repeat dose of 10 mg may be given after 30 min	Supraventricular tachyarrhythmias

CLASS IB DRUGS

Class Ib drugs share many characteristics with class Ia drugs but are grouped together because they act preferentially on ischemic myocardial tissue. They have little effect on conduction velocity in normal tissue. Class Ib agents have a weak depressive effect on phase 0 depolarization, the APD, and the ERP. They include lidocaine and mexiletine. Mexiletine is classified as a pregnancy category C agent and lidocaine is classified as a pregnancy category B agent.

▸▸ *lidocaine*

Lidocaine is the prototypical Ib agent. It is one of the most effective drugs for the treatment of ventricular dysrhythmias, but it can be administered only intravenously because it has an extensive first-pass effect (i.e., when taken orally, the liver metabolizes most of it to inactive metabolites).

Lidocaine exerts its effects on the conduction system of the heart by making it difficult for the ventricles to develop a dysrhythmia, an action called *raising the ventricular fibrillation threshold.* It does this by decreasing the sensitivity of the cardiac cell membrane to impulses and decreasing the cell's ability to depolarize on its own (decreasing automaticity). Many of these effects are accomplished by blockade of fast sodium channels.

Lidocaine is the drug of choice for treating the acute ventricular dysrhythmias associated with MI or during surgery or catheterization. Significant adverse effects include CNS toxicities such as twitching, convulsions, and confusion; respiratory depression or arrest; and the cardiovascular effects of hypotension, bradycardia, and dysrhythmias. It is contraindicated in clients who are hypersensitive to its use, who have severe SA or AV intraventricular block, or who have Stokes-Adams syndrome (syncope triggered by heart block). Lidocaine is available only in parenteral form for intramuscular injection (IM) or intravenous administration. It comes as 10- and 20-mg/mL solutions for intravenous and intramuscular injections. It is also available in dextrose solutions for intravenous use only in 2-, 4-, and 8-mg/mL and 200-, 400-, and 800-mg/100 mL solutions. Pregnancy category B. Common dosages are listed in the dosages table on p. 367.

PHARMACOKINETICS

Half-Life	Onset	Peak	Duration
IV/IM: 8 min, 1–2 hr (terminal)	IV/IM: 45–90 sec	IV/IM: 5–10 min	IV/IM: 10–20 min to 1.5 hr

mexiletine

Mexiletine is structurally and pharmacologically similar to lidocaine, and its effects on the conduction system of the heart are also similar. However, a response to parenteral lidocaine does not predict a response to mexiletine. Mexiletine effectively suppresses premature ventricular contractions (PVCs) in clients suffering from an acute MI, chronic coronary artery disease, or digitalis toxicity and in those undergoing cardiac surgery. It has proved particularly useful when taken in combination with selected class Ia or Ic agents or with beta-blockers.

The most frequent adverse effects are nausea, vomiting, dizziness, and tremor. These reactions are usually not serious, however, and are dose related and minimized by taking the drug with food or an antacid. Contraindications to its use include hypersensitivity, cardiogenic shock, and second- or third-degree AV block. It is available in oral form only as 100- and 200-mg tablets. Pregnancy category C. Common dosages are listed in the table on p. 368.

PHARMACOKINETICS

Half-Life	Onset	Peak	Duration
PO: 12 hr	0.5–2 hr	PO: 2–3 hr	Unknown

CLASS IC DRUGS

Class Ic drugs (flecainide, propafenone) have a more pronounced effect on sodium channel blockade than the Ia and Ib agents but have little effect on repolarization or the APD. These drugs markedly slow conduction in the atria, AV node, and ventricles. Because of their marked effect on conduction, these drugs strongly suppress PVCs, reducing or eliminating them in a large number of clients. All class Ic drugs are classified as pregnancy category C agents.

flecainide

Flecainide is a chemical analogue of procainamide. A large, multi-centre, double-blind, placebo-controlled study called the **Cardiac Arrhythmia Suppression Trial** (CAST Investigators, 1989) was conducted by the National Heart, Lung, and Blood Institute to determine whether the incidence of **sudden cardiac death** could be reduced in post-MI clients with asymptomatic non–life-threatening ectopy (displacement) through the use of flecainide. The findings showed that the mortality and non-fatal cardiac arrest rates in clients treated with this agent were actually comparable with or worse than those seen in clients who received placebo. Because of these findings, Health Canada required that the labelling for flecainide be revised to indicate that its use should be limited to the treatment of documented life-threatening ventricular dysrhythmias such as sustained ventricular tachycardia. Treatment with this agent should be initiated in the hospital. This drug is not indicated for the management of less severe dysrhythmias such as non-sustained ventricular tachycardia or frequent PVCs.

Although flecainide is better tolerated than quinidine or procainamide and is more effective than mexiletine, it is more proarrhythmic. It is this proarrhythmic potential that limits its use to the management of life-threatening dysrhythmias. Flecainide has a negative inotropic effect and depresses LV function. Less serious but more common non-cardiac adverse effects include dizziness, visual disturbances, headache, nausea, chest pain, palpitations, and dyspnea. Contraindications to its use include hypersensitivity, cardiogenic shock, second- or third-degree AV block, and non–life-threatening dysrhythmias. Flecainide is available in oral form as 50- and 100-mg tablets. Pregnancy category C. Common dosages are listed in the table on p. 367.

PHARMACOKINETICS

Half-Life	Onset	Peak	Duration
12–27 hr	30 min	3 hr	3–5 days*

*Therapeutic levels.

propafenone

Propafenone is similar in action to flecainide. It reduces the fast inward sodium current in Purkinje fibres and to a lesser extent in myocardial fibres. Unlike other class I drugs, propafenone has mild beta-blocking effects. This may contribute to its overall effects on the conduction system. It is also believed to have weak beta-blocking and calcium channel blocking effects, which may contribute to its mild negative inotropic effects.

Until recently propafenone's use has been limited to the treatment of documented life-threatening ventricular dysrhythmias such as sustained ventricular tachycardia. Although not officially approved for use in atrial fibrillation in Canada, at low doses it is believed to have benefit for this purpose. Treatment should also be started while the client is in the hospital. Unlike flecainide, however, propafenone can be used in clients with depressed LV function. It may be a better antidysrhythmic agent than disopyramide, procainamide, and quinidine in these clients. However, it should be used with caution in clients with heart failure because it has some beta-blocking properties and dose-dependent negative inotropic effects.

Propafenone is generally well tolerated. The most severe adverse effects are aggravation or induction of arrhythmia (4.7 percent), congestive heart failure (3.7 percent), and ventricular tachycardia (3.4 percent). The most commonly reported adverse reaction is dizziness. Clients may also complain of a metallic taste, constipation, and headache, along with nausea and vomiting. These GI side effects may be reduced by taking propafenone with food. Propafenone is contraindicated in clients with a known hypersensitivity to it and in those with bradycardia, bronchial asthma, significant hypotension, uncontrolled heart failure, cardiogenic shock, or various conduction disorders. It is available in oral form as 150- and 300-mg film-coated tablets. Pregnancy category C. Common dosages are listed in the dosages table on p. 368.

PHARMACOKINETICS

Half-Life	Onset	Peak	Duration
2–10 hr	Unknown	3–5 hr	3–4 days*

*Steady state.

CLASS II DRUGS

Class II antidysrhythmics are also known as *beta-blockers*. These agents work by reducing or blocking SNS stimulation to the heart and the heart's conduction system. By doing this, beta-blockers prevent catecholamine-mediated actions on the heart. The resulting cardiovascular effects include a reduced heart rate, delayed AV node conduction, reduced myocardial contractility, and decreased myocardial automaticity. The pharmacologically induced effects of the beta-blockers are especially beneficial after an MI because of the many catecholamines released at this time, making the heart hyperirritable and predisposed to many types of dysrhythmias. Beta-blockers offer protection from these potentially dangerous complications. Several studies have demonstrated a significant reduction (averaging 25 percent) in the incidence of sudden cardiac death after MI in clients treated with beta-blockers on an ongoing basis.

Although there are several beta-blockers, only a handful are used as antidysrhythmics: acebutolol, esmolol, propranolol, and sotalol (which has class II and III properties). The class II agents are classified as pregnancy category C agents except acebutolol, pindolol, and sotalol, which are all category B agents.

▶▶ atenolol

Atenolol is a cardioselective beta-blocker, which means that it preferentially blocks the beta$_1$-adrenergic receptors that are primarily located on the heart. Non-cardioselective beta-blockers block not only the beta$_1$-adrenergic receptors on the heart but also the beta$_2$-adrenergic receptors in the lungs, and therefore could exacerbate a pre-existing case of asthma or chronic obstructive pulmonary disease (COPD). In addition to having class II antidysrhythmic properties, atenolol is useful in the treatment of hypertension and angina. It is contraindicated in clients with severe bradycardia, second- or third-degree heart block, heart failure, cardiogenic shock, or a known hypersensitivity to it. Atenolol is available in oral form as 25-, 50-, and 100-mg tablets. Pregnancy category C. Common dosages are listed in the dosages table on p. 367.

PHARMACOKINETICS

Half-Life	Onset	Peak	Duration
PO: 6–7 hr	PO: 1 hr	PO: 2–4 hr	PO: ≥24 hr

esmolol

Esmolol is a short-acting beta-blocker with pharmacological and electrophysiological effects on the heart's conduction system similar to those of atenolol. Esmolol is also a cardioselective beta-blocker that primarily and preferentially blocks the beta$_1$-adrenergic receptors on the heart. It is used in the acute treatment of supraventricular tachyarrhythmias or dysrhythmias that originate above the ventricles and are fast instead of slow. It is also used to control hypertension and tachyarrhythmias that develop after an acute MI. Esmolol is contraindicated in clients with a known hypersensitivity to it or in those with hypotension, severe bradycardia, second- or third-degree heart block, heart failure, or cardiogenic shock. Esmolol is available only in parenteral form as a concentrated 250-mg/mL injection for intravenous infusion and a 10-mg/mL intravenous injection. Pregnancy category C. Common dosages are listed in the dosages table on p. 367.

PHARMACOKINETICS

Half-Life	Onset	Peak	Duration
IV: 9 min	IV: Rapid	IV: Rapid	IV: Short

▶ *metoprolol*

Metoprolol is another cardioselective beta-blocker commonly given after an MI to reduce the risk of sudden cardiac death. It is also used in the treatment of hypertension and angina. It is available in oral form as 100- and 200-mg extended-release tablets and as 25-, 50-, and 100-mg regular-release tablets. It is also available as a 1-mg/mL intravenous injection. In the treatment of hypertension it is combined with the thiazide diuretic hydrochlorothiazide in a product called Tenoretic. The contraindications to metoprolol use are the same as those to atenolol and esmolol. Pregnancy category C. Common dosages are listed in the dosages table on p. 367.

PHARMACOKINETICS

Half-Life	Onset	Peak	Duration
PO: 6–7 hr	PO: 1 hr	PO: 2–4 hr	PO: 24 hr

▶ *propranolol*

Propranolol was one of the first beta-blockers introduced into clinical practice, in 1968. It was then primarily used in the treatment of dysrhythmias. Propranolol is a non-specific beta-blocker that blocks both $beta_1$- and $beta_2$-adrenergic receptors on the heart and lungs. Its primary effect on the conduction system of the heart is the blockade of cardiac $beta_1$-adrenergic receptors, thereby preventing catecholamine-mediated stimulation of the heart. The resulting cardiovascular effects are a reduced heart rate, delayed AV node conduction, reduced myocardial contractility, and decreased myocardial automaticity. Propranolol is also believed to have membrane-stabilizing properties that may play a small role in its overall antidysrhythmic effect.

Because propranolol is the oldest of this class of drugs, there are now many indications for its use. Hypertension, angina, supraventricular dysrhythmias, ventricular tachycardia, the tachyarrhythmias associated with cardiac glycoside toxicity, hypertrophic subaortic stenosis, pheochromocytoma, thyrotoxicosis, migraines, post-MI, and essential tremor are just some of its uses. The contraindications to propranolol use are the same as those for atenolol. It is available in both oral and parenteral dosage forms. For oral administration it is available as 60-, 80-, 120-, and 160-mg extended-release capsules and 10-, 20-, 40-, 80-, 90-, and 120-mg tablets. For parenteral administration it is available as a 1-mg/mL injection. Pregnancy category C. Common dosages are listed in the dosages table on p. 368.

PHARMACOKINETICS

Half-Life	Onset	Peak	Duration
3–5 hr	IV: 2 min	IV: 15 min	IV: 3–6 hr
	PO: 30 min	PO: 1–1.5 hr	PO: 8–11 hr
	LA: 1–1.5 hr	LA: 6 hr	LA: 24 hr

▶ *sotalol*

Sotalol is another nonselective beta-blocker used to treat dysrhythmias. It is unique in that it possesses antidysrhythmic properties similar to those of the class III agents (such as amiodarone) while simultaneously exerting beta-blocker or class II effects on the conduction system of the heart. In addition, sotalol has pro-arrhythmic properties similar to those of the class Ic agents. This means that it can cause serious dysrhythmias such as torsades de pointes or a new ventricular tachycardia or fibrillation. For this reason, sotalol is usually reserved for the treatment of documented life-threatening ventricular dysrhythmias such as sustained ventricular tachycardia.

Contraindications to sotalol use include hypersensitivity to it, bronchial asthma, cardiogenic shock, and sinus bradycardia. Sotalol is available only in oral form as 80-, 160-, and 240-mg tablets. Pregnancy category C. Common dosages are listed in the dosages table on p. 368.

PHARMACOKINETICS

Half-Life	Onset	Peak	Duration
PO: 10–20 hr	PO: 1–2 hr	PO: 2.5–4 hr	PO: 12–24 hr

CLASS III DRUGS

Class III agents include amiodarone and bretylium. Amiodarone and bretylium control dysrhythmias by inhibiting repolarization and markedly prolonging refractoriness and the APD. Amiodarone and bretylium are indicated for the management of life-threatening ventricular tachycardia or ventricular fibrillation that is resistant to other drug therapy. Amiodarone and bretylium have also been effective in the treatment of sustained ventricular tachycardias. Amiodarone has recently been used more frequently to treat atrial dysrhythmias as well.

▶ *amiodarone*

Amiodarone markedly prolongs the APD and the ERP in all cardiac tissues. Besides these dramatic effects, it is also known to block both the alpha- and beta-adrenergic receptors of the SNS. Clinically it is one of the most effective antidysrhythmic agents for controlling supraventricular and ventricular dysrhythmias. It is indicated for the management of sustained ventricular tachycardia, ventricular fibrillation, and non-sustained ventricular tachycardia. Recently it has shown promise in the management of treatment-resistant atrial dysrhythmias. The results of the Canadian Amiodarone Myocardial Infarction Arrhythmia Trial (CAMIAT) (Cairns et al., 1997) and the European Myocardial Infarction Amiodarone Trial (EMIAT) (Julian et al, 1997), two large randomized, placebo-controlled, double-blind trials of amiodarone, along with some smaller controlled studies, showed an approximately 50 percent reduction of mortality two years post-MI using amiodarone.

However, amiodarone has many adverse effects attributable to its chemical properties. Amiodarone is lipophilic, or "fat loving." Therefore it can penetrate and concentrate in the adipose tissue of any organ in the body, where it may cause unwanted effects. It also has iodine in its chemical structure. One organ that sequesters iodine from the diet is the thyroid gland. As a result, amiodarone can cause either hypothyroidism or hyperthyroidism. Adverse reactions occur in approximately 75 percent of clients treated with this agent, but are more common and more severe when given at doses exceeding 400 mg/day over a prolonged period. The most common reaction is corneal microdeposits, which may cause visual halos, photophobia, and dry eyes. This occurs in virtually all adults who take the drug for more than 6 months.

The most serious adverse effect is pulmonary toxicity, which is fatal in about 10 percent of clients and involves a clinical syndrome of progressive dyspnea and cough accompanied by damage to the alveoli. The result can be pulmonary fibrosis. Another serious complication is that it may actually provoke dysrhythmias. Cirrhotic hepatitis is another potential adverse effect.

Amiodarone has an exceptionally long half-life, approaching many days. As a result, the therapeutic as well as any adverse effects of amiodarone may linger long after the drug has been discontinued. In fact, it may take as long as 2 to 3 months after the drug has been discontinued for some side effects to subside. For all these reasons, although it is effective, amiodarone is typically considered a drug of last resort. Therapy is usually started in the hospital and is closely monitored until the serum levels are within a therapeutic range.

Amiodarone is contraindicated in clients who have a known hypersensitivity to it and in those with severe sinus bradycardia, cardiogenic shock, or second- or third-degree heart block. Amiodarone is available in oral form as a 200-mg tablet and in a parenteral formulation in ampoules containing 3, 6, 9, and 18 mL of a 50-mg/mL solution. If long-term, orally administered amiodarone is indicated after IV administration, there are recommended conversions (see Table 22-7). Pregnancy category D. Common dosages are listed in the table on p. 367.

PHARMACOKINETICS

Half-Life	Onset	Peak	Duration
PO: 26–107 days	PO: 1–3 wk	PO: 3–12 hr	PO: 10–150 days

TABLE 22-7

RECOMMENDATIONS FOR ORAL DOSAGE AFTER IV INFUSION OF AMIODARONE

Duration of Amiodarone IV Infusion	Initial Daily Dose of Oral Amiodarone
<1 wk	800–1600 mg
1–3 wk	600–800 mg
>3 wk	400 mg

bretylium

Bretylium was initially marketed as an antihypertensive agent, but its effects on the conduction system were soon noted. It has both a direct and an indirect effect on cardiac conduction. The direct effect prolongs the APD of the Purkinje fibres and ventricular myocardium and the ERP. The indirect effect is due to an adrenergic-blocking effect, in that bretylium accumulates in the nerve endings of the SNS, where it displaces norepinephrine. This results in a short-term rise in blood pressure (BP); however, after this the further release of norepinephrine is blocked and ultimately the reuptake of norepinephrine is inhibited.

Bretylium is available only in parenteral form. It is used for the treatment of serious dysrhythmias such as life-threatening ventricular tachycardia or fibrillation. Therefore bretylium is most commonly used in intensive care unit settings and cardiac codes in clients who do not respond to lidocaine, quinidine, procainamide, or disopyramide treatment. This drug is rapidly falling into disuse, however, and does not appear on the latest Advanced Cardiac Life Support (ACLS) resuscitation guidelines. The major adverse effect associated with its use is postural hypotension, occurring in about 50 percent of clients. Other common side effects include nausea and vomiting. However, all of these side effects can be reduced by administering it by slow intravenous infusion. Bretylium is contraindicated in clients with a known hypersensitivity to it. It is available as 2- and 4-mg/mL injections for intravenous infusion and as a 50-mg/mL bolus injection. Pregnancy category C. Common dosages are listed in the dosages table on p. 367.

PHARMACOKINETICS

Half-Life	Onset	Peak	Duration
4–17 hr	6–20 min	IV: Rapid (<1 hr)	IV: 6–24 hr

CLASS IV DRUGS

Class IV antidysrhythmic drugs are CCBs. Although there are more than nine such agents currently available, only a few are commonly used as antidysrhythmics. Besides their effectiveness as antidysrhythmics, CCBs are effective in the treatment of hypertension and angina. Verapamil and diltiazem are the most commonly used CCBs to treat dysrhythmias, specifically those that arise above the ventricles (paroxysmal supraventricular tachycardia [PSVT]). They are also used to control the ventricular response to atrial fibrillation and flutter by slowing conduction and prolonging refractoriness of the AV node (i.e., not allowing the ventricles to beat as fast).

These agents block the slow inward flow of calcium ions into the slow (calcium) channels in cardiac conduction tissue. The conduction effects of these agents are limited to the atria and the AV node, where conduction is prolonged and the tissues are made more refractory to stimulation. These agents have little effect on the ventricular tissues.

▶▶ *diltiazem*

Diltiazem is primarily indicated for the temporary control of a rapid ventricular response in a client with atrial fibrillation or flutter and PSVT. Its use is contraindicated in clients with hypersensitivity, acute MI, pulmonary congestion, Wolff-Parkinson-White syndrome (a congenital abnormality associated with supraventricular tachycardia), severe hypotension, cardiogenic shock, sick sinus syndrome, or second- or third-degree AV block. Diltiazem is available in both oral and parenteral forms. In oral form it is available as 30- and 60-mg tablets usually taken 4 times a day; 60-, 90-, 120-, 180-, 240-, 300-, and 360-mg sustained-release, twice-a-day capsules; 120-, 180-, 240-, and 300-mg controlled delivery once-a-day capsules; and 120-, 180-, 240-, 300-, and 360-mg extended-release once-a-day tablets. In parenteral form it is available as a 5-mg/mL injection. Pregnancy category C. Common dosages are listed in the dosages table on p. 367.

PHARMACOKINETICS

Half-Life	Onset	Peak	Duration
PO: 3.5–6 hr	PO: 0.5–1 hr	2–4 hr	PO: 4–8 hr 12 hr*

*For extended-release product.

▶▶ *verapamil*

Verapamil has actions similar to those of diltiazem in that it also inhibits calcium ion influx across the slow calcium channels in cardiac conduction tissue. This results in dramatic effects on the AV node. Verapamil is used to prevent and convert recurrent PSVT and to control ventricular response in atrial flutter or fibrillation. It can also temporarily control a rapid ventricular response to these frequent atrial stimulations, usually decreasing the heart rate by at least 20 percent. Besides its use for the management of various dysrhythmias, verapamil is also used to treat angina, hypertension, and hypertrophic cardiomyopathy. The contraindications that apply to diltiazem apply to verapamil as well, and it is also available in both oral and parenteral forms. In oral form it is available as 80- and 120-mg film-coated tablets and 120-, 180-, and 240-mg extended-release capsules. In parenteral form it is available as a 2.5-mg/mL injection for intravenous administration. Pregnancy category C. Common dosages are listed in the dosages table on p. 368.

PHARMACOKINETICS

Half-Life	Onset	Peak	Duration
PO: 2.8–7.4 hr	PO: 30 min	PO: 1–2 hr	PO: 6–8 hr
IV: 2–5 hr	IV: 1–2 min	IV: 3–5 min	IV: 10–60 min

UNCLASSIFIED ANTIDYSRHYTHMICS
adenosine

Adenosine is a naturally occurring nucleoside that slows the electrical conduction time through the AV node and is indicated for the conversion of PSVT to sinus rhythm. It is particularly useful for the treatment of PSVT that has failed to respond to verapamil or when a client has coexisting conditions such as heart failure, hypotension, or LV dysfunction that limit the use of verapamil. It is contraindicated in clients with second- or third-degree heart block, sick sinus syndrome, bradycardia, atrial flutter or fibrillation, or ventricular tachycardia, as well as in those with a known hypersensitivity to it. It has an extremely short half-life of less than 10 seconds. For this reason, it is only administered intravenously and only as a fast intravenous push. It commonly causes asystole for a period of seconds. All other side effects are minimal because of its short duration of action. It is only available in parenteral form as a 3-mg/mL injection. Pregnancy category C. Common dosages are listed in the dosages table on p. 367.

PHARMACOKINETICS

Half-Life	Onset	Peak	Duration
<10 sec	1 min	Immediate	1–2 min

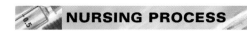

NURSING PROCESS

■ Assessment

Before administering any class I antidysrhythmics to a client, the nurse must obtain a thorough drug and medical history. Contraindications to the administration of these drugs include the following:

- Cardiogenic shock
- Heart failure
- Complete heart block
- Congenitally prolonged QT interval (class Ia agents)
- Hepatic or renal insufficiency
- Hypersensitivity to the local anaesthetic lidocaine
- Hypokalemia (class Ic agent)
- Hypotension
- Known hypersensitivity
- Myasthenia gravis
- Second- or third-degree heart block
- Urinary retention

Class Ia agents should be administered cautiously in clients with electrolyte imbalances, especially hypokalemia. Class Ib agents should be administered cautiously in geriatric clients and in clients with hepatic or renal disease, heart failure, bradycardia, or a markedly altered urinary pH (affects excretion) and in those who weigh less than 50 kg. The cautious administration of class Ic agents is required in clients with severe renal or liver disease, heart failure, prolonged QT intervals, and blood dyscrasias. The following are some of the drugs that interact with all class I antidysrhythmics:

- Anticholinergic drugs, which result in an increased anticholinergic effect
- Anticonvulsants, which interact with quinidine or disopyramide, resulting in increased metabolism of these antidysrhythmics

- Cimetidine, which interacts with procainamide, resulting in increased levels of the procainamide
- Cimetidine, which interacts with quinidine, resulting in increased serum quinidine
- Coumadin anticoagulants, which interact with quinidine, resulting in hypothrombinemia
- Digoxin and quinidine, which result in increased serum digoxin levels
- Neuromuscular blockers, which interact with quinidine, procainamide, and disopyramide, resulting in increased skeletal muscle relaxation
- Nifedipine, which interacts with quinidine, resulting in decreased serum quinidine levels

In addition, an increased urinary pH causes the serum levels of quinidine to be elevated. Class Ib antidysrhythmic drugs interact with other antidysrhythmics and with lidocaine. Lidocaine toxicity may result from the concurrent administration of propranolol or cimetidine. Class Ic agents interact with digoxin (which leads to an increase in serum digoxin levels and digoxin toxicity) and with flecainide and alkalinizing drugs (which leads to a decrease in the urinary excretion of flecainide). (See Table 22-6.)

Before administering any class II antidysrhythmics, the nurse needs to obtain a thorough drug and medical history. Contraindications to the administration of these drugs include a known hypersensitivity to them, asthma and other forms of COPD, sinus bradycardia, second- or third-degree heart block, diabetes mellitus, and peripheral vascular disease. Drugs that interact with the class II agents propranolol and acebutolol hydrochloride include phenothiazines and antihypertensive agents, with hypotension the effect. Propranolol also interacts with cimetidine, resulting in decreased metabolism of the propranolol.

Before administering either of the class III antidysrhythmic agents bretylium and amiodarone, the nurse should collect data regarding the client's medication history, present and past medical history, drug allergies, and specific laboratory test results. A thorough assessment is crucial to the safe use of these antidysrhythmics because of potentially severe adverse reactions. Because of these adverse reactions, they are not the first choice for antidysrhythmic therapy. Amiodarone must be administered cautiously in clients who have pre-existing bradycardia, conduction or sinus node disorders, severely depressed or compromised ventricular function, or marked cardiomegaly. Bretylium must be administered cautiously in clients with aortic stenosis, pulmonary hypertension, or digitalis-induced dysrhythmias. Drug interactions with these agents include digoxin, which results in increased digoxin levels, and warfarin, which results in increased clotting times with hypoprothrombinemia.

With class IV antidysrhythmic agents such as verapamil and diltiazem, the nurse should collect data on the client's medication history, present and past medical history, drug allergies, and specific laboratory results.

Cautious administration of these agents is warranted in clients with hypotension, heart failure, sick sinus syndrome, AV conduction disturbances, or hepatic impairment. Indications for their use include PSVT with rapid ventricular response rates. Drugs that interact with these agents include other antidysrhythmics and antihypertensive agents, which enhance the risk of hypotension and heart failure; digoxin, which increases the digoxin levels and causes digitalis toxicity; and highly protein-bound drugs such as hydantoin, acetylsalicylic acid, sulphonamide antibiotics, and sulphonylureas, which result in the adverse effects of verapamil, diltiazem, or the other medication.

Nursing Diagnoses

Nursing diagnoses related to the administration of antidysrhythmics include the following:
- Ineffective tissue perfusion related to the impact of the dysrhythmia.
- Risk for injury related to side effects of the medications.
- Deficient knowledge related to disease and medication therapy.
- Impaired gas exchange (decreased) related to adverse reaction to the medications.
- Diarrhea related to adverse reaction to the medications.
- Disturbed body image related to changes in lifestyle and sexual functioning due to side effects of the medications and impact of the disease process.

Planning

Therapeutic goals appropriate for clients receiving antidysrhythmic agents include the following:
- Client is free of further symptoms related to cardiac dysrhythmias once therapy is initiated.
- Client has improved tolerance to activity and improved general sense of well-being.
- Client is free of complications associated with nonadherence or with sudden withdrawal of medication.
- Client reports any increase in the symptoms of the dysrhythmia.
- Client demonstrates adequate knowledge of drug therapy and its side effects.

Outcome Criteria

Outcome criteria for clients receiving antidysrhythmics include the following:
- Client's dysrhythmia symptoms such as shortness of breath and chest pain are alleviated by the medication therapy.
- Client exhibits signs and symptoms of improved cardiac output, as evidenced by regular apical and radial pulses; vital signs within normal limits; and a decrease in weight, edema, crackles, and shortness of breath.
- Client states the importance of adhering with the medication regimen and of coming in for follow-up visits

with the physician (i.e., decreasing complications and manifestations of dysrhythmias).

- Client states the common side effects of the medication, such as constipation and dry mouth.

▨ Implementation

The administration of class I antidysrhythmics requires some specific nursing interventions. Initially the ECG and vital signs must be monitored closely because if the QT interval is prolonged by more than 50 percent, a variety of conduction disturbances may be precipitated. An intravenous pump is needed when administering procainamide intravenously. When switching from intravenous to oral forms, the infusion should be continued for 2 hours after the start of the oral agent, or as prescribed. Solutions of lidocaine containing epinephrine should not be used except as a local anaesthetic.

The administration of any of the class II and III antidysrhythmics also requires some specific nursing interventions. Initially the ECG and vital signs should be closely monitored because of the adverse cardiovascular effects they can precipitate, such as hypotension, bradycardia, and heart blocks. These problems usually occur when the drug is first given. Clients taking propranolol should be cautioned to report the appearance of any shortness of breath, edema, or skin rash. If the parenteral solution of any of these drugs appears discoloured, it should be discarded. Intravenous solutions should be administered over a 3-minute period or as per manufacturer guidelines—especially in geriatric clients—to minimize the risk of adverse effects. Clients should also be cautioned not to skip doses. Class III agents require cautious use, and BP and pulse rates must be checked because of side effects (especially with bretylium). The nurse should encourage the use of sun protection because of increased photosensitivity and be sure to have baseline data on the condition of the corneas and thyroid.

As with the remaining classes of antidysrhythmics, specific nursing interventions are required for class IV antidysrhythmics. Clients who are receiving such an agent initially or are having their doses altered must be monitored by ECG. In addition, BP and other vital signs need to be monitored frequently. Intravenous bolus doses should usually be administered over a 2-minute period, but should be administered over 3 minutes in geriatric clients to minimize adverse effects. It is crucial to remember that verapamil and beta-blockers cannot be administered intravenously at the same time or within a few hours of each other.

See the box on p. 376 for client teaching tips for antidysrhythmic agents.

▨ Evaluation

It is important to monitor clients receiving any class of antidysrhythmics to identify both therapeutic and adverse or toxic effects.

- *Class I:* Therapeutic effects include improved cardiac output; decreased chest discomfort; decreased fatigue; improved vital signs, skin colour, and urinary output; and improvement in irregularities to normal rhythm. Adverse effects include bradycardia, dizziness, headache, cinchonism, chest pain, heart failure, and peripheral edema. Toxic effects range from cardiac failure and bradycardia to CNS-related effects such as confusion or convulsions.
- *Class II:* Therapeutic effects include improved cardiac output; decreased chest discomfort; decreased fatigue; regular pulse rate or improvement in irregularities; and improved vital signs, skin colour, and urinary output. Adverse effects include bradycardia, dizziness, headache, and peripheral edema. Toxic effects consist of cardiac failure, bradycardia, bronchospasms, hypotension, and conduction problems.
- *Class III:* Therapeutic effects include improved cardiac output; more regular rhythm; decreased chest discomfort; decreased fatigue; and improved vital signs, skin colour, and urinary output. Adverse effects include peripheral neuropathies, extrapyramidal symptoms, headache, fatigue, lethargy, dizziness (bretylium use only), bradycardia, hypotension, dysrhythmias, severe orthostatic hypotension (bretylium use only), microdeposits on the cornea with visual disturbances, hypothyroidism or hyperthyroidism, nausea, vomiting, constipation, hepatic dysfunction with abnormal liver enzyme activity, electrolyte imbalances, photosensitivity, blue-grey skin colour, severe pulmonary changes with development of pneumonitis, alveolitis with high doses, pulmonary fibrosis, and pulmonary muscle weakness. The client's thyroid function should be monitored carefully during therapy so that abnormal function can be identified before any further adverse

COMMUNITY HEALTH POINTS

Antidysrhythmic Agents

- Clients taking antidysrhythmics at home need to be closely monitored by the community health nurse or by the physician or other healthcare provider. This should include frequent measurements of the blood levels of the medication and frequent monitoring of the BP and pulse. These measures are important, especially in geriatric clients, because of the toxic effects these agents can have.
- Client education is important because of the seriousness of the disease, the toxic effects of the medicines, and the risks of polypharmacy. Clients should be given as much reference material as possible: pamphlets, posters, journals, and other printed, video, or audio materials are often available free from pharmaceutical companies.
- The nurse should ensure that clients know to notify their physician or other healthcare provider of any worsening of their dysrhythmia and any shortness of breath, edema, chest pain, dizziness, or syncope. They should also know to report any adverse reactions or possible signs of toxicity of the particular agent they are taking.

effects appear. Toxic effects include hypotension or hypertension and bradycardia.

* *Class IV:* Therapeutic effects include improved cardiac output; decreased chest discomfort; decreased fatigue; and improved vital signs, skin colour, and urinary output. Adverse effects include bradycardia, heart failure, hypotension, AV conduction disorders, ventricular asystole, peripheral edema, and constipation. Toxic effects include hypotension, bradycardia, heart failure, and conduction disorders.

CLIENT TEACHING TIPS

Nurses should teach clients the following:

▲ This medicine must be taken cautiously. Do not skip doses, but if you do miss a dose, don't double up. Contact your physician if you miss a dose and aren't sure what to do.

▲ Don't crush or chew any of the oral sustained-release preparations. Don't be concerned if you notice portions of a tablet or capsule in your stool. This is usually just the wax matrix of the preparation; the medication has probably been extracted.

▲ Class I antidysrhythmics:
* (For Class Ia agents) You may experience ringing of the ears, dryness of the mouth, constipation, upset stomach, headache, fever, lightheadedness, or blurred vision. Report any of these signs. Overdose can cause you to faint or can make your heartbeat or breathing stop. Therefore, you need to take these drugs carefully, and keep track with a calendar or pillbox.
* (For Class Ib agents) You may experience confusion, tremors (shakiness), convulsions, lightheadedness, hypotension, dizziness, tinnitus, double vision, lethargy, and sensations of cold. Report any of these signs.
* (For Class Ic agents) You may experience dizziness, headaches, fatigue, shakiness, stomach upset, swelling, or chest pain. Report these signs. Report at once if you experience a slow heartbeat or heart failure. Heart failure can be recognized by shortness of breath, lethargy, less urination, swelling of feet, and weight gain of 1 kg (2 lb) or more in a week.

▲ Class II antidysrhythmics:
* Report to your physician if you experience increased lethargy and shortness of breath, swelling, a weight gain of 1 kg (2 lb) or more in a week, cough, decreased urinary output, dizziness, fainting spells, or heart palpitations.
* Take oral propranolol hydrochloride before meals and at bedtime, as ordered by the physician (i.e., if taken 3 to 4 times/day). Before taking the drug, always take your pulse at the wrist for 1 full minute. If the pulse is less than 60 beats per minute, notify your physician.

▲ Class III antidysrhythmics:
* Use sunscreen products when out in the sun because this medication makes you more likely to sunburn. Report any unusual tingling of the skin that is followed by blistering or reddened skin.
* (For amiodarone) Contact your physician if you experience either of the following patterns: lethargy, weight gain, cool and dry skin, slow heartbeat, low blood pressure, and/or intolerance to cold; or nervousness, palpitations, weight loss, warm and moist skin, and/or fast heartbeat.
* You may experience some of the following side effects: numbness and tingling of the hands and feet, uncontrolled shaking of the head and hands, headache, weakness, fatigue and loss of energy, dizziness, fainting spells (especially when going from lying to standing or sitting to standing or with sudden position changes such as stooping over), vision problems, nausea, vomiting, constipation, sunburn, blue-grey skin, or cough. Report any of these signs.

▲ Class IV antidysrhythmics:
* Make sure your physician knows about all other drugs you are taking. Do not take any over-the-counter drugs without checking with your physician, especially those containing ASA (Aspirin). If you need a prescription for an infection, make sure the physician knows that you are taking this medication.
* If you are taking diltiazem, you may experience dizziness, fatigue, headache, low blood pressure for a while, or constipation. Report any of these signs. Report immediately if you experience palpitations, skipped heartbeat, low blood pressure, slow heartbeat, or heart failure. Heart failure can be recognized by swelling, shortness of breath, cough, palpitations, less urination, and lethargy.

POINTS to REMEMBER

▼ The SA node, AV node, and bundle of His–Purkinje cells are all areas where there is automaticity (cells can depolarize spontaneously). The SA node is the pacemaker because it can spontaneously depolarize more easily and quickly than the others.

▼ Any disturbance or abnormality in the pattern of the heartbeat/pulse rate is termed a *dysrhythmia*. In the past, the term *arrhythmia* was used, but it properly means "without rhythm." The term *dysrhythmia* is more accurate for abnormal rhythms, but some sources use these terms interchangeably.

▼ Antidysrhythmic drugs are used to correct dysrhythmias; however, they may also cause dysrhythmias and for this reason are called *prodysrhythmic*. The Vaughan Williams classification system is most commonly used to classify antidysrhythmic drugs. Groups of drugs are classified according to where and how they affect cardiac cells and by their mechanisms of action:
  • *Class I:* Membrane-stabilizing agents (e.g., class Ia: quinidine; class Ib: lidocaine; class Ic: flecainide)
  • *Class II:* Beta-adrenergic blockers depress phase 4 depolarization (e.g., propranolol)
  • *Class III:* Prolong repolarization in phase 3 (e.g., bretylium, amiodarone, and sotalol)
  • *Class IV:* Depress phase 4 depolarization and prolong repolarization of phases 1 and 2 (e.g., CCBs such as verapamil)

▼ Nursing considerations for the various classes of antidysrhythmics include astute nursing assessment and close monitoring. Close monitoring generally requires ECGs, but it is also important to check heart rate, BP, heart rhythms, general well-being, skin colour, temperature, and heart and breath sounds. It is important to assess the plasma drug levels. Before using these agents, it is important to check for possible drug interactions and certain medical conditions and to measure serum potassium levels.

▼ The therapeutic response to antidysrhythmics includes a decrease in BP in hypertensive clients, a decrease in edema, and a regular (or more regular) pulse rate.

▼ Client education is important for safe and effective therapy; clients must understand the dosage schedule and the side effects they should report.

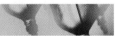

EXAMINATION REVIEW QUESTIONS

1 Which of the following should be reported immediately to the community health nurse for an 82-year-old client with heart failure who is taking oral procainamide?
  a. Rectal temperature of 38°C
  b. Mild nausea
  c. Muscle tetany
  d. Ventricular irregularities

2 Which of the following is a possible adverse reaction associated with procainamide?
  a. Glycosuria
  b. Dysphagia
  c. Leukopenia
  d. Hypothermia

3 Side effects associated with the use of quinidine include which of the following?
  a. Colitis
  b. Tinnitus
  c. Atrial ectopy
  d. Excessive thirst

4 Which of the following nursing interventions would be most appropriate for clients taking antidysrhythmics?
  a. Use of intravenous pumps at high drip rates might be used to avoid extravasation.
  b. Excess fluid volume should be encouraged to prevent conduction problems.
  c. Remember to use lidocaine with epinephrine.
  d. Intravenous solutions should be properly concentrated according to manufacturer guidelines.

5 Which of the following are contraindications for use of class I antidysrhythmics?
  a. Hyperkalemia
  b. Hypertension
  c. Incontinence
  d. Renal dysfunction

For answers see http://evolve.elsevier.com/Lilley/pharmacology/.

CRITICAL THINKING ACTIVITIES

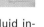

1 Mr. K. is a 68-year-old man who underwent coronary artery bypass grafting yesterday. He has developed some irregular heartbeats (dysrhythmias) and has been put on procainamide, infused at a rate of 4 mg/min. The nephrologist is concerned about the total volume the client is receiving because his urine output is low. He asks you to determine how much fluid per day Mr. K. is receiving from his procainamide infusion. The standard procainamide concentration at your hospital is 1 mg/mL.
  a. How many millilitres of fluid per day is Mr. K. receiving from his procainamide infusion?
  b. The nephrologist would like to keep Mr. K.'s fluid intake to less than 1000 mL/day. What concentration will accomplish this: 1, 2, 4, or 8 mg/mL?

2 What therapeutic response would you expect in a client prescribed a diuretic and antidysrhythmic to treat heart failure? Explain your answer.

3 Mrs. L. has been discharged to home on quinidine for the treatment of ventricular ectopy. What instructions are crucial for her to understand before her discharge?

4 Amiodarone has many precautions associated with its use. Discuss problems that you would warn your client about, especially in the summer in hot climates.

For answers see http://evolve.elsevier.com/Lilley/pharmacology/.

BIBLIOGRAPHY

Abrahams, P.H., Marks, S.C., & Hutchings, R. (2003). *McMinn's color atlas of human anatomy*. Philadelphia: Mosby.

Albanese, J., & Nutz, P. (2005). *Mosby's 2005 nursing drug cards.* St Louis, MO: Mosby.

Berne, R., & Levy, M. (2002). *Principles of physiology* (3rd ed.). St Louis, MO: Mosby.

Boron, W.F., & Boulpaep, E.L. (2003). *Medical physiology*. Philadelphia: Saunders.

Cairns, J.A., Connolly, S.J., Roberts, R.S., & Gent, M. for the Canadian Amiodarone Myocardial Infarction Arrhythmia Trial Investigators. (1997). Randomized trial of outcome after myocardial infarction in patients with frequent or repetitive premature depolarisations: CAMIAT. *Lancet, 349*, 675–82.

Canadian Pharmacists Association. *Therapeutic choices* (4th ed.). Ottawa, ON: Author.

Canadian Pharmacists Association. (2004). *Guide to drugs in Canada.* Toronto, ON: Dorling Kindersley.

Canadian Pharmacists Association. (2005). *Compendium of pharmaceuticals and specialties. The Canadian drug reference for health professionals.* Ottawa, ON: Author. [The subscription-based e-CPS is available at http://www.pharmacists.ca.]

Cardiac Arrhythmia Suppression Trial (CAST) Investigators. (1989). Preliminary report of the Cardiac Arrhythmia Suppression Trial (CAST): Effect of encainide and flecainide on mortality in a randomized trial of arrhythmia suppression after myocardial infarction. *New England Journal of Medicine, 321*(6), 406–412.

Facts and Comparisons. (2004). *Drug facts and comparisons pocket version* (9th ed.). St Louis, MO: Wolters Kluwer Health.

Gillis, A. (2001). Management of cardiac arrhythmias. [Electronic version]. *The Canadian Journal of CME*, 167–179. Retrieved August 26, 2005, from http://www.stacommunications.com/journals/cme/images/cmepdf/oct01/arrhythmia.pdf

Goldberger, J.J. (2000). Therapeutic developments in sudden cardiac death. *Expert Opinion on Investigational Drugs, 9*(11), 2543–2554.

Hardman, J.G., & Limbird, L.E. (2002). *Goodman and Gilman's the pharmacological basis of therapeutics* (10th ed.). New York: McGraw-Hill.

Haugh, K.H. (2002). Antidysrhythmic agents at the turn of the twenty-first century: A current review. *Critical Care Nursing Clinics North America, 14*(1), 53–69.

Health Canada. (2005). Drug product database (DPD). Retrieved August 8, 2005, from http://www.hc-sc.gc.ca/hpb/drugs-dpd/

Heart and Stroke Foundation of Canada. (2000). *Advanced cardiac life support guidelines.* Retrieved August 8, 2005, from http://209.5.25.171/ClientImages/1/Guidelines%20ACLS%202000.pdf

Heart and Stroke Foundation of Canada. (2000). Guidelines 2000 pediatrics. Retrieved August 8, 2005, from http://209.5.25.171/ClientImages/1/Guidelines_PALS_NRP_2000.pdf

Humphries, K.H., Kerr, C.R., Steinbuch, M., Dorian, P., & The Canadian Registry of Atrial Fibrillation (CARAF) Investigators. (2004). Limitations to anti-arrhythmic drug use in patients with atrial fibrillation. [Electronic version]. *Canadian Medical Association Journal, 171*(7), 752–753.

Joglar, J.A. (2001). Antiarrhythmic drugs in pregnancy. *Current Opinion in Cardiology, 16*(1), 40–45.

Johns Hopkins Hospital, Gunn, V.L., & Nechyba, C. (2002). *The Harriet Lane handbook* (17th ed.). St Louis, MO: Mosby.

Julian, D.G., Camm, A.J., Frangin, G., Janse, M.J., Schwartz, P.J., & Simon, P. (1997). Randomised trial of effect of amiodarone on mortality in patients with left-ventricular dysfunction after recent myocardial infarction: EMIAT. European Myocardial Infarct Amiodarone Trial Investigators. *Lancet, 349*(9053), 667–674.

Lacy, C.F., Armstrong, L.L., Goldman, M.P., & Lance, L.L. (2003). *Drug information handbook* (11th ed.). Hudson, OH: Lexi-Comp.

Lehne, R.A. (2004). *Pharmacology for nursing care* (5th ed.). St Louis, MO: Saunders.

Mancini, M.E., & Kaye, W. (1999). AEDs: Changing the way you respond to cardiac arrest. *American Journal of Nursing, 99*(5), 26.

Mosby. (2005). *Mosby's drug consult 2005: The comprehensive reference for generic and brand name drugs* (15th ed.). St Louis, MO: Mosby.

Naccarella F., Naccarelli, G.V., Maranga, S.S., Lepera, G., Grippo, M.C., Melandri, F., et al. (2002). Do ACE inhibitors or angiotensin II antagonists reduce total mortality and arrhythmic mortality? A critical review of controlled clinical trials. *Current Opinion in Cardiology, 17*(1), 6–18.

Sager, P.T. (2001). New advances in Class III antiarrhythmic drug therapy. *Current Opinion in Cardiology, 15*(1), 41–53.

Skidmore-Roth, L. (2006). *Mosby's 2006 nursing drug reference* (19th ed.). St Louis, MO: Mosby.

Tierney, L.M., McPhee, S.J., & Papadakis, M.A. (2002). *2002 Current medical diagnosis and treatment: Adult ambulatory and inpatient management.* New York: McGraw-Hill.

Woods, S.L., Sivarajan Froelocher, E.S., Underhill Motzer, S., & Bridges, E.J. (2005). *Cardiac nursing* (5th ed.). Philadelphia: Lippincott Williams & Wilkins.

Anti-Anginal Agents

OBJECTIVES

After reading this chapter, the successful student will be able to do the following:

1 Summarize the pathophysiology related to myocardial ischemia.

2 Explain how cellular ischemia is responsible for causing angina, including the precipitating factors and measures that decrease its occurrence.

3 Contrast the various anti-anginals, such as nitrates, beta-blockers, and calcium channel blockers in regard to their mechanisms of action, dosage forms, routes of administration, cautions, contraindications, side effects, tolerance, and toxicity.

4 Develop a nursing care plan related to nursing process and the administration of any of the anti-anginals, such as nitrates, beta-blockers, and calcium channel blockers.

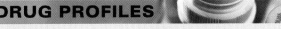

e-LEARNING ACTIVITIES

Student CD-ROM
- Review Questions: see questions 142–159
- Animations
- Medication Administration Checklists
- IV Therapy Checklists

evolve Web site (http://evolve.elsevier.com/Lilley/pharmacology/)
- Online Chapter Worksheet • Frequently Asked Questions
- Learning Tips and Content Updates • WebLinks • Online Appendices and Supplements • Mosby/Saunders ePharmacology Update • Access to *Mosby's Drug Consult*

DRUG PROFILES

▸▸ **atenolol,** p. 385
▸▸ **diltiazem,** p. 387
▸▸ **isosorbide dinitrate,** p. 382
▸▸ **isosorbide mononitrate,** p. 382

▸▸ **metoprolol,** p. 385
▸▸ **nifedipine,** p. 387
▸▸ **nitroglycerine,** p. 383
▸▸ **verapamil,** p. 387

▸▸ Key drug.

GLOSSARY

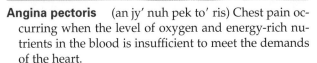

Angina pectoris (an jy' nuh pek to' ris) Chest pain occurring when the level of oxygen and energy-rich nutrients in the blood is insufficient to meet the demands of the heart.

Chronic stable angina Chest pain that has atherosclerosis as its primary cause, resulting in a long-term but relatively stable level of obstruction in one or more coronary arteries.

Coronary arteries Arteries that deliver oxygen to the heart muscle.

Coronary artery disease (CAD) Any one of the abnormal conditions that can affect the arteries of the heart and produce various pathological effects, especially a reduced supply of oxygen and nutrients to the myocardium.

Ischemia (is kee' mee uh) Poor blood supply to an organ.

Ischemic heart disease Poor blood supply to the heart via the coronary arteries.

Reflex tachycardia (tak' i kar' dee uh) A rapid heart sinus rhythm caused by a variety of autonomic nervous system effects, such as blood pressure changes, fever, or emotional stress.

Unstable angina Early stage of progressive coronary artery disease.

Variant angina Ischemia-induced myocardial chest pain caused by spasm of the coronary arteries.

ANGINA AND CORONARY ARTERY DISEASE

The heart is an efficient organ, but it is demanding in an aerobic sense because it requires a large supply of oxygen to meet the incredible demand placed on it. Pumping blood to all the tissues and organs of the body is a difficult job. The heart's much-needed oxygen supply is delivered to the heart muscle by means of the **coronary arteries.** However, when the supply of oxygen and energy-rich nutrients in blood is insufficient to meet the demands of the heart, the heart muscle (or myocardium) aches. This is called **angina pectoris,** or chest pain. Poor blood supply to an organ is referred to as **ischemia.** When the organ involved is the heart, the condition is called **ischemic heart disease.**

Ischemic heart disease is the number one killer in Canada today, and the primary cause is disease of the coronary arteries resulting from atherosclerosis. When atherosclerotic plaques form in the lumens (channels) of these vessels, they become narrow. The supply of oxygen and energy-rich nutrients to the heart is then decreased. This disorder is called **coronary artery disease (CAD).** An acute result of CAD and of ischemic heart disease is myocardial infarction (MI), or heart attack. It occurs when blood flow through the coronary arteries to the myocardium is completely blocked so that the heart muscle cannot receive any of the blood nutrients (especially oxygen) necessary for normal function. If this process is not reversed immediately, that area of the heart will die and become necrotic and non-functioning.

The rate at which the heart pumps and the strength of each heartbeat (contractility) also place oxygen demands on this organ. There are many substances and situations that can increase heart rate and contractility and thus increase oxygen demand. These include caffeine, exercise, and stress. These substances or situations result in stimulation of the sympathetic nervous system (SNS), which results in increased heart rate and contractility. In an already overburdened heart, such as in a person with CAD, this can worsen the balance between myocardial oxygen supply and demand and result in angina. Some drugs that are used to treat angina are aimed at correcting the imbalance between myocardial oxygen supply and demand by decreasing heart rate and contractility. Beta-blockers and calcium channel blockers (CCBs) are two examples.

The pain of angina results from the following process. Under ischemic conditions when the myocardium is deprived of oxygen, the heart shifts to anaerobic metabolism to meet its energy needs. One of the by-products of anaerobic metabolism is lactic acid. The accumulation of lactic acid and other metabolic by-products causes the pain receptors surrounding the heart to be stimulated, producing the heart pain known as *angina.* It is the same pathophysiological mechanism responsible for causing the soreness in skeletal muscles after vigorous exercise.

There are three classic types of chest pain, or angina pectoris. **Chronic stable angina** has atherosclerosis as its primary cause. *Classic angina* and *effort angina* are other names for it. Chronic stable angina can be triggered by either exertion or stress (cold, fear, or emotions). The nicotine in tobacco, or the consumption of alcohol, coffee, or other drugs that stimulate the SNS can exacerbate it. The pain of chronic stable angina is commonly intense but subsides within 15 minutes of either rest or appropriate anti-anginal drug therapy. **Unstable angina** is usually the early stage of progressive CAD. There are three presentations of unstable angina. It is generally described as (1) new onset angina that is severe or frequent (more than three times per day); (2) angina that is increasing in severity, frequency, or duration, or is brought on by less activity than before; or (3) angina at rest. It is important to categorize whether the client that presents with chest pain is low or high risk for myocardial ischemia so that MI can be prevented. **Variant angina**, a less common form, results from spasm of the layer of smooth muscle that surrounds the atherosclerotic coronary arteries. This pain often happens at rest and without any precipitating cause. The pain is usually severe, prolonged, and not relieved by nitroglycerine. It does, however, seem to follow a regular pattern, usually occurring at the same time of day. This type of angina is also called *Prinzmetal's angina.* Dysrhythmias and electrocardiogram (ECG) changes often accompany these different types of anginal attacks.

ANTI-ANGINAL DRUGS

Recent advances in pharmacotherapy have resulted in the development of a host of new anti-anginal agents that have been approved for clinical use. The three main classes of drugs used to treat angina pectoris are the nitrates/nitrites, beta-blockers, and CCBs. Their various therapeutic effects are summarized in Table 23-1. Anti-anginal drug therapy has three main therapeutic objectives: (1) to reduce the frequency, duration, and intensity of the anginal pain; (2) to improve the client's functional capacity with as few side effects as possible; and (3) to prevent or delay the worst possible outcome, MI. The overall goal of anti-anginal drug therapy is to increase blood flow to ischemic myocardium, decrease myocardial oxygen demand, or both. Figure 23-1 illustrates how drug therapy works to alleviate angina.

NITRATES/NITRITES

Nitrates, and in particular nitroglycerine, have long been the mainstay of both the prophylaxis and treatment for angina and other cardiac problems. This class of anti-anginal agents was first discovered by Sir Thomas Lauder Brunton in England, who noted that amyl nitrite was just as effective as venesection (venipuncture) in the management of angina. A few years later a chemically related substance, glyceryl trinitrate (nitroglycerine), was successfully isolated and used for this purpose. Today there are several chemical derivatives of these early precursors, all of which are organic nitrate esters. They are available in a wide variety of preparations, including sublingual (SL), chewable, and oral (PO) tablets; capsules; ointments; patches; a translingual spray; and intravenous (IV) solutions. The following nitrates are available for clinical use:

- Rapid-acting agents
  - amyl nitrite
  - nitroglycerine

TABLE 23-1

ANTI-ANGINAL AGENTS: THERAPEUTIC EFFECTS

Therapeutic Effect	Nitrates	Beta-Blockers*	Calcium Channel Blockers		
			Nifedipine	Verapamil	Diltiazem
SUPPLY					
Blood flow	↑↑	↑	↑↑↑	↑↑↑	↑↑↑
Duration of diastole	0	↑↑↑	0/↑	↑↑↑	↑↑
DEMAND					
Pre-load†	↓↓↓	↑	↓/0	0	0/↓
Afterload	↓	0/↓	↓↓↓	↓↓	↓↓
Contractility	0	↓↓↓	↓	↓↓↓	↓↓
Heart rate	0/↑	↓↓↓	0/↑	↓↓	↓↓

*In particular those that are cardioselective and do not have intrinsic sympathomimetic activity (ISA).
†*Pre-load* is pressure in the heart caused by blood volume. The nitrates effectively move part of this blood out of the heart and into blood vessels, thereby decreasing pre-load or filling pressure.
↓, Decrease; ↑, increase; 0, little or no effect.

- Long-acting agents
  - isosorbide dinitrate
  - isosorbide mononitrate

Mechanism of Action and Drug Effects

Medicinal nitrates and nitrites, more commonly referred to as simply *nitrates,* dilate all blood vessels and have a predominant effect on venous vascular beds. However, they also have a dose-dependent arterial vasodilator effect. These vasodilatory effects are the result of relaxation of the smooth muscle cells that are part of the wall structure of veins and arteries. Particularly notable, however, is the potent dilating effect of nitrates on the coronary arteries.

If the nitrate-induced venodilation just described occurs rapidly, the cardiovascular system overcompensates and increases its heart rate, a condition referred to as **reflex tachycardia.** This occurs because the venodilation causes a large shift in blood volume toward the venous circulation and away from the heart. Baroreceptors (blood pressure receptors) in the heart then falsely sense that there has been a dramatic loss of blood volume. At this point, the heart begins beating more rapidly to move the apparent smaller volume of blood more quickly throughout the body, especially toward the vital organs (including the heart itself). However, the same baroreceptors soon sense that there has not been a loss of blood volume but that the volume of blood missing in the heart is now in the periphery (e.g., venous system) and the heart rate slows back to normal.

Indications

Nitrate-induced vasodilation has many therapeutic effects (see Table 23-1). By causing venodilation, the nitrates bring about a decrease in venous return and in turn a lower left ventricular end-diastolic volume (LVEDV, or pre-load), resulting in a lower left ventricular (LV) pressure. LV systolic wall tension is thus reduced, as is myocardial oxygen demand.

The nitrates cause both large and small coronary vessels to dilate. The end result is a redistribution of blood and therefore oxygen to previously ischemic myocardial

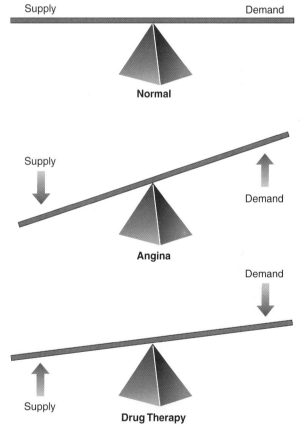

FIG. 23-1 Benefit of drug therapy for angina with increasing oxygen supply and decreasing oxygen demands.

tissue. The nitrates also alleviate coronary artery spasm (variant or Prinzmetal's angina). In addition, coronary arteries that are diseased and that have been narrowed by atherosclerosis can also be dilated as long as there is still smooth muscle surrounding the coronary artery and the atherosclerotic plaque is not complete. Exercise-induced constriction or spasms of atherosclerotic coronary arteries can be reversed or even prevented by nitrates, encouraging healthy physical activity in clients.

Contraindications

Contraindications to the use of nitrates include known drug allergy, severe anemia, closed-angle glaucoma, hypotension, or severe head injury.

Side Effects and Adverse Effects

Nitrates are well tolerated, and most side effects are usually transient and involve the cardiovascular system. The most common undesirable effect is headache, which usually diminishes in intensity and frequency soon after the start of therapy. Other cardiovascular effects include tachycardia and postural hypotension that occur secondary to vasodilation. Methemoglobinemia is an extremely rare adverse effect and usually occurs in clients with an inherited genetic propensity for the condition. (In this condition, the iron in hemoglobin is oxidized from the ferrous to the ferric state, resulting in an inability to transport oxygen normally. Symptoms can include headache, fatigue, shortness of breath, and potentially shock and seizures.) Topical nitrate dosage forms can produce various contact dermatitides (skin inflammations), but these are actually reactions not to the nitroglycerine itself but to the dosage delivery system.

Tolerance to the anti-anginal effects of nitrates can occur in some clients, especially those on long-acting formulations or taking nitrates around the clock. To prevent this, a regular nitrate-free period allows certain enzymatic pathways to replenish themselves. A common regimen with transdermal patches is to remove them at night for 8 hours and apply a new patch in the morning. This has been shown to prevent tolerance to the beneficial effects of nitrates.

Interactions

Nitrate anti-anginal drugs can produce additive hypotensive effects when taken in combination with alcohol, beta-blockers, CCBs, phenothiazines, and sildenafil.

Dosages

The organic nitrates are available in an array of forms and doses. See the dosages table below for more information. See Appendix B for some of the common brands available in Canada.

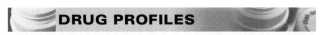

DRUG PROFILES

◤ isosorbide dinitrate

Isosorbide dinitrate is an organic nitrate and therefore a powerful explosive. It exerts the same effects as the other nitrates. When isosorbide dinitrate is metabolized in the liver, it is broken down into two active metabolites, both of which have the same therapeutic actions as isosorbide dinitrate itself. Isosorbide dinitrate is used for the acute relief of angina pectoris, for prophylaxis in situations likely to provoke angina attacks (e.g., exercise), and for the long-term prophylaxis of angina pectoris. The contraindications to isosorbide dinitrate use are the same as those to nitroglycerine. Isosorbide dinitrate is available only in oral form as 20- and 60-mg extended-release tablets, 10- and 30-mg tablets, and 5-mg sublingual tablets. Pregnancy category C. Refer to the table below for the recommended dosages.

PHARMACOKINETICS

Half-Life	Onset	Peak	Duration
Variable	20–40 min	Unknown	4–6 hr

◤ isosorbide mononitrate

Isosorbide mononitrate is one of the two active metabolites of isosorbide dinitrate, but itself has no active metabolites. As a result, it produces a more consistent, steady therapeutic response, with less variation in response over time and among clients. Its contraindications are the same as those of nitroglycerine. It is available only in oral formulations: two regular-release products, one sustained-release product, and one sublingual product. The regular-release products are taken twice a day, with 7 hours the recommended interval between the first and second doses. This 7-hour interval is believed to delay the development of nitrate tolerance, a limitation to long-term nitrate therapy. They are available as 10- and 30-mg tablets. The sublingual form is a 5-mg tablet, dissolved under the tongue, and is for the relief of acute pain. The sustained-release product is available as 20-, 40-, and 60-mg tablets, taken only once a day, usually in the morning for long-term prophylaxis of angina. Pregnancy category C. Refer to the table below for dosage recommendations.

DOSAGES	Selected Anti-Anginal Nitrate Coronary Vasodilators

Agent	Pharmacological Class	Usual Dosage Range	Indications
◤ isosorbide dinitrate		**Adult** SL: 5–10 mg × 3 PO: 10–30 mg tid and 20–40 mg bid given 7 hr apart for SR formulations	
◤ isosorbide mononitrate	Anti-anginal nitrate coronary vasodilator	**Adult** PO SR: 30–120 mg/day am	Angina
◤ nitroglycerine		**Adult** Ointment: 2.5–5 cm ribbon q6–8h, up to 10–12.5 cm ribbon q4h Spray: 0.4–0.8 mg onto or under the tongue prn SL: 0.3–0.6 mg q5min, 3 times Transdermal: daily in am, leave on 12–14 hr (0.2–0.8 mg/hr)	

SR, Sustained-release.

PHARMACOKINETICS

Half-Life	Onset	Peak	Duration
5 hr	15–30 min	0.5–1 hr	5–12 hr

▸ *nitroglycerine*

Nitroglycerine is the prototypical nitrate and is made by many pharmaceutical companies; therefore it goes by many trade names. It has traditionally been the most important drug used in the symptomatic treatment of ischemic heart conditions such as angina. Nitroglycerine is contraindicated in clients with a known hypersensitivity to it and in those suffering from increased intracranial pressure, inadequate cerebral perfusion, constrictive pericarditis, pericardial tamponade, severe hypotension, or severe anemia.

When given orally, nitroglycerine goes to the liver to be metabolized before it can be active in the body. During this process the majority of the nitroglycerine is removed from the circulation. For this reason, nitroglycerine is administered by many other routes to bypass the first-pass effect. It is also available in many formulations and has proved useful for the treatment of a variety of cardiovascular conditions. The sublingual and buccal routes of administration are employed for the treatment of chest pain or angina of acute onset, or for the prevention of angina when clients find themselves in situations likely to provoke an attack. These routes are advantageous for ameliorating these acute conditions because the area under the tongue and inside the cheek is highly vascular. This means that the nitroglycerine is absorbed quickly and directly into the bloodstream and hence its therapeutic effects occur rapidly.

Sublingual nitroglycerine is available as 0.3- and 0.6-mg tablets. Nitroglycerine also comes as a 0.4-mg/metered dose aerosol that is sprayed on or under the tongue. Nitroglycerine is available in an intravenous form that is used for BP control in the perioperative hypertensive client; for the treatment of ischemic pain, heart failure, pulmonary edema associated with acute MI; and in hypertensive emergency situations. Intravenous infusions are available in concentrations of 0.1, 0.2, or 0.4 mg/mL in 250 mL of 5 percent dextrose solution and in 1 mg/mL injection. Topical dosage formulations are used for the long-term prophylactic management of angina pectoris. Topical formulations offer the same advantages as the sublingual and buccal formulations in that they also bypass the liver and the first-pass effect. They also allow for the continuous slow delivery of nitroglycerine, which supplies a steady dose of nitroglycerine to the client. The transdermal delivery system forms are available as a 2 percent ointment or as 0.2-, 0.3-, 0.4-, 0.6-, and 0.8-mg/hr patches. To reduce the effects of tolerance, a patch is worn for 12 to 14 hours, and then removed to allow for a patch-free interval of 10 to 12 hours. Pregnancy category C. See the table on p. 382 for the recommended dosages.

PHARMACOKINETICS

Half-Life	Onset	Peak	Duration
1–4 min	SL: 1–3 min	Unknown	10–30 min

BETA-BLOCKERS

Beta-adrenergic blockers, more commonly referred to as beta-blockers, have become the mainstay in the treatment of a wide range of cardiovascular diseases. Most available beta-blockers demonstrate anti-anginal efficacy, although not all have been approved for this use. Those beta-blockers approved as anti-anginal agents are atenolol, metoprolol, nadolol, and propranolol.

The main beneficial effect of beta-blockers in the treatment of angina is slowing the heart rate (negative chronotropic effect) and decreasing myocardial contractility (negative inotropic effect). These two effects have two favourable physiological results. First, decreasing the heart rate decreases myocardial oxygen demand because a rapidly beating heart requires more energy and oxygen than a slowly or normally beating heart. In addition, this negative chronotropic effect increases oxygen delivery to the myocardium. Second, by decreasing contractility, the beta-blockers help conserve energy, or decrease demand. As mentioned in previous chapters, beta-blockers bind to and thus block the beta-adrenergic receptors, which would otherwise be stimulated by the binding of the neurotransmitters epinephrine and norepinephrine. These catecholamines would ordinarily be released in greater quantities during times of exercise or stress to stimulate the heart muscle to contract further, and the physiological act of contractility requires energy in the form of adenosine triphosphate (ATP), oxygen, and many other vital substances. Therefore any decrease in the energy demands on the heart is beneficial for alleviating conditions such as angina, in which the supply of these vital substances is already deficient because of the ischemia.

Beta-blockers are most effective in the treatment of typical exertional angina. This is because the usual physiological increase in the heart rate and systolic BP that occurs during exercise or stress is blunted, thereby decreasing the myocardial oxygen demand.

Mechanism of Action and Drug Effects

The primary drug effects of the beta-blockers are related to the cardiovascular system. As covered in previous chapters, the predominant beta-adrenergic receptors in the heart are the beta$_1$-adrenergic receptors. They are responsible for the conduction effects of the conduction system. When they are blocked by beta-blockers, the rate at which the pacemaker (sinoatrial [SA] node) fires decreases, and the time it takes for the node to recover increases. The result is a decrease in heart rate. Beta-blockers slow conduction through the atrioventricular (AV) node as well, which contributes to slowing the heart rate.

Beta-blockers may also suppress renin activity and the renin–aldosterone–angiotensin system. Renin is a potent vasoconstrictor that the kidneys release when they sense they are not being adequately perfused and receiving enough blood. When beta-blockers inhibit its release, the blood vessels to and in the kidney dilate, which decreases BP.

Beta-blockers are effective in the treatment of angina because they slow the heart rate and decrease contractility by binding to and blocking the beta-adrenergic receptors located on the heart's conduction system and throughout the myocardium. This has the ultimate effect of decreasing the workload of the heart. Slowing the heart rate is beneficial in a client with ischemic heart disease because the coronary arteries have more time to fill with oxygen- and nutrient-rich blood when the heart is relaxed during diastole and to deliver these vital substances to the myocardium. At a normal heart rate of 60 to 80 beats/min, the heart spends 60 to 70 percent of its time in diastole. As the heart rate increases during stress or exercise, the heart spends more and more time in systole and less and less time in diastole. The physiological consequence is that the coronary arteries receive increasingly less blood and eventually the myocardium becomes ischemic. In an ischemic heart the increased demand of increasing contractility also leads progressively to even more ischemia and chest pain. By blocking this mechanism, a beta-blocker reduces myocardial contractility and therefore the energy needs of the heart. This shifts the supply and demand back toward a more balanced (homeostatic) ratio.

There are many therapeutic effects of beta-blockers after an MI. After an MI, there is a high level of circulating catecholamines (norepinephrine and epinephrine), the release of which has been triggered by the myocardial damage resulting from the infarction. These catecholamines will produce several harmful consequences if their actions go unopposed. They essentially irritate the heart. They cause the heart rate to increase, causing a further imbalance in the supply and demand ratio, and they irritate the conduction system of the heart to the point at which potentially fatal dysrhythmias may ensue. The beta-blockers block all of these harmful effects and have been shown to improve the chances for survival in such clients. Unless contraindicated, they should be given to all clients in the acute stages after an MI.

Indications

As mentioned earlier, indications for the use of beta-blockers include angina and MI. They are also commonly used in hypertension (see Chapter 24), cardiac dysrhythmias (as described in Chapter 22), and essential tremor. Some non–Health Canada-approved but common uses include migraine headache and, in low doses, even the tachycardia associated with "stage fright."

Contraindications

There are a number of contraindications to the use of beta-blockers, including bronchial asthma and serious conduction disturbances. They should be used with caution in clients with systolic heart failure. Additionally, several common yet sometimes subtle conditions in geriatric clients may be exacerbated by beta-blockers. These include mental depression, diabetes mellitus, and peripheral vascular disease. The decision to initiate anti-ischemic therapy with a beta-blocker in any client should therefore be made carefully, weighing both the risks and the benefits.

Side Effects and Adverse Effects

The side effects of the beta-blockers result from their ability to block beta-adrenergic receptors in areas where they are not intended to. For example, the smooth muscle that surrounds many blood vessels throughout the circulation and the airways in the lungs has beta$_2$-adrenergic receptors on its surface. When these beta$_2$-adrenergic receptors are stimulated, they cause the smooth muscle to relax. When this occurs in blood vessels, they dilate and BP decreases. When this occurs in the airways of the lungs, they dilate and oxygen delivery increases. A beta-blocker that blocks beta$_2$-adrenergic receptors thus causes the opposite of these physiological actions, such that blood vessels constrict and hypertension occurs or the airways constrict and the delivery of oxygen decreases. This may in turn exacerbate a client's underlying asthma or chronic obstructive pulmonary disease (COPD). Another drawback to the use of beta-blockers is their negative effect on physical performance. Fatigue and lethargy are the most common client complaints and may be due to either a decreased cardiac output or a direct central nervous system (CNS) effect. The most common beta–blocker-related side effects and adverse effects are listed in Table 23-2.

Interactions

There are many drug interactions that involve the beta-blockers. The more common and important of these are listed in Table 23-3.

TABLE 23-2
BETA-BLOCKERS: ADVERSE EFFECTS

Body System	Side/Adverse Effects
Cardiovascular	Bradycardia, hypotension, second- or third-degree heart block, heart failure
Central nervous	Dizziness, fatigue, mental depression, lethargy, drowsiness, unusual dreams
Metabolic	Alter glucose and lipid metabolism
Other	Wheezing, dyspnea, erectile dysfunction

TABLE 23-3
BETA-BLOCKERS: COMMON DRUG INTERACTIONS

Drug	Mechanism	Result
Anticholinergics	Antagonize	Decrease beta-blocker
cimetidine	Decreases metabolism	Increases propranolol and metoprolol levels and pharmacodynamic effects
Diuretics and antihypertensives	Additive	Hypotension
phenothiazine	Additive hypotensive effects	Hypotension and cardiac arrest

Dosages

For information on the dosages of selected beta-blockers, see the dosages table below. See Appendix B for some of the common brands available in Canada.

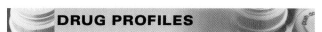

DRUG PROFILES

Beta-blockers are the mainstay in the treatment of a wide range of cardiovascular diseases, mainly hypertension, angina, and the acute stages of MI. The beta-blockers are all classified as pregnancy category C agents except acebutolol, pindolol, and sotalol. Contraindications to their use include hypersensitivity to the particular agent, cardiac failure or shock, second- or third-degree heart block, bronchospastic disease (primarily pertains to the use of non-specific beta-blockers), and hypotension. The three most commonly used beta-blockers are carvedilol, metoprolol, and bisoprolol. The drug profile for carvedilol is in Chapter 18 on p. 311.

⟩⟩ atenolol

Atenolol is a cardioselective beta$_1$-adrenergic receptor blocker and is indicated for the prophylactic treatment of angina pectoris. Atenolol's use after an MI has been shown to lead to a decrease in mortality. It is available in oral form as 25-, 50-, and 100-mg tablets. Pregnancy category C. Refer to the table below for the recommended dosages.

PHARMACOKINETICS*

Half-Life	Onset	Peak	Duration
6–7 hr	1 hr	2–4 hr	24 hr

*All values are for oral atenolol.

⟩⟩ metoprolol

Metoprolol is also a cardioselective beta$_1$-adrenergic receptor blocker that is used for the prophylactic treatment of angina and has many of the same characteristics as atenolol. It has shown similar efficacy in reducing mortality in the victims of MI and in treating angina. It is available in both oral and parenteral forms. In oral form it is available as 50- and 100-mg tablets and as 100- and 200-mg extended-release tablets. In parenteral form it is available as a 1-mg/mL injection. Pregnancy category C. Refer to the table below for recommended dosages.

PHARMACOKINETICS

Half-Life	Onset	Peak	Duration
3.5 hr	1 hr	1.5–2 hr	13–19 hr

CALCIUM CHANNEL BLOCKERS

CCBs are the most recent anti-anginal drugs to become available. The two main classes are dihydropyridines (nifedipine, amlodipine, felodipine, and nimodipine) and non-dihydropyridines that include diltiazem (a benzothiazepine) and verapamil (a phenylalkylamine). Although they all block calcium channels, their chemical structures and therefore their mechanisms of action differ slightly. There are many CCBs available today, with more on the way. Those that are used for the treatment of chronic stable angina are amlodipine, diltiazem, nifedipine, and verapamil.

Mechanism of Action and Drug Effects

CCBs affect both myocardial oxygen demand and supply. They decrease myocardial oxygen demand by causing peripheral arterial vasodilation and by a negative inotropic action (i.e., reduced myocardial contractility). CCBs may be particularly effective for the treatment of coronary artery spasm secondary to the relaxation of the smooth muscles in the vessel walls. However, they may not be as effective as beta-blockers in blunting exercise-induced elevations in heart rate and BP.

Other cardiovascular effects of CCBs include depressing the automaticity of and conduction through the SA and AV nodes, decreasing myocardial contractility, and decreasing peripheral and coronary artery tone. Verapamil and diltiazem also decrease heart rate. Their most dramatic anti-anginal effects are secondary to their effects on myocardial contractility and the smooth muscle tone of peripheral and coronary arteries.

Calcium plays an important role in the excitation–contraction coupling process that occurs in the heart and vascular smooth muscle cells. It is a vital component in the contraction of any muscle, whether it is smooth muscle or skeletal muscle. Preventing calcium from entering into and interacting in the contraction process therefore prevents muscle contraction, and the result is relaxation. Relaxation of the smooth muscles that surround the coronary arteries causes them to dilate. This increases blood flow to the heart, which in turn increases the oxygen supply and helps shift the supply and demand ratio back to normal. This also occurs in the arteries throughout the body, resulting in a decrease in the force (systemic vascular resistance) that the heart has to exert itself against when delivering blood to the body (afterload). Decreasing afterload reduces the workload of the heart and therefore reduces myocardial oxygen demand. This is the

DOSAGES Selected Beta-Adrenergic Agents			
Agent	**Pharmacological Class**	**Usual Dosage Range**	**Indication**
⟩⟩atenolol	Beta$_1$-blocker	**Adult** PO: 50–200 mg/day as a single dose	Angina
⟩⟩metoprolol	Beta$_1$-blocker	**Adult** PO: 100–400 mg/day in 2–3 divided doses	Angina

primary beneficial anti-anginal effect of the dihydropyridine CCBs and of nifedipine in particular.

Both diltiazem and verapamil have dramatic effects on the cells of the cardiac conduction system, or calcium channels, which are discussed in depth in Chapter 22. It is these channels that are blocked when these CCBs are given. The electrophysiological effect of this blockade is a slowing of AV node conduction and a prolonging of the refractory period, also discussed in Chapter 22. This is beneficial, especially with atrial fibrillation or flutter, because if these rapidly firing impulses are allowed to pass unhindered to the ventricles, the result could be life-threatening ventricular fibrillation or tachycardia.

Indications

The therapeutic benefits of the CCBs are numerous. Because of their acceptable side effect and safety profile, they are considered first-line agents for the treatment of such conditions as angina, mild to moderate hypertension, and supraventricular tachycardia. They are also used for the short-term management of atrial fibrillation and flutter, migraines, Raynaud's disease, and subarachnoid hemorrhage. (Their use in these other conditions is described in the corresponding chapters.)

Contraindications

Contraindications to the use of CCBs include known drug allergy, acute MI, second- or third-degree AV block (unless pacemaker present), cardiogenic shock, sick sinus syndrome, marked bradycardia, and hypotension.

Side Effects and Adverse Effects

The side effects of the CCBs are limited and primarily related to overexpression of their therapeutic effects. The most common of the CCB-related adverse effects are listed in Table 23-4.

Interactions

The drug interactions that can occur with CCBs vary with the particular agent, although there are not actually many such interactions. One of particular note because of its beneficial effect is the interaction that occurs between cyclosporin and diltiazem. Because diltiazem interferes with the metabolism and elimination of cyclosporin (slowing the breakdown of cyclosporin), smaller doses of cyclosporin are needed. This is advantageous because one of cyclosporin's most common and devastating effects is that it can destroy the kidney and cause renal failure. Other important drug interactions that involve CCBs are listed in Table 23-5.

TABLE 23-4

CALCIUM CHANNEL BLOCKERS: ADVERSE EFFECTS

Body System	Side/Adverse Effects
Cardiovascular	Hypotension, palpitations, tachycardia or bradycardia, heart failure
Central nervous system	Dizziness, headache, fatigue
Gastrointestinal	Constipation, nausea
Other	Dermatitis, dyspnea, rash, flushing, peripheral edema, wheezing

TABLE 23-5

CALCIUM CHANNEL BLOCKERS: COMMON DRUG INTERACTIONS

Drug	Mechanism	Result
Beta-blockers	Additive effects	Bradycardia and AV block
Digoxin	Interferes with elimination	Can increase digoxin levels; prolonged AV conduction
H₂ blockers	Decrease clearance	Elevated levels of CCBs

AV, Atrioventricular.

DOSAGES Selected Calcium Channel–Blocking Agents

Agent	Pharmacological Class	Usual Dosage Range	Indications
►►amlodipine besylate		**Adult** PO: Initial dose 5 mg/day; titrate upwards to max 10 mg/day	
►►diltiazem	Calcium channel blocker	**Adult** PO: Initial dose 30 mg qid ac and at bedtime; range of 240–360 mg divided in 3–4 doses Sustained-released capsule: 120–360 mg q 12 hr Controlled-delivery capsule: 120–360 mg once daily	Angina
►►nifedipine		**Adult** PO: 30–90 mg XL (extended release) daily; 10–20 mg (immediate release) tid (max 120 mg/day)	
►►verapamil		**Adult** PO: Initial dose 180 mg, titrate upwards at bedtime; range 180–480 mg qd; do not exceed 480 mg/day	

Dosages

For information on the dosages of selected CCBs, see the dosages table on p. 386. See Appendix B for some of the common brands available in Canada.

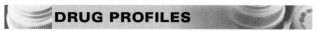

DRUG PROFILES

CCBs are beneficial, highly effective agents used to treat angina. Because they have a greater affinity for peripheral vascular smooth muscle, the dihydropyridines are more suited than other CCBs for the treatment of hypertension that occurs in the setting of exertional angina. This class of CCBs has grown enormously. As a class they are safe and effective. However, because of their potent peripheral vasodilating properties, they have a greater propensity than others to cause peripheral edema and reflex tachycardia. They are effective in the treatment of angina because they are potent decreasers of afterload. The non-dihydropyridines (benzothiazepines and phenylalkylamines) have a greater affinity for the cells of the conduction system and the coronary arteries, making them more suited for the management of dysrhythmias and for the dilation of atherosclerotic coronary arteries. The various agents are listed in Table 23-6 according to their respective chemical category. Although all these agents have anti-anginal effects, not all are used as anti-anginal drugs.

CCBs are safe and effective drugs with few contraindications. Some of the contraindications are hypersensitivity to the drugs, second- or third-degree AV block, hypotension, acute MI, and cardiogenic shock. They are all classified as pregnancy category C agents.

» *diltiazem*

Diltiazem is the only benzothiazepine CCB. It has a particular affinity for the cardiac conduction system and is effective for the oral treatment of angina pectoris resulting from coronary insufficiency and hypertension. There are two sustained-delivery formulations of diltiazem that can be confused with each other. There is a sustained-release capsule, which is taken twice a day, and a controlled delivery capsule, which is taken once a day. Oral forms of diltiazem are available as 30- and 60-mg tablets and as 60-, 90-, and 120-mg sustained-release capsules. The once-a-day formulation is available in 120-, 180-, 240-, 300-, and 360-mg controlled-release capsules and extended-release capsules. Pregnancy category C. Refer to the table on p. 386 for recommended dosages.

PHARMACOKINETICS

Half-Life	Onset	Peak	Duration
4–9.5 hr	30 min	2–3 hr	Up to 24 hr*

*With extended-release dosage forms.

» *nifedipine*

Nifedipine was the first dihydropyridine CCB to be developed and introduced into clinical use. In the past the liquid-filled nifedipine capsules have been squeezed to release their liquid contents under the tongue. This practice is no longer recommended because several studies have shown that it increases the mortality rate. As well, nifedipine tablets should never be crushed, because it may alter the intended effect or even cause an adverse event. Nifedipine is available only in oral form as 5- and 10-mg gelatin capsules; as 20-, 30-, and 60-mg tablets; and as a 10-mg extended-release, film-coated tablet. Pregnancy category C. Refer to the table on p. 386 for recommended dosages.

PHARMACOKINETICS

Half-Life	Onset	Peak	Duration
2–5 hr	20 min	30–60 min	IR: 6 hr XL: 24 hr

IR, Immediate release; *XL*, extended release.

» *verapamil*

Verapamil is the only phenylalkylamine CCB. Like diltiazem, it has a greater affinity for the conduction system of the heart than dihydropyridine CCBs such as nifedipine, and is therefore effective in treating such rhythm disturbances as PSVTs. Verapamil is also used for the treatment of angina, hypertension, and hypertrophic cardiomyopathy. The most common side effects of verapamil are constipation, dizziness, and nausea, occurring in less than 9 percent of clients. Verapamil is available in many oral dosage formulations and is also available in a parenteral preparation. Verapamil is available in oral form as 80- and 120-mg film-coated tablets; 120-, 180-, 240-mg slow-release tablets; and 180- and 240-mg film-coated, controlled onset, extended-release tablets. It is available in parenteral form as a 2.5-mg/mL injection. Pregnancy category C. Refer to the table on p. 386 for recommended dosages.

PHARMACOKINETICS

Half-Life	Onset	Peak	Duration
4.5–12 hr	0.5–2 hr	1–2 hr	Unknown

SUMMARY OF ANTI-ANGINAL PHARMACOLOGY

In clients with CAD, the clinical symptoms result from inadequate delivery of blood and the attendant oxygen and nutrients to the heart, which results in ischemic heart

TABLE 23-6
CLASSIFICATION OF CALCIUM CHANNEL BLOCKERS

Generic Name	Available Routes
BENZOTHIAZEPINES	
diltiazem	PO/IV
DIHYDROPYRIDINES	
amlodipine	PO
felodipine	PO
nifedipine	PO
nimodipine	PO
PHENYLALKYLAMINES	
verapamil	PO/IV

disease. Anti-anginal agents such as nitrates, nitrites, beta-blockers, and CCBs are used to reduce ischemia by increasing the delivery of oxygen- and nutrient-rich blood to cardiac tissues or by reducing oxygen consumption by the coronary vessels. Either of these mechanisms can reduce ischemia and lead to a decrease in anginal pain. Nitrates and nitrites work mainly by decreasing venous return to the heart (pre-load) and decreasing systemic vascular resistance (afterload). CCBs decrease calcium influx into the smooth muscle, causing vascular relaxation. This either reverses or prevents the spasms of coronary vessels that cause the anginal pain associated with Prinzmetal's or variant angina and with chronic anginal pain. Beta-blockers help by slowing the heart rate and decreasing contractility, thereby decreasing oxygen demands. Even though these groups of drugs have similar clinical effects, the nursing process required for each is somewhat specific in terms of the characteristics and effects of the agents and the indications for and contraindications to their use.

NURSING PROCESS

■ Assessment

Before administering any nitrates or nitrites, the nurse must obtain a complete health history to determine whether the client has any contraindications or cautions to the use of these medications. Information is needed on altered liver, kidney, or circulatory functioning, as well as on other medications taken, including OTC, prescription, herbal, and vitamins. The nurse must also inquire about any symptoms such as chest pain due to ischemia (angina), dizziness, lightheadedness, and/or syncope. Clients experiencing angina should be encouraged to describe their anginal attacks, including what precipitates them, because this will help in the selection of the appropriate therapy. The nurse must also assess the client's vital signs, including respiratory patterns and rate, BP readings (including orthostatic BPs), and pulse rates. It is important for the nurse to remember that cross-tolerance may develop when nitrates and nitrites are taken simultaneously.

Contraindications to the use of nitrates and nitrites include hypersensitivity to these agents, severe anemia, acute MI, increased intracranial pressure, hypertension, and cerebral hemorrhage. Cautious use is called for in clients suffering from head injuries or postural hypotension, as well as with pregnancy or lactation. Drug interactions include beta-blockers, narcotics, diuretics, antihypertensives, anticoagulants, alcohol (results in increased hypotension and even cardiovascular collapse), sympathomimetics (may antagonize the effects of nitrates and nitrites), and tricyclic antidepressants (their effect is enhanced when they are taken with nitrates). Cold temperature and tobacco use may reduce the effectiveness of nitrates. Nitrates also interact with sildenafil (discussed in Chapter 34).

CCBs used as anti-anginal agents require the same degree of assessment with attention to any disease process, conditions, symptoms, and other medications being taken simultaneously. Contraindications to the use of CCBs include sick sinus syndrome, second- or third-degree heart block, hypotension (with a systolic BP of <90 mm Hg), and cardiogenic shock. Cautious use is called for in pregnant or lactating women, children, and clients with renal or liver disease, hypotension, or heart failure. Specifically, amlodipine, a CCB commonly used for treatment of angina, should be used with caution in clients with bradycardia or heart failure. It is also used with caution in clients who have decreased renal and hepatic functioning, which affect excretion and metabolism. Drug interactions for CCBs as a group include beta-blockers, digitalis glycosides, and antidysrhythmic

---

RESEARCH

Nitrates and Related Concerns

Dosing of nitroglycerine has always been affected by the type of infusion set used for nitroglycerine injection. Although the usual starting adult dose range reported in clinical studies (*Mosby's Drug Consult*, 2005) was 25 μg/min or more, these were in clients in whom PVC tubing was used. With the use of non-PVC, nonabsorbing intravenous tubing, the dosage of nitroglycerine should be reduced. When a non-absorbing set is used, some sources recommend an initial dose of 5 μg/min through an infusion pump. Titration with dose increments of 5 μg/min (every 3–5 min) may occur until a positive clinical response is noted. Cyanide toxicity is worthy of discussion. Sodium nitroprusside infusions at rates above 2 μg/kg/min generate cyanide ion faster than the normal bodily functions can dispose of it. However, when clients are given sodium thiosulphate, the body's capacity for cyanide ion elimination is greatly increased. The true rates of clinically significant cyanide toxicity cannot be assessed from spontaneous reports or published data. Most clients who experience such toxicity have received prolonged infusions, with reported deaths being attributed to nitroprusside infusions at rates much greater than those recommended (e.g., 30–120 μg/kg/min). However, elevated cyanide levels, metabolic acidosis, and significant clinical deterioration have been reported in clients who received infusions at recommended rates for short periods. Cyanide toxicity results in venous hyperoxemia (bright red venous blood), metabolic acidosis, air hunger, confusion, and death. Every nurse working in an emergency room, surgical suite, cardiac care unit, or intensive care unit must be aware of the signs of cyanide toxicity, because astute assessment and early identification of the symptoms may prevent irreversible damage and possible death. Clients always react individually and professional nurses need to continually keep informed of drug therapies and negative as well as positive consequences.

agents. Amlodipine also interacts with theophylline, cimetidine, lithium, and quinidine.

Beta-blockers, also indicated for angina, are contraindicated in clients with asthma, heart failure, or serious conduction disturbances. Cautious use is recommended in geriatric clients. Drug interactions include the same medications mentioned for CCBs.

Nursing Diagnoses

Nursing diagnoses related to the administration of anti-anginal agents include the following:
- Acute pain related to the pathological impact of tissue ischemia.
- Impaired physical mobility related to the ischemia angina.
- Deficient knowledge related to first-time use of drugs used to treat angina.
- Risk for injury related to the side effects of anti-anginal drugs.

Planning

Goals of nursing care related to the administration of anti-anginals include the following:
- Client experiences fewer episodes of chest pain.
- Client is able to perform ADLs with increasing comfort and less chest pain.
- Client tolerates moderate, supervised exercise.
- Client states the actions to take when chest pain is unrelieved.
- Client states the side effects of therapy to report.

Outcome Criteria

Outcome criteria related to the administration of anti-anginals include the following:
- Client has increased comfort related to therapeutic effects of anti-anginals with fewer precipitating events and episodes.
- Client experiences increased tolerance for activity, with less chest pain with increasing exercise.
- Client states symptoms to report to the physician, such as syncope, excessive dizziness, severe headache, or chest pain.

Implementation

When a client first begins anti-anginal therapy, it is crucial for the nurse to review the client's baseline vital signs and any documentation of the client's anginal pain and precipitating factors. If taking sublingual forms of medication, the client should be told to take nitroglycerine in the supine position at the first sign of angina to prevent or decrease dizziness and fainting resulting from drug-induced hypotension. This dizziness may last for up to half an hour. When administering nitroglycerine intravenously, it must be diluted in 5 percent dextrose in water or 0.9 percent sodium chloride and must not be given with any other drugs or solutions because of incompatibilities. Intravenously administered nitroglycerine must be contained in specially designed non-polyvinyl-chloride (PVC)

plastic intravenous bags and tubing to avoid absorption and/or uptake of the nitrate by the intravenous tubing/bag, and decomposition of the nitrate into cyanide, which can be caused by exposure to light.

In the past, glass intravenous bottles were used, and any plastic tubing or bags were covered with aluminum foil to prevent light exposure and subsequent decomposition of the drug. Because PVC intravenous filters or volume-control chambers absorb the drug, they should not be used. Intravenous infusions should be administered only with the use of infusion pumps, and all specific manufacturer's instructions should be followed. Intravenous forms of nitroglycerine are stable for only 96 hours after preparation. Parenteral solutions that are not clear or are discoloured blue, green, or dark red should be discarded. If the client is on long-term treatment with sodium nitroprusside (administered only intravenously and in a hypertensive crisis), thiocyanate levels should be monitored daily to avoid thiocyanate toxicity. Amyl nitrite is highly flammable and should be kept away from flames or smoking materials. If clients are taking nitroglycerine (or any nitrate) at home, they should be reminded that the active ingredients in the oral or sublingual forms are easily destroyed, and should be stored in an airtight, dark glass bottle with a metal cap and without cotton filler, away from any area exposed to heat, steam, light, or moisture. For example, nitrates should not be stored in a medicine cabinet over the bathroom sink. Clients should also be told not to transfer sublingual or oral dosage forms of nitrates from the dark glass container it comes in to a plastic container, which may make the medication unstable.

The rapid-acting agents (amyl nitrite, sublingual nitroglycerine, and sublingual isosorbide dinitrate) are indicated for the relief of acute angina attacks. The longer-acting nitrates, along with the topical, transdermal, transmucosal, and oral sustained-release forms are used to prevent anginal attacks or decrease their frequency and severity and to prevent predictable anginal episodes. Skin exposure to ointment forms of nitrates should be avoided because of possible absorption of the drug. Isosorbide mononitrate is one of the two active metabolites of isosorbide. Isosorbide dinitrate has no active metabolites and therefore results in more consistent therapeutic responses.

The differences in these agents need to be emphasized to clients so that they fully understand the drug they are taking, including how it works and what to expect therapeutically and adversely. Oral CCBs should be taken before meals and as ordered. Some of the agents, such as diltiazem, must be stored in an airtight container at room temperature. It is important for the nurse to monitor for therapeutic blood levels of CCBs (e.g., diltiazem: 50 to 200 ng/mL). Beta-blockers should be given and taken exactly as ordered (as should any of these medications as anti-anginals). Measures to decrease constipation include eating a high-fibre diet and forcing fluids. If clients report parts of the sustained-release forms of anti-anginal medication are appearing in their stool, this may indicate that the medication is moving too quickly through the GI tract and clients may need to be switched to another dosage form. With CCBs, as with all anti-anginals (especially beta blockers), clients should be instructed to take their pulse daily before they take their medication. If their heart rate is 60 beats/min or lower, they should contact their healthcare provider for further instructions.

For client teaching tips for anti-anginal agents, see the box on p. 391.

■ Evaluation

Clients taking anti-anginal agents must be monitored carefully for an allergic reaction, which may be manifested by dyspnea, swelling of the face, or hives. Clients should be monitored both for improvement of symptoms and for adverse reactions such as headache, lightheadedness, decreased BP, and dizziness, which may indicate the need for a decreased dose. If the client is receiving intravenous nitrates, it is important for the nurse to evaluate for the degree of skin turgor, the development of pedal edema, nausea, vomiting, rales, dyspnea, and orthopnea (difficulty breathing except when sitting or standing straight). In addition, clients should be monitored for the therapeutic effects of the agents, such as relief of the angina and decreased BP. If the client is experiencing blurred vision or dry mouth, the drug should be discontinued and the physician notified immediately.

NURSING CARE PLAN | Chest Pain

Mr. L., a 59-year-old high school principal, was admitted to the ER with complaints of chest pain after a high school basketball game, which he attended after a 12-hour day at work. He was taken by ambulance to emergency where 12-lead ECG and serum enzyme studies were completed to rule out possible MI. Over the next 24 hours he was observed and monitored. All studies were negative, and there were no further complaints of chest pain. He was discharged on sublingual nitroglycerine and is scheduled for an ultrasound and stress test with thallium scan in 1 week.

ASSESSMENT	Subjective Data	Complaints of chest pain and palpitations
	Objective Data	• Smoker for 20 years, 2 packs/day
		• Occasional wine drinker
		• Principal of high school
		• Family history of MI
		• History of hypertension for 2 years
		• Minimal exercise and does not watch diet for fat intake
NURSING DIAGNOSIS		Deficient knowledge related to lack of experience with treatment of chest pain
PLANNING	Goals	Before discharge client will verbalize dosing, importance of adherence, side effects, and drug interactions to nitroglycerine
	Outcome Criteria	Client will demonstrate understanding of medication regimen by accurately explaining the following:
		• Use of nitroglycerine
		• Side effects of medication
		• Drug interactions
		• Symptoms and side effects to report to the physician immediately
		• When to call 911
		• How to minimize side effects
IMPLEMENTATION		Sublingual nitroglycerine is taken to abort acute attacks. Onset of action is 1–3 min and lasts only 30 min. Therefore, it is important to follow these guidelines:
		• Place sublingual tab under the tongue. Do not chew; let dissolve. Do not swallow until dissolved. Take one sublingual tab every 5 min until chest pain relieved, but no more than 3 tabs within 15 min. If chest pain is unrelieved, call 911.
		• Avoid alcohol and OTC drugs with this medication.
		• A headache may occur with the dose of drug, and you may develop tolerance to the headache as time goes on; however, a non-narcotic analgesic is recommended.
		• If the drug stings when in contact with the mucous membranes, it is still potent.

| **Chest Pain—cont'd**

IMPLEMENTATION —cont'd

- The drug loses potency within 6 months, so sublingual nitroglycerine prescriptions/drugs should be less than 6 months old; 3 to 5 months is a safe rule of thumb; always have fresh refills available.
- Keep the sublingual nitroglycerine container away from light, heat, and moisture because these decrease the drug's effectiveness.
- Once you take the nitroglycerine, lie down and be sure to change positions slowly to avoid falling or fainting.
- You may be instructed by the physician to take this medication before stressful activities such as exercise or sexual activity to prevent angina.
- Be sure to take the medication exactly as prescribed.

EVALUATION

- Client shows therapeutic response to nitroglycerine therapy as evidenced by decreased occurrence of chest pain
- Client is monitored for and reports minimal side effects such as
  - Headache
  - Dizziness
  - Nausea
  - Vomiting
  - Pallor
  - Sweating
  - Hypotension
  - Tachycardia
  - Fainting
  - Flushing of the face

CLIENT TEACHING TIPS

The nurse should instruct the client on the following points (as relevant):

▲ If you are taking a nitrate for acute chest pain, take one sublingual tablet as soon as possible after the pain begins, lie down immediately, remain calm, and rest. If there is no relief, take another one after five minutes, and then a third after another five minutes. If you still have no relief, call 911.

▲ Never chew or swallow the sublingual nitrate forms. This will interfere with the medicine's action and effectiveness. Place the tablet under your tongue and let it dissolve before swallowing. If it causes a burning sensation under your tongue, don't worry; that just means the drug is still potent.

▲ Do not chew, crush, or swallow transmucosal nitroglycerine tablets. Place the tablet inside the cheek or under the lip and allow it to dissolve slowly.

▲ Always keep a fresh supply of nitroglycerine on hand. Even when stored properly, this drug loses its strength within about three months after the bottle has been opened.

▲ You may experience flushing of the face, dizziness, fainting, brief throbbing headache, increase in heart rate, and lightheadedness. Headaches usually last no longer than 20 minutes and are generally relieved with analgesics such as acetaminophen. Don't use narcotics such as codeine.

▲ Keep all medications out of the reach of children.

▲ Keep a record of the how often you have anginal attacks, what they're like, anything that seems to bring them on, and the number of pills taken. Also record in your journal how you feel after taking the medicine, including relief from your symptoms as well as any side effects.

▲ Avoid things that can bring on your angina, such as stress, loss of sleep, overeating, heavy exercise, coffee, tea, chocolate, caffeinated soft drinks, and cigarettes or other tobacco products.

▲ Take this medicine with caution. While you are taking this medication, consuming alcohol and soaking in hot baths, saunas, or hot tubs may cause low blood pressure and possibly fainting or a risk of injury.

▲ If you are using nitrate ointment, spread it in a thin layer on the applicator paper provided with the product. Don't use the paper from another product; they are not interchangeable. Don't rub or massage the ointment into the skin. Wash off any residue before applying new ointment. You can apply ointment to any hairless site on your body—it doesn't have to be on the chest or over the heart. Cover the ointment with plastic wrap or the paper that comes with the product to seal it off. This prevents staining and makes sure you get the full dose. The person applying the topical ointment or transdermal patch should wear gloves to prevent skin contact with the nitrate.

▲ Apply transdermal nitrate patches to a hairless part of the body (not necessarily the chest), but only after removing the old patch and cleaning the old site. You can wear a patch while swimming or bathing, but if it comes off, try to find and discard it, then clean the old site and apply a new patch.

▲ Some people develop resistance or tolerance to the nitrates; this means they stop working as well as they used to. Contact your physician if you think this is happening, or if you have further questions.

▲ Because these medications can make your blood pressure drop, change positions slowly to make sure you don't fall or faint. Notify your physician if you experience blurred vision or a persistent headache.

▲ Take CCBs at the same time every day and be careful to take them as prescribed. Avoid hazardous activities (such as climbing, driving a car, or operating heavy equipment) until the drug effects have stabilized and dizziness is no longer a problem. If you're on mainte-nance therapy, take and record your pulse rate before each dose and keep notes about any chest pain.

▲ Don't take any OTC medications unless your physician says it's okay.

▲ If you gain 1 kg of weight in 1 day or 2.5 kg or more in 1 week, notify your healthcare provider.

▲ If you're taking a beta-blocker, this is for long-term prevention of angina, not for immediate relief.

▲ If you're taking beta-blockers, drink plenty of fluids and eat a diet high in fibre (e.g., fresh figs, prunes, raisins, bran, wheat germ) to prevent constipation, unless you've been told not to.

▲ Do not discontinue your medicine abruptly; you could develop very high blood pressure and be at risk. If you are having problems with the medication, contact your physician.

▲ Report to your physician any chest pain, palpitations, excessive dizziness, fainting episodes, pulse rate less than 60 beats/min, swelling, or difficulty breathing.

POINTS to REMEMBER

▲ Angina pectoris (chest pain) occurs because of a mismatch between the oxygen supply and oxygen demand, with either too much oxygen demand or too little oxygen delivery.

▲ The heart is an aerobic (oxygen-requiring) muscle, and when it does not receive enough oxygen it becomes ischemic and produces pain (angina). When the coronary arteries that deliver oxygen to the heart muscle become blocked, a heart attack (myocardial infarct) occurs.

▲ Coronary artery disease is an abnormal condition of the arteries (blood vessels) that deliver oxygen to the heart muscle. These arteries may become narrowed, resulting in reduced flow of oxygen and nutrients to the myocardium.

▲ Nitrates, CCBs, and beta-blockers may be used to treat the symptoms of angina.

▲ Nitroglycerine is the drug prototype for the nitrates. Nitrates dilate constricted coronary arteries, helping to increase oxygen and nutrient supply to the heart muscle. Venous dilation results in a decrease of blood return to the heart (decreased pre-load), whereas arterial dilation results in a decrease of peripheral resistance (decreased afterload—what the left ventricle has to work against).

▲ Isosorbide dinitrates were the first group of oral agents used for angina; isosorbide mononitrates are the new and improved nitrates used for angina. Nitroglycerine is the main intravenous nitrate used for angina and for hypertensive crises.

▲ CCBs relieve angina by reducing afterload (the force the ventricles must push against to eject their blood), thus reducing the workload of the heart and therefore the oxygen demand. These drugs relax the smooth muscle surrounding the blood vessels, causing them to dilate, thereby decreasing BP.

▲ Beta-blockers relieve angina by decreasing the heart rate, which helps reduce the workload of the heart and decreases oxygen demand on the heart.

▲ Nursing considerations for the use of all anti-anginals include the following:
- Intravenous administration of nitrates should be done in accordance with manufacturer's guidelines and institutional policies.
- Various dosage forms of nitrates cannot be used interchangeably.
- Beta-blockers may exacerbate conditions in clients with respiratory disease such as COPD.
- CCBs may be ordered for angina and are associated with side effects of hypotension, headache, dizziness, and edema.

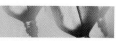

EXAMINATION REVIEW QUESTIONS

1 Transdermal nitroglycerine patches are most appropriately used or indicated in which of the following?
a. To abort any type of angina
b. For use with ventricular irregularity
c. To prevent the occurrence of angina
d. For use with atrial irregularities

2 Which of the following statements reflects adequate knowledge by the nurse about the administration of parenteral nitroglycerine?
a. Give the intravenous form by bolus injection.
b. Because the oral and intravenous forms are short-lived, the dosing must be every 2 hours.
c. Intravenous nitroglycerine must be protected from exposure to light through use of special tubing.
d. Nitroglycerine is compatible, in solution, with many drugs.

3 Which of the following statements by the client reflects the need for additional client education about diltiazem?
a. I can take this drug to abort acute anginal attacks.
b. I understand that food and antacids alter this drug's absorption orally.

c. When taking the sustained-release forms, the drug cannot be crushed.
d. When taking any oral form, I know to follow directions closely.

4 Which of the following is a contraindication for calcium channel blockers (CCBs)?
a. Temperature of 38.1°C
b. Heart failure and use of digitalis
c. BP of 130/84 mm Hg
d. Angina and use of nitrates

5 Which of the following would be the best to tell a client being placed on an anti-anginal drug?
a. Chew any extended-release preparations and follow with 420 mL of fluid.
b. Common side effects include hypertension, confusion, and vomiting.
c. Do not be too concerned if you abruptly withdraw the drug.
d. Chest pain, excessive dizziness, edema, and/or shortness of breath should be reported to your healthcare provider immediately.

For answers see http://evolve.elsevier.com/Lilley/pharmacology/.

CRITICAL THINKING ACTIVITIES

1 Mr. J. is a 45-year-old man with stable angina who has recently been prescribed sublingual nitroglycerine tablets for the relief of his anginal attacks. What teaching instructions does Mr. J. require in order to take the nitroglycerine appropriately?

2 Mr. J. has been switched from sublingual nitroglycerine to a transdermal form. What instructions does the nurse need to give him regarding the difference in his therapeutic regimen?

3 Mr. F. has just suffered an MI, for which he has received a thrombolytic agent, aspirin, heparin, oxygen, and now a nitroglycerine infusion. The infusion is running at a rate of 33 mg/min, and the concentration of the infusion is 200 mg/mL. At what rate should the infusion pump be set in millilitres per hour?

For answers see http://evolve.elsevier.com/Lilley/pharmacology/.

BIBLIOGRAPHY

Albanese, J., & Nutz, P. (2005). *Mosby's 2005 nursing drug cards.* St Louis, MO: Mosby.

Anderson, P.O., Knoben, J.E., & Troutman, W.G. (2002). *Handbook of clinical drug data* (10th ed.). New York: McGraw-Hill/Appleton & Lange.

Berne, R., & Levy, M. (2002). *Principles of physiology* (3rd ed.). St Louis, MO: Mosby.

Boron, W.F., & Boulpaep, E.L. (2003). *Medical physiology.* Philadelphia: Saunders.

Braunwald, E. & The Committee on the Management of Patients with Unstable Angina. (2002). ACC/AHA 2002 guideline update for the management of patients with unstable angina and non-ST-segment elevation myocardial infarction. [Electronic version]. Retrieved August 8, 2005, from http://www.acc.org/clinical/guidelines/unstable/incorporated/UA_incorporated.pdf

Canadian Pharmacists Association. (2003). *Therapeutic choices* (4th ed.). Ottawa, ON: Author.

Canadian Pharmacists Association. (2004). *Guide to drugs in Canada.* Toronto, ON: Dorling Kindersley.

Canadian Pharmacists Association. (2005). *Compendium of pharmaceuticals and specialties. The Canadian drug reference for health professionals.* Ottawa, ON: Author. [The subscription-based e-CPS is available at http://www.pharmacists.ca.]

Cornish, P. (2005). "Avoid the crush": Hazards of medication administration in patient with dysphagia or a feeding tube. *Canadian Medical Association Journal, 172*(7), 871–872. Retrieved November 11, 2005, from http://www.cmaj.ca/cgi/content/full/172/7/871

Hamm, C. W., & Braunwald, E. (2000). A classification of unstable angina revisited. *Circulation, 102,* 120.

Health Canada. (2005). Drug product database (DPD). Retrieved August 9, 2005, from http://www.hc-sc.gc.ca/hpb/drugs-dpd/

Johns Hopkins Hospital, Gunn, V.L., & Nechyba, C. (2002). *The Harriet Lane handbook* (17th ed.). St Louis, MO: Mosby.

Lacy, C.F., Armstrong, L.L., Goldman, M.P., & Lance, L.L. (2003). *Drug information handbook* (11th ed.). Hudson, OH: Lexi-Comp.

Lehne, R.A. (2004). *Pharmacology for nursing care* (5th ed.). St Louis, MO: Saunders.

Mosby. (2005). *Mosby's drug consult 2005: The comprehensive reference for generic and brand name drugs* (15th ed.). St Louis, MO: Mosby.

Skidmore-Roth, L. (2006). *Mosby's 2006 nursing drug reference* (19th ed.). St Louis, MO: Mosby.

Woods, S.L., Sivarajan Froelocher, E.S., Underhill Motzer, S., & Bridges, E.J. (2005). *Cardiac nursing* (5th ed.). Philadelphia: Lippincott Williams & Wilkins.

Antihypertensive Agents

OBJECTIVES

After reading this chapter, the successful student will be able to do the following:

1 Briefly discuss the normal anatomy and physiology of the autonomic nervous system, including the events that take place during synaptic transmission within the sympathetic and parasympathetic divisions that have an impact on the long-term as well as short-term control of blood pressure.

2 Define hypertension and compare primary and secondary hypertension and related manifestations.

3 Examine the various parameters for mm Hg pressure for hypertension outlined in the Canadian Hypertension Education Program Guidelines.

4 Contrast the older means of treating hypertension using a stepped-care approach and the newer method of treating hypertension.

5 Discuss the rationale for the non-pharmacological management of hypertension.

6 Compare the various drugs used in the pharmacological management of hypertension in terms of mechanisms of action, specific indications, side effects, toxic effects, cautions, contraindications, dosages, and routes of administration.

7 Develop a nursing care plan that includes all phases of the nursing process for clients receiving antihypertensive agents.

GLOSSARY

Alpha₁-blockers Drugs that primarily cause arterial and venous dilation through action on peripheral sympathetic neurons.

Antihypertensive agents Medications used to treat hypertension.

Cardiac output Amount of blood ejected from the left ventricle, measured in litres per minute.

Centrally acting adrenergic agents Drugs that modify the function of the sympathetic nervous system in the brain by stimulating alpha₂-receptors, which has a reverse sympathetic effect, causing decreased blood pressure.

Essential hypertension An elevated systemic arterial pressure for which no cause can be found and that is often the only significant clinical finding; also called *primary* or *idiopathic hypertension.*

Ganglionic-blocking agents (gang glee on' ik) Agents that prevent nerves from responding to the action of acetylcholine by occupying the receptor sites for acetylcholine (i.e., nicotinic receptors) on sympathetic and parasympathetic nerve endings.

Hypertension A common, often asymptomatic disorder in which blood pressure persistently exceeds 140/90 mm Hg.

Nicotinic receptor (nik o tin' ik) The receptor and site of action for acetylcholine in both the parasympathetic and sympathetic nervous systems. Nicotinic receptors are located at the junction of the pre- and post-ganglionic neurons of both of these systems.

Orthostatic hypotension (or tho stat' ik) A common side effect of adrenergic drugs involving a sudden drop in blood pressure when clients change position, especially when rising from a seated or horizontal position.

Pro-drug A drug that is inactive in its present form and must be biotransformed in the liver to its active form.

Secondary hypertension High blood pressure associated with one of several primary diseases, such as renal, pulmonary, endocrine, and vascular diseases.

Significant advancements have been made in the detection, evaluation, and treatment of high blood pressure (BP), or **hypertension.** Over the past 40 years the development of new antihypertensive medications has greatly enhanced the quality of life of affected people by reducing the incidence of the various complications associated with hypertension and improving the side effect profiles of the medications. Drug therapy for hypertension first became available in the early 1950s with the introduction of **ganglionic-blocking agents**. However, side effects and inconsistent therapeutic effects were common problems with these agents. Then in 1953 the vasodilator hydralazine was introduced and in 1958, the thiazide diuretics. These agents offered important advantages over the existing antihypertensive drug therapies. In addition, with the discovery of these newer drugs came a better understanding of the disease process itself. Now a myriad of antihypertensive drugs are available, the newer ones commonly being more effective, more versatile, and better tolerated than the older agents. These agents can be used either alone or in combination with other **antihypertensive agents.** The classes of drugs that can be employed are diuretics, beta-blockers (beta-receptor antagonists), angiotensin converting enzyme (ACE) inhibitors, alpha₁-antagonists, alpha₂-agonists, angiotensin II receptor blockers (ARBs), and calcium channel blockers (CCBs). Although some of the medications mentioned in this chapter represent older classes of drugs, all are current therapeutic options recommended by the treatment guidelines for hypertension published by the Canadian Hypertension Education Program (CHEP). For this reason selected examples from both older and newer drug classes are discussed in this chapter.

HYPERTENSION

By the year 2025, it is expected that 1.56 billion adults over 18 years of age worldwide will have hypertension. In Canada, as many as 5 million people have some form of hypertension. Many of them are undiagnosed. In addition, many of those under medical management do not achieve normal blood pressure. Untreated hypertension has many severe consequences; hypertension is the most common and the major risk factor for coronary artery disease (CAD), cardiovascular disease, and death resulting from cardiovascular causes. It is the most important risk factor for stroke and heart failure, and it is also a major risk factor for renal failure and peripheral vascular disease (PVD).

Guidelines for diagnosis, treatment, and management of hypertension have varied considerably over the years, resulting in a great deal of misunderstanding. In January 2005, the Canadian Hypertension Education Program (CHEP) and the Heart and Stroke Foundation of Canada released recommendations for the management of hypertension assembled by the 43 members of the CHEP Evidence-Based Recommendations Task Force. CHEP's intent is to educate both healthcare professionals and the general public about the dangers of hypertension and the importance of its treatment.

Since 2000, CHEP has produced yearly updated evidence-based hypertension management recommendations (Box 24-1). Each year the recommendations focus on a change from previous guidelines or an important initiative. In 2003, the Joint National Committee of the National High Blood Pressure Education Program and the Guidelines Committee of the World Health Organization and the International Society of Hypertension (WHO/ISH) developed new guidelines (JNC 7) for defining normal and elevated levels of blood pressure. This report adopts a stricter classification system for BP, because the previously applied term *mild hypertension* did not adequately reflect the serious nature of this condition: most of the morbidity and mortality occurs in the so-called "mild hypertension" group, which includes the vast majority of individuals with hypertension.

TABLE 24-1

TARGET VALUES FOR BLOOD PRESSURE

Condition	Target (SBP/DBP mm Hg)
Diastolic ± systolic hypertension	<140/90
Isolated systolic hypertension	<140
Diabetes	<130/80
Renal disease	<130/80
Proteinuria >1 g/day	<125/75

Useful Antihypertensive Drug Combinations

For additive hypotensive effect in dual therapy, combine an agent from Column 1 with any in Column 2.

Column 1	Column 2
Thiazide diuretic	Beta-blocker*
Long-acting calcium channel blocker*	ACE Inhibitor, ARB

*Caution should be exercised in combining a non-dihydropyridine calcium channel blocker (DHP-CCB) and a beta-blocker.
Source: Canadian Hypertension Education Program Recommendations, 2005.

In the 1970s, the stepped-care pharmacological approach to treating the illness was advocated to manage hypertension. Treatment regimens consisted of a thiazide diuretic as a first step, with sympatholytic agents and vasodilators added sequentially, if needed, to achieve the goal blood pressure. In Canada beta-blockers became widely used, and by November 1983 the Canadian Hypertension Society's Consensus Conference on the Management of Mild Hypertension recommended starting therapy with either a diuretic or a beta-blocker. Once angiotensin-converting enzyme (ACE) inhibitors and calcium antagonists were introduced, they received widespread attention as possible first-line therapy. The traditional stepped-care approach no longer adequately reflected the scope of pharmacological alternatives nor the scientific understanding of hypertension. Individualized therapy was deemed a more appropriate treatment strategy than stepped care. Some clients may require two or more medications, even as initial therapy, depending on their individual set of related cardiovascular risk factors, such as obesity, diabetes, and family history. Healthcare providers are therefore encouraged, in planning drug therapy, to take into consideration the client's demographic characteristics, the presence of concomitant diseases, the use of concurrent therapies, and the client's quality of life.

The classification scheme used to categorize individual cases of hypertension in Canada is based on target values, which are presented in detail in Table 24-1.

Hypertension can also be defined by its cause. When the specific cause for hypertension is unknown, it may be called *essential, idiopathic,* or *primary hypertension.* About 90 percent of the cases of hypertension are of this type. **Secondary hypertension** makes up the other 10 percent. It is most commonly the result of another disease such as pheochromocytoma, the eclampsia of pregnancy, or renal artery disease. It may also result from the use of certain medications. If the cause of secondary hypertension can be eliminated, the BP usually returns to normal.

BP is determined by the product of **cardiac output** and systemic vascular resistance (SVR). Cardiac output is the amount of blood that is ejected from the left ventricle and is measured in litres per minute. Normal cardiac output is 4 to 8 L/min. SVR is the force (resistance) the left ventricle has to overcome to eject its volume of blood. Numerous factors interact to regulate these two major variables and keep the BP within normal limits, as illustrated in Fig. 24-1. These same factors can be responsible for causing high blood pressure and are the sites of action of many of the antihypertensive drugs.

ANTIHYPERTENSIVE AGENTS

Drug therapy for hypertension should be individualized to accommodate or complement the specific needs or concerns of the client. Important considerations in planning drug therapy are whether the client has concomitant medical problems and the expected effect of drug therapy on the client's quality of life. Demographic factors, ethnocultural implications, the ease of medication administration (e.g., a once-a-day dosing schedule or transdermal administration), and cost are other important considerations.

There are six main categories of pharmacological agents: diuretics, adrenergic agents, vasodilators, ACE inhibitors, ARBs, and CCBs. These may be used either

New Hypertension Guidelines

In 1999, a steering committee composed of members from the Canadian Hypertension Society, the Canadian Coalition for High Blood Pressure Prevention and Control, Health Canada, and the College of Family Physicians of Canada collaborated to develop *Canadian Recommendations for the Management of Hypertension*. This document introduced changes that directly affect the detection, evaluation, and treatment of hypertension. One change was the introduction of individualized therapy, as discussed above. Healthcare providers were encouraged to consider not only demographics, concurrent therapies, and quality of life, but also ethnicity and ethnoculture. In 2005, the Canadian Hypertension Education Program, a group that meets annually to update evidence-based recommendations for the management of hypertension, introduced its sixth report with the following significant changes:

- The optimum level for blood pressure is reduced to <140/90 mm Hg for the general population and <130/80 mm Hg for clients with diabetes or renal disease.
- Screening for hypertension should be more frequent than the previously recommended six months, especially when the patient is at increased risk.
- Any of three validated technologies may be used to diagnose hypertension, including home monitoring.
- First-line monotherapy may use any of five validated classes of drugs: thiazide (and thiazide-like) diuretics; beta-adrenergic antagonists (in clients younger than 60 years); ACE inhibitors (in non-Black clients); longer-acting dihydropyridine calcium channel blockers; and angiotensin II receptor blockers. Also included for 2005 are the longer-acting non-dihydropyridine calcium channel blockers (verapamil and diltiazem).

The report also reinforced messages from previous recommendations:

- The overall management plan for clients with hypertension must be based on their overall cardiovascular risk.
- Lifestyle modifications are crucial and must be reinforced.
- Both lifestyle and drug management is necessary to achieve an optimum blood pressure.
- A varied approach can promote adherence.

Source: Hemmelgarn, B.R., McAllister, F.A., Myers, M.G., McKay, D.W., Bolli, P., Abbott, C., et al. (2005). The 2005 Canadian Hypertension Education Program recommendations for the management of hypertension: Part 1—Blood pressure measurement, diagnosis and assessment of risk. *Canadian Journal of Cardiology, 21*(8), 645–656.

Dietary Intake and Heart Disease

Diet and lifestyle are two of the most touted ways to reduce the risk of coronary heart disease (CHD). All Canadians need to make better food choices and to exercise more to reduce cardiovascular risk factors. The Heart and Stroke Foundation of Canada bases its recommendations for healthy eating on *Canada's Food Guide* and foods from each of the four food groups (grain products, vegetables and fruit, milk products, and meat and alternatives). Guidelines continue to recommend that fat intake be no more than 20 to 35 percent of total calories, with an emphasis on eating more polyunsaturated fats, especially monounsaturated fat, and avoiding trans fats. More recent is the recommendation that fish high in omega-3 oils (fatty fish), such as mackerel, albacore tuna, lake trout, sardines, salmon, and herring, should be part of a heart-healthy diet. Omega-3 oils are also found in walnuts. Omega-3 fatty acid consumption has been shown to improve the overall health of arteries and to reduce BP, triglyceride levels, atherosclerotic plaque growth, thrombosis, and sudden death. Both the Mediterranean Diet and the Dietary Approaches to Stop Hypertension (DASH) diet have also been found to have benefits to the heart. Research suggests that following the DASH diet can lower both systolic and diastolic blood pressure because of its diuretic effect. This diet emphasizes fruits and vegetables and low-fat dairy and meats, but also limits sodium intake. The Mediterranean diet is also primarily vegetarian with few meat and dairy products. However, diet is only part of a combination of diet, exercise, social support, and moderate intake of wine that may lower the incidence of heart disease in individuals who live in Mediterranean countries.

Sources: Hu, F. (2003). The Mediterranean diet and mortality—olive oil and beyond. *New England Journal of Medicine, 348*(26), 2599–2608; Heart and Stroke Foundation.

Antihypertensive Drug Therapy

Important generalizations about demographics and the drugs used to treat hypertension include the following:

- Beta-blockers and ACE inhibitors have been found to be more effective in white clients than in Black clients.
- CCBs and diuretics have been shown to be more effective in geriatric and Black clients than in white clients.

These findings help us to better understand the dynamics of pharmacological treatment in clients of different ethnic groups with a diagnosis of hypertension. It also allows us to appreciate individual responses to drug therapy and thus to more successfully treat the disease process. Many healthcare providers use these generalizations to select first-line therapy.

alone or in combination, and the various antihypertensive agents in each category are listed in Box 24-2. The diuretics are discussed in detail in Chapter 25 and therefore are not discussed here.

NICOTINIC RECEPTORS

The stimulation of the two divisions of the autonomic nervous system (ANS), the parasympathetic (PSNS) and sympathetic (SNS) nervous systems, is controlled by the neurotransmitters acetylcholine (ACh) and norepinephrine. The receptors for both divisions of the ANS are located throughout the body in a variety of tissues. ANS physiology can be reviewed in greater detail in the introductory sections of Chapters 17 through 20. The preganglionic

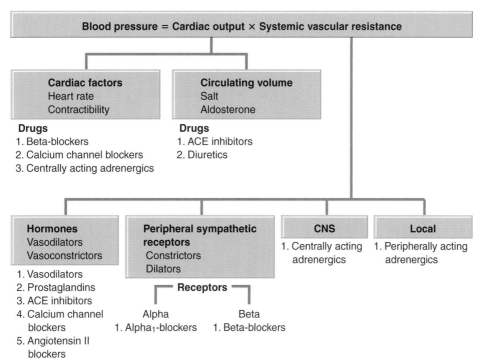

FIG. 24-1 Normal regulation of blood pressure and corresponding mechanisms.

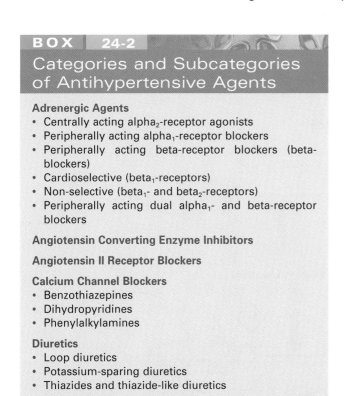

BOX 24-2

Categories and Subcategories of Antihypertensive Agents

Adrenergic Agents
- Centrally acting alpha$_2$-receptor agonists
- Peripherally acting alpha$_1$-receptor blockers
- Peripherally acting beta-receptor blockers (beta-blockers)
- Cardioselective (beta$_1$-receptors)
- Non-selective (beta$_1$- and beta$_2$-receptors)
- Peripherally acting dual alpha$_1$- and beta-receptor blockers

Angiotensin Converting Enzyme Inhibitors

Angiotensin II Receptor Blockers

Calcium Channel Blockers
- Benzothiazepines
- Dihydropyridines
- Phenylalkylamines

Diuretics
- Loop diuretics
- Potassium-sparing diuretics
- Thiazides and thiazide-like diuretics

Vasodilators
Act directly on vascular smooth muscle cells, *not* through alpha- or beta-receptors.

receptor for ACh in both the SNS and PSNS is the **nicotinic receptor.** It gets its name from the fact that it was the administration of the ganglionic stimulant nicotine that first revealed its existence. In both systems this receptor is located between the preganglionic and post-ganglionic fibres. The receptor located between the post-ganglionic fibre and the effector cells (i.e., the post-ganglionic receptor) is called the *muscarinic or cholinergic receptor* in the PSNS and the *adrenergic or noradrenergic receptor* (i.e., alpha- or beta-receptor) in the SNS. Physiological activity at muscarinic receptors is stimulated by ACh and cholinergic agonist drugs (Chapter 19) and is inhibited by cholinergic antagonists (anticholinergic drugs, Chapter 20). Similarly, physiological activity at adrenergic receptors is stimulated by norepinephrine and epinephrine and adrenergic agonist drugs (Chapter 17) and inhibited by anti-adrenergic drugs (adrenergic blockers, i.e., alpha- or beta-receptor blockers, Chapter 18). Figure 24-3 shows how these various receptors are arranged in both the PSNS and SNS, along with their corresponding neurotransmitters.

ADRENERGIC AGENTS

Adrenergic agents are a large group of antihypertensive agents, as shown in Box 24-2. The beta-blockers and combined alpha-beta blockers have been discussed in detail in Chapter 17. The adrenergic agents discussed here have different sites where they exert their antihypertensive action.

Mechanism of Action and Drug Effects

Five specific drug categories are included among the adrenergic antihypertensive agents, as indicated in Box 24-2. Each of these categories of drugs can be described as having central (in the brain) or peripheral (in the heart and blood vessels) action. These drugs include the adrenergic neuron blockers (central and peripheral), the alpha$_2$-receptor agonists (central), the alpha$_1$-receptor

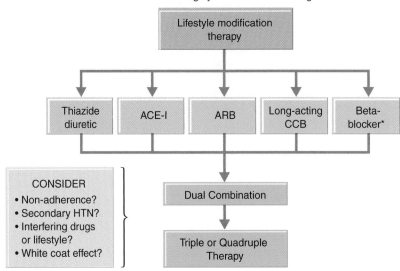

FIG 24-2 Treatment of systolic-diastolic hypertension without other compelling indications. Source: Canadian Hypertension Society. (2005). Management of Hypertension: Pamphlets, Slides and Summaries. CHEP 2005 Treatment slides. Retrieved from http://www.hypertension.ca/index2.html. Reproduced with permission.

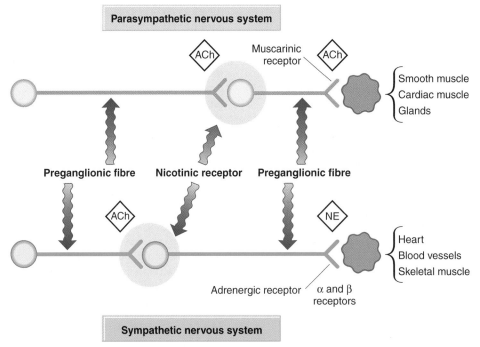

FIG. 24-3 Location of the nicotinic receptors within the parasympathetic and sympathetic nervous systems. *ACh,* Acetylcholine; *NE,* norepinephrine.

blockers (peripheral), beta-receptor blockers (peripheral), and the combination alpha$_1$- and beta-receptor blockers (peripheral).

The centrally acting alpha$_2$-adrenergic agents clonidine and methyldopa act by modifying the function of the SNS. Because SNS stimulation leads to an increased heart rate and force of contraction, the constriction of blood vessels, and the release of renin from the kidney, the result is hypertension. The **centrally acting adrenergic agents** work by stimulating the alpha$_2$-adrenergic receptors in the brain. The alpha$_2$-adrenergic receptors are unique in that receptor stimulation actually reduces sympathetic outflow, in this case from the CNS. The resulting lack of norepinephrine production reduces BP. This stimulation of the alpha$_2$-adrenergic receptors also affects the kidneys by reducing the activity of renin. Renin is the hormone and enzyme that converts the protein precursor angiotensinogen to the protein angiotensin I, the precursor of angiotensin II (AII), a potent vasoconstrictor that raises BP.

In the periphery, the **alpha$_1$-blockers** doxazosin, prazosin, and terazosin also modify the function of the SNS. However, they do so by blocking the alpha$_1$-adrenergic receptors, which, when stimulated by circulating norepinephrine, produce increased BP. Thus when these receptors are blocked, BP is decreased. The drug effects of the alpha$_1$-blockers are primarily related to their ability to dilate arteries and veins, with reduced peripheral vascular resistance and subsequent decrease in BP. This produces a marked decrease in the systemic and pulmonary venous pressures and an increase in cardiac output. Alpha$_1$-blockers also increase urinary flow rates and decrease outflow obstruction by preventing smooth muscle contractions in the bladder neck and urethra. This can be beneficial in cases of benign prostatic hypertrophy (BPH).

Beta-blockers also act in the periphery and include such agents as propranolol, atenolol, and several others. These drugs are discussed in more detail in Chapter 22 because they also have antidysrhythmic properties. Their antihypertensive effects are related to their reduction of the heart rate due to beta$_1$-receptor blockade. Two dual-action alpha$_1$- and beta-receptor blockers are currently available: labetalol and the newer drug carvedilol, which is growing in use. They have the dual antihypertensive effects of vasodilation (alpha$_1$-receptor blockade) and reducing heart rate (beta$_1$-receptor blockade). Figure 24-4 illustrates the site and mechanism of action for the various antihypertensive agents.

Indications

All of the agents mentioned are primarily used for the treatment of hypertension, either alone or in combination with other antihypertensive agents. Various forms of glaucoma may also respond to treatment with some of these agents. Clonidine also has several unlabelled uses (that is, uses not approved by Health Canada but still

common), including prophylaxis against migraine headaches and the treatment of severe dysmenorrhea or menopausal flushing. It is also useful in managing withdrawal symptoms in opioid-, nicotine-, or alcohol-dependent persons. The alpha$_1$-blockers doxazosin, prazosin, and terazosin have been used to relieve the symptoms associated with BPH. They have also proved effective in the management of severe heart failure when used with cardiac glycosides (Chapter 21) and diuretics (Chapter 25).

Contraindications

Contraindications to the use of the adrenergic antihypertensive agents include known drug allergy and may also include acute heart failure, concurrent use with monoamine oxidase inhibitors (MAOIs; Chapter 15), severe depression, peptic ulcer, colitis, and severe liver or kidney disease. As mentioned in Chapter 21, vasodilating agents may also be contraindicated in cases of heart failure secondary to diastolic dysfunction.

Side Effects and Adverse Effects

As with all drug classes, adrenergic drugs can cause side effects and adverse effects. The most common side effects include postural and post-exercise hypotension, dry mouth, drowsiness, sedation, and constipation. Other effects include headaches, sleep disturbances, nausea, rash, peripheral pooling of blood, and cardiac disturbances such as palpitations. There is also a high incidence of **orthostatic hypotension**, a condition in which BP drops suddenly during changes in position. In addition, the abrupt discontinuation of the centrally acting alpha$_2$-receptor agonists can result in rebound hypertension. However, this may also be true for other antihypertensive drug classes. Any change in the dosing regimen for cardiovascular medications should be undertaken gradually and with appropriate client monitoring and follow-up. Although this is also true for most classes of medications, abrupt dosage changes in cardiovascular medications, either up or down, can be especially hazardous for the client.

Interactions

Adrenergic agents interact primarily with CNS depressants such as alcohol, benzodiazepines, and opioids. The additive effects of these combinations of agents increase CNS depression. Other drug interactions that can occur with selected adrenergic agents are summarized in Table 24-2. This list is merely representative and is not exhaustive. The nurse should always keep a drug information handbook available to check if a specific drug interaction is suspected.

Dosages

For information on the dosages of selected adrenergic antihypertensive agents, see the table on p. 403. See Appendix B for some of the common brands available in Canada.

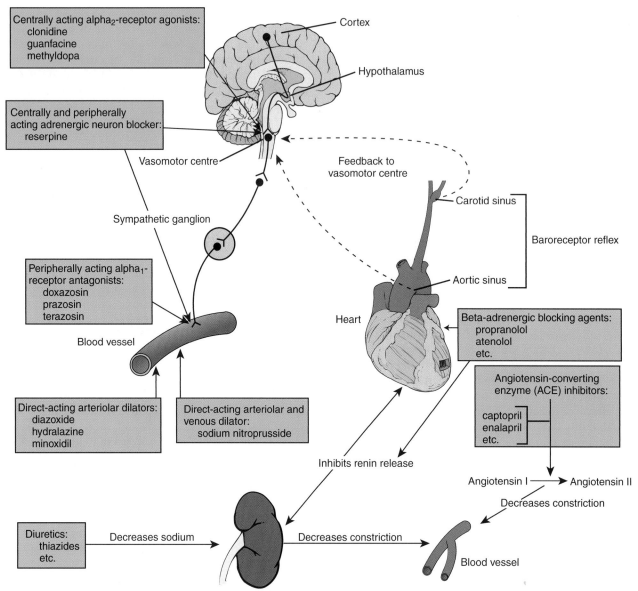

FIG 24-4 Site and mechanism of action for the various antihypertensive agents. Note: Reserpine is not available in Canada. Source: U.S. Department of Health and Human Services. (1997). *The sixth report of the Joint National Committee on detection, evaluation, and treatment of high blood pressure (JNC-VI).* Washington, DC: National Institutes of Health. In S.M. Lewis, M.M. Heitkemper, & S.R. Dirksen. (2004). *Medical-surgical nursing: Assessment and management of clinical problems* (6th ed.). St Louis, MO: Mosby.

DRUG PROFILES

ALPHA₂-ADRENERGIC RECEPTOR STIMULATORS (AGONISTS)

Of the available alpha₂-receptor agonists clonidine and methyldopa, clonidine is by far the most commonly used and the prototype agent for this drug class. Methyldopa is also used in the treatment of hypertension and is the drug of choice for treating hypertension in pregnancy. However, these agents are not typically prescribed as first-line antihypertensive agents because their use is associated with a high incidence of side effects such as orthostatic hypotension, fatigue, and dizziness. They may be used as adjunct agents in the therapy for hypertension

after other agents have failed or may be used in conjunction with other antihypertensives such as diuretics.

▶▶ clonidine

Clonidine is primarily used for its ability to decrease BP. As previously noted, clonidine is also useful in the management of opioid withdrawal. It has a better safety profile than the other centrally acting adrenergics. Clonidine is available in oral form as 0.1- and 0.2-mg tablets. Clonidine should not be abruptly discontinued because of severe rebound hypertension. Its use is contraindicated in clients who have shown hypersensitivity reactions to it. Pregnancy category C. See the table on p. 403 for recommended dosages.

TABLE 24-2

ADRENERGIC AGENTS: DRUG INTERACTIONS

Drug	Interacts With	Mechanism	Result
Clonidine	Opioids, sedatives, hypnotics, anaesthetics, alcohol	Additive	Increased CNS depression
	Tricyclic antidepressants (TCAs), monoamine oxidase inhibitors (MAOIs), appetite suppressants, amphetamines	Opposing actions	Decreased hypotensive effects
	Diuretics, other antihypertensive agents	Additive	Increased hypotensive effects
	Beta-blockers, cardiac glycosides	Additive	May potentiate bradycardia and increase the rebound hypertension in clonidine withdrawal
Prazosin	Diuretics, other hypotensive agents	Additive	Increased hypotension
	indomethacin	Opposing effects	Decreased hypotensive effect
	verapamil	Increased serum prazosin levels	Increased hypotension

DOSAGES   Selected Antihypertensive Agents: Adrenergic Agonists and Antagonists

Agent	Pharmacological Class	Usual Dosage Range	Indications
carvedilol	Peripherally acting alpha$_1$, beta$_1$, and beta$_2$-receptor antagonist (blocker)	PO: 3.125 to 25 mg bid	Hypertension (also used in heart failure)
▸▸clonidine	Centrally acting alpha$_2$-receptor agonist	PO: Initial dose 0.1 mg qd–bid; may titrate up to a maximum of 0.6 mg/day, divided bid–qid	Hypertension (may have other unlabelled uses including psychiatric, cardiovascular, and GI problems)
prazosin	Peripherally acting alpha$_1$, receptor antagonist	PO: Initial dose 1 mg bid–tid; may titrate up to maximum of 20 mg/day, divided bid–qid	Hypertension

PHARMACOKINETICS

Half-Life	Onset	Peak	Duration
12–16 hr	30–60 min	3–5 hr	8 hr

ALPHA$_1$-BLOCKERS

The alpha$_1$-blockers—doxazosin, prazosin, tamsulosin, and terazosin—are the newest of the adrenergics and have the best safety and efficacy profiles, but they are not free of adverse effects. They are contraindicated in clients who have shown a hypersensitivity to them and are classified as pregnancy category C agents. They are available only in oral preparations. Tamsulosin is not used to control BP but is indicated solely for symptomatic control of BPH. This use is described further in Chapter 34.

prazosin

Prazosin is the oldest of the alpha$_1$-blockers and the prototype. It reduces both peripheral vascular resistance and BP by dilating both arterial and venous blood vessels. It has been shown beneficial in the treatment of hypertension, the relief of the symptoms of obstructive BPH, and as an adjunct to cardiac glycosides and diuretics in the treatment of severe heart failure. Prazosin is available as 1-, 2-, and 5-mg tablets. Recommended dosages are given in the table above.

PHARMACOKINETICS

Half-Life	Onset	Peak	Duration
2–4 hr	2 hr	2–4 hr	<24 hr

DUAL-ACTION ALPHA$_1$- AND BETA-RECEPTOR BLOCKERS

carvedilol

Carvedilol, a newer agent, was approved by Health Canada in 1996. It is growing in use and seems to be well tolerated by most clients. It is beginning to be recognized for its use in hypertension but it is only currently indicated for use in mild to severe heart failure in conjunction with digoxin, diuretics, and ACE inhibitors. Its contraindications include known drug allergy, cardiogenic shock, severe bradycardia or heart failure, primary obstructive valve disease, hepatic impairment, bronchospastic conditions such as asthma, and various cardiac problems involving the conduction system. It is currently available only in oral form in 3.125-, 6.25-, 12.5-, and 25-mg tablets. Pregnancy category C. Dosage information appears in the table above.

PHARMACOKINETICS

Half-Life	Onset	Peak	Duration
7–10 hr	1–2 hr	1–2 hr	Unknown

ANGIOTENSIN CONVERTING ENZYME INHIBITORS

The ACE inhibitors represent a large group of antihypertensive agents. There are currently 10 ACE inhibitors available for clinical use, in addition to various combination drug products in which a thiazide diuretic or a CCB is combined with an ACE inhibitor. Currently available ACE inhibitors are captopril, benazepril, cilazapril, enalapril, fosinopril, lisinopril, perindopril, quinapril, ramipril, and trandolapril. These agents are safe and efficacious and are often used as the first-line agents in the treatment of both heart failure and hypertension. Some of the distinguishing characteristics of the various agents that make up this large class of antihypertensives are summarized in Table 24-3. The ACE inhibitors as a class are similar and differ in only a few of their chemical properties, but show some significant differences in clinical properties. Knowing these differences can be helpful in selecting the proper agent for a particular client.

Captopril has the shortest half-life and therefore must be dosed more frequently than any of the other ACE inhibitors. This may be an important drawback to its use in a client who has a history of non-adherence. On the other hand, it may be best to start with a drug that has a short half-life in a client who is still critically ill and may not tolerate medications well, so that if problems arise they will be short lived. Captopril is administered three times a day, while enalapril is administered two times a day.

Captopril and lisinopril are the only two ACE inhibitors that are not pro-drugs. A **pro-drug** is a drug that is inactive in its present form and must be biotransformed in the liver to its active form to be effective. This is an important advantage in a client with liver dysfunction because all of the other ACE inhibitors are pro-drugs and their transformation to active form in such clients would be hindered.

Enalapril is the only ACE inhibitor that is available in a parenteral preparation. All other agents are available only in oral formulations. All of the newer ACE inhibitors, such as benazepril, fosinopril, lisinopril, quinapril, and ramipril, have long half-lives and durations of action, allowing them to be given only once a day. This is particularly beneficial in a client who is taking many other medications and may have difficulty keeping track of the various dosing schedules for each. A once-a-day medication regimen promotes better client adherence.

All ACE inhibitors have detrimental effects on the unborn fetus and neonate. They are classified as pregnancy category C agents for women in their first trimester and as pregnancy category D agents for women in their second or third trimester. ACE inhibitors should be used in pregnant women only if there are no safer alternatives. Fetal and neonatal morbidity and mortality have been reported in at least 50 women who were receiving ACE inhibitors during their pregnancies. All ACE inhibitors are contraindicated in clients with a known hypersensitivity to them, lactating women, and children.

Many of the ACE inhibitors are combined with either a diuretic or a CCB. Often an individual with hypertension or heart failure must take many medications, including an ACE inhibitor, to control high BP. The convenience of combination products increases client adherence. The only new combination ACE inhibitor–CCB product available currently in Canada is trandolapril and verapamil.

Mechanism of Action and Drug Effects

As is often the case with pharmaceutical discoveries, the development of the ACE inhibitors was spurred by the discovery of an animal substance found to have beneficial effects in humans. This particular animal substance was the venom of the South American viper, which was found to inhibit kininase activity. Kininase is an enzyme that normally breaks down bradykinin, a potent vasodilator in the human body.

The ACE inhibitors have several beneficial cardiovascular effects. As their name implies, they inhibit the angiotensin converting enzyme, which is responsible for converting angiotensin I (AI) to angiotensin II (AII), the latter a potent vasoconstrictor and stimulator of aldosterone secretion by the adrenal glands. Aldosterone

TABLE 24-3

ACE INHIBITORS: DISTINGUISHING CHARACTERISTICS

Generic Name	Combination with Hydrochlorothiazide	Interval	Route	Pro-drug
benazepril	None	Once a day	PO	Yes
captopril	None	Multiple	PO	No
cilazapril	Inhibace Plus	Once a day	PO	Yes
enalapril	Vaseretic	Multiple	PO/IV	Yes
fosinopril	None	Once a day	PO	Yes
lisinopril	Prinzide 12.5 and 25	Once a day	PO	No
lisinopril	Zestoretic 12.5 and 25	Once a day	PO	No
perindopril	None	Once a day	PO	Yes
quinapril	Accuretic	Once a day	PO	Yes
ramipril	None	Once to twice daily	PO	Yes
trandolapril	None	Once a day	PO	Yes

TABLE 24-4

ACE INHIBITORS: THERAPEUTIC EFFECTS

Body Substance	Effect in Body	ACE Inhibitor Action	Resulting Hemodynamic Effect
Aldosterone	Causes sodium and water retention	Prevents its secretion	Diuresis = ↓ plasma volume = ↓ filling pressures or ↓ pre-load
Angiotensin II	Potent vasoconstrictor	Prevents its formation	↓ SVR = ↓ afterload
Bradykinin	Potent vasodilator	Prevents its breakdown	↓ SVR = ↓ afterload

ACE, Angiotensin converting enzyme; ↓, decreased; *SVR,* systemic vascular resistance.

stimulates sodium and water resorption, which can raise BP. This whole system is referred to as the renin angiotensin–aldosterone system (RAAS).

The primary effects of the ACE inhibitors are cardiovascular and renal. Their cardiovascular effects are due to their ability to reduce BP by decreasing SVR. They do this by preventing the breakdown of the vasodilating substance bradykinin and the formation of AII. These combined effects decrease afterload, or the resistance against which the left ventricle must eject its volume of blood during contraction. The ACE inhibitors are beneficial in the treatment of heart failure because they prevent sodium and water resorption by inhibiting aldosterone secretion. This causes diuresis, which decreases blood volume and return to the heart. This in turn decreases pre-load, or the left ventricular end-diastolic volume, and the demand on the heart.

Indications

The therapeutic effects of the ACE inhibitors are related to their potent cardiovascular effects. They are excellent antihypertensives and adjunctive agents for the treatment of heart failure. They may be used alone or in combination with other agents such as diuretics in the treatment of hypertension or heart failure.

The beneficial hemodynamic effects of the ACE inhibitors have been studied extensively. Because of their ability to decrease SVR (a measure of afterload) and preload, ACE inhibitors can stop the progression of left ventricular hypertrophy, which is sometimes seen after a myocardial infarction (MI). This pathological process is known as *ventricular remodelling.* The ability of ACE inhibitors to prevent it is known as a *cardioprotective effect.* ACE inhibitors have been shown to decrease morbidity and mortality rates in clients with heart failure. They should be considered the drugs of choice for hypertensive clients with heart failure. ACE inhibitors also have been shown to have a protective effect on the kidneys, and this is one reason for their being among the cardiovascular drugs of choice in diabetic clients. The various therapeutic effects of the ACE inhibitors are listed in Table 24-4.

Contraindications

Contraindications to the use of ACE inhibitors include known drug allergy, especially a previous reaction of angioedema (laryngeal swelling) with an ACE inhibitor.

Clients with a baseline potassium of 5.0 mmol/L or greater may not be suitable candidates for ACE inhibitor therapy because these drugs can promote hyperkalemia (see later).

Side Effects and Adverse Effects

Hypotension may occur in clients taking ACE inhibitors, usually during initial therapy. It usually disappears within a month. Other cardiovascular effects such as chest pain, tachycardia, palpitations, angina, and MI are rare. A characteristic dry, non-productive cough thought to be due to accumulation of kinins in the respiratory tract is reversible with discontinuation of the therapy. Other side effects include loss of taste, proteinuria, hyperkalemia, rash, pruritus, anemia, neutropenia, thrombocytosis, and agranulocytosis. In clients with severe heart failure whose renal function may depend on the activity of the RAAS, treatment with ACE inhibitors may cause acute renal failure (ARF). ACE inhibitors tend to promote potassium resorption in the kidney, even though they also promote sodium excretion because of their reduction of aldosterone secretion. For this reason serum potassium levels should be regularly monitored. This is especially true in cases of concurrent therapy with potassium-sparing diuretics, though many clients tolerate both types of drug therapy with no major problems.

Toxicity and Management of Overdose

The most pronounced symptom of an overdose of an ACE inhibitor is hypotension. Treatment is symptomatic and supportive and includes the administration of intravenous (IV) fluids to expand the blood volume. Hemodialysis is known to be effective for the removal of captopril, enalapril, lisinopril, and perindopril.

Interactions

ACE inhibitors cause decreased aldosterone production that can lead to increased potassium retention by the kidney. When combined with potassium-sparing diuretics, severe hyperkalemia can occur. The antihypertensive effect of ACE inhibitors can be antagonized by nonsteroidal anti-inflammatory drugs (NSAIDs), leading to reduced therapeutic effect. ACE inhibitors, when given with other antihypertensives or diuretics, have additive effects, resulting in increased therapeutic effects.

Lithium and ACE inhibitors, when given together, can result in lithium toxicity. Potassium supplementation, when given with ACE inhibitors, may result in hyperkalemia. As noted earlier, monitoring of serum potassium becomes especially important in these cases. Acetone may be falsely detected in the urine of clients taking captopril.

Dosages

For information on the dosages for selected ACE inhibitors, see the table below. See Appendix B for some of the common brands available in Canada.

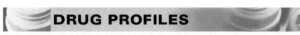

DRUG PROFILES

ACE INHIBITORS

▶▶ captopril

Captopril was the first ACE inhibitor to become available and is considered the prototypical agent for the class. Several large multi-centre studies have shown its clinical efficacy in minimizing or preventing the left ventricular dilation and dysfunction (also called *ventricular remodelling*) that can arise in the acute period after an MI, thereby improving the client's chances of survival. It can also reduce the risk of heart failure in these clients and thus the need for subsequent hospitalizations. Because it has the shortest half-life of all of the currently available ACE inhibitors, captopril is an excellent agent to give to hospitalized clients who are in a fragile condition but need afterload and pre-load reduction. Such a reduction will decrease the workload of a failing heart. A long-acting agent may reduce these hemody-

namic variables too much and have lingering effects that may be difficult to compensate for. Captopril is available only in oral form as 12.5-, 25-, 50-, and 100-mg tablets. Recommended dosages are given in the table below.

PHARMACOKINETICS

Half-Life	Onset	Peak	Duration
<2 hr	15 min	1–2 hr	2–6 hr

enalapril

Enalapril is the only currently available ACE inhibitor that is available in both oral and parenteral preparations. The parenteral formulation (enalaprilat) is an active drug. It offers the hemodynamic benefit of inhibiting ACE activity in an acutely ill client who cannot tolerate oral medications. Although its half-life is slightly longer than that of captopril, it may in some instances be given every 6 hours for effect. The oral form of enalapril is a pro-drug and relies on a functioning liver to be converted to its active form. Like captopril, it has been shown in many large studies to improve a client's chances of survival after an MI and to reduce the incidence of heart failure and the need for subsequent hospitalizations. Enalapril can also be used in children. The oral form of enalapril is available as 2.5-, 5-, 10-, and 20-mg tablets. The parenteral form is available as a 1.25-mg/mL injection. Recommended dosages are given in the table below.

PHARMACOKINETICS*

Half-Life	Onset	Peak	Duration
<2 hr	1 hr	4–6 hr	12–24 hr

*For oral enalapril.

DOSAGES Selected Antihypertensive Agents: ACE Inhibitors and Angiotensin II Receptor Blockers

Agent	Pharmacological Class	Usual Dosage Range	Indications
▶▶ captopril		**Adult** PO: 25–150 mg bid–tid	Hypertension, heart failure
enalapril	ACE inhibitor	**Adult** PO: 10–40 mg/day as a single dose or in 2 equal doses PO: 5–20 mg/day as a single or divided dose with digoxin and diuretic; max 40 mg/day IV: 1.25 mg q6h over a 5-min period (In fixed combination tablet with hydrothiazide) PO: Usual dose 1–2 tabs/day or higher based on the ratio of the 2 drugs **Pediatric <4 wks** PO: 0.08–0.58 mg/kg/day	Hypertension Heart failure Hypertension Hypertension
ramipril		**Adult** PO: 2.5–10 mg/day (max 20 mg) single dose PO: 2.5–5 mg bid	Hypertension Post-MI
▶▶ losartan	ARB	**Adult** PO: 50–100 mg in 1–2 doses	Hypertension, heart failure
valsartan		**Adult** PO: 80–160 mg in a single dose	

ACE, Angiotensin converting enzyme; *ARB,* angiotensin II receptor blocker.

ANGIOTENSIN II RECEPTOR BLOCKERS

ARBs, one of the newest classes of antihypertensives, include losartan, eprosartan, valsartan, irbesartan, candesartan, and telmisartan.

Mechanism of Action and Drug Effects

ARBs block the binding of AII to type 1 AII receptors (AT1 receptors). ACE inhibitors such as enalapril block conversion of AI to AII, but AII may also be formed by other enzymes that are not blocked by ACE inhibitors. In addition, ACE inhibitors block the breakdown of bradykinins and substance P, which accumulate and may cause adverse effects such as cough but might also contribute to the drugs' antihypertensive and cardiac and nephroprotective effects. Bradykinins are potent vasodilators and help to reduce BP by dilating arteries and decreasing systemic vascular resistance.

The drug effects of ARBs are primarily seen on vascular smooth muscle and the adrenal gland. By selectively blocking the binding of AII to the AT1 receptor, ARBs block vasoconstriction and the secretion of aldosterone. AII receptors have been found in other tissues throughout the body, but the effects of blocking these with an ARB are unknown.

Clinically, ACE inhibitors and ARBs appear to be equally effective for the treatment of hypertension. Both are well tolerated, but ARBs do not cause cough. It is not yet clear whether ARBs are as effective as ACE inhibitors in decreasing mortality rates after an MI, in treating heart failure (cardioprotective effects), or in their nephroprotective effects, as in diabetes. Both types of drugs are contraindicated for use in the second or third trimester of pregnancy. Because these drugs are relatively new, the possibility of adverse effects with long-term use is unknown.

Indications

The therapeutic effects of ARBs are related to their potent vasodilating properties. They are excellent antihypertensives and adjunctive agents for the treatment of heart failure. They may be used alone or in combination with other agents such as diuretics in the treatment of hypertension or heart failure. The beneficial hemodynamic effects of ARBs are their ability to decrease SVR (a measure of afterload). Their use is rapidly growing, and more and more studies are verifying their beneficial effects. Currently these agents are used primarily in clients who have been intolerant of ACE inhibitors.

Contraindications

The only usual contraindication to the use of ARBs is known drug allergy.

Side Effects and Adverse Effects

The most common side effects of ARBs are upper respiratory infections and headache. Occasionally dizziness, inability to sleep, diarrhea, dyspnea, heartburn, nasal congestion, back pain, and fatigue can occur. Rarely, anxiety, muscle pain, sinusitis, cough, and insomnia can also occur. Hyperkalemia is also much less likely to occur than with the ACE inhibitors.

Toxicity and Management of Overdose

Overdose may manifest as hypotension and tachycardia; bradycardia occurs less often. Treatment is symptomatic and supportive and includes the administration of intravenous fluids to expand the blood volume.

Interactions

ARBs can interact with cimetidine, lithium, phenobarbital, and rifampin (see Table 24-5).

Dosages

For information on the dosages for selected ARBs, see the table on p. 406. See Appendix B for some of the common brands available in Canada.

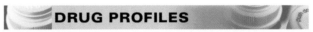

DRUG PROFILES

▶▶ *losartan*

Losartan has been shown to be beneficial in clients with hypertension and heart failure. It is not entirely clear whether ARBs are superior or equivalent to ACE inhibitors in decreasing mortality rates after an MI, in treating heart failure (cardioprotective effects), or in their nephroprotective effects, as in diabetes. More and more studies are showing the beneficial effects of ARBs, including losartan, in the treatment of heart failure. These studies are showing ARBs to be better tolerated and to produce a marginally lower mortality rate than treatment with ACE inhibitors. In clinical trials losartan has also been shown to delay the progression of renal disease in individuals with type 2 diabetes with proteinuria and hypertension.

The use of losartan is contraindicated in clients who are hypersensitive to any component of this product. It should be used with caution in clients with renal or hepatic dysfunction and in clients with renal artery

TABLE 24-5		
ANGIOTENSIN II RECEPTOR BLOCKERS: DRUG INTERACTIONS		
Drug	Mechanism	Result
cimetidine	Competes with metabolism	Increased ARB effect
lithium	Inhibits lithium elimination	Increased lithium concentrations
phenobarbital, rifampin	Increases metabolism	Decreased ARB effect

stenosis. Breastfeeding women should not take losartan because it can cause serious adverse effects on the nursing infant. Losartan is available as 25-, 50-, and 100-mg tablets and as a combination product (Hyzaar) that has 12.5 mg of hydrochlorothiazide and 50 mg of losartan or 25 mg of hydrochlorothiazide and 100 mg of losartan. It is classified as a pregnancy category C agent during the first trimester of pregnancy and a pregnancy category D agent during the second and third trimesters. Recommended dosages are given in the table on p. 406.

PHARMACOKINETICS

Half-Life	Onset	Peak	Duration
6–9 hr	Unknown	3–4 hr	24 hr

valsartan

Valsartan is indicated for the treatment of hypertension. It has also been shown to be effective in the treatment of heart failure; however, some research suggests that it should be reserved for clients intolerant of ACE inhibitors, which appear to be associated with fewer severe cardiac events (including sudden death). It may be used alone or in combination with other antihypertensive agents. It is generally well tolerated, with few side effects.

Valsartan has contraindications and precautions similar to those of losartan. Valsartan is available as 80- and 160-mg tablets and as a combination product in tablet form that has 12.5 mg of hydrochlorothiazide and either 80 or 160 mg of valsartan. Valsartan is classified as a pregnancy category C agent during the first trimester and a pregnancy category D agent during the second and third trimesters. Recommended dosages are given in the table on p. 406.

PHARMACOKINETICS

Half-Life	Onset	Peak	Duration
6 hr	2 hr	2–4 hr	24 hr

CALCIUM CHANNEL BLOCKERS

CCBs have been discussed in some detail in the two previous chapters as antidysrhythmic agents (Chapter 22) and anti-anginal agents (Chapter 23). As a class of medications, they are used for several indications and have many beneficial effects and relatively few side effects. CCBs are primarily used for the treatment of hypertension and angina. Their effectiveness in treating hypertension is related to their ability to cause smooth muscle relaxation by blocking the binding of calcium to its receptors, thereby preventing contraction. Because of their effectiveness and safety, they have been added to the list of first-line agents for the treatment of hypertension. CCBs are used for many other indications as well. They are effective antidysrhythmics and they can prevent the cerebral artery spasms that can occur after a subarachnoid hemorrhage (nimodipine). They are also sometimes used in the treatment of Raynaud's disease and migraine headache.

DIURETICS

The diuretics are a highly effective class of antihypertensive agents. They are listed as one of the current first-line antihypertensives in the CHEP guidelines for treatment of hypertension. They may be used as monotherapy (single-drug therapy) or in combination with other antihypertensive classes. Their primary therapeutic effect is decreasing the plasma and extracellular fluid volumes, which results in decreased pre-load. This leads to a decrease in cardiac output and total peripheral resistance, all of which decrease the workload of the heart. This large group of antihypertensives is discussed in detail in Chapter 25.

VASODILATORS

Vasodilators act directly on arteriolar smooth muscle to cause relaxation. They do not work through adrenergic receptors. Sodium nitroprusside is particularly useful in the management of hypertensive emergencies when the BP is severely, or even only moderately, elevated. However, there is a threat of impending end-organ damage, particularly of the brain, heart, or eyes.

Mechanism of Action and Drug Effects

These agents directly elicit peripheral vasodilation thus reducing systemic vascular resistance. In general, the most notable effect of the vasodilators is their hypotensive effect. However, in recent years minoxidil (in its topical

RESEARCH

The ALLHAT Study

Results from the Antihypertensive and Lipid-Lowering Treatment to Prevent Heart Attack Trial (ALLHAT), one of the largest hypertension clinical trials conducted in North America, revealed that the less expensive thiazide diuretics are more effective than the more expensive newer antihypertensives on the market. The ALLHAT, a double-blind trial, involved 42 418 participants from Canada and the United States in a five-year study to compare the impact of four antihypertensive drugs: chlorthalidone (a thiazide diuretic), amlodipine (a CCB), lisinopril (an ACE inhibitor), and doxazosin (an alpha blocker). Forty-seven percent of the participants were women. Early on, the study involving doxazosin was terminated because of adverse CV events. Although the benefits of the three remaining drugs turned out to be quite similar, overall chlorthalidone had fewer adverse CV events and lowered systolic blood pressure better than the other two drugs. The pragmatic message is that the diuretic chlorthalidone should be the first-line drug used in the management of hypertension.

Source: ALLHAT Officers and Coordinators for the ALLHAT Collaborative Research Group. (2002). Major outcomes in high-risk hypertensive patients randomized to angiotensin-converting enzyme inhibitor or calcium channel blocker vs. diuretic: The Antihypertensive and Lipid-Lowering Treatment to Prevent Heart Attack Trial (ALLHAT). *Journal of the American Medical Association, 288,* 2981–97.

form) has also received increasing attention because of its effectiveness in restoring hair growth. This is described further in Chapter 55.

Indications

All of the vasodilators can be used to treat hypertension, either alone or in combination with other antihypertensives. Sodium nitroprusside is reserved for the management of hypertensive emergencies. Minoxidil in its topical form is used to restore hair growth.

Contraindications

Contraindications include known drug allergy, and may also include hypotension, cerebral edema, head injury, acute MI, or coronary artery disease.

As mentioned in Chapter 21, vasodilating agents may also be contraindicated in cases of heart failure secondary to diastolic dysfunction.

Side Effects and Adverse Effects

The adverse effects of hydralazine include dizziness, headache, anxiety, tachycardia, edema, nasal congestion, dyspnea, anorexia, nausea, vomiting, diarrhea, anemia, agranulocytosis, hepatitis, peripheral neuritis, lupus erythematosus, and rash. Minoxidil's adverse effects include T-wave electrocardiogram (ECG) change, pericarditis, pericardial effusion or tamponade, angina, breast tenderness, rash, leucopenia and thrombocytopenia. Sodium nitroprusside's adverse effects include bradycardia, decreased platelet aggregation, rash, hypothyroidism, hypotension, and possible cyanide toxicity.

Toxicity and Management of Overdose

Hydralazine toxicity or overdose produces hypotension, tachycardia, headache, and generalized skin flushing. Treatment is supportive and symptomatic and includes the administration of intravenous fluids, digitalization if needed, and the administration of beta-blockers for the control of tachycardia.

Minoxidil overdose or toxicity can precipitate excessive hypotension. Treatment is supportive and symptomatic and includes the administration of intravenous fluids. Norepinephrine and epinephrine should not be used

to reverse the hypotension because of the possibility of excessive cardiac stimulation.

The main symptom of sodium nitroprusside overdose or toxicity is excessive hypotension. This drug is normally only administered to clients receiving intensive care. Under these conditions the infusion rate is usually carefully titrated to immediately visible results on a cardiovascular monitor that provides constant measurements of BP from centrally placed venous or arterial catheters. For this reason excessive hypotension is usually avoidable. When it does occur, discontinuation of the infusion has an immediate effect because the drug is metabolized rapidly (half-life 10 minutes). Treatment for the hypotension is supportive and symptomatic; if necessary, pressor agents can be infused to quickly raise BP. The chemical structure of nitroprusside contains cyanide groups, which are released upon its metabolism in the body. This can theoretically result in cyanide toxicity, although this is extremely rare. In the unlikely event of such toxicity, there are standard cyanide antidote kits that include sodium nitrite and sodium thiosulphate for injection and amyl nitrite for inhalation. However, the release of cyanide ions is rarely, if ever, of sufficient concentration to paralyze respiration, as can be the case with concentrated occupational or wartime exposure to cyanide.

Interactions

The incidence of drug interactions with the direct-acting vasodilators (especially sodium nitroprusside) is low. Drug interactions are summarized in Table 24-6.

Dosages

For dosage information for selected vasodilator agents, see the table on p. 410. See Appendix B for some of the common brands available in Canada.

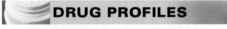

DRUG PROFILES

▸▸ *hydralazine hydrochloride*

Hydralazine is less commonly used than when it first became available, but it is still effective for selected clients. It can be taken orally for routine cases of **essential hypertension** and it is also available in

TABLE 24-6

DIRECT-ACTING VASODILATORS: DRUG INTERACTIONS

Drug	Mechanism	Result
HYDRALAZINE		
Adrenergics	Antagonism	Decreased hypotensive effect
Antihypertensives	Additive effects	Increased hypotensive effect
MAOIs	Altered biotransformation	Increased hypotensive effect
MINOXIDIL		
Antihypertensives/thiazides	Additive effects	Increased hypotensive effect
guanethidine	Additive effects	Significant hypotensive effect
SODIUM NITROPRUSSIDE		
Ganglionic-blocking agents	Additive effects	Increased hypotensive effect

DOSAGES	Selected Antihypertensive Agents: Vasodilators			
Agent	**Pharmacological Class**	**Usual Dosage Range**		**Indications**
▶▶ hydralazine hydrochloride	Direct-acting peripheral vasodilator	**Pediatric** PO: 0.75–7.5 mg/kg/day to a max of 200 mg/day **Adult** PO: 10 mg qid for 2–4 days, followed by 25 mg qid for balance of week; second and subsequent weeks 50 mg qid, then adjust to lowest effective dose for maintenance IV: 20–40 mg prn		Hypertension
minoxidil		**Pediatric <12 yr** PO: 0.25–1 mg/kg/day divided; do not exceed 50 mg/day **Pediatric <12 yr and adult** PO: 10–40 mg/day divided; do not exceed 100 mg/day		
sodium nitroprusside		**Pediatric and adult** IV: 0.3–10 μg/kg/min		

injectable form for hypertensive emergencies. However, its currently listed contraindications, in addition to drug allergy, include CAD and mitral valve dysfunction, such as that related to childhood rheumatic fever. Available tablet strengths are 10-, 25-, and 50-mg, and the injectable form is 20 mg/mL. Pregnancy category C. See the table above for dosage information.

PHARMACOKINETICS

Half-Life	Onset	Peak	Duration
3–7 hr	IV: 5–20 min PO: 20–30 min	IV: 30–45 min PO: 1–2 hr	IV: 2–4 hr PO: 6–12 hr

minoxidil

Minoxidil is now usually reserved for resistant cases of hypertension that have failed other drug therapies. It is contraindicated in cases of known drug allergy, pheochromocytoma, acute MI, and aortic aneurysm. In oral form it is available only in 2.5- and 10-mg tablets. Topical forms (Rogaine) are also used to treat hair loss (Chapter 55) in men and women. Pregnancy category C. See the table above for oral dosage information.

PHARMACOKINETICS

Half-Life	Onset	Peak	Duration
4.2 hr	30 min	2–8 hr	2–5 days

sodium nitroprusside

Sodium nitroprusside is normally used in the intensive care setting for severe hypertensive emergencies and is titrated to effect by intravenous infusion. It is contraindicated in clients with a known hypersensitivity to it and in those with the compensatory hypertension associated with coarctation (constriction) of the aorta or arteriovenous shunt, severe heart failure, and known inadequate cerebral perfusion (especially during neurosurgical procedures). It is also contraindicated in clients with congenital Leber's optic atrophy (which involves a loss of central vision) or tobacco amblyopia (which first manifests with blurring or loss of central vision); both of these conditions may predispose the client to cyanide toxicity. Because of the risk for cyanide toxicity at maximal doses (up to 10 μg/kg/min) for extended

periods, sodium nitroprusside at such doses is used for no more than 10 minutes. This drug is available only in injectable form for intravenous infusion in 50-mg vials of powder for reconstitution. Pregnancy category C. See the table above for dosage information.

PHARMACOKINETICS

Half-Life	Onset	Peak	Duration
2 min	<2 min	2–5 min	1–10 min

MISCELLANEOUS ANTIHYPERTENSIVE AGENTS

DRUG PROFILES

Three newer medications exemplify some of the most recent antihypertensive drugs to be made available in Canada. These include epoprostenol, bosentan, and treprostinil.

epoprostenol

Epoprostenol is a naturally occurring prostaglandin that lowers blood pressure through a combined mechanism of action by direct dilation of both pulmonary and systemic arterial blood vessels and by inhibiting platelet aggregation. Epoprostenol is indicated specifically for long-term treatment of pulmonary artery hypertension in clients with moderate to severe heart failure who do not respond to traditional therapy. Its use is contraindicated in clients with known drug hypersensitivity and in clients with congestive heart failure with severe left ventricular systolic function. Epoprostenol is administered with a portable pump through a surgically implanted central venous catheter via the subclavian or jugular vein. Intense client education and access to medical care is required because of potential problems with the drug delivery system. The most common adverse effects noted during clinical trials were dizziness (83 percent), headache (83 percent), nausea/vomiting (67 percent), jaw pain (54 percent), flushing (42 percent), flu-like symptoms (25 percent), and anxiety/

DOSAGES Miscellaneous Antihypertensive Agents

Agent	Pharmacological Class	Usual Dosage Range	Indications
bosentan	Endothelin-receptor antagonist	**Adult only** PO: Initial dose of 62.5 mg bid × 4 wk, then increase as tolerated to maintenance dose of 125 mg bid	Pulmonary artery hypertension in clients with moderate to severe heart failure
epoprostenol	Vasodilator and platelet aggregation inhibitor	**Adult only** IV: 2 ng/kg/min continuous infusion, may increase by 1–2 ng/kg/min until effect	Long-term IV management of pulmonary hypertension
treprostinil	Vasodilator and platelet aggregation inhibitor	**Adult only** Continuous subcutaneous infusion: 0.625–2.5 mg/kg/min	

nervousness (21 percent). Thrombocytopenia has also been reported. There have been no adequate well-controlled studies demonstrating risk to pregnant women. The drug is available in 0.5 mg freeze-dried powder to be reconstituted in 50 mL specific sterile diluent. Recommended dosages are given in the table above.

bosentan

Bosentan is currently the single novel drug in a new drug class, non-selective endothelin-receptor antagonist, and works by blocking the receptors of the hormone endothelin. Normally this hormone acts to stimulate the narrowing of blood vessels by binding to endothelin receptors (ET_A and ET_B) in the endothelial (innermost) lining of blood vessels and in vascular smooth muscle. Bosentan reduces blood pressure by blocking this action. However, it is currently specifically indicated only for pulmonary artery hypertension in clients with moderate to severe heart failure. It is contraindicated in clients with known drug allergy, pregnancy, or significant liver impairment, and in clients receiving concurrent drug therapy with cyclosporine or glyburide. Pregnancy category X. The drug is currently available in oral tablet form in strengths of 62.5 and 125 mg. Recommended dosages are given in the table above.

treprostinil

Treprostinil lowers blood pressure through a combined mechanism of action by dilating both pulmonary and systemic blood vessels and by inhibiting platelet aggregation. Like bosentan, treprostinil is indicated specifically for pulmonary artery hypertension in clients with moderate to severe heart failure. Its only current contraindication is known drug allergy. Pregnancy category B. The drug is currently available only in injectable form in the concentration of 5 mg/mL. Recommended dosages are given in the table above.

NURSING PROCESS

Although much of the nursing process is similar for all classes of antihypertensives, there are some considerations specific to particular classes.

It is important for the nurse to understand the newly developed guidelines for the evaluation, classification, diagnosis, risk factors, and identifiable causes of hypertension. These guidelines will hopefully encourage earlier identification and management, both pharmacological and non-pharmacological.

■ Assessment

Before administering any antihypertensive agent to a client, the nurse should obtain a thorough health history and perform a head-to-toe physical examination, which are crucial for ensuring safe drug therapy. Parameters to measure and document include BP, pulse, and respirations. Laboratory values related to fluid and electrolyte imbalance (blood urea nitrogen [BUN], creatinine, potassium, sodium, and chloride) should be assessed. It is also important for the nurse to look for underlying causes of the hypertension, such as the following:
- Addison's disease
- Coarctation of the aorta
- Cushing's disease
- PVD
- Pheochromocytoma
- Renal artery stenosis
- Renal or liver dysfunction
- Stressful lifestyle

Many of these causes demand cautious administration of the antihypertensive agent or may even constitute a contraindication to its use. Cautious use of antihypertensives is also necessary in geriatric clients and in clients who have chronic illnesses. Any of the agents, including diuretics, should be used with extreme caution in geriatric clients and in clients with hypotension suffering from fluid and electrolyte disturbances because of their exacerbation of hypotension.

Alpha-blockers, such as prazosin, should be used cautiously in clients with dizziness and syncope because this drug class may cause hypotension and exacerbate such symptoms. Other cautions include lactation and pregnancy. Contraindications include conditions that hypotension could exacerbate, such as myocardial, cerebrovascular, and other organ ischemia. Drug interactions include alcohol, beta-blockers, other alpha-receptor blockers, diuretics, and other classes of antihypertensives. Central-acting alpha-blockers, such as clonidine, must be used with caution in severe coronary insufficiency, conduction disorders, recent myocardial infarcts, coronary insufficiency, Raynaud's disease, history of depression, cerebrovascular disease, renal failure, pregnancy, and lactation. Methyldopa should not be used in clients with active liver disease. All of the cautions listed for clonidine apply to methyldopa, and in addition it should be used cautiously in clients with hemolytic anemia. Contraindications to methyldopa use are similar to those of clonidine. Drug interactions for methyldopa include tricyclic antidepressants, general anaesthetics, CNS depressants, and other antihypertensive agents. It is important for the nurse to be aware if the client is undergoing surgery because these agents, as well as other antihypertensives, require a "weaning-off" period before surgery to avoid interactions with general anaesthetics.

Beta-blockers may be non-selective or cardioselective. The non-selective agents block *both* beta$_1$ and beta$_2$; the cardioselective agents have more beta$_1$-receptor blocking action. Non-selective beta-blockers, such as propranolol, should be used cautiously in clients with diabetes mellitus, renal and/or hepatic diseases, hyperthyroidism, hyperlipidemia, or systemic lupus erythematosus (SLE). They should also be used cautiously in geriatric clients and in pregnant or lactating women. Contraindications include COPD, asthma, and heart failure (because of the negative inotropic effects of the beta non-specific blocking action). Drug interactions include alcohol, CNS depressants, antithyroid drugs, barbiturates, sedative hypnotics, NSAIDs, antituberculin drugs, CCBs, digitalis, and theophylline.

ACE inhibitors are indicated as first-line agents in the treatment of hypertension. They also delay the progression of nephropathy in type 1 diabetics. Because of their potentially serious side effects, ACE inhibitors should be used cautiously in clients with hyperkalemia, salt or water depletion, heart failure, or reduced renal function, and in pregnant or lactating women. Contraindications include a history of ACE-inhibitor–associated angioedema and second- or third-trimester pregnancy. Drug interactions include potassium supplements, potassium-sparing diuretics, salt substitutes that are high in potassium, diuretics, and lithium.

ARBs such as losartan should be used cautiously in geriatric clients and in clients with renal function impairment. Other cautions include volume depletion, renal dysfunction, and renal insufficiency. Drug interactions include potassium salts or supplements, cimetidine, phenobarbital, rifampin, and lithium. Contraindications include the second and third trimesters of pregnancy, hyperaldosteronism, and renal artery stenosis. Common drug interactions include NSAIDs (decrease antihypertensive effects of the ARB), potassium-sparing diuretics, potassium-containing salt substitutes, potassium supplements, and sympathomimetics.

Vasodilators, such as hydralazine, should be used cautiously in clients with impaired cerebral or cardiac circulation. Arterial and venous dilator drugs should not be used in clients with inadequate cerebral circulation and should be used cautiously in clients suffering from impaired renal or hepatic function or vitamin B$_{12}$ deficiency. Contraindications include gastrointestinal disorders, hypotensive states, dizziness, syncope, and edema. Drug interactions include other antihypertensive agents or any type of drug that constricts blood vessels leading to a decrease in perfusion (e.g., sympathomimetics).

CCBs should be used cautiously in clients suffering from severe aortic stenosis, bradycardia, heart failure, or cardiogenic shock. Cautious use is recommended in geriatric clients and pregnant or lactating women and in those with aortic stenosis, angina, obstructive coronary artery disease, or heart failure. Contraindications include severe degrees of aortic stenosis, sick sinus syndrome, heart blocks, acute MI, hypotension, and pulmonary congestion. Drug interactions include digoxin, beta-blockers, benzodiazepines, cimetidine, rifampin, and anaesthetics.

The nurse should encourage clients to learn to monitor themselves and their response to their drug therapy, including taking their own BP and pulse rates. Some of the baseline parameters the nurse should assess include BP, pulse rates, heart sounds, breath sounds, respiratory rate and rhythm, weight, intake and output, and laboratory studies such as serum levels of potassium, sodium, chloride, calcium, magnesium, creatinine, BUN, and urinalysis with specific gravity. (These are just a few of the laboratory studies that should be collected before beginning treatment. These and other studies may also be collected during and after treatment.)

Nursing Diagnoses

Nursing diagnoses appropriate to clients receiving antihypertensive agents include, but are not limited to, the following:

- Deficient knowledge related to a newly prescribed treatment with medications and lifestyle changes.
- Non-adherence with the therapy related to lack of familiarity with or acceptance of the disease process.
- Sexual dysfunction related to side effects of some antihypertensive drugs.
- Risk for injury related to side effects of the antihypertensive agent such as dizziness, orthostatic hypotension, and syncope.
- Acute pain related to headache as a side effect of some antihypertensive agents.
- Ineffective tissue perfusion related to the impact of the disease process.
- Excess fluid volume related to side effects of some of the antihypertensive agents and treatment protocol.
- Imbalanced nutrition, less than body requirements, related to side effects of the antihypertensive agent.
- Constipation related to the side effects of antihypertensive agents.
- Risk for injury related to possible excessive CNS effects such as sedation, tremors, weakness, seizures, or paraesthesia (burning, prickling, tickling, or tingling).

- Risk for injury to mucous membranes related to dry mouth effects of drug.
- Disturbed body image related to side effects of hypertension medication (e.g., impotence, sexual dysfunction, weight gain, fatigue).

■ Planning

Nursing goals for antihypertensive therapy should focus on educating the client and the client's family on the need for adequate management to prevent end-organ damage. These goals include making sure the client understands the nature of the disease, its symptoms and treatment, and the importance of adhering with the treatment regimen. The client must also come to terms with the diagnosis as well as with the fact that there is no cure for the disease and treatment will be lifelong. The influence of chronic illness and the importance of non-pharmacological therapy, stress reduction, and follow-up care must also be underscored. The nurse needs to plan for ongoing assessment of BP, weight, diet, exercise, smoking habits, alcohol intake, adherence with therapy, and sexual function in such clients.

Specific client goals include the following:
- Client takes the drug exactly as prescribed.
- Client experiences relief of symptoms (if any) for which the medication was prescribed.
- Client demonstrates an adequate knowledge about the use of the specific medication, its side effects, and the appropriate dosing at home.
- Client is free of self-injury resulting from adverse effects of the medication.
- Client states the rationale and importance of medication therapy.
- Client records any side effects.
- Client reports any change in sexual patterns and function, bowel habit, or activity intolerance.
- Client implements measures to decrease the occurrence of side effects.
- Client remains adherent to therapy.

■ *Outcome Criteria*

Outcome criteria related to the use of antihypertensive agents are as follows:
- Client states the risks and complications of potent antihypertensive agents, such as tremors, decreased sweating, tachycardia, and hypotension.
- Client states conditions that the physician should be notified of, such as fainting and chest pain.
- Client states the importance of lifelong adherence to the pharmacological treatment of hypertension to decrease end-organ damage and complications to every organ system.
- Client follows instructions to change position slowly, monitor BP, keep follow-up appointments with the physician, and keep a journal to help decrease injury from drug side effects.
- Client communicates openly with nurses and other members of the healthcare team regarding the disease

and the treatment prescribed and any concerns related to changes in body image or function.
- Client reports to the physician immediately any edema or weight gain of more than 1 kg in 1 week.
- Client maintains normal nutritional status through adherence to a prescribed diet high in fibre and fluids and avoidance of alcohol.

■ Implementation

Nursing interventions generally can help the client achieve stable BPs and can minimize adverse effects. Many clients have problems adhering with treatment

---

COMMUNITY HEALTH POINTS

Antihypertensive Agents

One of the major side effects of antihypertensive agents is orthostatic hypotension. One of your clients has been discharged after a 6-day hospitalization for hypertensive crises and to rule out stroke. At 78 years of age, she is somewhat fragile and weakened, lives alone, and has an order for a community health nurse to visit twice weekly to monitor her BP and the success of the prescribed antihypertensive regimen. On one of your first visits she complains of lightheadedness and dizziness. After doing a complete head-to-toe assessment and taking supine and standing BP measurements, you determine that she is most likely suffering from postural hypotension. You report the symptoms to the physician and make the client aware of the problem, its signs and symptoms, contributing factors, and other educational information for safe medication use at home. Client teaching in the home in this situation should include the following information:

- This medication can make your blood pressure drop when you move from sitting or lying to standing. This can cause dizziness, lightheadedness, lethargy, weakness, and even fainting.
- Hot climates, saunas, hot showers or baths, alcohol, exercise, and dehydration can make this reaction worse.

The client can do several things at home to increase her safety and minimize injury:
- Drink fluids regularly (as determined by your physician; generally 6–8 glasses of water a day is recommended), especially during the summer months or whenever you are exposed to hot temperatures or are perspiring a lot.
- Move from one position to another slowly and always hold onto rails, a bar, or any other stationary aide when moving from lying or sitting to standing.
- Take cooler showers or baths and make sure to have adequate safety bars in the bathroom.
- Avoid alcohol because it may increase episodes of fainting and/or dizziness.
- Wear support stockings and try calf muscle exercises.
- Keep a journal of your blood pressure, your weight, any symptoms or side effects, and situations that make you feel better or worse. Update it several times a week.

because the disease itself is silent but the medication often has altering effects on self-concept and sexual function. Any symptoms clients experience may well be side effects of the medication.

Alpha-blockers such as prazosin are to be taken at bedtime, if possible. With prazosin in particular the postural hypotensive side effects may be severe enough to result in syncope and subsequent potential self-injury. Taking this medication at bedtime allows the client to sleep through these hypotensive side effects. The first-dose effect decreases with time or with a reduction in the dose, as ordered by the physician. It may take 4 to 6 weeks for this drug to work at its full potential. Daily weights are important while taking these and other antihypertensive medications.

It is important for nurses to be aware of the action of *all* of the antihypertensives and their related potency. Often if more than one medication is used, agents such as alpha-blockers have their dosage decreased.

Centrally acting alpha-blockers, such as methyldopa, have the same type of nursing interventions as other alpha-blockers; however, these agents may cause more pronounced hypotension, sedation, bradycardia, and edema. These central agents may also affect the client's sexual functioning (erectile dysfunction and/or decreased libido). Clients should be informed of the possibility of these side effects and should be encouraged to speak with their healthcare provider regarding other treatment options, if available. If a client is scheduled for surgery, the drug may be discontinued 4 hours before surgery with resumption of the drug as soon as possible after surgery.

Beta-blockers are either non-selective (block both beta$_1$- and beta$_2$-receptors; e.g., propranolol) or cardioselective (block mainly beta$_1$-receptors; e.g., atenolol). Careful adherence is crucial to client safety. Clients taking a non-selective beta-blocker may experience an exacerbation of respiratory diseases such as asthma, bronchospasm, and COPD, or an exacerbation of heart failure because of the drug's negative inotropic (decreased contractility) effects and bronchoconstricting effects. Clients should be weaned off beta-blockers for approximately 1 to 2 weeks and closely watched for adverse effects during that period.

ACE inhibitors must be taken exactly as prescribed. If angioedema occurs, the physician should be contacted immediately. Usually the drug is discontinued; however, in most situations it is recommended that the client be weaned slowly. Salt and water levels/volume should be monitored closely to help prevent any adverse effects, especially in clients taking an ACE inhibitor and a diuretic. Lozenges or hard candy may help with the dry hacking cough many clients complain about while taking an ACE inhibitor.

ARBs must be taken exactly as prescribed. They are often tolerated best with meals. As with all other antihypertensives (and all other medications) the dosage should not be changed nor the medication discontinued unless prescribed by the physician. With any of the ARBs, if the client has hypovolemia (abnormally low blood volume) or hepatic dysfunction, the dosage may need to be reduced. A diuretic such as hydrochlorothiazide (HCTZ) may be ordered in combination with an ARB for clients who have hypertension with left ventricular hypertrophy. Losartan is also an option for clients at risk for stroke and for those who are hypertensive and have left ventricular hypertrophy.

Vasodilators, such as hydralazine and sodium nitroprusside, have additional nursing considerations. Injected hydralazine must never be given without adequate monitoring and frequent assessment, because it may lower BP within 10 to 80 minutes and because ECG changes, cardiovascular inadequacies, and hypotension may create pronounced effects on the client's cardiac status. If signs and symptoms of systemic lupus erythematosus (SLE) occur, the drug should be discontinued and the physician contacted immediately. Pyridoxine may help to diminish associated peripheral neuritis.

Sodium nitroprusside must always be diluted per manufacturer guidelines. Because it is a potent vasodilator, there may be extreme decreases in the client's BP; therefore proper and astute monitoring is crucial to prevent injury to the client, such as irreversible ischemic injuries to organ systems and even possible death. To avoid severe and even life-threatening complications, sodium nitroprusside should never be infused at the maximum dose rate for more than 10 minutes. (The usual dose rate is 0.5 to 10 μg/kg/min.) If this drug does not control a client's BP after 10 minutes, then it should be discontinued and further orders sought from the physician. In addition, the metabolism of this drug may lead to the conversion of hemoglobin (Hgb) into methemoglobin and cyanide (cyanmethemoglobin), resulting in thiocyanate toxicity and/or methemoglobinemia. To avoid this the nurse should do the following: (1) dilute the medication properly and avoid use of any solution that has turned blue, green, or red; (2) infuse only through a "volumetric" infusion pump, not through ordinary intravenous sets; (3) continuously monitor BP during the infusion—preferably by invasive measures. Infusing more than 500 μg/kg of sodium nitroprusside faster than 2 μg/kg/min may produce cyanide faster than the "unaided" client can eliminate it.

CCBs such as verapamil are to be taken exactly as prescribed with the warning *not* to puncture, open, or crush the extended-release and sustained-release tablets and capsules. Because these are negative inotropic drugs (used to decrease cardiac contractility) they may induce more signs of heart failure if given with drugs that increase cardiac contractility, such as digitalis. Monitoring BP and pulse rate before and during therapy will help to prevent or to identify early any problems related to the negative inotropic effects (decreased contractility), negative chronotropic effects (decreased heart rate), and negative dromotropic effects (decreased conduction).

Ethnocultural diversity must be considered with regard to the treatment of hypertension. Some ethnic groups respond less favourably to certain drugs than to others. As with any disease process, clients need to be managed and dealt with holistically, with their physical and psychosocial needs taken under consideration (see Ethnocultural Implications box earlier in this chapter).

Client teaching tips for antihypertensive agents are listed on p. 418.

■ Evaluation

Because clients with hypertension are at high risk for cardiovascular injury, it is critical for them to be adherent with both their pharmacological and non-pharmacological treatment. Monitoring clients for the adverse effects (e.g., orthostatic hypotension, dizziness, fatigue) and toxic effects of the various types of antihypertensive agents helps the nurse to identify potentially life-threatening complications. The most important aspect of the evaluation process is collecting data and monitoring clients for evidence of controlled BP. BP should be maintained at less than 140/90 mm Hg. BP monitoring should be at periodic intervals, and education about self-monitoring is important to the safe use of these drugs. In addition, the physician needs to examine the fundus of the client's eyes because this is a more reliable indicator of the long-term effectiveness of treatment than BP readings. The client must constantly be monitored for the development of end-organ damage and for specific problems that the medication can cause. Men receiving an antihypertensive agent should be questioned about erectile dysfunction because they often are not aware that this is an expected side effect of most antihypertensive agents. Follow-up visits to the physician are important for monitoring client adherence, the effectiveness of or problems with treatment, and complications of the hypertension.

Therapeutic effects of antihypertensives in general include an improvement in BP and in the disease process. Clients should report a return to a normal baseline of BP with improved energy levels and reduced signs and symptoms of hypertension, such as less edema, improved breath sounds, no abnormal heart sounds, capillary refill less than 5 seconds, and less shortness of breath (dyspnea). Side effects for which to monitor include all of the specific side effects listed with each category of antihypertensives.

CASE STUDY

Hypertension

Hypertension was diagnosed in G.S. when she was 33 years old. Both her mother and sister suffer from hypertension, and both were also in their 30s when it was diagnosed. G.S.'s most current BP is 150/96 mm Hg, and for this reason the nurse practitioner has recommended that she see her primary care provider. After examining her, the physician prescribes atenolol and relaxation therapy. After 14 days of this therapy G.S.'s BP is found to be 145/86 mm Hg. Stress reduction has been the biggest obstacle in her treatment because she is a lawyer in a prominent law firm and has found that her BP is consistently elevated (diastolic blood pressure >100 but <110 mm Hg) whenever she measures it at work.

- What should G.S. know about the expected therapeutic effects and side effects of atenolol?
- Discuss the differences between an agent such as atenolol and the agent propranolol.
- What lifestyle changes would you recommend? What information would you give to help her change her lifestyle and more effectively reduce stress?

For answers see http://evolve.elsevier.com/Lilley/pharmacology/.
BP, Blood pressure.

RESEARCH

Thiocyanate and Cyanide Toxicity

Most of the cyanide produced during the metabolism of sodium nitroprusside is excreted in the form of thiocyanate. The steady state of thiocyanate after prolonged sodium nitroprusside infusions is increased with an increased infusion rate and when there is coinfusion of thiosulphate. Thiocyanate toxicity is life threatening at levels of 200 mg/L. To keep the steady state level of thiocyanate below 1 mmol/L, a prolonged infusion of sodium nitroprusside should be *no more* than 3 μg/kg/min and down to 1 μg/kg/min in those clients who are anuric (unable to pass urine). Altering the pH of urine is *not* known to increase thiocyanate excretion; however, dialysis may help with thiocyanate clearance. Signs and symptoms of thiocyanate toxicity include dizziness, headache, muscle twitching, retrosternal discomfort (behind the breastbone), and abdominal pain; these have all been noted when BP is reduced too rapidly.

Overdosage of nitroprusside results in excessive hypotension or cyanide toxicity. Cyanide levels are identifiable by laboratory testing, and blood gas draws may show acidosis. However, acidosis may not appear until an hour or more after the appearance of dangerous cyanide levels. Treatment includes the following:

1. Discontinue sodium nitroprusside.
2. Provide a buffer for cyanide by using sodium nitrite to convert hemoglobin into methemoglobin but only as much as the client can tolerate.
3. *Then* infuse sodium thiosulphate to convert cyanide into thiocyanate. Necessary medications are currently found in commercially available cyanide antidote kits.

Hemodialysis is ineffective in removing cyanide but it *will* eliminate most thiocyanate. The cyanide antidote kits contain both amyl nitrite and sodium nitrite to induce methemoglobinemia.

Sources: Mosby. (2005). *Mosby's drug consult 2005: The comprehensive reference for generic and brand name drugs* (15th ed.). St. Louis, MO: Mosby; and Facts and Comparisons. (2004). *Drug facts and comparisons pocket version* (9th ed.). St Louis, MO: Wolters Kluwer Health.

NURSING CARE PLAN | Hypertension

Mr. C., a 58-year-old man of Jamaican heritage, reports to the doctor's office today and is newly diagnosed as hypertensive. He has never taken any medications for any disorder and has been extremely healthy until this recent bout with headaches and chest pain. His BP at the office today is 172/98, his pulse is 92, his respiration rate is 22, and he is somewhat anxious about his BP and taking any medication. His wife of 25 years is supportive and has attended each visit to the doctor's office with him. He is an executive vice-president for a local computer company and is a hardworking individual. He denies smoking and drinking, and his weight and height are within normal limits. Nursing assessment is negative for any edema, chest pain, distress, dyspnea, palpitations, or other problems. He exercises regularly and will be instructed on a low-fat diet and supervised at a local cardiac rehabilitation centre for appropriate exercise and stress management. The main concern today, however, is education about his medication, enalapril maleate.

ASSESSMENT

Subjective Data
- "I really am not sure about how to take this new BP medicine or anything about its side effects."
- "Are there any medications I can't take when I'm taking this BP medicine?"

Objective Data
- New diagnosis of hypertension
- Addition of enalapril maleate to treatment regimen
- Vital signs: BP 168/106, P 88, RR 22
- Electrolyte panel within normal limits
- Renal and liver function studies within normal limits

NURSING DIAGNOSIS

Deficient knowledge related to lack of experience with medications

PLANNING

Goals
Client will remain adherent and with minimal side effects to enalapril maleate therapy within 1 month

Outcome Criteria
Client will demonstrate an understanding of the following before leaving the physician's office:
- How to take the medication (including not skipping or doubling up on missed doses)
- How to measure and record BPs with pulse
- Side effects associated with therapy
- Ways to maximize the effects of the medication
- Side effects to report to the physician immediately
- The importance of adherence to therapy
- Drug interactions and the importance of a holistic approach to therapy (e.g., exercise and relaxation techniques)

IMPLEMENTATION

Client education should focus on the following instructions:
- Take medication at least 1 hour before meals as ordered.
- Avoid OTC cold preparations because of their vasoconstricting properties, which in turn elevate BP, and avoid any other products (e.g., OTCs, vitamins, natural health products) that may elevate BP.

NURSING CARE PLAN | Hypertension—cont'd

IMPLEMENTATION (cont'd)

- Take this medication exactly as prescribed, without missing any doses or doubling up on doses. Don't stop taking your medicine if you feel better. Stopping this medication abruptly could raise your blood pressure dangerously.
- Lightheadedness may occur for the first few days of therapy and usually subsides after this time; however, you should always rise slowly from lying to sitting or standing position to avoid fainting from low blood pressure.
- Make sure you adhere with dosage schedule, even if you are feeling better.
- Photosensitivity may occur; therefore avoid sunlight or wear sunscreen if outdoors.
- You may develop a dry cough; if so, let the physician know.
- Contact your physician if you have problems with mouth sores, fever, swelling of hands or feet, palpitations, or irregular heartbeats and chest pain.
- If you perspire heavily or suffer from dehydration, vomiting, or diarrhea your blood pressure could drop, resulting in fainting, dizziness, or falling. Contact your physician should this occur.
- Record in a journal your BPs at least 3 times a week. Take them yourself or stop by a local pharmacy.

EVALUATION

Client will display therapeutic response to medication. Evidence includes the following:
- Client is taking medications as prescribed.
- Client's BP is within normal limits, with DBP consistently $\leq$90 mm Hg.
- Client is avoiding medications that may adversely interact with drug therapy.
- Client is contacting the physician appropriately with problems or concerns, including when ill and possibly dehydrated or if concerned about medication, treatment program, or lifestyle.
- Client is positioning self slowly from lying or sitting to standing without fainting or falls.
- After several months of therapy, client reports improved health, increased energy levels, and a sense of well-being.
- Client has normal appetite.
- Client is without weight gain, edema, dyspnea, wet rales, and signs and symptoms of heart failure.
- Client is monitored for side effects but experiences minimal problems.
- Client is suffering minimal side effects and does not have mouth sores, edema, or irregular heartbeats or chest pain.

CLIENT TEACHING TIPS

The nurse should instruct the client as follows:

All Antihypertensive Agents

▲ Take your medication exactly as prescribed by the physician. An overdose can be life threatening; therefore if you miss a dose, check with your physician for instructions. Never double up on doses.

▲ *Never* stop taking your medication without your physician's approval because this may lead to dangerous increases in blood pressure and life-threatening complications such as stroke. If you are having troublesome side effects, contact your physician.

▲ Medication is only part of a treatment program. You need to watch your diet intake of fatty foods and monitor your stress level. It's also important to avoid smoking and excessive alcohol.

▲ Keep your medication out of the reach of children.

▲ Wear a medical alert tag or bracelet and carry a medical identification card specifying your condition and listing all medications (prescribed, OTC, natural health products).

▲ When you are taking this medication, some things may make your blood pressure go too low. These things include hot tubs, hot showers or baths, saunas, hot weather, prolonged sitting or standing, physical exercise, and alcohol. If you experience dizziness, get some assistance and sit or lie down until you feel better.

▲ Weigh yourself daily at the same time and with the same clothing (e.g., bath robe or night clothes) and keep a daily journal of weight, blood pressure, and other important information.

▲ If you experience dizziness when you move, try to change positions slowly, with ease and with purposeful movement.

▲ Inform all healthcare providers (e.g., dentist, surgeon) that you are taking antihypertensive agents.

▲ Check with your healthcare provider before taking any other medications, OTC drugs, or natural health products; some may cause high blood pressure.

▲ Always keep an adequate supply of medications on hand, especially while travelling.

▲ Have your eyes examined periodically (every six months).

▲ Keep regular appointments with your physician; they are important to your health and overall well-being.

Centrally Acting Alpha-Blockers and Beta-Blockers

▲ (Especially for older clients) Your medication may make you feel dizzy or light-headed, or even make you faint. This usually happens when you change positions suddenly.

▲ It is especially dangerous to stop taking this drug abruptly. If you are experiencing serious side effects or feel you need a change of medicine or dose, contact your physician immediately.

▲ If you are taking an alpha-blocker, you may not get the whole benefit for 4 to 6 weeks.

ACE Inhibitors

▲ You may not experience the full benefits of your medication for several weeks.

▲ Report any signs of infection or easy bruising or bleeding.

▲ Your sense of taste may be impaired; this usually goes away in 2 to 3 months.

▲ Don't take potassium supplements or increase your intake of potassium.

Angiotensin II Receptor Blockers (ARBs)

▲ Take your medication at the same time every day.

▲ Be careful while exercising or in hot weather. These situations may cause your blood pressure to go too low when you stand up, and could possibly cause fainting.

▲ Report any unusual shortness of breath, difficulty breathing, weight gain, chest pain, or palpitations to your healthcare provider.

Vasodilators

▲ Take your pulse and blood pressure frequently and report any changes to your physician.

▲ Weigh yourself daily and report an increase of 1 kg or more within 24 hours or 2 kg or more within a week to your physician.

▲ Report any shortness of breath, chest pain, cough, or fatigue to your physician.

POINTS to REMEMBER

▼ BP is the product of cardiac output (CO) multiplied by the SVR.

▼ All antihypertensives in some way affect CO and/or SVR.
- *CO:* Amount of blood ejected from the left ventricle measured in litres per minute.
- *SVR:* Force the left ventricle must overcome to eject its end-diastolic volume.

▼ Main groups of antihypertensives: diuretics (see Chapter 25), alpha-blockers, central alpha-blockers, beta-blockers, ACE inhibitors, vasodilators, and CCBs.

▼ ACE inhibitors work by blocking a critical enzyme system responsible for the production of angiotensin II (a potent vasoconstrictor). They prevent the following: (1) vasoconstriction caused by angiotensin II, (2) aldosterone secretion and therefore sodium and water resorption, and (3) bradykinin (a potent vasodilator) from being broken down by angiotensin II.

▼ ARBs work by blocking angiotensin at the receptors; therefore the end result is a blocking of angiotensin and thus a decrease in BP.

▼ CCBs may be used to treat angina, dysrhythmias, and hypertension and help to reduce BP by causing smooth muscle relaxation and dilation of blood vessels. If calcium is not present then the smooth muscle of the blood vessels cannot contract.

▼ Nursing considerations for antihypertensives include the following:
- A thorough nursing assessment should include finding out whether the client has any underlying causes of hypertension, such as renal or liver dysfunction, a stressful lifestyle, Cushing's disease, Addison's disease, renal artery stenosis, PVD, or pheochromocytoma.
- The nurse should always check for the existence of contraindications, cautions, and drug interactions before administering any of the antihypertensive agents.
- Clients should be managed by both pharmacological and non-pharmacological means. They should be encouraged to consume a diet low in fat, make any other necessary modifications in their diet (such as a possible decrease in the intake of sodium, ingestion of "good" carbohydrates, and increase in fibre), engage in regular, supervised exercise, and reduce the amount of stress in their life.
- Contraindications include a history of MI or chronic renal disease. Cautious use is recommended for clients with renal insufficiency and glaucoma.

▼ Drug interactions for antihypertensive agents include other antihypertensive agents, anaesthetics, and diuretics.

▼ Therapeutic effects include fewer hypertensive-related symptoms such as chest pain, severe headaches, and high BP readings.

▼ Side effects to constantly monitor for include tachycardia, confusion, hallucinations, CNS depression, and constipation.

EXAMINATION REVIEW QUESTIONS

1 Which of the following is a goal for hypertension drug therapy?
a. Preventing end-organ damage
b. Enhancing cerebrovascular perfusion
c. Elevating HDLs and lowering LDLs
d. Avoiding renal damage

2 Which of the following side effects is of most concern for the older adult client taking antihypertensive agents?
a. Erectile dysfunction
b. Increased libido
c. Hyperplasia
d. Hypotension

3 Your female client is 45 years of age, smokes three packs of cigarettes per day, and is taking oral contraception. She also has a 2-year history of untreated hypertension. Which of the following complaints or abnormalities would be of most concern?
a. Polyuria
b. Systolic BP of 150 mm Hg
c. Weight gain
d. Increased BUN and creatine

4 Which of the following drugs requires a dosing at bedtime with the first dose?
a. magnesium citrate
b. furosemide
c. prazosin
d. diabenase

5 Mr. L.P. informs you of some problems with sexual intercourse. Which of the following would be your most appropriate response?
a. "Not to worry. Tolerance will develop."
b. "The physician can work with you on changing the dose and/or drugs."
c. "Sexual dysfunction happens and you must learn to accept it."
d. "Ephedra or adrenalin can help decrease this problem."

For answers see http://evolve.elsevier.com/Lilley/pharmacology/.

CRITICAL THINKING ACTIVITIES

1 Primary hypertension has been diagnosed in J.M., a 53-year-old woman. What is the current thinking regarding antihypertensive therapy? Before initiating antihypertensive therapy, what past medical conditions should you inquire about during the nursing assessment?

2 B.T. is a 78-year-old woman who has been admitted to the emergency room for the treatment of a possible acute MI and acute hypertensive crisis. One of the physician's orders is to start a sodium nitroprusside infusion. What is the purpose for using sodium nitroprusside?

3 You are caring for a client who needs rapid reduction of BP and is in a hypertensive crisis. An immediate reduction is needed, and a fairly high dosage of sodium nitroprusside is ordered. Are there any concerns for this scenario and, if so, what are they and what is the treatment for possible toxicity?

For answers see http://evolve.elsevier.com/Lilley/pharmacology/.

BIBLIOGRAPHY

Albanese, J., & Nutz, P. (2005). *Mosby's 2005 nursing drug cards.* St Louis, MO: Mosby.

Anderson, P.O., Knoben, J.E., & Troutman, W.G. (2002). *Handbook of clinical drug data,* (10th ed.). New York: McGraw-Hill/Appleton & Lange.

Berne, R., & Levy, M. (2002). *Principles of physiology* (3rd ed.). St Louis, MO: Mosby.

Boron, W.F., & Boulpaep, E.L. (2003). *Medical physiology.* Philadelphia: Saunders.

Brenner, B.M., Cooper, M.E., De Zeeuw, D., Keane, W.F., Mitch, W.E., Parving, H.H., et al. (2001). Effects of losartan on renal and cardiovascular outcomes in patients with type 2 diabetes and nephropathy. *New England Journal of Medicine, 345,* 861–869.

Canadian Diabetes Association & The Clinical Practice Guidelines Expert Committee. (2003). Macrovascular complications, dyslipidemia, and hypertension. *2003 Clinical Practice Guidelines.* Retrieved August 11, 2005, from http://www.diabetes.ca/cpg2003/downloads/macrovascular.pdf

Canadian Hypertension Society. (2002). *Hypertension therapeutic guide* (2nd ed.). Montreal, QB: Author.

Canadian Hypertension Society. (2005). Management of Hypertension: Pamphlets, Slides and Summaries. CHEP 2005 Treatment slides. Retrieved August 11, 2005, from http://www.hypertension.ca/index2.html

Canadian Pharmacists Association. (2003). *Therapeutic choices* (4th ed.). Ottawa, ON: Author.

Canadian Pharmacists Association. (2004). *Guide to drugs in Canada.* Toronto, ON: Dorling Kindersley.

Canadian Pharmacists Association. (2005). *Compendium of pharmaceuticals and specialties. The Canadian drug reference for health professionals.* Ottawa, ON: Author. [The subscription-based e-CPS is available at http://www.pharmacists.ca.]

Cohn, J.N., Tognoni, G., & Valsartan Heart Failure Trial Investigators. (2001). A randomized trial of the angiotensin-receptor blocker valsartan in chronic heart failure. *New England Journal of Medicine, 345,* 1667–1675.

Facts and Comparisons. (2004). *Drug facts and comparisons pocket version* (9th ed.). St Louis, MO: Wolters Kluwer Health.

Health Canada. (2005). Drug product database (DPD). Retrieved August 11, 2005, from http://www.hc-sc.gc.ca/hpb/drugs-dpd/

Hemmelgarn, B.R., McAllister, F.A., Myers, M.G., McKay, D.W., Bolli, P., Abbott, C., et al. (2005). The 2005 Canadian Hypertension Education Program recommendations for the management of hypertension: Part 1—Blood pressure measurement, diagnosis and assessment of risk. *Canadian Journal of Cardiology, 21*(8), 645–656.

Inspra information Web site. Retrieved August 11, 2005, from http://www.inspra.com/pdf/pi.pdf

Johns Hopkins Hospital, Gunn, V.L., & Nechyba, C. (2005). *The Harriet Lane handbook* (17th ed.). St Louis, MO: Mosby.

Joint National Committee on Detection, Evaluation, and Treatment of High Blood Pressure. (2003). *The seventh report of the Joint National Committee on Detection, Evaluation, and Treatment of High Blood Pressure (JNC-7),* National Institutes of Health.

Julius, S., Kjeldsen, S.E., Weber, M., Brunner, H.R., Ekman, S., Hansson, L., et al. (2004). Outcomes in hypertensive patients at high cardiovascular risk treated with regimes based on valsartan or amlodipine: the VALUE randomized trial. *Lancet, 363,* 2022–2031.

Katzung, B.G. (2004). *Basic and clinical pharmacology* (9th ed.). New York: McGraw-Hill.

Kearney, P.M., Whelton, M., Reynolds, K., Munter, P., & He, J. (2005). Global burden of hypertension: Analysis of worldwide data. *Lancet, 365*(9455), 217–223.

Kohli, S., & Joneja, A. (2004). Should thiazide diuretics be first-line therapy for high-risk hypertensive patients? [Electronic version]. *Canadian Family Physician.* Retrieved August 11, 2005, from http://www.cfpc.ca/cfp/2004/May/vol50-may-critical-1.asp

Lacy, C.F., Armstrong, L.L., Goldman, M.P., & Lance, L.L. (2003). *Drug information handbook* (11th ed.). Hudson, OH: Lexi-Comp.

Leenen, F.H.H. (2004). ALLHAT. What has it taught us so far? *Canadian Medical Association Journal, 171*(7), 719–720.

Lehne, R.A. (2004). *Pharmacology for nursing care* (5th ed.). St Louis, MO: Saunders.

McKenry, L.M., & Salerno, E. (2003). *Mosby's pharmacology in nursing—revised and updated* (21st ed.). St Louis, MO: Mosby.

Mosby. (2005). *Mosby's drug consult 2005: The comprehensive reference for generic and brand name drugs* (15th ed.). St Louis, MO: Mosby.

Pulmonary Hypertension Society of Canada. Treatment. Retrieved August 11, 2005, from http://www.phscanada.com/treatment.html

Sica, D.A. (2003). Combination angiotensin-converting enzyme inhibitor and angiotensin receptor blocker therapy: its role in clinical practice. *Journal of Clinical Hypertension, 5*(6), 414–420.

Skidmore-Roth, L. (2006). *Mosby's 2006 nursing drug reference* (19th ed.). St Louis, MO: Mosby.

Tracleer information Web site. Retrieved August 11, 2005, from http://www.tracleer.com/TRALibrary/TRALib001/L001/TRALib001L001Overview.html

Woods, S.L., Sivarajan Froelocher, E.S., Underhill Motzer, S., & Bridges, E.J. (2005). *Cardiac nursing* (5th ed.). Philadelphia: Lippincott Williams & Wilkins.

Wright, J.T., Dunn, J.K., Cutler, J.A., Davis, B.R., Cushman, W.C., Ford, C.E., et al. (2005). Outcomes in hypertensive blacks and nonblack patients treated with chlorthalidone, amlodipine, and lisinopril. *Journal of the American Medical Association, 293*(13), 1595–1607.

CHAPTER

25 Diuretic Agents

OBJECTIVES

After reading this chapter, the successful student will be able to do the following:

1 Summarize the various indications for diuretics.

2 Distinguish among the different diuretics by classes and mechanisms of action, cautions, contraindications, dosages, routes of administration, side effects, toxicity, and rationale.

3 Contrast the various groups of diuretics as related to drug interactions.

4 Develop a nursing care plan that includes all phases of the nursing process for the client receiving diuretics.

e-LEARNING ACTIVITIES

Student CD-ROM
- Review Questions: see questions 175–189
- Animations
- Medication Administration Checklists
- IV Therapy Checklists

evolve Web site (http://evolve.elsevier.com/Lilley/pharmacology/)
- Online Chapter Worksheet • Frequently Asked Questions
- Learning Tips and Content Updates • WebLinks • Online Appendices and Supplements • Mosby/Saunders ePharmacology Update • Access to *Mosby's Drug Consult*

DRUG PROFILES

acetazolamide, p. 425   ▸▸mannitol, p. 428
amiloride, p. 430   metolazone, p. 432
▸▸ furosemide, p. 427   ▸▸pironolactone, p. 430
▸▸ hydrochlorothiazide, p. 432   triamterene, p. 430

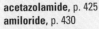 Key drugs.

GLOSSARY

Afferent arteriole The small blood vessel approaching the glomerulus (proximal part of the nephron).

Aldosterone (al dos' tər own) A mineralocorticoid steroid hormone produced by the adrenal cortex that mediates the actions of the renal tubule in the regulation of sodium and potassium balance in the blood.

Ascites (uh sigh teez) An abnormal intraperitoneal accumulation of fluid (defined as a volume of 500 mL or greater) containing large amounts of protein and electrolytes.

Collecting duct The most distal part of the nephron between the distal convoluted tubule and the ureters, which lead to the urinary bladder.

Distal convoluted tubule The part of the nephron immediately distal to the ascending loop of Henle.

Diuretic (dye' ə ret' ik) Drug or other substance that tends to promote the formation and excretion of urine.

Efferent arteriole The small blood vessel exiting the glomerulus. At this point blood has completed its filtration in the glomerulus.

Glomerular filtration rate (GFR) (glow mare' oo lər) The amount of ultrafiltrate formed per unit of time by the plasma flowing through the glomeruli of the kidney.

Glomerulus (glow mare'oo ləs) The cluster of capillaries that marks the beginning of the nephron and is immediately proximal to the proximal convoluted tubule.

Kaliuretic diuretics (ka lee yoo ret' ik) Agents that induce potassium loss in the urine.

Loop of Henle Part of the nephron immediately distal to the proximal convoluted tubule.

Nephron (nef' ron) The microscopic functional filtration unit of the kidney, consisting of (in anatomical order from proximal to distal) the glomerulus; proximal convoluted tubule; loop of Henle; distal convoluted tubule; and the collecting duct, which empties urine into the ureters. There are approximately one million nephrons in each kidney.

Open-angle glaucoma (glaw koe' muh) Elevated pressure in an eye because of obstruction of the outflow of aqueous humor.

Proximal convoluted tubule Part of the nephron that is immediately distal to the glomerulus and proximal to the loop of Henle.

The drugs that accelerate the rate of urine formation are termed **diuretics,** and they accomplish this through a variety of mechanisms. The result is that they remove sodium and water from the body.

Diuretics were discovered by accident when it was noticed that a mercury-based antibiotic had a potent diuretic effect. Thus began the early developmental stages of diuretics. All the major classes of diuretic drugs in use today were developed between 1950 and 1970, and they remain among the most commonly prescribed drugs in the world. Diuretics, especially the thiazides, play a key role as first-line agents in the treatment of hypertension. The hypotensive activity of diuretics is due to many different mechanisms. They cause direct arteriolar dilation, decreasing peripheral vascular resistance. They also decrease extracellular fluid volume, plasma volume, and cardiac output, which may account for the decrease in blood pressure (BP). They have long been the mainstay of therapy not only for hypertension but also for heart failure. Two of their advantages are their relatively low cost and a good safety profile compared with many other drug classes. The main problem is the metabolic side effects that can result from excessive fluid and electrolyte loss. These effects are usually dose related and therefore controllable with dosage titration (careful adjustment).

This chapter reviews the essential properties and actions of the following important classes of diuretic agents: carbonic anhydrase inhibitors (CAIs), loop diuretics, osmotic diuretics, potassium-sparing diuretics, and thiazide and thiazide-like diuretics. However, before these are discussed in detail, it is important to quickly review kidney function.

KIDNEY FUNCTION

The kidney serves an important role in the day-to-day functioning of the body. It filters out toxic waste products from the blood while simultaneously saving essential ones. This delicate balance between toxins and essential chemicals is maintained by the **nephron.** This is the main structural element in the kidney, and each kidney contains approximately one million of them. It is in the nephron that diuretic agents exert their effect. The initial filtering of the blood takes place in the **glomerulus,** a cluster of capillaries surrounded by the glomerular capsule. The rate at which this occurs is referred to as the **glomerular filtration rate (GFR),** and it is used as a gauge of how well the kidneys are functioning as filters. Normally about 180 L of blood are filtered through them per day. The GFR, which can also be

thought of as the rate at which blood flows into and out of the glomerulus, is regulated by the small blood vessels approaching the glomerulus (**afferent arterioles**) and the small blood vessels exiting the glomerulus (**efferent arterioles**). A mnemonic (memory aid) for remembering which arteriole is which is to think "A for approach and afferent" and "E for exit and efferent." Alterations in blood flow such as those that occur in a client in shock would therefore have a dramatic effect on kidney (renal) function. When blood flow is reduced the kidney receives less blood, and therefore less diuretic gets to its site of action. For this reason diuretics may have diminished effects, though they are often used to promote renal blood flow and glomerular filtration in such situations. This is especially true of the loop diuretics.

The **proximal convoluted** (twisted) **tubule** or, more simply, *proximal tubule,* anatomically follows the glomerulus and serves to resorb 60 to 70 percent of the sodium and water from the filtered fluid (ultrafiltrate) back into the bloodstream. Blood vessels surround the nephrons and allow substances to be directly absorbed from or secreted into the bloodstream. This process is an active one that requires energy (active transport) in the form of adenosine triphosphate (ATP) molecules. As sodium and potassium ions are actively transported back into the blood, this causes the passive resorption of chloride and water. The chloride ions (Cl^-) and water simply follow the sodium ions (Na^+) and, to a lesser extent, potassium ions (K^+). Another 20 to 25 percent of sodium is resorbed back into the bloodstream in the ascending **loop of Henle**. This is a passive process that does not require energy because here it is the chloride that is actively resorbed and the sodium that passively follows it.

The remaining 5 to 10 percent of sodium resorption takes place in the **distal convoluted tubule**, or more simply, the *distal tubule,* which anatomically follows the ascending loop of Henle. Here sodium is actively filtered in exchange for potassium or hydrogen ions, a process regulated by the hormone **aldosterone**. The **collecting duct** is the final common pathway for the filtrate that started in the glomerulus. It is here that antidiuretic hormone acts to increase the absorption of water back into the bloodstream, thereby preventing it from being lost in the urine. This entire process, along with the sites of action of the different classes of diuretics, is shown in Fig. 25-1.

DIURETIC AGENTS

The various diuretics are classified according to their sites of action within the nephron, their chemical structure, and their diuretic potency. The sites of action of the various diuretics are determined by the way in which they affect the various solute (electrolyte) and water transport systems located along the nephron (see Figure 25-1). The commonly used classes of agents and the individual

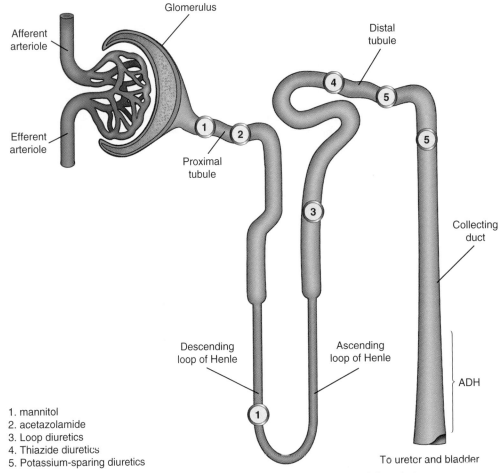

1. mannitol
2. acetazolamide
3. Loop diuretics
4. Thiazide diuretics
5. Potassium-sparing diuretics

FIG. 25-1 The nephron and diuretic sites of action. *ADH,* Antidiuretic hormone.

drugs in these classes are listed in Table 25-1. The most potent diuretics are the loop diuretics, followed by mannitol, metolazone (a thiazide-like diuretic), the thiazides, and the potassium-sparing diuretics. Their potency is a function of where they work in the nephron to inhibit sodium and water resorption. The more sodium and water they inhibit from resorption the greater the amount of diuresis and therefore the greater the potency.

CARBONIC ANHYDRASE INHIBITORS

Carbonic anhydrase inhibitors (CAIs) are chemical derivatives of sulphonamide antibiotics. As their name implies, CAIs inhibit the enzyme carbonic anhydrase, which exists in the kidneys, eyes, and other parts of the body. The site of action of the CAIs is the location of the carbonic anhydrase enzyme system along the nephron, primarily in the proximal tubule. For instance, acetazolamide acts principally in the proximal tubule, which, as previously described, is directly behind the glomerulus.

Mechanism of Action and Drug Effects

As previously noted, the carbonic anhydrase system in the kidney is located just distal to the glomerulus in the proximal tubules, where roughly two-thirds of all sodium and water is resorbed into the blood. Here a specific transport system operates that exchanges sodium for hydrogen ions. For sodium and thus water to be resorbed back into the blood, hydrogen must be exchanged for it. Without the hydrogen this cannot occur, and the sodium and water are eliminated with the urine. The carbonic anhydrase helps make the hydrogen ions available for this exchange. When its actions are inhibited with a CAI such as acetazolamide, little sodium and water can be resorbed into the blood and they are eliminated with the urine. The CAIs reduce the formation of hydrogen (H^+) and bicarbonate (HCO_3^-) ions from carbon dioxide and water by the non-competitive, reversible inhibition of carbonic anhydrase. This results in a reduction in the availability of these ions, mainly hydrogen, for active transport systems.

CAIs' reduction of the formation of bicarbonate and hydrogen ions can have many effects on other parts of the body. The metabolic acidosis induced by CAIs is beneficial in preventing certain seizure conditions. In addition, CAIs may induce respiratory and metabolic acidosis, which may in turn increase oxygenation during hypoxia by increasing ventilation and cerebral blood flow and dissociating oxygen from oxyhemoglobin. An undesirable effect of CAIs is that they elevate the blood glucose level and cause glycosuria in diabetic clients. This may be due in part to CAI-enhanced potassium loss through the urine.

Indications

The therapeutic applications of CAIs are wide and varied. They are commonly used in the treatment of glaucoma, edema, epilepsy, and high-altitude sickness.

CAIs are used principally as adjunct agents in the long-term management of **open-angle glaucoma** that cannot be controlled by topical miotic (pupil-contracting) agents or epinephrine derivatives alone. These agents together can increase the outflow of aqueous humor, the obstruction of which is responsible for the glaucoma. They are also used short term in conjunction with miotics to lower intra-ocular pressure in preparation for ocular surgery in clients with acute ocular disorders or narrow-angle glaucoma and as an adjunct in the treatment of secondary glaucoma.

CAIs, particularly acetazolamide, are used to manage edema secondary to heart failure that has become resistant to other diuretics. However, as a class, CAIs are much less potent diuretics than loop diuretics or thiazides, and the metabolic acidosis they induce diminishes their diuretic effect in 2 to 4 days.

Acetazolamide may be a useful adjunct to other anticonvulsants in the prophylactic management of various forms of epilepsy. However, tolerance to the anticonvulsant effects of CAIs develops quickly, and they may be ineffective for prolonged therapy. Acetazolamide is also effective in both preventing and treating the symptoms of acute mountain or high-altitude sickness, including headache, nausea, shortness of breath, dizziness, drowsiness, and fatigue.

Contraindications

Contraindications to the use of CAIs include known drug allergy and may include hyponatremia, hypokalemia, hyperchloremic acidosis, severe renal or hepatic dysfunction, adrenal gland insufficiency, and cirrhosis.

Side Effects and Adverse Effects

The more common undesirable effects of CAIs are metabolic abnormalities such as acidosis. They may also cause drowsiness, anorexia, paraesthesia, hearing disturbances or tinnitus, urticaria, photosensitivity, hematuria (blood in urine), and melena (blood in stool).

Interactions

Significant drug interactions include an increase in digitalis toxicity stemming from the hypokalemia that CAIs may induce. Concomitant use with corticosteroids may cause hypokalemia, and use with oral hypoglycemic agents and quinidine induces greater activity or toxicity of the latter agents.

Dosages

For information on the dosages of acetazolamide, see the following drug profile. See Appendix B for some of the common brands available in Canada.

TABLE 25-1
CLASSIFICATION OF DIURETICS

Class	Drugs
Carbonic anhydrase inhibitors	acetazolamide, methazolamide
Loop diuretics	bumetanide, ethacrynic acid, furosemide
Osmotic diuretics	mannitol
Potassium-sparing diuretics	amiloride, spironolactone, triamterene
Thiazide and thiazide-like diuretics	chlorthalidone, hydrochlorothiazide, indapamide, metolazone, trichlormethiazide

PEDIATRIC CONSIDERATIONS

Diuretic Therapy

- Pediatric dosages of these medications should be calculated carefully. Overdose can result in fluid volume and electrolyte loss, hypotension, shock, and possibly death. Weight should be recorded on admission and daily, so that a possible overdose can be identified.
- To make sure the child is responding appropriately and to identify possible adverse reactions or complications, intake and output should be checked daily, along with vital signs, including the rate, depth, and rhythm of respirations.
- The oral forms of these drugs may be taken with food or milk and should be taken early in the day.
- Sunscreen containing PABA should be avoided and clothing should be worn to protect the child from the sun during even brief exposure. Lengthy exposure to either heat or sun should be avoided because it may precipitate heat stroke, exhaustion, and fluid volume loss.
- Thiazide diuretics can cross the placenta and pass through to the fetus. They are also secreted in breast milk. Therefore they can produce exaggerated and even toxic or lethal effects in the fetus or neonate of women taking them.
- CAI diuretics are for adult use only.
- Potassium-sparing diuretics are contraindicated in pregnant women because of the effects on the mother and on the fetus.

DRUG PROFILES

Of the two available CAIs (see Table 25-1), by far the most widely prescribed is acetazolamide, and it is thus the only CAI profiled here.

acetazolamide

Acetazolamide is contraindicated in clients who have a known hypersensitivity to it and to sulphonamides, as well as in those with significant liver or kidney dysfunction, low serum potassium or sodium levels, acidosis, and adrenal gland failure. Acetazolamide is available only in oral form as a 500-mg extended-release capsule and a 250-mg tablet. The parenteral form, a Special Access Programme drug requiring Health Canada approval, is available in a pediatric solution of 100 mg/mL in a syringe. The adult formulation is available as 250 mg/50 mL D5W or as a 500-mg vial. A recommended dosage for pediatric clients is oral administration of 4–5 mg/kg/day. A common oral dosage for adults is 250 to 375 mg/day given on alternate days. Pregnancy category C.

PHARMACOKINETICS

Half-Life	Onset	Peak	Duration
10–15 hr	1 hr	2–4 hr	8–12 hr

LOOP DIURETICS

Loop diuretics (bumetanide, ethacrynic acid, and furosemide) are potent diuretics. Bumetanide and furosemide are chemically related to the sulphonamide antibiotics.

Mechanism of Action and Drug Effects

Loop diuretics have renal, cardiovascular, and metabolic effects, with renal effects being their major mechanism of action. These agents act primarily along the thick ascending limb of the loop of Henle, blocking chloride and, secondarily, sodium resorption. They are also believed to activate renal prostaglandins, resulting in dilation of the blood vessels of the kidneys, the lungs, and the rest of the body (i.e., reduction in renal, pulmonary, and systemic vascular resistance). The beneficial hemodynamic effects of loop diuretics are a reduction in both the pre-load and central venous pressures, which are the filling pressures of the ventricles. These actions make them valuable in the treatment of the edema associated with heart failure, hepatic cirrhosis, and renal disease.

Loop diuretics are particularly useful when rapid diuresis is needed because of their rapid onset of action. In addition, the diuretic effect lasts at least 2 hours. A distinct advantage over thiazide diuretics is that their diuretic action continues even when the creatinine clearance decreases below 25 mL/min. This means that even when the function of the kidney diminishes, loop diuretics can still work. Because of their potent diuretic effect and the duration of this effect, loop diuretics are effective in a single daily dose. This allows the renal tubule time to partially compensate for the potassium depletion and other electrolyte disturbances that often accompany around-the-clock diuretic therapy. Despite this, the major side effect of loop diuretics is electrolyte disturbances. Rarely, prolonged high doses can also result in hearing loss stemming from ototoxicity.

Summary of Major Drug Effects of Loop Diuretics

As previously noted, loop diuretics produce a potent diuresis and subsequent loss of fluid. The resulting decreased fluid volume leads to a decreased return of blood to the heart, or decreased filling pressures. This has the following cardiovascular effects:

- Reduces BP
- Reduces pulmonary vascular resistance
- Reduces systemic vascular resistance
- Reduces central venous pressure
- Reduces left ventricular end-diastolic pressure

The metabolic effects of the loop diuretics are secondary to the electrolyte losses resulting from the potent diuresis. Major electrolyte losses include sodium and potassium and, to a lesser extent, calcium. Observed changes in the plasma insulin, glucagon, and growth hormone levels have been associated with loop diuretic therapy.

Indications

As indicated earlier, loop diuretics are used to manage the edema associated with heart failure and hepatic or renal disease, to control hypertension, and to increase the renal excretion of calcium in clients with hypercalcemia. As with certain other classes of diuretics, they may also be indicated in cases of heart failure resulting from diastolic dysfunction.

Contraindications

Contraindications to the use of loop diuretics include known drug allergy and may include allergy to sulphonamide antibiotics, anuria (inability to urinate), hepatic coma, or severe electrolyte loss.

Side Effects and Adverse Effects

Common undesirable effects of the loop diuretics are listed in Table 25-2. Those commonly associated with bumetanide therapy are muscle cramps, dizziness, dry mouth, arthritic pain, and encephalopathy. These are especially common in clients with pre-existing liver disease. Rarely, ethacrynic acid may cause severe neutropenia and episodes of Henoch-Schönlein purpura (indicated by purple spots, joint pain, and gastrointestinal symptoms). Furosemide can produce urticaria, erythema multiforme, exfoliative dermatitis, pruritus, photosensitivity, and rare cases of hemolytic anemia and aplastic anemia.

Toxicity and Management of Overdose

Electrolyte loss and dehydration, which can result in circulatory failure, are the main toxic effects of loop diuretics that require attention. Treatment involves electrolyte and fluid replacement.

TABLE 25-2
LOOP DIURETICS: COMMON ADVERSE EFFECTS

Body System	Side/Adverse Effect
Central nervous	Dizziness, headache, tinnitus, blurred vision
Gastrointestinal	Nausea, vomiting, diarrhea
Hematological	Agranulocytosis, thrombocytopenia, neutropenia
Metabolic	Hypokalemia, hyperglycemia, hyperuricemia

Interactions

Loop diuretics exhibit both neurotoxic and nephrotoxic properties, and they produce additive effects when given in combination with drugs that have similar toxicities. The drug interactions are summarized in Table 25-3.

Loop diuretics also affect certain laboratory results. They cause increases in the serum levels of uric acid, glucose, alanine aminotransferase (ALT), and aspartate aminotransferase (AST). Because their combined use with a thiazide (especially metolazone) results in the blockade of sodium and water resorption at multiple sites in the nephron, a property referred to as *sequential nephron blockade,* their effectiveness is increased. The reduction of vascular resistance induced by loop diuretics may be impeded when these drugs are taken concurrently with non-steroidal anti-inflammatory drugs (NSAIDs) because these two drug classes have opposite effects on prostaglandin activity.

Dosages

For the recommended dosages of loop diuretics, see the dosages table on p. 428. See Appendix B for some of the common brands available in Canada.

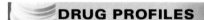

DRUG PROFILES

The currently available loop diuretics are bumetanide, ethacrynic acid, and furosemide. As a class they are potent diuretics, but potency varies. The equipotent doses for these various agents are as follows:

Bumetanide	Ethacrynic acid	Furosemide
1 mg	50 mg	40 mg

⇢ *furosemide*

Furosemide is by far the most commonly used loop diuretic in clinical practice and the prototype agent in this class. Structurally it is related to the sulphonamide antibiotics (Chapter 37). It has all the therapeutic and adverse characteristics of the loop diuretics mentioned earlier. It is primarily used in the management of pulmonary edema and the edema associated with heart failure, liver disease, nephrotic syndrome, and **ascites**

(the accumulation of fluid in the peritoneal area). It has also been used in the treatment of hypertension, usually that caused by heart failure.

Furosemide is contraindicated in clients who have shown a hypersensitivity to sulphonamides; in infants and lactating women; and in clients suffering from anuria, hypovolemia, and electrolyte depletion. It is available in oral form as a 40-mg/5 mL and a 10-mg/mL solution. It is also available as 20-, 40-, and 80-mg tablets and as a special 500-mg high-dosage formulation for specific use in clients with a glomerular filtration rate of less than 20 mL/min but greater than 5 mL/min who did not respond to traditional doses of furosemide. In parenteral form it is available as a 10-mg/mL injection. Pregnancy category C. Recommended dosages are given in the dosages table on p. 428.

PHARMACOKINETICS

Half-Life	Onset	Peak	Duration
1–2 hr	1 hr	1–2 hr	4–8 hr

OSMOTIC DIURETICS

The osmotic diuretics include mannitol, urea, organic acids, and glucose. Mannitol, a non-absorbable solute, is the most commonly used of these agents.

Mechanism of Action and Drug Effects

Mannitol works along the entire nephron. Its major site of action, however, is the proximal tubule and descending limb of the loop of Henle. Because it is non-absorbable, it produces an osmotic pressure in the glomerular filtrate that in turn pulls fluid, primarily water, into the renal tubules from the surrounding tissues. This process also inhibits the tubular resorption of water and solutes, producing a rapid diuresis. Ultimately this reduces cellular edema and increases urine production, causing diuresis. However, it produces only a slight loss of electrolytes, especially sodium. Therefore mannitol is not indicated for clients in an edematous state because it does not promote sufficient sodium excretion.

Mannitol may induce vasodilation and in doing so increases both glomerular filtration and renal plasma flow. This makes it an excellent agent for preventing kidney

TABLE 25-3

LOOP DIURETICS: COMMON DRUG INTERACTIONS

Drug	Mechanism	Results
Aminoglycosides chloroquine vancomycin	Additive effect	Increased neurotoxicity, especially ototoxicity
Corticosteroids digoxin	Hypokalemia	Additive hypokalemia Increased digoxin toxicity
lithium	Decreases renal excretion	Increased lithium toxicity
NSAIDs	Inhibit renal prostaglandins	Decreased diuretic activity
Sulphonylureas	Decrease glucose tolerance	Hyperglycemia

DOSAGES	Selected Loop Diuretics and Osmotic Diuretics		
Agent	**Pharmacological Class**	**Usual Dosage Range**	**Indications**
bumetanide		**Adult** PO: 0.5–2 mg/day as a single dose; max 10 mg/day	Edema
ethacrynic acid		**Pediatric** PO: Initial dose 25 mg/day; careful titration 25 mg increases to effect **Adult** PO: 0.5–1 mg/day; max 200 mg/day IV: 0.5–1 mg/kg	
▸▸furosemide	Loop diuretic	**Pediatric** IM/IV: 1 mg/kg/dose; do not exceed 2 mg/kg/ dose PO: 0.5–1 mg/kg q4h; do not exceed 2 mg/kg/day divided **Adult** IM/IV: 20–40 mg/dose; max 200 mg/day; administer high-dose IV therapy as a controlled infusion at a rate ≤4 mg/mL PO: 40–80 mg/day as a single dose; max 200 mg/day	Heart failure, hyperten-sion, renal failure, pul-monary edema, cirrhosis
▸▸mannitol	Osmotic diuretic	**Adult** IV infusion: 50–200 g/day, 1.5–2 g/kg over 30–60 min Suggested loading dose of 25 g, followed by an infusion rate to produce a urine flow of at least 100 mL/hr	Renal failure; reduction of intra-ocular and intracra-nial pressure; drug in-toxication

damage during acute renal failure (ARF). It is also often used to reduce intracranial pressure and cerebral edema resulting from head trauma. In addition, mannitol treat-ment may be tried when elevated intra-ocular pressure is unresponsive to other drug therapies.

Indications

Mannitol is the osmotic diuretic of choice. It is com-monly used in the treatment of clients in the early, olig-uric (reduced urination) phase of ARF. However, for it to be effective in this setting, enough renal blood flow and glomerular filtration must exist to enable the drug to reach the tubules. Increased renal blood flow result-ing from the dilation of blood vessels supplying blood to the kidneys is another therapeutic benefit of manni-tol therapy in such clients. It can also be used to pro-mote the excretion of toxic substances, reduce intracra-nial pressure, and treat cerebral edema. In addition, it can be used as a genitourinary irrigant in the prepara-tion of clients for transurethral surgical procedures and as supportive treatment in clients with edema induced by other conditions.

Contraindications

Contraindications to the use of mannitol include known drug allergy, severe renal disease, pulmonary edema (loop diuretics used instead), and intracranial bleeding unless intra-operative.

Side Effects and Adverse Effects

The significant undesirable effects of mannitol include convulsions, thrombophlebitis, and pulmonary conges-tion. Other less significant effects are headaches, chest pains, tachycardia, blurred vision, chills, and fever.

Interactions

There are no drugs that interact significantly with mannitol.

Dosages

For the recommended dosages of mannitol, see the dosages table above. See Appendix B for some of the common brands available in Canada.

DRUG PROFILES

▸▸ mannitol

Mannitol is the prototypical osmotic diuretic. It is con-traindicated in clients with a hypersensitivity to it as well as in those suffering from anuria, severe dehydration, pulmonary congestion, or cerebral hemorrhage. Treat-ment should be terminated if severe cardiac or renal im-pairment develops after the initiation of therapy. It is available only in parenteral form as 10 percent, 15 per-cent, 20 percent, and 25 percent solutions for intra-venous (IV) injection. Mannitol may crystallize when exposed to low temperatures. This is more likely to oc-cur when concentrations exceed 15 percent. Therefore,

Diuretic Therapy

- The nurse should always obtain baseline measurements of the client's height, weight, intake and output amounts, and serum sodium, potassium, and chloride levels.
- Diuretics should be taken early in the day to prevent nocturia (voiding at night), which could lead to lack of sleep and possible injury because of the need to get out of bed during the night.
- If the geriatric client is living alone and has minimal or no assistance with medications, visits from a home health or public health professional may help ensure the safety of the therapy and adherence with the therapy and diet.
- Caution should be taken with the use of diuretics in geriatric clients because these clients are more sensitive to the therapeutic effects of diuretics and more likely to experience dehydration, electrolyte loss, dizziness, and syncope.
- Encourage geriatric clients to change positions slowly because of the risk of orthostatic hypotension and the high risk for falls.

mannitol should always be administered intravenously through a filter, and vials of the drug are often stored in a warmer in the pharmacy. Pregnancy category C. Recommended dosages are given in the dosages table on p. 428.

PHARMACOKINETICS

Half Life	Onset	Peak	Duration
>1.5 hr	0.5–1 hr	0.25–2 hr	6–8 hr

POTASSIUM-SPARING DIURETICS

The currently available potassium-sparing diuretics are amiloride, spironolactone, and triamterene (which in Canada is available only in combination with hydrochlorothiazide). These diuretics are also referred to as aldosterone-inhibiting diuretics because they block the aldosterone receptors. In fact, spironolactone is a competitive antagonist of aldosterone and for this reason causes sodium and water to be excreted and potassium to be retained. It is the most commonly used of the three agents.

Mechanism of Action and Drug Effects

These agents work in the collecting ducts and distal convoluted tubules, where they interfere with sodium–potassium exchange. As noted earlier, spironolactone competitively binds to aldosterone receptors and therefore blocks the resorption of sodium and water that is induced by aldosterone secretion. These receptors occur primarily in the distal tubule. Amiloride and triamterene do not bind to aldosterone receptors. However, they inhibit both aldosterone-induced and basal sodium reabsorption, working in both the distal tubule and collecting

Body System	Side/Adverse Effects
Central nervous	Dizziness, headache
Gastrointestinal	Cramps, nausea, vomiting, diarrhea
Other	Urinary frequency, weakness, hyperkalemia

TABLE 25-4

POTASSIUM-SPARING DIURETICS: COMMON ADVERSE EFFECTS

ducts. They are often prescribed in children with heart failure because pediatric cardiac problems are often accompanied by an excess secretion of aldosterone and the loop and thiazide diuretics are often ineffective in their management.

Because around 3 percent of the total filtered urine volume reaches the collecting ducts, the potassium-sparing diuretics are relatively weak compared with the thiazide and loop diuretics. When diuresis is needed, they are generally used as adjuncts to thiazide treatment. This combination is beneficial in two respects. First, it has synergistic diuretic effects; second, the two agents counteract each other's adverse metabolic effects. The thiazide diuretics cause potassium, magnesium, and chloride to be lost in the urine, and the potassium-sparing diuretics counteract this by elevating the potassium and chloride levels.

Indications

The therapeutic applications of the potassium-sparing diuretics vary depending on the particular agent. Spironolactone and triamterene are used in the treatment of hyperaldosteronism and hypertension and for reversing the potassium loss caused by the **kaliuretic diuretics** or other potassium-losing drugs. The uses for amiloride are similar, but amiloride is less effective in the long term. It may, however, be more effective than spironolactone or triamterene in the treatment of metabolic alkalosis. It is primarily used in the treatment of heart failure. As with certain other classes of diuretics, potassium-sparing diuretics may also be indicated in cases of heart failure due to diastolic dysfunction.

Contraindications

Contraindications to the use of potassium-sparing diuretics include known drug allergy, hyperkalemia (e.g., serum potassium level greater than 5.5 mmol/L), and severe renal failure or anuria. Triamterene may also be contraindicated in cases of severe hepatic failure.

Side Effects and Adverse Effects

Potassium-sparing diuretics have several common undesirable effects, which are listed in Table 25-4. There are also some significant adverse effects specific to the individual agents. Spironolactone can cause gynecomastia in men; in women, it can cause amenorrhea, irregular menses, and postmenopausal bleeding. Triamterene may reduce folic acid levels and cause the formation of kidney stones and urinary casts. It may

DOSAGES | Selected Potassium-Sparing Diuretic Agents

Agent	Pharmacological Class	Usual Dosage Range	Indications
amiloride		**Adult** PO: 5–20 mg/day	Edema and as an adjunct to kaliuretic diuretics
▸▸spironolactone	Potassium-sparing diuretics	**Pediatric** PO: 3 mg/kg/day single or divided; 1–2 mg/kg maintenance **Adult** PO: 50–200 mg/day	Edema, hypertension, heart failure, ascites
triamterene 50 mg/ hydrochlorothiazide 25 mg		**Adult** PO: 1–4 tablets daily after meals	Diuretic-antihypertensive

also precipitate megaloblastic anemia. Hyperkalemia also may occur when triamterene is used alone or in combination with other diuretics. Side effects from triamterene use are rare.

Interactions

The concomitant use of potassium-sparing diuretics with lithium, angiotensin converting enzyme (ACE) inhibitors, or potassium supplements can result in significant drug interactions. The combined use of ACE inhibitors or potassium supplements with potassium-sparing diuretics can result in hyperkalemia. When given together, lithium and potassium-sparing diuretics can result in lithium toxicity. NSAIDs can inhibit renal prostaglandins, decreasing blood flow to the kidneys and therefore decreasing the delivery of diuretic drugs to this site of action. This in turn can lead to a diminished diuretic response.

Dosages

For the recommended dosages of potassium-sparing diuretics, see the dosages table above. See Appendix B for some of the common brands available in Canada.

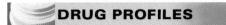

DRUG PROFILES

amiloride

Amiloride is generally used in combination with a thiazide or loop diuretic in therapy for heart failure. Hyperkalemia may occur in as many as 10 percent of clients who take amiloride alone. It should be used with caution in clients suffering from renal impairment or diabetes mellitus and in geriatric clients. It has only weak antihypertensive properties. It is available only in oral form as a 5-mg tablet. It is also available in combination with hydrochlorothiazide. Pregnancy category B. Recommended dosages are given in the dosages table above.

PHARMACOKINETICS

Half-Life	Onset	Peak	Duration
6–9 hr	2 hr	6–10 hr	24 hr

▸▸spironolactone

Structurally, spironolactone is a synthetic steroid that blocks aldosterone receptors. It is used in high doses for the treatment of ascites. This condition is commonly associated with cirrhosis of the liver. The serum potassium level should be monitored frequently in clients who have impaired renal function or who are currently taking potassium supplements because hyperkalemia is a common complication of spironolactone therapy. It is the potassium-sparing diuretic most commonly prescribed for children who have heart failure because pediatric heart failure often causes excess aldosterone to be secreted, which in turn causes increased sodium and water resorption. Recently spironolactone has been shown to reduce morbidity and mortality rates in clients with severe heart failure when added to standard therapy. Of the three commonly used potassium-sparing diuretics, spironolactone has the greatest antihypertensive activity. It is available only in oral form as 25- and 100-mg tablets. It is also available in combination with hydrochlorothiazide. Pregnancy category D. Recommended dosages are given in the dosages table above.

PHARMACOKINETICS

Half-Life	Onset	Peak	Duration
13–24 hr	1–3 days	2–3 days	2–3 days

triamterene

Like amiloride, triamterene acts directly on the distal renal tubule of the nephron to depress the resorption of sodium and the excretion of potassium and hydrogen, processes otherwise stimulated at that site by aldosterone. It has little or no antihypertensive effect. It is available only in combination with hydrochlorothiazide. The advantage of this combination of triamterene/hydrochlorothiazide is that triamterene helps the body to retain the potassium that hydrochlorothiazide causes to be lost, eliminating the need for potassium supplements. Pregnancy category D. Recommended dosages are given in the dosages table above.

PHARMACOKINETICS

Half-Life	Onset	Peak	Duration
2–3 hr	2–4 hr	6–8 hr	12–16 hr

THIAZIDES AND THIAZIDE-LIKE DIURETICS

Thiazide and thiazide-like diuretics are generally considered equivalent in their effects. Thiazide diuretics, like several of the loop diuretics, are chemical derivatives (benzothiadiazines) of sulphonamide antibiotics. However, chlorthalidone is somewhat different because of its long duration of action. Metolazone, which is commonly prescribed, may be more effective than other agents of this class in the treatment of clients with renal dysfunction. Hydrochlorothiazide is one of the most commonly used and the least expensive of the generic preparations. The thiazide diuretics include hydrochlorothiazide and trichlormethiazide. The thiazide-like diuretics are similar in action and include chlorthalidone, indapamide, and metolazone. Hydrochlorothiazide and metolazone are by far the most commonly prescribed in practice.

Mechanism of Action and Drug Effects

Thiazides are used as adjunct agents in the management of heart failure, hepatic cirrhosis, and edema of various origins. The primary site of action of thiazides and thiazide-like diuretics is the distal convoluted tubule, where they inhibit sodium, potassium, and chloride resorption. This results in osmotic water loss as well. Thiazides also cause direct relaxation of the arterioles (small blood vessels), reducing peripheral vascular resistance (afterload). Decreased pre-load (filling pressures) and decreased afterload (the force the ventricles must overcome to eject the volume of blood they contain) are the beneficial hemodynamic effects. This makes them effective for the treatment of both heart failure and hypertension.

As renal function decreases, the efficacy of thiazides diminishes, probably because delivery of the drug to the active site is impaired. Thiazides generally should not be used if the creatinine clearance is less than 30 to 50 mL/min. Normal creatinine clearance is 125 mL/min. The only exception is metolazone, which remains effective to a creatinine clearance of 10 mL/min. The major side effects of the agents stem from the electrolyte disturbances they produce. They are noted for precipitating hypokalemia and hypercalcemia, as well as metabolic disturbances such as hyperlipidemia, hyperglycemia, and hyperuricemia.

Indications

The thiazide and thiazide-like diuretics are also approved by Health Canada for the treatment of hypertension and edematous states. Any of these drugs can be used either as a sole agent or in combination with other agents. This group of diuretics may also be useful as adjunct agents in the treatment of edema related to heart failure, hepatic cirrhosis, and corticosteroid or estrogen therapy. As with certain other classes of diuretics, they may also be indicated in cases of heart failure due to diastolic dysfunction.

TABLE 25-5

THIAZIDE AND THIAZIDE-LIKE DIURETICS: POTENTIAL ADVERSE EFFECTS

Body System/ Process	Side/Adverse Effects
Central nervous	Dizziness, headache, blurred vision, paraesthesia, restlessness, insomnia, vertigo, reduced libido
Gastrointestinal	Abdominal pain, anorexia, constipation, nausea, vomiting, diarrhea, pancreatitis, cholecystitis
Genitourinary	Erectile dysfunction
Hematological	Jaundice, leukopenia, purpura, agranulocytosis, aplastic anemia, thrombocytopenia
Integumentary	Urticaria, photosensitivity
Metabolic	Hypokalemia, glycosuria, hyperglycemia, hyperuricemia, hypochloremic alkalosis
Musculoskeletal	Muscle cramps, muscle spasm

Contraindications

Contraindications to the use of thiazides and thiazide-like diuretics include known drug allergy, hepatic coma (metolazone), anuria, and severe renal failure.

Side Effects and Adverse Effects

Major side effects of the thiazide and thiazide-like diuretics relate to the electrolyte disturbances they cause. These mainly comprise reduced potassium levels and elevated levels of calcium, lipids, glucose, and uric acid. Other effects, such as gastrointestinal disturbances, skin rashes, photosensitivity, thrombocytopenia, pancreatitis, and cholecystitis, are less common. Dizziness and vertigo are common side effects of metolazone therapy and are attributed to sudden shifts in the plasma volume brought about by the agent. Headache, erectile dysfunction, and reduced libido are other important side effects of these agents. Many of these side effects are dose related and are seen at higher doses, especially those above 25 mg. The more common side effects of the thiazide and thiazide-like diuretics are listed in Table 25-5.

Toxicity and Management of Overdose

An overdose of these drugs can lead to an electrolyte imbalance resulting from hypokalemia. Symptoms include anorexia, nausea, lethargy, muscle weakness, mental confusion, and hypotension. Treatment involves electrolyte replacement.

Interactions

There are many drug interactions associated with thiazides and related agents. Corticosteroids, diazoxide, digitalis, and oral hypoglycemics, as well as some natural health products, specifically coltsfoot, Siberian ginseng, ginkgo, and ma huang, may affect the efficacy of the thiazides and related agents. The mechanisms and results of these interactions are summarized in Table 25-6. Excessive consumption of licorice can lead to an additive hypokalemia in clients taking these drugs.

Dosages

For information on the dosages for thiazide and thiazide-like diuretics, see the dosages table below. See Appendix B for some of the common brands available in Canada.

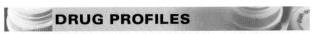

DRUG PROFILES

Thiazide and thiazide-like diuretics fall into several pregnancy categories. Hydrochlorothiazide, indapamide, and metolazone are category B agents. Trichlormethiazide is a category C agent. Chlorthalidone is not classified in any pregnancy category.

↠ hydrochlorothiazide

Hydrochlorothiazide, which is considered the prototypical thiazide diuretic, is a commonly prescribed and inexpensive thiazide diuretic. It is also a safe and effective diuretic. Hydrochlorothiazide is used in combination with many other drugs: amiloride, angiotensin II receptor antagonists, methyldopa, propranolol, spironolactone, triamterene, hydralazine, ACE inhibitors, beta-blockers, and labetalol. Daily doses exceeding 50 mg/day rarely produce additional clinical results and may only increase drug toxicity. This property is known as a *ceiling effect*.

Hydrochlorothiazide is contraindicated in clients with a known hypersensitivity to thiazides or sulphonamides and in those suffering from anuria, renal decompensa-tion, or hypomagnesemia. It is available only in oral form as 25-, 50-, and 100-mg capsules and tablets. Pregnancy category B. Recommended dosages are given in the dosages table below.

PHARMACOKINETICS

Half-Life	Onset	Peak	Duration
5.6–14.8 hr	2 hr	4–6 hr	6–12 hr

metolazone

Metolazone is a thiazide-like diuretic that appears to be more potent than the thiazide diuretics. This is most visible in clients with renal dysfunction. One striking advantage of metolazone is that it remains effective to a creatinine clearance as low as 10 mL/min. It may also be given in combination with loop diuretics to obtain a potent diuresis in clients with severe symptoms of heart failure. Metolazone is contraindicated in clients with a known hypersensitivity to thiazides or sulphonamides, in those with anuria, and in pregnant or lactating women. It is available only in oral form as a 2.5-mg tablet. Brands cannot be interchanged because the bioavailability of each is different. Pregnancy category B. Recommended dosages are given in the dosages table below.

PHARMACOKINETICS

Half-Life	Onset	Peak	Duration
6–20 hr	1 hr	2 hr	12–24 hr

NURSING PROCESS

■ Assessment

Before administering any type of diuretic, the nurse should obtain a thorough client history. A physical examination must also be completed and the findings documented. Because fluid volume levels and electrolyte concentrations are affected by diuretics, the client's baseline fluid volume status, intake and output measurements, serum electrolyte values, weight, and vital signs should be documented. Skin turgor, the serum creatinine level, arterial blood gas values, blood pH, and the uric acid level should also be documented before the start of diuretic therapy. Often it is necessary to measure postural

TABLE 25-6

THIAZIDE AND THIAZIDE-LIKE DIURETICS: COMMON DRUG INTERACTIONS

Drug	Mechanism	Results
Corticosteroids	Additive effect	Hypokalemia
diazoxide	Additive effect	Hyperglycemia, hyperuricemia
digoxin	Hypokalemia	Increased digoxin toxicity
lithium	Decreases clearance	Increased lithium toxicity
NSAIDs	Inhibit renal prostaglandins	Decreased diuretic activity
Oral antidiabetic agents	Antagonism	Reduced therapeutic effect

DOSAGES **Thiazide and Selected Thiazide-Like Diuretic Agents**

Agent	Pharmacological Class	Usual Dosage Range	Indications
↠ hydrochlorothiazide	Thiazide diuretic	**Pediatric** PO: 2–4 mg/kg/day q12h **Adult** PO: 25–200 mg/day, usually divided PO: 25–100 mg/day **Geriatric** 12.5–25 mg/day	Edema, hypertension, heart failure, nephrotic syndrome
metolazone	Thiazide-like diuretic	**Adult** PO: 2.5–20 mg/day	

BPs (lying and standing) in clients who are to receive these agents because they cause fluid to be lost from the intravascular spaces first, and this may precipitate BP changes (both a decrease and postural changes).

Cautious use of diuretics, with close monitoring of fluid volume status, electrolytes, and vital signs, is recommended in clients with hypokalemia, hypovolemia, renal disease, liver disease, lupus, diabetes, chronic obstructive pulmonary disease (COPD), and gout. Potassium-sparing diuretics should be used cautiously in clients who are dehydrated, those with renal disease, and lactating women. Cautious use of osmotic diuretics is recommended in clients with severe renal disease or heart failure, those who are dehydrated, and pregnant or lactating women.

Contraindications to the use of diuretics include allergies to the specific medication or to sulphonamides in the case of furosemide and thiazide diuretic treatment, anuria, dehydration, hypovolemia, hypotension, and electrolyte disturbances. Their use is also contraindicated in infants and in breastfeeding women. Thiazide diuretics are contraindicated in clients suffering from altered renal function or hypomagnesemia. Potassium-sparing diuretics are contraindicated in clients suffering from hyperkalemia and in pregnant women. Osmotic diuretics are contraindicated in clients with severe pulmonary edema, severe edema, active intracranial bleeding, and severe dehydration.

Nursing Diagnoses

Nursing diagnoses associated with the use of diuretics include the following:
- Decreased cardiac output related to adverse effects of diuretics.

CASE STUDY

Diuretic Therapy

Primary hypertension has been diagnosed in S.G., a 47-year-old woman. Her BPs have been ranging between 158 and 172 mm Hg systolic and 94 and 110 mm Hg diastolic. Her average BP over the past month has been 156/98 mm Hg. She has a strong family history of hypertension and is a single parent of two adolescents. She is also trying to keep up with her responsibilities as a full-time assistant professor of education at a local urban university. There is no evidence of renal insufficiency or cardiac damage at this time, nor is there evidence of retinopathy or other signs and symptoms of end-organ disease. No other problems are reported, and S.G. is begun on 50 mg of hydrochlorothiazide daily.

- Discuss the antihypertensive effects of hydrochlorothiazide.
- What sort of guidelines must you give this client so that she does not have adverse reactions to the diuretic therapy?
- What non-pharmacological measures should you suggest to help the client control her BP?

For answers see http://evolve.elsevier.com/Lilley/pharmacology/.

- Deficient fluid volume related to effects of diuretics.
- Risk for injury related to postural hypotension and dizziness.
- Deficient knowledge related to new use of diuretic therapy and lack of experience.
- Acute headache from adverse effects of diuretics.
- Non-adherence to treatment related to lack of information about side effects of medications.

Planning

Goals related to the administration of diuretics include the following:
- Client regains fluid and electrolyte balance.
- Client remains free of the complications associated with diuretic use.
- Client remains free of injury while on diuretics.
- Client remains adherent with therapy.

Outcome Criteria

The outcome criteria in clients receiving diuretics are as follows:
- Client maintains normal electrolyte values (sodium, potassium, and chloride values) while on diuretics.
- Client continues to show or regain normal cardiac output while on diuretic therapy as evidenced by vital signs, adequate intake, and output within normal limits (pulse <100, >60; BP 120/80; urine output ≥30 mL/hr).
- Client's skin is pliable and without edema or dryness.
- Client rises slowly and changes positions slowly and cautiously while receiving diuretics.
- Client states the importance and rationale for follow-up visits with the physician, such as monitoring for adverse effects, dehydration, and fluid and electrolyte imbalances.
- Client reports dizziness, fainting, palpitations, tingling, confusion, or disorientation to the physician immediately.

Implementation

If possible, diuretics should be taken in the morning to avoid frequent urination interfering with sleep. Potassium supplements are generally not recommended when potassium levels exceed 3.0 mmol/L except per physician's advice.

More detailed information is presented in the client teaching tips on p. 435.

Evaluation

The therapeutic effects of diuretics include resolution of or reduction in edema, fluid volume overload, heart failure, or hypertension or a return to normal intraocular pressures. The client must also be monitored for the occurrence of adverse reactions such as metabolic alkalosis (monitor arterial blood gas values), drowsiness, lethargy, hypokalemia, tachycardia, hypotension, leg cramps, restlessness, and a decrease in mental alertness.

NURSING CARE PLAN

Diuretic Therapy

Mr. P. is a 59-year-old lawyer who is a partner in a prestigious law firm. His typical workday begins at 7:30 am and lasts until about 8 pm. He exercises two to three times a week, but not regularly. However, he is in good health and his cholesterol and lipid profiles are within normal limits. He has been diagnosed with hypertension and needs to lose about 10 kg per physician's orders. He is to begin taking hydrochlorothiazide at a dosage of 50 mg twice daily and is to follow up in 1 week with the physician and dietician for further consultation. He has been asked to take his BP three times a week and to keep a daily journal of any symptoms, as well as to record BP readings.

ASSESSMENT	Subjective Data	Complaint of severe headaches
	Objective Data	• Lawyer for 24 years
		• History of stress ulcers
		• Family history of hypertension
		• BP at physician's office was 180/98 mm Hg
NURSING DIAGNOSIS		Deficient knowledge related to new treatment of hypertension and lack of experience with medication
PLANNING	Goals	Client will remain adherent to diuretic therapy within 1 month
	Outcome Criteria	Client will verbalize safe and accurate means of taking diuretic medication as evidenced by: • Fewer side effects • Increased therapeutic effects within 1 month of therapy

IMPLEMENTATION

Client education should include the following statements:
- Hydrochlorothiazide is a diuretic that will help eliminate water to help decrease your BP. It also eliminates through urine sodium, chloride, potassium, and magnesium, which means we monitor electrolytes frequently, along with BPs.
- Weigh yourself weekly and report a gain in weight of 1 kg or more in 1 week.
- Take plenty of fluids, up to 2–3 L/day, or as per physician's advice.
- Change positions slowly when you rise from sitting or standing to avoid dizziness and/or fainting.
- If applicable, take your medication with food.
- Take the diuretic medication early in the morning to prevent urination at nighttime.
- Eat a diet high in potassium, including foods such as strawberries, orange juice, apricots, and bananas, to help counter the potassium lost in the urine, as applicable.
- Contact your physician should you experience muscle cramps, dizziness, nausea, or muscle weakness, because this may indicate possible side effects from an electrolyte disorder or deficit.
- Record and monitor your BPs at least 3 times a week until you receive further instructions from the healthcare provider.
- Changes in blood pressure may indicate therapeutic effects or adverse effects (changes in blood pressure when you change position are an adverse effect).

EVALUATION

Client shows a therapeutic response to diuretic therapy as evidenced by
- Improved BP
- Less edema in feet and hands
- Improved energy levels

Client is monitored for side effects such as
- Dizziness
- Drowsiness
- Postural hypotension, nausea, vomiting, anorexia
- Muscle cramps
- Fatigue
- Headache
- Hyperglycemia
- Hypokalemia
- Polyuria
- Blurred vision

CLIENT TEACHING TIPS

The nurse should instruct clients as follows:
▲ Always eat a proper diet and drink adequate fluids.
▲ (For any but the potassium-sparing diuretics) Eat more potassium-rich foods, such as apricots, bananas, citrus fruits, dates, raisins, plums, fresh vegetables, potatoes (especially potato skins), meat, and fish.
▲ If you are also taking a digitalis preparation, monitor your pulse rate. Call the physician at the first signs of toxicity. Symptoms include anorexia, nausea, vomiting, and a pulse rate of <60 beats/min.
▲ If you are diabetic and are taking thiazide and/or loop diuretics, monitor your blood sugar levels closely, because these drugs can raise them.
▲ Change positions slowly and rise slowly after sitting or lying to prevent dizziness and possible fainting.
▲ Return to your physician for follow-up visits and laboratory tests.
▲ Keep a journal or log of your daily weight.

▲ If you have gout, it may get worse with this medication; notify the physician if it does.
▲ Don't drink excessive alcohol, which may increase dizziness and make fainting more likely. If you are prescribed a sedative or painkiller, make sure the physician knows you are taking this medication.
▲ Report cramps in the legs or elsewhere, muscle weakness, constipation, irregular heart rate, and an overall feeling of lethargy. These symptoms may mean you need more potassium-rich foods.
▲ If you are ill and have experienced vomiting or diarrhea, notify your physician and ask whether you need to replace the lost fluid.
▲ Notify your physician immediately if you experience rapid heart rate or fainting.
▲ If you gain 1 kg in a day or 2 kg in a week, notify your physician immediately.

POINTS to REMEMBER

▼ The main types of diuretics are CAIs and loop, osmotic, potassium-sparing, thiazide, and thiazide-like diuretics.
▼ The loop, potassium-sparing, thiazide, and thiazide-like diuretics are the most commonly used.
▼ The purpose of diuretics is to cause a net loss of certain electrolytes and thus water from the body; therefore they increase urinary output.
▼ The nephron is the main structural element in the kidney and is the main site of action for diuretics. The nephron is composed of the glomerulus, afferent and efferent arterioles, proximal and distal tubules, loop of Henle, and collecting ducts.
▼ Loop diuretics, the most potent class, work in the loop of Henle, where most of the sodium is reabsorbed. The most commonly used loop diuretics are furosemide and bumetanide. Ethacrynic acid is seldom used. Equipotent doses are as follows: 1 mg of bumetanide = 40 mg of furosemide = 50 mg of ethacrynic acid.
▼ Thiazide diuretics are the most commonly used and the least expensive because several generic preparations are available. Hydrochlorothiazide is considered

the prototypical thiazide diuretic and is used as adjunctive therapy to manage hepatic cirrhosis, edema, and heart failure. Adverse metabolic effects include hypokalemia, hypercalcemia, hyperlipidemia, hyperglycemia, and hyperuricemia.
▼ Combination products and potassium-sparing diuretics are not as potent as other diuretics. With potassium-sparing diuretics, hyperkalemia may be a side effect.
▼ Fluid volume status should be monitored in clients receiving diuretics because of the serious excess and deficit states they can cause.
▼ Methods of monitoring for excess and deficit states include assessing skin and mucous membrane status and sodium, potassium, and chloride levels. Intake and output amounts should be monitored in clients receiving diuretics. The nurse should always be concerned about more vulnerable clients, such as geriatric clients, who are more susceptible to the effects of diuretics.
▼ Adverse reactions to diuretics include metabolic alkalosis, drowsiness, lethargy, hypokalemia, tachycardia, hypotension, leg cramps, restlessness, and decreased mental alertness.

EXAMINATION REVIEW QUESTIONS

1 Which of the following do loop diuretics have a cross-sensitivity with?
   a. Vitamins E and K
   b. Antacids
   c. Sulpha drugs
   d. NSAIDs

2 Use of loop and thiazide diuretics may result in which of the following?
   a. Decreased serum levels of sodium and diuresis
   b. Increased levels of mannitol from the nephron and oliguria
   c. Decreased serum glucose levels and gross osmotic diuresis
   d. Increased serum levels of sodium and polyuria

3 Hyperkalemia would occur more commonly with which of the following drugs?
a. spironolactone
b. Beta-blockers
c. CAI diuretics
d. furosemide

4 Which of the following statements should be included in client education for an 81-year-old female with heart failure taking daily doses of spironolactone?
a. Check weight monthly and report it to the physician.
b. Avoid foods that are high in potassium.

c. Change positions slowly because this drug causes severe hypertensive-induced syncope.
d. A weight gain of 1–1.25 kg in 24 hours is a normal finding.

5 Which of the following may occur with daily dosing of 80 mg oral furosemide?
a. Increased BUN
b. Hypokalemia
c. Decreased urine creatinine
d. Hyperkalemia

For answers see http://evolve.elsevier.com/Lilley/pharmacology/.

CRITICAL THINKING ACTIVITIES

1 Mr. G. is a 64-year-old man who has been admitted to the coronary care unit because he is suffering from heart failure. He has been given 80 mg of furosemide q6h, but with no relief of his pulmonary and peripheral edema. The physician would like to change him to bumetanide. What is the equivalent daily dose of bumetanide?

2 What type of caution would you give a client who is beginning treatment with a potassium-sparing diuretic?

3 Describe the antihypertensive effects of loop diuretics in the treatment of hypertension.

For answers see http://evolve.elsevier.com/Lilley/pharmacology/.

BIBLIOGRAPHY

Albanese, J., & Nutz, P. (2005). *Mosby's 2005 nursing drug cards.* St Louis, MO: Mosby.

Anderson, P.O., Knoben, J.E., & Troutman, W.G. (2002). *Handbook of clinical drug data* (10th ed.). New York: McGraw-Hill/Appleton & Lange.

Berne, R., & Levy, M. (2002). *Principles of physiology* (3rd ed.). St Louis, MO: Mosby.

Boron, W.F., & Boulpaep, E.L. (2005). *Medical physiology* (2nd ed.). Philadelphia: Saunders.

Canadian Pharmacists Association. (2003). *Therapeutic choices* (4th ed.). Ottawa, ON: Author.

Canadian Pharmacists Association. (2004). *Guide to drugs in Canada.* Toronto, ON: Dorling Kindersley.

Canadian Pharmacists Association. (2005). *Compendium of pharmaceuticals and specialties. The Canadian drug reference for health professionals.* Ottawa, ON: Author. [The subscription-based e-CPS is available at http://www.pharmacists.ca.]

Cheng, A., Williams, B.A., & Sivarajan, B.V. (Eds.). *The HSC handbook of pediatrics* (10th ed.). Toronto, ON: Elsevier.

Health Canada. (2005). Drug product database (DPD). Retrieved August 12, 2005, from http://www.hc-sc.gc.ca/hpb/drugs-dpd/

Khan, N.A., & Campbell, N.R.C. (2004). Thiazide diuretics in the management of hypertension. *Canadian Journal of Clinical Pharmacology, 11*(1), e41–e44.

Lacy, C.F., Armstrong, L.L., Goldman, M.P., & Lance, L.L. (2003). *Drug information handbook* (11th ed.). Hudson, OH: Lexi-Comp.

Lehne, R.A. (2004). *Pharmacology for nursing care* (5th ed.). St Louis, MO: Saunders.

Mosby. (2005). *Mosby's drug consult 2005: The comprehensive reference for generic and brand name drugs* (15th ed.). St Louis, MO: Mosby.

Skidmore-Roth, L. (2006). *Mosby's 2006 nursing drug reference* (19th ed.). St Louis, MO: Mosby.

Woods, S.L., Sivarajan Froelocher, E.S., Underhill Motzer, S., & Bridges, E.J. (2005). *Cardiac nursing* (5th ed.). Philadelphia: Lippincott Williams & Wilkins

Fluids and Electrolytes

OBJECTIVES

After reading this chapter, the successful student will be able to do the following:

1 Identify the various fluid and electrolyte solutions commonly used in the management of fluid and electrolyte disorders.

2 Discuss the mechanisms of action, indications, dosages, contraindications, cautions, side effects, toxicity, and drug interactions related to fluid and electrolyte solutions.

3 Compare the various solutions used to expand a client's fluid volume and restore fluid status.

4 Develop a nursing care plan that includes all phases of the nursing process for the client receiving fluid and electrolyte solutions.

e-LEARNING ACTIVITIES

Student CD-ROM
- Review Questions: see questions 190–193
- Animations
- Medication Administration Checklists
- IV Therapy Checklists

evolve Web site (http://evolve.elsevier.com/Lilley/pharmacology/)
- Online Chapter Worksheet • Frequently Asked Questions
- Learning Tips and Content Updates • WebLinks • Online Appendices and Supplements • Mosby/Saunders ePharmacology Update • Access to *Mosby's Drug Consult*

DRUG PROFILES

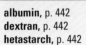

albumin, p. 442
dextran, p. 442
hetastarch, p. 442

sodium chloride, p. 441, 447
sodium polystyrene
sulphonate, p. 446

GLOSSARY

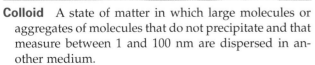

Colloid A state of matter in which large molecules or aggregates of molecules that do not precipitate and that measure between 1 and 100 nm are dispersed in another medium.

Colloid oncotic pressure (COP) (ong kot′ ik) The osmotic pressure exerted by a colloid in solution, such as that produced when the concentration of protein in the plasma on one side of a cell membrane is higher than that in the neighbouring interstitial fluid (ISF).

Crystalloids A substance in a solution that diffuses through a semi-permeable membrane.

Dehydration Excessive loss of water from the body tissues. It is accompanied by an imbalance in the essential electrolyte concentrations, particularly sodium, potassium, and chloride.

Edema (ə dee′ muh) The abnormal accumulation of fluid in interstitial spaces, such as in the pericardial sac, intrapleural space, peritoneal cavity, and joint capsules.

Extracellular fluid (ECF) (eks′ truh sel′ yoo lər) That portion of the body fluid comprising the ISF and blood plasma. The adult body contains about 11.2 L of ISF, constituting about 16 percent of the body weight, and about 2.8 L of plasma, constituting about 4 percent of the body weight.

Extravascular fluid (EVF) (eks′ truh vas′ kyoo lər) Fluids in the body that are outside the blood vessels. Examples include lymph and cerebrospinal fluid.

Hydrostatic pressure (HP) (hy′ droe stat′ ik) The pressure exerted by a liquid.

Hypokalemia (hy′ poe kuh lee′ mee uh) A condition in which there is an inadequate amount of potassium, the major intracellular cation (positively charged particle), in the bloodstream.

Hyponatremia (hy′ poe nuh tree′ mee uh) A condition in which there is an inadequate amount of sodium in

437

the blood, caused either by inadequate excretion of water or by excessive water in the bloodstream.

Interstitial fluid (ISF) (in tər stish' əl) ECF that fills in the spaces between most of the cells of the body and provides a substantial portion of the liquid environment of the body.

Intracellular fluid (ICF) Fluid located within cell membranes throughout most of the body. It contains dissolved solutes that are essential to maintaining electrolyte balance and healthy metabolism.

Intravascular fluid (IVF) The fluid inside blood vessels.

Isotonic (eye' soe ton' ik) Having the same concentration of a solute as another solution, hence exerting the same osmotic pressure as that solution, such as an isotonic saline solution that contains an amount of salt equal to that found in the intracellular and ECF.

Osmotic pressure The pressure exerted on a semi-permeable membrane separating a solution from a solvent; the membrane being impermeable to the solutes in the solution and permeable only to the solvent.

Plasma The watery, straw-coloured fluid component of lymph and blood in which the leukocytes, erythrocytes, and platelets are suspended.

Fluid and electrolyte management is one of the cornerstones of client care. Most disease processes, tissue injuries, and surgical procedures greatly influence the physiological status of fluids and electrolytes in the body. A prerequisite to understanding fluid and electrolyte management is knowledge of the extent and composition of the various body fluid compartments.

PHYSIOLOGY OF FLUID BALANCE

About 60 percent of the adult human body is water. This is referred to as the *total body water* (TBW), and it is distributed to the three main compartments in the following proportions: **intracellular fluid (ICF)**, 67 percent; **interstitial fluid (ISF)**, 25 percent; and plasma volume (PV), 8 percent. This distribution is illustrated in Figure 26-1. Typical fluid volumes are shown in Table 26-1.

The terms used to identify the various spaces within which the TBW is distributed can be quite confusing, and there are two basic approaches to distinguishing among the locations of the fluid. The TBW can be described as being in or out of the blood vessels, or vasculature. If this terminology is used, then the term **intravascular fluid (IVF)** describes fluid inside the blood vessels and the term **extravascular fluid (EVF)** describes the fluid outside the blood vessels. The term **plasma** is used to describe the fluid that flows through the blood vessels (intravascular). Fluid can also be described as being within or outside of cells. Using this terminology, fluid can be intracellular fluid (ICF) or **extracellular fluid (ECF)**. ECF includes both plasma and interstitial fluid (ISF). ISF is the fluid that is in the space between cells, tissues, and organs. Both plasma and ISF make up *extracellular* volume. Both ISF and ICF

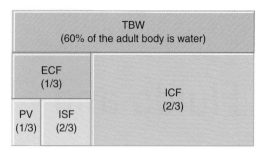

FIG. 26-1 Distribution of total body water (TBW). *ECF,* Extracellular fluid; *ICF,* intracellular fluid; *ISF,* interstitial fluid; *PV,* plasma volume.

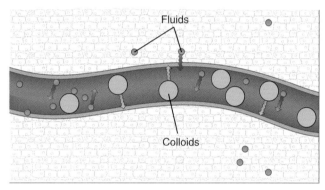

FIG. 26-2 Colloid osmotic pressure (oncotic pressure). As shown, the colloids inside the blood vessel are too large to pass through the vessel wall. The resulting oncotic pressure exerted by the colloids draws fluid from the surrounding tissues and other extravascular spaces into the blood vessels and also keeps fluid inside the blood vessel.

make up *extravascular* volume. These terms are often confused and misused. Table 26-1 lists these definitions for further clarity and understanding.

What keeps fluid inside the blood vessels? All the fluid outside the cells, the *extracellular fluid (ECF)* (plasma and ISF), has about the same concentration of electrolytes. However, there is one big difference between the plasma and the ISF. The plasma has a protein concentration, primarily consisting of albumin but also including globulin and fibrinogen, four times greater than that of the ISF. The reason for this higher concentration of protein is that these solutes (proteins) have a molecular weight that exceeds 69 000 daltons, and this makes them too large to pass through the walls of the blood vessels. Because of the difference in this concentration of plasma proteins (also known as **colloids**), fluid flows from the area of low protein concentration in the interstitial compartment to the area of high concentration inside the blood vessel to try to create an **isotonic** environment. (*Isotonic* means an equal concentration of solutes.) The protein in the blood vessels therefore exerts a constant **osmotic pressure** that prevents the leakage of too much plasma through the capillaries into the tissues. This pressure is called **colloid oncotic pressure (COP),** and normally it is 24 mm Hg. The opposing pressure, that exerted by the ISF, is called **hydrostatic pressure (HP),** and normally it is 17 mm Hg, which, of course, is less than the COP. The phenomenon of COP is illustrated in Figure 26-2.

TABLE 26-1
FLUID LOCATION: DESCRIPTIVE TERMS AND ACTUAL VOLUMES

Name	Location	Actual Volumes
		(In a 70-kg man with a total body water content of 60% of his total body weight)
IF THE POINT OF REFERENCE IS THE CELLS, THEN THESE TERMS ARE USED:		
Intracellular fluid (ICF)	Inside of cells	28 000 mL
Extracellular fluid (ECF)	Outside of cells	14 000 mL (composed of both intravascular plasma and ISF)
IF THE POINT OF REFERENCE IS THE BLOOD VESSELS, THEN THESE TERMS ARE USED:		
Intravascular fluid or plasma volume (PV)	In blood vessels	3500 mL
Extravascular fluid (EVF)	Out of blood vessels	38 500 mL
IF THE POINT OF REFERENCE IS THE TISSUES, THEN THESE TERMS ARE USED:		
Interstitial fluid (ISF)	In the spaces between cells, tissues, and organs but not in the plasma or the cells	10 500 mL

TABLE 26-2
TYPES OF DEHYDRATION

Type of Dehydration	Characteristics
Hypertonic	Caused when water loss is greater than sodium loss, resulting in a concentration of solutes outside the cells and causing the fluid inside the cells to move to the extracellular space, thus dehydrating the cells. *Example:* Elevated temperature resulting in perspiration.
Hypotonic	Caused when sodium loss is greater than water loss, resulting in higher concentrations of solute inside the cells, thus pulling fluid from outside the cells (plasma and interstitial spaces) into the cells. *Examples:* Renal insufficiency and inadequate aldosterone secretion.
Isotonic	Caused by a loss of sodium and water from the body, resulting in a decrease in the volume of ECF. *Examples:* Diarrhea and vomiting.

Osmotic pressure can also be measured in terms of osmolality or osmolarity. *Osmolality* is the osmole concentration of dissolved substances in a solution, expressed in millimoles of solute particles, such as sodium or glucose, per kilogram of solvent, such as water (mmol/kg). *Osmolarity* is likewise an osmole concentration but expressed in millimoles of solute particles per litre of solvent (mmol/L) instead. Both concentration measures are essentially the same, but osmolality is thermodynamically more precise than omolarity because the latter measures the solvent in terms of volume, which may vary with temperature shifts. Changes in both osmolality and osmolarity values can influence the movement of solute or solvent particles across a semi-permeable membrane.

The regulation of the volume and composition of body water is essential for life because it is the medium in which all metabolic reactions occur. The body keeps the volume and composition remarkably constant by maintaining a balance between intake and excretion. The amount of water gained each day is kept equal to the amount of water lost. When for some reason the body cannot maintain this equilibrium, therapy with various agents becomes necessary. If the amount of water gained exceeds the amount of water lost, a water excess or overhydration occurs. This is referred to as **edema.** If the quantity of water lost exceeds that gained, a water deficit,

TABLE 26-3
CONDITIONS LEADING TO FLUID LOSS AND ASSOCIATED SYMPTOMS*

Condition	Associated Symptoms
Bleeding	Tachycardia and hypotension
Bowel obstruction	Reduced perspiration and mucous secretions
Diarrhea	Reduced urine output (oliguria)
Fever	Dry skin and mucous membranes
Vomiting	Reduced lacrimal (tears) and salivary secretions

*Note: There may be overlap involving more than one of the symptoms depending on the client's specific condition.

or **dehydration,** occurs. It has been estimated that death usually occurs when 20 to 25 percent of the TBW is lost.

Dehydration leads to a disturbance in the balance between the amount of fluid in the extracellular compartment and that in the intracellular compartment. In the initial stages of dehydration, water is lost first from the extracellular compartments. The nature of further fluid losses, COP changes, or both depends on the type of clinical dehydration (see Table 26-2). Clinical conditions that can result in dehydration and fluid loss, as well as the symptoms of dehydration and fluid loss, are listed in Table 26-3.

TABLE 26-4

CRYSTALLOIDS

Product	Composition (mmol/L)						Volume (mL)	Cost*
	Na	Cl	K	Ca	Mg	Lactate		
NS	154	154	0	0	0	0	1000	1
Hypertonic saline	513	513	0	0	0	0	500	1
Lactated Ringer's	130	109	4	3	0	28	1000	2.5×
D5W	0	0	1	0	0	0	1000	2×
Plasma-Lyte	140	103	10	5	3	8	1000	5×

*Relative cost; example: D5W is two times the cost of hypertonic saline.
Na, Sodium; *Cl,* chloride; *K,* potassium; *Ca,* calcium; *Mg,* magnesium; *NS,* normal saline; *D5W,* 5 percent dextrose in water.

Three categories of agents can be used to replace lost fluid: crystalloids, colloids, and blood products. The clinical situation dictates which category is most appropriate.

CRYSTALLOIDS

Crystalloids are fluids that supply water and sodium to maintain the osmotic gradient between the extravascular and intravascular compartments. Their PV-expanding capacity is related to the sodium concentration. The different crystalloids are listed in Table 26-4.

Mechanism of Action and Drug Effects

As previously mentioned, crystalloids supply sodium and water to maintain the osmotic gradient between the fluid outside the blood vessels (EVF) and the fluid inside the blood vessels (IVF). This capacity to expand the PV is related to the sodium content. Therefore hypertonic saline (3 percent sodium chloride) is more efficient than normal saline (NS) (0.9 percent sodium chloride) for expanding the PV.

Crystalloid solutions contain fluids and electrolytes that are normally found in the body. They do not contain proteins (colloids), which are necessary to maintain the COP and prevent water from leaving the plasma compartment. In fact, the administration of large quantities of crystalloid solutions for fluid resuscitation decreases the COP. Crystalloids are also distributed faster than colloids into the interstitial and intracellular compartments, which makes them better for treating dehydration than for expanding the PV, such as is needed in hypovolemic shock. Crystalloids cannot expand the PV as well as colloids and require much larger initial quantities.

Indications

Crystalloid solutions are most commonly used as maintenance fluids. They are used to replace fluids when there are body fluid deficits, to manage specific fluid and electrolyte disturbances, and to compensate for insensible fluid losses. *Insensible* fluid loss, so called because people are usually unaware of it, is fluid lost through evaporation from the skin and the respiratory tract. Crystalloids also promote urinary flow. They are much less expensive than colloids and blood products. In addition, there is no risk of viral transmission or anaphylaxis and no alteration in the coagulation profile associated with their use.

The choice whether to use a crystalloid or colloid depends on the severity of the condition. Following are the common indications for either crystalloid or colloid replacement therapy:
• Acute liver failure
• Acute nephrosis
• Adult respiratory distress syndrome
• Burns
• Cardiopulmonary bypass
• Hypoproteinemia
• Reduction of the risk of deep vein thrombosis (DVT)
• Renal dialysis
• Shock

Contraindications

Contraindications to the use of crystalloids include known drug allergy to a specific product, hypervolemia, and may include severe electrolyte disturbance.

Side Effects and Adverse Effects

Crystalloids are a safe and effective means of replacing needed fluid. They do, however, have some unwanted effects. Because they contain no large particles such as proteins, they do not stay within the blood vessels and can leak out of the plasma into the tissues and cells. This may result in edema anywhere in the body. Peripheral edema and pulmonary edema are two common examples. Crystalloids also dilute the proteins that are in the plasma, further reducing the COP. Because crystalloids cannot carry oxygen as the blood products do, their use may result in decreased oxygen tension. Typically, large volumes (litres of fluid) are required for them to be effective. As a result, large or prolonged infusions may worsen tissue acidosis or adversely affect central nervous system (CNS) function in clients suffering from hepatic insufficiency, renal failure, or hypovolemic shock. Another disadvantage of crystalloids is that their effects are transient (short lived).

Interactions

Interactions with crystalloid solutions are rare because they are similar if not identical to normal physiological substances. Certain electrolytes contained in lactated Ringer's solution may interact with other electrolytes, forming a complex that results in the formation of a precipitate. However, this would be an incompatibility rather than a true interaction.

TABLE 26-5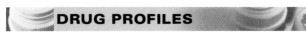
CRYSTALLOIDS AND COLLOIDS: DOSING GUIDELINES

	Crystalloids and Colloids			
	0.9% NS	3% NS	5% Colloid*	25% Colloid†
To raise plasma volume by 1 L, administer:				
	5–6 L	1.5–2 L	1 L	0.5 L
Fluid compartment distributed to:				
Plasma	25%	25%	100%	200%–300%
Interstitial space	75%	75%	0	Decreased fluid levels
Intracellular space	0	0	0	Decreased fluid levels

*Iso-oncotic solutions such as 5% albumin, dextran 70, and hetastarch.
†Hyperoncotic solutions such as 25% albumin.
NS, Normal saline.

Dosages

For the recommended dosages of crystalloids, see Table 26-5.

DRUG PROFILES

The most commonly used crystalloid solutions are NS (0.9 percent sodium chloride) and lactated Ringer's solution. The available crystalloid solutions and their compositions are summarized in Table 26-4.

sodium chloride

Sodium chloride (salt, NaCl) is available in several concentrations, the most common being 0.9 percent. This is the normal concentration of sodium chloride, and for this reason it is referred to as *normal saline* (NS). Other commonly used concentrations are 0.45 percent (half-NS) and 3 percent (hypertonic saline). These solutions have different indications, and they are used in different situations depending on how urgently fluid volume restoration is needed and/or the extent of the sodium loss.

Sodium chloride is a physiological fluid that is present throughout the body. For this reason there are no hypersensitivity reactions to it. It is safe to administer it during any stage of pregnancy, but it is contraindicated in clients with conditions in which the administration of sodium and chloride would be detrimental. Hypertonic saline injections (3 percent and 5 percent) are contraindicated in the presence of increased, normal, or only slightly decreased serum electrolyte concentrations. Sodium chloride is available as 0.45 percent, 0.9 percent, 3 percent, and 5 percent solutions.

PHARMACODYNAMICS

Plasma Volume Expansion	Colloid Oncotic Pressure	Duration of Expansion
60–70 mL*	30 mm Hg	Few hours

*500 mL of NS will expand the plasma volume by 60 to 70 mL.

The dose of sodium chloride administered depends on the clinical situation. The percentages of crystalloid or colloid needed to expand the PV by 1 L, or 1000 mL, are given in Table 26-5, and this can be used as a general guide to dosing.

TABLE 26-6
COMMONLY USED COLLOIDS

	Composition (mmol/L)		
Product	Na	Cl	Volume (mL)
Dextran 70*	154	154	500
Dextran 40*	154	154	500
Hetastarch	154	154	500
5% Albumin	145	145	500
25% Albumin	145	145	100

*Dextran is available in NaCl, which has 154 mmol/L of both Na and Cl. It is also available in 5% dextrose in water (D5W), which contains no Na or Cl.
Na, Sodium; *Cl,* chloride.

COLLOIDS

Colloids are substances that increase the COP and effectively move fluid from the interstitial compartment to the plasma compartment by pulling the fluid into the blood vessels. Normally this task is performed by the three blood proteins: albumin, globulin, and fibrinogen. However, for them to be effective, the total protein level must be in the range of 74 g/L. If this level drops below 53 g/L, the COP then becomes less than the HP and fluid shifts into the tissues. When this happens, colloid replacement therapy is required to reverse this process by increasing the COP. The COP decreases with age and also with hypotension and malnutrition. The commonly used colloids are listed in Table 26-6.

Mechanism of Action and Drug Effects

The mechanism of action of colloids is related to their ability to increase the COP. As previously explained, because the colloids cannot pass into the extravascular space, there is ordinarily a higher concentration of solutes (solid particles) inside the blood vessels (intravascular space) than outside the blood vessels. Fluid thus moves toward this hypertonic area in an attempt to make it isotonic. The result is that fluid is pulled from the extravascular space to the intravascular space, thereby increasing the blood volume. Because colloids increase the blood volume, they are sometimes called *plasma expanders.* They also make up part of the total PV.

Colloids increase the COP and move fluid from outside the blood vessels to inside the blood vessels. They can maintain the COP for several hours. They are naturally occurring products and consist of proteins (albumin), carbohydrates (dextrans or starches), and animal collagen (gelatin). Usually they contain a combination of both small and large particles. The small particles are eliminated quickly and promote diuresis and perfusion of the kidneys; the larger particles maintain the PV. Albumin is the one exception in that it contains particles that are all the same size.

Indications

Colloids are used to treat a wide variety of conditions (see list on p. 440). Clinically colloids are superior to crystalloids in their ability to expand the PV. However, crystalloids are less expensive and are less likely to promote bleeding. On the other hand, crystalloids are more likely to cause edema because of the larger volumes needed to achieve the desired clinical effect.

Contraindications

Contraindications to the use of colloids include known drug allergy to a specific product, hypervolemia, and may include severe electrolyte disturbance.

Side Effects and Adverse Effects

Colloids are relatively safe agents, although there are some disadvantages to their use. They can alter the coagulation system, resulting in impaired coagulation and possibly bleeding. They have no oxygen-carrying ability and contain no clotting factors. They may also dilute the plasma protein concentration, which may impair the function of platelets. Rarely, dextran therapy precipitates anaphylaxis or renal failure. All of these undesirable effects should be closely monitored for.

Interactions

Because colloid solutions are so compatible with drugs, they are sometimes used as the medium for delivering them. The drug propofol is such an example. It is delivered in a 10 percent lipid emulsion.

Dosages

For the recommended dosages of colloids, see Table 26-5. See Appendix B for some of the common brands available in Canada.

DRUG PROFILES

The specific colloid used for replacement therapy varies from institution to institution. The three most commonly used are dextran 40, hetastarch, and 5 percent albumin. They are all quick in onset and have a long duration of action. They are metabolized in the liver and excreted by the kidneys, with albumin the one

exception. It is metabolized by the reticulo-endothelial system and excreted by the kidneys and the intestines.

albumin

Albumin is a natural protein that is normally produced by the liver. It is responsible for generating about 70 percent of the COP. Human albumin is a sterile solution of serum albumin prepared from pooled venous plasma obtained from healthy human donors. It is pasteurized (heated at 60°C for 10 hours) to destroy any contaminants.

Albumin is contraindicated in clients with a known hypersensitivity to it and in those with heart failure, chronic anemia, or renal insufficiency. Albumin is available only in parenteral form in concentrations of 5 percent and 25 percent. Pregnancy category C. See Table 26-5 for the dosing guidelines.

PHARMACOKINETICS

Half-Life	Onset	Peak	Duration
16 hr	<1 min	Unknown	<24 hr

dextran

Dextran is a solution of glucose. It is available in two concentrations, dextran 40 and the more concentrated dextran 70, and it has a molecular weight similar to that of albumin. Dextran 40 is the more commonly used of the two and is a low-molecular-weight polymer of glucose. It is a derivative of sugar that has actions similar to those of human albumin in that it expands the PV by drawing fluid from the interstitial space to the intravascular space.

Dextran is contraindicated in clients with hypersensitivity to it and in those with heart failure, renal insufficiency, and extreme dehydration. It is available only in parenteral form in either a 5-percent dextrose solution or a 0.9-percent sodium chloride solution. Pregnancy category C. See Table 26-5 for the dosing guidelines.

PHARMACOKINETICS

Half-Life	Onset	Peak	Duration
2–6 hr (D-40)	<5 min	Unknown	4–6 hr
12 hr (D-70)	1 hr	Unknown	12 hr

hetastarch

Hetastarch is a synthetic colloid derived from cornstarch. Its molecular weight is similar to that of albumin, and the colloidal properties of the 6-percent hetastarch solution resemble those of human albumin and dextran. It is similar to dextran in that it is a synthetic colloid and has no protein-binding properties. Hetastarch is contraindicated in clients who have shown a hypersensitivity to hydroxyethyl starch and in those with severe bleeding disorders, heart failure, or renal insufficiency. It is not used for treatment of lactic acidosis. Hetastarch is available only in parenteral form as a 6 percent concentration in a 0.9-percent sodium chloride solution. Pregnancy category C. See Table 26-5 for dosing guidelines.

PHARMACOKINETICS

Half-Life	Onset	Peak	Duration
17–48 days	<1 min	Unknown	24–36 hr

BLOOD PRODUCTS

Blood products are also known as *oxygen-carrying resuscitation fluids*. They can be thought of as biological drugs and are the only class of fluids that are able to carry oxygen because they are the only class of fluids that contains hemoglobin. They not only can increase the PV but also can improve tissue oxygenation. They are also the most expensive and least available of the three types of fluids (crystalloids, colloids, and blood products) because they are natural products and require human donors. The available blood products are listed in Table 26-7. Their use is called for when more than 25 percent of blood volume is lost.

Mechanism of Action and Drug Effects

The mechanism of action of blood products is related to their ability to increase the COP, and hence the PV. They do so in the same manner as colloids and crystalloids, by pulling fluid from the extravascular space to the intravascular space. Because of this they are also considered plasma expanders. Red blood cell (RBC) products also have the ability to carry oxygen. They can maintain the COP for several hours to days, and because they come from human donors they have all the effects that human blood products have. They are administered when a person's body is deficient in these products.

Indications

Blood products are used to treat a wide variety of clinical conditions, and the blood product used depends on the specific indication. The available blood products

TABLE 26-7
BLOOD PRODUCTS

Product	Dosage	Cost*
Cryoprecipitate		1
FFP		1.7×
PRBCs	1 unit	2.2×
PPF		1
Whole blood		3.3×

*Using the cost of cryoprecipitate as the means of comparison.
FFP, Fresh frozen plasma; *PRBCs,* packed red blood cells; *PPF,* plasma protein fractions.

TABLE 26-8
BLOOD PRODUCTS: INDICATIONS

Blood Product	Indication
Cryoprecipitate and PPF	To manage acute bleeding (>50% blood loss slowly or 20% acutely)
FFP	To increase clotting factor levels in clients with a demonstrated deficiency
PRBCs	To increase oxygen-carrying capacity in clients with anemia, in clients with substantial hemoglobin deficits, and in clients who have lost >25% of their total blood volume
Whole blood	Same as for PRBCs

PPF, Plasma protein fraction; *FFP,* fresh frozen plasma; *PRBCs,* packed red blood cells.

and specific conditions they are used to treat are listed in Table 26-8.

Contraindications

There are no absolute contraindications to the use of blood products. However, because they carry a remote risk of transfer of infectious disease, their use should be based on careful clinical evaluation of the client's condition.

Side Effects and Adverse Effects

Blood products can produce undesirable effects, some potentially serious. Because these products come from other humans, they can be incompatible with the recipient's immune system. These incompatibilities are tested for before the administration of the particular blood product by determining the respective blood types of the donor and recipient and by doing cross-matching tests. This helps reduce the likelihood of the recipient rejecting the blood products, which would in turn precipitate transfusion reactions and anaphylaxis. These products can also transmit pathogens such as hepatitis and HIV from the donor to the recipient. Various preparation techniques are now used to reduce this risk of pathogen transmission, resulting in a drastic reduction in the incidence of such problems. More recently the Centers for Disease Control is studying the possible transmission of the West Nile virus through blood transfusions. Another virus that has a remote possibility of transmission via blood products is Creutzfeldt-Jakob disease (better known as *Mad Cow Disease*).

Interactions

As with crystalloids and colloids, blood products are similar if not identical to normal physiological substances; therefore they interact with few substances. Calcium and drugs such as acetylsalicylic acid that normally affect coagulation may interact with these substances when infused in the body in much the same way they interact with the body's own blood products.

Dosages

For the dosage guidelines pertaining to blood products, see Table 26-9.

TABLE 26-9
SUGGESTED GUIDELINES FOR BLOOD PRODUCTS: MANAGEMENT OF BLEEDING

Amount of Blood Loss	Fluid of Choice
≤20% (slow loss)	Crystalloids
20%–50% (slow loss)	Non-protein plasma expanders (dextran and hetastarch)
>50% (slow loss) or 20% (acutely)	Whole blood or PPF and FFP
≥80% lost	As above, but for every 5 units of blood given, administer 1–2 units of FFP and 1–2 units of platelets to prevent the hemodilution of clotting factors and bleeding

PPF, Plasma protein fraction; *FFP,* fresh frozen plasma.

DRUG PROFILES

Whole blood and PRBCs are currently the most commonly used oxygen-carrying resuscitation fluids. They should be used in clients who have lost more than 25 percent of their total blood volume. All of the blood products are derived from pooled human blood donors. For this reason they can carry oxygen, increase the PV, and improve tissue oxygenation.

PLASMA PROTEIN FRACTION

Plasma protein fraction (PPF) is obtained using a process similar to the one used to obtain albumin. It involves the fractionation of human plasma with ethanol and its pasteurization at 60°C for 10 hours. More than 83 percent of PPF is albumin and more than 1 percent is gamma-globulin. PPF and albumin are similar in that both have similar colloidal properties. The primary advantages to the use of PPF over albumin are that it is simpler to manufacture and greater amounts of protein per unit of plasma are yielded. The disadvantage to its use is that it is more antigenic than albumin. The suggested guidelines are given in Table 26-9.

FRESH FROZEN PLASMA

Fresh frozen plasma (FFP) is obtained by centrifuging whole blood and thereby removing the cellular elements. The resulting plasma is then frozen at −18°C. FFP is not recommended for routine fluid resuscitation, but it may be used as an adjunct to massive blood transfusion in the treatment of clients with underlying coagulation disorders. The plasma-expanding capability of FFP is similar to that of dextran but slightly less than that of hetastarch. The disadvantage to FFP use is that it can transmit pathogens. The suggested guidelines are given in Table 26-9.

PACKED RED BLOOD CELLS

Packed red blood cells (PRBCs) are obtained by centrifuging whole blood to separate red blood cells from plasma and the other cellular elements. PRBCs have better oxygen-carrying capacity than that of the other blood products, and they are less likely to cause cardiac fluid overload. They are small, compact oxygen carriers. However, they have a poor shelf life, their availability fluctuates, they can transmit viruses, they can cause allergic reactions, they can precipitate bleeding abnormalities, and they are expensive. The suggested guidelines are given in Table 26-9.

WHOLE BLOOD

Whole blood is a complete and physiological volume expander. One unit provides hemoglobin, protein, and water that not only restores lost oxygen-carrying capacity but also expands the PV. The advantages and disadvantages of whole blood transfusion are the same as those associated with PRBC use. The suggested guidelines are given in Table 26-9.

PHYSIOLOGY OF ELECTROLYTE BALANCE

The chemical composition of the fluid compartments varies from compartment to compartment. The principal electrolytes in the ECF are sodium cations (Na^+) and chloride anions (Cl^-); the major electrolyte of the ICF is the potassium cation (K^+). A cation is a positively charged ion, or atomic-level particle; an anion is a negatively charged ion. Other important electrolytes are calcium, magnesium, and phosphorus. These different chemical compositions are vital to the normal function of all systems in the body, and they are controlled by the renin–angiotensin–aldosterone system, antidiuretic hormone (ADH) system, and sympathetic nervous system (SNS). When these compositions are imbalanced, adverse consequences occur.

POTASSIUM

Potassium is the most abundant cationic (positively charged) electrolyte inside cells (the intracellular space), where the normal concentration is approximately 150 mmol/L. Approximately 95 percent of the potassium in the body is intracellular. In contrast, the potassium content outside the cells in the plasma ranges from 3.5 to 5.0 mmol/L. These plasma levels are critical to normal body function and are maintained by the adrenal gland hormone aldosterone.

Potassium is obtained from a variety of foods, the most common being fruit and juices, fish, vegetables, poultry, meats, and dairy products. It has been estimated that for normal body functions to be maintained, a person must consume 5 to 10 mmol of potassium per day. Fortunately the average adult daily diet usually provides 40 to 80 mmol of potassium, which is well above the required daily amount. Excess dietary potassium is usually excreted by the kidneys in the urine. However, if the kidneys lose their ability to filter and secrete waste products, potassium can accumulate, leading to toxic levels, and these in turn can precipitate ventricular fibrillation and cardiac arrest. Hyperaldosteronism and potassium-sparing diuretics can alter normal potassium balance as well. *Hyperkalemia* is the term for an excessive serum potassium level, and it is defined as a serum potassium level exceeding 5 mmol/L. There are several causes of hyperkalemia. One, renal failure, was just mentioned. Others are as follows:

- Angiotensin converting enzyme (ACE) inhibitors
- Burns
- Excessive loss from cells
- Infections
- Metabolic acidosis
- Potassium supplements
- Potassium-sparing diuretics
- Trauma

The opposite of hyperkalemia is **hypokalemia,** or a deficiency of potassium. This condition is more a result of excessive potassium loss than of poor dietary intake.

Hypokalemia can be caused by a multitude of clinical conditions, including

- Alkalosis
- An increased secretion of mineralocorticoids (hormones of the adrenal cortex)
- Burns*
- Corticosteroids
- Crash diets
- Diarrhea
- Hyperaldosteronism
- Ketoacidosis
- Large amounts of licorice
- Loop diuretics
- Malabsorption
- Prolonged laxative misuse
- Thiazide diuretics
- Thiazide-like diuretics
- Vomiting

Too little serum potassium can also greatly increase the toxicity associated with digitalis preparations, and this can precipitate serious ventricular dysrhythmias.

The early detection of hypokalemia is important in the prevention of serious, life-threatening consequences. The key to early detection is recognizing its early symptoms, which are generally mild and can easily go undetected. Both the early (mild) symptoms and late (severe) symptoms of hypokalemia are listed in Box 26-1. The treatment of hypokalemia involves both identifying and treating the cause and restoring the serum potassium levels to normal (>3.5 mmol/L). The consumption of potassium-rich foods can usually correct mild hypokalemia, but clinically significant hypokalemia requires the oral or parenteral administration of a potassium supplement, which usually contains potassium chloride.

Mechanism of Action and Drug Effects

Potassium's importance as the primarily intracellular electrolyte is highlighted by the enormous number of life-sustaining reactions and everyday physiological functions that require it, functions that we take for granted. Muscle contraction, the transmission of nerve impulses, and the regulation of heartbeats (the pacemaker function of the heart) are just a few functions that would not be possible without potassium.

Potassium is also essential for the maintenance of acid–base balance, isotonicity, and the electrodynamic characteristics of the cell. It plays a role in many enzymatic reactions, and it is an essential component of gastric secretion, renal function, tissue synthesis, and carbohydrate metabolism.

Indications

Potassium replacement therapy is called for in the treatment or prevention of potassium depletion in clients whenever dietary measures prove inadequate. The potassium salt used for this purpose is potassium chloride. The chloride is required to correct the hypochloremia (low chloride) that commonly accompanies potassium deficiency.

Other therapeutic effects of potassium are related to its role in the contraction of muscles and the maintenance of the electrical characteristics of cells. Potassium salts may be used to stop irregular heartbeats (dysrhythmias) and to manage the tachyarrhythmias that can occur after cardiac surgery. Potassium may also be used to treat thallium poisoning and to help increase muscular strength in some clients with myasthenia gravis.

Contraindications

The only usual contraindications to the use of potassium replacement products are known drug allergy to a specific product and hyperkalemia.

Side Effects and Adverse Effects

The adverse effects of potassium therapy are primarily limited to the gastrointestinal (GI) tract and occur with the oral administration of potassium preparations. These GI effects include diarrhea, nausea, and vomiting. More significant ones include GI bleeding and ulceration. The parenteral administration of potassium usually produces pain at the injection site. Cases of phlebitis have been associated with intravenous (IV) administration, and the excessive administration of potassium salts can lead to hyperkalemia and toxic effects.

Toxicity and Management of Overdose

The toxic effects of potassium are the result of hyperkalemia. Symptoms include nausea, vomiting, diarrhea, abdominal cramps, muscle weakness, paraesthesia, paralysis, convulsions, cardiac rhythm irregularities that can result in ventricular fibrillation, and cardiac arrest. The treatment instituted depends on the degree of the hyperkalemia and ranges from regimens for reversing life-threatening problems to simple dietary restrictions. In the event of severe hyperkalemia, the intravenous administration of 10 percent glucose with insulin is implemented. Acidosis is corrected with sodium bicarbonate. Calcium gluconate is

BOX   26-1

Symptoms of Hypokalemia

Early
Anorexia
Hypotension
Lethargy
Mental confusion
Muscle weakness
Nausea

Late
Cardiac dysrhythmias
Neuropathy
Paralytic ileus
Secondary alkalosis

---

*Burn clients can exhibit either hyperkalemia or hypokalemia.

also administered under continuous ECG monitoring. This should be followed by the cation exchange resin, sodium polystyrene sulphonate (e.g., Kayexalate), by retention enema, or by hemodialysis to eliminate the extra potassium from the body. Less critical levels can be reduced with ion-exchange resins and by means of dietary restrictions.

Interactions

The use of potassium-sparing diuretics and ACE inhibitors can produce a hyperkalemic state. The use of diuretics, amphotericin B, and mineralosteroids can produce a hypokalemic state.

Dosages

Fluid and electrolyte therapy involves replacing any losses leading to deficits and/or maintaining levels for specific client requirements. Accordingly, specific dosage amounts of fluids or electrolytes depend on several clinical factors:

- Specific client losses
- Efficacy of client physiological systems involved in fluid and electrolyte metabolism, especially adrenal, cardiovascular, and kidney functions
- Current drug therapy for pathological conditions that complicate the amount and duration of replacement
- Selection of oral or parenteral replacement formulations
  Suggested dosage guidelines with subsequent adjustments for potassium are 10 to 20 mmol administered orally several times a day or parenteral administration of 30 to 60 mmol every 24 hours.

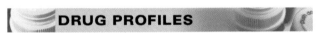

DRUG PROFILES

POTASSIUM SUPPLEMENTS

Potassium supplements are administered to prevent or treat potassium depletion. The acetate, bicarbonate, chloride, citrate, and gluconate salts of potassium are available for oral (PO) administration. The parenteral salt forms of potassium for intravenous administration are acetate, chloride, and phosphate.

The dosage of potassium supplements is usually expressed in millimoles of potassium and depends on the requirements of the individual client. The different salt forms of potassium deliver varying amounts of potassium (see Table 26-10).

Potassium is contraindicated in clients with severe renal disease, severe hemolytic disease, or Addison's disease and in those suffering from hyperkalemia, acute

TABLE 26-10
POTASSIUM: VARIOUS SALT FORMS

Salt Form	Amount (g) Needed to Yield 40 mmol of Potassium
Acetate	3.9
Chloride	3.0
Citrate	4.3
Dibasic phosphate	3.5
Gluconate	9.4
Monobasic phosphate	5.4

dehydration, or extensive tissue breakdown stemming from multiple traumas. Potassium is available in many different oral and intravenous formulations. It is available in oral form as a tablet and powder for solution, an extended-release capsule and tablet, and an elixir and solution. It is also available as an injection for intravenous use. Potassium should never be administered by intravenous push. Pregnancy category A.

PHARMACOKINETICS

Half-Life	Onset	Peak	Duration
IV: Variable	IV: Immediate	IV: Rapid	IV: Variable
PO: Variable	PO: 30 min	PO: 30 min	PO: Variable

sodium polystyrene sulphonate (potassium exchange resin)

Sodium polystyrene sulphonate is known as a *cation exchange resin* and is used to treat hyperkalemia. For this purpose it is usually administered orally, via nasogastric tube, or as an enema. It has no listed contraindications per se, but it can cause disturbances in electrolytes other than potassium, such as calcium and magnesium. For this reason clients' electrolytes should be closely monitored during treatment with SPS. It is typically dosed in multiples of 15 to 30 g until the desired effect on serum potassium is achieved. It is available in a powder for reconstitution. Pregnancy category C.

SODIUM

Sodium is the counterpart to potassium: potassium is the principal cation (positively charged substance) inside cells, and sodium is the principal cation outside cells. The normal concentration of sodium outside cells is 135 to 145 mmol/L, and it is maintained through the dietary intake of sodium in the form of sodium chloride, which is obtained directly from salt added to food; from fish, seafood, and meats; and from foods flavoured, seasoned, or preserved with salt. Inadequate dietary sodium is unlikely; most North Americans consume many times the required amount of sodium.

Hyponatremia is the condition of sodium loss or deficiency and occurs when the serum levels decrease below 135 mmol/L. It is manifested by lethargy, hypotension, stomach cramps, vomiting, diarrhea, and seizures. Some of the same conditions that cause hypokalemia can also cause hyponatremia, and these are listed on p. 445. Other causes of hyponatremia are excessive perspiration, occurring during hot weather or physical work; prolonged diarrhea or vomiting, especially in young children; renal disorders; and adrenocortical impairment.

Hypernatremia is the condition of sodium excess and occurs when the serum levels of sodium exceed 145 mmol/L. Some of the symptoms are water retention (edema) and hypertension. The most common cause is poor renal excretion stemming from kidney malfunction. Inadequate water consumption and dehydration are other causes. Symptoms of hypernatremia include red, flushed skin; dry, sticky mucous membranes; increased thirst; temperature elevation; and decreased or absent urination.

Mechanism of Action and Drug Effects

As one of the body's electrolytes, sodium performs many physiological roles necessary for the normal function of the body. It is the major cation in ECF and is principally involved in the control of water distribution, fluid and electrolyte balance, and osmotic pressure of body fluids. Sodium also participates along with both chloride and bicarbonate in the regulation of acid–base balance. Chloride, the major extracellular anion (negatively charged substance), closely complements the physiological action of sodium. Sodium is also capable of causing diuresis.

Indications

Sodium is primarily administered in the treatment or prevention of sodium depletion when dietary measures have proved inadequate. Sodium chloride is the primary salt used for this purpose. Mild hyponatremia is usually treated with the oral administration of sodium chloride tablets and/or fluid restriction. Pronounced sodium depletion is treated with NS or lactated Ringer's solution administered intravenously. These agents are discussed earlier in this chapter.

Contraindications

The only usual contraindications to the use of sodium replacement products are known drug allergy to a specific product and hypernatremia.

Side Effects and Adverse Effects

The oral administration of sodium chloride can cause gastric upset consisting of nausea, vomiting, and cramps. Venous phlebitis can be a consequence of its parenteral administration.

Toxicity and Management of Overdose

Hypernatremia leads to hypertension, edema, thirst, tachycardia, weakness, convulsions, and possibly coma. Treatment consists of increased fluid intake and dietary restrictions. The intravenous administration of dextrose solution may be required in more serious cases to help promote renal excretion.

Interactions

Sodium is not known to interact significantly with any drugs.

Dosages

Fluid and electrolyte therapy involves replacing any deficit losses and/or maintaining levels for specific client requirements. Accordingly, specific dosage amounts of fluids or electrolytes depend on several clinical factors:
- Specific client losses
- Efficacy of client physiological systems involved in fluid and electrolyte metabolism, especially adrenal, cardiovascular, and kidney functions
- Current drug therapy for pathological conditions that complicate the amount and duration of replacement
- Selection of oral or parenteral replacement formulations

Suggested dosage guidelines with subsequent adjustments for sodium chloride are 1 to 2 g administered orally several times a day or parenteral administration of 1 L of sodium chloride injection (NS).

DRUG PROFILES

sodium chloride

Sodium chloride is primarily used as a replacement electrolyte for either the prevention or treatment of sodium loss. It is also used as a diluent for the infusion of compatible drugs and in the assessment of kidney function after a fluid challenge. Sodium chloride is contraindicated in clients who are hypersensitive to it. It is available in many intravenous preparations. Pregnancy category C.

PHARMACOKINETICS

Half-Life	Onset	Peak	Duration
Unknown	Immediate	Rapid	Variable

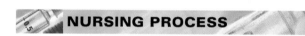

NURSING PROCESS

■ Assessment

Parenterally administered hydrating solutions, such as 5 percent dextrose in water (D5W), are used mainly for the prevention of dehydration. Isotonic solutions such as NS are customarily used to augment extracellular volumes diminished as the result of blood loss, severe vomiting, or any condition that leads to a chloride loss equal to or greater than the sodium loss. NS is also used as the medium for blood transfusions because D5W results in the hemolysis of RBCs. Hypertonic solutions such as 3 percent sodium chloride are used to treat hypotonic expansion, such as that resulting from water intoxication. Plasma-Lyte 56 and Plasma-Lyte 148 are maintenance solutions used to replace electrolytes and water lost as the result of severe diarrhea or vomiting.

Although the physician prescribes the specific solution to be administered, the nurse, by monitoring and assessing the client, helps in the diagnosis of the problem and complications of the therapy and also helps determine the appropriateness of the therapy. Today many clients needing replacement therapy are in home care settings, making the nurse even more accountable and responsible for ensuring adequate assessment. Registered dieticians are generally a resource for assessing and giving suggestions for replacements.

The assessment of a client who is to receive any parenteral replacement solutions should focus on the client's medical history, including diseases and GI, renal, cardiac, or hepatic dysfunction or disorders. The nurse should question clients about prescription and over-the-counter (OTC) medications they are taking and their dietary habits. Clients' fluid volume and electrolyte status and baseline vital signs should be determined and laboratory studies performed. The skin, mucous membranes, daily weights, and intake and output measurement should also be assessed and the skin turgor noted in clients being treated for a fluid or electrolyte disorder. Pediatric and geriatric clients may be more sensitive to the effects of potassium chloride.

Before administering potassium to clients, it is important to assess the ECG for the presence of peaking T waves, depressed R waves, a prolonged Q-R interval, or a widening QRS complex, as well as the potassium levels and intake and output amounts. Contraindications to the use of potassium include renal disease, severe hemolytic disease, hyperkalemia, Addison's disease, acute dehydration, and multiple traumas that involve severe tissue breakdown. Potassium supplementation should be avoided or used with extreme caution in clients taking ACE inhibitors. Cautious use is recommended in clients suffering from cardiac disease or systemic acidosis and those taking potassium-sparing diuretics. The client's pulse rate, BP, and evidence of edema also need to be documented.

Albumin and other colloids are contraindicated in clients with heart failure or severe anemia and in those who have shown a hypersensitivity to it. Cautious use is called for in clients with decreased salt intake, decreased cardiac reserve, hepatic disease, and pregnancy, as well as in the absence of an albumin-deficient state. The hematocrit (Hct), hemoglobin (Hgb) levels, and serum protein levels should be documented. Baseline BP, pulse rate, respiratory status, and intake and output amounts should also be documented and any dyspnea or hypoxia noted.

Before administering blood or blood components, the nurse should obtain a thorough history regarding transfusions. If the client has any history of adverse reactions, this should be reported to the physician and blood bank or laboratory and the nature of these reactions documented. It is also important to assess venous access as well as to check the client's laboratory values (e.g., Hct, Hgb, white blood cells [WBCs], RBCs, clotting factors) and baseline vital signs before infusing the blood or blood product. Even the general appearance of the client and the client's mood can be a source of early evidence of adverse reactions to a transfusion or infusion of blood components.

Nursing Diagnoses

Nursing diagnoses relevant to the client who is to receive blood products, blood components, or related agents include the following:
- Risk for falls related to fluid and electrolyte imbalances.
- Risk for imbalanced fluid volume related to drug-induced fluid and electrolyte disorders.
- Deficient knowledge about treatment regimen related to lack of client education about electrolyte disturbances and influence of treatment.
- Risk for injury related to complications of the transfusion or infusion of blood products, blood components, or related agents.

Planning

Following are the goals related to the administration of fluids, electrolytes, and blood components:
- Client has minimal problems with volume overload related to the transfusion or infusion.
- Client begins minimal exercise and shows increased tolerance daily.
- Client participates in activities as he or she can tolerate them.
- Client states measures to implement to minimize self-injury related to altered blood component levels or altered fluid and electrolyte levels.
- Client states the rationale for treatment and the side effects of replacement agents.
- Client states symptoms and problems to report to the physician.

Outcome Criteria

Following are the outcome criteria for clients receiving fluids, electrolytes, or blood components:
- Client remains free of self-injury as the result of allergic reaction or adverse reactions (dizziness, volume overload, hypersensitivity) to the transfusion or infusion.
- Client regains the ability to engage in normal or near-normal exercise, showing increased tolerance daily as evidenced by walking small distances and increasing to regular supervised exercise.
- Client participates in activities according to his or her ability to tolerate them without dyspnea or chest pain.
- Client demonstrates a return to normal or near-normal values of blood components or fluid and electrolyte levels.
- Client sees the physician for follow-up as ordered to monitor laboratory values pertinent to treatment.

Implementation

Continued monitoring and reassessment of the client during therapy is crucial to ensure safe and effective treatment and to prevent the complications of overzealous treatment and/or undertreatment, which may be life threatening. Serum electrolyte levels should not exceed normal ranges (sodium, 135–145 mmol/L; chloride, 95–108 mmol/L; potassium, 3.5–5.0 mmol/L; calcium, 4.5–5.8 mmol/L; magnesium, 1.5–2.5 mmol/L) and should be watched carefully after the conclusion of treatment as well. It is important for the nurse to document all changes in the client and any changes in assessment findings. Besides monitoring the infusion rate, the appearance of the fluid or solution, and the infusion site, the nurse must also constantly watch for infiltration of the solution, thrombosis, thrombophlebitis, pain at the intravenous catheter site, pulmonary edema, fever, and air emboli.

With the administration of any fluid and electrolyte solution, a steady and even flow rate must be maintained to prevent complications. If for some reason the nurse cannot administer the solution ordered or cannot administer it in the amount or at the rate specified, this must be dealt with immediately, the situation resolved, the physician notified, an incident report filed, and the matter documented. Special prudence is required with geriatric or pediatric clients because they are more sensitive to changes in fluid and electrolyte levels.

When administering potassium replacements parenterally, the nurse should carefully monitor the dosage during infusion. When given intravenously, potassium must always be given in diluted form and administered slowly and only to clients with a documented urine output. It is generally recommended that intravenous solutions not contain more than 40 mmol/L of potassium and the rate not exceed 20 mmol/hr. When intravenous potassium chloride is ordered for a client, the nurse must remember the danger associated with potassium infusions. Potassium chloride should never be given as an intravenous bolus or given undiluted because cardiac arrest may occur. When adding potassium chloride to a litre bag of intravenous solution, the nurse must mix the bag thoroughly to prevent areas of uneven concentration. To avoid errors, many hospitals now use commercially prepared ready-to-use diluted potassium solutions; others have specific preparation guidelines. Potassium should never be administered by intravenous push. Oral preparations of potassium should be prescribed whenever possible and in conjunction with a high potassium diet so as to avoid the need for intravenous administration. Potassium chloride is the salt customarily used for intravenous infusions.

Oral forms of potassium are usually prepared in doses of 10, 20, or 40 mmol/15 mL and must be diluted in water or fruit juice to minimize GI distress or irritation. Powder or effervescent forms should be prepared according to the package guidelines. Both enteric-coated and uncoated forms can cause GI ulcers with bleeding; therefore their use should always be closely monitored. Any complaints of nausea, vomiting, GI pain, or GI bleeding should be assessed, noted, and reported to the physician immediately and all doses withheld until further orders are received.

Symptoms of hyponatremia include lethargy, hypotension, stomach cramps, vomiting, diarrhea, and seizures. Treatment with Ringer's solution or NS is usually helpful in alleviating these symptoms, but sodium can also be taken in by consuming a diet high in salt, obtained from such sources as ketchup, mustard, cured meats, cheeses, potato chips, peanut butter, popcorn, and table salt. Careful administration with constant monitoring of the intravenous solution and the rate and site of administration is recommended in any client undergoing electrolyte replacement therapy.

Intravenous infusion of albumin and other colloids should always be done slowly and cautiously and with careful monitoring to prevent fluid overload and possible heart failure, especially in clients at particular risk for heart failure. The Hct and Hgb values should also be determined in advance so that any anemia can be detected

LEGAL and ETHICAL PRINCIPLES

Infiltrating IV

Nurses often encounter an infiltrating IV in the routine care of many of their clients. Every action taken is important to the standard of care of the client and in ensuring that the nurse has acted as any prudent nurse would. The assessment and action taken by the nurse can be important for the client, as in the case of **Macon-Bibb Hosp. Authority vs. Ross** (335 S.E. 2d 633-GA). Although this is an American example, it is relevant for Canadian nurses.

Situation
Ms. Ross was brought to the emergency room of the hospital with dyspnea, bradycardia, and a BP of 250/150 mm Hg. She went into respiratory arrest at 2:55 pm; she was intubated with an endotracheal tube, and nitroprusside was administered intravenously to decrease her BP. Because of the rapid drop in BP, an intravenous administration of dopamine was started at 3:28 pm in her right wrist to increase her BP. When her BP was stable, she was transferred to the cardiac care unit at 4:30 pm. At midnight, a nurse noted that the intravenous catheter site had a "bruise bluish in colour." The next notation was at 11:00 am the following day, in which it was recorded that the client's right arm was swollen and painful with a large blistered area around the intravenous catheter site. The same notation was made at 4:00 pm. It was not until 6:50 pm that a note indicated that a physician was informed of the infiltration. As a result of the extravasation of dopamine, the client's lower right arm was permanently scarred. On a jury verdict, the court entered judgement for the client. The hospital appealed.

The court of appeals affirmed the judgement of the lower court. It was noted that, although an infiltration may result from an improper technique, it may also be due to the size of the needle, the status of the client's veins, or specific intolerance to an intravenous catheter. However, according to the expert nurse's testimony, supported by suitable references, dopamine should be infused into a "large vein," such as in the antecubital fossa, to minimize the risk of extravasation. In addition, dopamine should be monitored continuously for free flow. If extravasation of dopamine occurs, the recommended treatment of the site is infiltration with a saline solution of phentolamine within 12 hr.

The nurses were criticized for not being sufficiently knowledgeable regarding dopamine, which resulted in their failure to notify a physician of the client's impaired tissue integrity.

From McKenry, L.M., & Salerno, E. (2003). *Mosby's pharmacology in nursing—revised and updated* (21st ed.). St Louis, MO: Mosby.

and care taken not to overload the heart pump with an increased volume. Albumin and any blood products should be infused at room temperature.

The client should be carefully assessed and all data/findings documented at the beginning of the administration of a blood product, solution, or component (e.g., PPF, platelets, and FFP). The client should then be assessed and the findings documented every 15 minutes, or more frequently if needed, thereafter. At this point the product should be infused at a rate of about 20 drops/min. Vital signs should be checked and recorded every 15 minutes, or more frequently if possible. Should a reaction occur, the transfusion should be stopped immediately. The nurse should implement appropriate nursing measures, notify the physician, and document the nature of the event, the measures taken, and the client's response. The physician should be notified immediately of any restlessness, flushed skin, increased pulse and respirations, dyspnea, rash, swelling, fever and chills (a febrile reaction beginning 1 hour after the start of administration and lasting up to 10 hours), nausea, weakness, or jaundice. The expiration date of blood components should be checked to make sure they are fresh. No outdated blood or blood components should be used.

See the box below for client teaching tips for these agents.

■ Evaluation

The therapeutic response to fluid, electrolyte, and blood or blood component therapy includes normalized laboratory values for RBCs, WBCs, Hgb, Hct, sodium, potassium, and calcium. In addition, the fluid levels, volume status, and cardiac function should return to normal, and the client should be able to resume normal or near-normal activities. The client should also show an increased tolerance to activity; improved skin colour; and minimal to no dyspnea, chest pain, weakness, or fatigue. The therapeutic response to albumin therapy includes increased BP, decreased edema, and increased serum albumin levels. The evaluation process must also include monitoring for side effects and for conditions stemming from either an excess or deficit of the particular product. Any such findings should be reported to the physician and documented. Adverse reactions to albumin include distended neck veins; shortness of breath; anxiety; insomnia; expiratory rales; frothy, blood-tinged sputum; and cyanosis.

CLIENT TEACHING TIPS

The nurse should give clients the following instructions, as appropriate to their situation:

▲ Consume foods high in potassium to take in the recommended daily allowance, which is between 40 and 50 mmol for adults and 2 to 3 mmol/kg of body weight for infants. Two medium-sized bananas or an 8-oz glass of orange juice contains 45 mmol; 20 large dried apricots contain 40 mmol; and a level teaspoon of salt substitute (KCl) contains 60 mmol of potassium. If you are taking an oral potassium supplement, it will usually be increased gradually over about 1 week to make sure your potassium level doesn't go too high.

▲ Sodium may be lost as the result of major injury, vomiting, your body's inability to produce enough of certain hormones, diuretic use, tap water enemas, wound

drainage, or excessive perspiration. Follow replacement instructions carefully and as the physician prescribed.

▲ If you are taking any type of fluid or electrolyte substance, colloid, or blood component, report any unusual side effects immediately to your physician. Such complaints include chest pain, dizziness, weakness, shortness of breath, or any unusual symptom.

▲ It's important to drink enough water. Water is the medium in which all metabolic reactions occur and it is needed to control the volume and composition of body fluid, both of which are essential for life. It is especially important to make sure you drink enough water if you are older, if the weather is hot and humid, or if you are losing fluids as the result of perspiration or drainage.

POINTS to REMEMBER

▼ TBW is divided into intracellular (inside the cell) and extracellular (outside the cell) compartments. Fluid volume outside cells is either in the plasma (intravascular volume) or between the tissues, cells, or organs (ISF).

▼ COP is the concentration of colloids such as albumin and is four times greater inside blood vessels than outside them.

▼ Colloids are large protein particles that cannot leak out of the blood vessels. Because of their greater concentration inside blood vessels, fluid is pulled into the blood vessels. Examples of colloids that can be administered are albumin, hetastarch, and dextran.

▼ Crystalloids are fluids that supply water and sodium to maintain the osmotic gradient between extravascular and intravascular compartments. Their PV expanding capacity is related to the sodium concentration. These agents contain fluids and electrolytes that are normally found in the body.

▼ Blood products are also known as *oxygen-carrying resuscitation fluids.* They are the only class of fluids that are able to carry oxygen because they are the only fluids that contain hemoglobin.

▼ Blood products increase the oxygen-carrying capabilities as well as the COP.

▼ Solutions including 0.45 percent, 0.9 percent, or higher saline in water (hypertonic solutions: 3 percent and 5 percent) are used to hydrate clients and prevent dehydration. Caution: Hypertonic solutions should be given slowly (<100 mL/hr) because of the risk of hypervolemia due to overzealous replacement.

▼ Dehydration may be hypotonic, resulting from the loss of salt; hypertonic, resulting from fever with perspiration; or isotonic, resulting from diarrhea or vomiting. Each form of dehydration is treated differently.

▼ Potassium-related problems: Symptoms of hypokalemia include lethargy, weakness, fatigue, respiratory difficulty, paralysis, and even possible paralytic ileus. Caution: When replacing potassium via intravenous infusions, the nurse should never give undiluted KCl because it can result in ventricular fibrillation and cardiac arrest due to hyperkalemia. Nursing units should only use diluted potassium (e.g., 1000 mL of intravenous fluids premixed by the manufacturer of the drug and intravenous fluids). The nurse should never give undiluted KCl intravenously and never exceed recommended dosages of KCl. The usual dose per 1000 mL of intravenous fluids is 40 to 60 mmol.

▼ Hyponatremia is manifested by lethargy, hypotension, stomach cramps, vomiting, diarrhea, and possibly seizures. Hypernatremia is manifested by red, flushed skin; dry, sticky mucous membranes; increased thirst; temperature elevation; and a decrease in or absence of urination.

▼ Blood products may cause hemolysis of RBCs and therefore adverse reactions such as fever, chills, and back pain should be watched for continually. Hematuria may occur if the hemolysis reaction is present. If noted, the intravenous infusion should be discontinued, the physician should be notified immediately, and the nature of the reactions and all actions taken should be documented. Vital signs and frequent monitoring of the client before, during, and after infusions is critical to client safety. Blood products should be given only with NS 0.9 percent because D5W will cause hemolysis of the blood product.

▼ During the infusion of albumin and like products, the client should be constantly monitored for the development of increased central venous pressure, as manifested by the occurrence of distended neck veins; shortness of breath; expiratory rales; anxiety; and frothy, blood-tinged sputum.

EXAMINATION REVIEW QUESTIONS

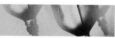

1 Which of the following statements is true about administration of blood?
   a. Intravenous infusion rates of blood may safely exceed 150–200 mL/hr in any client.
   b. When giving intravenous blood products it is crucial to *always* give it with dextrose.
   c. Most blood products contain more than 20 mmol KCl/mL and are safe.
   d. Normal saline is preferred with blood transfusions to prevent RBC hemolysis.

2 Absolute contraindications for use of KCl include which of the following?
   a. BP of 130/84, P 78
   b. Diarrhea for 5 days
   c. Extremely poor turgor
   d. Addison's disease

3 Albumin should be used cautiously in clients in which of the following situations?
   a. Normal cardiac reserve
   b. Cardiac contractility
   c. Hepatic disease
   d. Volume excess

4 KCl should not be administered to clients with which of the following potassium levels?
   a. 2
   b. 3.8
   c. 5
   d. 6.2

5 Which of the following may result when hypertonic solutions are given intravenously?
   a. Diaphoresis
   b. Hypertension
   c. Decreased turgor with pitting edema
   d. Fluid overload and possible heart failure

For answers see http://evolve.elsevier.com/Lilley/pharmacology/.

CRITICAL THINKING ACTIVITIES

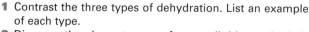

1 Contrast the three types of dehydration. List an example of each type.
2 Discuss the importance of crystalloids and their therapeutic effectiveness. Provide examples of crystalloids and the conditions for which they would be ordered.
3 Compare the use of crystalloids with that of colloids.

For answers see http://evolve.elsevier.com/Lilley/pharmacology/.

BIBLIOGRAPHY

Albanese, J., & Nutz, P. (2005). *Mosby's 2005 nursing drug cards.* St Louis, MO: Mosby.

Canadian Pharmacists Association. (2003). *Therapeutic choices* (4th ed.). Ottawa, ON: Author.

Canadian Pharmacists Association. (2005). *Compendium of pharmaceuticals and specialties. The Canadian drug reference for health professionals.* Ottawa, ON: Author. [The subscription-based e-CPS is available at http://www.pharmacists.ca.]

Cheng, A., Williams, B.A., & Sivarajan, B.V. (Eds.). *The HSC handbook of pediatrics* (10th ed.). Toronto, ON: Elsevier.

Facts and Comparisons. (2004). *Drug facts and comparisons pocket version* (9th ed.). St Louis, MO: Wolters Kluwer Health.

Health Canada. (2005). Drug product database (DPD). Retrieved August 13, 2005, from http://www.hc-sc.gc.ca/hpb/drugs-dpd/

Lehne, R.A. (2004). *Pharmacology for nursing care* (5th ed.). St Louis, MO: Saunders.

Malick, L.B. (2004). Fluid, electrolyte, and acid-base imbalances. In S.L. Lewis., M.M. Heitkemper, and S.R. Dirksen (Eds.), *Medical-surgical nursing. Assessment and management of clinical problems* (6th ed., pp. 330–338). St. Louis, MO: Mosby.

McKenry, L.M., & Salerno, E. (2003). *Mosby's pharmacology in nursing—revised and updated* (21st ed.). St Louis, MO: Mosby.

Mosby. (2005). *Mosby's drug consult 2005: The comprehensive reference for generic and brand name drugs* (15th ed.). St Louis, MO: Mosby.

Skidmore-Roth, L. (2006). *Mosby's 2006 nursing drug reference* (19th ed.). St Louis, MO: Mosby.

White, B. (2005). Clients with fluid imbalances. In J.M. Black and J.H. Hawks (Eds.), *Medical-surgical nursing. Clinical management for positive outcomes* (7th ed., pp. 205–221). St. Louis, MO: Saunders.

White, B. (2005). Clients with electrolyte imbalances. In J.M. Black and J.H. Hawks (Eds.), *Medical-surgical nursing. Clinical management for positive outcomes* (7th ed., pp. 223–245). St. Louis, MO: Saunders.

Coagulation Modifier Agents

OBJECTIVES

After reading this chapter, the successful student will be able to do the following:

1   Discuss the mechanisms of action of coagulation modifiers such as anticoagulants, antiplatelet agents, antifibrinolytics, and thrombolytics.

2   Compare the indications for and cautions and contraindications to the use of the various coagulation modifiers.

3   Discuss the administration procedures for the various coagulation modifiers.

4   Identify the drug interactions associated with the use of coagulation modifiers, specific observations related to their use, and the antidotes for an overdose.

5   Develop a nursing care plan that includes all phases of the nursing process for clients receiving anticoagulants, antiplatelet agents, antifibrinolytics, and thrombolytics.

e-LEARNING ACTIVITIES

Student CD-ROM
- Review Questions: see questions 194–208
- Animations
- Medication Administration Checklists
- IV Therapy Checklists

evolve **Web site** (http://evolve.elsevier.com/Lilley/pharmacology/)
- Online Chapter Worksheet • Frequently Asked Questions
- Learning Tips and Content Updates • WebLinks • Online Appendices and Supplements • Mosby/Saunders ePharmacology Update • Access to *Mosby's Drug Consult*

DRUG PROFILES

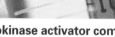

▸▸ alteplase, p. 467
   aminocaproic acid, p. 465
▸▸ acetylsalicylic acid (ASA), p. 463
▸▸ clopidogrel, p. 464
   desmopressin, p. 466

▸▸ enoxaparin, p. 460
▸▸ eptifibatide p. 464
▸▸ heparin, p. 460
   pentoxifylline, p. 464
▸▸ streptokinase, p. 468
▸▸ warfarin sodium, p. 459

▸▸ Key drug.

GLOSSARY

Anisoylated plasminogen streptokinase activator complex (APSAC)   A plasminogen–streptokinase complex that has been chemically modified by acylation, allowing a prolonged half-life.

Anticoagulant   (an' tee koe ag' yoo lənt) A substance that prevents or delays coagulation of the blood.

Antifibrinolytic   (an' tee fy' bri noe lit' ik) A drug that prevents the lysis of fibrin and in so doing promotes clot formation.

Antiplatelet drug   (an' tee plate' lət) A substance that prevents platelet plugs from forming, which can be beneficial in defending the body against heart attacks and strokes.

Antithrombin III   (an' tee throm' bin) A substance that turns off the three main activating factors: activated II (thrombin), activated X, and activated IX.

Beta-hemolytic streptococci (group A)   The pyogenic (pus-forming) streptococci of group A that cause hemolysis of red blood cells in blood agar in the laboratory setting. These organisms cause most of the acute streptococcal infections seen in human beings.

Clot specific   Refers to whether a thrombolytic agent will lyse clots only in coronary arteries or throughout the body.

Deep vein thrombosis (DVT)   (throm boe' sis) The formation of a thrombus in one of the deep veins of the

453

body. The deep veins most commonly affected are the iliac and femoral veins.

Embolus (em′ boe ləs) A blood clot that has been dislodged from the wall of a blood vessel and is travelling throughout the bloodstream. Emboli that lodge in critical blood vessels can result in ischemic injury to a vital organ (e.g., heart, lung, brain), leading to disability or death.

Fibrin (fy′ brin) A stringy, insoluble protein produced by the action of thrombin on fibrinogen during the clotting process.

Fibrinogen A plasma protein that is converted into fibrin by thrombin in the presence of calcium ions.

Fibrinolysis (fy′ bri nol′ ə sis) The continual process of fibrin decomposition produced by the actions of fibrinolysin. It is the normal mechanism for removing small fibrin clots and is stimulated by anoxia, inflammatory reactions, and other kinds of stress.

Fibrinolytic system A system undergoing fibrinolysis.

Hemorrheological drug (hee′ moe ree′ ol oj′ ik əl) A drug that alters the function of platelets without preventing them from working.

Hemostasis (hee′ moe stay′ sis) The termination of bleeding by mechanical or chemical means or by the complex coagulation process of the body, consisting of vasoconstriction, platelet aggregation, and thrombin and fibrin synthesis.

Hemostatic agent A procedure, device, or substance that arrests the flow of blood.

Plasmin (plaz′ min) The enzyme that breaks down fibrin into fibrin degradation products.

Plasminogen (plaz min′ ə jən) A plasma protein that is converted to plasmin and promotes fibrinolysis.

Pulmonary embolus (pul′ mən are ee) The blockage of a pulmonary artery by foreign matter such as fat, air, tumour, or a thrombus that usually arises from a peripheral vein.

Streptokinase (SK) (strep′ toe ki′ nase) A fibrinolytic activator that enhances the conversion of plasminogen to the fibrinolytic enzyme plasmin. It is used in the treatment of certain cases of pulmonary and coronary embolism.

Stroke Occlusion of the blood vessels of the brain by an embolus, thrombus, or cerebrovascular hemorrhage, resulting in ischemia of the brain tissue normally perfused by the damaged blood vessels.

Thromboembolic event An event in which a blood vessel is blocked by an embolus carried in the bloodstream from the site of its formation. The area supplied by an obstructed artery may tingle and become cold, numb, and cyanotic.

Thrombolytic drug (throm′ boe lit′ ik) A drug or other agent that dissolves thrombi.

Thrombus (throm′ bəs) An aggregation of platelets, fibrin, clotting factors, and the cellular elements of the blood that is attached to the interior wall of a vein or artery, sometimes occluding the lumen of the vessel.

Tissue plasminogen activator A naturally occurring plasminogen activator secreted by vascular endothelial cells (the walls of the blood vessels).

COAGULATION

The process that halts bleeding after injury to a blood vessel is called **hemostasis**. Normal hemostasis involves the complex interaction of substances that promote clot formation and substances that either inhibit coagulation or dissolve the formed clot. The drugs discussed in this chapter aid the body in achieving hemostasis, and they can be broken down into several main categories based on their actions. **Anticoagulants** inhibit the action or formation of clotting factors and thereby prevent clots from forming. **Antiplatelet drugs** prevent platelet plugs from forming by inhibiting platelet aggregation, which can be beneficial in preventing heart attacks and strokes. Other agents alter platelet function without preventing them from working. These are sometimes referred to as **hemorrheological drugs**. Sometimes clots form and totally block a blood vessel. When this happens in one of the coronary arteries, a heart attack occurs, and the clot blocking the blood vessel must be lysed to prevent or minimize damage to the myocardial muscle. The **thrombolytic drugs** lyse (break down) such preformed clots. This is a unique difference between thrombolytics and the anticoagulants, which can only prevent the formation of a clot. **Hemostatic agents** have the opposite effect of these other classes of agents; they promote blood coagulation and are helpful in the management of conditions in which excessive bleeding would be harmful. The various agents in each category of coagulation modifiers are listed in Table 27-1. Understanding the individual coagulation modifiers and their mechanisms of action requires a basic working knowledge of the coagulation pathway and coagulation factors, explained in the next section.

HEMOSTASIS

Normal hemostasis involves a complex relationship between substances that promote clot formation (platelets, von Willebrand factor, activated clotting factors, and tissue thromboplastin) and substances that either inhibit coagulation (prostacyclin, antithrombin III, protein C and S) or dissolve a formed clot (**tissue plasminogen activator**). Each of these systems is discussed, along with the actions of the various classes of coagulation modifiers.

The coagulation system is called a *cascade* because each activated factor serves as a catalyst that amplifies the next reaction. The result is a large concentration of a clot-forming substance called **fibrin**. The coagulation cascade is typically divided into the intrinsic and extrinsic pathways, which are activated simultaneously by distinct mechanisms. When blood vessels are damaged, thromboplastin, a substance contained in the walls of blood vessels, is released. Thromboplastin activates the extrinsic pathway by activating factors VIIa and X. The intrinsic system is activated when factors XI and XII come in contact with exposed collagen in damaged blood vessels. Activated factors XI and XII amplify the activation of factor X. The

TABLE 27-1

COAGULATION MODIFIERS: CATEGORIES AND AGENTS

Type of Coagulation Modifier	Drug Class	Individual Agents
PREVENT CLOT FORMATION		
Inhibit certain clotting factors	Anticoagulants	anagrelide, dalteparin, enoxaparin, fondaparinux, nadroparin, nicoumalone, tinzaparin, heparin, warfarin
Prevent platelets from working	Antiplatelet drugs	abciximab, aspirin, clopidogrel, dipyridamole, eptifibatide, pentoxifylline, ticlopidine, tirofiban
PROMOTE CLOT FORMATION		
Prevent lysis of fibrin	Antifibrinolytics	aminocaproic acid, tranexamic acid, aprotinin
LYSE A PREFORMED CLOT		
Directly lyse the clot	Thrombolytics	alteplase, reteplase, streptokinase, tenecteplase
REVERSAL AGENTS	Heparin antagonist	protamine sulphate
	Warfarin sodium antagonist	vitamin K

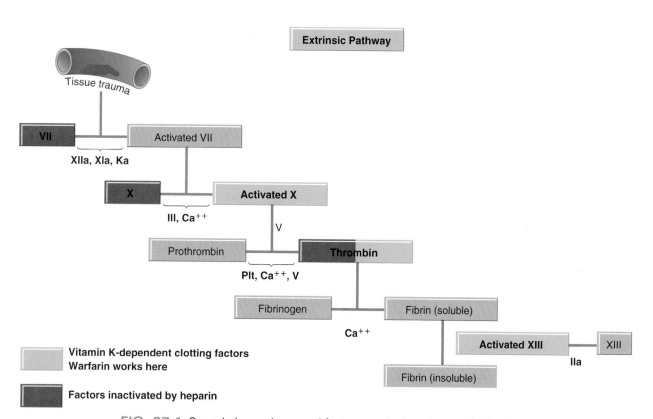

FIG. 27-1 Coagulation pathway and factors: extrinsic pathway. *Plt*, Platelets.

extrinsic and intrinsic pathways converge into the common pathway at the activation of factor X, which converts prothrombin to thrombin. Figures 27-1 and 27-2 illustrate the steps that occur in the extrinsic and intrinsic pathways, respectively, and the factors involved. They also show where in these pathways the various coagulation modifiers work.

Once a clot is formed and fibrin is present, the **fibrinolytic system** is activated. This is the system that regulates the breakdown of clots and keeps the coagulation system from going out of control. **Fibrinolysis** is the mechanism by which formed thrombi are lysed to prevent excessive clot formation and blood vessel blockage. **Plasmin** is the enzyme that eventually breaks fibrin down into the fibrin degradation products, although it must first be activated by **plasminogen.** It is the fibrin in the clot that binds to circulating plasminogen, which in turn activates plasmin and keeps the clot localized. Figure 27-3 illustrates the fibrinolytic system.

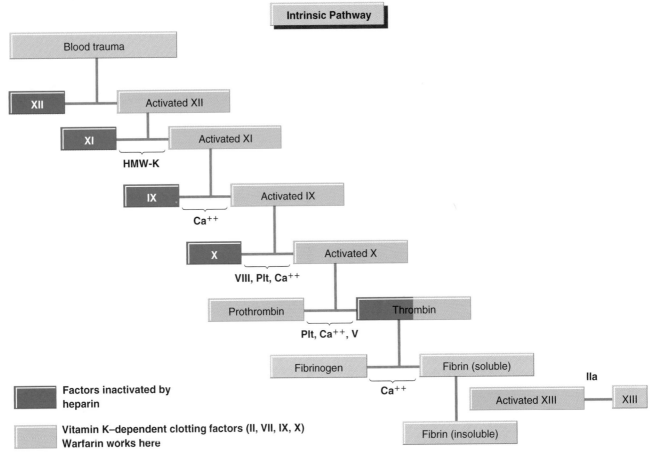

FIG. 27-2 Coagulation pathway and factors: intrinsic pathway. *HMW-K*, High-molecular weight kininogen; *Plt*, platelets.

COAGULATION MODIFYING AGENTS

ANTICOAGULANTS

Drugs that prevent the formation of a clot by inhibiting certain clotting factors are called anticoagulants. These agents are given only prophylactically; they have no direct effect on a blood clot that has already formed or on ischemic tissue injured as the result of an inadequate blood supply caused by the clot. By decreasing blood coagulability, anticoagulants prevent intravascular thrombosis. Their uses vary from preventing clot formation to preventing the extension of a preformed clot, or a **thrombus.**

Once a clot forms on the wall of a blood vessel, it may dislodge and travel through the bloodstream. This is referred to as an **embolus.** If it goes to the brain, it causes a **stroke;** if it goes to the lungs, it is a **pulmonary embolus;** and if it goes to the veins in the legs, it is a **deep vein thrombosis (DVT).** Collectively these complications are called **thromboembolic events** because they involve a thrombus becoming an embolus and causing an "event." Used correctly, anticoagulants can prevent all of these

from occurring. There are both orally and parenterally administered anticoagulants, and each agent has a slightly different mechanism of action and indications. All of them have their own risks, mainly the risk of bleeding.

Mechanism of Action and Drug Effects

The mechanisms of action of the anticoagulants vary depending on the agent. Although other anticoagulants exist (e.g., low molecular-weight heparins such as dalteparin and enoxaparin), this chapter focuses on heparin and warfarin, which are by far the most commonly used. All anticoagulants work in the clotting cascade but do so at different points. As shown in Figures 27-1 and 27-2, heparin works by binding to a substance called **antithrombin III,** which turns off three main activating factors: activated II (also called *thrombin*), activated X, and activated IX. (Factors XI and XII are also inactivated but do not play as important a role.) Of these, the thrombin is the most sensitive to the actions of heparin. The overall effect of heparin is that it turns off the coagulation pathway and prevents clots from forming. As previously noted, however, it cannot lyse a clot that already exists. The low molecular weight heparins (LMWHs) such as enoxaparin and dalteparin work in a similar way.

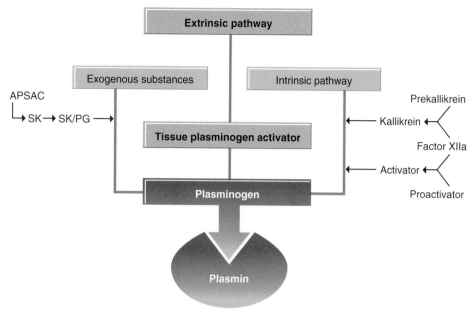

FIG. 27-3 The fibrinolytic system. *APSAC*, Anisoylated plasminogen streptokinase activator complex; *PG*, plasminogen; *SK*, streptokinase.

Heparin binds primarily to activated factors II, X, and IX. LMWHs are much more specific for activated factor X (Xa) than for activated factor II (IIa). Unlike heparin, LMWHs have a much more predictable anticoagulant response, and thus do not require frequent laboratory monitoring of bleeding times such as activated partial thromboplastin times (APTTs).

Warfarin also works by inhibiting certain clotting factors, in particular clotting factors II, VII, IX, and X. These factors rely heavily on vitamin K for their synthesis, a process that takes place in the liver. Warfarin specifically works by interfering with the production of vitamin K. The result is that the vitamin K needed for the production of clotting factors II, VII, IX, and X is dysfunctional, causing the clotting factors to be dysfunctional. As with heparin, the final effect is the prevention of clot formation. Figures 27-1 and 27-2 show where in the clotting cascade this occurs.

Oral direct thrombin inhibitors (DTIs) such as ximelagatran are being investigated as a new class of anticoagulant drug that may be used as alternatives to warfarin. DTIs easily penetrate the clot to directly inhibit thrombin and block its interaction with its substrates.

Indications

The ability of anticoagulants to prevent clot formation is of benefit when there is a high likelihood of clot formation. Clot formation is a risk with myocardial infarction (MI), unstable angina, atrial fibrillation, indwelling devices such as mechanical heart valves, and conditions in which blood flow may be slowed and blood may pool, such as major orthopedic surgery. The ultimate benefit is the prevention of a stroke, heart attack, DVT, or pulmonary embolism (PE).

TABLE 27-2	
ANTICOAGULANTS: ADVERSE EFFECTS	
Body System	**Side/Adverse Effects**
Gastrointestinal	Nausea, vomiting, diarrhea, abdominal cramps, ulcerations, bleeding
Hematological	Bleeding, thrombocytopenia, thrombosis, vasculitis
Other	Osteoporosis, skin necrosis, hypoaldosteronism, anaphylactic reactions, priapism, rebound hyperlipidemia

Contraindications

Contraindications to the use of anticoagulants include known drug allergy to a specific product and usually include any acute bleeding process or high risk of bleeding. Some examples include leukemia, pregnancy, and gastrointestinal (GI) obstruction or serious inflammation (e.g., colitis).

Side Effects and Adverse Effects

Bleeding is the main complication of anticoagulation therapy, and the risk increases with increasing dosages. It also depends on the nature of the client's underlying clinical disorder and is increased in clients also taking high doses of ASA or other drugs that impair platelet function. Some of the possible side effects of anticoagulant therapy are listed in Table 27-2.

Interactions

The drug interactions involving the oral anticoagulants are profound and complicated (see Table 27-3). Anticoagulant activity is increased by the following mechanisms:

TABLE 27-3

ANTICOAGULANTS: DRUG INTERACTIONS

Drug	Mechanism	Result
WARFARIN SODIUM		
acetaminophen (high doses) amiodarone	Displaces from inactive protein-binding sites	Increased anticoagulant effect
ASA/other NSAIDs Broad-spectrum antibiotics cephalozin	Decreases platelet activity	
Mineral oil Vitamin E	Interferes with vitamin K	
Barbiturates carbamazepine rifampin	Enzyme inducer	Decreased anticoagulant effect
amiodarone cimetidine ciprofloxacin erythromycin ketoconazole metronidazole omeprazole Sulphonamides	Enzyme inhibitor	Increased anticoagulant effect
cholestyramine sucralfate	Impairs absorption of warfarin	Decreased anticoagulant effect
HEPARIN ASA/other NSAIDs Oral anticoagulants	Decrease platelet activity Additive	Increased anticoagulant effect
Thrombolytics Cephalosporins Penicillins	Additive	

NSAID, Non-steroidal anti-inflammatory drug.

- Enzyme inhibition of biotransformation
- Displacement of the agent from inactive protein-binding sites
- Decrease in vitamin K absorption or synthesis by the bacterial flora of the large intestine
- Alteration in platelet count or activity

Drugs that can increase the activity of heparin include salicylates and other NSAIDS, GP IIb-IIIa antagonists, and the oral anticoagulants. Antihistamines, quinine, ACTH, digitalis, and insulin may partially antagonize the anticoagulant effects of heparin. The main interaction mechanism responsible for decreasing anticoagulant activity is an increase in the biotransformation of the oral agents (enzyme inducers). Heparin can alter the serum levels of lipids, glucose, thyroxine, aspartate aminotransferase (AST), and alanine aminotransferase (ALT), and also affect triiodothyronine (T_3) uptake.

Toxicity and Management of Overdose

Treatment of the toxic effects of anticoagulants is aimed at reversing the underlying cause. Although the toxic effects of heparin, LMWHs, and warfarin are hemorrhagic in nature, the management of each is different. Symptoms that may be attributed to toxicity or an overdose of anticoagulants are hematuria, melena (black stools), petechiae (pinpoint-sized hemorrhages in the skin), ecchymoses (blotchy areas of hemorrhage in the skin), and gum or mucous membrane bleeding. In the event of either heparin or warfarin toxicity, the anticoagulant should be discontinued. In the case of heparin this may be enough to reverse the toxic effects because of the short half-life of the drug (approximately 90 minutes). In severe cases or when large doses have been given intentionally (i.e., during cardiopulmonary bypass for heart surgery), a reversal agent may need to be given. If large amounts of blood have been lost, replacement with packed red blood cells (PRBCs) may be necessary. The anticoagulant effects of heparin can be reversed with protamine sulphate. The protamine forms a complex with heparin, which completely reverses the heparin's anticoagulant properties in as few as 5 minutes. As a rule of thumb, 1 mg of protamine can reverse the effects of 100 units of heparin. In theory, however, the protamine dosing should vary depending on the source of the heparin given, as heparin comes from three different sources and each has a different anticoagulant potency. Recommended doses are 1 mg of protamine for 90 units of heparin sodium from bovine lung tissue, 100 units of heparin calcium from porcine intestinal mucosa, and 115 units of heparin sodium from porcine intestinal mucosa. Decreasing amounts of protamine are required as the time

DOSAGES Selected Anticoagulant Agents

Agent	Pharmacological Class	Usual Dosage Range	Indications
▸▸enoxaparin	LMWH	**Adult** SC: 15 mg bid or 30 mg qd for DVT prophylaxis; 1 mg/kg bid or 1.5 mg/kg daily for treatment of DVT; 1 mg/kg bid (max 100 mg/dose) for unstable angina and non–Q-wave MI	
▸▸heparin	Natural anticoagulant	**Pediatric Neonates** IV: Initial 50–100 units/kg, then 20–30 units/kg/hr **Infants and older** IV: Initial 75 units/kg, then 20–28 units/kg/hr **Adult*** SC: Initial IV bolus of 5000 units followed by 15 000–20 000 units bid IV infusion: 20 000–40 000 units/day ACT or APTT determines maintenance dose	Anticoagulant
▸▸warfarin sodium	Coumarin anticoagulant	PT or INR determines maintenance dose, usually 2–10 mg/day	

LMWH, Low-molecular-weight heparin; *DVT,* deep vein thrombosis; *ACT,* activated clotting time; *APTT,* activated partial thromboplastin time; *PT,* prothrombin time; *INR,* International Normalization Ratio.
*IV and SC dosage ranges vary depending on client variables and diagnosis, platelet and clotting laboratory values, and prevention versus treatment.

period from the heparin administration lengthens. Protamine administration should not exceed 20 mg/min or more than 50 mg in any 10-minute period. Protamine may also be used to reverse the effects of LMWHs. A dose of protamine equal to the dose of the LMWH should be used (e.g., 1 mg protamine/1000 U enoxaparin).

In the event of warfarin sodium toxicity or overdose, the first step is to discontinue the anticoagulant. However, therapy after discontinuation differs from treatment of heparin toxicity. As with heparin, the toxicity associated with sodium warfarin use is an extension of its therapeutic effects on the clotting cascade. However, because sodium warfarin functionally inactivates the vitamin K-dependent clotting factors and because these clotting factors are synthesized in the liver, it may take 36 to 42 hours before the liver can resynthesize enough clotting factors to reverse the warfarin effects. Treatment with warfarin's reversal agent, vitamin K (phytonadione), can hasten the return to normal coagulation. The dose and route of administration of the vitamin K depend on the clinical situation and its acuity (i.e., how quickly the sodium warfarin-induced effects must be reversed). High doses of vitamin K (10 to 15 mg) given intravenously should reverse the anticoagulation within 6 hours. If the warfarin therapy must be reinstated, resistance to its effect will be encountered because the large dose of vitamin K will maintain its reversal effects for up to 1 week. Low doses of vitamin K may minimize the resistance to warfarin therapy when warfarin must be restarted. If bleeding is too severe to wait for the vitamin K to take effect, it may be necessary to administer plasma or factor concentrates.

Dosages

For the dosages of anticoagulants, see the dosages table on this page. See Appendix B for some of the common brands available in Canada.

DRUG PROFILES

All the anticoagulants discussed here (enoxaparin, heparin sodium, and warfarin sodium) are prescription medications. Warfarin is available in tablets and an injection. Heparin can be given only by subcutaneous (SC) or intravenous injection. Four LMWHs are currently available: enoxaparin, dalteparin, tinzaparin, and nadroparin. All are administered by subcutaneous injection only (not intramuscular [IM]) with the exception of dalteparin, which can be administered by intermittent or continuous IV infusion. The prototype drug for this newer class of heparins is enoxaparin, the first to come onto the market in Canada. These products are made by taking heparin and enzymatically removing part of the heparin molecule, making a smaller, more accurate heparin. They are presently used for preventing and treating various thromboembolic events in high-risk clients, including those undergoing total hip or knee surgery and high-risk general surgery. They are also being recognized for their use in treatment of unstable angina or non–Q-wave MI, concurrently with acetylsalicylates. There are occasions when it is appropriate to use an oral anticoagulant such as warfarin with an intravenous anticoagulant such as heparin (e.g., while waiting for the full anticoagulant effect of warfarin to take place).

▸▸ *warfarin sodium*

Warfarin sodium is a coumarin derivative. Warfarin is one of the most commonly prescribed oral (PO) anticoagulants. Warfarin is contraindicated in clients who have shown a hypersensitivity to it and in those with subacute bacterial endocarditis or any type of potential or actual bleeding condition. Because warfarin can pass the placental barrier, it is also contraindicated in pregnant women. Warfarin sodium is available as an injection (5 mg per vial) and as 1-, 2-, 2.5-, 3-, 4-, 5-, 6-, and

10-mg tablets. It is pregnancy category X. See the table on p. 459 for dosage information.

PHARMACOKINETICS

Half-Life	Onset	Peak	Duration
0.5–3 days	12–24 hr	3–4 days	2–5 days

▸▸ enoxaparin

Enoxaparin is an LMWH obtained by enzymatically cleaving large unfractionated heparin molecules into small fragments. These smaller fragments of heparin have a greater affinity for factor Xa than for factor IIa and have a higher degree of bioavailability and a longer elimination half-life than unfractionated heparin. Laboratory monitoring, as done for heparin, is not necessary with enoxaparin because of its high bioavailability and greater affinity for factor Xa. Enoxaparin is currently indicated for the prevention and treatment of DVT, which may lead to PE after knee or hip replacement surgery. There is new evidence that LMWHs are also effective for the prevention of thromboembolic events in high-risk general surgery clients and clients with unstable angina. Enoxaparin is contraindicated in clients with active major bleeding; thrombocytopenia associated with enoxaparin; or hypersensitivity to enoxaparin, heparin, or other porcine products. Enoxaparin is available only in parenteral form as 30-, 40-, 60-, 80-, and 100-mg prefilled syringes and a multi-dose vial. Pregnancy category B. See the table on p. 459 for dosage information.

PHARMACOKINETICS

Half-Life	Onset	Peak	Duration
3–4.5 hr	3–5 hr	3 hr	12 hr

▸▸ heparin

Heparin is a natural mucopolysaccharide anticoagulant obtained from the lungs, intestinal mucosa, or other suitable tissues of animals, primarily sheep and cows. One brand name for some of the commonly used heparin products is Hepalean-Lok. However, this brand name refers only to small vials of aqueous heparin intravenous flush solutions used to maintain patency of heparin lock intravenous insertion sites. This type of use is fundamentally different from the systemic use of heparin for its anticoagulant cardiovascular effects, as discussed in this chapter. Furthermore, heparin solutions used for such heparin lock flushes are usually in a lower concentration than heparin used for systemic cardiovascular purposes. In fact, some institutions routinely used normal saline (0.9 percent sodium chloride) as a flush for heparin lock intravenous ports and have moved away from using heparin flush solutions for this purpose.

Heparin is contraindicated in clients with hypersensitivity to it and those with any potential or actual bleeding condition. It is available in the following concentrations and strengths: 10-, 100-, 1000-, 10 000-, and 25 000-units/mL injections; 1000-, 10 000-, and 25 000-units/mL vials; and infusions of 1000-, 20 000-, and 25 000-units/500 mL and 2000-units/1000 mL. Heparin can be given either subcutaneously or intravenously.

See the dosages table on p. 459 for dosage recommendations. Note that most institutions have adopted nomograms for the dosing of heparin. Pregnancy category C.

PHARMACOKINETICS

Half-Life	Onset	Peak	Duration
1–2 hr	SC: 20–60 min IV: Immediate	SC: 2–4 hr	Dose-dependent

ANTIPLATELET AGENTS

Another class of coagulation modifiers that prevent clot formation is the antiplatelet drugs, but they accomplish this in an entirely different manner. The anticoagulants work in the clotting cascade, whereas the antiplatelet drugs work at the initial step of the coagulation process, preventing platelet adhesion. An understanding of the role of platelets in the clotting process is essential to understanding how antiplatelet drugs work.

Platelets normally flow through blood vessels without adhering to their surfaces. When blood vessels are injured by a disruption to blood flow, trauma, or the rupture of plaque from the vessel wall, substances present in the walls of blood vessels such as collagen and fibronectin are exposed. Collagen is a potent stimulator of platelet adhesion, as is a prevalent component of the platelet membranes themselves, known as *glycoprotein IIb/IIIa* (GP IIb/IIIa). Once platelet adhesion occurs, stimulators (adenosine diphosphate [ADP], thrombin, thromboxane A2 [TXA_2], and prostaglandin H_2) are released from the damaged blood vessels. These cause the platelets to aggregate at the site of injury. Once there, they change shape and release their contents, which include ADP, serotonin, and platelet factor 4 (PF4). The hemostatic function of these substances is twofold. First, they attract platelets to the site of injury (platelet recruiters); second, they are potent vasoconstrictors. Vasoconstriction limits blood flow to the damaged blood vessel, thus also decreasing blood loss.

A platelet plug that has formed at a site of injury to plug the damaged blood vessel is not stable and can be dislodged. The clotting system is therefore stimulated to form a more permanent fibrin plug. The role of the platelet and the relationship between platelets and the clotting cascade in the generation of a stabilized fibrin clot are illustrated in Figure 27-4.

Mechanism of Action and Drug Effects

The mechanisms of action of the antiplatelet drugs vary depending on the agent. Acetylsalicylic acid (ASA), clopidogrel, dipyridamole, pentoxifylline, and ticlopidine all affect the normal function of platelets. Many of the antiplatelet drugs affect the cyclo-oxygenase pathway, which is one of the common final enzymatic pathways in the complex arachidonic acid pathway that operates in platelets and on blood vessel walls. This pathway as it

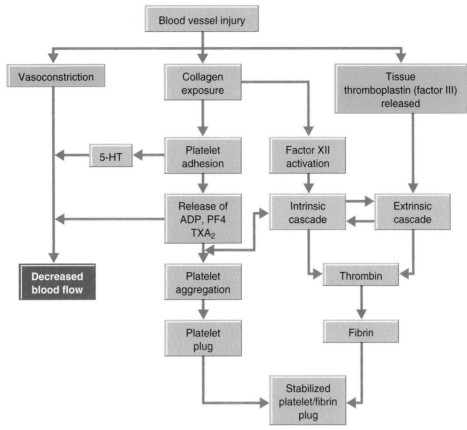

FIG. 27-4 Relationship between platelets and the clotting cascade. *ADP*, Adenosine diphosphate; *5-HT*, serotonin; *PF4*, platelet factor 4; *TXA₂*, thromboxane A₂.

functions in both platelets and blood vessel walls is illustrated in Figure 27-5.

ASA acetylates and inhibits cyclo-oxygenase in the platelet irreversibly, so that the platelet cannot regenerate this enzyme. Therefore the effects of ASA last the life span of a platelet, or 7 to 10 days. This inhibition of cyclo-oxygenase prevents the formation of thromboxane (TX), a substance that causes blood vessels to constrict and platelets to aggregate. By preventing TX formation, ASA prevents these actions, resulting in dilation of the blood vessels and prevention of platelets from aggregating or forming a clot. This system also exists in the blood vessel. However, much higher doses of ASA (>80 mg/day) are needed to inhibit the cyclo-oxygenase pathway in the blood vessels. This has the drawback of also preventing the formation of prostacyclin, a beneficial substance that causes blood vessel dilation and inhibits platelet aggregation. If prostacyclin is prevented from forming, vasoconstriction and platelet aggregation occur. By interfering with the function of the coagulation pathway, ASA may also have a hematological action. This is believed to consist of altering the hepatic synthesis of blood coagulation factors VII, IX, and X. ASA accomplishes this in much the same way that warfarin does, by interfering with the action of vitamin K.

Dipyridamole, another antiplatelet agent, also works by inhibiting platelet aggregation, which it does by preventing the release of ADP, PF4, and TXA₂, substances that stimulate platelets to aggregate or form a clot. Figure 27-4 shows how these substances accomplish this. Dipyridamole may also directly stimulate the release of prostacyclin and inhibit the formation of TXA₂ (see Figure 27-5).

Clopidogrel and ticlopidine belong to one of the newest classes of antiplatelet drugs, called the *ADP inhibitors*. Their mechanism of action is entirely different from that of ASA. They inhibit platelet aggregation by altering the platelet membrane so that it can no longer receive the signal to aggregate and form a clot. This signal is usually sent by **fibrinogen,** which attaches to a glycoprotein receptor (GP IIb/IIIa) on the surface of the platelet. Ticlopidine, tirofiban, and clopidogrel inhibit the activation of this receptor. It may take 24 to 48 hours for this action to take effect, which suggests that these therapeutic effects may be produced by ticlopidine metabolites rather than by the ticlopidine itself. Clopidogrel is a new antiplatelet drug, similar to ticlopidine in its actions, that has shown much promise. It has been shown to be significantly better than ASA at reducing the number of heart attacks, strokes, and vascular deaths in at-risk clients. It is also used in combination with ASA after angioplasty and stent insertion.

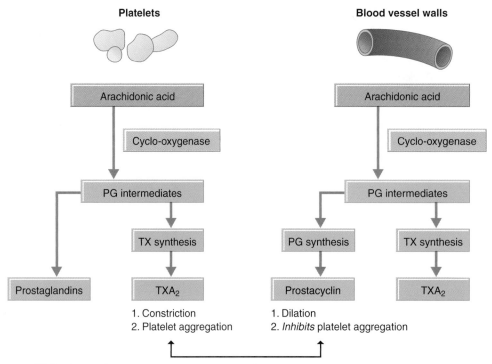

FIG. 27-5 Cyclo-oxygenase pathway. *PG*, Prostaglandin; *TXA₂*, thromboxane A₂.

Pentoxifylline, another antiplatelet agent, is a methyl-xanthine derivative with properties similar to those of theobromine, caffeine, theophylline, and other methyl-xanthines. Unlike other methylxanthines, it has few car-diac effects. However, it has many effects on blood. It can both increase the flexibility of red blood cells (RBCs) and reduce the aggregation of platelets. It is sometimes re-ferred to as a *hemorrheological agent,* or a drug that alters the normal function of the blood. It affects the RBCs by increasing the flexibility (deformability) of the cells and reducing the viscosity of whole blood, which it appears to do by facilitating the ability of the RBCs to maintain their integrity. Pentoxifylline inhibits platelet aggregation by inhibiting ADP, serotonin, and platelet factor 4 (see Fig-ure 27-4). Pentoxifylline also stimulates the synthesis and release of prostacyclin from blood vessels (see Figure 27-5). In addition, it may stimulate the fibrinolytic system, to in-crease the breakdown of fibrin by raising the plasma con-centrations of the tissue plasminogen activator (see Fig-ure 27-3).

The newest available antiplatelet class of drugs is the GP IIb/IIIa inhibitors. They work by blocking the recep-tor protein of the same name that occurs in the platelet wall membranes. This protein plays a role in promoting the aggregation of platelets in preparation for fibrin clot formation. Currently available agents in this class are tirofiban, eptifibatide, and abciximab. Their purpose is to prevent the formation of thrombi during acute cardiovas-cular events (e.g., MI). This is known as *thromboprevention.* It is easier and less risky to prevent a thrombus from forming than to lyse a formed thrombus.

Indications

The therapeutic effects of the antiplatelet drugs depend on the particular agent. ASA has multiple therapeutic ef-fects, but many of them vary depending on the dose. ASA has analgesic, anti-inflammatory, and antipyretic properties. It also has potent antithrombotic and hema-tological effects. Dipyridamole is used as an adjunct to warfarin in the prevention of post-operative throm-boembolic complications. It is also used to decrease platelet aggregation in a number of other thromboem-bolic disorders. Ticlopidine's therapeutic effects are sim-ilar to a few of the therapeutic effects of ASA. It has an-tithrombotic effects and is useful for reducing the risk of fatal and non-fatal thrombotic stroke. The GP IIb/IIIa inhibitors are used to treat acute unstable angina and during percutaneous coronary angioplasty (PTCA) pro-cedures. Their purpose is to prevent platelet aggrega-tion and the formation of any kind of thrombus or em-bolus (moving thrombus).

Contraindications

Contraindications to the use of antiplatelet agents include known drug allergy to a specific product, thrombocy-topenia, active bleeding, leukemia, traumatic injury, and recent stroke.

Side Effects and Adverse Effects

The potential adverse effects of the various antiplatelet drugs can be serious, and they all pose a risk for inducing a serious bleeding episode. Ticlopidine can produce ele-vations in alkaline phosphatase activity, bilirubin level,

DOSAGES   Selected Antiplatelet Agents

Agent	Pharmacological Class	Usual Dosage Range	Indications
▸▸ASA	Salicylate antiplatelet	**Adult** PO: 81–325 mg/day PO: 75–1300 mg/day	MI prophylaxis TIA prophylaxis
▸▸clopidogrel	Antiplatelet	**Adult** PO: 75 mg daily; 300–375 mg may be given as a one-time loading dose after coronary stent implantation	Reduction of atherosclerotic events; acute coronary syndrome without ST-segment elevation
▸▸eptifibatide	GP IIb/IIIa inhibitor	IV: Single bolus 180 μg/kg followed by continuous infusion 2 μg/kg for 96 hr total; specific doses are based on client weight from 37 to 121 kg*	Unstable angina/Non–ST-segment elevation MI
pentoxifylline	Antiplatelet/hemorrheological	**Adult** PO: 400 mg bid–tid with meals	Claudication associated with peripheral arterial disease

*See manufacturer's directions for specific dose.
TIA, transient ischemic attack; *GP*, glycoprotein.

TABLE 27-4
ANTIPLATELET AGENTS: ADVERSE EFFECTS

Body System	Side/Adverse Effects
ASA	
Central nervous	Stimulation, drowsiness, dizziness, confusion, flushing
Gastrointestinal	Nausea, vomiting, GI bleeding, diarrhea, heartburn
Hematological	Thrombocytopenia, agranulocytosis, leukopenia, neutropenia, hemolytic anemia, bleeding
CLOPIDOGREL	
Cardiovascular	Chest pain, hypertension, edema
Central nervous	Flu-like symptoms, headache, dizziness, fatigue
Gastrointestinal	Abdominal pain, dyspepsia, diarrhea, nausea, vomiting
Miscellaneous	Epistaxis (severe nosebleed) and integumentary disorders, including rash and pruritus (itching)
PENTOXIFYLLINE	
Cardiovascular	Angina, dysrhythmias, palpitation, hypotension, chest pain, dyspnea, flushing
Central nervous	Headache, anxiety, tremors, confusion, dizziness
Gastrointestinal	Nausea, vomiting, bloating, dyspepsia, constipation, dry mouth, thirst, bad taste

and transaminase activity. The most common adverse effects are listed in Table 27-4.

Interactions

Potentially dangerous drug interactions can occur with antiplatelet agents. Co-administration of ticlopidine with antacids results in its decreased absorption. Its use with digoxin causes the plasma levels of the digoxin to be decreased. Concurrent use with ASA is not recom-

mended. The concurrent use of dipyridamole and ASA produces additive antiplatelet activity. ASA, when given with non-steroidal anti-inflammatory drugs (NSAIDs), can potentiate bleeding. Also, a client who is allergic to ASA may also be allergic to NSAIDs. When ASA is given with oral antidiabetic agents the client can experience a loss of diabetic control. The combined use of steroids or NSAIDs with ASA can increase the ulcerogenic effects of ASA. The combined use of ASA and heparin with GP IIb/IIIa inhibitors also further enhances antiplatelet activity and increases the likelihood of a serious bleeding episode.

Dosages

For information on the dosages of selected antiplatelet agents, see the dosages table above. See Appendix B for some of the common brands available in Canada.

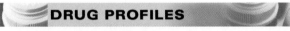

DRUG PROFILES

Antiplatelet drugs are extremely useful in the management of thromboembolic disorders. Each has unique pharmacological properties.

▸▸ ASA

ASA is available in many combinations with other prescription and non-prescription drugs and goes by many product names. ASA is contraindicated in clients with a known hypersensitivity to salicylates, those with asthma, those with GI bleeding or bleeding disorders, peptic ulcer disease, or a vitamin K deficiency. It is also contraindicated in lactating women, children under 12, and teenagers or young adults with chicken pox, influenza, or flu-like symptoms. It is available in both oral and rectal forms. Orally it is available in many doses and dosage forms: chewing gum containing 227 mg per stick; 80-, 81-, 162-, 325-, 500-, and 650-mg enteric-coated tablets; 325-, 500-, and 650-mg tablets; 80- and

81-mg chewable tablets; and 81-, 325-, and 500-mg film-coated tablets. Pregnancy category D. For commonly recommended dosages, see the table on p. 463.

PHARMACOKINETICS

Half-Life	Onset	Peak	Duration
3.5–4.5 hr	15–30 min	1–2 hr	4–6 hr

▶▶ clopidogrel

Clopidogrel and ticlopidine are the only two ADP inhibitors on the market. They are potent antiplatelet agents. Ticlopidine is primarily used to reduce the risk of fatal and non-fatal thrombotic stroke in clients who have suffered either a completed thrombotic stroke or stroke precursors (e.g., transient ischemic attacks, reversible ischemic neurological deficit, or minor stroke). Clopidogrel is indicated for the reduction of MI, stroke, or vascular death in clients with atherosclerosis documented by recent stroke, established peripheral arterial disease, or acute coronary syndrome without ST segment elevation. They are also used after intracoronary stent implantation to reduce the risk of stent thrombosis.

Because ticlopidine can precipitate life-threatening neutropenia and agranulocytosis, it should be reserved for clients unable to tolerate ASA therapy. Clopidogrel has not been shown to cause this side effect to the same degree. Clopidogrel can be dosed once a day; ticlopidine must be dosed twice a day. Clopidogrel is contraindicated in clients with a known hypersensitivity to it and in those with active pathological bleeding such as peptic ulcer or intracranial hemorrhage. Clopidogrel is available as a 75-mg tablet. Pregnancy category B. Recommended dosages are given in the table on p. 463.

PHARMACOKINETICS

Half-Life	Onset	Peak	Duration
8 hr	1–2 hr*	1 hr*	7–10 days

*Onset and peak values can be reduced by giving a loading dose of 300–375 mg.

▶▶ eptifibatide

Eptifibatide is a GP IIb/IIIa inhibitor, along with tirofiban, and abciximab. These agents are indicated primarily for thromboprevention during acute episodes of unstable angina or MI. They are also useful during interventional cardiac procedures such as PTCA. They are usually administered in intensive care settings where continuous cardiovascular monitoring is the norm. These agents may be administered by intravenous bolus, followed by continuous infusion. All are available only in injectable form, with eptifibatide provided in concentrations of 0.75 mg/mL and 2 mg/mL. Pregnancy category B. Dosage information appears in the table on p. 463.

PHARMACOKINETICS

Half-Life	Onset	Peak	Duration
2–2.5 hr	1 hr	Unknown	4 hr

pentoxifylline

Pentoxifylline is the sole agent currently approved for treatment of intermittent claudication (cramping, aches, or burning pain in the legs) caused by occlusive peripheral arterial disease. Pentoxifylline improves erythrocyte flexibility, microcirculatory flow, and tissue oxygenation concentration and reduces blood viscosity. It is a prescription-only medication. Pentoxifylline is contraindicated in clients with a known hypersensitivity to it or to any methylxanthine. It is available only in oral form as a 400-mg film-coated, extended-release tablet. Pregnancy category C. For commonly recommended dosages see the table on p. 463.

PHARMACOKINETICS

Half-Life	Onset	Peak	Duration
0.5–1 hr	Unknown	2–3 hr	Unknown

ANTIFIBRINOLYTIC AGENTS

The individual antifibrinolytic agents have varying mechanisms of action, but all prevent the lysis of fibrin, the substance that helps make the platelet plug insoluble and anchors the clot to the damaged blood vessel (see Figures 27-1 and 27-2). The term **antifibrinolytic** refers to what these drugs do, which is to prevent the lysis of fibrin; in doing so, they promote clot formation. They have the opposite effects of anticoagulant and antiplatelet agents, which prevent clot formation. There are two synthetic antifibrinolytics, aminocaproic acid and tranexamic acid; one natural antifibrinolytic agent, aprotinin; and another antifibrinolytic with a different mechanism of action, desmopressin. Other drugs used to stop excessive bleeding are referred to as *hemostatic agents*. These agents, including thrombin, microfibrillar collagen, absorbable gelatin, and oxidized cellulose, are not discussed here.

Mechanism of Action and Drug Effects

Antifibrinolytics vary in several ways, depending on the particular agent. The various antifibrinolytic agents and their proposed mechanisms of action are described in Table 27-5.

The drug effects of the antifibrinolytics are specific and limited. They do not have many effects outside of their hematological ones. Aminocaproic acid, tranexamic acid, and aprotinin prevent the breakdown of fibrin, which prevents the destruction of the formed platelet clot. Desmopressin increases the resorption of water by the collecting ducts in the kidneys, resulting in increased urine osmolality and a decreased urinary flow rate. It also causes a dose-dependent increase in the concentration of von Willebrand factor, along with an increase in the plasma concentration of tissue plasminogen activator. The overall effect of this is increased platelet aggregation and clot formation.

Indications

Antifibrinolytics are useful in both the prevention and treatment of excessive bleeding resulting from systemic hyperfibrinolysis or surgical complications. They have

TABLE 27-5
ANTIFIBRINOLYTICS: MECHANISMS OF ACTION

Antifibrinolytic Agent	Mechanism of Action
Synthetic agents: aminocaproic acid and tranexamic acid	Form a reversible complex with plasminogen and plasmin. By binding to the lysine-binding site of plasminogen, these agents displace plasminogen from the surface of fibrin. This prevents plasmin from lysing the fibrin clot. Therefore these drugs can only work if a clot has formed.
Natural agent: aprotinin	Inhibits the proteolytic enzymes trypsin, plasmin, and kallikrein, which lyse proteins that destroy fibrin clots. By inhibiting these enzymes, aprotinin prevents the degradation of the fibrin clot. It is also thought to inhibit the action of the complement system.
Other: desmopressin (DDAVP)	Works by increasing von Willebrand factor, which anchors platelets to damaged vessels via the GP IIb platelet receptor. It appears that desmopressin acts as a general endothelial stimulant, stimulating factor VIII, prostaglandin I_2, and plasminogen-activated release.

GP, Glycoprotein.

also proved successful in arresting excessive oozing from surgical sites such as chest tubes, as well as in reducing the total blood loss and the duration of bleeding in the post-operative period.

Desmopressin's therapeutic effects exceed those of the antifibrinolytics. It can be given either intranasally or parenterally to prevent or control polydipsia, polyuria, and dehydration in clients with diabetes insipidus caused by a deficiency of endogenous posterior pituitary vasopressin and in clients with polyuria and polydipsia stemming from trauma or surgery in the pituitary region. It may also be used in clients who have hemophilia A or type I von Willebrand's disease. Desmopressin increases the levels of clotting factors in which these clients are deficient.

Contraindications

Contraindications to the use of antifibrinolytic agents include known drug allergy to a specific product and disseminated intravascular coagulation (DIC).

Side Effects and Adverse Effects

The adverse effects of antifibrinolytic drugs are uncommon and generally mild. However, there have been rare reports of these agents causing thrombotic events such as acute cerebrovascular thrombosis and acute MI. The common side effects of antifibrinolytics are listed in Table 27-6.

Interactions

The concurrent use of drugs such as estrogens or oral contraceptives with aminocaproic acid, tranexamic acid, and aprotinin may have an additive effect, resulting in increased coagulation. Few specific interactions have been reported for desmopressin, although it should be given cautiously in clients receiving lithium, large doses of epinephrine, demeclocycline, heparin, or alcohol because these combinations may lead to a reduced antidiuretic response to the desmopressin. Drugs such as chlorpropamide and fludrocortisone may potentiate the antidiuretic response.

TABLE 27-6
ANTIFIBRINOLYTICS: ADVERSE EFFECTS

Body System	Side/Adverse Effects
Cardiovascular	Dysrhythmias, orthostatic hypotension, bradycardia
Central nervous	Headache, dizziness, fatigue, hallucinations, psychosis, convulsions
Gastrointestinal	Nausea, vomiting, abdominal cramps, diarrhea

Dosages

For information on the dosages for aminocaproic acid and desmopressin, see the dosages table on p. 466. See Appendix B for some of the common brands available in Canada.

DRUG PROFILES

Antifibrinolytics have a limited use in preventing the lysis of fibrin, thus promoting clot formation. The prototypical antifibrinolytic is aminocaproic acid. The effects of tranexamic acid and aprotinin are similar to those of aminocaproic acid, but desmopressin's effects are totally different.

aminocaproic acid

Aminocaproic acid is a synthetic antifibrinolytic agent used to prevent and control the excessive bleeding that can result from surgery or overactivity of the fibrinolytic system. Its use is contraindicated in clients who have had a hypersensitivity to it, as well as in clients with postpartum bleeding, disseminated intravascular coagulation, upper urinary tract bleeding, and new burns. It is available in oral form as a 500-mg tablet. Pregnancy category C. For commonly recommended dosages, see the dosages table on p. 466.

PHARMACOKINETICS

Half-Life	Onset	Peak	Duration
2 hr	Unknown	1.2 hr	unknown

DOSAGES	Aminocaproic Acid and Desmopressin			
Agent	**Pharmacological Class**	**Usual Dosage Range**		**Indications**
aminocaproic acid	Hemostatic	***Adult*** IV infusion: 5 g during first hr, then 1–1.25 g at 1-hr intervals up to a daily max of 30 g		Excessive bleeding caused by systemic hyperfibrinolysis or urinary fibrinolysis
desmopressin	Synthetic posterior pituitary hormone	***Adult*** IV: 0.3 μg/kg infused over 15–30 min; pre-op use: agent is administered 30 min before surgery		Surgical and post-op hemostasis and management of bleeding in clients with hemophilia A or type I von Willebrand's disease

desmopressin

Desmopressin is a synthetic polypeptide. It is structurally similar to vasopressin, which is antidiuretic hormone (ADH), the natural human posterior pituitary hormone. Because of these physical characteristics, it is often used to increase the resorption of water by the collecting ducts in the kidneys to prevent or control polydipsia, polyuria, and dehydration in clients with diabetes insipidus caused by a deficiency of endogenous posterior pituitary vasopressin or in clients with polyuria and polydipsia resulting from trauma or surgery in the pituitary region.

Desmopressin also causes a dose-dependent increase in von Willebrand factor along with an increase in tissue plasminogen activator, resulting in increased platelet aggregation and clot formation. Desmopressin is contraindicated in clients with a known hypersensitivity to it and in those with nephrogenic diabetes insipidus. It is available as a 0.1-mg/mL intranasal solution, 0.1- and 0.2-mg tablets, and a 4-μg/mL parenteral injection. Desmopressin nasal spray and tablets are used for primary nocturnal enuresis and diabetes insipidus. Pregnancy category B. For commonly recommended dosages, see the dosages table above.

PHARMACOKINETICS

Half-Life	**Onset**	**Peak**	**Duration**
<2 hr	15–30 min	1.1–2 hr	8–12 hr

THROMBOLYTIC AGENTS

Thrombolytic drugs are coagulation modifiers that break down, or lyse, preformed clots (thrombi) in the blood vessels that supply the heart with blood, the coronary arteries. This re-establishes blood flow to the blood-starved heart muscle. If the blood flow is re-established early, the heart muscle and left ventricular function can be saved. If not, the heart muscle becomes ischemic, then necrotic, and eventually non-functional.

Thrombolytic therapy made its debut in 1933 when a substance that would break down fibrin clots was isolated from a client's blood. This substance was observed to be produced by a bacterium growing in the client. The bacterium was found to be group A **beta-hemolytic strepto-**cocci, and the substance was eventually called **streptokinase (SK)**. SK was first used in a client in 1947 to dissolve a clotted hemothorax (blood in the pleural cavity), but it was not until 1958 that the first client with an acute MI received it. In 1960 a naturally occurring human plasminogen activator called *urokinase* became available that was found to exert fibrinolytic effects on pulmonary emboli (clots in the lungs). However, the results of the early thrombolytic trials, conducted during the 1960s and 1970s on clients who had had an acute MI, were not taken seriously by the medical community. It was not until the 1980s, when DeWood (DeWood, Spores, Notske, Mouser, Burroughs, Golden, et al, 1980) and colleagues demonstrated that the underlying cause of acute MIs was a coronary artery occlusion that the use of thrombolytics for the early treatment of acute MIs took off.

During the past decade new thrombolytics have been developed and launched. Tissue plasminogen activator and **anisoylated plasminogen streptokinase activator complex (APSAC)** are two of these agents. With the advent of these new thrombolytics came several large landmark thrombolytic research studies, which showed that early thrombolytic therapy could bring about a 50 percent reduction in mortality, a reduction in the infarct size, an improvement in left ventricular function, and a reduction in the incidence and severity of congestive heart failure. These findings and developments, along with a better understanding of the pathogenesis of acute MIs, have led the way in the advancements made in the treatment of acute MIs.

Mechanism of Action and Drug Effects

There is a fine balance between the formation and dissolution of a clot. The coagulation system is responsible for forming the clot, whereas the fibrinolytic system is responsible for dissolving the clot. The natural fibrinolytic system within blood takes days to break down a clot. This is of little value in the case of a clotted blood vessel supplying blood to the heart muscle. Necrosis of the myocardium would not be prevented by these natural means, but thrombolytic therapy can activate the fibrinolytic system to break down the clot (thrombus) in the blood vessel quickly so that the delivery of blood to the heart muscle via the coronary arteries is quickly re-established. This prevents myocardial tissue (heart muscle) and heart function from being destroyed. Thrombolytics accomplish this by activating the conversion of plasminogen to plasmin, which breaks down, or lyses, the thrombus (see Figure 27-3). Plasmin is a *proteolytic* enzyme, which means that it breaks down proteins. It is a relatively non-specific serine protease that is capable of degrading such proteins as fibrin, fibrinogen, and other pro-coagulant proteins such as factors V, VIII, and XII. In other words, the substances that form clots are destroyed by plasmin. Essentially these drugs work by mimicking the body's own process of clot destruction. Although the individual thrombolytic agents are somewhat diverse in their actions, they all have this common result.

SK binds with plasminogen to form an SK–plasminogen complex, which then acts on other plasminogen molecules to form plasmin. The plasmin formed then lyses the clots. SK is not **clot specific**. Not only does it break down the thrombus in the coronary artery, but it also breaks down clots anywhere in the body. It activates fibrinolysis throughout the body. APSAC is an SK–plasminogen complex that has been chemically modified by acylation, allowing a prolonged half-life. Like SK it is not clot specific; therefore systemic fibrinolysis is induced with its use.

Tissue plasminogen activator (t-PA) is a naturally occurring plasminogen activator secreted by vascular endothelial cells (the walls of blood vessels). However, the amount secreted naturally is not sufficient to dissolve a coronary thrombus quickly enough to restore circulation to the heart and save the heart muscle. This substance is now made through recombinant DNA techniques and can be administered in quantities sufficient to dissolve a coronary thrombus quickly. It is fibrin specific and also clot specific, meaning that only the fibrin clot stimulates t-PA to convert plasminogen to plasmin. Therefore it does not induce a systemic lytic state.

The drug effects of the thrombolytics are primarily related to their action on the fibrinolytic system. They stimulate the fibrinolytic system to lyse preformed clots, and their action is limited solely to the fibrinolytic system.

Indications

The purpose of all the thrombolytic agents is to activate the conversion of plasminogen to plasmin, the enzyme that breaks down a thrombus. The presence of a thrombus that interferes significantly with normal blood flow on either the venous or the arterial side of the circulation is an indication for the use of thrombolytic therapy. An exception may be a thrombus that has formed in blood vessels that connect directly with the central nervous system (CNS). The indications for thrombolytic therapy include acute MI, arterial thrombosis, DVT, occlusion of shunts or catheters, and PE. Its use for other thrombotic disorders is currently being evaluated.

Contraindications

Contraindications to the use of thrombolytic agents include known drug allergy to the specific product and any preservatives, and concurrent use with other drugs that alter clotting.

Side Effects and Adverse Effects

The most common undesirable effect of thrombolytic therapy is internal, intracranial, and superficial bleeding. Other problems include hypersensitivity, anaphylactoid reactions, nausea, vomiting, and hypotension. These drugs can also induce dysrhythmias. Urokinase, a drug no longer available in Canada, is associated with the development of a Guillain–Barré-type syndrome (in which the body's immune system attacks part of the peripheral nervous system).

Toxicity and Management of Overdose

Acute toxicity primarily causes an extension of the side effects of the thrombolytic agent. Treatment is symptomatic and supportive.

Interactions

The most common effect of drug interactions is an increased bleeding tendency resulting from the concurrent use of anticoagulants and anti-platelet drugs or drugs that affect platelet function.

Laboratory Test Interactions

Thrombolytic agents can reduce laboratory plasminogen and fibrinogen levels.

Dosages

For information on the dosages for SK and alteplase, see the dosages table on p. 468. See Appendix B for some of the common brands available in Canada.

DRUG PROFILES

All thrombolytic agents exert their effects by activating plasminogen and converting it to plasmin, which is capable of digesting fibrin, a major component of clots. The four thrombolytic agents currently approved for intravenous use in the management of acute MIs are streptokinase, alteplase, reteplase, and tenecteplase. In Canada, tenecteplase is the preferred thrombolytic agent in many areas. Urokinase, used for many years, is no longer available.

▸▸ alteplase

Alteplase is a naturally occurring t-PA secreted by vascular endothelial cells. The pharmaceutically available t-PA is made through recombinant DNA techniques, using modified hamster ovary cells. It is clot (fibrin) specific and therefore does not produce a systemic lytic state. In addition, because it is present in the human body in a natural state, it does not induce an antigen–antibody reaction. Therefore it can be readministered immediately in the event of reinfarction. Alteplase has a brief half-life of under 5 minutes. It is believed to open the clogged artery faster, but its action is short-lived. Therefore it is given concomitantly with heparin to prevent re-occlusion of the infarcted blood vessel. The contraindications to alteplase use are the same as those for SK. Alteplase is available only in parenteral form as 50- and 100-mg injections for intravenous infusion. Pregnancy

DOSAGES   Selected Thrombolytic Agents

Agent	Pharmacological Class	Usual Dosage Range	Indications
▸▸ alteplase	Thrombolytic enzyme	**Adult** IV: 100 mg over 90 min given as a 15-mg IV bolus, then 50 mg over 30 min, then 35 mg over 60 min	Acute MI
		IV: 100 mg over 2 hr or 30–50 mg over 1.5–2 hr via pulmonary artery	PE
		IV: 0.9 mg/kg (total dose not to exceed 90 mg) given as an IV bolus over 1 min, given within 3 hr of onset of symptoms	Acute ischemic stroke
▸▸ streptokinase	Thrombolytic enzyme	**Adult** IV: 1.5 million units infused over 60 min or intracoronary infusion initiated with a bolus of 20 000 units followed by 2000 units/min for 1 hr	Acute MI
		IV: Loading dose of 250 000 units over 30 min followed by a maintenance infusion of 100 000 units/hr for 24–72 hr	DVT, arterial thrombosis and embolism, PE
		IV: 250 000 units into each occluded limb of the cannula over 25–35 min and clamped for 2 hr followed by aspiration of the infusion cannula with saline and reconnection of the cannula	Arteriovenous cannula occlusion

DVT, deep vein thrombosis; *PE,* pulmonary embolism.

category C. For the commonly recommended dosages, see the table above.

PHARMACOKINETICS

Half-Life	Onset	Peak	Duration
5 min	Unknown	Varies with dose	Unknown

▸▸ *streptokinase*

SK is the oldest thrombolytic agent, the one produced from beta-hemolytic streptococci. It binds with plasminogen, and this SK–plasminogen complex then acts on other plasminogen molecules to form plasmin. As mentioned previously, SK is not clot specific. Because it is made from a non-human source, it is antigenic and may provoke allergic reactions. This happens because the body's immune system recognizes it as a foreign substance (an antigen) and launches an antibody against it, resulting in an antigen–antibody reaction. These antibodies develop approximately 5 days after SK therapy and persist for 6 months to 1 year. It is recommended that clients not be retreated with SK or APSAC during this period. Hypotension secondary to vasodilation occurs in approximately 10 percent to 15 percent of clients given SK. SK is contraindicated in clients with a known hypersensitivity to it, in clients who have recently undergone surgery, and those with active internal bleeding, aneurysm, uncontrolled hypotension, intracranial or intraspinal neoplasm, and trauma. It is available only in parenteral form in doses of 250 000, 750 000, and 1 500 000 IU per vial. Pregnancy category C. For the commonly recommended dosages, see the table above.

PHARMACOKINETICS

Half-Life	Onset	Peak	Duration
18 min, then 83 min	1 hr	Varies with dose	24–36 hr

NURSING PROCESS

A variety of conditions warrant the use of coagulation modifiers. These conditions range from venous or arterial thromboembolism to vessel injury, and any of the coagulation modifiers, such as heparin, warfarin, ASA, dipyridamole, and streptokinase, may be required for treatment. These agents with their different mechanisms of action and indications require some specific nursing processes and are addressed as a drug class and as specific drugs.

■ Assessment

The nursing assessment of clients receiving anticoagulants and other blood clotting–altering drugs requires astute assessment of
- Medical history
- Family history
- Dieting and changes in body weight over time
- Exercise habits
- Employment activities
- Success with previous medication and treatment regimens
- Parameters such as BP, pulse, respirations, body weight, and height
- Laboratory values for lipoprotein fractionation, triglyceride levels, and cholesterol levels
- All medications
- Signs and symptoms such as chest pain, difficulty breathing, altered circulation, and poor circulation in lower extremities

■ *Heparin*

Assessment of the client is essential to safe and efficient use of heparin. It is important to obtain a prior medical and medication history, including any hypersensitivity reactions, such as reactions to benzyl alcohol, which is present in heparin sodium preparations. Contraindications include severe thrombocytopenia, bleeding, and active and/or uncontrollable GI bleeding. Other conditions in which there is a risk of hemorrhage, such as severe hypertension, ulcer disease, ulcerative colitis, aneurysms, malignant hypertension, alcoholism, and head injuries, are also contraindications. Heparin should not be used if it will not be possible to monitor closely the client's condition and laboratory values. Caution should be used when administering this drug to women who are pregnant or breastfeeding. (Note: If a drug is needed for its anticoagulant effects during pregnancy then heparin is used, not warfarin sodium). Extreme caution is necessary when heparin is used in clients undergoing major surgery or in clients receiving any other agents that may precipitate bleeding, such as those listed in Table 27-1. Other cautions include bacterial endocarditis, heparin resistance, and women over the age of 60 years. It is *crucial* to client safety that nurses remember that heparin is NOT interchangeable unit for unit with LMWH and that it is a pregnancy category C drug. Drug interactions include other agents that may potentiate the effects of heparin such as other anticoagulants, antiplatelets, and any other drug that decreases clotting or increases bleeding, such as NSAIDs and ASA. The herbs ginkgo and ginseng may affect blood coagulation and are considered drug interactions. Heparin's effects are antagonized by digitalis, tetracyclines, nicotine, and antihistamines.

LMWHs

Although their use leads to fewer adverse reactions in some clients and scenarios, LMWHs still have contraindications and cautions. Dalteparin, enoxaparin, and other LMWHs such as tinzaparin are not recommended for children as their safety and efficacy have not been established. They are contraindicated in clients with active bleeding, unstable angina, thrombocytopenia, and an allergy to heparin and/or pork. Cautious use is recommended in clients with epidural catheters and/or spinal anaesthesia. Other cautions include renal or hepatic defects, retinopathy, GI bleeding, pregnancy, lactation, and platelet dysfunction. Drug interactions include oral anticoagulants, antiplatelets, and thrombolytics. LMWHs also contain sulphites and/or benzyl alcohol; therefore allergies to these need to be assessed.

Warfarin

Warfarin sodium should not be used in clients under the age of 18 years or in clients with a history of abnormal or GI bleeding, hemorrhagic conditions, malignant hypertension, blood dyscrasias, psychosis, or senile dementia. It also should not be used in unsupervised clients with alcoholism, in uncooperative clients, or during pregnancy and lactation. Other contraindications include surgery to the eye, CNS and/or traumatic surgery, and regional or lumbar block anaesthesia. Cautious use is recommended in geriatric or debilitated clients and in clients with renal or liver diseases, diabetes, hypertension, heart failure,

edema, hyperlipidemia, thyroid disorders, cancer, vasculitis, fever, dental procedures, and allergic disorders in general. Drug interactions include: hepatic enzyme inhibitors, NSAIDs, ASA, and any other type of drug that alters clotting, such as the thrombolytics. Warfarin sodium's effects are potentiated by other highly protein-bound drugs, acetaminophen, antibiotics, hepatic enzyme inhibitors, anabolic steroids, flu vaccines, vitamin K deficits, thyroid disorders, polycythemia vera (an abnormal increase in red blood cells), and collagen vascular disease. Warfarin sodium should be withdrawn with dental procedures and if there is tissue necrosis, gangrene, diarrhea, intestinal flora imbalances, and steatorrhea (large amounts of fat in feces).

Antiplatelet Drugs

A nursing assessment should be performed before initiation of therapy. Possible drug interactions include anticoagulants and antiplatelet agents or any agent altering platelet function. Contraindications and cautions for the use of these drugs are similar to those for other classes of coagulation modifiers. Thrombolytics are contraindicated with active internal bleeding, severe uncontrolled hypertension, and recent stroke. Baseline vital signs and related clotting laboratory studies (thrombin time, prothrombin time [PT], APTT, Hct, and platelet counts) should be monitored.

Antifibrinolytic Agents

Clients receiving desmopressin or aminocaproic acid, as well as any blood-altering or clotting-altering drugs, should have vital signs and appropriate laboratory values assessed. Aminocaproic acid is *not* to be used when there is evidence of intravascular clotting, postpartum bleeding, disseminated intravascular coagulation (DIC), new burns, and upper urinary tract bleeding, or if there is uncertainty as to whether the bleeding is from primary fibrinolysis or DIC. Cautious use is recommended in clients with upper urinary tract bleeding, hematuria, and other bleeding disorders. Desmopressin is contraindicated in clients with hypersensitivity to it and those with nephrogenic diabetes insipidus. Cautious use is recommended in clients receiving lithium, heparin, or large doses of epinephrine and with alcoholic beverages. Drug interactions include concurrent use of oral contraceptives and other blood clotting–altering drugs such as NSAIDs, ASA, and antiplatelet agents.

Thrombolytics

Alteplase and other thrombolytics are contraindicated in the presence of active internal bleeding, history of stroke, cerebral neoplasms, arteriovenous malformation, aneurysm, known bleeding disorders, severe uncontrolled hypertension, and intracranial or intraspinal surgery or trauma within the past 2 months. Cautious use is recommended in the presence of internal bleeding, superficial or surface bleeding (such as venous cutdown sites, arterial punctures), intramuscular injections, concomitant use of heparin, history of stroke, blood clotting defects, liver dysfunction, diabetic "hemorrhagic" retinopathies or other eye-related hemorrhagic disorders, pericarditis, cerebrovascular disease, organ biopsy, and major surgery within the past 10 days. Drug interactions include other clotting-related drugs, heparin, vitamin K antagonists, and platelet-altering drugs such as ASA or dipyridamole.

■ *Antiplatelet Drugs*

Eptifibatide, tirofiban, and abciximab are drugs within a new drug classification group termed *GP IIb/IIIa inhibitors.* Commonly used for thromboprevention during acute episodes of unstable angina or MI and during interventional cardiac procedures such as PTCA, they are preg-

nancy category B drugs. Contraindications include a history of bleeding disorders or active abnormal bleeding within the past 30 days, severe hypertension, major surgery within the past 6 weeks, history of stroke within the past 30 days, any hemorrhagic event or stroke, renal dialysis, or allergy to any of the drug's components. Cautious use is recommended in those with renal dysfunction, platelet counts less than 100×10^9/L (because these drugs are inhibitors to platelet aggregation), bleeding disorders and sites of bleeding, thrombocytopenia, and with geriatric clients. Drug interactions include other drugs in the same category, thrombolytics, anticoagulants, and other antiplatelet drugs.

Dipyridamole and dipyridamole in combination with ASA as antiplatelet drugs are contraindicated in clients with ASA or NSAID allergies, clotting disorders, or bleeding disorders; in children or teenagers with viral infections; and in the third trimester of pregnancy. ASA is contraindicated in clients with any bleeding disorder, in children younger than 16 years of age, in children with flu-like symptoms, in pregnant or lactating women, and in clients with a vitamin K deficiency or peptic ulcer disease. Cautious use is recommended in clients with a history of asthma, peptic ulcer disease, bleeding disorders, severe coronary artery disease, liver or renal dysfunction, or hypotension. Caution is recommended during lactation and pregnancy (dipyridamole is pregnancy category B; ASA is pregnancy category D). Drug interactions include any drug that increases the risk of GI bleeding such as alcohol and NSAIDs, anticoagulants, warfarin, oral hypoglycemics, methotrexate, ACE inhibitors, beta-blockers, uricosurics, phenytoin, valproic acid, and other anticonvulsants. ASA regimens and Ecotrin are used for their antiplatelet activity; therefore this information applies to these drugs as well. Several drugs interact with ASA (see Table 27-3). With use of the antiplatelet agents baseline vital signs need to be determined in all clients. It is important for the nurse to monitor lying and standing BPs because of the orthostatic hypotension these agents may precipitate.

Clopidogrel, ticlopidine HCl, and pentoxifylline are used as platelet aggregation inhibitors and are contraindicated in clients with blood disorders, neutropenia, thrombocytopenia, history of thrombocytopenic purpura (TTP), active bleeding disorders, and severe liver disorders. Cautious use is recommended in clients with neutropenia, other blood-related changes, disorders with bleeding risks (peptic ulcer disease), or hyperlipidemic disorders, and in those who take hyperlipidemic drugs. Cautious use also recommended during pregnancy (category B) and lactation. In addition, these drugs should be discontinued 10 to 14 days before surgery. Drug interactions include all agents discussed with the antiplatelet drugs plus antacids, cimetidine, digoxin, and drugs metabolized by CYP450 (including many of the benzodiazepines, most calcium channel blockers, HIV protease inhibitors, HMG-CoA-reductase inhibitors, cisapride, and most antihistamines).

Nursing Diagnoses

Nursing diagnoses that pertain to clients receiving anticoagulants include the following:

- Ineffective tissue perfusion related to the clotting disorder or thrombus formation.
- Impaired physical mobility related to tissue injury or decreased tissue perfusion from coagulation disorders.
- Risk for injury related to possible adverse reactions to any of the drugs that alter blood clotting.
- Acute pain related to symptoms of underlying disorder or ischemia.
- Deficient knowledge related to new medication regimen and need for altered lifestyle.
- Activity intolerance related to underlying tissue disorder or ischemia.

Planning

Goals for the client receiving anticoagulants include the following:

- Client experiences increased comfort and relief of pain.
- Client exhibits improved blood flow as the result of the therapeutic effects of the anticoagulants.
- Client remains free from injury stemming from either the disease or the medication.
- Client is adherent with the lifestyle changes required and with the medication therapy.
- Client demonstrates adequate knowledge regarding medication therapy and its potential side effects.

Outcome Criteria

Outcome criteria pertaining to the use of anticoagulants include the following:

- Client experiences relief of symptoms such as decreased pain, swelling, and edema once tissue perfusion is regained as the result of medication therapy.
- Client shows improved circulation with warm extremities or strong pedal pulses or experiences a return to pre-disease state of tissue perfusion.
- Client is free of bruising, bleeding problems, or any other adverse reaction to the medication.
- Client states the rationale for the use of the medication regimen, such as decreased clotting or clot formation.

- Client states the nature of and rationale for the lifestyle changes needed, such as improved diet, exercise, and no smoking.
- Client states the side effects, how to monitor for complications of the anticoagulants, the importance of coming in for follow-up appointments with the physician and of frequent laboratory studies, and when to contact the physician to prevent complications such as hemorrhage.

Implementation

Vital signs are routinely monitored in all clients during both the initiation and maintenance of anticoagulant therapy. Various laboratory values should also be monitored (see Table 27-7 for the laboratory values for drugs that alter clotting). The physician should be notified immediately of any change in pulse rate or rhythm, BP, or level of consciousness, or any unexplained restlessness. These changes may indicate bleeding or hemorrhage.

Knowledge of the proper techniques of administration is crucial for the safe and effective use of any of the clotting-altering drugs. With heparin, a "second check" by a registered nurse is required to ensure the "5 Rights": right drug, right dose, right route, right time, and right client. Heparin injections should be given only subcutaneously or intravenously, *not* intramuscularly. Inadvertent intramuscular injection can be avoided if the nurse uses only subcutaneous syringes that have a ½-inch needle. (No major harm would result from a subcutaneous dose inadvertently being given intravenously, but it is important for the nurse to prevent intramuscular heparin injection.) Subcutaneous sites of injection include areas of deep subcutaneous fat, such as the fatty layer of the abdomen 5 cm away from the umbilicus or the area near the iliac crest. Sites need to be rotated. Subcutaneous injections should not be given within 5 cm of abdominal incision areas or unhealed wounds, and they should not be aspirated because of the risk for hematoma formation. Massage of subcutaneous sites should be avoided. Box 27-1 lists the procedure for subcutaneous heparin administration.

When rapid anticoagulation is needed, the physician generally orders intravenous heparin, either by continuous or intermittent infusion. During continuous intravenous heparin infusion, blood levels may be maintained

TABLE 27-7

LABORATORY VALUES FOR DRUGS THAT ALTER CLOTTING

Laboratory Study	Normal Value	Indications
APTT	24–36 sec; therapeutic range is 1½–2 × normal; 36–72 range would indicate that the heparin is working.	To monitor effectiveness of heparin and monitor therapeutic vs. toxic blood levels
PT	Pre-treatment levels are 10–14 sec. This used to be reported in ratio with the longer ratio representing effective treatment. Now it is reported in terms of an INR with a desired range of 2–3, and in some clients warrant a range of 3–4.5 is preferred. With warfarin, INRs cannot be altered quickly.	To monitor effectiveness of warfarin and monitor therapeutic vs. toxic blood levels

APTT, Activated partial thromboplastin time; *PT,* prothrombin time; *INR,* international normalized ratio.

BOX 27-1

Subcutaneous Heparin Administration

- After thoroughly checking the physician's order, assess the client for the existence of any allergies, contraindications, or cautions.
- Wash your hands thoroughly. Check the heparin bottle for the proper dilution of the agent, the expiration date, and the clarity of the solution. Using a tuberculin syringe, especially for small doses, draw up the exact dose of heparin. Always double-check with another registered nurse to ensure the right dose. Replace the needle with a new sterile ½-inch, 26- to 28-gauge needle to ensure adequate sharpness and to avoid residue.
- Check the client's identification band to make sure you have the correct client.
- Put on disposable gloves and select the injection site outside a 5-cm area around the umbilicus. Although the abdominal area or the area around the iliac crest is the preferred site of injection, any of the subcutaneous sites may be used. Always check where previous injections have been administered so that you can rotate the sites appropriately.
- Cleanse the site thoroughly with antiseptic but be careful not to massage or rub the site before or after the injection. Let the antiseptic dry before giving the injection.
- Grasp the subcutaneous tissue firmly to form a fat pad, then quickly insert the needle at a 90-degree angle. *Do not aspirate*, and be careful not to pinch the skin. Release the skin gently, and slowly inject the heparin. Count for 10 seconds, then withdraw the needle without changing its angle. Press a sterile 5 × 5-cm gauze pad or sponge over the area and maintain gentle but firm pressure for 10 seconds. *Be careful not to massage, rub, or traumatize the skin.*
- Check the site for bleeding or bruising and document the site, time, dose, and any other pertinent information on the client's chart and/or medication record. Make sure your client is comfortable, then remove your gloves and wash your hands.

BOX 27-2

Intravenous Heparin Administration

- For the continuous intravenous administration of heparin, an intravenous pump must be used to ensure a steady and precise rate of infusion.
- Always double-check the physician's order for the dose, rate, time, and route before initiating therapy. Generally, about a 6- to 12-hour supply is ordered.
- No other medication should be administered with the heparin or through the heparin line.
- For intermittent infusions, a heparin lock was used in years past. Now in most institutions heparin locks are called *intermittent infusion locks* and they are generally flushed with NS. Some institutions still use heparin locks and administer 10–100 units of heparin per millilitre of a flushing solution.
- Intermittent infusions of heparin are usually ordered to be given every 4–6 hours because of heparin's short half-life. The drug should be infused slowly and given either undiluted or diluted with 50–100 mL of isotonic saline solution, though the latter practice is preferred.
- Guidelines for intermittent infusions include injection through the lock after cleansing the diaphragm with 70 percent alcohol and using a 25- to 27-gauge needle, which helps the diaphragm to reseal after repeated injections.
- Regardless of whether the injection is given through an intravenous pump or by intermittent or continuous intravenous infusion, it is crucial to always check the site to determine whether infiltration has occurred to prevent a hematoma from forming there. Should this occur, the lock should be removed and replaced in a new site before the next scheduled infusion. Document your actions appropriately in the nurse's notes.

and monitored by daily laboratory studies, and the effects can be easily reversed with the intravenous administration of protamine sulphate. Protamine sulphate can also reverse subcutaneous heparin, but several doses may be needed because the rate of absorption of subcutaneous forms varies. See Box 27-2 for the procedure for the intermittent or continuous intravenous administration of heparin. In addition, various dosages of heparin are available in Tubex forms or multi-dose vials, ranging from 5000 units up to 10 000 units.

Currently LMWHs are used in high-risk clients (thromboembolic events). These new agents, such as enoxaparin, have a more predictable anticoagulant response. They may also be given by subcutaneous injection in the abdominal area using the same techniques as with heparin. Like heparin, the LMWHs are often used as

prophylaxis for post-operative thrombus formation; for post-hip replacement or surgery; or in clients at a high risk for thromboembolitis, such as those with malignancies. They are administered subcutaneously, and some forms are preservative-free. Rotation of sites is recommended for both heparin and the LMWHs when given subcutaneously.

When oral anticoagulants such as warfarin sodium are prescribed, therapy is often initiated while dosing with heparin and continued until the PTs indicate an adequate therapeutic response. This overlap in dosing is necessary because the full therapeutic effect of oral anticoagulants does not appear until 4 to 5 days after the first dose. The administration procedures for the oral anticoagulants are outlined in Box 27-3. For conversion from heparin to an oral anticoagulant such as warfarin sodium, the dose of the oral drug should be the usual initial amount and thereafter the PT should be determined at the usual intervals. To ensure continuous therapeutic anticoagulation coverage it is generally recommended that heparin therapy be continued at the full dosage (for the particular client and situation) for several days (sometimes 3 to 5 days) while initiating oral anticoagulant therapy and

BOX 27-3
Oral Anticoagulant Administration

- Recheck the physician's orders and the client's medication and medical history before administering the agent. Always check to make sure the client has no known hypersensitivity to the agent.
- Many more drugs can interact with oral anticoagulants than with heparin, especially those that are highly protein bound such as the ones listed in Table 27-3. Always check the client's medication list before initiating therapy with warfarin sodium.
- The dose of the medication is calculated on the basis of the client's clotting values.
- Administer oral anticoagulants at the same time every day to maintain steady blood levels.
- Document the dose, time of administration, and any other pertinent facts.

allowing for the onset of therapeutic effects with the oral drug. Heparin is then discontinued without tapering.

Client education is a vital part of the nursing care plan for clients receiving anticoagulants. Not only do clients need to understand the reason they are receiving anticoagulants, but they also need to understand the importance of laboratory testing to monitor the therapeutic, side, and toxic effects of these drugs. Should uncontrolled bleeding occur, the nurse must institute emergency measures to stabilize the client's condition. Laboratory values should be reported to the physician. The antidote to hemorrhage or uncontrolled bleeding resulting from heparin and to reverse effects of LMWH therapy is protamine sulphate. The antidote to oral anticoagulant (warfarin sodium) therapy is vitamin K, which may be administered intravenously, intramuscularly, or orally.

Concerns about and teaching tips for antiplatelet drugs, platelet aggregation inhibitors, and antifibrinolytics are the same as those for anticoagulants. These drugs should be administered as ordered and taken exactly as prescribed, with no omission of doses. Clients should watch for drug–drug and drug–food interactions and they should contact their healthcare provider should bleeding occur while on the medication. It is important for the nurse to monitor vital signs, laboratory values for liver and renal function, and clotting studies to prevent possible adverse reactions. It is also important for the nurse to remind clients taking any clotting-altering drug that they need to carefully check the ingredients of any natural health or over-the-counter (OTC) products they are taking for possible interactions. Capsicum pepper, feverfew, garlic, ginger, ginkgo, and ginseng have potential interactions, especially to warfarin. Clients should avoid activities that pose a risk for injury to prevent bleeding that may occur in the tissue. Also, clients should be monitored for possible infection and bleeding resulting from the side effects of neutropenia and agranulocytosis.

Safe and effective treatment with antiplatelet agents requires that the nurse have an adequate knowledge about these agents, including knowledge of the drug interactions that can occur and the lifestyle changes the client must make, such as the following:

- For maximal absorption, dipyridamole should be taken either on an empty stomach or 1 hour before or 2 hours after meals. ASA should be taken 30 minutes before or 2 hours after meals to minimize GI upset.
- Clients taking these agents should quit smoking because the vasoconstriction induced by the nicotine alters the therapeutic effectiveness of the drug.
- ASA and other antiplatelets interfere with the results of certain laboratory tests, such as coagulation studies, liver function tests, serum uric acid levels, and serum potassium and cholesterol levels.
- With clopidogrel, clients need to be aware of the adverse reactions that must be reported immediately to their healthcare provider, such as respiratory difficulty, back pain, skin rash, GI bleeding, bleeding disorders, diarrhea, acute severe headache, or change in vision (blurred vision or loss of vision).
- Clients must be continually cautious about abnormal bleeding and watch for bleeding from a specific site (e.g., hematemesis, hematuria) or any abnormal amount.
- Before administering aminocaproic acid intravenously, check the rate of infusion and dilutional factor because too rapid infusion may result in bradycardia or hypotension.
- Desmopressin should be infused intravenously over 15 to 30 minutes for doses of 0.3 mg/kg. Intranasal dosage forms should be administered exactly as ordered.

Nursing considerations related to thrombolytics are similar for these agents. Specifically, their intravenous administration should be prepared per manufacturer guidelines and per protocol. Intravenous infusion sites should be monitored frequently for bleeding, redness, and pain. Intramuscular injections are contraindicated with the use of these agents. Any bleeding from gums or mucous membranes or the occurrence of epistaxis and increased pulse (>100 beats/min) should be reported to the physician immediately. All vital signs should be monitored frequently as well. Other nursing considerations include monitoring for decreased BP and restlessness, which should be reported to the physician immediately. Clients should be instructed to report pink, red, or cloudy urine; black, tarry stools or frank red blood in the stools; abdominal or chest pain; dizziness; or severe headache. Reconstitution of intravenous streptokinase should be done slowly with 5 mL NaCl or D5W. This should be rolled gently and not shaken.

Client teaching tips for the anticoagulant agents are listed in the box on p. 475.

■ Evaluation

Monitoring for the therapeutic and adverse effects of clotting-altering drugs is crucial for their safe use. Because these drugs are used for a variety of purposes, therapeutic responses vary. Some of the therapeutic effects include decreased chest pain and a decrease in dizziness and other neurological symptoms. Adverse effects of these drugs include elevated BP, headache, hematoma formation, irritation and pain at the injection site, hemorrhage, thrombocytopenia, shortness of breath, chills, and fever. Early signs of drug overdose for any of the clotting-altering drugs include bleeding gums while brushing teeth, unexplained nosebleeds or bruising, and heavier-than-usual menstrual bleeding. Abdominal pain, back pain, bloody or tarry stools, bloody urine, constipation, blood in the sputum, severe or continuous headaches, and the vomiting of frank red blood or a "coffee ground" substance (old blood) are all indications of internal bleeding. The adverse effects of ASA use include GI upset or bleeding, heartburn, headache, hepatitis, thrombocytopenia, agranulocytosis, leukopenia, neutropenia, hemolytic anemia, prolonged PT, tinnitus, hearing loss, rapid pulse, wheezing, hypoglycemia, hyponatremia, and hypokalemia. Adverse effects of dipyridamole use include postural hypotension, headache, weakness, syncope, GI upset, rash, flushing of the face, and dizziness. It is necessary to continually monitor liver, renal, and clotting function with laboratory studies in clients on long-term ASA therapy. It is also critical to the safe care of clients receiving these medications that the nurse reassess, monitor and document the client's response to the treatment. Continuous monitoring of the client for signs of internal or external bleeding is of utmost importance both during the initiation of therapy and during ongoing therapy.

CASE STUDY

Heparin Therapy

In the past 2 years, Mr. L., a 56-year-old lawyer, has suffered three episodes of deep vein thrombosis (DVT). All occurred without complications and all were treated successfully with anticoagulant therapy and bedrest. He now arrives at the urgent care centre because of increased pain and swelling in his left calf that has lasted for the past 3 days. Initially he is given 5000 units of heparin. On admission to the hospital for anticoagulant therapy he is started on a continuous infusion of 25 000 units of heparin in 1000 mL of 0.9 percent sodium chloride, to be run at 850 units/hour.
• Calculate how many millilitres of solution will be infused per hour.
• What nursing actions should be implemented to ensure the accuracy and safety of the continuous heparin infusion?
• What client findings would indicate a therapeutic response to the heparin therapy?
• If Mr. L. suddenly complains of numbness and tingling in his lower extremities with accompanying changes in muscle strength and sensation 12 hr after the initiation and continuation of heparin therapy, what would be the most appropriate nursing action(s) to implement?

For answers see http://evolve.elsevier.com/Lilley/pharmacology/.

Therapeutic effects of clopidogrel and ticlopidine include a decrease in the occurrence of clotting events such as transient ischemic attacks (TIAs) and strokes. Side effects for which to monitor with these agents include increased bleeding tendencies, flu-like symptoms, headache, fatigue, chest pain, and epistaxis.

Therapeutic levels of anticoagulants and other clotting-altering drugs are also monitored by laboratory tests. The standard tests for determining the effects of heparin therapy are the clotting times, measured through Lee-White whole blood clotting time, whole blood activated partial thromboplastin time (WBAPTT), or APTT, with the latter most commonly used.

Dosage of heparin is considered to be adequate when the APTT is 1.5 to 2 times normal or WBAPTT is elevated 2.5 to 3 times the control value. A whole blood clotting time of 2.5 to 3 times the control value indicates that therapeutic levels have been reached. With intravenous heparin administration, especially continuous intravenous infusions, coagulation studies should be performed every 4 hours. PTs are used to determine the dose of warfarin sodium. Prothrombin times are determined daily in clients just starting warfarin sodium therapy until a value of 1.5 to 2.5 times the normal control value is reached, which indicates a therapeutic effect. Once the level of the particular agent stabilizes, the times may be determined at 1- to 4-week intervals depending on the client's response and physical condition. The international normalized ratio (INR) is a standardized system of reporting PT based on a reference calibration model and calculated by comparing the client's PT with a control value. When using the INR to monitor anticoagulant therapy, it should be maintained between 2.0 and 3.0 regardless of the actual PT in seconds. An INR of 2–2.5 is usually desirable for short term prophylactic treatment of deep vein thrombosis (DVT); an INR of 2–3 is desirable for prophylactic treatment for hip surgery and treatment of DVT and pulmonary embolism (PE); an INR of 3-4.5 is indicated for treatment of recurrent DVT and PE and long-term treatment of clients with prosthetic heart valves.

Should a heparin overdose occur, the antidote is protamine sulphate, given intravenously over 1 to 3 minutes. Vitamin K, or phytonadione, is the antidote to oral anticoagulant overdose and can be given intramuscularly, subcutaneously, intravenously, or orally, depending on the client's condition.

Because of the complexity and life-threatening nature of the conditions for which anticoagulants and clotting-altering drugs are used, the nurse must continually reassess and monitor the client's response to the treatment and document the response accordingly. Continuous monitoring for the signs and symptoms of internal or external bleeding is crucial during both the initiation and maintenance of therapy. Therapeutic effects of antifibrinolytics include the arrest of oozing of blood from a surgical site or a decrease in blood loss. In addition, desmopressin may result in control or prevention of polyuria, polydipsia, and dehydration in clients with diabetes insipidus.

CLIENT TEACHING TIPS

The nurse should instruct the client as follows:

▲ Report any abnormal bleeding, such as nosebleeds, excessive bleeding from cuts or wounds, excessive menstrual bleeding, or any unusual bleeding from anywhere on the body. Also report severe headache; blurred vision; blood-tinged urine, vomit, or mucus; red, dark brown, or black stools; dizziness; fever; muscular or limb weakness; or rash.

▲ If you have any bleeding, apply pressure to the site immediately. If the bleeding continues after 10 minutes, call your physician.

▲ Avoid intramuscular injections, brushing with a hard-bristled toothbrush, shaving with a straight razor, or engaging in any activity that could cut or bruise you. Be careful when shaving, trimming your nails, gardening, and participating in rough or contact sports. Your physician may prefer you to avoid such activities altogether. Take care to avoid hazardous activities until you are stabilized on your therapy.

▲ Take your medication exactly as prescribed. If you miss a dose, don't double up on the next one. If you miss a dose and aren't sure what to do, call your physician.

▲ Carry or wear a medical alert bracelet or tag and carry information in your wallet naming your disorder and the medication you are taking.

▲ Inform your dentist and any other physician you are seeing of the type of medication you are taking and why.

▲ Avoid eating foods high in vitamin K, such as tomatoes, dark leafy vegetables, bananas, and fish.

▲ Avoid smoking and alcohol.

▲ If you are taking ASA or salicylate products, report any of the following symptoms to your physician: decrease in urination; constant ringing in the ears; swelling of the feet, ankles, or legs; dark urine; clay-coloured stools; abdominal pain; and blurred vision or the perception of halos around objects. If a rash occurs, discontinue use and call your physician.

▲ Keep this medication out of the reach of children.

▲ This medication is not a cure and you may need to take it long term.

▲ If you are taking ticlopidine or dipyridamole, don't take ASA unless your physician tells you to do so; this combination can precipitate bleeding.

▲ Don't taking antacids with this medication. If your physician says it's okay to take antacids, space the dosing of the two at least 2 hours apart.

POINTS to REMEMBER

▼ Coagulation modifiers work by (1) preventing clot formation, (2) promoting clot formation, (3) lysing a preformed clot, or (4) reversing the action of anticoagulants.

▼ Anticoagulants, antiplatelet agents, antifibrinolytics, thrombolytics, and reversal agents are all examples of coagulation modifiers.

▼ Clot formation takes place concurrently with clot destruction. Clot destruction is governed by the fibrinolytic system; clot formation is accomplished by the coagulation pathway, which includes an extrinsic and an intrinsic pathway.

▼ Warfarin prevents clot formation by inhibiting vitamin K–dependent clotting factors (II, VII, IX, and X) and is used prophylactically to prevent clots from forming; it cannot lyse preformed clots.

▼ The degree of anticoagulation (for any of the medications) is monitored by the PT.

▼ Heparin prevents clot formation by binding to antithrombin III and by doing so turns off certain activating factors. The overall effect is to turn off the coagulation pathway and prevent clots from forming. Heparin does not lyse (break down) a clot.

▼ Antiplatelet drugs (ASA, dipyridamole, pentoxifylline, and ticlopidine) prevent clot formation by preventing platelet involvement in clot formation. All of these drugs affect normal platelet function.

▼ Antifibrinolytics prevent lysis of fibrin, thus promoting clot formation, and have the opposite effects to anticoagulants. Examples of these agents are aminocaproic acid, tranexamic acid, aprotinin, and desmopressin. These drugs work in opposition to anticoagulants, antiplatelets, and thrombolytics and are often used to arrest the oozing of blood from surgical sites such as chest tubes and to reduce blood loss post-operatively.

▼ Thrombolytics are able to break down or lyse preformed clots in blood vessels that supply the heart with blood. Examples of agents include SK and APSAC. SK is derived from group A beta-hemolytic streptococci and converts plasminogen to plasmin, which breaks down thrombi. Therapeutic effects include improved tissue perfusion, decreased chest pain, and prevention of further myocardial damage. Adverse effects include nausea, vomiting, hypotension, and bleeding.

▼ The therapeutic effects of most coagulation modifier agents include improved circulation, tissue perfusion, decreased pain, and prevention of further tissue damage. Before using any of these agents it is important for the nurse to perform a thorough physical assessment and record findings, as well as monitor any pertinent laboratory values.

▼ Clients should be monitored for bleeding from all orifices as well as for easy bruising.

EXAMINATION REVIEW QUESTIONS

1 Which of the following would be of most concern in a client taking oral warfarin?
   a. Nausea and vomiting
   b. Diaphoretic reactions
   c. Prolonged bleeding times
   d. Increased urine output
2 Which of the following is contraindicated with warfarin therapy?
   a. Vitamin A
   b. Acetaminophen
   c. Codeine sulphate
   d. NSAIDs
3 LMWHs are not to be administered in which of the following?
   a. Clients with pneumonia
   b. Clients with heat or cold intolerance
   c. Pediatric clients
   d. Clients with intolerance to oral warfarin
4 The effects of warfarin sodium are potentiated by which of the following?
   a. Vitamin C
   b. Low-degree, protein-bound drugs
   c. Potassium sulphate
   d. Anabolic steroids
5 Platelet counts of less than 100×10^9/L reflect which of the following?
   a. Anti-inflammatory effects of the antiplatelet drugs
   b. The need for caution and further assessment of the client
   c. The need for more antiplatelet drugs
   d. Anti-autoimmune activity

For answers see http://evolve.elsevier.com/Lilley/pharmacology/.

CRITICAL THINKING ACTIVITIES

1 Mrs. P. is a 69-year-old woman who has just had hip replacement surgery. Her orthopedic surgeon has prescribed 5000 units of subcutaneous heparin to be given bid for 7 days because she is at high risk for the development of a PE. The concentration of heparin for subcutaneous injections is 2500 units/mL and it comes in a 10-mL vial. How many vials of subcutaneous heparin will be needed to complete Mrs. P.'s 7-day course of therapy?

2 There are many side effects of the anticoagulant heparin. One of your clients has been on intravenous heparin for 72 hours. She is complaining of numbness and tingling of the extremities and fell when you got her out of bed, an activity she had no trouble with 6 hours earlier. What would your first action be and why? What other data would you collect on this client?

3 Explain the rationale for a client to receive warfarin and heparin.

For answers see http://evolve.elsevier.com/Lilley/pharmacology/.

BIBLIOGRAPHY

Albanese, J., & Nutz, P. (2005). *Mosby's 2005 nursing drug cards*. St Louis, MO: Mosby.

Ageno, W., & Turpie, G.G. (2002). New advances in the management of acute coronary syndromes: 4. Low molecular-weight heparins. *Canadian Medical Association Journal, 166*(7), 919–924.

Anderson, P.O, Knoben, J.E., & Troutman, W.G. (2002). *Handbook of clinical drug data* (10th ed.). New York: McGraw-Hill/ Appleton & Lange.

Berne, R., & Levy, M. (2003). *Principles of physiology* (3rd ed.)., St Louis, MO: Mosby.

Boron, W.F., & Boulpaep, E.L. (2005). *Medical physiology* (2nd ed.). Philadelphia: Saunders.

Buller, C.E., & Carere, R.G. (2002). New advances in the management of acute coronary syndromes: 3. The role of catheter-based procedures. *Canadian Medical Association Journal, 166*(1), 51–61.

Canadian Pharmacists Association. (2003). *Therapeutic choices* (4th ed.). Ottawa, ON: Author.

Canadian Pharmacists Association. (2004). *Guide to drugs in Canada*. Toronto, ON: Dorling Kindersley.

Canadian Pharmacists Association. (2005). *Compendium of pharmaceuticals and specialties. The Canadian drug reference for health professionals*. Ottawa, ON: Author. [The subscription-based e-CPS is available at http://www.pharmacists.ca.]

Cheng, A., Williams, B.A., & Sivarajan, B.V. (Eds.). *The HSC handbook of pediatrics* (10th ed.). Toronto, ON: Elsevier.

DeWood, M.A., Spores, J., Notske, R., Mouser, L.T., Burroughs, R., Golden, M.S., et al. (1980). Prevalence of total coronary occlusion during the early hours of transmural myocardial infarction. *New England Journal of Medicine, 30*, 897–902.

Di Nisio, M., Middeldorp, S., & Büller, H.R. (2005). Direct thrombin inhibitors. *New England Journal of Medicine, 353*(10), 1028–1040.

Hardman, J.G., & Limbird, L.E. (2002). *Goodman and Gilman's the pharmacological basis of therapeutics* (10th ed.). New York: McGraw-Hill.

Health Canada. (2005) Drug product database (DPD). Retrieved August 14, 2005, from http://www.hc-sc.gc.ca/hpb/ drugs-dpd/

Hill, M.D., Buchan, A.M. for The Canadian Alteplase for Stroke Effectiveness Study (CASES) Investigators. (2005). Thrombolysis for acute ischemic stroke: Results of the Canadian Alteplase for Stroke Effectiveness Study. *Canadian Medical Association Journal, 172*(10), 1307–1312.

Institute for Clinical Evaluation Studies. (2002). Stenosis diagnosis. The detection and treatment for peripheral artery disease. *Informed, 8*(2), 1–2.

Katzung, B.G. (2004). *Basic and clinical pharmacology* (9th ed.). New York: McGraw-Hill.

Lacy, C.F., Armstrong, L.L., Goldman, M.P., & Lance, L.L. (2003). *Drug information handbook* (11th ed.). Hudson, OH: Lexi-Comp.

Lehne, R.A. (2004). *Pharmacology for nursing care* (5th ed.). St Louis, MO: Saunders.

Mosby. (2005). *Mosby's drug consult 2005: The comprehensive reference for generic and brand name drugs* (15th ed.). St Louis, MO: Mosby.

Skidmore-Roth, L. (2006). *Mosby's 2006 nursing drug reference* (19th ed.). St Louis, MO: Mosby.

Woods, S.L., Sivarajan Froelocher, E.S., Underhill Motzer, S., & Bridges, E.J. (2005). *Cardiac nursing* (5th ed.). Philadelphia: Lippincott Williams & Wilkins.

Antilipemic Agents

After reading this chapter, the successful student will be able to do the following:

1 Explain the nature of hyperlipidemia.

2 Discuss the different types of lipoproteins and their role in cardiovascular diseases.

3 Compare the various antilipemic agents commonly used to treat hyperlipidemia, including the rationale for treatment, mechanism of action, dosages, routes of administration, side effects, toxicity, cautions, contraindications, and associated drug interactions.

4 Develop a nursing care plan that includes all phases of the nursing process for the client receiving an antilipemic agent.

e-LEARNING ACTIVITIES

Student CD-ROM
- Review Questions: see questions 209–223
- Animations
- Medication Administration Checklists
- IV Therapy Checklists

evolve **Web site** (http://evolve.elsevier.com/Lilley/pharmacology/)
- Online Chapter Worksheet • Frequently Asked Questions
- Learning Tips and Content Updates • WebLinks • Online Appendices and Supplements • Mosby/Saunders ePharmacology Update • Access to *Mosby's Drug Consult*

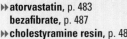

DRUG PROFILES

▸▸**atorvastatin**, p. 483
bezafibrate, p. 487
▸▸**cholestyramine resin**, p. 485
colestipol hydrochloride, p. 485

ezetimibe, p. 487
fenofibrate, p. 487
gemfibrozil, p. 487
▸▸**niacin**, p. 486

▸▸ Key drug.

GLOSSARY

Antilipemic (an′ tee li pee′ mik) A drug that reduces lipid levels.

Apolipoprotein (ap′ o lip′ o proe′ teen) The protein component of a lipoprotein.

Cholesterol (kə les′ tər ol) A fat-soluble crystalline steroid alcohol found in animal fats, oils and egg yolk and widely distributed in the body, especially in the bile, blood, brain tissue, liver, kidneys, adrenal glands, and myelin sheaths of nerve fibres.

Chylomicrons (ky′ loe my′ kronz) Minute droplets of lipoproteins; the form in which dietary fats are absorbed from the small intestine. Chylomicrons consist of about 90 percent triglycerides and small amounts of cholesterol, phospholipids, and proteins.

Exogenous lipids (ek soj′ ə nəs lip′ idz) Lipids originating outside the body or an organ (e.g., dietary fats) or produced as the result of external causes, such as a disease caused by a bacterial or viral agent foreign to the body.

Foam cells The characteristic initial lesion of atherosclerosis, also known as the *fatty streak*.

HMG–CoA reductase inhibitors A class of cholesterol-lowering drugs that work by inhibiting the rate-limiting step in cholesterol synthesis; also commonly referred to as *statins* (see *statins*).

Hypercholesterolemia (hy′ pə r kə les′ tər ol ee′ mee uh) A condition in which greater-than-normal amounts of cholesterol are present in the blood. High levels of cholesterol and other lipids may lead to the development of atherosclerosis and serious illnesses such as coronary heart disease.

Lipoproteins (lip′ oe proe′ teenz) Conjugated proteins in which lipids form an integral part of the molecule. They are synthesized primarily in the liver; contain varying amounts of triglycerides, cholesterol, phospholipids, and protein; and are classified according to their composition and density.

Statins A class of cholesterol-lowering drugs that are more formally known as *HMG–CoA reductase inhibitors*.

Triglycerides (try glis' ə rydz) A compound consisting of a fatty acid (oleic, palmitic, or stearic) and a type of alcohol known as *glycerol*. Triglycerides make up most animal and vegetable fats and are the principal lipids in the blood, where they circulate bound to a protein, forming high- and low-density lipoproteins (HDLs and LDLs).

An understanding of **antilipemic** drugs begins with an understanding of how **cholesterol** and **triglycerides** are transported and used in the human body and how lipoproteins, apolipoproteins, receptors, and enzyme systems are involved in these processes. Also essential is an understanding of the basic mechanisms underlying lipid abnormalities and the link between hyperlipidemia and coronary heart disease (CHD). Armed with this knowledge, the clinician can develop and implement a rational approach to treatment using both non-pharmacological and pharmacological interventions. Some clients also use garlic-containing dietary supplements for control of hyperlipidemia (see Natural Health Therapies box on p. 488).

LIPIDS AND LIPID ABNORMALITIES

PRIMARY FORMS OF LIPIDS

Triglycerides and cholesterol are the two primary forms of lipids in the blood. Triglycerides function as an energy source and are stored in adipose (fat) tissue. Cholesterol is primarily used to make steroid hormones, cell membranes, and bile acids. Triglycerides and cholesterol are both water-insoluble fats that must be bound to specialized lipid-carrying proteins called **apolipoproteins.** This combination of triglycerides and cholesterol with an apolipoprotein is referred to as a **lipoprotein.** Lipoproteins transport lipids via the blood. They are made up of a lipid core of triglycerides or cholesterol esters, or both, which is surrounded by a thin layer of phospholipids, apolipoproteins, and cholesterol. There are various types of lipoproteins, and they are classified according to their density and the type of apolipoproteins they contain. These various types of lipoproteins and their classification are listed in Table 28-1.

TABLE 28-1
LIPOPROTEIN CLASSIFICATION

Lipid Content	Lipoprotein Classification	Protein Content
Most ↑ ⎮ ↓ Least	Chylomicron VLDL LDL IDL HDL	Least ↑ ⎮ ↓ **Most**

VLDL, Very-low-density lipoprotein; *LDL,* low-density lipoprotein, *IDL,* intermediate-density lipoprotein; *HDL,* high-density lipoprotein.

CHOLESTEROL HOMEOSTASIS

A complex array of biochemical factors and reactions contribute to physiological (normal) cholesterol homeostasis. Figure 28-1 summarizes the major components. Fats are taken into the body through the diet and are broken down in the small intestine to form triglycerides. These triglycerides are in turn incorporated into **chylomicrons** in the cells of the intestinal wall, which are then absorbed into the lymphatic system. The primary purpose of chylomicrons is to transport lipids obtained from dietary sources **(exogenous lipids)** from the intestines to the liver to be used to make steroid hormones, lipid structural components for peripheral body cells, and bile acids.

The liver is the major organ where lipid metabolism occurs. The liver produces very-low-density lipoprotein (VLDL) from both endogenous and exogenous sources. The major role of VLDL is the transport of endogenous lipids to peripheral cells. Once VLDL is circulating, it is enzymatically cleaved by lipoprotein lipase and loses triglycerides. This creates intermediate-density lipoprotein (IDL), which is soon also cleaved by lipoprotein lipase, creating low-density lipoprotein (LDL). Cholesterol is almost all that is left in LDL after this process. Any tissues that require LDL, such as endocrine cells, possess LDL receptors. LDL and about half of IDL are reabsorbed from the circulation into the liver by means of LDL receptors on the liver.

High-density lipoprotein (HDL) is produced in the liver and intestines and is also formed when chylomicrons are broken down. Lipids that are not used by peripheral cells are transferred as cholesterol esters to HDL. HDL then transfers the cholesterol esters to IDL to be returned to the liver. HDL is responsible for the "recycling" of cholesterol. HDL is sometimes referred to as the good lipid (or "good cholesterol") because it is believed to be cardioprotective.

If the liver has an excess amount of cholesterol, the number of LDL receptors on the liver decreases, resulting in an accumulation of LDL in the blood. One explanation for **hypercholesterolemia** (cholesterol in the blood) therefore is this down-regulation (reduced production) of hepatic LDL receptors. A major function of the liver is to manufacture cholesterol, a process that requires acetyl coenzyme A (CoA) reductase. Inhibition of this enzyme thus results in decreased cholesterol production by the liver.

ATHEROSCLEROTIC PLAQUE FORMATION

Fundamental to the study of hyperlipidemia is an understanding of the processes by which lipids and lipoproteins participate in the formation of atherosclerotic plaque and subsequently the development of CHD. When serum cholesterol levels are elevated, circulating monocytes adhere to the smooth endothelial surface of the coronary vasculature. These monocytes burrow into the next layer of the blood vessel (subendothelial tissue) and change into macrophage cells, which then take up cholesterol from circulating lipoproteins until they become filled with fat. Soon they become what are known as **foam cells,** the characteristic precursor lesion of atherosclerosis, also known as the *fatty streak.* Once this process is established, it is usually present throughout the coronary and systemic circulation.

LINK BETWEEN CHOLESTEROL AND CORONARY HEART DISEASE

Numerous epidemiological trials have shown that as blood cholesterol levels increase in the members of a population, the incidence of death and disability related to CHD also increases. The risk of CHD in clients with cholesterol levels of 5.2 mmol/L is three to four times greater than that in clients with levels lower than 4.0 mmol/L. The absolute incidence of CHD in premenopausal women and women on estrogen replacement therapy is approximately 25 percent lower than in men. This is thought to be secondary to the effects of estrogen because the risk of CHD climbs considerably in postmenopausal women. There has been emerging controversy, however, regarding this long-standing belief because two recent estrogen replacement therapy (ERT) trials did not demonstrate prevention of cardiovascular events in women receiving ERT. Other experimental studies that looked for any benefits of low-dose estrogen therapy in *male* clients also did not demonstrate significant cardioprotective efficacy.

Approximately 70 000 heart attacks occur in Canada each year. In 2001 (the latest year for which statistics are available from Statistics Canada), 19 000 Canadians died from heart attacks. It is the leading cause of death for both men and women. The thrust of treatment is two-pronged: primary prevention of cardiac events in clients with risk factors and secondary prevention of subsequent cardiac events in individuals who have previously suffered a cardiac event (e.g., myocardial infarction [MI]). The benefits of primary prevention as it refers to cholesterol reduction have been illustrated in a variety of recent trials. Some of the larger and more recent trials are the Lipid Research Clinics (LRC) Coronary Primary Prevention Trial, the Helsinki Heart Study, and the West of Scotland Coronary Prevention Study (WOS). The LRC trial used the drug cholestyramine, the Helsinki study used the drug gemfibrozil, and the WOS used the hydroxymethylglutaryl (HMG)–CoA reductase inhibitor pravastatin. These studies help reinforce the belief that in clients with known risk factors for CHD, drug therapy with an antilipemic agent can reduce the occurrence of CHD. First-time heart attack and death caused by heart disease can be reduced with drug therapy.

The benefits of secondary prevention as it refers to cholesterol reduction have been illustrated in a variety of recent trials as well. Some of the larger trials are the Cholesterol Lowering Atherosclerosis Study (CLAS), the Familial Atherosclerosis Treatment Study, the Scandinavian Simvastatin

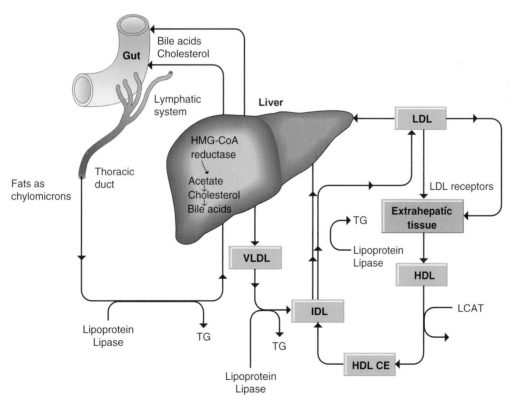

FIG. 28-1 Cholesterol homeostasis. *CE,* Cholesterol ester; *HDL,* high-density lipoprotein; *HMG-CoA,* hydroxymethylglutaryl-coenzyme A; *IDL,* intermediate-density lipoprotein; *LCAT,* lecithin cholesterol acetyltransferase; *LDL,* low-density lipoprotein; *TG,* triglyceride; *VLDL,* very-low-density lipoprotein.

Survival Study (4S trial), and the Treating to New Targets (TNT) trial (LaRosa, Grundy, Waters, & The Treating to New Targets Investigators, et al, 2005). CLAS used the drugs colestipol and niacin, the Familial Atherosclerosis Treatment Study used the drugs niacin/colestipol and lovastatin/colestipol, and the 4S trial used the drug simvastatin. The completion of the TNT trial produced evidence that the aggressive reduction of LDL levels to less than 2.2 mmol/L reduces the risk of cardiovascular events by 22 percent. These secondary prevention trials showed that in clients with documented CHD, treatment with a cholesterol-lowering drug has many positive outcomes. Three of these are decreased coronary events, regression of coronary atherosclerotic lesions, and prolonged survival.

Measures taken early in a person's life to reduce and maintain cholesterol levels in a desirable range should have a dramatic effect in terms of preventing CHD and the death and disability it causes. These include lifestyle modifications related to diet, weight, and activity level. Diets lower in saturated fat and higher in fibre and plant chemicals known as sterols and stanols and possibly the substitution of soy-based proteins for animal proteins appear to promote healthier lipid profiles. These are among the latest dietary recommendations by the third National Cholesterol Education Program Adult Treatment Panel III (NCEP ATP III) from the National Institutes of Health. The eating of fatty fish or dietary supplements containing omega-3 fatty acids appears to have beneficial effects on triglyceride and HDL levels and is currently recommended by the Heart and Stroke Foundation of Canada. The Heart and Stroke Foundation also strongly emphasizes the substantial therapeutic benefits of even modest weight reduction and exercise in both improvement of lipid profiles and reduction of the likelihood of heart disease. The Canadian Clinical Practice Guidelines for the Management of Dyslipidemia and the Prevention of Cardiovascular Disease reinforce that therapeutic lifestyle measures such as diet, exercise, smoking cessation, and weight loss along with medications are necessary to achieve target cholesterol-level goals.

HYPERLIPIDEMIAS AND TREATMENT GUIDELINES

The decision to prescribe hyperlipemic drugs as an adjunct to diet therapy in clients with an elevated cholesterol level should be based on the client's clinical profile. This includes the client's age, sex, menopausal status for women, family history, and response to dietary treatment, as well as the presence of risk factors (other than hyperlipidemia) for premature CHD and the cause, duration, and phenotypic pattern of the client's hyperlipidemia.

As mentioned earlier, major sources of guidance for antilipemic treatment at the disposal of healthcare professionals in Canada and the United States have been the Clinical Practice Guidelines for the Management of Dyslipidemia and the Prevention of Cardiovascular Disease and the U.S. National Cholesterol Education Program (NCEP). These programs have two main thrusts, both aimed at reducing the total risk of CHD in the North American population. One is focused on the entire population and consists of gen-

---

BOX 28-1

High Blood Cholesterol: Screening Risk Factors

The new recommendations state that clients of any age may be screened for dyslipidemia at the discretion of their physician, particularly when lifestyle changes are indicated. The recommendations also specifically promote screening for dyslipidemia in individuals with the following characteristics:

- Age over 40 years (for men)
- Age over 50 years (for women) or post-menopause
- Diabetes mellitus
- Risk factors such as hypertension, smoking or abdominal obesity
- A strong family history of premature cardiovascular disease
- Manifestations of hyperlipidemia, such as xanthelasma (yellowish fatty plaques under the skin), xanthoma (plaques on the eyelids) or arcus corneae (a white or grey opaque region at the edge of the cornea)
- Evidence of symptomatic or asymptomatic atherosclerosis

TABLE 28-2

TARGET LIPID LEVELS

Risk Categories and Target Lipid Levels			
		Target Level	
Risk Category	10-Year Risk	LDL-C (mmol/L)	Total Cholesterol: HDL–C ratio
High	≥20%	<2.5 *and*	<4.0
Moderate	11–19%	<3.5 *and*	<5.0
Low	≤10%	<4.5 *and*	<6.0

Note: Although specific targets for triglyceride levels are no longer recommended, the guidelines emphasize that a plasma triglyceride concentration of less than 1.7 mmol/L is optimal. Canada's target lipid levels are based on LDL-C levels. In addition, the total-cholesterol to HDL ratio is considered to be of greater importance than HDL levels alone.
HDL, high-density lipoprotein; *LDL*, low-density lipoprotein.

---

eral guidelines for the prevention of CHD. It emphasizes the appropriate dietary intake of total cholesterol and saturated fat, weight control, physical activity, and the control of other lifestyle risk factors. The other aspect is focused on the management of individual clients who are at increased risk for CHD. In these guidelines the selection of diet and drug therapy options is determined by whether certain risk factors are present. In an effort to standardize risk assessment across North America, the most recent Canadian guidelines are the first to include CHD risk equivalents. There are three levels of risk: high, intermediate, and low. These risk factors allow a physician to estimate the 10-year risk of a major coronary event (e.g., MI) for clients who do not currently have CHD. New target lipid levels are identified for those at high, intermediate, and low risk of developing CHD. These risk factors are listed in Box 28-1 and target lipid levels are given in Table 28-2. Increasingly

TABLE 28-3
TYPES OF HYPERLIPIDEMIAS

Phenotype	Lipoprotein Elevated	Lipid Composition	
		Cholesterol (mmol/L)	Triglyceride
I	Chylomicrons	>7.8	>34.2
IIa	LDL	>7.8	Normal ≅ 1.7
IIb	LDL, VLDL	>7.8	Normal ≅ 1.7
III	IDL	>10.6	>6.8 (1–3 × higher than cholesterol)
IV	VLDL	Normal or mildly elevated >6.5	>4.6
V	VLDL, chylomicrons	>7.8	>22.8

LDL, Low-density lipoprotein; VLDL, very-low-density lipoprotein; IDL, intermediate-density lipoprotein.

BOX 28-2
High Blood Cholesterol: Metabolic Risk Factors

There are now three categories of risk recognized: high, intermediate and low.
- High-risk individuals include:
  - those with established coronary artery disease, cerebrovascular disease, or peripheral arterial disease
  - those with chronic kidney disease
  - adults with diabetes
  - asymptomatic individuals in whom the 10-year risk of death from coronary artery disease or non-fatal MI is 20 percent or higher
- Intermediate-risk individuals have a 10-year risk between 11 and 19 percent
- Low-risk individuals have a 10-year risk of 10 percent or lower

BOX 28-3
The Metabolic Syndrome

- Abdominal obesity
  - Men: Waist circumference >102 cm
  - Women: Waist circumference >88 cm
- Triglyceride level ≥1.7 mmol/L
- HDL-C
  - Men: <1 mmol/L
  - Women: <1.3 mmol/L
- Blood pressure ≥130/85 mm Hg
- Fasting blood glucose level 6.2–7.0 mmol/L

recognized as a significant health issue is a cluster of cardiovascular risk factors referred to as the metabolic syndrome (see Boxes 28-2 and 28-3). Other potential risk factors include levels of apolipoprotein B, lipoprotein(a), homocysteine, and C-reactive protein.

When the decision to institute drug therapy has been made, the choice of drug should then be determined by the specific lipid profile of the client. There are five identified patterns or phenotypes of hyperlipidemia, and these are determined by the nature of the plasma (serum) concentrations of total cholesterol, triglycerides, and lipoprotein fractions (HDL, LDL, IDL, VLDL). These various types of hyperlipidemia are listed in Table 28-3. The process of characterizing a client's specific lipid profile in this way is referred to as *phenotyping*.

One of the basic tenets of the Canadian and NCEP guidelines is that all reasonable non-pharmaceutical means of controlling the blood cholesterol level (diet, exercise, etc.) should be tried for at least six months and found to fail before drug therapy is considered. However, some experts recommend that those at high risk start treatment with lipid-lowering medications as well as diet and exercise. Because drug therapy for hyperlipidemia entails a long-term commitment to the therapy, before initiation of therapy several factors should be considered: the type and magnitude of dyslipidemia, the age and lifestyle of the client, the

relative indications and contraindications of different drugs and drug categories for a given client, potential drug interactions, side effects, and the overall cost of therapy.

Four established classes of drugs are currently used to treat dyslipidemia: HMG–CoA reductase inhibitors (statins), bile acid sequestrants, the B-vitamin niacin (vitamin B3, also known as *nicotinic acid*), and the fibric acid derivatives (fibrates). In addition to all of these agents, a new medication called ezetimibe has just recently become available. It is a cholesterol absorption inhibitor.

HMG–CoA REDUCTASE INHIBITORS

The rate-limiting enzyme in cholesterol synthesis is known as HMG–CoA reductase. The class of medications that competitively inhibit this enzyme, the **HMG–CoA reductase inhibitors**, are the most potent of the drugs available for reducing plasma concentrations of LDL cholesterol and are the most prescribed drug class in Canada. Lovastatin was the first agent in this drug class to be approved for use. Since that time five other HMG–CoA reductase inhibitors have become available on the Canadian market: pravastatin, simvastatin, atorvastatin, rosuvastatin, and fluvastatin. Because of the shared suffix of their generic names, these drugs are often collectively referred to as *statins*. In August of 2001, Bayer Corporation voluntarily recalled from the market its drug cerivastatin because of increasing numbers of serious adverse effects. Medications may not achieve their maximum effect until 6 to 8 weeks after the start of therapy. Few direct comparisons of the statins have been published. However, the authors of the published account of one such study concluded that the following doses of agents would yield the same reduction in the LDL cholesterol level: simvastatin, 10 mg; pravastatin, 20 mg; and lovastatin, 20 mg. This particular study did not assess fluvastatin, rosuvastatin, or atorvastatin.

The role of HMG–CoA reductase inhibitors in lowering LDLs and the resulting cardiovascular protection is well established. However, in October 2005, Health Canada issued an advisory pointing to conflicting evidence in the current literature on the effect of statins on cognitive function. Health Canada received 19 reports of amnesia suspected of being associated with statins and recommends monitoring changes in cognitive status in clients receiving statin therapy.

Mechanism of Action and Drug Effects

Statins lower the blood cholesterol level by decreasing the rate of cholesterol production. The liver requires HMG–CoA reductase to produce cholesterol. It is the rate-limiting enzyme in the reactions needed to make cholesterol. The statins inhibit this enzyme, thereby decreasing cholesterol production. When less cholesterol is produced, the liver increases the number of LDL receptors to augment the recycling of LDL from the circulation back into the liver, where it is required for the synthesis of other needed substances such as steroids, bile acids, and cell membranes. There is also evidence that statins may have many other positive effects. They may also reduce the risk of cardiovascular events by promoting plaque stability, reducing inflammation around the plaque, reducing coro-

nary artery calcification, and suppressing the production of thrombin. Lovastatin and simvastatin are inactive drugs or pro-drugs that must be biotransformed into their active metabolites in the liver. In contrast, pravastatin is administered in its active form. Atorvastatin and fluvastatin are synthetic preparations.

Indications

The statins are still recommended as first-line drug therapy for hypercholesterolemia (elevated LDL cholesterol, or LDL-C), the most common and dangerous form of dyslipidemia. More specifically, they are indicated for the treatment of type IIa and IIb hyperlipidemia and have been shown to reduce the plasma concentrations of LDL cholesterol by 30 to 40 percent. Their cholesterol-lowering properties are dose dependent. A 10 to 30 percent decrease in the concentrations of plasma triglycerides has also been observed in clients receiving any of these drugs. Another frequent therapeutic effect of the statins is an increase of 2 to 15 percent in the HDL cholesterol level, which is known to reduce the risk of cardiovascular disease. See the Research box below for more information on statins.

These drugs also appear to be equally effective in their ability to reduce LDL cholesterol concentrations. Simvastatin and atorvastatin are more potent per milligram, although rosuvastatin is emerging as being more effective in lowering LDL-C levels and raising HDL-C levels. Atorvastatin appears to be more effective in lowering triglycerides than other HMG–CoA reductase inhibitors. Combined drug therapy with more than one class of antilipemic agents may be necessary for desired results and the statins are often combined with niacin or fibrates for this purpose, though this combination can increase the risk of adverse drug effects (see Side Effects and Adverse Effects).

Contraindications

Contraindications to the use of HMG–CoA reductase inhibitors (statins) include known drug allergy, pregnancy, and lactation. Other contraindications may include liver disease or elevation of liver enzymes.

Side Effects and Adverse Effects

The common undesirable effects of the HMGs are listed in Table 28-4. Generally speaking, however, the HMG–CoA reductase inhibitors available for clinical use have proved to be well tolerated, with significant side effects being fairly uncommon. Mild, transient gastrointestinal (GI) disturbances, rash, and headache have been the most common problems.

RESEARCH

Statin Drugs Have Positive Effects on Cardiovascular System and Hypertension

The Heart Protection Study was a multi-centre, randomized, double-blind, placebo-controlled study of some 20 000 clients ages 40 to 80 years, who had non-fasting total blood cholesterol concentrations of at least 3.5 mmol/L. Trial participants had heart disease or were likely to develop heart disease because of a pre-existing disease such as diabetes or history of stroke. A dose of 40 mg of simvastatin or placebo was administered for an average of five years. Outcomes showed major benefits of simvastatin in reducing the risks of fatal and non-fatal heart attacks and strokes as well as reducing the need for bypass surgery and angioplasty. The likelihood of stroke was reduced by 2.5 percent and the likelihood of death from coronary heart disease was reduced by 18 percent. Benefits of statin therapy were demonstrated for a range of individuals, including clients with cardiovascular disease, diabetes, and peripheral vascular disease.

These effects were found two years after initiation of medication and continued while drug therapy continued.

Source: Heart Protection Collaborative Study Group. (2002). MRC/BHF heart protection study of cholesterol lowering with simvastatin in 20 536 individuals: A randomized placebo-controlled trial. *Lancet, 360,* 7–22.

TABLE 28-4

HMG-CoA REDUCTASE INHIBITORS: ADVERSE EFFECTS

Body System	Side/Adverse Effects
Gastrointestinal	Constipation, diarrhea, heartburn, nausea/vomiting, flatulence, taste perversion, abdominal pain/cramps
Other	Dry mouth, dizziness, insomnia, headache, paraesthesia, rash/pruritus

Elevations in liver enzymes may also occur and the client should be monitored for excessive elevations, which may indicate the need for alternative drug therapy. Dose-dependent elevations in liver enzyme activity to values greater than 3 times the upper limit of normal have been noted in approximately 1 to 2 percent of clients taking HMG–CoA reductase inhibitors. The serum creatine kinase (CK) concentrations may be increased by more than 10 times the normal level in clients receiving these agents. Most of these clients have remained asymptomatic, however.

A less common but still clinically important side effect is myopathy (muscle pain), which may progress to a serious condition known as *rhabdomyolysis.* This is a condition involving the breakdown of muscle protein leading to myoglobinuria, which is the urinary elimination of the muscle protein myoglobin, the oxygen-carrying pigment of muscle tissue that is similar to a single subunit of hemoglobin (Hgb). This abnormal urinary excretion of protein can place a severe strain on the kidneys, possibly leading to acute renal failure and even death. This myopathy is uncommon (0.1–0.2 percent) during monotherapy for dyslipidemia with statins alone, but it appears to be dose dependent and is more common in clients receiving a statin in combination with cyclosporine, niacin, gemfibrozil (a fibrate), or erythromycin. Clients receiving statin therapy should be advised to report immediately to their healthcare provider any unexplained muscular pain or discomfort. When recognized reasonably early, rhabdomyolysis is usually reversible with discontinuation of the statin agent.

Toxicity and Management of Overdose

Limited data are available on the nature of toxicity and overdose in clients taking HMG–CoA reductase inhibitors. Treatment, if needed, is supportive and based on presenting symptoms.

Interactions

HMG–CoA reductase inhibitors should be used cautiously in clients taking oral anticoagulants. In addition, the co-administration of these drugs with fibric acid derivatives (bezafibrate, fenofibrate, gemfibrozil), or niacin has been observed to lead to the development of rhabdomyolysis in rare cases.

Dosages

For dosage information on atorvastatin, see the following drug profile. See Appendix B for some of the common brands available in Canada.

DRUG PROFILES

HMG–CoA REDUCTASE INHIBITORS (STATINS)

The HMG–CoA reductase inhibitors, or statins, are all potent inhibitors of the enzyme that catalyzes the rate-limiting step in the synthesis of cholesterol. There are currently six statins on the market in Canada: atorva-

statin, fluvastatin, lovastatin, pravastatin, rosuvastatin, and simvastatin. There are some minor differences between agents in this class of antilipemics; the most dramatic difference is that of potency. All six agents are prescription-only drugs and are contraindicated in pregnant or lactating women and in those suffering from active liver dysfunction or with elevated serum transaminase levels of unknown cause. There is little evidence to recommend one agent over another, with the exception of fluvastatin, which may be somewhat less effective than the others.

▶▶ atorvastatin

Atorvastatin has become the most commonly used agent in this class of cholesterol-lowering drugs. It is used primarily to lower total and LDL cholesterol as well as triglycerides. It is indicated for the treatment of type IIa and IIb hyperlipidemia. Atorvastatin has also been shown to raise "good cholesterol," the HDL component. All statins are generally dosed once daily, usually with the evening meal or at bedtime, thought to be the time to coincide with cholesterol synthesis. One particular advantage of atorvastatin is that it can be dosed at any time of day. The recommended dosage for atorvastatin is 10 to 80 mg daily. It is available only in tablet form in strengths of 10, 20, 40, and 80 mg. Pregnancy category X.

PHARMACOKINETICS

Half-Life	Onset	Peak	Duration
14 hr	1–2 hr	2 wk*	Unknown

*Maximum therapeutic effect.

OTHER ANTILIPEMIC AGENTS

BILE ACID SEQUESTRANTS

Bile acid sequestrants, also called *bile acid–binding resins* and *ion-exchange resins,* include cholestyramine and colestipol. Both of these agents have been used widely for more than 20 years and have been evaluated extensively in well-controlled clinical trials. They were actually the original anticholesterol prescription drugs. However, they are now considered second-line agents in most cases, except, for example, in clients intolerant of the statins. Generally these drugs lower the plasma concentrations of LDL cholesterol by 15 to 30 percent. They also increase the HDL cholesterol level by 3 to 8 percent and increase hepatic triglyceride and VLDL production, which may result in a 10 to 50 percent increase in the triglyceride level.

Mechanism of Action and Drug Effects

Bile acid resins bind and absorb bile acids, preventing the resorption of the bile acids from the small intestine. Bile acids are necessary for the absorption and entero-hepatic resorption of cholesterol. The hepatic synthesis of bile acids from cholesterol is stimulated by the depletion of the bile acid pool, resulting in a decreased pool of cholesterol in the liver. To compensate for this, both cholesterol biosynthesis and the number of high-affinity LDL receptors expressed on the liver's surface are increased, resulting in an increased rate of LDL catabolism (increased removal of LDL from the bloodstream). In this way the bile acid sequestrants lower the plasma LDL levels by enhancing the efficiency of the receptor-mediated removal of LDL from plasma. The result of ion-exchange resin binding to bile acids is an insoluble resin–bile acid complex that is excreted in the feces.

Indications

Bile acid sequestrants are used as adjuncts in the management of type II hyperlipoproteinemia. In addition, cholestyramine is used to relieve the pruritus associated with partial biliary obstruction.

Contraindications

Contraindications to the use of bile acid sequestrants include known drug allergy, bowel obstruction, and complete biliary obstruction.

Side Effects and Adverse Effects

The adverse effects of colestipol and cholestyramine are similar; constipation is a common problem and may be accompanied by abdominal discomfort, heartburn, nausea, flatulence, and bloating. These adverse effects tend to disappear over time, however. Many clients require extra education and support to help them deal with the GI effects and adhere with the medication regimen. It is important that therapy is initiated with low doses and clients instructed to take the drugs with meals to reduce the side effects. Constipation and bloating may be relieved by increasing the dietary fibre intake or taking a fibre supplement such as psyllium (Metamucil and others),

as well as increasing fluid intake. These drugs may also cause mild increases in the triglyceride levels as well as bleeding tendencies due to vitamin K deficiency. The most common side effects and adverse effects of the bile acid sequestrants are listed in Table 28-5.

Toxicity and Management of Overdose

Because the bile acid sequestrants are not absorbed, an overdose could cause obstruction of the GI tract. Therefore treatment of an overdose involves restoring gut motility.

Interactions

The significant drug interactions associated with the use of bile acid sequestrants are limited to the absorption of concurrently administered drugs. All drugs should be taken at least 1 hour before or 4 to 6 hours after the

TABLE 28-5

BILE ACID SEQUESTRANTS: POTENTIAL ADVERSE EFFECTS

Body System	Side/Adverse Effects
Central nervous	Headache, anxiety, vertigo, dizziness, tinnitus, syncope, blurred vision, night blindness, fatigue, drowsiness, paraesthesia
Gastrointestinal	Constipation, cramps, diarrhea, nausea/vomiting, abdominal discomfort, flatulence, rectal bleeding, hemorrhoidal bleeding, sour taste
Renal	Hematuria, dysuria, burnt odour of urine, diuresis
Other	Myalgia, skin rashes, weight loss or gain, edema, increased libido, swollen glands, dental caries

DOSAGES   Selected Antilipemic Agents

Agent	Pharmacological Class	Usual Dosage Range	Indications
▸▸ atorvastatin	HMG–CoA reductase inhibitor	**Adult** PO: 10–80 mg/day	
▸▸ cholestyramine	Antilipemic ion-exchange resin	**Adult** PO: Powder, 4 g 1–6 ×/day	
bezafibrate	Fibric acid derivative	**Adult** PO: 400 mg/day	
colestipol hydrochloride	Antilipemic ion-exchange resin	**Adult** PO: Granules: 5–30 g/day once or in divided doses; tabs: 2–16 g/day	Hyperlipidemia
ezetimibe	Cholesterol absorption inhibitor	**Adult** PO: 10 mg 1 ×/day	
fenofibrate	Fibric acid derivative	**Adult** PO: 67 mg/day initial dose; max 200 mg/day	
gemfibrozil	Fibric acid derivative	**Adult** PO: 600 mg bid 30 min ac in A.M. and P.M.	
simvastatin	HMG–CoA reductase inhibitor	**Adult** PO: 10–40 mg/day; max 80 mg/day	

administration of ion-exchange resins. In addition, high doses of a bile acid sequestrant will decrease the absorption of fat-soluble vitamins (A, D, E, and K).

Dosages

For dosage information on cholestyramine and colestipol hydrochloride, see the table on p. 484. See Appendix B for some of the common brands available in Canada.

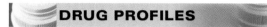

DRUG PROFILES

BILE ACID SEQUESTRANTS

The bile acid sequestrants cholestyramine and colestipol are indicated for the treatment of type IIa and IIb hyperlipidemia. They lower the cholesterol level, in particular the LDL cholesterol level, by increasing the destruction of LDL. However, their use may result in increases in the VLDL cholesterol level. Because of the high incidence of GI side effects in clients taking these agents, adherence with the prescribed dosage schedules is often poor. However, educating clients about the purpose and expected side effects of therapy can improve adherence. Clients must be warned not to take bile acid sequestrants concurrently with other drugs because the drug interactions can be pronounced. Other drugs must be taken at other times of the day. This caution cannot be overemphasized.

▸▸ cholestyramine

Cholestyramine is a prescription-only drug that is contraindicated in clients with a known hypersensitivity to it and in those suffering from complete biliary obstruction. It may interfere with the distribution of the proper amounts of fat-soluble vitamins to the fetus or nursing infant of pregnant or nursing women taking the agent. It is therefore classified as pregnancy category C. The drug is available only in oral (PO) form as 4- and 9-g packets of powder to be taken as an oral suspension. The recommended dosages are given in the table on p. 484.

colestipol hydrochloride

Colestipol hydrochloride is a prescription-only drug. It is contraindicated in clients who have shown a hypersensitivity reaction to it and in those suffering from complete biliary obstruction. It may interfere with the distribution of the proper amounts of fat-soluble vitamins to the fetus or nursing infant of pregnant or nursing women taking the agent. This drug is available in 5-g packets or 1-g film-coated tablets. Pregnancy category B. The recommended dosages of colestipol are given in the table on p. 484.

NIACIN

Niacin, or nicotinic acid, is not only a unique lipid-lowering agent, it is also a vitamin—specifically, vitamin B_3. Much larger doses are required to achieve its lipid-lowering properties than are commonly given when it is used as a vitamin. It is an effective and inexpensive medication that exerts favourable effects on the plasma concentrations of all lipoproteins. Niacin is often given in combination with other antilipemic drugs to enhance the lipid-lowering effects.

Mechanism of Action and Drug Effects

Although the exact mechanism of action of niacin is unknown, the beneficial effects are believed to be related to its ability to inhibit lipolysis in adipose tissue, decrease esterification of triglycerides in the liver, and increase the activity of lipoprotein lipase. The drug effects of niacin are primarily limited to its ability to reduce the metabolism or catabolism of cholesterol and triglycerides. Niacin decreases the LDL levels moderately (10 to 20 percent), decreases the triglyceride levels (20 to 30 percent), decreases cholesterol levels (10 to 15 percent), and increases the HDL levels moderately (20 to 35 percent). Niacin is also a vitamin needed for many bodily processes. In large doses it may produce vasodilation that is limited to the cutaneous vessels. This effect seems to be induced by prostaglandins. Niacin also causes the release of histamine, resulting in an increase in gastric motility and acid secretion. Niacin may also stimulate the fibrinolytic system to break down fibrin clots.

Indications

Niacin has been shown to be effective in lowering lipid levels. This includes triglyceride, total serum cholesterol, and LDL cholesterol levels. It also brings about an increase in the HDL cholesterol levels. Niacin may also lower the lipoprotein (a) level, except in clients with severe hypertriglyceridemia. It has been shown to be effective in the treatment of types IIa, IIb, III, IV, and V hyperlipidemia.

Niacin's effects on triglyceride levels begin to be noticed after 1 to 4 days of therapy, with the decrease in the levels ranging from 20 to 30 percent. The decline in the LDL levels is less, with the maximum decrease ranging from 10 to 15 percent. The maximum effects of niacin are seen after 3 to 5 weeks of continuous therapy.

Contraindications

Contraindications to the use of niacin include known drug allergy and may include liver disease, hypertension, peptic ulcer, and any active hemorrhagic process.

Side Effects and Adverse Effects

Niacin can cause flushing, pruritus, and GI distress. Small doses of aspirin or non-steroidal anti-inflammatory drugs (NSAIDs) may be taken 30 minutes before niacin to minimize the cutaneous flushing. These undesirable effects can also be minimized by starting clients on a low initial dosage and increasing it gradually and by having clients take the drug with meals. The most common side effects and adverse effects associated with niacin therapy are listed in Table 28-6.

Interactions

The major drug interactions associated with niacin are minimal. Niacin reportedly potentiates the hypotensive effects of ganglionic blockers (discussed in Chapter 24). In addition, when niacin is taken concomitantly with an

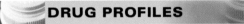

TABLE 28-6
NICOTINIC ACID: POTENTIAL ADVERSE EFFECTS

Body System	Side/Adverse Effects
Gastrointestinal	Abdominal discomfort, nausea, vomiting, bloating, flatulence, heartburn, diarrhea; GI distress
Integumentary	Cutaneous flushing, rash, pruritus, hyperpigmentation
Other	Blurred vision, glucose intolerance, hyperuricemia, dry eyes (rare), hepatotoxicity

GI, Gastrointestinal.

HMG–CoA reductase inhibitor, the likelihood of myopathy developing is greatly increased.

Dosages

For dosage information on niacin, see the following drug profile for this agent. See Appendix B for some of the common brands available in Canada.

DRUG PROFILES

▸▸ niacin (nicotinic acid, vitamin B₃)

Used alone or in combination with other lipid-lowering drugs, niacin is an effective, inexpensive medication that, as previously mentioned, has beneficial effects on LDL cholesterol, triglyceride, and HDL cholesterol levels. Drug therapy with niacin is usually initiated at a small daily dose taken with or after meals to minimize the side effects previously discussed. Liver dysfunction has been observed in individuals taking sustained-release (SR) forms of niacin, not immediate-release (IR) dosage forms. However, newer extended-release (ER) dosage forms, which dissolve more slowly than the IR forms but faster than the SR forms, appear to have even better side effect profiles, including less hepatotoxicity and flushing of the skin. Niacin is contraindicated in clients who have shown a hypersensitivity to it, in those with peptic ulcer, gallbladder disease, hepatic disease, hemorrhage, or severe hypotension, and in lactating women. It is also not recommended for clients with gout. Niacin can also elevate blood glucose levels in clients with diabetes so insulin and oral antidiabetic dosages may need adjustment. Niacin is available over the counter (OTC) as regular 50- and 500-mg tablets and in a flush-free formulation of 500-mg tablets. It is available by prescription as 500-, 750-, and 1000-mg ER tablets (Niaspan). Pregnancy category C. Niacin is commonly given in 2 to 4 divided doses of 1.5 to 6 g/day.

PHARMACOKINETICS

Half-Life	Onset	Peak	Duration
20–60 min	Unknown	30–70 min	Unknown

FIBRIC ACID DERIVATIVES

Until recently clofibrate and gemfibrozil were the only two fibric acid antilipemics approved for clinical use in Canada. Fenofibrate and bezafibrate have since been added to this drug class, and clofibrate is now no longer available in Canada. These agents primarily affect the triglyceride levels but may also lower the total cholesterol and LDL cholesterol levels and raise the HDL cholesterol level. They are often collectively referred to as *fibrates*.

Mechanism of Action and Drug Effects

Fibric acid agents are believed to work by activating lipoprotein lipase, an enzyme responsible for the breakdown of cholesterol. This enzyme usually cleaves off a triglyceride molecule from VLDL or LDL, leaving behind lipoproteins. Fibric acid derivatives can also suppress the release of free fatty acid from adipose tissue, inhibit the synthesis of triglycerides in the liver, and increase the secretion of cholesterol into bile. Fibric acid derivatives have been shown to reduce triglyceride levels. They have also been shown to reduce serum VLDL and LDL concentrations. Independent of their lipid-lowering actions, fibric acid derivatives can also induce changes in blood coagulation. This involves a tendency for them to decrease platelet adhesiveness. They can also increase plasma fibrinolysis, the process that causes fibrin—and therefore clots—to be broken down.

Indications

The fibric acid derivatives bezafibrate, gemfibrozil, and fenofibrate all decrease the triglyceride levels and increase the HDL cholesterol level by as much as 25 percent. Both decrease the LDL concentrations in clients with type IIa and IIb hyperlipidemia but increase the LDL levels in clients with type IV and V hyperlipidemia. They are indicated for the treatment of type III, IV, and V hyperlipidemia, and in some cases the type IIb form, though other classes of antilipemics are usually attempted first.

Contraindications

Contraindications to the use of fibrates include known drug allergy and may include severe liver or kidney disease, cirrhosis, or gallbladder disease.

Side Effects and Adverse Effects

As a class, the most common adverse effects of the fibric acid derivatives are abdominal discomfort, diarrhea, nausea, headache, blurred vision, increased risk of gallstones, and prolonged prothrombin time. Liver function tests may also show increased function. The more common side effects and adverse effects are listed in Table 28-7.

Toxicity and Management of Overdose

The management of fibrate overdose, which is uncommon, is supportive care based on presenting symptoms.

Interactions

Gemfibrozil and bezafibrate can enhance the action of oral anticoagulants, thus also necessitating careful dose adjustments of these latter agents. When it is given in conjunction with an HMG–CoA reductase inhibitor, the risk for myositis, myalgia, and rhabdomyolysis is increased.

TABLE 28-7
FIBRIC ACID DERIVATIVES: POTENTIAL ADVERSE EFFECTS

Body System	Side/Adverse Effects
Gastrointestinal	Nausea, flatulence, dyspepsia, abdominal pain, diarrhea, constipation, gallstones
Genitourinary	Impotence
Other	Drowsiness, dizziness, rash, erythema, pruritus, alopecia (pattern baldness), decreased libido, eczema, blurred vision, vertigo, headache

Clients taking gemfibrozil may have altered laboratory results, including a decrease in the Hgb level, hematocrit (Hct) value, and white blood cell count. These usually stabilize with long-term administration. In addition, bilirubin levels can be increased. Clofibrate may increase AST, alanine aminotransferase (ALT), alkaline phosphatase, CK, and LDH, which return to normal when the drug is discontinued.

Dosages

For dosage information on bezafibrate, gemfibrozil and fenofibrate, see the table on p. 484. See Appendix B for some of the common brands available in Canada.

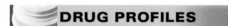 **DRUG PROFILES**

FIBRIC ACID DERIVATIVES (FIBRATES)

The fibric acid derivatives bezafibrate, gemfibrozil, and fenofibrate are prescription-only drugs. They are pregnancy category C agents and are contraindicated in clients with hypersensitivity, pre-existing gallbladder disease, significant hepatic or renal dysfunction, and primary biliary cirrhosis. These agents decrease the triglyceride and to a lesser extent the LDL levels and increase the HDL levels by as much as 25 percent. They are good agents for the treatment of mixed hyperlipidemia.

bezafibrate

Bezafibrate, a fibric acid derivative, decreases LDL and VLDL levels and increases the HDL levels. In the 5-year double-blind, placebo-controlled Bezafibrate Coronary Atherosclerosis Intervention Trial (BECAIT; Ericsson et al, 1997), bezafibrate was effective in slowing or preventing the progression of atherosclerosis in post-infarction clients under 45 years of age. Bezafibrate is contraindicated in those with a known hypersensitivity to it. Pregnancy category C. Bezafibrate is available as a 400-mg sustained release tablet to be taken once daily with the main meal. The recommended dose is given in the table on p. 484.

PHARMACOKINETICS

Half-Life	Onset	Peak	Duration
1–2 hr	Unknown	3–4 hr	Unknown

fenofibrate

Fenofibrate, a fibric acid derivative structurally similar to the now discontinued drug clofibrate, has been approved by Health Canada for treatment of hypertriglyceridemia. The new micronized form is more rapidly and completely absorbed, especially when taken with food. It may be easier to take than gemfibrozil because of smaller tablet size and may have more favourable effects on LDL cholesterol; however, more direct comparisons are needed. Fenofibrate is contraindicated in clients with a known hypersensitivity to it. Fenofibrate is currently available as 100- and 200-mg micro-coated tablets; 67-, 100-, and 200-mg gelatin capsules; and 67- and 200-mg micronized capsules. Pregnancy category C. Recommended dosages are given in the table on p. 484.

PHARMACOKINETICS

Half-Life	Onset	Peak	Duration
20 hr	Unknown	6–8 hr	Unknown

gemfibrozil

Gemfibrozil is a fibric acid derivative that decreases the synthesis of apolipoprotein B (Apo B) and lowers the VLDL level. It can also increase the HDL level and lower the LDL level. In addition, it is highly effective for lowering plasma triglyceride levels and total cholesterol. In a large trial, the Helsinki study, the triglyceride levels of the group receiving gemfibrozil were reduced by as much as 43 percent compared with the control group. The total cholesterol and LDL levels were reduced by 11 percent and 10 percent, respectively, and the HDL level was increased by 10 percent. Gemfibrozil is indicated for the treatment of extremely high triglyceride levels, type IV and V hyperlipidemia and the type IIa and IIb mixed hyperlipidemia. Gemfibrozil is available only in oral form as a 300-mg gelatin capsule and a 600-mg film-coated tablet. Pregnancy category C. The specific dosing recommendations are given in the table on p. 484.

PHARMACOKINETICS

Half-Life	Onset	Peak	Duration
1.3–1.5 hr	Unknown	1–2 hr	Unknown

CHOLESTEROL ABSORPTION INHIBITOR
ezetimibe

Ezetimibe is currently the only member of a brand new class of drugs used to treat dyslipidemia, having been approved by Health Canada in 2003. It is so new that much remains to be learned about the drug and its clinical benefits. Ezetimibe has a novel mechanism of action in that it selectively inhibits absorption in the small intestine of cholesterol and related sterols. The result is a reduction in several blood lipid parameters: total cholesterol, LDL cholesterol (LDL-C), Apo B, and triglycerides. However, the serum level of HDL cholesterol (HDL-C), the so-called "good cholesterol," has been shown to actually increase with the use of ezetimibe. These beneficial effects thus far appear to be further enhanced when ezetimibe is taken with a statin agent, though ezetimibe may be used as monotherapy. In several small studies ezetimibe was not shown to interact significantly with cimetidine, warfarin, digoxin, oral contraceptives, glipizide, or antacids. However, fibric acid derivatives (fibrates) have been shown to significantly increase the serum levels of ezetimibe. It is not yet known whether this is harmful, but at the present time concurrent use of ezetimibe with fibrates is not recommended. The use of ezetimibe with bile acid sequestrants has been shown thus far to reduce the serum level of ezetimibe by 55 percent and 80 percent in two small studies. Concurrent use of these two types of agents it not yet contraindicated, but it should be recognized that the extent of LDL reduction normally promoted by ezetimibe is likely to be reduced with this drug combination. Ezetimibe does not yet have a pregnancy category, but the manufacturer recommends following the guidelines for the use of statins, which are all contraindicated in pregnancy. Ezetimibe is contraindicated in cases of demonstrated allergy to the drug, active liver disease or unexplained elevations in serum liver enzymes. The drug is currently available only as a 10-mg tablet for once-daily dosing. It may be taken with or without food and for client convenience may be dosed at the same time as a statin agent if prescribed.

PHARMACOKINETICS

Half-Life	Onset	Peak	Duration
22 hr	Unknown	4–12 hr	Unknown

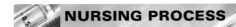

NURSING PROCESS

■ Assessment

Before initiating antilipemic therapy in a client, the nurse should obtain a thorough health and medication history, including any OTC drugs, natural health products, and prescription drugs. Hypersensitivity to any of these drugs is also important to document. It is important for the nurse to assess the client's dietary patterns, exercise program and

NATURAL HEALTH THERAPIES

GARLIC (*allium sativum*)

Overview
Garlic obtains its pharmacological effects from the active ingredient allinin.

Common Uses
Antispasmodic, antiseptic, antibacterial and antiviral, antihypertensive, antiplatelet, lipid-lowering

Adverse Effects
Dermatitis, vomiting, diarrhea, anorexia, flatulence, antiplatelet activity

Potential Drug Interactions
May inhibit iodine uptake, warfarin, diazepam, and protease inhibitors

Contraindications
Contraindicated in clients about to undergo surgery within 2 weeks and in clients with HIV or diabetes

frequency, weight, height, and vital signs, and use of tobacco, alcohol, or social drugs. Food intake should be documented over several weeks. A thorough family history should be taken, since some of the lipid disorders are hereditary. Risk factors for CHD include the following:
- Age (male 45 years old or older; female 55 years old or older)
- Smoking
- HDL levels of 0.9 mmol/L or lower
- Diabetes mellitus
- Family history of premature CHD

RESEARCH

Antilipemic Therapy and Related Cautions

The use of HMG–CoA reductase inhibitors, a class of antilipemics also known as *statins,* is contraindicated in clients with active liver disease or unexplained elevated serum transaminase and in pregnant or lactating women, and cautious use is required in any client with altered liver function. Should liver function studies become elevated during therapy with HMG–CoA reductase inhibitors (e.g., simvastatin), immediate intervention is needed. The physician should be contacted. A decrease in dose or change in drug therapy is the usual recommendation. It is well documented in the current pharmacological literature that these types of antilipemics are associated with dose-dependent elevations in liver enzymes up to three times the upper normal limit, although the client may remain asymptomatic. A clinically important side effect is myopathy (muscle pain), which may lead to a serious condition known as *rhabdomyolysis.* This condition involves the actual breakdown of the muscle protein myoglobin. Myoglobin is the oxygen-carrying pigment of muscle tissue the urinary excretion of which has been found to place an unusual strain on the kidneys, with possible progression to acute renal failure or even death (Talbert, 2003; CPA, 2005). Unless this kidney damage is identified early it may be irreversible and even require dialysis. Rhabdomyolysis may occur more commonly when the drug simvastatin is given with cyclosporin, niacin, gemfibrozil (another antilipemic), or erythromycin. Clients taking simvastatin should know to contact their physician immediately if they experience any unexplained muscular pain or discomfort because, if recognized early, rhabdomyolysis may be reversible with discontinuation of the statin drug. Another concern for clients taking the statin antilipemics is the clinical picture portrayed, because certain liver enzymes are elevated (e.g., creatine kinase) that are also elevated in acute MI. Often the client has to be further evaluated by the physician to rule out any cardiac concerns.

Data from Talbert, R.L. (2003). Role of the National Cholesterol Education Program Adult Treatment Panel III guidelines in managing dyslipidemia. *American Journal of Health-System Pharmacy.* 60(Suppl2), S3–S8; Lehne, R.A. (2004). *Pharmacology for nursing care* (5th ed.). St Louis, MO: Saunders; and Canadian Pharmacists Association. (2005). *Compendium of pharmaceuticals and specialties. The Canadian drug reference for health professionals.* Ottawa, ON: Author; and http://www.mosbysdrugconsult.com

Generally speaking, contraindications to the use of antilipemics include hypersensitivity, biliary obstruction, liver dysfunction, and active liver or gallbladder disease. Cautious use is indicated in children and in pregnant or lactating women. Major drug interactions may occur with other antilipemics, insulin, oral antidiabetic agents, oral anticoagulants, and any drugs with activity or adverse effects in the liver.

Any antilipemic must be discontinued if elevated serum transaminase, myopathy, or rhabdomyolysis develops. See the Research box on p. 488 for more information on these drugs.

HMG–CoA reductase inhibitors (the statins) must not be used in clients under 10 years of age. Contraindications include liver dysfunction, unexplained elevated serum transaminase (unexplained elevations of liver function studies), pregnancy, and lactation. Cautious use is recommended with altered liver function, elevated AST or ALT, and substantial alcohol consumption (because of the impact of alcohol on the liver, with the risk of cirrhosis).

Drug interactions for the statins include erythromycin; the calcium channel blockers diltiazem, digoxin, warfarin, cimetidine, ketoconazole, clarithromycin (discontinue these drugs if simvastatin must be used); other CYP3A4 inhibitors (this includes human immunodeficiency virus [HIV] protease inhibitors, particularly ritonavir, nefazodone, and grapefruit juice); fibric acid derivatives bezafibrate, fenofibrate, and gemfibrozil; niacin (if these drugs *must* be used, then the antilipemic may be discontinued or the dosage decreased); itraconazole and cyclosporin.

Bile acid sequestrants are contraindicated in those clients under the age of 18 years and in those with liver dysfunction, jaundice, and GI obstruction. Cautious use includes triglycerides above 7.7 mmol/L; susceptibility to deficiencies in vitamins A, D, E, and K (fat soluble vitamins); GI motility disorders; and pregnancy and lactation (these are pregnancy category B drugs). Some other cautions include constipation, secondary causes of hyperlipidemia such as hypothyroidism, and hemorrhoids. Drug interactions include thiazides, furosemide, tetracycline, penicillin G, gemfibrozil, digitalis, and propranolol.

Niacin is contraindicated in active peptic ulcer disease or bleeding. It is not to be used in clients under the age of 21 years. Cautions, in addition to those listed previously, include hepatobiliary disease, jaundice, renal dysfunction, cardiovascular disease, gout, surgery, diabetes, pregnancy, and lactation. Drug interactions include other products containing alcohol, nitrates, antihypertensive agents, vasoactive drugs, HMG–CoA reductase inhibitors (may precipitate higher risk for rhabdomyolysis), CCBs, anticoagulants, and antidiabetic agents.

Fibric acid derivatives, such as fenofibrate, are contraindicated in children and in clients with hepatic dysfunction, renal disease, and gallbladder disease. Cautious use is recommended in clients with any type of GI, hepatic, or biliary dysfunctions. In addition, the client's complete blood count (CBC) and liver function levels must be monitored closely for the first year. Should ab-

normalities in liver function studies (such as ALT, CK) occur, the antilipemic drug should be discontinued.

Nursing Diagnoses

Nursing diagnoses in the client receiving an antilipemic agent include the following:

- Imbalanced nutrition, more than body requirements, related to poor dietary habits of high fat intake.
- Deficient knowledge related to a lack of knowledge about the disease and related complications
- Deficient knowledge related to a lack of understanding of drug therapy and the need for lifestyle changes.
- Impaired home maintenance related to lack of experience with lifestyle changes and unfamiliar medication therapy.

Planning

Goals for the client receiving antilipemics include the following:

- Client remains adherent with both non-pharmacological and pharmacological therapy.
- Client remains free of the complications associated with antilipemics because of appropriate use of the drug.
- Client sees physician regularly and as indicated for the treatment of hyperlipidemia and to repeat laboratory studies.

Outcome Criteria

Outcome criteria related to the administration of antilipemics include the following:

- Client states the importance of pharmacological and non-pharmacological therapy to his or her overall health and safety, such as for decreasing the risk of CHD.
- Client states the rationale of therapy as well as its side effects and expected therapeutic effects (i.e., decreasing lipid levels, GI side effects, and therapeutic response of improved lipid profile).
- Client states conditions of which the physician should be notified, such as jaundice and abdominal pain.
- Client states the importance of follow-up care with the physician to monitor for changes in liver function studies as well as the lipid levels.

Implementation

Clients who are taking antilipemics for a long period may have altered levels of the fat-soluble vitamins and may then require supplementation of vitamins A, D, and K. Antilipemics may also cause problems with the liver and biliary systems, and they may cause GI tract problems such as constipation. To avoid or minimize constipation, clients should increase fibre and fluids. Blood levels should be monitored per the healthcare provider's instructions; serum transaminase and other serum liver function studies are especially important. HMG–CoA reductase inhibitors (statin drugs) should not be discontinued abruptly or without contacting the healthcare provider. These drugs should be stored away from heat and moisture and should be taken with meals. Clients need to inform other healthcare providers, including dentists, that they are taking these medications.

Bile acid sequestrants such as cholestyramine and colestipol come in powder form and should be mixed thoroughly with fruit (e.g., crushed pineapple) or other food or fluids (at least 120 to 180 mL of fluid). The powder may not mix completely at first, but clients should be sure to mix the dose as much as possible and then dilute any undissolved portion with additional fluid. The powder should be dissolved for at least 1 full minute without stirring. (Stirring is not recommended with most powders because it causes them to clump.) Powder and/or granule dosage forms are *never* to be taken dry.

It is important that colestipol be taken 1 hour before or 4 to 6 hours after any other oral medication and/or meals because of the high risk for drug–drug or drug–food interactions. Cholestyramine should be taken just before or with meals. Clients with phenylketonuria must not take the cholestyramine "Questran Light" because it contains aspartame.

To prevent injuries from falls, clients should be encouraged to change positions slowly and to lie down should they get dizzy (from orthostatic changes). Also, they should know to contact their healthcare provider immediately should their stools appear black and tarry.

The nurse should advise clients that niacin may lead to flushing of the face. Postural hypotensive side effects demand that the client change positions slowly and with caution, as well as lie down should dizziness or syncope occur. Many antilipemics take weeks to reach therapeutic levels. When the HMG–CoA reductase inhibitors atorvastatin, fluvastatin, lovastatin, pravastatin, and simvastatin are prescribed to be taken once a day they should be administered in the evening.

Client teaching tips for each classification are listed in the box below.

■ **Evaluation**

Clients receiving an antilipemic agent need to be monitored for therapeutic and side effects during their therapy. The therapeutic effects of both non-pharmacological and pharmacological measures would be evidenced by a decrease in cholesterol and triglyceride levels. The non-pharmacological measures include a low-fat, low-cholesterol diet; supervised moderate exercise; weight loss; cessation of smoking and drinking; and relaxation therapy. If there is no response to pharmacological therapy after about 3 months, then the medication is generally withdrawn. Fenofibrate may be increased at 4- to 8-week intervals depending on the triglyceride levels. Adverse effects for which to monitor include GI upset, dyspepsia, increased liver enzyme levels, hepatomegaly (enlarged liver), flatulence, weight gain, cholelithiasis (gallstones), rash, fatigue, leukopenia, anemia, bleeding, dizziness, decreased libido, erectile dysfunction, hematuria, myalgia, angina, and pulmonary emboli. Clients should also be closely monitored for the development of liver or renal dysfunction.

CLIENT TEACHING TIPS

The nurse should instruct the client as follows:

▲ Take your medication as ordered; do not change dosing without the physician's approval.

▲ Do not stop taking these medications without the physician's approval.

▲ Follow recommendations on diet and nutrition. (If this has not been provided, the nurse should arrange for counselling.) This is an important part of your therapy.

▲ Eat less animal fat and red meat.

▲ Eat lots of raw vegetables, fruit, and bran and drink at least 2 L of fluids a day. This will help prevent the constipation that this medication sometimes causes; it will also help lower your cholesterol levels.

▲ If your physician has given approval, get moderate daily exercise.

▲ If your medication comes in a powder, take it with liquid. Mix thoroughly but do not stir.

▲ Notify your physician if you have any new or troublesome symptoms; persistent upset stomach, constipation, gas, bloating, heartburn, nausea, or vomiting; abnormal or unusual bleeding; or yellowish skin. Also report decreased sex drive, erectile dysfunction, and difficulty urinating.

▲ Keep this medication out of the reach of children.

▲ If you take oral contraceptives, check with your physician about possible drug interactions.

▲ Make sure you know when to take your medication (some medications are best taken with meals; others must not be taken with meals). Once-a-day medications are often best taken with the evening meal.

▲ Check with your physician before taking any other medication. This includes herbal products; some of these can interact with your medications.

POINTS to REMEMBER

- There are two primary forms of lipids: triglycerides and cholesterol.
- Triglycerides function as an energy source and are stored in adipose (fat) tissue.
- Cholesterol is used primarily to make steroid hormones, cell membranes, and bile acids.
- Lipoproteins transport lipids via the blood.
- Lipids and lipoproteins participate in the formation of atherosclerotic plaque, which leads to CHD.
- Plaque forms in the blood vessels that supply the heart with needed oxygen and nutrients, eventually decreasing the lumen size of these blood vessels and reducing the amount of oxygen and nutrients that can reach the heart.
- Antilipemic drugs are used to lower the high levels of lipids within the blood (triglycerides and cholesterol).
- The major classes of antilipemics are as follows:
  - HMG–CoA reductase inhibitors
  - Bile acid sequestrants
  - Niacin
  - Fibric acid derivatives
- The mechanisms of action vary with each class and each drug.
- HMG–CoA reductase inhibitors (a newer group of antilipemics) lower blood cholesterol levels by decreasing the rate of cholesterol production and inhibiting the enzyme necessary for the liver to produce cholesterol. There are six agents in this group: lovastatin, pravastatin, simvastatin, fluvastatin, rosuvastatin, and atorvastatin.
- Contraindications to the use of antilipemics include hypersensitivity, biliary obstruction, liver dysfunction, and active liver disease.
- While taking a nursing history it is important to assess the client for any possible drug interactions with the various antilipemics, such as insulin, oral antidiabetic agents, or oral anticoagulants.
- Fat-soluble vitamins may need to be prescribed for clients taking these medications long term because the antilipemics have long-term effects on the liver's production of these vitamins.
- Powder or granule forms must be mixed with noncarbonated liquids and *never* taken dry.
- Liver and renal functions must be monitored.
- The statins have gained much attention for their side effects of muscle aches and pain due to breakdown of muscle tissue. Some clients suffer irreversible renal damage and severe pain and may have to switch dosages or drugs as ordered by their healthcare provider.

EXAMINATION REVIEW QUESTIONS

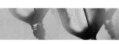

1 The statin drugs are most likely to result in which of the following?
   a. Hyperlipidemias, types IV and V
   b. Hypercholesterolemia
   c. Postural changes in pulse rates
   d. Changes in bowel function

2 Which of the following are side effects of nicotinic acid?
   a. Cutaneous flushing
   b. Low back pain
   c. Glycosuria
   d. Polycythemia

3 Which of the following points is important to emphasize to a client taking an antilipemic medication?
   a. Take with food at bedtime. If GI upset occurs, try taking Prilosec OTC.
   b. The medications elevate protein and albumin levels.

   c. It is important to report muscle pain as soon as possible.
   d. Renal toxicity is not common.

4 Which of the following is a contraindication for antilipemic medications?
   a. Diabetes insipidus
   b. Pulmonary fibrosis
   c. Liver malfunction
   d. Fatty deposits in the skin

5 Rhabdomyolysis occurs more commonly when simvastatin is given concurrently with which of the following?
   a. Amino acid derivatives
   b. Multivitamins
   c. Gemfibrozil
   d. Insulin

For answers see http://evolve.elsevier.com/Lilley/pharmacology/.

CRITICAL THINKING ACTIVITIES

1 Flushing of the face and neck may occur with the administration of nicotinic acid. What would you suggest to a client to help decrease these reactions and their unpleasantness?

2 Is the following statement true or false? Explain your answer.

Antilipemics may be safely taken without concern for other medications, especially prescribed medications, and may be discontinued abruptly.

3 Your client has just informed you that he was told that it was okay to take his colestipol powder without fluids. Are you concerned about this? Explain your answer.

For answers see http://evolve.elsevier.com/Lilley/pharmacology/.

BIBLIOGRAPHY

Albanese, J., & Nutz, P. (2005). *Mosby's 2005 nursing drug cards.* St Louis, MO: Mosby.

Anderson, P.O., Knoben, J.E., & Troutman, W.G. (2002). *Handbook of clinical drug data* (10th ed.). New York: McGraw-Hill/Appleton & Lange.

Berne, R., & Levy, M. (2002). *Principles of physiology* (3rd ed.). St Louis, MO: Mosby.

Canadian Pharmacists Association. (2003). *Therapeutic choices* (4th ed.). Ottawa, ON: Author.

Cheng, A.Y.Y., & Leiter, L.A. (2003). Clinical use of ezetimibe. *The Canadian Journal of Clinical Pharmacology, 10*(A), 21A–25A.

Collins, R., Armitage, J., Parish, S., Sleigh, P., & Peto, R. (2003). MRC/BHF Heart Protection Study of cholesterol-lowering with simvastatin in 5963 people with diabetes: A randomised placebo-controlled trial. *Lancet, 361,* 2005–2016.

Ericsson, C.G., Nilsson, J., Grip, L., Swane, B., & Hamsten, A. (1997). Effect of bezafibrate treatment over five years on coronary plaques causing 20% to 50% diameter narrowing (The Bezafibrate Coronary Atherosclerosis Intervention Trial). *American Journal of Cardiology, 80,* 1125–1129.

Expert Panel on Detection, Evaluation, and Treatment of High Blood Cholesterol in Adults (Adult Treatment Panel III): *Brief summary,* 2001, National Guideline Clearinghouse. Retrieved August 30, 2005, from http://www.guideline.gov.

Expert Panel on Detection, Evaluation, and Treatment of High Blood Cholesterol in Adults (Adult Treatment Panel III). (2002). Third Report of the National Cholesterol Education Program (NCEP) Expert Panel on Detection, Evaluation, and Treatment of High Blood Cholesterol in Adults (Adult Treatment Panel III): Final report. *Circulation 106,* 3143–3421.

Facts and Comparisons. (2004). *Drug facts and comparisons pocket version* (9th ed.). St Louis, MO: Wolters Kluwer Health.

Fung, M.A. & Frolich, J.J. (2002). Common problems in the management of hypertriglyceridemia. *Canadian Medical Association Journal, 167*(11), 1261–1266.

Genest, J., Frolich, J., Fodor, G. & McPherson, G. (The Working Group on Hyperlipidemia and other dyslipidemias). (2003). Recommendations for the management of dyslipidemia and the prevention of cardiovascular disease: 2003 update. [Electronic version]. *Canadian Medical Association Journal, 169*(9).

Heart and Stroke Foundation of Canada. (2003). *The growing burden of heart disease and stroke in Canada 2003.* Ottawa, ON: Author.

Health Canada. (2001). Warning. Voluntary withdrawal of Baycol. Retrieved August 14, 2005, from http://www.hc-sc.gc.ca/ahc-asc/media/advisories-avis/2001/2001_89_e.html

Health Canada. (2005). Statins and memory loss. *Canadian Adverse Reaction Newsletter, 15*(4). Retrieved November 13 from http://www.hc-sc.gc.ca/dhp-mps/medeff/bulletin/carn-bcei_v15n4_e.html

Heart Protection Study Collaborative Group. (2002). MRC/BHF Heart Protection Study of cholesterol lowering with simvastatin in 20 536 high-risk individuals: A randomised placebo-controlled trial. *Lancet, 360*(9326), 7–22

Hulley, S., Grady, D., Bush, T., Furberg, K., Herrington, D., Riggs, B., et al. for the Heart and Estrogen Replacement Study (HERS) Research Group. (1998). Randomized trial of estrogen plus progestin for secondary prevention of coronary heart disease in postmenopausal women. *Journal of the American Medical Association, 280,* 605–613.

Jenkins, D.J., Kendall, C.W., Marchie, A., Jenkins, A.L., Augustin, L.S., Ludwig, D.S., et al. (2003). Effects of a dietary portfolio of cholesterol-lowering foods vs. lovastatin on serum lipids and C-reactive protein. *Journal of the American Medical Association, 290,* 502–510.

Kasper, D.L., Braunwald, D., Faci, A., Hauser, S., Longo, D., & Jameson, J.L. (2005). *Harrison's principles of internal medicine* (16th ed.). New York: McGraw-Hill.

Lacy, C.F., Armstrong, L.L., Goldman, M.P., & Lance, L.L. (2003). *Drug information handbook* (11th ed.). Hudson, OH: Lexi-Comp.

LaRosa, J.C., Grundy, S.M., Waters, D.D., & The Treating to New Targets (TNT) Investigators. (2005). Intensive lipid lowering with atorvastatin in patients with stable coronary disease. *New England Journal of Medicine, 352*(14).

Merck/Schering Plough Pharmaceuticals. (2005). Zetia prescribing information. Retrieved August 15, 2005, from http://www.zetia.com/ezetimibe/zetia/hcp/index.jsp

Mosby. (2005). *Mosby's drug consult 2005: The comprehensive reference for generic and brand name drugs* (15th ed.). St Louis, MO: Mosby.

Skidmore-Roth, L. (2006). *Mosby's 2006 nursing drug reference* (19th ed.). St Louis, MO: Mosby.

Talbert, R.L. (2003). Role of the National Cholesterol Education Program Adult Treatment Panel III guidelines in managing dyslipidemia. *American Journal of Health-System Pharmacy, 60*(2), S3–S8.

Writing Group for the Women's Health Initiative Investigators. (2002). Risks and benefits of estrogen plus progestin in healthy postmenopausal women: Principal results from the Women's Health Initiative randomized controlled trial. *Journal of the American Medical Association, 288,* 321–333.

PART FIVE

Drugs Affecting the Endocrine System: Study Skills Tips

- QUESTIONING STRATEGY

QUESTIONING STRATEGY

One of the most important activities for learning is to become actively involved with the text. The best way to achieve this involvement is to develop the habit of asking questions. These questions can be generated using a number of different cues and structures that are part of the part and chapter structure. Some of what you anticipate as related material will not be correct. You will adjust your expectations as you read the material. For now focus on asking a lot of questions and making use of everything you know, which can help start the process of answering your questions.

Part Title

As you begin each new part, ask a question to focus your attention. What do all the chapters in this part have in common? In Part Five this question is: "What is the endocrine system?" This same question could be asked of Parts Two through Nine by simply replacing "endocrine" with the appropriate system for the specific part. Looking at the chapter titles in the part tells us that the endocrine system has to do with the pituitary agents, thyroid and antithyroid agents, antidiabetic agents, adrenal agents, women's health agents, and men's health agents. Although this answer is far too general to demonstrate any real understanding of the endocrine system, it is a beginning and helps keep you aware of what you need to learn from each chapter.

Chapter Titles

Chapter titles provide the first mechanism to generate questions. The first question to ask about each chapter is a basic one. What is this chapter about? That question is also answered immediately. "What is Chapter 29 about?" It is about pituitary agents.

The next question is equally obvious but also extremely important. The question to ask next is: "To what do pituitary (Chapter 29), thyroid and antithyroid (Chapter 30), antidiabetic and hypoglycemic (Chapter 31), adrenal (Chapter 32), women's health (Chapter 33), and men's health (Chapter 34) refer?" Take the chapter title and state it as a question. What do you know about these subjects?

Chapter Objectives

To enhance your study, turn each chapter objective into one or more questions. Here are some possible questions using the objectives from Chapter 31.

Objective 1

Discuss the normal actions and functions of the pancreas and the feedback system that regulates it.
- What are the normal actions and functions of the pancreas?
- What is the feedback system for the pancreas?

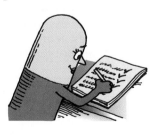

Objective 2

Contrast type 1 and type 2 diabetes mellitus.
- What is type 1 diabetes mellitus?
- What is type 2 diabetes mellitus?
- How do types 1 and 2 diabetes mellitus differ?

Since the objectives tell you what the authors expect you to know at the end of the chapter, starting out with questions based on the objectives will improve your learning and probably save you time.

Chapter Headings

The same principle can be applied to each of the topic headings set out in the chapter. Continuing to use Chapter 31 as a model, here are some samples of questions that might be useful as preparation for reading.

Type 1 Diabetes Mellitus

- What is type 1 diabetes?
- What is mellitus?

As you start to process the chapter headings, you should also notice that they begin to answer some of the questions from the chapter objectives. This is a good time to begin setting up vocabulary cards.

Mechanism of Action and Drug Effects

- What is the mechanism of action of insulin?
- Is there more than one mechanism?
- What are the most important drug effects of insulin?
- Where do these effects take place?
- What is the evidence of these effects?

The idea is to focus on the major content of the chapter and establish a guide for learning as you read.

Print Conventions Within the Body of the Chapter

Print conventions are useful in this study skills strategy. The use of *italics*, **bold,** underlining, and multiple colours of ink are examples of print conventions. They are designed to catch your attention. Use them as a basis for questions.

Chapter 31

In the first paragraph of this chapter, the first obvious print convention is the word **glucose.** It is printed in bold. If you let your eyes float down the page and do not read anything, this word stands out. It must be important.

- What is glucose?
- What is the relationship between glucose and type 1 diabetes mellitus?

There are more words on the first page of the chapter text that are in the same print style. Apply the same procedure to these terms. Also, notice that two of the terms, *glycogen* and *glycogenolysis*, must have some direct rela-

tionship, since the second term contains the first word. The basic question in each case is, "What does the term mean?" However, there should be more to your questions than just the basics. Glycogenolysis seems to mean that there is some operation or activity taking place. Ask yourself the following:

- What happens in glycogenolysis?
- Where does glycogenolysis occur?
- When does glycogenolysis occur?
- How does it relate to type 1 diabetes mellitus?

Chapter Tables

Tables serve as a summary of information discussed in the chapter. You can learn a great deal from tables if you take the time.

Look at Table 31-1. The table summarizes characteristics of type 1 and type 2 diabetes. There are two obvious questions for each type.

- What is type 1 (type 2) diabetes?
- What are its characteristics?

Use these questions to study Table 31-1 and you will find that all the information you need to respond to these questions is found here. It may be useful to make a first pass throughout the chapter focusing only on the tables before you begin to read. You will learn a great deal about some of the topics, and you will have established background information that will help you ask better questions and read with better understanding.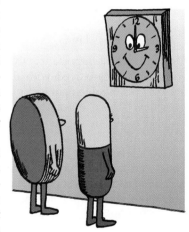

The time you spend asking questions makes the reading and learning go more quickly. Another benefit is that some of the questions you ask will appear on tests. These questions will be easy for you to answer. This promotes test-taking confidence, and better scores result in better grades. If you have not been using questioning strategy up to this point in your text, begin now. After you use the strategy for two or three chapters, you will find that the benefits far outweigh the time it takes.

Pituitary Agents

OBJECTIVES

After reading this chapter, the successful student will be able to do the following:

1 Describe the normal function of the anterior and posterior aspects of the pituitary gland.

2 Contrast the various pituitary agents in terms of their indications, mechanisms of action, side effects, cautions, contraindications, and drug interactions.

3 Develop a nursing care plan that includes all phases of the nursing process for clients receiving pituitary agents.

e-LEARNING ACTIVITIES

Student CD-ROM
- Review Questions: see questions 224–229
- Animations
- Medication Administration Checklists
- IV Therapy Checklists

evolve Web site (http://evolve.elsevier.com/Lilley/pharmacology/)
- Online Chapter Worksheet • Frequently Asked Questions
- Learning Tips and Content Updates • WebLinks • Online Appendices and Supplements • Mosby/Saunders ePharmacology Update • Access to *Mosby's Drug Consult*

DRUG PROFILES

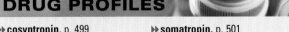

▸▸**cosyntropin**, p. 499   ▸▸**somatropin**, p. 501
desmopressin, p. 499   ▸▸**vasopressin**, p. 501
octreotide, p. 499

▸▸ Key drug.

GLOSSARY

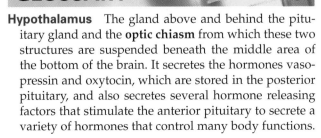

Hypothalamus   The gland above and behind the pituitary gland and the **optic chiasm** from which these two structures are suspended beneath the middle area of the bottom of the brain. It secretes the hormones vasopressin and oxytocin, which are stored in the posterior pituitary, and also secretes several hormone releasing factors that stimulate the anterior pituitary to secrete a variety of hormones that control many body functions.

Negative feedback loop   In endocrinology, a system in which the production of one hormone by its source gland is controlled by the levels of a second hormone, which is produced by a second gland after being stimulated by the hormone from the first gland. The source gland of the first hormone then reduces production of that hormone, until blood levels of the second hormone fall below a certain minimum level needed for specific hormonal effects; then the cycle begins again.

Neuroendocrine system   (nyur′ oh en′ də krən) The system that regulates the reactions of the organism to both internal and external stimuli and involves the integrated activities of the endocrine glands and nervous system.

Optic chiasm   The part of the hypothalamus formed by the crossing of optic nerve fibres from the medial half of each retina.

Pituitary gland   (pi too′ ə tare′ ee) An endocrine gland suspended beneath the brain that supplies numerous hormones that control many vital processes.

ENDOCRINE SYSTEM

The maintenance of physiological stability is the main goal of the endocrine system, and it must accomplish this task despite constant changes in the internal and external environments. Every cell, and hence organ, in the body comes under its influence. The endocrine system communicates with the nearly 50 million target cells in the body using a chemical "language" called *hormones.* These are a large group of natural substances with chemical structures that are highly specific for causing physiological effects in the cells of their target tissues. They are secreted into the bloodstream in response to the body's needs and travel through the blood to their site of action—the target cell.

For decades the pituitary gland was believed to be the master gland that regulated and controlled the other endocrine glands in this diverse system. However, this belief has been discarded in the face of strong evidence that the central nervous system (CNS), specifically the **hypothalamus**, controls the pituitary. The hypothalamus and pituitary are now viewed as functioning together as an integrated unit, with the primary direction coming from the hypothalamus. For this reason the system is now commonly referred to as the **neuroendocrine system**. In fact, the endocrine system can be considered in much the same way as the CNS. Each is basically a system for signalling, and each operates in a stimulus-and-response manner. Together these two systems essentially govern all bodily functions.

The **pituitary gland** is made up of two distinct glands—the anterior pituitary (adenohypophysis) and posterior pituitary (neurohypophysis). They are individually linked to and communicate with the hypothalamus, and each gland secretes its own different set of hormones. These various hormones are listed in Box 29-1 and shown in Figure 29-1.

Hormones are either water or lipid soluble. The water-soluble hormones are protein-based substances such as the catecholamines norepinephrine and epinephrine. The receptors for these hormones are usually located on cell membranes. These hormones bind to their receptors on the cell surface, whereupon they either directly activate the cell

---

BOX 29-1

Hormones of the Anterior and Posterior Pituitary

Anterior Pituitary Adenohypophysis
Adrenocorticotropic hormone (ACTH)
Follicle-stimulating hormone (FSH)
Growth hormone (GH)
Luteinizing hormone (LH)
Prolactin (PH)
Thyroid-stimulating hormone (TSH)

Posterior Pituitary (Neurohypophysis)
Antidiuretic hormone (ADH)
Oxytocin

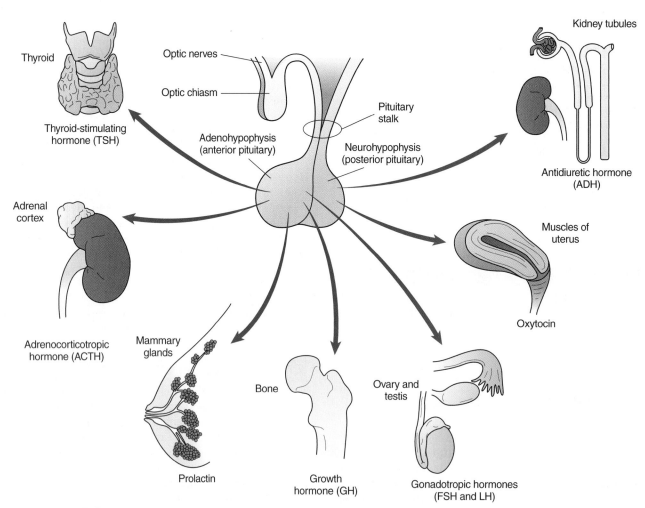

FIG. 29-1 Pituitary hormones. (From L.M. McKenry, & E. Salerno (2003). *Mosby's pharmacology in nursing—revised and updated* (21st ed.). St Louis, MO: Mosby.)

to perform a function or cause a chemical signal to be sent by means of a "second messenger" to generate an appropriate cellular response. The lipid-soluble hormones consist of the steroid and thyroid hormones. They are capable of crossing the plasma membrane through the process of simple diffusion and of binding with receptors within the cell nucleus, where they stimulate a specific cellular response.

The activity of the endocrine system is regulated by a system of surveillance and signalling usually dictated by the body's ongoing needs. Hormone secretion is commonly regulated by the **negative feedback loop.** This is best explained using a simplified example: When gland X releases hormone X, this stimulates target cells to release hormone Y. When there is an excess of hormone Y, gland X "senses" this and inhibits its release of hormone X.

PITUITARY AGENTS

A variety of drugs affect the pituitary gland. They are used as replacement therapy to make up for a hormone deficiency, as drug therapy to produce a particular hormone response in clients with hormone deficiencies, and as diagnostic aids to determine whether the client's hormonal functions are overactive or underactive. The currently identified anterior and posterior pituitary hormones and the drugs that mimic or antagonize their actions are listed in Table 29-1. Many of these hormones have been synthesized, and some of them have already been discussed in other chapters.

The anterior pituitary drugs discussed in this chapter include cosyntropin, somatropin, and octreotide; the posterior pituitary drugs discussed in this chapter are vasopressin and desmopressin.

Mechanism of Action and Drug Effects

The mechanisms of action of the various pituitary agents differ depending on the agent, but overall they either augment or antagonize the natural effects of the pituitary hormones. Exogenously administered cosyntropin elicits all of the same pharmacological responses as those elicited by the endogenous *adrenocorticotropic hormone,* or *ACTH.* Regardless of whether it is exogenous or endogenous in origin, cosyntropin travels to the adrenal cortex located just above the kidneys and stimulates the secretion of the mineralocorticoid cortisol (the drug form of which is hydrocortisone), corticosterone, several weakly androgenic (masculinizing) substances, and to a limited extent, aldosterone.

The drug that mimics growth hormone (GH) is somatropin. This agent promotes growth by stimulating various anabolic (tissue-building) processes. A drug that

TABLE 29-1
ANTERIOR AND POSTERIOR PITUITARY HORMONES AND DRUGS

Hormone	Function/Mimicking Drug
ANTERIOR PITUITARY	
Adrenocorticotropic hormone	Targets adrenal gland; mediates adaptation to physical and emotional stress and starvation; redistributes body nutrients; promotes synthesis of adrenocortical hormone (glucocorticoids, mineralocorticoids, androgens); involved in skin pigmentation.
	Cosyntropin: Diagnosis of adrenocortical insufficiency
Follicle-stimulating hormone	Stimulates oogenesis and follicular growth in females and spermatogenesis in males.
	Menotropins: Same pharmacological effects as FSH; many of the other gonadotropins also stimulate FSH (see Chapter 33).
Growth hormone	Regulates anabolic processes related to growth and adaptation to stressors; promotes skeletal and muscle growth; increases protein synthesis; increases liver glycogenolysis (convergence of glycogen to glucose); increases fat mobilization.
	Somatropin: Human GH for hypopituitary dwarfism.
	Octreotide: A synthetic polypeptide structurally and pharmacologically similar to GH release-inhibiting factor; it inhibits GH.
Luteinizing hormone	Stimulates ovulation and estrogen release by ovaries in females; stimulates interstitial cells in males to promote spermatogenesis and testosterone secretion
	Gonadotropins: Many of the agents discussed in Chapter 33 stimulate LH.
Prolactin	Targets mammary glands; stimulates lactogenesis (milk production) and breast growth.
	Bromocriptine: Inhibits action of PH and therefore inhibits lactogenesis (see Chapter 14).
Thyroid-stimulating hormone	Stimulates secretion of thyroid hormones T_3 and T_4 by the thyroid.
	Thyrotropin: Increases the production and secretion of thyroid hormones (see Chapter 30).
POSTERIOR PITUITARY	
Antidiuretic hormone	Increases water resorption in distal tubules and collecting duct of nephron; concentrates urine; causes potent vasoconstriction.
	Vasopressin: ADH; performs all the physiological functions of ADH.
	Desmopressin: A synthetic vasopressin.
Oxytocin	Targets mammary glands; stimulates ejection of milk and contraction of uterine smooth muscle.
	Pitocin: Has all the physiological actions of oxytocin (see Chapter 33).

FSH, Follicle-stimulating hormone; *GH,* growth hormone; *LH,* luteinizing hormone; *PH,* prolactin; T_3, tri-iodothyronine; T_4, thyroxine; *ADH,* antidiuretic hormone.

antagonizes the effects of the natural GH is octreotide, and it does so by inhibiting GH release. It is a synthetic polypeptide that is structurally and pharmacologically similar to GH release-inhibiting factor, which is also called *somatostatin.*

The drugs that affect the posterior pituitary, such as vasopressin and desmopressin, mimic the actions of the naturally occurring antidiuretic hormone (ADH). Exogenous vasopressin elicits all of the same pharmacological responses as those elicited by endogenous vasopressin (ADH). It increases water resorption in the distal tubules and collecting ducts of the nephrons, concentrates urine, and is a potent vasoconstrictor.

The drug effects of the various pituitary drugs differ depending on the agent. Many of the effects are the same as those of the pituitary hormones. Cosyntropin mimics the effects of ACTH. Clinically its use is limited to diagnostic screening of clients with adrenocortical insufficiency. It has a rapid effect on the adrenal cortex such that the plasma cortisol response and hence adrenal functioning can be quickly determined.

When the cortex of the adrenal gland is stimulated to secrete cortisol, sodium is retained, resulting in edema and hypertension. Cortisol can decrease inflammation by preventing the release of destructive substances from leukocytes, and it also inhibits macrophage accumulation in inflamed areas, reduces leukocyte adhesion to capillary walls, and reduces capillary wall permeability and edema formation. Other effects are a decrease in the level of complement components, the antagonism of histamine activity, reduction in fibroblast proliferation, the deposition of collagen, and the subsequent formation of scar tissue following a tissue injury.

Somatropin has pharmacological effects equivalent to those of human GH. It promotes linear growth in children who lack normal amounts of the endogenous hormone. In addition, it causes increased cellular protein synthesis, nitrogen retention, liver glycogenolysis, impaired glucose tolerance, lipid mobilization from body fat stores, and increased plasma levels of fatty acids. GH derivatives also cause the retention of sodium, potassium, and phosphorus.

Octreotide is a synthetic octapeptide that is structurally and pharmacologically related to somatostatin (GH release-inhibiting factor), but with a prolonged duration of action. It can eliminate or alleviate certain symptoms of carcinoid tumours (e.g., severe diarrhea, flushing). It is also effective in the management of the potentially life-threatening hypotension associated with a carcinoid crisis. Octreotide decreases the stool volume, electrolyte loss, and plasma concentrations of vasoactive intestinal polypeptide (VIP), a substance secreted by a type of tumour known as *VIPoma* that causes profuse watery diarrhea. It is used to reduce blood levels of growth hormone in clients with acromegaly (a disorder that results in unusual height and enlarged hands, feet, and head). It is also used after high-risk pancreatic surgery to prevent post-operative complications such as fistulas, abscesses, sepsis, and acute pancreatitis. Octreotide is also used, along with sclerotherapy (injecting a hardening substance) for clients with bleeding esophageal ulcers to control bleeding and improve survival.

The synthetically made hormones that are structurally identical or similar to ADH are vasopressin and desmopressin. By increasing the resorption of sodium and water in the distal tubules and collecting duct of the nephron, they decrease the urinary flow rate, thereby causing as much as 90 percent of the water that might otherwise be excreted in the urine to be conserved. In large doses, vasopressin directly stimulates the contraction of smooth muscle, particularly of the capillaries and small arterioles, causing vasoconstriction. Desmopressin causes a dose-dependent increase in the plasma levels of factor VIII (antihemophilic factor), von Willebrand's factor (acts closely with factor VIII), and tissue plasminogen activator.

Indications

The primary therapeutic effect of cosyntropin is the stimulation of the release of cortisol from the adrenal cortex, making it an excellent agent in the diagnosis of, but not usually the treatment of, adrenocortical insufficiency. Upon diagnosis the actual drug therapy for treating adrenocortical insufficiency generally involves replacement hormonal therapy using drug forms of the deficient corticosteroid hormones. These agents are discussed in more detail in Chapter 32. Synacthen Depot is a long-acting formulation of cosyntropin combined with zinc hydroxide that has been used for collagen diseases such as rheumatoid arthritis and systemic lupus erythematosus, acute exacerbations of multiple sclerosis, ulcerative colitis, and others.

Somatropin is a human GH made through recombinant DNA. It is effective in stimulating skeletal growth in clients suffering from an inadequate secretion of normal endogenous GH, such as those with hypopituitary dwarfism. Octreotide is a synthetic polypeptide that is structurally and pharmacologically related to somatostatin (GH release-inhibiting factor). It is of benefit in alleviating or eliminating certain symptoms of carcinoid tumours stemming from the secretion of VIP. (These symptoms were described in the previous section.)

Vasopressin and desmopressin are used to prevent or control polydipsia (excessive thirst), polyuria, and dehydration in clients with diabetes insipidus caused by a deficiency of endogenous ADH. (Note that this is an entirely different disease from diabetes mellitus, usually referred to simply as diabetes). Because of their vasoconstrictor properties, vasopressin and desmopressin are useful in treating various types of bleeding, in particular gastrointestinal (GI) hemorrhage. Because of its unique ability to increase the plasma level of factor VIII (von Willebrand's factor) and tissue plasminogen activator, desmopressin is especially useful in the treatment of hemophilia A and type I von Willebrand's disease. Vasopressin and desmopressin are also occasionally used after cranial surgery that may involve the pituitary gland.

Contraindications

Contraindications for the use of pituitary agents vary with each individual drug and are listed in the drug profiles in this chapter. Because even small amounts of these agents can initiate major physiological changes, all of them should be used with special caution in clients with acute or chronic illnesses such as migraine headaches, epilepsy, and asthma.

Side Effects and Adverse Effects

Many of the adverse effects of the pituitary drugs are specific to the individual agents. Agents possessing similar hormonal effects generally have similar adverse effects. The most common adverse effects of the pituitary drugs described here are listed in Tables 29-2 to 29-4.

Interactions

Desmopressin when given with carbamazepine or chlorpropamide may result in additive therapeutic effects of desmopressin. Co-administration of desmopressin with lithium, alcohol, demeclocycline, or heparin may result in decreased therapeutic effects of desmopressin.

Dosages

For the recommended dosages of pituitary agents, see the dosages table on p. 500. See Appendix B for some of the common brands available in Canada.

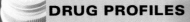

DRUG PROFILES

▶▶ cosyntropin

Cosyntropin is contraindicated in clients who have shown a hypersensitivity to it. Cosyntropin is intended for short-term use only. The longer acting depot form is contraindicated in those with Cushing's syndrome, osteoporosis, heart failure, peptic ulcer disease, hypertension or primary adrenocortical insufficiency or hyperfunction, untreated infections, acute psychosis, and in those who have undergone recent surgery. Cosyntropin

is available in two parenteral forms: a regular form that may be given by intravenous (IV), intramuscular (IM), or subcutaneous (SC) injection; and a repository (depot) form that may be given intramuscularly or subcutaneously and that has a more prolonged effect. The parenteral form is available in 250-µg/mL strength, and the repository form of 1 mg cosyntropin as a zinc hydroxide complex. Pregnancy category C. Common dosages are listed in the table on p. 500.

PHARMACOKINETICS

Half-Life	Onset	Peak	Duration
Unknown	Rapid	1 hr	N/A

desmopressin

Desmopressin is a synthetically made hormone that is structurally related to the endogenous hormone arginine vasopressin (ADH), but its effects differ slightly from those of the natural vasopressin (see the Mechanisms of Action and Drug Effects and Indications sections). It is contraindicated in clients who have shown a hypersensitivity to it and in those with nephrogenic diabetes insipidus. It is available as 0.1-mg/mL and 1.5-mg/mL metered-dose nasal sprays, 4- and 15-µg/mL parenteral injections, and most recently 0.1- and 0.2-mg oral tablets. For optimal control of the client's disease, consistent timing of their intranasal dose is important. Pregnancy category B. Common dosages are listed in the table on p. 500.

PHARMACOKINETICS

Half-Life	Onset	Peak	Duration
IV/SC/IN: 3.2–3.6 hr	IV: 30 min	IV: 1.5–2 hr	IN*: 12 hr

*IN, Intranasal.

octreotide

Octreotide is contraindicated only in clients who have shown a hypersensitivity to it or to similar drugs. In clinical trials octreotide biliary tract abnormalities occurred in 63 percent of clients. Because of the tendency for biliary abnormalities to occur especially in clients on long-term octreotide, periodic ultrasound of the gallbladder and biliary tract is recommended. It is available only in parenteral form as 50-, 100-, 200-, and 500-µg/mL injections and as 10-, 20-, and 30-mg/2 mL depot injections. Pregnancy category B. Common dosages are listed in the table on p. 500.

PHARMACOKINETICS

Half-Life	Onset	Peak	Duration
1.7 hr	Unknown	15–30 min	12 hr

TABLE 29-2
COSYNTROPIN-ZINC HYDROXIDE: COMMON ADVERSE EFFECTS

Body System	Side/Adverse Effects
Central nervous	Convulsions, dizziness, euphoria, insomnia, headache, depression, psychosis
Gastrointestinal	Nausea, vomiting, peptic ulcer perforation, pancreatitis, abdominal distension, ulcerative esophagitis
Genitourinary	Water and sodium retention, hypokalemia, alkalosis, calcium loss
Other	Sweating, acne, hyperpigmentation, weakness, muscle atrophy, myalgia, arthralgia

TABLE 29-3
DESMOPRESSIN AND VASOPRESSIN: COMMON ADVERSE EFFECTS

Body System	Side/Adverse Effects
Central nervous	Drowsiness, headache, lethargy, flushing
Gastrointestinal	Nausea, heartburn, cramps
Genitourinary	Vulvar pain
Other	Bronchial constriction, nasal irritation and congestion, tremor, sweating, vertigo

TABLE 29-4
DRUGS THAT AFFECT GROWTH HORMONE: COMMON ADVERSE EFFECTS

Body System	Side/Adverse Effects
Central nervous	Headache
Endocrine	Hyperglycemia, ketosis, hypothyroidism
Genitourinary	Hypercalciuria
Other	Rash, urticaria, antibodies to GH, inflammation at injection site

DOSAGES Selected Pituitary Agents

Agent	Pharmacological Class	Usual Dosage Range	Indications
▸▸cosyntropin	Adrenal cortex stimulating hormone	**Adult*** IV: 250 μg in 500 mL of D5W over 6 hr IM depot injection: 0.5–1 mg q48–72h	Diagnosis of adrenocortical insufficiency Exacerbation of multiple sclerosis
desmopressin	ADH, antihemophilic hormone	**Adult and pediatric ≥6 yr** Intranasal spray: 10–40 μg at bedtime PO: 0.2 mg at bedtime, titrated upward as needed to max 0.6 mg/day based on diurnal response **Adult** Intranasal: 10–40 μg divided daily–tid IV/SC: 0.3 μg/kg; max IV 20 μg **Pediatric 3 mo–12 yr** Intranasal spray: 5–30 μg divided daily, bid–tid **Adult and pediatric** PO: Initial dose, both adult and pediatric, is 0.1 mg tab tid with careful titration upward to max 1.2 mg/day as needed based on diurnal response **Pediatric** IV infusion: 0.3 μg/kg, diluted in 50 mL of NS (use 10 mL of saline diluent in clients weighing <10 kg) **Adult** IV infusion: 10.0 μg/m², diluted in 50 mL of NS to max 20 μg	Primary nocturnal enuresis Central cranial diabetes insipidus Hemophilia A and type 1 von Willebrand's disease
octreotide	Somatostatin (GH inhibitor) analogue	**Adult†** IV/SC: Initial dose of 100–300 μg bid–tid; may titrate up to 1500 μg tid Depot IM: 20–30 mg q4 wk IV/SC: 100–750 μg/day divided bid–qid Depot IM: 20–30 mg q4 wk IV/SC: 200–450 μg/day divided bid–qid Depot IM: 10–30 mg q4wk	Acromegaly Metastatic carcinoid tumours (to control flushing and diarrhea symptoms) VIPomas
▸▸somatropin	GH analogue	**Adult and pediatric** Dosages vary widely among the many products on the market; a typical dosage regimen is 0.16–0.24 mg/kg/wk divided into 6–7 daily IM or SC injections; consult product insert.	Growth failure; AIDS-related wasting syndrome
▸▸vasopressin	Natural or synthetic ADH	**Adult and pediatric** IM/SC 0.25–0.5 mL q3–4 hr	Diabetes insipidus; prevention or treatment of post-operative abdominal distension; dispersal of abdominal gas to improve imaging in abdominal X-ray studies

*Pediatric dosage must be carefully individualized and should be followed by a pediatric endocrinologist.
†Normally used only in adults.
D5W, 5 percent dextrose in water; *ADH,* antidiuretic hormone; *NS,* normal saline; *GH,* growth hormone.

▶▶ somatropin

Somatropin is made by recombinant DNA techniques. It is contraindicated in anyone whose bones have stopped growing (i.e., those with closed epiphyses, which typically occurs in late adolescence). It also should not be used in any client showing evidence of an active malignancy. Somatropin is usually given only by subcutaneous injection. It is a pregnancy category C agent. Common dosages are listed in the table on p. 500.

PHARMACOKINETICS

Half-Life	Onset	Peak	Duration
<30 min	SC: 3–6 hr	SC: 3–5 hr	Variable

▶▶ vasopressin

Vasopressin is a synthetic arginine vasopressin that is structurally identical to endogenous vasopressin (ADH) and produces all of the same effects as the endogenous hormone. It is contraindicated in clients who have shown a hypersensitivity to it and in those with chronic nephritis or vascular disease. It is available only as a 20-unit/mL injection. Pregnancy category B. Common dosages are listed in the table on p. 500.

PHARMACOKINETICS

Half-Life	Onset	Peak	Duration
10–35 min	Unknown	Unknown	2–8 hr

NURSING PROCESS

■ Assessment

Before administering any of the pituitary agents, the nurse should perform a thorough nursing assessment, obtain a complete medication history, and document the findings. Contraindications and cautions for the use of pituitary agents vary with each individual drug and are listed in each of the drug profiles included in this chapter, but a few examples are as follows:

- Cosyntropin depot is contraindicated in clients with osteoporosis, heart failure, peptic ulcer disease, hypertension, or dysfunction of the adrenocortex.
- Somatropin is contraindicated in clients with closed epiphyseal plates of the long bones.
- Octreotide is contraindicated in clients who have shown allergic reactions to it or similar drugs.
- Desmopressin should be given cautiously in clients with chronic migraines, seizures, and asthma.

Small doses of these drugs may initiate major physiological changes and should therefore be used with special caution in clients with such acute or chronic illnesses as migraine headache, epilepsy, asthma, and other chronic disease processes. Drug interactions for these agents are as follows:

- *Desmopressin:* carbamazepine and chlorpropamide (result in additive effects of the desmopressin); lithium,

alcohol, demeclocycline, and heparin (may result in decreased therapeutic effects of the desmopressin)
- *Cosyntropin:* potassium-lowering drugs such as diuretics

The other GH agents should be avoided with those drugs that antagonize the effects of these drugs. A hypersensitivity reaction to any of these medications is a contraindication to its use. For further assessment data, see Box 29-2.

■ Nursing Diagnoses

Nursing diagnoses related to the administration of pituitary agents include the following:

- Disturbed body image related to specific disease processes or drug side effects and their influence on physical characteristics.
- Excess fluid volume related to side effects of various pituitary agents.
- Fatigue related to the side effects associated with the various pituitary agents.
- Acute pain related to gastrointestinal side effects of the various pituitary agents.
- Deficient knowledge related to new treatment with various pituitary agents.

■ Planning

Goals pertaining to clients receiving pituitary medications include the following:

- Client maintains positive body image.
- Client maintains normal fluid volume and electrolyte status while on various pituitary agents.
- Client returns to normal or pre-therapy levels of activity.
- Client experiences little to no pain related to medication-induced GI upset or epigastric distress.
- Client remains adherent with medication therapy.
- Client is without self-injury related to adverse effects of medications.

■ Outcome Criteria

The outcome criteria for clients receiving pituitary agents include the following:

- Client openly verbalizes fears, anxieties, and concerns with healthcare professionals regarding body image changes related to disease process and medication therapy.
- Client's sodium level is within normal limits while on medication therapy.
- Client states ways, such as dietary precautions, to decrease edema caused by medication.
- Client experiences minimal GI upset and gastric distress by taking medication with food or at mealtimes.
- Client states measures to employ to diminish the risk of falls related to the musculoskeletal and neurological (seizures) side effects of medication.
- Client performs activities of daily living and other normal activity without difficulty.
- Client states the importance of follow-up visits to the physician for monitoring of adherence, therapeutic effects, and adverse reactions.

BOX 29-2

Pituitary Agents: Assessment Data

Assessment Parameters	Cautions	Drug Interactions	Contraindications
COSYNTROPIN			
Baseline vital signs	Pregnancy	Alcohol	Allergy
Electrolyte values	Lactation		Osteoporosis
Blood glucose levels	Liver disease		Heart failure
Chest X-ray study	Mental illness		Ulcer disease
CBC, I&O, weight	Myasthenia gravis		Fungal infections
Cortisol levels	Gout		Recent surgery
Allergy to pork because	Hypothyroidism		Adrenocortical hypo- and hyper-
of cross-sensitivity	Latent tuberculosis		function (primary)
DESMOPRESSIN			
Vital signs with BP lying	Depression or suicidal		Allergy to drug or to TCAs
and standing q4h	tendencies		Glaucoma
CBC: Leukocytes	Cystic fibrosis		Cardiac insufficiency
Cardiac enzymes	Narrow-angle glaucoma		Hypertension
Weight every wk	Increased intra-ocular		BPH
ECG	pressure		Seizure disorder
Urine volume, osmolality	Seizure disorder		Children <3 mos
	Children <3 mos		
SOMATROPIN			
Thyroid function studies	Diabetes mellitus	Glucocorticoids	Drug allergy
GH antibodies	Hypothyroidism	Androgens	Intracerebral lesions
	Pregnancy	Thyroid hormones	Closed epiphyseal plates
VASOPRESSIN			
Pulse and vital signs,	Coronary artery disease		Allergy
especially with IM/IV	Epilepsy		Chronic renal disease
dosage forms	Migraine		
I&O	Asthma		
Weight	Heart failure		
Edema	Pregnancy		

CBC, Complete blood count; *I&O,* intake and output; *TCA,* tricyclic antidepressant; *BP,* blood pressure; *ECG,* electrocardiogram; *BPH,* benign prostatic hypertrophy; *GH,* growth hormone; *IM,* intramuscular; *IV,* intravenous.

■ Implementation

Cosyntropin is available in intramuscular, subcutaneous, and intravenous forms and in a repository form. Intramuscular injections should be administered using a 21-gauge needle. Intravenous injections should be given over 2 minutes, or as designated in the packaging insert, and should be diluted with the recommended amounts of normal saline solution. The client's protein intake should be increased because of the protein loss and the potential negative nitrogen balance that can occur. Clients are usually encouraged to decrease their sodium intake and increase their potassium intake to counteract the side effects of the medication. Instructions should be given about the various forms of vasopressin (e.g., nasal spray). Vital signs should be monitored during administration of vasopressin. Injection sites for somatropin should be rotated; injections are usually given subcutaneously. Desmopressin should be administered per physician's orders because it may vary per indication (i.e., diabetes insipidus vs. other forms of pituitary dysfunction).

Teaching tips for clients receiving pituitary agents are presented in the box on p. 503.

■ Evaluation

Following are the therapeutic responses expected in clients receiving pituitary agents:
- Cosyntropin should eliminate the pain associated with inflammation and produce increased comfort and muscle strength in clients with myasthenia gravis.
- Somatropin should increase growth in children.
- Desmopressin and vasopressin should eliminate severe thirst and decrease urinary output.

It is crucial for the nurse to monitor not only for the therapeutic effects but also for the following side effects:
- For cosyntropin and somatropin, the side effects are dependent edema, moon face, pulmonary edema, infection, and mental status changes that include increased aggressive behaviour and irritability. Allergic reactions to cosyntropin include rash, urticaria, fever, and dyspnea. If these occur, the drug should be discontinued and the physician notified. Somatropin has the additional side effect of hypercalciuria.
- Desmopressin and vasopressin may cause similar side effects as cosyntropin and somatropin. Additional side effects include hypertension, nausea, GI upset, tremors, respiratory distress, and drowsiness.

CLIENT TEACHING TIPS

The nurse should instruct clients as follows, depending on the medication prescribed:

All Pituitary Agents

▲ Do not discontinue this medication abruptly. Because of the way hormones work, with levels of one hormone controlling another, stopping abruptly could cause serious imbalances.
▲ As with any medication or illness, a medical alert bracelet or tag should be worn at all times, naming the medication and the specific disease.
▲ Tell all of your healthcare professionals, including your dentist, that you are taking this medication.

Cosyntropin or Cosyntropin-like Drugs

▲ Drink plenty of fluids—up to 2000 mL per day, unless you have been told not to. Fluids should be low in sodium content (soft drinks may be high in salt), especially if you have heart problems.
▲ Avoid vaccinations.
▲ Do not take over-the-counter medications while you are on this drug.
▲ Do not drink alcohol while you are on this drug.

▲ This medication does not lead to a cure but can alleviate your symptoms.
▲ Notify your physician if you experience infection, fever, sore throat, joint pain, or muscular pain.

Somatropin

▲ It is important to take this drug as directed.
▲ Keep a journal of your (or your child's) measurements.

Desmopressin

▲ Use the nasal spray as demonstrated. Clear your nasal passages before using the spray. Do not inhale. (Note: The technique for nasal instillation of desmopressin should be demonstrated to the child and caregiver. The child's demonstration of the technique should be evaluated before discharge and re-evaluated at later visits, with repeat demonstrations from the nurse if necessary. Written instructions should always follow any verbal or taped instructions.)
▲ Do not take any over-the-counter medications for colds, cough, allergies, or hay fever because the epinephrine in these preparations may interact with this medication.

POINTS to REMEMBER

▼ The pituitary gland is composed of two distinct glands: anterior and posterior.
▼ Each distinct gland has its own set of hormones: *anterior:* thyroid-stimulating hormone (TSH), GH, ACTH, prolactin (PH), follicle-stimulating hormone (FSH), luteinizing hormone (LH); *posterior:* ADH, oxytocin.
▼ Pituitary drugs are used to either mimic or antagonize the action of endogenous pituitary hormones.
▼ Drugs that mimic the action of endogenous pituitary hormones include cosyntropin, somatropin, vasopressin, and desmopressin.
▼ Drugs that antagonize the actions of endogenous pituitary hormones include octreotide, which suppresses or inhibits certain symptoms related to carcinoid tumours and decreases plasma concentration of VIP.

▼ Nursing assessment for those clients receiving cosyntropin should include baseline vital signs, electrolyte values (sodium, potassium, chloride), blood glucose levels, chest X-ray studies, weight, and cortisol levels. Those clients receiving somatropin should have thyroid function and GH levels assessed and documented. Those receiving desmopressin should be assessed with documentation of vital signs, including both supine and standing blood pressure and pulse rates. Other assessment data should include complete blood count (CBC), cardiac and liver enzyme activity, electrocardiogram (ECG), and weight.
▼ Assessment in clients receiving vasopressin should include vital signs, intake and output amounts, weight, and presence and status of edema.

EXAMINATION REVIEW QUESTIONS

1 Which of the following nursing interventions is important with the use of cosyntropin?
a. Any lesions should be surgically removed and no further medications given once it is applied via a transdermal patch.
b. Medication should be abruptly discontinued to minimize overall effects.
c. Intravenous injection forms should be diluted with normal saline and given over at least 2 minutes.
d. Clients should increase their sodium and potassium intake.

2 Which of the following statements reflects the most accurate information about cosyntropin?
a. Use the nasal spray only when symptoms are present.
b. Intramuscular injections need to be given using an 18-gauge, 1½-inch needle.
c. After each nasal spray, be sure to take a deep breath with each inhalation of the dosage so that the lungs are covered.
d. Intramuscular, subcutaneous, intravenous, and repository dosage forms are available.

3 The hypothalamus is responsible for which of the following?
  a. Secretion of insulin
  b. Decrease in oxytocin level
  c. Secretion of vasopressin and oxytocin
  d. Decrease in testosterone level

4 Contraindications for the use of desmopressin include which of the following?
  a. Allergies to beef insulin
  b. White blood cell count of 8000

  c. Children under 3 months of age
  d. Nephrogenic diabetes insipidus

5 Growth hormones are associated with which of the following adverse effects?
  a. Hypoglycemia
  b. Hypocalciuria
  c. Hyperglycemia
  d. Hyperthyroidism

For answers see http://evolve.elsevier.com/Lilley/pharmacology/.

CRITICAL THINKING ACTIVITIES

1 Vasopressin and desmopressin are structurally identical or similar to what endogenous hormone?

2 Identify human GH products made by recombinant DNA techniques.

3 Your client is excited that he is beginning therapy with pituitary agents and is positive about a cure. What would be your most appropriate response and why?

For answers see http://evolve.elsevier.com/Lilley/pharmacology/.

BIBLIOGRAPHY

Albanese, J., & Nutz, P. (2005). *Mosby's 2005 nursing drug cards.* St Louis, MO: Mosby.

Canadian Pharmacists Association. (2003). *Therapeutic choices* (4th ed.). Ottawa, ON: Author.

Canadian Pharmacists Association. (2004). *Guide to drugs in Canada.* Toronto, ON: Dorling Kindersley.

Canadian Pharmacists Association. (2005). *Compendium of pharmaceuticals and specialties. The Canadian drug reference for health professionals.* Ottawa, ON: Author. [The subscription-based e-CPS is available at http://www.pharmacists.ca.]

Cheng, A., Williams, B.A., & Sivarajan, B.V. (Eds.). *The HSC handbook of pediatrics* (10th ed.). Toronto, ON: Elsevier.

Facts and Comparisons. (2004). *Drug facts and comparisons pocket version* (9th ed.). St Louis, MO: Wolters Kluwer Health.

Hardman, J.G., & Limbird, L.E. (2002). *Goodman and Gilman's the pharmacological basis of therapeutics* (10th ed.). New York: McGraw-Hill.

Health Canada. (2005). Drug product database (DPD). Retrieved August 16, 2005, from http://www.hc-sc.gc.ca/hpb/drugs-dpd/

Lacy, C.F., Armstrong, L.L., Goldman, M.P., & Lance, L.L. (2003). *Drug information handbook* (11th ed.). Hudson, OH: Lexi-Comp.

Larsen, P.R., Kronenberg, H.M., Melmod, S., & Polonsky, K.S. (2002). *Williams textbook of endocrinology* (10th ed.). Philadelphia: Saunders.

Lehne, R.A. (2004). *Pharmacology for nursing care* (5th ed.). St Louis, MO: Saunders.

Mosby. (2005). *Mosby's drug consult 2005: The comprehensive reference for generic and brand name drugs* (15th ed.) St Louis, MO: Mosby.

Skidmore-Roth, L. (2006). *Mosby's 2006 nursing drug reference* (19th ed.). St Louis, MO: Mosby.

Thyroid and Antithyroid Agents

CHAPTER 30

OBJECTIVES

After reading this chapter, the successful student will be able to do the following:

1 Discuss the normal actions and functions of the thyroid hormones.

2 Describe the differences in the diseases resulting from the hyposecretion and hypersecretion of the thyroid gland.

3 Identify the various drugs used to treat the hyposecretion and hypersecretion states of the thyroid gland.

4 Discuss the mechanisms of action, indications, contraindications and cautions, and side effects related to the various drugs used to treat hypo- and hyperthyroidism.

5 Develop a nursing care plan that includes all phases of the nursing process for clients receiving thyroid replacement as well as for clients receiving antithyroid agents.

e-LEARNING ACTIVITIES

Student CD-ROM
- Review Questions: see questions 230–235
- Animations
- Medication Administration Checklists
- IV Therapy Checklists

evolve Web site (http://evolve.elsevier.com/Lilley/pharmacology/)
- Online Chapter Worksheet • Frequently Asked Questions
- Learning Tips and Content Updates • WebLinks • Online Appendices and Supplements • Mosby/Saunders ePharmacology Update • Access to *Mosby's Drug Consult*

DRUG PROFILES

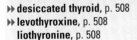

▶▶ desiccated thyroid, p. 508   methimazole, p. 510
▶▶ levothyroxine, p. 508   ▶▶ propylthiouracil, p. 510
    liothyronine, p. 508

▶▶ Key drug.

GLOSSARY

Hyperthyroidism (hy′ pər thy′ roid iz əm) A condition characterized by excessive production of the thyroid hormones. Also called *thyrotoxicosis*.

Hypothyroidism A condition characterized by diminished production of the thyroid hormones.

Thyroid-stimulating hormone (TSH) An endogenous substance secreted by the pituitary gland that controls the release of thyroid gland hormones and is necessary for the growth and function of the thyroid gland (also called *thyrotropin*). As a drug preparation, TSH increases the uptake of radioactive iodine in the thyroid and the secretion of thyroxine by the thyroid gland.

Thyroxine (T₄) (thy rok′ sən) The thyroid hormone that influences the metabolic rate.

Tri-iodothyronine (T₃) (try eye′ o do thy′ roe nin) The thyroid hormone that helps regulate growth, development, metabolism, and body temperature and inhibits the secretion of thyrotropin by the pituitary gland.

THYROID FUNCTION

The thyroid gland lies across the larynx in front of the thyroid cartilage ("Adam's apple"). Its lobes extend laterally on both sides of the front of the neck. It is responsible for the secretion of three hormones essential for the proper regulation of metabolism: **thyroxine (T₄)**, **tri-iodothyronine (T₃)**, and calcitonin. It is close to and communicates with the parathyroid gland, which lies just above and behind it. The parathyroid gland consists of two pairs of bean-shaped glands. These glands are made up of encapsulated cells, which are responsible for maintaining adequate levels of calcium in the extracellular fluid, primarily by mobilizing calcium from bone.

T_4 and T_3 are produced in the thyroid gland through the iodination and coupling of the amino acid tyrosine. The iodide (I, the ionized form of iodine) needed for this process is acquired from the diet, and for normal function to be maintained about 1 mg of iodide is needed per week. This iodide is sequestered by the thyroid gland, where it is trapped and concentrated to 20 times its potency in blood. It is here that it is also converted to iodine (I_2), which is combined with the tyrosine to make di-iodotyrosine. The combination of two molecules of di-iodotyrosine causes the formation of thyronine, which therefore has four iodine molecules in its structure (T_4). Tri-iodothyronine is formed by the coupling of one molecule of di-iodotyrosine with one molecule of monoiodotyrosine; thus it has three iodine molecules in its structure (T_3). The biological potency of T_3 is about four times greater than that of T_4, but T_4 is present in much greater quantities. After the synthesis of these two thyroid hormones, they are stored in a complex with thyroglobulin (a protein that contains tyrosine and an amino acid) in the follicles in the thyroid gland called the *colloid*. When the thyroid gland is signalled to do so, it enzymatically breaks down the thyroglobulin–thyroid hormone complex to release either T_3 or T_4 into the circulation. This entire process is triggered by **thyroid-stimulating hormone (TSH)**, also called *thyrotropin*. Its release from the anterior pituitary is stimulated when the blood levels of T_3 and T_4 are low.

The thyroid hormones are involved in a wide variety of bodily processes. They regulate lipid and carbohydrate metabolism; are essential for normal growth and development; control the heat-regulating system (thermoregulatory centre); and have multiple effects on the cardiovascular, endocrine, and neuromuscular systems. Therefore hyperfunction or hypofunction of the thyroid gland can lead to a wide range of serious consequences.

HYPOTHYROIDISM

A deficiency in thyroid hormones can be caused by a number of different diseases that affect the thyroid in different ways. There are two types of **hypothyroidism**. Primary hypothyroidism stems from an abnormality in the thyroid gland itself and occurs when the thyroid gland is not able to perform one or more of its many functions, such as releasing the thyroid hormones from their storage sites, coupling iodine with tyrosine, trapping iodide, or converting iodide to iodine. It is the most common of the two types of hypothyroidism. The most common cause of primary hypothyroidism is autoimmune thyroiditis, also known as Hashimoto's thyroiditis, an autoimmune disorder that causes inflammation and subsequent lessened function of the thyroid. Hypothyroidism may also result from surgical treatment of other thyroid disorders. Secondary hypothyroidism results when the pituitary gland is dysfunctional and does not secrete the TSH needed to trigger the release of the T_3 and T_4 stored there. Knowledge of the underlying cause of the hypothyroidism allows one to eliminate the deficiency.

Hypothyroidism can also be classified by when it occurs in life. Hyposecretion of thyroid hormone during youth may lead to cretinism. It usually occurs during infancy as a result of deficiencies of the thyroid gland during fetal or neonatal periods. Cretinism is a condition characterized by low metabolic rate, retarded growth and sexual development, and possibly mental retardation. Hyposecretion of thyroid hormone as an adult may lead to myxedema and typically affects women in their fifties but can occur at any age. Myxedema is a condition characterized by decreased metabolic rate but also involves loss of mental and physical stamina, gain in weight, loss of hair, firm edema, and yellow dullness of the skin.

Some forms of hypothyroidism may result in the formation of a goitre, which is an enlargement of the thyroid gland resulting from its overstimulation by elevated levels of TSH. The TSH level is elevated because there is little or no thyroid hormone in the circulation. Common symptoms of hypothyroidism are thickened skin, hair loss, lethargy, constipation, and anorexia.

HYPERTHYROIDISM

The excessive synthesis and secretion of thyroid hormones is a clinical syndrome often referred to as **hyperthyroidism**. Hyperthyroidism may be caused by several

---

RESEARCH

Hyperthyroidism in Women

Women with hyperthyroidism may experience irregular menstrual cycles and their fertility status has been found to be decreased. The frequency of irregular menstrual cycles has been shown to vary in many different studies and there remains little information about the appearance of the ovaries in these specific women. However, one recent study reported that of 18 women studied (mean age of 36 years and with newly diagnosed hyperthyroidism), 10 reported having irregular cycles before the onset of the symptoms of hyperthyroidism and the other eight were found to have regular cycles, although two had noted hypomenorrhea. Before medical treatment, 15 of these women had abnormal ovarian findings on their ultrasounds. The abnormalities varied and included the presence of multiple or single large follicles, irregular cysts, and two-compartment cysts. This particular study concluded that some women with hyperthyroidism have polycystic ovaries with a resolving of the changes during antithyroid drug treatment. A commentary on this same study stated that women with hyperthyroidism may have irregular menses, which is one part of the definition of polycystic ovarian syndrome, but that the clients in this study did *not* have evidence of hyperandrogenism, which is the other part of the definition.

Source: Skjoldebrand Sparre, L., Kollind, M., & Carlstrom, K. (2002). Ovarian ultrasound and ovarian and adrenal hormones before and after treatment for hyperthyroidism. *Gynecologic and Obstetric Investigation, 54*, 50–55. Visit the Thyroid Foundation of Canada at http://www.thyroid.ca/

different diseases and drugs. Some of the more common diseases are Graves' disease (also an autoimmune disorder, and the most common cause), *toxic nodular disease* (the least common cause), multinodular disease, thyroiditis, pituitary tumours, and thyroid cancer.

Hyperthyroidism can affect multiple body systems, resulting in an overall increase in metabolism. Commonly reported symptoms are diarrhea, flushing, increased appetite, muscle weakness, fatigue, palpitations, irritability, nervousness, sleep disorders, heat intolerance, and altered menstrual flow.

THYROID AGENTS

Both types of hypothyroidism are amenable to thyroid hormone replacement using various thyroid preparations. These agents can be either natural or synthetic in origin. The natural thyroid preparations are derived from the thyroids of animals such as cattle and hogs. There is currently only one such preparation available in Canada, which is called simply *thyroid* or *thyroid, desiccated*. Desiccation is the term for the drying process used to prepare this drug form, which basically consists of pulverized animal thyroid gland. All of the natural preparations are standardized according to their iodine content. These agents are used infrequently. The synthetic thyroid preparations are levothyroxine and liothyronine. The approximate clinically equivalent doses of the agents are given in Table 30-1. This information is useful for guiding dosage adjustments when switching a client from one thyroid hormone to another.

Mechanism of Action and Drug Effects

The thyroid preparations are given to replace what the thyroid gland itself cannot produce to achieve normal thyroid levels (euthyroid). The thyroid drugs work in the same manner as the endogenous thyroid hormone. At the cellular level they work to induce changes in the metabolic rate, stimulate the cardiovascular system, and increase oxygen consumption, body temperature, blood volume, growth, and overall cellular growth.

The drugs that are used to treat hypothyroid conditions affect many body systems, and they do this in the same way the endogenous thyroid hormones do. The principal pharmacological effect of these drugs is an increase in the rate of protein, carbohydrate, and lipid metabolism. Thyroid hormones are also involved in the regulation of cell growth and differentiation and have a

cardiostimulatory effect, which involves increasing the sensitivity of the heart to catecholamines or increasing the number of myocardial beta-adrenergic receptors, or both. In addition, thyroid hormones increase cardiac output, renal blood flow, and the glomerular filtration rate, which results in a diuretic effect.

Indications

The various thyroid preparations are used in the treatment of both forms of hypothyroidism, although levothyroxine is generally the preferred agent because its hormonal content is standardized and its effect is therefore predictable. The thyroid drugs can also be used for the diagnosis of suspected hyperthyroidism (as a TSH-suppression test) and in the prevention or treatment of various types of goitres. They are also used for replacement hormonal therapy in clients whose thyroid glands have been surgically removed or destroyed by radioactive iodine in the treatment of thyroid cancer or hyperthyroidism.

Contraindications

Contraindications to thyroid preparations include known drug allergy to a given drug product, recent myocardial infarction (MI), angina hypertension, adrenal insufficiency, or hyperthyroidism.

Side Effects and Adverse Effects

The adverse effects of thyroid medications are usually the result of overdose. The most significant adverse effect is cardiac dysrhythmia with the risk of life-threatening or fatal irregularities. Other more common undesirable effects are listed in Table 30-2.

Interactions

When thyroid preparations are taken in conjunction with oral anticoagulants, the activity of the oral anticoagulants may be increased, thus necessitating reduced anticoagulant doses. Thyroid preparations when taken concomitantly with digitalis glycosides may decrease serum digitalis levels. Cholestyramine binds to thyroid hormone in the gastrointestinal (GI) tract. This prevents the thyroid hormone from being absorbed into the bloodstream, which is necessary to produce its desired effect. Concurrent use of thyroid preparations with cholestyramine results in reduced oral

TABLE 30-1
THYROID DRUGS: CLINICALLY EQUIVALENT DOSES

Thyroid Drug	Approximate Equivalent Dose
NATURAL THYROID PREPARATION	
Desiccated thyroid	60–65 mg
SYNTHETIC THYROID PREPARATIONS	
Levothyroxine	0.1 mg
Liothyronine	25 μg

TABLE 30-2
THYROID DRUGS: COMMON ADVERSE EFFECTS

Body System	Side/Adverse Effects
Cardiovascular	Tachycardia, palpitations, angina, dysrhythmias, hypertension
Central nervous	Insomnia, tremors, headache, anxiety
Gastrointestinal	Nausea, diarrhea, increased or decreased appetite, cramps
Other	Menstrual irregularities, weight loss, sweating, heat intolerance, fever, thyroid storm (a rare, acute, life-threatening hypermetabolic state)

absorption of the antilipemic, and diabetic clients taking a thyroid agent may require increased doses of their hypoglycemic agents and insulin. In addition, the use of thyroid preparations with epinephrine in clients with coronary disease may induce coronary insufficiency.

Dosages

For the recommended dosages of the thyroid agents, see the dosages table below. See Appendix B for some of the common brands available in Canada.

DRUG PROFILES

The most commonly used agents for hypothyroidism are synthetic; the natural agents are seldom used today. Many factors must be considered before the initiation of drug therapy with a thyroid agent. These include the desired ratio of T_3 to T_4, the cost, and the desired duration of effect. The thyroid hormone replacement drugs are classified as pregnancy category A agents. They are all contraindicated in clients who have had a hypersensitivity reaction to them in the past and in those suffering from adrenal insufficiency, MI, or hyperthyroidism.

▸ desiccated thyroid

Desiccated thyroid is the cleaned, dried, and powdered thyroid gland of domesticated animals, usually hogs, and it is a combination of both T_3 and T_4 in a normal physiological ratio. Each 60 to 65 mg of thyroid is approximately equivalent to 100 μg or less of T_4 and 25 μg of T_3. Thyroid is not considered the drug of choice for treating hypothyroidism because of the lack of purity, uniformity, and stability in the formulation. It is the oldest of the available

preparations. Thyroid is available only in oral form as 30-, 60-, and 125-mg tablets. Pregnancy category A. Common dosages are given in the table below.

PHARMACOKINETICS

Half-Life	Onset	Peak*	Duration*
6–7 days	2 days	3–4 wk	1–3 wk

*Therapeutic effects.

▸ levothyroxine

Levothyroxine, or T_4, is the most commonly prescribed synthetic thyroid hormone. One advantage it has over the natural thyroid preparations is that it is chemically pure, being 100 percent T_4 (thyroxine). Its half-life is long enough that it needs to be administered only once a day. It is available in oral (PO) form as 25-, 50-, 75-, 88-, 100-, 112-, 125-, 137- 150-, 175-, 200-, and 300-μg tablets and in parenteral form as a 500-μg injection. Pregnancy category A. Common dosages are given in the table below.

PHARMACOKINETICS

Half-Life	Onset	Peak*	Duration*
6–7 days	2 days	3–4 wk	1–3 wk

*Therapeutic effects.

liothyronine

Like levothyroxine, liothyronine is also a chemically pure synthetic thyroid hormone preparation, but it is 100 percent T_3 (tri-iodothyronine) instead of T_4. Another way in which it differs from levothyroxine is that it has a rapid onset and a short duration of action. These pharmacokinetic differences are important because they make liothyronine the preferred agent when either

DOSAGES Selected Thyroid Agents

Agent	Pharmacological Class	Usual Dosage Range	Indications
▸▸ **desiccated thyroid**	Desiccated (dried) animal thyroid gland	***Adult*** PO: 30–125 mg/day PO: 30–180 mg/day ***Pediatric 0–12 yr*** 15–90 mg/day	Hypothyroidism Myxedema Congenital hypothyroidism
▸▸ **levothyroxine**	Synthetic levothyroxine (thyroid hormone T_4)	***Adult*** PO: 100–200 μg/day IM/IV: 50% of oral dose IV: 300–500 μg in a single dose; repeat next day 75–100 μg if necessary ***Pediatric 0–12 yr*** PO: 25–150 μg/day	Hypothyroidism Myxedema coma Congenital hypothyroidism
liothyronine*	Synthetic liothyronine (thyroid hormone T_3)	***Adult only*** PO: 25–100 μg/day PO: 50–100 μg daily PO: 5–50 μg qod	Hypothyroidism Myxedema Cretinism

*Liothyronine is synonymous with tri-iodothyronine (T_3).

a rapid effect or a rapidly reversible effect is desired, such as for diagnostic procedures requiring short-term thyrotropin suppression or for the treatment of myxedema coma. On the other hand, its more pronounced adverse cardiovascular effects, along with its short duration of action, make it less likely to be used for long-term use. It is available in oral form as 5- and 25-μg tablets. Pregnancy category A. Common dosages are given in the table on p. 508.

PHARMACOKINETICS

Half-Life	Onset	Peak*	Duration*
2.5 days	hours	48–72 hr	72 hr

*Therapeutic effects.

ANTITHYROID AGENTS

The treatment of hyperthyroidism may be aimed at treating either the primary cause or the symptoms of the disease. Antithyroid drugs, iodides, ionic inhibitors, and radioactive isotopes of iodine are used to treat the underlying cause, and drugs such as beta-blockers are used to treat the symptoms. The focus of the discussion here is on the antithyroid drugs called the *thioamide* derivatives, which mainly consist of methimazole and propylthiouracil. Besides the thioamides, radioactive iodine may be used to treat hyperthyroidism. Radioactive iodine (iodine 131, ^{131}I) works by destroying the thyroid gland. It does this by emitting destructive beta rays once it is taken up into the follicles of the thyroid gland. It may be used as a second- or third-line treatment for some cases of hyperthyroidism but is more commonly used to treat thyroid cancer (Chapter 46). Surgery is a non-pharmacological means of treating hyperthyroidism and involves removal of part of the thyroid gland. It is usually an effective way to treat hyperthyroidism. After either surgery or treatment by radioactive iodine, thyroid replacement may be necessary.

Mechanism of Action and Drug Effects

Methimazole and propylthiouracil act by inhibiting the incorporation of iodine molecules into the amino acid tyrosine, a process required to make both monoiodotyrosine and di-iodotyrosine, the precursors of T_3 and T_4. Doing so impedes the formation of thyroid hormone. Propylthiouracil has the added ability to inhibit the conversion of T_4 to T_3 in the peripheral circulation. Neither drug, however, can inactivate existing thyroid hormone.

The drug effects of methimazole and propylthiouracil are primarily limited to the thyroid gland, their overall effect being a decrease in the thyroid hormone level. The administration of these medications to clients suffering from hyperthyroidism lowers the high levels of thyroid hormone, thereby normalizing the overall metabolic rate.

Indications

Antithyroid agents are used to palliate hyperthyroidism and to prevent the surge in thyroid hormones that occurs after the surgical treatment of or during the radioactive iodine therapy for hyperthyroidism. In some types of hyperthyroidism, such as that seen in Graves' disease, the long-term administration of these agents (several years) may induce a spontaneous remission. However, most clients eventually require surgery or radioactive iodine therapy.

Contraindications

The only usual contraindications to the use of the two antithyroid agents is known drug allergy. These agents should be avoided in pregnancy whenever possible and are both rated pregnancy category D. However, they are sometimes used in the lowest effective dose to treat hyperthyroidism that is exacerbated by the metabolic demands of pregnancy.

Side Effects and Adverse Effects

The most damaging or serious adverse effects of the antithyroid medications are liver and bone marrow toxicity. These and the more common adverse effects of methimazole and propylthiouracil are listed in Table 30-3.

Interactions

Drug interactions that occur with antithyroid agents include an additive agranulocytosis when they are taken in conjunction with other bone marrow depressants and an increase in the activity of oral anticoagulants.

Dosages

See the dosages table on p. 511 for the recommended dosages of methimazole and propylthiouracil. See Appendix B for some of the common brands available in Canada.

TABLE 30-3
ANTITHYROID DRUGS: COMMON ADVERSE EFFECTS

Body System	Side/Adverse Effect
Central nervous	Drowsiness, headache, vertigo, fever, paraesthesia
Gastrointestinal	Nausea, vomiting, diarrhea, jaundice, hepatitis, loss of taste
Genitourinary	Smoky-coloured urine, decreased urine output
Hematological	Agranulocytosis, leukopenia, thrombocytopenia, hemolytic anemia, hypothrombinemia, lymphadenopathy, bleeding
Integumentary	Rash, pruritus, hyperpigmentation
Musculoskeletal	Myalgia, arthralgia, nocturnal muscle cramps
Renal	Increased BUN and serum creatinine
Other	Enlarged thyroid, nephritis, loss of hair

BUN, Blood urea nitrogen.

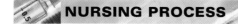

DRUG PROFILES

methimazole

Methimazole is one of the two thioamide antithyroid agents and is contraindicated in clients who have shown a hypersensitivity to it. It is available only in oral form as a 5-mg tablet. It is rated as a pregnancy category D agent but is sometimes used in minimally effective doses in cases of hyperthyroidism that are exacerbated by pregnancy. However, propylthiouracil is often preferred because it is less likely to cross the placenta and cause neonatal complications such as neonatal goitre. Common dosages are given in the table on p. 511.

PHARMACOKINETICS

Half-Life	Onset	Peak*	Duration
5–13 hr	5 days	7 wk	2–4 hr

*Therapeutic effects.

▶ *propylthiouracil*

Propylthiouracil (PTU) is the other thioamide antithyroid agent and is also rated as a pregnancy category D agent. The contraindications to its use are the same as those for methimazole. About 2 weeks of therapy with propylthiouracil may be necessary before symptoms improve. It is available only in oral form as 50- and 100-mg tablets. Common dosages are given in the table on p. 511.

PHARMACOKINETICS

Half-Life	Onset	Peak*	Duration
1–2 hr	10–21 days†	6–10 wk	weeks

*Therapeutic effects.
†Effects on serum thyroid hormone concentration may occur within 60 min of a single dose.

NURSING PROCESS

Assessment

Before thyroid therapy is initiated, the nurse should assess the client for contraindications, such as adrenal insufficiency, MI, and hyperthyroidism. Cautious use is recommended in clients with coronary heart disease, hypertension, angina, cardiac disease and in pregnant women. A female's menses may be affected by change in hormone levels and therefore a baseline assessment is important for women of childbearing age and women who are menstruating.

The antithyroid hormones methimazole and propylthiouracil are contraindicated in clients who have shown a hypersensitivity to the medication and in pregnant women during the third trimester. Cautious use is recommended in clients with liver disease, infections, or bone marrow disease (because of the agranulocytosis and other blood dyscrasias they can cause), and during the first and second trimesters of pregnancy.

Baseline weights, vital signs, and intake and output should be obtained and recorded in clients receiving either a thyroid or an antithyroid preparation.

Nursing Diagnoses

Nursing diagnoses appropriate to clients receiving a thyroid or antithyroid preparation include the following:

- Risk for injury related to the side effects of the medication.
- Risk for infection related to the bone marrow depression caused by antithyroid medication.
- Acute pain related to the side effects of the medication.
- Decreased cardiac output related to side effects of the thyroid agents.
- Deficient knowledge related to lack of experience with self-administration of the medication.

Planning

Goals pertaining to clients receiving a thyroid or an antithyroid preparation include the following:

- Client remains free from injury as the result of the side effects of the medication.
- Client is monitored closely (e.g., for thyroid levels) while taking the medication.
- Client remains free of infection while receiving antithyroid medication.
- Client maintains normal energy levels while on thyroid agents.
- Client experiences minimal side effects resulting from the medication.
- Client demonstrates an understanding of the use of the thyroid agent and its side effects and the need for adherence.

Outcome Criteria

Outcome criteria that pertain to clients receiving a thyroid or an antithyroid preparation include the following:

- Client states the measures to implement to decrease the likelihood of self-injury related to the drug's side effects, such as frequent laboratory checks and monitoring of vital signs.
- Client states the importance of follow-up appointments with the physician for frequent blood studies and monitoring of therapeutic effects.
- Client states ways to decrease the risk of infection while receiving an antithyroid medication, such as avoiding persons with infections, eating a proper diet, and getting adequate rest.
- Client uses relaxation techniques to deal with the nervousness and irritability caused by the agents or the diseases.

Implementation

When administering thyroid agents, it is important for the nurse to give the medication at the same time each day to maintain consistent blood levels of the agent. If possible it is best to administer thyroid agents taken once daily in the morning to decrease the likelihood of insomnia that may result from evening dosing. If administering levothyroxine intravenously, the nurse should follow the manufacturer's guidelines regarding the dilutional substances and the rate of administration.

DOSAGES   Selected Antithyroid Agents

Agent	Pharmacological Class	Usual Dosage Range	Indications
methimazole	Antithyroid	**Adult** PO: 15–60 mg/day divided tid **Pediatric** PO: 0.4 mg/kg/day divided tid	Hyperthyroidism
▸▸ propylthiouracil (PTU)	Antithyroid	**Adult** PO: 150–900 mg/day divided tid **Pediatric 6–10 yr** PO: 50–150 mg/day divided **Pediatric >10 yr** PO: 150–300 mg/day divided	

If the client is scheduled to undergo any radioactive isotope studies, the thyroid medication is usually discontinued about 4 weeks before the test, but only with a physician's order.

Antithyroid medications are better tolerated when taken with meals. These agents should also be given at the same time every day to maintain consistent blood levels of the agent, and they should never be withdrawn abruptly.

Teaching tips for clients receiving thyroid or antithyroid agents are presented in the box below.

■ Evaluation

A therapeutic response to thyroid agents is reflected by the disappearance of the symptoms of hypothyroidism, including depression, constipation, loss of appetite, weight gain, cold intolerance, syncope, and dry and brittle hair. Increased nervousness, irritability, mood changes, angina, and palpitations are side effects that need to be reported to the physician immediately. Clues that a client is receiving inadequate doses include a return of the symptoms of hypothyroidism (see previous discussion).

A therapeutic response to antithyroid medications would be characterized by weight gain, decreased pulse,

a return to a normal blood pressure, and decreased serum levels of T_4. Symptoms of overdose include cold intolerance, depression, and edema. The client should be encouraged to report the development of any swelling, sore throat, lesions, or other signs of inflammation. Clues that a client is not receiving adequate doses include tachycardia, insomnia, irritability, fever, and diarrhea.

CLIENT TEACHING TIPS

The nurse should instruct the client as follows:
▲ Never discontinue your medication without your physician's approval or order.
▲ It is important for clients taking thyroid agents to take the medication exactly as prescribed, at the same time every day, and not to switch brands unless approved by the physician.
▲ You may not get the full benefit of your medication for several months.
▲ Too high a dose of a thyroid agent may result in nervousness, irritability, and insomnia.
▲ Report any unusual symptoms, chest pain, or heart palpitations.

▲ Do not take any over-the-counter medications without your physician's approval.
▲ If you are taking antithyroid medications, you may be advised to avoid eating foods high in iodine, such as soy, tofu, turnip, seafood, and some breads. In addition, you should avoid using iodized salt.
▲ For the first few months of drug therapy, keep a log or journal of your pulse, weight, mood, daily energy levels, and appetite to help in evaluating the effectiveness of the medication.

POINTS to REMEMBER

▼ Thyroxine (T₄) and tri-iodothyronine (T₃) are the two hormones produced by the thyroid gland.

▼ Thyroid hormone is made by iodination and coupling with the amino acid tyrosine.

▼ T₄ is made by combining two molecules of di-iodotyrosine (it has four iodine molecules).

▼ T₃ is formed by coupling one molecule of di-iodotyrosine with one molecule of monoiodotyrosine (it has three iodine molecules).

▼ T₃ is about four times more biologically potent than thyroxine.

▼ Primary hypothyroidism is caused by an abnormality in the thyroid gland itself.

▼ Secondary hypothyroidism may result from a dysfunctional pituitary gland (lowered TSH level).

▼ Thyroid replacement is generally done carefully by a healthcare provider with frequent monitoring.

▼ Synthetic preparations include levothyroxine and liothyronine.

▼ Hyperthyroidism is caused by excessive secretion of thyroid hormone from the thyroid gland and may be attributed to different diseases (Graves' disease and multinodular disease) or drugs.

▼ Antithyroid drugs may be thioamide derivatives and consist mainly of methimazole and propylthiouracil.

▼ Surgery is the non-drug treatment for hyperthyroidism.

▼ Antithyroid drugs act by inhibiting the incorporation of iodine molecules into the amino acid tyrosine, thus preventing the formation of thyroid hormone.

▼ Children taking thyroid replacement hormones will show almost immediate behaviour and personality changes reflecting an improved thyroid state.

▼ Clients should report the occurrence of excitability, irritability, or anxiety to their healthcare provider because these symptoms may indicate toxicity.

▼ Hair loss in children taking thyroid replacements is temporary.

EXAMINATION REVIEW QUESTIONS

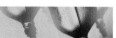

1 Which of the following side effects are associated with antithyroid drugs?
  a. Polyuria
  b. Decrease in or loss of taste
  c. Hyperactivity
  d. Temperature below 36.7°C

2 Which of the following may occur in women who are hyperthyroid?
  a. Sluggish feeling all the time
  b. Polycystic lungs
  c. Irregular menstrual cycles
  d. Polycythemia

3 Which of the following non-specific symptoms may represent hypothyroidism in the older adult client?
  a. Leukopenia, anemia
  b. Loss of appetite, polyuria
  c. Weight loss, dry cough
  d. Cold intolerance, depression

4 To help with the insomnia associated with thyroid hormone replacement therapy, the client may be encouraged to do which of the following?
  a. Take half the dose at lunch time and the other half 2 hours later.
  b. Take 75–150 mg of diphenhydramine every 4 hours or less.
  c. Always take the dose early in the morning and contact the physician if there is little improvement in the sleeping pattern.
  d. Be sure to add ephedra and ginseng to help with insomnia.

5 Which of the following are common side effects of thyroid drugs?
  a. Weight gain
  b. Excessive fatigue
  c. Bradycardia and hypotension
  d. Menstrual irregularities and tremors

For answers see http://evolve.elsevier.com/Lilley/pharmacology/.

CRITICAL THINKING ACTIVITIES

1 Your client has been taking thyroid agents for about 16 months and has recently noted palpitations and some heat intolerance. Should you be concerned about this or is this a fairly benign reaction to thyroid replacement? Explain your answer.

2 Your client has just had her thyroid gland removed. At 44 years of age she is now being placed on thyroid hormone replacement with levothyroxine at a dose of 200 μg once a day. How much levothyroxine in milligrams is found in this hormone replacement drug?

3 Your client, a new admission from the medical surgical unit to the step-down ICU, underwent a thyroidectomy 2 days ago. While reviewing the orders you note that the client is to be started on his thyroid medication upon transfer to your unit. The written orders specify that 25 μg of levothyroxine should be given once daily. However, the pharmacy has sent 25 μg of liothyronine, another thyroid replacement product. Because the dose of each is the same, is it okay to administer the liothyronine? Explain your answer.

For answers see http://evolve.elsevier.com/Lilley/pharmacology/.

BIBLIOGRAPHY

Albanese, J., & Nutz, P. (2005). *Mosby's 2005 nursing drug cards.* St Louis, MO: Mosby.

Canadian Pharmacists Association. (2003). *Therapeutic choices* (4th ed.). Ottawa, ON: Author.

Canadian Pharmacists Association. (2004). *Guide to drugs in Canada.* Toronto, ON: Dorling Kindersley.

Canadian Pharmacists Association. (2005). *Compendium of pharmaceuticals and specialties. The Canadian drug reference for health professionals.* Ottawa, ON: Author. [The subscription-based e-CPS is available at http://www.pharmacists.ca.]

Cheng, A., Williams, B.A., & Sivarajan, B.V. (Eds.). *The HSC handbook of pediatrics* (10th ed.). Toronto, ON: Elsevier.

Facts and Comparisons. (2004). *Drug facts and comparisons pocket version* (9th ed.). St Louis, MO: Wolters Kluwer Health.

Ginsberg, J. (2003). Diagnosis and management of Graves' disease. *Canadian Medical Association Journal, 168*(1), 575–585.

Health Canada. (2005). Drug product database (DPD). Retrieved August 16, 2005, from http://www.hc-sc.gc.ca/hpb/drugs-dpd/

Lacy, C.F., Armstrong, L.L., Goldman, M.P., & Lance, L.L. (2003). *Drug information handbook* (11th ed.). Hudson, OH: Lexi-Comp.

Mosby. (2005). *Mosby's drug consult 2005: The comprehensive reference for generic and brand name drugs* (15th ed.). St Louis, MO: Mosby.

Skidmore-Roth, L. (2006). *Mosby's 2006 nursing drug reference* (19th ed.). St Louis, MO: Mosby.

Skjoldebrand Sparre, L., Kollind, M., & Carlstrom, K. (2002). Ovarian ultrasound and ovarian and adrenal hormones before and after treatment for hyperthyroidism. *Gynecologic and Obstetric Investigation, 54,* 50–55.

Tierney, L.M., McPhee, S.J., & Papadakis, M.A. (2003). *Current medical diagnosis and treatment 2003.* New York: McGraw-Hill.

CHAPTER

31 Antidiabetic Agents

OBJECTIVES

After reading this chapter, the successful student will be able to do the following:

1 Discuss the normal actions and functions of the pancreas and the feedback system that regulates it.

2 Contrast type 1 and type 2 diabetes mellitus in terms of age of onset, signs and symptoms, treatment, drug therapy, incidence, and etiology.

3 Discuss the various factors influencing blood glucose in non-diabetic individuals and in clients with either type of diabetes mellitus.

4 Identify the various medications used to manage type 1 and type 2 diabetes mellitus.

5 Compare the signs and symptoms and related treatment of hypoglycemia and hyperglycemia.

6 Discuss the mechanisms of action, indications, contraindications, cautions, and side effects associated with the various categories of insulin and the various oral antihyperglycemic agents.

7 Compare rapid, regular, intermediate, and long-acting insulins in reference to their onset of action, peak effects, duration of action, indications, side effects, and cautions and contraindications.

8 Develop nursing care plans that include all phases of the nursing process for clients with type 1 or type 2 diabetes with a focus on medication regimens.

e-LEARNING ACTIVITIES

Student CD-ROM
- Review Questions: see questions 236–250
- *Animations*
- Medication Administration Checklists
- IV Therapy Checklists

evolve Web site (http://evolve.elsevier.com/Lilley/pharmacology/)
- Online Chapter Worksheet • Frequently Asked Questions
- Learning Tips and Content Updates • WebLinks • Online Appendices and Supplements • Mosby/Saunders ePharmacology Update • Access to *Mosby's Drug Consult*

DRUG PROFILES

acarbose, p. 526
chlorpropamide, p. 526
▸▸ extended insulin zinc suspension (Ultralente) and glargine, p. 522

glimepiride, p. 527
▸▸ gliclazide, p. 526
▸▸ glyburide, p. 527
▸▸ insulin lispro and insulin aspart, p. 521

▸▸ insulin zinc suspension (Lente) and insulin isophane suspension (NPH), p. 521

▸▸ metformin, p. 527
▸▸ regular insulin, p. 521
repaglinide, p. 527
▸▸ rosiglitazone, p. 527

▸▸ Key drugs.

GLOSSARY

Diabetes mellitus (dye ə bee' teez mel' lə təs) A complex disorder of carbohydrate, fat, and protein metabolism primarily resulting from the lack of insulin secretion by the beta cells of the pancreas or from defects of the insulin receptors; commonly referred to more simply as *diabetes*. There are two major types of diabetes: type 1 and type 2.

Diabetic ketoacidosis (DKA) (kee' to as' ə doe' sis) Severe metabolic complication of uncontrolled type 1 diabetes, which, untreated, eventually leads to diabetic coma and death.

514

Gestational diabetes   A type of glucose intolerance that develops during pregnancy. It may resolve after pregnancy but may also be a precursor of diabetes in later life.

Glucagon   (gloo′ kə gon) Hormone produced by the alpha cells in the islets of Langerhans that stimulates the conversion of glycogen to glucose in the liver.

Glucose   (gloo′ kose) One of the simple sugars found in fruits that serve as a major source of energy.

Glycogen   (gly′ koe jən) A polysaccharide that is the major carbohydrate stored in animal cells.

Glycogenolysis   (gly′ koe jə nol′ ə sis) The breakdown of glycogen to glucose.

Hemoglobin A1c   Hemoglobin molecules to which glucose molecules are bound; used as a diagnostic measurement of average daily blood glucose in the monitoring of diabetes; also called *glycosylated hemoglobin* or *glycated hemoglobin.*

Hyperglycemia   (hy′ pər gly see′ mee uh) A condition involving a fasting blood glucose level greater than or equal to 7 mmol/L or any blood glucose level greater than or equal to 11.1 mmol/L.

Hypoglycemia   A condition involving a blood glucose level less than 2.8 mmol/L.

Insulin   (in′ sə lin) A naturally occurring hormone secreted by the beta cells of the islets of Langerhans in the pancreas in response to increased levels of glucose in the blood.

Ketones   (kee′ tonez) An organic chemical compound produced through the oxidation of secondary alcohols, including dietary carbohydrates.

Nephropathy   (nə frop′ ə thee) A disorder of the kidney that includes inflammatory, degenerative, and sclerotic conditions; a long-term complication of uncontrolled diabetes.

Neuropathy   (nyoo rop′ ə thee) Inflammation or degeneration of the peripheral nerves; a long-term complication of uncontrolled diabetes.

Polydipsia   (pol′ ee dip′ see uh) Chronic excessive intake of water; a common symptom of diabetes.

Polyphagia   (pol′ ee fay′ jee uh) Excessive eating; a common symptom of diabetes.

Polyuria   (pol′ ee yur′ ee uh) Increased frequency of urinary output; a common symptom of diabetes.

Retinopathy   (ret′ i nop′ ə thee) A non-inflammatory eye disorder resulting from changes in the retinal blood vessels; a long-term complication of uncontrolled diabetes.

Type 1 diabetes mellitus   A genetically determined autoimmune disorder involving a complete or nearly complete lack of insulin production; most commonly arises in children or adolescents. Formerly referred to as *insulin-dependent diabetes mellitus (IDDM)* or *juvenile-onset diabetes;* however, "type 1" has been the official classification designated by the Canadian Diabetes Association (CDA) since 1995.

Type 2 diabetes mellitus (T2DM)   A type of diabetes that most commonly presents in middle age. The disease may be controlled by lifestyle modifications, oral drug therapy, and/or insulin, but clients are not necessarily dependent on insulin. May also be referred to as *non–insulin-dependent diabetes mellitus (NIDDM)* or *adult-onset diabetes;* however, "type 2" has been the official classification designated by the CDA since 1995.

THE PANCREAS

The pancreas is a large, elongated organ that is located behind the stomach. It is both an exocrine gland (secreting digestive enzymes through the pancreatic duct) and an endocrine gland (secreting hormones directly into the bloodstream and not through a duct). The endocrine functions of the pancreas are the focus of this chapter. The pancreas produces two main hormones: insulin and glucagon. Both hormones play an important role in the regulation of the endocrine system, specifically the use, mobilization, and storage of **glucose**, one of the primary sources of energy for the cells of the body. There is a normal amount of glucose that circulates in the blood to meet quick energy requirements. However, not all of the glucose we consume is needed. When the quantity of glucose in the blood is sufficient, the excess is stored as **glycogen** in the liver and, to a lesser extent, in skeletal muscle tissue, where it remains until the body needs it. Glucose is also stored in adipose tissue as triglyceride body fat stores.

When blood glucose is needed, the glycogen stored primarily in the liver is converted back to glucose through a process called **glycogenolysis.** The hormone responsible for initiating this process is **glucagon.** Glucagon has only minimal effects on muscle glycogen and adipose tissue triglyceride stores.

Glucagon is a protein hormone, consisting of a single chain of amino acids (polypeptide chain) with molecules about half the size of insulin. It is released from the alpha cells of the islets of Langerhans in the pancreas. The beta cells of these same islets secrete **insulin,** a protein hormone composed of two amino acid chains (acidic A chain and basic B chain) joined by a disulphide linkage.

Insulin serves several important metabolic functions in the body. It stimulates carbohydrate metabolism in skeletal and cardiac muscle and adipose tissue by facilitating the transport of glucose into these cells. In the liver, insulin facilitates the phosphorylation of glucose to glucose-6-phosphate, which is then converted to glycogen for storage. By causing glucose to be stored in the liver as glycogen, insulin keeps the kidney free of glucose. Without insulin the kidney would lose through urinary excretion large amounts of important substances such as glucose (a critical body nutrient and energy source), **ketones**, and other solutes. This loss of nutrient energy sources would eventually lead to **polyphagia**, weight loss, and malnutrition. The presence of these solutes in the distal renal tubules and collecting ducts would also osmotically draw large volumes of water into the urine, leading to **polyuria**, dehydration, and **polydipsia**.

Insulin also has a direct effect on fat metabolism. It stimulates lipogenesis and inhibits lipolysis and the release of fatty acids from adipose cells. In addition, insulin stimulates protein synthesis and promotes the intracellular shift of potassium and magnesium, thereby decreasing elevated blood concentrations of these electrolytes. There is a continuous homeostatic balance in the body between the actions of insulin and those of glucagon. This natural balance normally serves to maintain physiologically optimal blood glucose levels. The adrenocortical hormone cortisol and the adrenomedullary hormone epinephrine work synergistically with glucagon to counter the effects of insulin and cause increases in the blood glucose level. The actions of insulin are also antagonized by somatropin (growth hormone), the adrenomedullary hormone norepinephrine, the adrenocortical hormone aldosterone, thyroid hormones, and estrogens.

DIABETES MELLITUS

Hyperglycemia is a state involving excessive concentrations of glucose in the blood and results when the normal counterbalancing actions of glucagon and insulin go awry. The current key diagnostic criterion for **diabetes mellitus** is hyperglycemia consisting of a fasting plasma glucose (FPG) of greater than 7 mmol/L. Diabetes mellitus, more commonly referred to as simply *diabetes,* is primarily a disorder of carbohydrate metabolism that involves either a deficiency of insulin, a resistance to insulin, or both. Whatever the cause of the diabetes, the result is hyperglycemia. This can lead to serious short- and long-term adverse health effects if not controlled.

Diabetes mellitus has been recognized since 1552 BC, when Egyptians wrote of a malady they called *honeyed urine.* The first step toward discerning the cause of diabetes mellitus occurred in 1788 when Thomas Cawley, an English physician, voiced his suspicion that the source of the illness lay in the pancreas. However, it took over a century to prove this, and it took even longer to discover the substance, insulin, that is secreted from the pancreas, the lack of which is responsible for causing the disease. It was known that the substance, whatever it was, was needed by those afflicted with the illness, but the substance could not be isolated. It was not until the early 1920s that insulin was finally discovered by Canadians Dr. Fred Banting and Dr. Charles Best. Its discovery is now considered one of the greatest triumphs of twentieth-century medicine, and

its use in the therapy for diabetes mellitus has proved to be a life-saving remedy for millions of people afflicted with the disease.

Diabetes mellitus is not actually a single disease, however, but a group of diseases. This is why it is often regarded as a syndrome rather than a disease. The relative or absolute lack of insulin is believed to result from the destruction of beta cells in the pancreas such that insulin can be neither produced nor secreted. Hyperglycemia can also be caused by insulin receptor defects. When the receptor proteins in various tissues (e.g., liver, muscle, adipose tissue) that normally function in coordination with insulin to remove glucose from the blood are defective, they no longer respond normally to insulin molecules. The result is that glucose molecules remain in the blood, rather than being stored in the tissues. Two major types of diabetes mellitus are currently recognized and designated by the Canadian Diabetes Association (CDA): type 1 and type 2. Type 1 diabetes was previously also called *insulin-dependent diabetes mellitus (IDDM)* or *juvenile-onset diabetes.* Type 2 diabetes was previously also called *non–insulin-dependent diabetes mellitus (NIDDM)* or *adult-onset diabetes.* The older designations have been abandoned for a few reasons. One reason is that many clients with type 2 diabetes *do* eventually become dependent on insulin therapy for control of their illness. A second reason is that the current epidemic of both child and adult obesity in Canada is increasing the incidence of type 2 diabetes in children and adolescents. Obesity is one major risk factor for the development of type 2 diabetes. The differences between type 1 and type 2 diabetes mellitus are listed in Table 31-1. Less common types of diabetes included in the CDA classification are **gestational diabetes** (which emerges during pregnancy) and other specific types that consist primarily of genetically defined forms of diabetes or diabetes associated with other diseases or drug use. (Note that diabetes insipidus, mentioned in Chapter 29, is an unrelated disease.)

Type 1 Diabetes Mellitus

Type 1 diabetes mellitus is characterized by a lack of insulin production or by the production of defective insulin. Affected clients require exogenous insulin to treat and prevent its many complications. Common complications

TABLE 31-1

TYPE 1 AND TYPE 2 DIABETES: CHARACTERISTICS

Characteristic	Type 1	Type 2
Onset	Juvenile-onset diabetes, age <20 yr	Maturity-onset diabetes, generally age >40 yr but can occur at younger ages especially in certain ethnic groups such as First Nations populations
Endogenous insulin	Little or none	Normal
Treatment	Insulin	Weight loss, diet and exercise, oral antihyperglycemics; clients often require insulin
Incidence	10% of cases	90% of cases
Insulin receptors	Normal	Decreased or defective
Body weight	Usually non-obese	Obese (80%)
Etiology	Autoimmune destruction of beta cells in the pancreas	Multifactorial genetic defects; strong association with obesity and insulin resistance resulting from a reduction in insulin receptors

of the disorder are damage to the retina of the eye (**retinopathy**), damage to peripheral nerves (**neuropathy**), and damage to the nephrons of the kidney (**nephropathy**). Instead of the normal metabolic reactions taking place that lead to the storage of glucose, glucose may be broken down into fatty acids that are converted to ketones. If this happens in sufficient amounts, **diabetic ketoacidosis (DKA)** may result. This is a complex multisystem disorder and a common complication of uncontrolled type 1 diabetes mellitus that, unchecked, will lead to coma and death. The person experiencing DKA is suffering from extreme hyperglycemia, positive serum ketone levels, acidosis, dehydration, and electrolyte imbalances. Approximately 25 to 30 percent of clients with newly diagnosed type 1 diabetes mellitus present with DKA. The most common precipitator of DKA is some kind of physical or emotional stress. The stressor(s) trigger the release of the counter-regulatory hormones cortisol and epinephrine, which then mobilize glucagon and release glucose from the storage sites in the liver, further adding to the already elevated levels of glucose in the blood. At some point during this crisis cascade of events, an autoimmune reaction may be initiated that destroys the insulin-producing beta cells of the pancreatic islets of Langerhans. The result is essentially a complete lack of endogenous insulin production by the pancreas, necessitating chronic replacement insulin therapy. Oral antihyperglycemic agents, discussed later in this chapter, are not effective for type 1 diabetes.

Type 2 Diabetes Mellitus

Type 2 diabetes mellitus (T2DM), which was once thought to be a mild form of type 1 diabetes mellitus, is an important but poorly treated disorder. It is by far the most common form of diabetes mellitus, accounting for about 90 percent of all cases and affecting 10 percent of the population over 65 years of age. Of concern is the recent global increase in the number of children, adolescents, and young adults diagnosed with T2DM, as well as the estimated large number of young people with the disease who may not be aware of it. It is estimated that T2DM now represents at least 10 percent of all youth onset diabetes. High-risk populations in Canada include Latinos, people of East Asian and South Asian descent, and First Nations children. For example, in the Oji-Cree of northeastern Manitoba and northwestern Ontario, up to 4 percent of female adolescents are affected with T2DM. However, no ethnic group is immune to the development of T2DM. Weight gain, poor nutrition, and lack of exercise in the younger population are contributing factors to this disturbing trend. This population of young onset T2DM is at risk for significant morbidity and mortality because of the high risk of developing complications.

Type 2 diabetes mellitus is due to both insulin resistance and insulin deficiency, but there is not an absolute lack of insulin as with type 1 diabetes. As previously noted, one of the normal roles of insulin is to take circulating glucose and transport it to tissues to be used as energy. With type 2 diabetes all of the main target tissues of insulin (muscle, liver, and adipose tissue) are hyporesponsive (resistant) to the effects of the hormone. Not only is the absolute number of insulin receptors on these tissues reduced, but their individual sensitivity and responsiveness to insulin is reduced as well. Therefore it is possible for a client with type 2 diabetes mellitus to have normal or even elevated levels of insulin yet still have high blood glucose levels. Another reason for this paradoxical situation is that the altered insulin–receptor dynamics cause the liver to overproduce glucose, exacerbating the hyperglycemic condition. All of these processes also result in impaired post-prandial (after a meal) glucose metabolism, further contributing to a hazardous hyperglycemic state.

In addition to a reduced number and sensitivity of insulin receptors, type 2 diabetes involves reduced insulin secretion by the pancreas. This insulin deficiency results from a loss of the normal responsiveness of the beta cells in the pancreas to elevated blood glucose levels. When these beta cells do not recognize glucose, they do not secrete insulin, and glucose is not transported into cells or tissues, nor is it stored in the liver. Insulin resistance and insulin deficiency may induce or aggravate each other.

Type 2 diabetes is a multifaceted disorder. Although loss of blood glucose control is its primary hallmark, several other significant co-occurring conditions are strongly associated with the disease. These include impaired glucose tolerance, abdominal obesity, dyslipidemia (Chapter 28), hypertension (Chapter 24), insulin resistance, hyperinsulinemia, microalbuminuria (urinary "spilling" of protein), and conditions in the blood that increase the likelihood of thrombosis (blood clotting). The cluster of co-occurring conditions of abdominal obesity, elevated triglycerides, elevated high-density lipoproteins (HDL-C), and hypertension greater than 130/85 are strongly associated with the development of type 2 diabetes and are collectively referred to as *metabolic syndrome*. Roughly 90 percent of clients are obese at the time of its initial diagnosis. Obesity serves only to worsen the insulin resistance because adipose tissue is often the site of a large proportion of the body's defective insulin receptors. Therefore the initial treatment of type 2 diabetes mellitus should consist of weight loss and lifestyle changes. Weight loss not only lowers blood glucose and lipid levels, but also reduces another common co-occurring condition, hypertension. Commonly recommended lifestyle changes include improved dietary habits (e.g., a diet higher in protein, lower in fat and carbohydrates), smoking cessation, decreasing alcohol consumption, and regular physical exercise. Cigarette smoking doubles the risk of cardiovascular disease in diabetic clients, largely because of its effects on peripheral vascular circulation and respiratory function. In fact, smoking cessation would probably save far more lives than antihypertensive, antilipemic, and antidiabetic drug treatments all together!

There is also a strong correlation between diabetes and heart disease. Cardiovascular disease is responsible for 80 percent of deaths for those with diabetes. Microvascular problems are now recognized at FPG levels of greater than 7 mmol/L. The CDA and the Clinical Practice Guidelines Expert Committee recommend testing all adults 40 years of age and older for FPG levels every 3 years. Decreasing alcohol consumption is helpful because alcohol is broken down in the body to simple carbohydrates, which leads to increases in blood glucose. Regular exercise has tremendous benefit in that it increases insulin sensitivity, the loss of which is a primary problem in type 2 diabetes.

Gestational Diabetes

Gestational diabetes is a type of glucose intolerance that develops during pregnancy. It occurs in about 2 to 4 percent of all pregnancies. The use of insulin is necessary to decrease risks of birth defects. In most cases gestational diabetes subsides after delivery. However, as many as 30 percent of these women develop type 2 diabetes within 10 to 15 years, and this percentage is even higher in First Nations women. Issues associated with diabetes management during pregnancy are discussed further in the section *Insulins*.

Hypoglycemia

Hypoglycemia is the condition in which the blood glucose level is abnormally low (generally below 2.8 mmol/L). When the cause is organic and the effects are mild, treatment usually consists of dietary modifications, primarily a higher intake of protein and lower intake of carbohydrates, to prevent a rebound post-prandial hypoglycemic effect. Hypoglycemia can also be a side effect of the antidiabetic agents when the pharmacological effects of these agents are greater than expected. Because the brain needs a constant amount of glucose to function, early symptoms of hypoglycemia include the central nervous system (CNS) manifestations of confusion, irritability, and sweating. Later symptoms include tremor, hypothermia, and seizures. Without adequate restoration of normal blood and CNS glucose levels, coma and death will occur.

ANTIDIABETIC AGENTS

The two major classes of drugs used to treat diabetes mellitus are the insulins and the oral antihyperglycemic agents. These drugs are more broadly referred to as *antidiabetic agents* and they are aimed at producing a normoglycemic or euglycemic (normal blood sugar) state.

INSULINS

The primary treatment for type 1 diabetes mellitus is insulin therapy. Clients with type 2 diabetes are not generally prescribed insulin until other measures, namely lifestyle changes and oral drug therapy, no longer provide adequate glycemic control. There are currently two main sources of insulin. It can be extracted from domesticated animals or synthesized in laboratories using recombinant deoxyribonucleic acid (DNA) technology. Originally isolated from cattle, beef-derived insulin is no longer available on the Canadian market. Insulin isolated from pigs is known as *porcine insulin* and has a chemical structure that differs from human insulin by only one amino acid. Porcine insulin (i.e., all Iletin products) is available in Canada but is seldom used and is being discontinued in 2006 (see Drug Profiles). Beef insulin can be imported from the United Kingdom through Health Canada's Special Access Programme (SAP). Since the early 1990s, all newly diagnosed clients

TABLE 31-2

COMPARISON ACTIONS OF HUMAN INSULINS AND ANALOGUES

Insulin Preparation	Onset of Action	Peak Action	Duration of Action
lispro*/aspart*	10–15 min	60–90 min	4–5 hr
Human regular	30–60 min	2–4 hr	5–8 hr
Human NPH/Lente	1–3 hr	5–8 hr	10–18 hr
Ultralente	3–4 hr	8–15 hr	22–26 hr
glargine*	90 min	—	24 hr

From Canadian Diabetes Association.
*Insulin analogue.
Lente is the trade name for insulin zinc suspension; Ultralente is the trade name for insulin zinc suspension extended.

with diabetes who require insulin have been started on human insulins. The development of recombinant DNA technologies has led to widespread use of recombinant insulins that are based on the natural chemical structure of the human insulin molecule. This insulin is produced by feeding bacteria or yeast the genetic information necessary for them to reproduce an insulin that is exactly like human insulin. The pharmacokinetic properties of insulin (onset of action, peak effect, and duration of action) can also be altered by making various minor modifications to either the insulin molecule itself or the drug formulation (final product). This practice has led to the development of several different insulin preparations, including several combination insulin products that contain more than one type of insulin in the same solution. Chemical manipulation of insulin activity in this way helps to meet the often individualized time-oriented metabolic demands for insulin in diabetic clients. Table 31-2 compares the pharmacokinetic parameters of various commonly prescribed insulin products. Further modifications can be accomplished by mixing compatible insulin preparations in the syringe before administration. The latest syringe compatibility data for currently available insulin products appears in Table 31-3. Clients should be thoroughly educated regarding how, when, and whether they should (or should not) mix different types of insulin. Some combinations are chemically incompatible and can result in undesirable alteration of glycemic effects.

Many insulin regimens have been used to manage type 1 diabetes mellitus. Insulin regimens should be individualized to the client's treatment goals, lifestyle, diet, age, general health, motivation, capacity for hypoglycemia awareness and self-management, as well as social and financial circumstances. The fixed-dose regimen, once considered conventional therapy, may still be used occasionally but is no longer the preferred strategy. Instead, the goal is to mimic normal pancreatic secretion, which is most successfully achieved with intensive therapy. Intensive therapy generally consists of a *basal-bolus* regimen. Intermediate- or long-acting insulin, or extended long-acting insulin analogue is given once or twice daily as the *basal* insulin, and fast-acting insulin or rapid-acting insulin analogue is given as the *bolus* insulin for food intake at each meal. According to the Diabetes Control and Complications Trial (DCCT, 1993), intensive therapy delays the onset and slows the progression of microvascular complications.

TABLE 31-3

INSULIN MIXING COMPATIBILITIES

Type of Insulin	Compatible With
Regular (Humulin-R, Novolinge-Toronto)	All insulins except glargine, Lente, and Ultralente (see below). Recommended that Humulin-R be mixed with Humalin formulations and Novolinge-Toronto be mixed with Novolinge.
Regular	Lente or Ultralente*
Regular	NPH; may use mixture immediately or store for future use
Insulin lispro (Humalog), insulin aspart (NovoRapid)	Regular, NPH, Lente, and Ultralente; inject mixture 15 min before meal†
Insulin glargine (Lantus)	Must be given alone due to low pH of diluent
Premixed insulin combinations of regular and NPH (Humulin 20/80, 30/70); Novolinge (10/90, 20/80, 30/70, 40/60, 50/50)	Already premixed; do not mix with other insulins
Premixed NPH 50 units and regular insulin 50 units (Novolinge 50/50)	
Premixed insulin lispro protamine suspension 75 units and insulin lispro 25 units cartridges (Humalog Mix 25)	

*These combinations are not normally recommended unless the client is already adequately controlled on this mixture. If so, the client should standardize the length of time between mixing and injection because of chemical interactions that delay the onset of action of the regular insulin. For this reason this mixture must be used soon after preparation; it is not suitable for storage for future use.
†Normally used as an alternative to regular insulin and therefore not usually given with it.
NPH, Isophane insulin suspension.

Pediatric clients and pregnant women require especially careful insulin therapy. Insulin doses for both are calculated by weight as they are for the general adult population. The usual dosage range is 0.3 to 0.6 units/kg/day as a total daily dose. However, there are a few important differences to be aware of regarding the use of the more "exotic" insulin products for children. The rapid-acting insulin lispro product is often used concurrently with oral sulphonylurea therapy (discussed later in this chapter). However, the combination lispro product Humalog Mix 25, which is 75 percent insulin lispro protamine (an intermediate-acting insulin) and 25 percent insulin lispro (a rapid-acting insulin) is currently available in cartridges approved for children. The other rapid-acting product, insulin aspart, is also approved for pediatric use. Glargine is the only insulin available with a 24-hour duration and a peakless profile. It is currently recommended for subcutaneous use in clients over 17 years of age. Any insulin prescriptions that fall outside of standard dosing guidelines should generally be prescribed by a trained pediatric endocrinologist, who must monitor the client carefully. Children need age-appropriate education and supervision, from both healthcare professionals and parents, that includes a safe and gradual transfer of responsibility for self-management of their illness.

Gestational diabetes reportedly occurs in 2 to 4 percent of pregnancies in the non-Aboriginal population and 8 to 18 percent in the Aboriginal populations in Canada. Women of Latino, South Asian, East Asian, or African descent are also at higher risk. Although most of these mothers will revert to a normal glycemic state after pregnancy, they also have an increased risk of developing diabetes again in later life. All currently available oral antidiabetic agents are contraindicated for pregnant clients. Therefore insulin therapy is the only currently recommended drug therapy. Roughly 15 percent of women who develop gestational diabetes require insulin therapy during pregnancy. All insulin products are classified as pregnancy category B agents except for the glargine and aspart products, which are pregnancy category

C agents. Insulins, both endogenous and exogenous, do not normally cross the placenta. However, insulin is normally excreted into human milk. Because this is a natural process, nursing mothers may still receive insulin therapy. However, it is currently not known whether glargine is excreted in breast milk and so it should not be used while breastfeeding. Optimization of insulin and diet is especially important for a nursing mother because inadequate or excessive glycemic control may reduce milk production. Nonetheless, effective glycemic control during pregnancy is essential because infants born to women with gestational diabetes have a two- to threefold risk of congenital anomalies. In addition, the incidence of stillbirths is directly related to the degree of hyperglycemia in the mother. Weight reduction is generally *not* advised for these women because it can jeopardize fetal nutritional status.

All pregnant women should have blood glucose screenings at regular prenatal visits. Women who develop gestational diabetes should be screened for type 2 diabetes within 6 months postpartum. They should also be advised of their increased risk for recurrent diabetes and of the importance of regular medical checkups. Finally, women who are known to be diabetic before pregnancy should ideally have detailed pre-pregnancy counselling (and therefore preferably a planned pregnancy) and prenatal care from a physician experienced in diabetic pregnancies.

Mechanism of Action and Drug Effects

Exogenously administered insulin functions as a substitute for the endogenous hormone. It serves to replace the insulin that is either not made at all or is made defectively in the body of a diabetic client. The drug effects of exogenously administered insulin are many and affect many body systems. They are the same as those of normal endogenous insulin. That is, exogenously administered insulin restores the diabetic client's ability to metabolize carbohydrates, fats, and proteins; to store glucose in the liver; and to convert glycogen to fat stores.

Indications

All insulin preparations can be indicated for both type 1 and type 2 diabetes, keeping in mind that each client requires careful customization of the dosing regimen for optimal glycemic control. Additional factors such as lifestyle modifications (e.g., dietary and exercise habits) and oral medications may also be indicated, especially in type 2 diabetes.

Contraindications

Contraindications to the use of all insulin products include known drug allergy to a specific product. Insulin should never be administered to an already hypoglycemic client.

Side Effects and Adverse Effects

Hypoglycemia resulting from an insulin overdose can result in shock and possibly death. This is the most immediate and serious adverse effect of insulin. Other more common adverse effects of insulin therapy are listed in Table 31-4.

Interactions

Significant drug interactions can occur with the insulins. Chlorthalidone, corticosteroids, diazoxide, epinephrine, ethacrynic acid, furosemide, phenytoin, thiazides, and thyroid hormones can all antagonize the hypoglycemic effects of insulin. Alcohol, anabolic steroids, guanethidine, monoamine oxidase inhibitors (MAOIs), propranolol, and the salicylates can all increase insulin's hypoglycemic effects.

Dosages

See the dosages table below for the recommended dosages of the various insulin agents. Some common brands available in Canada are also shown.

TABLE 31-4

INSULIN: COMMON ADVERSE EFFECTS

Body System	Side/Adverse Effect
Cardiovascular	Tachycardia, palpitations
Central nervous	Headache, lethargy, tremors, weakness, fatigue, delirium, sweating
Metabolic	Hypoglycemia, hypokalemia
Other	Blurred vision, dry mouth, hunger, nausea, flushing, rash, urticaria, anaphylaxis, lipodystrophy

DOSAGES **Human-Based Insulin Products**

Agent	Pharmacological Class	Usual Dosage Range	Indications
Rapid-Acting			
▸▸insulin aspart (NovoRapid) ▸▸insulin lispro (Humalog)	Human recombinant rapid-acting insulin analogues	SC: 0.5–1 unit/kg/day; doses are highly individualized to desired glycemic control; rapid-acting insulins are best given 15 min before a meal	
Short-Acting			
▸▸regular insulin (Humulin-R, Novolinge-Toronto)	Human recombinant short-acting insulin	SC only: Same dosage as insulin aspart and insulin lispro; SC doses of regular insulin are best given 30 to 60 min before a meal; regular insulin is also the only insulin that can be given IV as a continuous infusion	
Intermediate-Acting			
▸▸isophane insulin suspension (NPH, Humulin-N, Novolinge NPH) insulin zinc suspension (Humulin-L)	Human recombinant intermediate-acting insulin analogues	SC only: Same dosage as insulin aspart, insulin lispro, and regular insulin	Diabetes mellitus, type 1 and type 2
Long-Acting			
▸▸insulin glargine (Lantus) insulin zinc suspension, extended (Humulin-U)	Human recombinant long-acting insulin analogues	SC only: Same dosage as others but is approved only for once-daily dosage at bedtime	
Combination Insulin Products			
regular insulin 20% (30%) and NPH 80% (70%) (Humulin 20/80, 30/70. Also available in various combinations, regular and NPH, respectively (Novolinge 10/90, 20/80, 30/70, 40/60, 50/50)	Human recombinant intermediate-acting and short-acting combination insulin products	SC only: Same dosage as others	
insulin lispro protamine suspension 75% and insulin lispro 25% (Humalog Mix 25)	Human recombinant intermediate-acting and rapid-acting combination insulin product		

DRUG PROFILES

INSULINS

The primary treatment for both type 1 diabetes and gestational diabetes is insulin therapy. There are currently four major classes of insulin, as determined by their pharmacokinetic properties: rapid-acting, short-acting, intermediate-acting, and long-acting. Management regimes for type 2 diabetes more frequently are including insulin in combination with antihyperglycemic agents in order to achieve target blood glucose levels. The insulin dosage regimen for all diabetic clients is highly individualized and may consist of one or more types of insulin administered at either fixed doses or variable doses in response to self-measurements of blood glucose. The three remaining porcine (pork-derived) insulin products (Table 31-5) have actions comparable to those of the corresponding human-based insulins and analogues. However, because they are derived from a different animal species they are more likely to be allergenic. For this reason they are seldom used today in developed countries, except in the unusual case of a client who is intolerant of other insulins or demonstrates better glycemic control with a porcine product. Regular insulin, insulin lispro, and insulin glargine normally appear as clear, colourless solutions; the rest are white opaque (cloudy) solutions. The nurse should avoid using insulin products that appear to be inappropriately coloured or cloudy. All of the Lente insulin products have been largely eclipsed in practice by other types of insulin, including lispro and glargine. The Lente products are included here since they currently remain on the Canadian market and are still used occasion-

ally. Comparative pharmacokinetic parameters for several commonly used insulin products appear in Table 31-2.

RAPID-ACTING INSULINS

⇥ insulin lispro and insulin aspart

There are currently two insulin products that are classified as rapid acting. These have the most rapid onset of action (roughly 15 minutes) but often also a shorter duration of action than other insulin categories. These products include insulin lispro and insulin aspart. Their effects are most like those of the endogenous insulin produced from the pancreas in response to a meal. After a meal, the glucose that is ingested stimulates the pancreas to secrete insulin. This insulin then takes the excess glucose and stores it in the liver as glycogen. In people with diabetes mellitus, the insulin response to meals is deficient; therefore a rapid-acting insulin product is often used within 15 minutes of mealtime. This corresponds with the time required for the onset of action of these products.

Insulin lispro was approved by Health Canada in 1998. Unlike regular insulin, insulin lispro and insulin aspart are human insulin analogues with synthetic alterations to their chemical structures that alter their onset or duration of action. They have a faster onset of action and a shorter time to peak plasma level than regular insulin, but also a shorter duration. Produced with recombinant DNA technology, both insulin lispro and insulin aspart mimic the body's natural rapid insulin output after eating a meal more closely than previous insulin products. For this reason both are usually dosed within 15 minutes of beginning a meal. Both of these products are available in concentrations of 100 units/mL. Pregnancy category B for insulin lispro and category C for insulin aspart. The usually recommended doses are given in the table on p. 520.

SHORT-ACTING INSULIN

⇥ regular insulin

Regular insulin is currently the only insulin classified as short-acting. Some references still classify it as a rapid-acting insulin. However, it does not have as fast an onset as insulin lispro and insulin aspart. Regular insulin is the only insulin product that can be administered via intravenous (IV) bolus, intravenous infusion, or even intramuscularly (IM). These routes, especially the intravenous infusion route, are often used in cases of DKA or coma associated with uncontrolled type 1 diabetes.

Regular insulin solution was the first medicinal insulin product developed and was originally isolated from bovine (cow) and porcine (pig) sources. It is now primarily made with recombinant DNA technology (though one pork-derived product is still available until 2006) and, unlike the rapid-acting analogues discussed above, is essentially identical in structure to the human insulin hormone. Pregnancy category B for all regular insulin products. Table 31-2 lists these differences in more detail.

INTERMEDIATE-ACTING INSULINS

⇥ insulin zinc suspension and insulin isophane suspension

Currently available intermediate-acting insulin products include the two basic types: insulin zinc suspension, or Lente insulin; and insulin isophane suspension, more commonly called *NPH insulin* (for Neutral Protamine

TABLE 31-5

SOURCES OF AVAILABLE INSULIN PRODUCTS

Activity Classification	Human Recombinant Insulins	Purified Pork Insulins*
RAPID-ACTING		
insulin lispro	Humalog	N/A
insulin aspart	NovoRapid	N/A
SHORT-ACTING		
regular	Humulin-R, Novolinge-Toronto	Iletin II Pork Regular
INTERMEDIATE-ACTING		
isophane insulin suspension (NPH)	Humulin-N, Novolinge NPH	Iletin II Pork NPH
insulin zinc suspension (Lente)	Humulin-L	Iletin II Pork Lente
LONG-ACTING		
insulin glargine	Lantus	N/A
insulin zinc suspension extended (Ultralente)	Humulin-U	N/A

*The three pork-derived insulin products above are currently available but seldom used since the advent of recombinant DNA technology and its ability to produce human recombinant insulin products (based on the structure of the human insulin hormone) in quantities sufficient to treat large human populations on even a global scale. Beef-derived insulin products are no longer commercially available in Canada.

Hagedorn). As the experience with the regular insulins grew, a search was mounted for a longer-acting insulin that required less frequent dosing. It was found that the duration of the effects of insulin could be prolonged through the addition of a basic protein such as protamine or a substance such as zinc. This led to the development in the late 1930s and 1940s of protamine zinc insulin (PZI) and NPH insulin. PZI is no longer available in Canada, replaced by extended insulin zinc suspension (Ultralente), discussed in the next section.

Lente insulin is an intermediate-acting insulin that contains zinc, 70 percent of which is long-acting insulin zinc (crystalline insulin suspension, or Ultralente) and 30 percent of which is a more rapid-acting amorphous (non-crystalline) insulin suspension. The result is a cloudy insulin suspension with a usual onset of action of about 1 to 2 hours. NPH insulin, also known as *isophane insulin,* is a sterile suspension of zinc insulin crystals and protamine sulphate in buffered water for injection. It also appears cloudy or opaque.

The effects of these insulins are slower in onset and more prolonged than those of endogenous insulin. Both of these intermediate-acting insulins are available in strengths of 100 units/mL. Both are pregnancy category B. The usual recommended dosages are given in the table on p. 520.

LONG-ACTING INSULINS
» *extended insulin zinc suspension (Ultralente) and glargine*

Two long-acting insulin products are now available: extended insulin zinc suspension (Ultralente) and insulin glargine. The duration of action of Ultralente was prolonged through the addition of even more zinc than with Lente, specifically zinc chloride. Ultralente, like the Lente and NPH insulins, appears as a white, opaque suspension. In contrast, insulin glargine is normally a clear colourless solution. This is a recombinant-DNA-produced insulin analogue and is unique in that it provides a flat, constant level of insulin in the body. It is dosed once daily at bedtime, whereas Ultralente may sometimes be dosed more than once daily. Pregnancy category B for Ultralente insulin and pregnancy category C for insulin glargine. The usually recommended dosages are given in the table on p. 520.

Often for those being switched from twice-daily NPH, the initial glargine dose is reduced to 80 percent of the previous total NPH dose, with a range of 2 to 100 units.

Convenient cartridge-filled pens (FlexPens) are available for use with the following dosages: Novolin NR 70/30; NPH and regular insulin 70/30 (InnoLet); Novo-Rapid Mix 70/30.

FIXED-COMBINATION INSULINS

Currently available fixed combination insulin products include Humulin (20/80, 30/70), Novolinge (10/90, 20/80, 30/70, 40/60, 50/50), and Humalog Mix 25. The numerical designations indicate the relative percentages of each of the two components in the product. Notice that in each case the numbers add to up 100 (percent). Each of these products contains two different insulins, with one faster-acting and one slower-acting type of insulin that act simultaneously in the body to optimize glycemic control. These products were developed to more closely simulate the varying levels of endogenous insulin that

occur normally in non-diabetic people. To maintain constant blood glucose levels both after and between meals, insulin must be present. In most insulin regimens, clients take a combination of a rapid-acting insulin to deal with the surges in glucose that occur after meals and an intermediate or long-acting insulin for the period between meals when glucose levels are lower. However, this requires the mixing and use of different types of insulins. Fixed-combination products were developed in an attempt to simplify the dosage process. The percentage compositions of each of the available combination insulin products are specified in the table on p. 520. The insulin lispro protamine component of Humalog Mix 25 is a modified insulin lispro molecule with a longer duration of action. Humalog Mix 25 and Humulin (20/80, 30/70) are available in cartridges for use only with the Lilly pen. Novolinge premixed insulins are available in Penfill cartridges. Pregnancy category B for all combination insulin products.

SLIDING-SCALE INSULIN DOSING

An important method for dosing insulin is referred to as the *sliding-scale method.* With this method, subcutaneous (SC) regular insulin doses are adjusted according to blood glucose test results. They are typically used in hospitalized diabetic clients whose insulin requirements may vary drastically because of stress (e.g., infections, surgery, acute illness), inactivity, or variable caloric intake. Sliding-scale insulin may also be used in type 1 clients on intensive insulin therapy. When an individual is on a sliding-scale insulin regimen, blood glucose concentrations are determined several times a day (e.g., every 4 hours; every 6 hours; or at specified times, such as 7 am, 11 am, 4 pm, and midnight). This enables the client to obtain fasting blood glucose values and values before meals. Subcutaneously administered regular insulin is then ordered in an amount that increases with the increase in blood glucose. For example,
- No insulin for a blood glucose value of less than 11.1 mmol/L
- 4 units for a blood glucose value of 11.1 to 13.7 mmol/L
- 6 units for a blood glucose value of 13.8 to 16.6 mmol/L
- 8 units for a blood glucose value of 16.7 mmol/L or greater

Sliding-scale dosing is also now used in a similar fashion with insulin lispro, based on the value of a blood glucose level measured by the client just before a meal.

ORAL ANTIHYPERGLYCEMIC AGENTS

Type 2 diabetes is usually a complex illness. Effective treatment involves several elements, including lifestyle modifications (e.g., diet, exercise, smoking cessation), careful monitoring of blood glucose, and possibly therapy with multiple drugs. The need to treat co-occurring conditions may further complicate the process.

The *Canadian Diabetes Association 2003 Clinical Practice Guidelines for the Prevention and Management of Diabetes in Canada* maps out clear strategies for managing T2DM such as early treatment with medication (Figure 31-1). New research recommends that the sooner glycosylated hemoglobin (A1c) level targets are achieved (A1c of less than

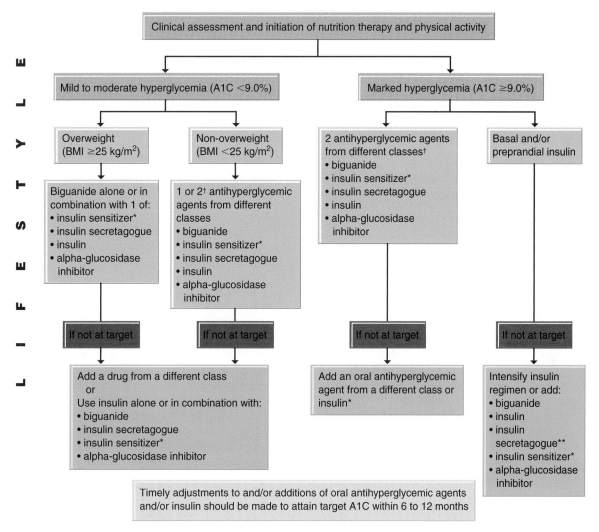

FIG. 31-1 Management of Hyperglycemia in Type 2 Diabetes. Source: *Canadian Diabetes Association 2003 Clinical Practice Guidelines.* Reproduced with permission from the Canadian Diabetes Association.

*When used in combination with insulin, insulin sensitizers may increase the risk of edema or congestive heart failure. The combination of an insulin sensitizer and insulin is currently not an approved indication in Canada.

**If using preprandial insulin, do not add an insulin secretagogue

†May be given as a combined formulation: rosiglitazone and metformin (Avandamet)

7 percent is considered normal), the better the long-term outcomes. The A1c measures the average blood glucose level over the past three months and can be used to predict the risk for diabetes complications. As a result, one of the recommended guidelines is starting combination therapy using 2 agents from 2 different classes of oral antihyperglycemics if the A1c exceeds 9 percent. However, the client should be clearly advised that the ability of any drug therapy to improve health is aided by appropriate changes in diet and activity level. Drug therapy may fail or become inadequate if the client does not make behavioural changes.

Mechanism of Action and Drug Effects

The insulin secretagogues are a group of oral antihyperglycemic agents (OHAs) made up of 2 subclasses, sulphonylureas and non-sulphonylureas, which are able to stimu-

late insulin secretion from the beta cells of the pancreas. This increased insulin then helps to transport the glucose out of the blood and into the tissues, cells, and organs where it is needed.

The sulphonylureas have been the backbone of the oral pharmacological therapy for type 2 diabetes mellitus for more than 30 years. The commonly used sulphonylurea drugs and their comparative durations of action are listed in Table 31-6. Sulphonylurea compounds exert their antihyperglycemic activity by stimulating the beta cells of the pancreas to secrete insulin. In clients with type 2 diabetes this forces the extra glucose out of the blood (the site of its harmful effects) and into cells, tissues, and organs (where it can be used as energy or stored as fuel). For these drugs to work there must be functioning beta cells to stimulate. Thus these drugs work best during the early stages of the disease

TABLE 31-6

SULPHONYLUREA AGENTS: QUALITATIVE COMPARISON OF PHARMACOKINETIC PROPERTIES

Agent	Potency	Onset of Action	Duration of Action	Active Metabolite?
FIRST GENERATION				
chlorpropamide	Low	Fast	Very long	Yes
tolbutamide	Low	Fast	Short	No
SECOND GENERATION				
glimepiride	High	Intermediate	Long	Yes
gliclazide	High	Fast	Long	No
glyburide	High	Slow	Long	Yes

when there is preserved beta cell function. The sulphonylureas have many other beneficial effects besides their ability to stimulate insulin release from the pancreas. The compounds also increase the sensitivity of the insulin receptor proteins in the cells of the muscles, liver, and fat to the effects of insulin, allowing these tissues to take up and store glucose more easily as a later source of energy. They may also increase the availability of insulin by preventing the liver from breaking insulin down as fast as it ordinarily would (reduced hepatic clearance). In summary, the overall effect of the sulphonylureas is that they improve both insulin secretion and the sensitivity to insulin in tissues.

The non-sulphonylureas, repaglinide and nateglinide, are structurally different from the sulphonylureas but share similar mechanisms of action with them. Repaglinide and nateglinide also increase insulin secretion from the pancreas by binding to adenosine triphosphate (ATP)-sensitive potassium channels on pancreatic beta cells.

Another group of OHAs used to treat type 2 diabetes mellitus are called *biguanides*, and include metformin. Metformin differs significantly from the sulphonylureas in that it does not increase insulin secretion from the pancreas and thus does not cause hypoglycemia. The biguanide metformin is believed to exert its beneficial effects via three mechanisms: (1) it decreases glucose production by the liver; (2) it decreases intestinal absorption of glucose; and (3) it improves insulin receptor sensitivity in the liver, skeletal muscle, and adipose tissue. This results in increased peripheral glucose uptake and use and decreased hepatic production of triglycerides and cholesterol. In May 2005, a once-daily extended-release formulation of metformin became available on the Canadian market.

Two newer drug categories have more recently emerged for the oral treatment of type 2 diabetes mellitus. The first of these is the alpha-glucosidase inhibitors, of which acarbose is the sole agent approved in Canada. The other new drug category is the thiazolidinediones (TZDs).

Acarbose is indicated for the management of hyperglycemia secondary to type 2 diabetes mellitus. It works by reversibly inhibiting an enzyme called *alpha-glucosidase*. This enzyme is found in the brush border (villi) of the small intestine. The alpha-glucosidase is responsible for the hydrolysis of oligosaccharides and disaccharides to glucose and other monosaccharides. Blocking this enzyme

delays glucose absorption. The timing of administration of the alpha-glucosidase inhibitor is important. Taking an alpha-glucosidase inhibitor with meals can blunt excessive post-prandial blood glucose elevation.

Thiazolidinediones (TZDs), better known as insulin-sensitizing agents, work to decrease insulin resistance by enhancing the sensitivity to insulin of insulin receptors. This results in enhanced glucose uptake and storage. TZDs work at two of the primary sites in the body that are abnormal in clients with type 2 diabetes mellitus: the liver and the skeletal muscle. In the presence of endogenous or exogenous insulin, TZDs reduce gluconeogenesis (formation of glycogen from non-carbohydrates such as protein and fat by converting them to glucose), glucose output, and triglyceride synthesis in the liver. They increase glucose uptake and use in skeletal muscle, and they increase glucose uptake and decrease fatty acid output in adipose tissue. TZDS have no known effect on insulin secretion. The first TZD agent to receive approval for use in Canada was troglitazone in 1997 but it was never marketed. It has recently been removed from the market in the United States over concerns of liver toxicity. The two newest TZDs are pioglitazone and rosiglitazone. They offer efficacy similar to that of troglitazone with less risk of toxicity. A combined formulation of rosiglitazone and metformin is also available.

Indications

The decision about which class of antihyperglycemic drug to use is based on the initial assessment and initiation of diet and exercise, weight, and baseline blood glucose and glycosylated hemoglobulin (see guidelines in Figure 31-1). A more aggressive approach to reach target blood glucose levels is indicated to reduce long-term complications. Sulphonylurea drugs are used to lower the blood glucose levels often as first-line therapy in combination with antihyperglycemics from other classes, although beta cell function must be preserved for this to happen. The biguanide metformin may be given alone or in combination for clients who are overweight. The alpha-glucosidase inhibitor may be indicated as monotherapy in clients who are not overweight or in combination in clients with marked hyperglycemia. The TZDs are most commonly used alone or with a sulphonylurea, metformin, or insulin in clients with type 2 diabetes mellitus. The goal is to achieve target glycemic control, as indicated by the glycosylated hemoglobulin, within 6 to 12 months.

Contraindications

Contraindications to the use of all antihyperglycemic agents generally include known drug allergy and active hypoglycemia. They may also include severe liver or kidney disease, depending on the required metabolic pathways of the drug in question. These oral agents are generally not used during pregnancy; insulin therapy is both safer for the fetus and provides closer glycemic control, which is critical during pregnancy.

Side Effects and Adverse Effects

The most serious adverse effects of sulphonylureas involve the hematological system and include agranulocytosis, hemolytic anemia, thrombocytopenia, and cholestatic jaundice. Effects on the gastrointestinal (GI) system include nausea, epigastric fullness, and heartburn. Other undesirable effects include hypoglycemia, photosensitivity, and skin eruptions, which may be erythematous (red and inflamed), morbilliform (red and bumpy, like measles), or maculopapular (flat reddish areas with bumps in the middle).

The biguanide metformin primarily affects the GI tract. The most common side effects of therapy with metformin are abdominal bloating, anorexia, nausea, cramping, a feeling of fullness, flatulence, and diarrhea. These effects are usually self-limiting, transient, and can be lessened by starting with low doses, titrating up slowly, and taking the medication with food. Less common side effects with metformin are metallic taste and reduction in vitamin B_{12} levels. Lactic acidosis is a rare but serious complication that can occur with metformin and is lethal in 50 percent of the cases. Unlike sulphonylureas, metformin does not cause hypoglycemia.

The alpha-glucosidase inhibitor acarbose also has side effects that primarily involve the GI tract and are dose-dependent. It can cause flatulence, diarrhea, abdominal pain, abdominal distention, nausea, vomiting, dyspepsia, constipation, and headache. At high doses it may also elevate hepatic enzymes (transaminases). Unlike sulphonylureas, acarbose does not cause hypoglycemia, hyperinsulinemia, or weight gain.

Rosiglitazone and pioglitazone both may cause moderate weight gain, edema, and mild anemia, possibly as a result of fluid retention. The safe use of the TZDs during pregnancy, in children, and in clients with heart failure has not been established. There is concern that hepatic toxicity may be a class effect of TZDs. For this reason liver enzymes should be measured prior to beginning treatment and regularly thereafter. If alanine aminotransferase (ALT) levels are two-and-a-half times as high as upper normal limits, then treatment should not be started.

Interactions

Significant potential drug interactions can occur with sulphonylureas. Their hypoglycemic effect is increased when taken concurrently with ACE inhibitors, alcohol, anabolic steroids, allopurinol, chloramphenicol, fibric acid derivatives, fluconazole, H_2 antagonists, MAOIs, NSAIDs, quinine, salicylates, and sulphonamides.

Drugs that are capable of reducing the hypoglycemic effect of sulphonylureas include adrenergics, corticosteroids, thiazides, estrogens, rifampin, and oral contraceptives. Concentrations of sulphonylurea can be increased when given concomitantly with anticoagulants. Metformin concentrations can be increased when it is given together with furosemide and nifedipine. When it is given with cationic drugs such as cimetidine or digoxin, competition for renal tubular secretion occurs, resulting in increased metformin concentrations. Alpha-glucosidase inhibitors potentially interact with intestinal absorbents (e.g., charcoal) and digestive enzyme preparations containing carbohydrase-splitting enzymes (e.g., amylase, pancreatin). When these drugs are concomitantly administered with an alpha-glucosidase inhibitor, they may reduce the effect of the alpha-glucosidase inhibitor. Cholestyramine given concomitantly with acarbose may enhance the effects of acarbose while digoxin bioavailability may be affected by acarbose. Clinically important interactions between rosiglitazone and other drugs have not been reported. Total cholesterol, low-density lipoprotein (LDL), and high-density lipoprotein (HDL) cholesterol increased between 12 and 19 percent in individuals taking rosiglitazone, and there may be decreases in free fatty acids. Pioglitazone, on the other hand, is partly metabolized by CYP3A4. Serum concentrations of pioglitazone may be increased if taken concurrently with a 3A4 inhibitor such as ketoconazole. However, pioglitazone significantly raises the HDL cholesterol, lowers serum triglyceride concentrations, and increases the particle size of LDL cholesterol.

Dosages

For the recommended dosages of oral antihyperglycemic agents, see the table on p. 526. See Appendix B for some of the common brands available in Canada.

DRUG PROFILES

Over the past few years several new oral agents have been approved for the treatment of type 2 diabetes mellitus. Within the larger class of the insulin secretagogues, the sulphonylureas are the oldest class of agents. There are two generations of sulphonylurea drugs. The first-generation sulphonylureas are the older, low-potency drugs tolbutamide and chlorpropamide, still available in Canada but rarely used. The second-generation sulphonylureas are the newer, high-potency drugs gliclazide, glyburide, and glimepiride, which are more commonly used but are associated with hypoglycemia. The subclass of non-sulphonylureas, a fairly new class, is currently represented by nateglinide and repaglinide. They function similarly to the sulphonylureas but with a faster onset and shorter half-life.

There are also several new drug categories of oral agents used to treat clients with type 2 diabetes mellitus, including the biguanides, alpha-glucosidase inhibitors, and thiazolidinediones. Currently the only biguanide used in Canada is metformin. Acarbose is the only available alpha-glucosidase inhibitor in Canada. The newest drug class to treat clients with type 2 diabetes mellitus is the insulin sensitizers, the thiazolidinediones. Pioglitazone and rosiglitazone are currently the only thiazolidinediones available. Although not clinically an OHA, orlistat, an intestinal lipase inhibitor (Chapter 16), was added to the list of OHAs for the treatment of diabetes in the 2003 Canadian Diabetes Association clinical practice guidelines. Its use is limited to overweight or obese clients and it is used with other antihyperglycemic agents as its blood glucose lowering effect is minimal.

acarbose

Acarbose is the sole currently available alpha-glucosidase inhibitor. Acarbose works by blunting elevated blood sugar levels after a meal. To work optimally it is taken with the first bite of each meal. It may also be taken concomitantly with sulphonylurea agents or with metformin. Acarbose is contraindicated in clients with a hypersensitivity to alpha-glucosidase inhibitors, diabetic ketoacidosis, cirrhosis, inflammatory bowel disease, colonic ulceration, partial intestinal obstruction, or chronic intestinal disease. It is available only in oral (PO) form as 50- and 100-mg tablets. Common dosages are listed in the table below.

PHARMACOKINETICS

Half-Life	Onset	Peak	Duration
2–3 hr	1–1.5 hr	14–24 hr	9–15 hr

chlorpropamide

Chlorpropamide is an insulin secretagogue of the sulphonylurea subclass. It is a first-generation sulphonylurea agent that is structurally similar to the other first-generation agent, tolbutamide. It is the most common of the first-generation agents but used infrequently now because of the newer drugs available. Unlike tolbutamide, it has a long duration of action. The chlorpropamide-induced decrease in the blood glucose level may be prolonged in clients with decreased renal function because the drug is dependent on the kidneys for elimination. Like tolbutamide, it has active metabolites that can accumulate if they are not eliminated by the kidneys, resulting in a prolongation of their effects and possible toxicity. This would be manifested by hypoglycemia.

Chlorpropamide is contraindicated in clients with a known hypersensitivity to sulphonylureas, clients with type 1 diabetes mellitus, and clients experiencing renal failure. Profound flushing of the skin and in particular the face occurs if it is taken with alcohol. Although this can occur with any of the sulphonylurea compounds, it is most prominent with chlorpropamide use and is called the *chlorpropamide–alcohol flush*. Facial temperature can also increase. Chlorpropamide is available in oral form as 100- and 250-mg tablets. Common dosages are listed in the table below.

PHARMACOKINETICS

Half-Life	Onset	Peak	Duration
36 hr	1 hr	2–4 hr	24–72 hr

▶ gliclazide

Gliclazide, also an insulin secretagogue, is a second-generation sulphonylurea agent with a potency much greater than that of the first-generation agents. In contrast to the other second-generation agent, glyburide, gliclazide has a rapid onset and short duration of action, with no active metabolites. This confers many benefits. The rapid onset of action allows it to function much like the body's normal response to meals when greater levels of insulin are rapidly required to deal with the increased glucose in the blood. When a client with type 2 diabetes mellitus takes gliclazide, it rapidly stimulates the pancreas to release

DOSAGES	Selected Oral Antihyperglycemic Agents		
Agent	**Pharmacological Class**	**Usual Dosage Range**	**Indications**
acarbose	Alpha-glucosidase inhibitor	PO: 50–100 mg tid, taken at start of meal	
chlorpropamide	Insulin secretagogue: First-generation sulphonylurea	PO: 100–500 mg divided once to twice daily	
glimepiride	Insulin secretagogue: Second-generation sulphonylurea	PO: 1–8 mg daily	
▶ gliclazide	Insulin secretagogue: Second-generation sulphonylurea	PO: 80–320 mg once to twice daily (doses above 160 mg bid, divided) MR: 30–120 mg once daily	
▶ glyburide	Insulin secretagogue: Second-generation sulphonylurea	PO: 2.5–20 mg/day divided once to twice daily	Type 2 diabetes mellitus
▶ metformin	Biguanide	PO: 500 mg bid or 850 mg daily; max daily dose 2550 mg for adults and 2000 mg for pediatric clients age 10–16 yr	
repaglinide	Insulin secretagogue: Non-sulphonylurea	PO: 0.5–4 mg tid; best taken with meals	
▶ rosiglitazone	Thiazolidinedione	PO: 4–8 mg divided once to twice daily	
Combination Oral Agents			
rosiglitazone/ metformin	Combination thiazolidinedione/ biguanide	PO: 4 mg /500 mg–8 mg/2000 mg bid	

insulin and transport the extra glucose in the blood to the muscles, liver, and adipose tissues.

Its short duration of action prevents the long-term stimulation of the beta cells in the pancreas, which may otherwise cause the beta cells to become resistant to the effects of the sulphonylurea agents. It may also cause them to make too much insulin, thereby inducing hyperinsulinemia, which can cause the muscle, liver, and fat tissues to become resistant to the effects of insulin. Gliclazide also reduces platelet adhesiveness and aggregation.

Gliclazide has the same contraindications as chlorpropamide. It works best if taken with meals. Generally, it is advantageous to begin with a low dose and titrate upward every 1 to 2 weeks to achieve the desired glycemic control and avoid hypoglycemia, particularly in elderly clients. It is available only in oral form as 80-mg regular-release and 30-mg extended-release tablets. Common dosages are listed in the table on p. 526.

PHARMACOKINETICS

Half-Life	Onset	Peak	Duration
10.4 hr	1–1.5 hr	4–6 hr	10–24 hr

glimepiride

Glimepiride is the newest of the sulphonylurea agents. It has properties comparable to those of the older second-generation sulphonylureas, except that it has an onset of action that is intermediate to that of gliclazide and glyburide, as indicated in Table 31-6. It is available in 1-, 2-, and 4-mg tablets. Common dosages are listed in the table on p. 526.

PHARMACOKINETICS

Half-Life	Onset	Peak	Duration
5–9 hr	2–3 hr	2–3 hr	24 hr

⤷ glyburide

Glyburide is another second-generation sulphonylurea drug. It differs from the first-generation oral hypoglycemic agents in its greater potency, slower onset and longer duration of action and the fact that it has active metabolites. These differences can have significant consequences. Because of its relatively slow onset of action, glyburide is less desirable for the treatment of the short-term elevations in the blood glucose levels that occur after meals. However, its longer duration of action makes it better for the long-term, constant stimulation of the pancreas, causing it to release a constant amount of insulin. This may be beneficial in controlling blood glucose levels during the night and/or throughout the day.

Glyburide is available only in oral form as 2.5- and 5-mg tablets. It is a pregnancy category B drug with the same contraindications as gliclazide. Common dosages are listed in the table on p. 526.

PHARMACOKINETICS

Half-Life*	Onset	Peak	Duration
2–4 hr	1–1.5 hr	4 hr	20–24 hr

*When assays have been performed to measure the metabolite levels, the terminal elimination half-life has been found to average 10 hr.

⤷ metformin

Metformin is a biguanide, oral antihyperglycemic agent. It works primarily by inhibiting hepatic glucose production and increasing the sensitivity of peripheral tissue to insulin. Because its mechanism of action differs from that of the sulphonylurea agents, it may be given concomitantly with these agents.

Metformin is available only in oral form as 500- and 850-mg tablets. It is a pregnancy category B drug and is contraindicated in clients with a hypersensitivity to biguanides, hepatic or renal disease, alcoholism, or cardiopulmonary disease. Common dosages are listed in the table on p. 526.

PHARMACOKINETICS

Half-Life	Onset	Peak	Duration
1.7–3 hr	<1 hr	1–3 hr	24 hr

repaglinide

Repaglinide is one of two antihyperglycemic agents in the insulin secretagogues subclass of non-sulphonylureas, the other being nateglinide. These agents have a comparable mechanism of action to the sulphonylureas in that they stimulate the release of insulin from pancreatic beta cells. They are used because some clients simply respond better to them and have better glycemic control. Contraindications include known drug allergy. Dosage information for repaglinide appears in the table on p. 526. Repaglinide is currently available in 0.5-, 1- and 2-mg tablets.

PHARMACOKINETICS

Half-Life	Onset	Peak	Duration
2–3 hr	15–60 min	1 hr	4–6 hr

⤷ rosiglitazone

Rosiglitazone is classified as an insulin sensitizer or a thiazolidinedione. It is marketed for the treatment of clients with type 2 diabetes. Rosiglitazone and pioglitazone are used alone or with a sulphonylurea, metformin, or insulin. The insulin sensitizer agents work by increasing insulin sensitivity in the muscle and adipose tissue.

The safe use of glitazones during pregnancy, in children, and in clients with heart failure has not been established. There is concern that hepatic toxicity may be a class effect of thiazolidinediones. For this reason it is recommended to check liver enzymes, especially ALT, before beginning treatment and to maintain frequent monitoring thereafter. Rosiglitazone is available as 2-, 4-, and 8-mg unscored tablets. It is classified as a pregnancy category C agent. Recommended dosages are given in the table on p. 526.

PHARMACOKINETICS

Half-Life	Onset	Peak	Duration
3–4 hr	Unknown	1 hr	Unknown

GLUCOSE-ELEVATING DRUGS

Two drugs are used for the treatment of hypoglycemia. Glucagon, a natural hormone secreted by the pancreas, has also been synthesized in the laboratory and is now

Potential Combinations of OHAs for the Treatment of Type 2 Diabetes

Metformin plus
- Sulphonylurea
- Non-sulphonylurea insulin secretagogue
- Thiazolidinedione
- Alpha-glucosidase inhibitor
- Insulin

Thiazolidinedione plus
- Metformin
- Sulphonylurea
- Non-sulphonylurea insulin secretagogue
- Alpha-glucosidase inhibitor

Alpha-glucosidase Inhibitor plus
- Metformin
- Thiazolidinedione
- Sulphonylurea
- Non-sulphonylurea insulin secretagogue
- Insulin

Do **not** combine:
- Sulphonylurea + non-sulphonylurea insulin secretagogue
- Insulin secretagogue + preprandial insulin
- Thiazolidinedione + insulin

Source: Dr. I. George Fantus, Mount Sinai Hospital. Reproduced with permission.

available as a tablet to be given when a quick response to hypoglycemia is needed. Diazoxide is another agent that may be given to correct abnormally low blood glucose levels. It works by inhibiting the release of insulin from the pancreas and is most commonly given to clients with long-term illnesses that are causing hypoglycemia. An example of such an illness is pancreatic cancer, which may cause the pancreas to oversecrete insulin, resulting in too much insulin in the blood, or hyperinsulinemia. The oral form of diazoxide is used for the treatment of hypoglycemia. The intravenous form is used for the treatment of hypertensive emergencies (extremely high blood pressures). Oral forms of concentrated glucose are also available for clients to use in the event of a hypoglycemic crisis. Dosage forms of these include rapidly dissolving buccal tablets and semisolid gel forms designed for oral use and rapid buccal absorption.

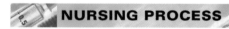

NURSING PROCESS

■ Assessment

■ Insulin

Before administering any type of insulin it is important for nurses to assess their own knowledge about the disease processes and recommended treatment. Insulin is always used to treat type 1 diabetes, and may be used to treat type 2 diabetics who do not achieve the desired results with oral agents. For type 2 diabetes (see Research box on p. 531),

oral antihyperglycemic agents are recommended. It is important to examine an insulin order carefully to ensure the correct route, type of insulin (e.g., clear [rapid or regular] or cloudy [intermediate or NPH]), dose, and timing. Because various types of insulin are available, it is critical to client safety to assess the type, dose, and timing of the dosage before giving the drug. Contraindications generally are allergy to the specific type of insulin, such as pork; fewer problems have been encountered with humalin insulins because of their close similarity to endogenous insulin. The nurse must always check for allergies to the insulin product before administering the dose. Cautious use is recommended in geriatric clients and in those who have labile blood glucose levels, other illnesses, and renal, hepatic, and/or cardiac dysfunction. Drug interactions with all types of insulin include those drugs that may increase the effects of the insulin (thereby causing more hypoglycemia), such as MAOIs, alcohol, sulpha drugs, some angiotensin converting enzyme (ACE) inhibitors, and drugs affecting pancreatic function. Drugs that antagonize the effects of insulin and thus result in hyperglycemia include beta-blockers, corticosteroids, isoniazid (an antituberculin drug), niacin, thiazide diuretics, and sympathomimetics.

■ Insulin Secretagogues

Oral antihyperglycemic agents are contraindicated in clients with allergies to the medication proper. Cautious use of the sulphonylureas, such as chlorpropamide, glyburide, gliclazide, and others, is indicated for clients with impaired renal, hepatic, pituitary, or adrenal functioning; clients under stress; geriatric clients; debilitated or malnourished clients; and pregnant women (category C; insulin preferred in pregnancy). Contraindications include clients with ketoacidosis; lactating women; and clients with type 1 diabetes. Oral agents will not work with type 1 diabetics; they have no functioning beta cells in the pancreas to stimulate. A significant contraindication is drug allergy, and not just to the sulphonylurea: cross-allergy may occur with loop diuretics and sulphonamide antibiotics, because they have similar chemical structures. These sulphonylurea agents should be administered with caution to geriatric clients, who often tend to be on multiple medications, or to anyone with cardiac, renal, hepatic, or thyroid disease. Drug interactions include warfarin sodium, acetylsalicylate, digoxin, insulin, diuretics, beta-blockers, calcium channel blockers (CCBs), corticosteroids, phenobarbital, phenytoin, sulphonamides, chloramphenicol, MAOIs, and non-steroidal anti-inflammatory drugs (NSAIDs). Use of these drugs with alcohol can result in a highly unpleasant reaction similar to that with disulfiram (Antabuse): flushing, throbbing, palpitations, headache, severe vomiting, and sometimes respiratory depression.

■ Biguanides

With the sole biguanide, metformin, contraindications include pregnancy, lactation, renal disease, heart failure, acidosis and ketoacidosis, and drug allergy. Cautious use is recommended in geriatric clients and in clients who are malnourished, use alcohol, or have adrenal and/or pituitary dysfunction, altered renal function, or hepatic disease.

Drug interactions include ranitidine, digoxin, furosemide, quinidine, procainamide, nifedipine, diuretics, alcohol, CCBs, and steroids.

There are several drug interactions for which to assess before administering metformin. Cimetidine may increase metformin levels, and anticoagulant levels may be decreased if oral anticoagulants are given concurrently with metformin. If a client taking metformin needs to have a procedure performed with contrast media (such as an angiogram), there may be increased risk for renal dysfunction; therefore the metformin should be discontinued just before the procedure and restarted as ordered only after renal function has been re-evaluated.

Alpha-glucosidase Inhibitors

The alpha-glucosidase inhibitor acarbose and other related oral antihyperglycemics are contraindicated in children, lactating women, clients with ketoacidosis, and clients who have inflammatory bowel disease, colon ulcerations, or chronic intestinal diseases and/or conditions. Cautions include significant renal dysfunction, stress, and pregnancy. Drug interactions include drugs that may cause hyperglycemia, such as diuretics, steroids, estrogens, phenothiazines, thyroid products, phenytoin, niacin (used as an antilipemic), sympathomimetics, CCBs, digoxin, isoniazid, and intestinal absorbents. Overdosage of the agent may not necessarily cause hypoglycemia, but it may lead to GI tract symptoms that may require medical treatment; therefore these drugs should be used with extra caution in clients who have a history of GI disorders.

Thiazolidinediones

Contraindications to pioglitazone and rosiglitazone include use in children under the age of 18 years, heart failure, history of thiazolidinedione-related jaundice, lactation, pregnancy, type 1 diabetes, and allergy to the drug. Cautious use is recommended for those with hepatic disease or with elevated alanine aminotransferase (ALT) levels. It is advisable to measure liver enzymes (especially ALT) before beginning treatment and to maintain frequent monitoring thereafter. Drug interactions include ketoconazole and drugs used for heart failure.

General

In summary, it is important for the nurse to ask questions about the client's medical history to determine whether the client's diabetes is well controlled or the client has problems with polyuria, polydipsia, polyphagia, weight loss, visual changes, or fatigue. The nurse should ask about both symptoms of hypoglycemia, such as the acute onset of nervousness, sweating, lethargy, weakness, cold and clammy skin, and a change in sensorium, and symptoms of hyperglycemia, such as tachycardia, blood glucose levels that exceed 8.3 mmol/L, and Kussmaul's breathing: rapid, deep, laboured breaths. The nurse must also be aware that overall concerns for any diabetic client (type 1 or type 2) increase when the client is pregnant, under stress, or has any infection, illness, or trauma. Before administering any glucose-elevating drug, the nurse should always obtain and document a thorough history, plus vital signs and blood glucose level.

Nursing Diagnoses

Nursing diagnoses appropriate for clients receiving insulin or the oral antihyperglycemic agents include the following:
- Risk for injury related to changes in sensorium from the pathology of diabetes.
- Risk for infection related to diabetes and its pathological impact on every cell in the body.
- Imbalanced nutrition, more than body requirements, related to the disease process.
- Deficient knowledge related to diabetes mellitus, its management, and the prevention of its complications.
- Ineffective therapeutic regimen management related to lack of experience with a significant daily treatment regimen.

Planning

Goals for clients receiving insulin or oral antihyperglycemic agents include the following:
- Client remains free from self-injury and complications of diabetes.
- Client remains free from infection.
- Client maintains adequate weight control and dietary habits in the overall management of diabetes.
- Client states the effects of diabetes on body function.
- Client remains adherent with the medical regimen.
- Client states the importance of adherence to medication regimens, lifestyle changes, dietary restrictions, and high-risk behaviours.
- Client states the action and side effects of insulin or the oral antihyperglycemic agents.

Outcome Criteria

Outcome criteria for clients receiving insulin or oral antihyperglycemic agents include the following:
- Client performs self-assessment and foot care as directed and as needed to maintain healthy skin.
- Client immediately reports elevated temperature, difficult-to-heal lesions or sores, and any unusual redness of an area to the healthcare provider.
- Client observes the diet recommended by the CDA or other dietary consultant per the physician's orders or nutritional consult.
- Client eats a healthy diet, gets sufficient rest and relaxation, and notifies the physician should any unusual problems occur with changes in usual activity (problems such as nausea and vomiting).
- Client keeps all scheduled appointments with healthcare providers to monitor therapeutic effectiveness or for complications of therapy.
- Client takes medication as scheduled, monitors blood glucose levels, and watches for any signs and symptoms of hyperglycemia or hypoglycemia.

Implementation

Insulin

With any client who is to receive insulin or the oral antihyperglycemic agents, it is critical for the nurse to check the blood glucose levels (and other related laboratory values) before administering the agent so that accurate baseline levels are documented. The nurse should always check any medication order at least three times before administering the drug, and with insulin (as well as heparin) there should be an additional check of the order and prepared dosage by another registered nurse. Insulin is *not* to be shaken. Instead it should be rolled between one's hands before withdrawing the prescribed dosage to avoid air in the syringe, which may lead to an inaccurate dose. Insulin may be stored at room temperature if it is to be used within 1 month; otherwise it needs to be refrigerated.

Refrigeration is recommended if the environmental temperature is warm. Insulin that is discoloured or past its expiration date should never be used. Insulin should be administered subcutaneously at a 90-degree angle unless the client is emaciated, in which case it is administered at a 45-degree angle. Only regular insulin may be administered intravenously; however, this route is controversial because of absorption of the insulin into the intravenous bag and/or tubing. A 25- to 28-gauge, $\frac{1}{2}$- to $\frac{5}{8}$-inch needle should be used with subcutaneous injections of insulin, and *only* insulin syringes should be used because of their calibration in *units.* When mixing insulins, the nurse should always withdraw the regular or rapid-acting (unmodified) insulin first and then the intermediate-acting or NPH (modified) insulin so that there is no contamination of the rapid-acting insulin by the intermediate-acting insulin. The nurse should educate the client about the type of insulin; its source; whether it is rapid, intermediate, or long acting; and related pharmacokinetics. For example, subcutaneous lispro insulin is absorbed more rapidly than regular insulin, with an onset of 15 minutes and a peak effect of 30 to 90 minutes. As a result lispro must be given 15 minutes before meals, whereas regular insulin is given 30 to 60 minutes before meals. Lispro mixtures with Humulin-N or Humulin-U should be given 15 minutes before meals and immediately after the agents are mixed. Two important points to remember with regard to lispro administration: (1) Food needs to be eaten quickly after lispro is administered. (2) One unit of lispro has the same glucose lowering effect as 1 unit of regular insulin; however, lispro has a more rapid onset and shorter duration of action than regular insulin. The physician may order an increase in carbohydrate intake and a decrease in fat intake to avoid post-prandial hypoglycemia.

Regardless of the composition of the insulin (pork or recombinant human), it is the peak, onset, and duration that helps the nurse to adequately judge when the insulin and food should be administered, but always following the physician's order. The intermediate-acting insulins, such as NPH and the numerous combination products of regular and intermediate insulin (e.g., Humulin 30/70, Humulin 50/50, and Novolinge 30/70),* have an onset of between 30 minutes and 1 to 2 hours. The nurse should ensure that the meal is available at or right before the onset of action.

The nurse should always be sure that the meal trays are on the unit before giving insulin, or have other forms of allowed foods available to the client just in case meals are delayed and insulin has already been administered. Clients must eat the right amount and types of carbohydrates after insulin administration, otherwise complications from hypoglycemia will occur. If the client needs mixed insulins, the unmodified or clear and rapid-acting insulin is always drawn up first and the intermediate, NPH, or cloudy insulin drawn up last (see Table 31-3). This occurs only after the correct amount of air (in units) is appropriately injected into each vial of insulin, with air first going into the NPH and then into the regular insulin, then first withdrawing the regular insulin. Some insulin products are premixed. A newer insulin, insulin glargine, is used when basal or longer-acting insulin action is needed.

Clients taking insulin injections should be instructed to rotate sites within the same location for about 1 week before moving to a new location (e.g., all injections for a week in the upper right thigh before moving a little lower on the right thigh). Injections should be at least 1.5 to 2.5 cm away from the previous injection. This allows approximately up to 6 weeks before having to switch or rotate to a totally new area of the body. In years past it was the standard to shift to a completely different area with each injection, but the system described above provides better insulin absorption. Thigh areas (front and back) and outer areas of the upper arm (middle third area of the upper arm between the shoulder area and the elbow) are used, but some practitioners may recommend only using the abdomen because of more complete absorption.

■ *Oral Antihyperglycemics*

Oral antihyperglycemic agents are usually administered at least 30 minutes before meals. Some of the sulphonylureas are to be taken with breakfast, alpha-glucosidase inhibitors are always to be taken with the first bite of each main meal, and the thiazolidinediones are to be given once daily or in two divided doses. Biguanides are sometimes taken with the morning meal or both the morning and evening meals; the meglitinide analogue is to be taken 30 minutes before breakfast, and the dose is skipped if the meal is skipped. Metformin should be taken with meals to minimize nausea or diarrhea. With metformin it is important (as with any antihyperglycemic agent or insulin) for both the nurse and client to know what to do if symptoms of hypoglycemia occur, such as using glucagon; eating glucose tablets or gel, corn syrup, or honey; drinking fruit juice or a non-diet soft drink; or eating a small snack such as crackers or half of a sandwich. It is crucial to the safe and efficient use of oral antihyperglycemics to be sure that food will be or is being tolerated before giving the dose. The nurse must always assess the client's ability to consume food and ask about any nausea or vomiting because if there is no food intake there will be complications from hypoglycemia. If the oral agent and/or insulin is taken without any meal consumption or at a meal time later than the usual, hypoglycemia may develop, causing negative health consequences and even unconsciousness. Because rosiglitazone and pioglitazone may both cause moderate weight gain, edema, and mild anemia, it is also important to educate the client about the need for monitoring and documenting weight

---

*The numerator represents the units of rapid or regular insulin; the denominator represents the units of intermediate or NPH insulin.

Diabetes Mellitus

B.G. is a 58-year-old male with a diagnosis of type 2 diabetes mellitus for the last 10 years. He has needed to take insulin for the last 2 years. He has been recovering, without complications, from a laparoscopic cholecystectomy, but his blood glucose levels have had some wide fluctuations over the last 24 hours. The physician has changed his insulin to lispro to see if there is any better control of his blood glucose levels.

- What is the rationale for the use of oral antihyperglycemic agents in a client with type 2 diabetes? Why is it that some clients with type 2 diabetes have to begin taking insulin?
- What are the pharmacokinetics related to lispro?
- What, if any, special instructions should B.G. be given about the lispro before he is discharged?

For answers see http://evolve.elsevier.com/Lilley/pharmacology/.

Treatment of Type 2 Diabetes

More than 60 000 Canadians are diagnosed annually with type 2 diabetes mellitus. Type 2 diabetes has reached epidemic proportions in Canada and worldwide. Prevalence rates are estimated at 4.8 percent in Canadians over 20 years of age but it is estimated to be greater than 7 percent, as many cases go undiagnosed. Demographic trends such as an aging population, increased immigration from high-risk populations, and growth in the Aboriginal population will contribute to an increased prevalence in the future. In recent years many new oral medications have been introduced that offer better glycemic control than the older medications. Metformin has been available in Canada for many years and is first-line treatment for overweight clients with type 2 diabetes, and for children. However, metformin is not recommended for use in clients with impaired renal function (creatinine clearance <60 mL/min) or decreased hepatic function or in those at risk for developing these system dysfunctions because of the risk of lactic acidosis. Thiazolidinediones have the benefit of vascular smooth muscle reactivity. They are contraindicated for use in clients with New York Heart Association class III and intravenous heart failure because of their side effects of fluid retention and slight anemia. Troglitazone was removed from the market owing to severe hepatotoxicity; therefore clients on the thiazolidinediones should have frequent liver function tests performed and documented. The insulin secretagogues, the non-sulphonylureas, are a newer group of oral antihyperglycemic agents and provide a short-term (4-hour) burst of insulin. They are used before meals to help prevent post-prandial hyperglycemia. The latest group of agents, alpha-glucosidase inhibitors, act by inhibiting and decreasing the digestion of carbohydrates and often cause flatulence and diarrhea.

Several new insulins are available. Insulin glargine provides fewer peaks of action and is given once daily for basal insulin levels for 24 hr, but it cannot be mixed with any other insulin in the same syringe. Insulin aspart has a rapid insulin rise about 15 minutes after administration and may be given alone or in combination.

References: Cheng, A.Y.Y., & Fantus, I.G. (2005). Oral antihyperglycemic therapy for type 2 diabetes mellitus. *Canadian Medical Association Journal, 172*(2), 213–226; Canadian Diabetes Association Clinical Practice Guidelines Expert Committee. (2003). Canadian Diabetes Association 2003 clinical practice guidelines for the prevention and management of diabetes in Canada. *Canadian Journal of Diabetes, 27*(suppl 2).

and maintaining regular follow-up appointments with the physician or healthcare provider to make sure that weight is maintained at or near normal levels. All of the oral agents are to be taken exactly as prescribed. (See the Research box to the right for more information.)

If a client on antihyperglycemics needs a procedure that requires NPO (nothing by mouth), the nurse must follow the physician's orders regarding drug administration. If there are no written orders, the nurse must contact the physician to clarify what to do with regard to the client's antihyperglycemic drug therapy. If a client is NPO but is also receiving an intravenous solution of dextrose, the physician may order insulin for the specific situation. The physician should also be contacted when a client becomes ill at home and is unable to take the usual dosage of insulin or oral antihyperglycemic agent. Clients who are diabetic and on drug therapy need to wear a medical alert bracelet or tag that identifies the type of diabetes and the prescribed medications, as well as allergies.

Client education is crucial to ensure the safe and effective use of insulin and oral antihyperglycemic agents. Client teaching tips for these agents are listed in the box on p. 532.

Evaluation

The therapeutic response to insulin and any of the oral antihyperglycemic agents is a decrease in the blood glucose levels to the level prescribed by the physician or to near normal levels. Most often, fasting blood glucose levels (>4 and <7 mmol/L, or a level designated by the physician) are used to measure the degree of glycemic control. To get a picture of adherence for several months prior, a **hemoglobin A1c** measurement is performed. This measurement provides the healthcare provider with information on how well the client has been doing with diet and drug therapy. Clients with diabetes need to be monitored to make sure they are adhering to therapy. The nurse needs to watch the client for manifestations of hypoglycemia or hyperglycemia and monitor for insulin allergy, which is manifested by local swelling, itching, and redness at the injection site. With insulin lispro, because the onset is more rapid than with regular insulin and there is a shorter duration of action, it is crucial for the nurse and the client to monitor blood glucose levels more closely until the dosage is regulated and blood glucose is at the target level. Should a client be switched from one insulin or oral antihyperglycemic agent to another, it is important for glucose levels to be monitored closely.

CLIENT TEACHING TIPS

Clients need to have a thorough understanding of their type of diabetes and its specific management, including special diets and exercise, as ordered by the physician. The nurse should provide the client with any available literature, pamphlets, and videos on diabetes. The CDA can also provide the client with information on diabetes and other resources available. The nurse should instruct the client as follows:

▲ Always carry an identification card and wear a medical alert bracelet or tag that identifies you as diabetic.

▲ Make sure you know the signs and symptoms of hyperglycemia, such as an increased pulse rate, abnormal breathing, and a fruity, acetone odour to your breath.

▲ Make sure you know the signs and symptoms of hypoglycemia, such as weakness, nervousness, cold and clammy skin, sweating, paleness of the skin, and shallow, rapid breathing. Notify your physician if any of these symptoms occur.

▲ Make sure you know how to measure your blood glucose level with a glucometer. Do this as ordered by your physician.

▲ Notify your physician if you note yellow discoloration of the skin, dark urine, fever, sore throat, weakness, or any unusual bleeding or easy bruising.

▲ Notify your physician if you are ill, have an infection, are vomiting or not able to eat, or are under stress. Any of these conditions may require a change in your treatment.

▲ You may consume alcohol in moderate amounts (1 to 2 standard drinks) with food without causing problems or changing your meal plan. Be aware, however, that alcohol may mask the symptoms of hypoglycemia.

▲ Many drugs can interact with your medication. Make sure you have written information about your medication and drugs that should not be taken with it. If in doubt, check with your physician before taking any new drug, including an over-the-counter drug.

For Clients Taking Insulin

▲ Always keep an extra supply of medication, syringes, needles, alcohol or antiseptic swabs, and supplies of "quick" glucose at home, and carry them with you when travelling.

▲ Make sure you understand how your particular type of insulin works, including onset of action (when it begins to work), peak action (when it acts the most), and duration (how long it acts).

POINTS to REMEMBER

▼ Insulin normally takes glucose from the blood and puts it in the liver to be stored.

▼ Beef insulins are no longer used; pork and human insulins are now used. Pork insulin in Canada will no longer be available after 2006.

▼ Oral antihyperglycemics stimulate insulin secretion from the beta cells of the pancreas as well as enhance insulin's effectiveness.

▼ Glucagon is the second hormone secreted by the pancreas and is responsible for initiating glycogenolysis. Glycogenolysis opposes the action of insulin; it increases the blood glucose level.

▼ Glycogen is the storage form of glucose, and most of it is stored in the liver. Glycogen is broken down by the synergistic actions of glucagon, cortisol, and epinephrine.

▼ In type 1 diabetes mellitus, the pancreas produces little or no endogenous insulin. It is much less common than T2DM, affecting only about 10 percent of all diabetics. Clients are usually not obese.

▼ In type 2 diabetes mellitus, the pancreas usually secretes a normal amount of insulin. T2DM is much more common than type 1 diabetes, affecting about 90 percent of all diabetics. Eighty percent of clients are obese.

▼ Gestational diabetes is a type of glucose intolerance that develops during pregnancy. It is important to follow postpartum because of the risk of developing T2DM.

▼ Complications associated with diabetes include retinopathy, neuropathy, nephropathy, hypertension, cardiovascular disease, and coronary artery disease.

▼ A severe complication of uncontrolled diabetes is diabetic ketoacidosis (DKA). DKA results when the body uses sources of energy other than glucose, such as fatty acids. Fatty acids are broken down into ketones, which leads to acidosis.

▼ Nursing considerations:
  • The nurse should always check for allergies to specific medications and to pork insulins before initiating therapy.
  • Clients need to learn about their disease and the type of insulin they are taking—its onset of action, peak effect, and duration of action—as well as the importance of always having a rapidly active form of glucose available.
  • Clients need to learn the signs and symptoms of hypoglycemia and hyperglycemia and the methods of treating them at home, as well as when to contact their physician.
  • Information on foot care and the prevention of infection should be part of the client education given to diabetics.
  • Drug interactions for troglitazone include oral contraceptives; troglitazone may reduce their efficacy by as much as 30 percent.

EXAMINATION REVIEW QUESTIONS

1 Which of the following statements is true about Humulin-N?
  a. It is a rapid-acting insulin.
  b. It is an intermediate-acting insulin.
  c. There are no reactions associated with this synthetic insulin.
  d. There are no problems with hypoglycemia with these forms of insulin.

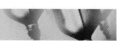

2 Which of the following statements would be important to include in the client teaching for type 2 diabetics?
  a. Because you have insulin injections with your diabetes, you can eat unlimited amounts of carbohydrates.
  b. Insulin injections are *never* used with type 2 diabetes.
  c. Alcohol should not be consumed with your diabetes and/or oral antihyperglycemic agents.
  d. Oral agents must be refrigerated at all times.
3 A therapeutic response to oral antihyperglycemic agents would include which of the following?
  a. Fewer episodes of DKA
  b. Weight gain of 23 kg
  c. Hemoglobin A1c levels within normal limits
  d. Elevation of glucose levels to at least 15.6 mmol/L
4 Which of the following drugs should *not* be used with insulin?
  a. Acetaminophen products
  b. MAOIs
  c. Vitamin C
  d. Zinc supplements
5 Diabetes is associated with which of the following?
  a. Decrease in HDLs
  b. Microvascular regeneration
  c. Renal hyperplasia
  d. Retinopathies

For answers see http://evolve.elsevier.com/Lilley/pharmacology/.

CRITICAL THINKING ACTIVITIES

1 Type 1 diabetes mellitus has recently been diagnosed in a 109-kg, 45-year-old woman. When she is admitted to your unit for additional testing and control of her diabetes, she is placed on a 1500-calorie diabetic diet and on 30 units of Humulin-N insulin to be given every day at 7:30 AM. At 4 PM on the first day of therapy she becomes diaphoretic, weak, and pale. How would you explain these symptoms to this client?

2 Which of the following substances would eliminate the polydipsia, polyuria, and a low specific gravity of urine in a diabetic client: insulin, glucagon, ADH, or aldosterone? Explain your answer.

3 What actions would be necessary in the nursing care of the type 1 diabetes mellitus client who is NPO for surgery but with orders for the usual AM (before breakfast) regular and NPH insulin? Explain your answer.

For answers see http://evolve.elsevier.com/Lilley/pharmacology/.

BIBLIOGRAPHY

Albanese, J., & Nutz, P. (2005). *Mosby's 2005 nursing drug cards.* St Louis, MO: Mosby.

Anderson, P.O., Knoben, J.E., & Troutman, W.G. (2002). *Handbook of clinical drug data* (10th ed.). New York: McGraw-Hill/Appleton & Lange.

Berne, R., & Levy, M. (2002). *Principles of physiology* (3rd ed.). St Louis, MO: Mosby.

Boron, W.F., & Boulpaep, E.L. (2003). *Medical physiology.* Philadelphia: Saunders.

Canadian Diabetes Association Clinical Practice Guidelines Expert Committee. Canadian Diabetes Association 2003 clinical practice guidelines for the prevention and management of diabetes in Canada. *Canadian Journal of Diabetes, 27*(suppl 2).

Canadian Pharmacists Association. (2003). *Therapeutic choices* (4th ed.). Ottawa, ON: Author.

Canadian Pharmacists Association. (2004). *Guide to drugs in Canada.* Toronto, ON: Dorling Kindersley.

Canadian Pharmacists Association. (2005). *Compendium of pharmaceuticals and specialties. The Canadian drug reference for health professionals.* Ottawa, ON: Author. [The subscription-based e-CPS is available at http://www.pharmacists.ca.]

Cheng, A., Williams, B.A., & Sivarajan, B.V. (Eds.). (2003). *The HSC handbook of pediatrics* (10th ed.). Toronto, ON: Elsevier.

Cheng, A.Y.Y., & Fantus, I.G. (2005). Oral antihyperglycemic therapy for type 2 diabetes mellitus. *Canadian Medical Association Journal, 172*(2), 213–226.

GlaxoSmithKline. (2005). Avandamet (rosiglitazone maleate/metformin HCL). About avandamet. Retrieved August 18, 2005, from http://www.avandamet.com

Hardman, J.G., & Limbird, L.E. (2002). *Goodman and Gilman's the pharmacological basis of therapeutics* (10th ed.). New York: McGraw-Hill.

Health Canada. (2005). Drug product database (DPD). Retrieved August 18, 2005, from http://www.hc-sc.gc.ca/hpb/drugs-dpd/

Jones, K.L., Arslanian, S, Peterokova, V.A., Park, J.S., & Tomlinson, M.J. (2002). Effect of metformin in pediatric patients with type 2 diabetes: A randomized controlled trial. *Diabetes Care, 25,* 89–94.

Kasper, D.L., Braunwald, D., Faci, A., Hauser, S., Longo, D., & Jameson, J.L. (2005). *Harrison's principles of internal medicine* (16th ed.). New York: McGraw-Hill.

Katzung, B.G. (2004). *Basic and clinical pharmacology* (9th ed.). New York: McGraw-Hill.

Lacy, C.F., Armstrong, L.L., Goldman, M.P., & Lance, L.L. (2003). *Drug information handbook* (11th ed.). Hudson, OH: Lexi-Comp.

Larsen, P.R., Kronenberg, H.M., Melmod, S., & Polonsky, K.S. (2003). *Williams textbook of endocrinology* (10th ed.). Philadelphia: Saunders.

Lehne, R.A. (2004). *Pharmacology for nursing care* (5th ed.). St Louis, MO: Saunders.

McKenry, L.M., & Salerno, E. (2003). *Mosby's pharmacology in nursing—revised and updated* (21st ed.). St Louis, MO: Mosby.

Mosby. (2005). *Mosby's drug consult 2005: The comprehensive reference for generic and brand name drugs* (15th ed.). St Louis, MO: Mosby.

Skidmore-Roth, L. (2006). *Mosby's 2006 nursing drug reference* (19th ed.). St Louis, MO: Mosby.

The Diabetes Control and Complications Trial Research Group. (1993).The effect of intensive treatment of diabetes on the development and progression of long-term complications in insulin-dependent diabetes mellitus. *New England Journal of Medicine, 329,* 977–986.

UK Prospective Diabetes Study (UKPDS) Group. (1998). Intensive blood-glucose control with sulphonylureas or insulin compared with conventional treatment and risk of complications in patients with type 2 diabetes (UKPDS 33). *Lancet, 352,* 837–853.

CHAPTER

32 Adrenal Agents

OBJECTIVES

After reading this chapter, the successful student will be able to do the following:

1 Discuss the normal actions and functions of the adrenal system and its feedback mechanism of hormonal control.

2 Contrast the mechanism and end result of hyposecretion and hypersecretion of adrenal hormones.

3 Discuss the pathology of the diseases attributed to the hyposecretion and hypersecretion of the adrenal system.

4 Identify the various agents used to manage the hyposecretion and hypersecretion of adrenal hormones, as well as other indications for the use of adrenal agents.

5 Discuss the mechanisms of action, indications, contraindications, cautions, side effects, and toxicity of medications affecting the adrenal system.

6 Develop a nursing care plan that includes all phases of the nursing process for clients receiving adrenal medications.

e-LEARNING ACTIVITIES

Student CD-ROM
- Review Questions: see questions 251–256
- Animations
- Medication Administration Checklists
- IV Therapy Checklists

evolve Web site (http://evolve.elsevier.com/Lilley/pharmacology/)
- Online Chapter Worksheet • Frequently Asked Questions
- Learning Tips and Content Updates • WebLinks • Online Appendices and Supplements • Mosby/Saunders ePharmacology Update • Access to *Mosby's Drug Consult*

DRUG PROFILES

▶▶ **dexamethasone**, p. 539   ▶▶ **hydrocortisone**, p. 539
▶▶ **fludrocortisone**, p. 539   ▶▶ **prednisone**, p. 539

▶▶ Key drug.

GLOSSARY

Addison's disease Life-threatening condition caused by failure of adrenocortical function.

Adrenal cortex (uh dre' nəl kor' teks) Outer portion of the adrenal gland.

Adrenal medulla (uh dre' nəl mə dul' ə) Inner portion of the adrenal gland.

Aldosterone (al dos' tər own) Mineralocorticoid hormone produced by the adrenal cortex that acts on the renal tubule to regulate sodium and potassium balance in the blood.

Cortex Outer layer of a body organ or other structure.

Corticosteroid (kor' tə koe ster' oid) Any one of the natural or synthetic adrenocortical hormones, i.e., those produced by the cortex of the adrenal gland.

Cushing's syndrome Metabolic disorder characterized by abnormally increased secretion of the adrenocortical steroids caused by any one of several sources: adrenocorticotropic hormone (ACTH)-dependent adrenocortical hyperplasia or tumour, ectopic ACTH-secreting tumour, or excessive administration of steroids.

Epinephrine (ep' i nef' rin) Endogenous hormone secreted into the bloodstream by the adrenal medulla; also a synthetic drug that is an adrenergic vasoconstrictor. Epinephrine also increases cardiac output.

Norepinephrine (nor' ep i nef' rin) Adrenergic hormone, also secreted by the adrenal medulla, that increases blood pressure by causing vasoconstriction but does not affect cardiac output.

ADRENAL SYSTEM

The adrenal gland is an endocrine organ that sits on top of the kidneys like a cap. It is composed of two distinct parts, called the **adrenal cortex** and the **adrenal medulla**, that differ both structurally and functionally. The adrenal cortex comprises roughly 80 to 90 percent of the entire adrenal gland, with the remainder being the medulla. The adrenal cortex is made up of regular endocrine tissue, and the adrenal medulla is made up of neurosecretory tissue. Therefore the adrenal gland actually functions as two different endocrine glands, with each secreting different hormones.

The adrenal medulla secretes two important hormones, both of which are catecholamines. These are **epinephrine**, or adrenaline, which accounts for about 80 percent of the secretion, and **norepinephrine**, or noradrenaline, which accounts for the other 20 percent. (Both of these hormones are discussed in Chapter 17 and are not discussed further in this chapter in any detail.) The differences between the adrenal cortex and the adrenal medulla and the various hormones secreted by each are listed in Table 32-1.

The hormones secreted by the adrenal cortex, which are the focus of this chapter, are broadly referred to as **corticosteroids** because they arise from the cortex and they are made from the crystalline steroid alcohol cholesterol. There are two types of corticosteroids—glucocorticoids and mineralocorticoids. These are secreted by two different layers, or zones, of the **cortex**. The zona glomerulosa, which is the outer layer, secretes the mineralocorticoids, and the zona fasciculata, which lies under the zona glomerulosa, secretes the glucocorticoids. A third, inner layer, the zona reticularis, secretes small amounts of sex hormones. All the hormones secreted by the adrenal cortex are steroid hormones.

The mineralocorticoids get their name from the fact that they play an important role in regulating mineral salts (electrolytes) in the body. In humans the only physiologically important mineralocorticoid is **aldosterone**. Its primary role is to maintain normal levels of sodium in the blood (sodium homeostasis) by causing sodium to be resorbed from the urine back into the blood in exchange for potassium and hydrogen ions. In this way aldosterone not only regulates the blood sodium levels but also influences the potassium levels of the blood and its pH.

Overall the corticosteroids are necessary for many vital bodily functions, and some of the important ones are listed in Box 32-1. Without these hormones, life-threatening consequences may arise.

Adrenal corticosteroids are synthesized as needed; the body does not store them as it does other hormones. The body levels of these hormones are regulated by the hypothalamus–pituitary–adrenal (HPA) axis in much the same way as the levels of hormones secreted by the previously discussed endocrine glands (pancreas, thyroid, and pituitary) are regulated. As the name implies, this axis consists of a highly organized system of communication between the adrenal gland, the pituitary, and the hypothalamus and, as is the case for the other endocrine glands, uses hormones as the messengers and a negative feedback mechanism as the controller and maintainer of the process. This feedback process operates as follows: When the level of a particular corticosteroid is low, corticotropin-releasing hormone is released from the hypothalamus into the bloodstream and travels to the anterior pituitary, where it triggers the release of adrenocorticotropic hormone (ACTH). The corticotropin is then transported in the blood to the adrenal cortex, where it stimulates the production of the corticosteroid. The corticosteroid is then released into the bloodstream. When it reaches a peak level, a signal (negative feedback) is sent to the hypothalamus, and the HPA axis is inhibited until the level of the corticosteroid is depleted, whereupon the axis is stimulated once again.

BOX 32-1

Adrenal Cortex Hormones: Biological Functions

Glucocorticoids
Anti-inflammatory actions
Carbohydrate and protein metabolism
Fat metabolism
Maintenance of normal BP
Stress effects

Mineralocorticoids
BP control
Potassium levels and pH of blood
Sodium and water resorption

TABLE 32-1

ADRENAL GLAND: CHARACTERISTICS

Type of Tissue	Type of Hormone	Specific Drugs/Hormones
ADRENAL CORTEX		
Endocrine	Glucocorticoids	Adrenocorticotropic hormone (ACTH), betamethasone, cortisone, dexamethasone, hydrocortisone, methylprednisolone, prednisolone, triamcinolone
	Mineralocorticoids	aldosterone, desoxycorticosterone, fludrocortisone
ADRENAL MEDULLA		
Neuroendocrine	Catecholamines	epinephrine, norepinephrine

TABLE 32-2

AVAILABLE SYNTHETIC CORTICOSTEROIDS

Hormone Type	Method of Administration	Individual Drugs
Adrenal steroid inhibitor	Systemic	mitotane, ketoconazole
Glucocorticoid	Topical	alclometasone dipropionate, amcinonide, betamethasone benzoate, betamethasone dipropionate, betamethasone valerate, clobetasol 17-propionate, clobetasol 17-butyrate, clocortolone pivalate desonide, desoximetasone, diflucortolone valerate, flumethasone, fluocinolone acetonide, fluocinonide, halcinonide, halobetasol propionate, hydrocortisone acetate, hydrocortisone valerate, methylprednisolone acetate, mometasone furoate, prednicarbate, triamcinolone acetonide
	Systemic	beclomethasone, cortisone, dexamethasone, fludrocortisone, hydrocortisone, methylprednisolone, prednisolone, prednisone, triamcinolone
	Inhaled	beclomethasone, budesonide, fluticasone
	Nasal	beclomethasone dipropionate, budesonide, flunisolide, fluticasone, mometasone, triamcinolone acetonide
Mineralocorticoid	Systemic	fludrocortisone acetate

The oversecretion (hypersecretion) of adrenocortical hormones can lead to a collection of signs and symptoms called **Cushing's syndrome**. The hypersecretion of glucocorticoids results in the redistribution of body fat from the arms and legs to the face, shoulders, trunk, and abdomen, resulting in the "moon face" characteristic. The hypersecretion of aldosterone, or primary aldosteronism, leads to increased water retention and muscle weakness resulting from the potassium loss.

The undersecretion (hyposecretion) of adrenocortical hormones causes a condition referred to as **Addison's disease**. It is associated with decreased blood sodium levels and decreased blood glucose, increased potassium levels, dehydration, and weight loss. The combination of a mineralocorticoid (fludrocortisone) and a glucocorticoid (prednisone or some other suitable agent) are used for treatment.

ADRENAL AGENTS

All the naturally occurring corticosteroids are available as exogenous agents, and there are also higher-potency synthetic analogues. The adrenal glucocorticoids are an extremely large group of steroids, classified in various ways. They may be classified by natural or synthetic origin, by the method of administration (e.g., systemic, topical), by their salt and water retention potential (mineralocorticoid activity), by their duration of action (short, intermediate, or long acting), or by some combination of these schemes. The only corticosteroid with exclusive mineralocorticoid activity is fludrocortisone. The currently available synthetic adrenal hormones are listed in Table 32-2.

Mechanism of Action and Drug Effects

The action of the corticosteroids is related to their involvement in the synthesis of specific proteins. There are several steps to this process. Initially the steroid hor-

mones bind to a receptor on the surface of a target cell to form a steroid–receptor complex, which is then transported to the nucleus of that target cell. Once inside the nucleus of the target cell, the complex stimulates the cell's deoxyribonucleic acid (DNA) to produce messenger ribonucleic acid (mRNA), which is then used as a template for the synthesis of a specific protein. It is these proteins that exert specific drug effects.

Most of the corticosteroids exert their effects by modifying enzyme activity; therefore their role is more intermediary than direct. As previously mentioned, the naturally occurring mineralocorticoid aldosterone affects electrolyte and fluid balance by working on the distal renal tubule to promote sodium resorption from the nephron into the blood, which pulls water and fluid along with it. In doing so it causes fluid and water retention, which leads to edema and hypertension. It may also promote potassium and hydrogen excretion.

The naturally occurring glucocorticoids hydrocortisone (cortisol) and cortisone have some mineralocorticoid activity and therefore have some of the same effects as aldosterone (i.e., fluid and water retention). Their other main effect is the inhibition of inflammatory and immune responses. Glucocorticoids primarily inhibit or help control the inflammatory response by stabilizing the cell membranes of inflammatory cells called *lysosomes*, decreasing the permeability of capillaries to the inflammatory cells and decreasing the migration of white blood cells (WBCs) into already inflamed areas. They may also lower fever by reducing the release of interleukin-1 (IL-1) from WBCs. They do this by stimulating the cells that eventually become red blood cells (RBCs) called *erythroid cells*. The stimulation of these cells in the bone marrow prolongs the survival of erythrocytes (RBCs and platelets). Glucocorticoids inhibit phospholipase A_2 and thus block the production of both prostaglandins and leukotrienes, exerting a potent anti-inflammatory effect. The glucocorticoids also promote

TABLE 32-3
SYSTEMIC GLUCOCORTICOIDS: A COMPARISON

Drug	Origin	Duration of Action	Equivalent Dose (mg)	Salt and Water Retention Potential
betamethasone	Synthetic	Long	0.6	Minimal
cortisone	Natural	Short	25.0	High
dexamethasone	Synthetic	Long	0.75	Minimal
hydrocortisone	Natural	Short	20.0	High
methylprednisolone	Synthetic	Intermediate	4.0	Low
prednisone	Synthetic	Intermediate	5.0	Low
prednisolone	Synthetic	Intermediate	5.0	Low
triamcinolone	Synthetic	Intermediate	4.0	Minimal

the breakdown (catabolism) of protein, the production of glycogen (gluconeogenesis), and the redistribution of fat from peripheral to central areas of the body.

Indications

All of the systemically administered glucocorticoids have a similar clinical efficacy but differ in their potency and duration of action and in the extent to which they cause salt and fluid retention (Table 32-3). They are indicated for the following:

- Adrenocortical deficiency
- Adrenogenital syndrome
- Bacterial meningitis
- Cerebral edema
- Collagen diseases (e.g., systemic lupus erythematosus)
- Dermatological diseases (e.g., exfoliative dermatitis, pemphigus)
- Endocrine disorders (thyroiditis)
- Gastrointestinal (GI) diseases (ulcerative colitis, regional enteritis)
- Exacerbations of chronic respiratory illnesses such as asthma and chronic obstructive pulmonary disease (COPD)
- Hematological disorders (reduce bleeding tendencies)
- Ophthalmic disorders (non-pyogenic inflammations)
- Organ transplant (decrease immune response)
- Palliative management of leukemias and lymphomas
- Remission of proteinuria in nephrotic syndrome
- Tuberculosis meningitis
- Spinal cord injury

Glucocorticoids are also administered by inhalation for the control of steroid-responsive bronchospastic states. Nasally administered glucocorticoids are used in the management of allergic rhinitis and to prevent the recurrence of polyps after surgical removal. The topical steroids are the largest group and are used in the management of inflammations in the eye, ear, and skin.

Contraindications

Contraindications to the administration of glucocorticoids include drug allergy and any serious infection, including septicemia, systemic fungal infections, and vari-

TABLE 32-4
CORTICOSTEROIDS: COMMON ADVERSE EFFECTS

Body System	Side/Adverse Effects
Cardiovascular	Heart failure, cardiac edema, hypertension—all due to electrolyte imbalances
Central nervous	Convulsions, headache, vertigo, mood swings, psychic impairment, nervousness, insomnia
Endocrine	Growth suppression, Cushing's syndrome, menstrual irregularities, carbohydrate intolerance, hyperglycemia, HPA axis suppression
Gastrointestinal	Peptic ulcers with possible perforation, pancreatitis, ulcerative esophagitis, abdominal distension
Integumentary	Fragile skin, petechiae (hemorrhagic spots), ecchymoses (hemorrhagic patches), facial erythema (redness), increased risk of infection and delayed wound healing, hirsutism, urticaria (hives)
Musculoskeletal	Muscle weakness, loss of muscle mass, osteoporosis
Ocular	Increased intra-ocular pressure, glaucoma, exophthalmos (protrusion of the eyeballs), cataracts
Other	Weight gain

cella (chicken pox). One exception to this rule is a diagnosis of tuberculous meningitis, in which glucocorticoids may be used to prevent inflammatory central nervous system (CNS) damage.

Side Effects and Adverse Effects

The potent metabolic, physiological, and pharmacological effects of the corticosteroids can influence every body system, with the result that they can produce a wide variety of significant undesirable effects. The more common of these are summarized in Table 32-4.

Interactions

The systematically administered corticosteroids can interact with many agents:

- Their use with non–potassium-sparing diuretics (e.g., thiazides, loop diuretics) can lead to severe hypocalcemia and hypokalemia.
- Their use with acetylsalicylic acid (ASA), other nonsteroidal anti-inflammatory drugs (NSAIDs), and other ulcerogenic drugs produces additive GI effects. Corticosteroids may increase the renal clearance of ASA, which may result in decreased efficacy or toxicity.
- Their use with anticholinesterase drugs produces weakness in clients with myasthenia gravis.
- Their use with immunizing biologicals inhibits the immune response to the biological.
- Their use with antidiabetic agents may reduce the hypoglycemic affect.
- Their use with oral antihyperglycemics or insulin may require dose adjustments of these drugs.

Dosages

For information on the recommended dosages of adrenal agents, see the table below. See Appendix B for some of the common brands available in Canada.

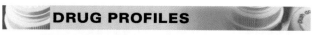

DRUG PROFILES

CORTICOSTEROIDS

The systemic corticosteroids consist of chemically different but pharmacologically similar hormones. They all exert varying degrees of glucocorticoid and mineralo-

DOSAGES Selected Anti-Adrenal and Corticosteroid Agents			
Agent	**Pharmacological Class**	**Usual Dosage Range**	**Indications**
▸▸ dexamethasone	Synthetic long-acting glucocorticoid	**Adult** PO/IV/IM: 0.75–9 mg/day divided bid–qid **Pediatric** PO/IV: 0.5–2 mg/kg/day divided q6h	Wide variety of endocrine (including adrenocortical insufficiency), rheumatic, collagen, dermatological, allergic, ophthalmic, respiratory, hematological, neoplastic, GI, and nervous system disorders; edematous states
methylprednisolone	Short-term glucocorticoid	**Adult only** IM: 8–16 mg q1–3wk	Same as dexamethasone
methylprednisolone sodium succinate	Rapid-acting systemic glucocorticoid	IV: 30 mg/kg bolus dose over 15 min, 15 min pause, then continuous infusion 5.4mg/kg/h over 23 h Retention enema: 40–120 mg Continuous IV: 40-120 mg 3–7 times/wk for 2 or more wks Intralesional: 0.8–1.6 mg Intra-articular and soft tissue: 5–30 mg 3–4/yr	Acute spinal cord injury Adjunctive treatment for ulcerative colitis Anti-inflammatory Anti-inflammatory
▸▸ fludrocortisone	Synthetic mineralocorticoid	**Adult and pediatric (including infant)** PO: 0.05–0.2 mg q24h	Addison's disease; salt-losing adrenogenital syndrome
▸▸ hydrocortisone	Natural, short-acting glucocorticoid	**Adult** PO: 20–240 mg/day **Pediatric** PO: 2.5–10 mg/kg/day divided q6–8h	Adrenocortical insufficiency; many inflammatory conditions
hydrocortisone sodium succinate	Natural, water-soluble, short-acting glucocorticoid	**Adult** IV/IM: 100–500 mg q2–6h, depending on condition and client response **Pediatric** IV/IM: 1.5 mg/kg/day divided qd–bid	Adrenocortical insufficiency; many inflammatory conditions
▸▸ prednisone	Synthetic intermediate-acting glucocorticoid	**Adult** PO: 0.55–30 mg/kg/day **Pediatric** PO: 0.05–2 mg/kg/day divided once daily–qid	Wide variety of endocrine (including adrenocortical insufficiency), rheumatic, collagen, dermatological, allergic, ophthalmic, respiratory, hematological, neoplastic, GI, and nervous system disorders; edematous states

corticoid effects. Their differences arise out of slight changes in their chemical structures.

Corticosteroids can cross the placenta and produce fetal abnormalities. For this reason they are classified as pregnancy category C agents. They may also be secreted in breast milk and cause abnormalities in the nursing infant. They are contraindicated in clients who have exhibited hypersensitivity reactions to them in the past as well as in clients with fungal or bacterial infections. Short- or long-term use can lead to a condition known as *steroid psychosis.* In addition, the cessation of long-term treatment with these agents requires a tapering of the daily dose because the administration of the exogenous hormones causes the endogenous production of the hormones to stop. Tapering daily doses allows the HPA axis the time it needs to recover and start to stimulate the normal production of the endogenous hormones.

▶▶ dexamethasone

Dexamethasone is one of the two long-acting glucocorticoids, the other being betamethasone. These agents have half-lives that range from 36 to 54 hours and durations of action of 32 to 48 hours. Usually dexamethasone and the other long-acting corticosteroids are used for anti-inflammatory or immunosuppressant purposes. They have only minimal mineralocorticoid properties and therefore alone are inadequate for the management of adrenocortical insufficiency. A dexamethasone suppression test may be performed to establish the diagnosis of Cushing's syndrome or an adrenal adenoma. Dexamethasone inhibits the release of ACTH from the pituitary gland and decreases the output of endogenous corticosteroids. Dexamethasone has also been shown to be effective in preventing the nausea and vomiting associated with cancer chemotherapy. It is administered intravenously (IV) before chemotherapy or orally after chemotherapy for this purpose; however, for control of cerebral edema in neurosurgical situations such as head trauma, dexamethasone would be used intravenously.

Dexamethasone is available in oral (PO) form as a 0.5-mg/5 mL oral elixir; as a 0.5-mg/5 mL solution; and as 0.5-, 0.75-, and 4-mg tablets. Dexamethasone sodium phosphate is given intramuscularly; intra-articularly (into a joint space); or intravenously as a 1-, 4-, or 10-mg/mL injection. Pregnancy category C. Recommended dosages are given in the table on p. 538.

PHARMACOKINETICS

Half-Life	Onset	Peak	Duration
36–54 hr	Unknown	1–2 hr	32–48 hr

▶▶ fludrocortisone

Fludrocortisone is a synthetic analogue of aldosterone. It is classified as a glucocorticoid but is used more for its potent mineralocorticoid activity. It is used for oral replacement therapy in clients suffering from an adrenocortical insufficiency such as Addison's disease. It has also been used to increase systolic and diastolic blood pressure (BP) in clients suffering from chronic severe postural hypotension. It is available only in oral form as a 0.1-mg tablet. Pregnancy category C. Recommended dosages are given in the table on p. 538.

PHARMACOKINETICS

Half-Life	Onset	Peak	Duration
18–36 hr	10–20 min	PO: 1.7 hr	Unknown

▶▶ hydrocortisone

Hydrocortisone is a short-acting adrenocortical steroid. It and cortisone are the only two short-acting agents. Compared with other glucocorticoids they have the strongest mineralocorticoid actions (potassium excretion and sodium and water retention) and the weakest glucocorticoid actions (anti-inflammatory, immunosuppressant, and metabolic-type effects). They have relatively short half-lives (0.5 to 2 hours) and therefore short durations of action. Because they have both glucocorticoid and mineralocorticoid properties, either hydrocortisone or cortisone is usually the corticosteroid of choice for replacement therapy in clients with adrenocortical insufficiency.

Hydrocortisone is available in oral, injectable, and topical preparations. It is available in oral form as 10- and 20-mg tablets and as a 1-mg/mL suspension in Act-O-Vials of powdered drug containing 100-, 250-, 500-, and 1000-mg for injection. It is also available in a variety of topical preparations of various strengths, including creams, ointments, a gel, a spray, a lotion, a liquid, and even a roll-on stick as well as hydrocortisone enema, rectal aerosol, suppository, and eye drop formulations. Pregnancy category C. Recommended dosages are given in the table on p. 538.

PHARMACOKINETICS

Half-Life	Onset	Peak	Duration
0.5–2 hr	Unknown	1 hr	30–36 hr

▶▶ prednisone

Prednisone is one of the four intermediate-acting glucocorticoids, the others being methylprednisolone, prednisolone, and triamcinolone. These agents have half-lives that are more than double those of the short-acting corticosteroids (2 to 5 hours), and therefore they have much longer durations of action. Prednisone is the preferred oral glucocorticoid for anti-inflammatory or immunosuppressant purposes. Along with methylprednisolone and prednisolone, it is also used for exacerbations of chronic respiratory illnesses such as asthma and chronic bronchitis. This agent has only minimal mineralocorticoid properties and therefore alone is inadequate for the management of adrenocortical insufficiency (Addison's disease).

Prednisone is available in oral form as a 5-mg/5 mL solution; and 1-, 5-, and 50-mg tablets. Pregnancy category C. Recommended dosages are given in the table on p. 538.

PHARMACOKINETICS

Half-Life	Onset	Peak	Duration
18–36 hr	Unknown	1–2 hr	36 hr

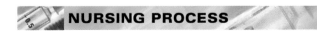 **NURSING PROCESS**

■ Assessment

Before administering any of the adrenal agents, the nurse should perform a thorough physical assessment to determine the client's baseline weight, intake and output status, vital signs (especially BP), hydration status, skin condition, and immune status. Important baseline laboratory values include the serum Na, K, blood urea nitrogen (BUN), and hemoglobin (Hgb) levels and hematocrit (Hct). Because glucocorticoids may elevate a client's blood glucose level, a baseline level must be determined. All this is crucial for ensuring the safest and most effective use of these adrenal agents, for identifying any cautions or contraindications, and for monitoring the client's response to treatment. Any edema or electrolyte imbalances need to be documented and brought to the attention of the physician. Because corticosteroids often aggravate peptic ulcer disease, the nurse should find out whether the client has a history of ulcer disease, gastritis, or heartburn or is taking any other medication that could cause ulcers.

Many drugs interact with corticosteroids (see previous discussion); therefore the nurse should always find out what prescription and OTC medications the client is currently taking.

■ Nursing Diagnoses

Nursing diagnoses appropriate for the client receiving adrenal agents include the following:

- Imbalanced nutrition, more than body requirements, related to changes in appetite resulting from corticosteroid therapy.
- Disturbed body image related to the physiological influence of diseases of the adrenal gland on the body.
- Excess fluid volume related to increased cardiac output from increased volume and/or fluid retention associated with mineralocorticoids.
- Risk for infection related to side effects of glucocorticoid therapy.
- Impaired skin integrity related to side effects of glucocorticoids.
- Risk for injury stemming from changes in sensorium and possible confusion related to side effects of corticosteroid therapy.

■ Planning

The goals for clients receiving corticosteroids include the following:

- Client describes the healthy diet to observe during treatment.
- Client experiences minimal body image disturbances.
- Client exhibits minimal complications resulting from the fluid retention caused by mineralocorticoid therapy.
- Client is free of infection during corticosteroid therapy.
- Client's skin and mucous membranes remain intact during treatment.
- Client maintains normal electrolyte levels.
- Client remains free of changes in sensorium and possible confusion or dizziness from adrenal therapy.
- Client states symptoms to report immediately to the physician should they occur.

■ *Outcome Criteria*

Outcome criteria for clients receiving adrenal agents include the following:

- Client eats adequate foods according to the food guide pyramid and maintains weight within normal range with adequate menu planning.
- Client openly verbalizes fears about body image disturbances to healthcare providers.
- Client experiences minimal problems with fluid volume excess and does not gain more than 1 kg/wk.
- Client notifies the physician if fever (>38° C) occurs.
- Client performs frequent mouth and skin care to prevent infections and maintain intactness.
- Client drinks plenty of fluids, and restricts salt or additives if ordered, to minimize major electrolyte imbalances during corticosteroid or mineralocorticoid therapy.
- Client changes positions slowly and walks carefully to prevent injuries resulting from dizziness or syncope.
- Client identifies symptoms to report to the physician, such as a weight gain of more than 1 kg/wk, shortness of breath, edema, dizziness, and syncope.
- Client experiences minimal problems when being weaned off corticosteroids.

■ Implementation

Some of the systemic forms of adrenal agents, such as hydrocortisone and prednisone, may be given by the oral, intramuscular, intravenous, or rectal route. Parenteral forms of these agents should be diluted according to the manufacturer's guidelines and administered over the recommended time span; for example, hydrocortisone should be given at a rate of 25 mg or less per minute. All liquid and parenteral forms should be mixed thoroughly before administration. Intramuscular forms should always be administered in a large muscle (e.g., gluteal) site as opposed to the deltoid muscle, and the sites should be rotated to prevent tissue trauma and damage. Oral forms should be given with food or milk to minimize GI upset. Injections should not be given subcutaneously (SC) because this may lead to tissue damage.

Topical agents should be applied as ordered and only according to the instructions in the package insert, which, for example, may specify the use of an occlusive dressing. The skin should be clean and dry before application, and the nurse should wear gloves and apply the medication with either a sterile tongue depressor or cotton-tipped applicator if the skin is intact. *A sterile technique should be used if the skin is not intact.*

Beclomethasone is a nasally administered synthetic corticosteroid that should be used as ordered. Any written instructions that come with the product should be read and followed carefully. Before administering a nasal corticosteroid the client should clear the nasal passages, and this may require a decongestant, which the physician may need to prescribe. See Chapter 9 for more instructions on nasal sprays.

Steroid inhalers should be used as ordered and the client adequately taught the technique for administration (also covered in Chapter 9). It is important to tell the client to rinse with mouthwash after using the inhaler to prevent oral fungal infections.

Clients receiving fludrocortisone should take it with food or milk to minimize GI upset. Weight gain of more than 2.25 kg in a week or 1 kg over a 24-hour period during mineralocorticoid or corticosteroid therapy should be reported to the physician as soon as possible. Abrupt withdrawal is not recommended because this may precipitate an adrenal crisis due to the negative feedback loop system.

See the box below for additional teaching tips for clients receiving adrenal agents.

Evaluation

A therapeutic response to corticosteroids includes a resolution of the underlying manifestations of the disease, such as a decrease in inflammation. Adverse effects for which to monitor include weight gain, increased BP, pulse irregularities, electrolyte disturbances, elevated glucose levels, decreased healing, GI upset and ulcer-related symptoms, and mental status changes such as aggression, depression, or psychosis. The systemic agents may cause potassium depletion; this is manifested by fatigue, nausea, vomiting, muscle weakness, and dysrhythmias.

CLIENT TEACHING TIPS

Nurses should instruct clients as follows (as applicable):

▲ Because your immune system is not functioning properly, avoid contact with people with infections and report any fever, increased weakness and lethargy, or sore throat.

▲ Report any unpleasant side effects or changes in appearance.

▲ Get adequate rest, exercise, and nutrition.

▲ During therapy, it is important that we keep track of your nutritional status, weight, fluid volume, electrolytes (sodium, potassium, and calcium), skin condition, and glucose levels.

▲ Keep a daily log of your general feelings of well-being and any response to the medication, along with any questions for the physician.

▲ Do not discontinue your medication without checking with your physician. Stopping this medication suddenly could cause your levels of cortisone hormone to drop sharply, which could cause a health crisis.

▲ Keep all medications out of the reach of children.

▲ Take your medication exactly as prescribed and at the same time every day. If you are taking oral medication, take it with meals or food.

▲ If you are using a cream or ointment, follow the physician's and manufacturer's instructions. Make sure the skin is clean and dry before applying the ointment. Often the site needs to be covered with a dressing; make sure you know the proper way to do this.

▲ If you are taking hydrocortisone or prednisone, take it exactly as ordered.

▲ Notify your physician of any weakness, joint pain, difficulty breathing, fever, irregular heartbeat, depression, swelling, or any other unusual symptom.

▲ If you are taking a nasal spray, follow the manufacturer's guidelines and the physician's orders. Make sure you know the proper way to take the spray. (See Chapter 9 for more information on the administration of nasal agents.)

▲ Wear a medical alert tag or bracelet at all times, identifying any disease and specific medication(s).

POINTS to REMEMBER

▼ The adrenal gland is an endocrine organ that is located on top of the kidneys and is composed of two distinct tissues: the adrenal cortex and the adrenal medulla. The adrenal medulla secretes two important hormones: epinephrine (80 percent) and norepinephrine (20 percent); the adrenal cortex secretes hormones known as *corticosteroids*: glucocorticoids and mineralocorticoids.

▼ Glucocorticoid functions include anti-inflammatory actions; maintenance of normal BP; carbohydrate, protein, and fat metabolism; and stress effects.

▼ Mineralocorticoid functions include sodium and water resorption, BP control, and control of potassium levels and pH of blood.

▼ Adrenal agents may be administered orally, intramuscularly, or intravenously; some are also administered by means of a rectal enema.

▼ Parenteral forms should be diluted and administered according to the manufacturer's guidelines.

▼ Intramuscular forms of adrenal agents should be administered deep into a large muscle, such as in the gluteal area.

▼ Steroid inhalers should be used as ordered and only after adequate client education, with rinsing of the mouth after their use to avoid oral fungal infections (oral candidiasis).

▼ Adverse effects to monitor for include weight gain (if more than 2.25 kg in a week), increase in BP, pulse irregularities, mental status changes such as aggression or depression, electrolyte disturbances, elevated glucose levels, decreased healing, GI tract upset, and ulcer-related symptoms.

▼ Clients should be monitored frequently for weight gain, changes in nutritional status, electrolyte imbalances, and fluid volume excess.

▼ Clients should not withdraw from these agents abruptly.

▼ Adrenal suppression from corticosteroid therapy may be minimized if the dose is given between 6 and 9 A.M.; however, this would only apply to once-a-day dosing. The importance of timing should be explained to the client.

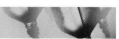

EXAMINATION REVIEW QUESTIONS

1 Which of the following statements is correct regarding corticosteroids?
  a. They have few side effects.
  b. They are often used for their anti-inflammatory effects.
  c. They may be administered only by inhalant dosage forms.
  d. They may be used long term without major complications.

2 Which of the following actions is associated with glucocorticoids?
  a. Antiplatelet activity
  b. Protein catabolism
  c. Blood pressure maintenance
  d. Electrolyte suppression

3 Which of the following is considered one of the classical features or characteristics of increased levels of corticosteroids or Cushing's syndrome?
  a. Weight loss
  b. Moon face

  c. Muscle thickening
  d. Increased thoracic subcutaneous tissue

4 Which of the following may occur with the administration of fludrocortisone?
  a. Elevated blood pressure
  b. Dysphagia
  c. Weight loss
  d. Severe bradycardia

5 Which of the following is an adverse effect of a corticosteroid?
  a. Excessive sedation
  b. Weight loss
  c. Osteoporosis
  d. Addison's disease

For answers see http://evolve.elsevier.com/Lilley/pharmacology/.

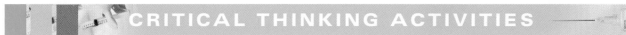

CRITICAL THINKING ACTIVITIES

1 A 19-year-old man is admitted through the emergency room after a motorcycle accident. He is conscious upon admission, has stable vital signs, and has minimal cuts and abrasions on the left side of his body. You perform a thorough neurological examination and find absence of sensation to light touch and pinprick and lower extremity paralysis. Reflexes are absent below the groin area. The physician orders a high-dose intravenous methylprednisolone. What is the purpose of this medication and

what should you, as the nurse, watch for while the client is receiving this medication?

2 You are caring for a client who is taking 100 mg of hydrocortisone orally. The physician decides that he is more familiar with prednisone and wants to change the client over to the equivalent oral dose of prednisone. What should you recommend?

3 Discuss the influence of hyperaldosteronism on the body and the indicated treatment.

For answers see http://evolve.elsevier.com/Lilley/pharmacology/.

BIBLIOGRAPHY

Albanese, J., & Nutz, P. (2005). *Mosby's 2005 nursing drug cards.* St Louis, MO: Mosby.

Berne, R., & Levy, M. (2003). *Principles of physiology* (3rd ed.). St Louis, MO: Mosby.

Canadian Pharmacists Association. (2003). *Therapeutic choices* (4th ed.). Ottawa, ON: Author.

Canadian Pharmacists Association. (2004). *Guide to drugs in Canada.* Toronto, ON: Dorling Kindersley.

Canadian Pharmacists Association. (2005). *Compendium of pharmaceuticals and specialties. The Canadian drug reference for health professionals.* Ottawa, ON: Author. [The subscription-based e-CPS is available at http://www.pharmacists.ca.]

Cheng, A., Williams, B.A., & Sivarajan, B.V. (Eds.). (2003). *The HSC handbook of pediatrics* (10th ed.). Toronto, ON: Elsevier.

Facts and Comparisons. (2004). *Drug facts and comparisons pocket version* (9th ed.). St Louis, MO: Wolters Kluwer Health.

Hardman, J.G. & Limbird, L.E. (2002). *Goodman and Gilman's the pharmacological basis of therapeutics* (10th ed.). New York: McGraw-Hill.

Health Canada. (2005). Drug product database (DPD). Retrieved August 21, 2005, from http://www.hc-sc.gc.ca/hpb/drugs-dpd/

Lacy, C.F., Armstrong, L.L., Goldman, M.P., & Lance, L.L. (2003). *Drug information handbook* (11th ed.). Hudson, OH: Lexi-Comp.

Lehne, R.A. (2004). *Pharmacology for nursing care* (5th ed.). St Louis, MO: Saunders.

Mosby. (2005). *Mosby's drug consult 2005: The comprehensive reference for generic and brand name drugs* (15th ed.). St Louis, MO: Mosby.

Skidmore-Roth, L. (2006). *Mosby's 2006 nursing drug reference* (19th ed.). St Louis, MO: Mosby.

CHAPTER

33 Women's Health Agents

OBJECTIVES

After reading this chapter, the successful student will be able to do the following:

1 Discuss the variety of disorders that are treated with estrogens and progestins.

2 Discuss the normal hormonally mediated feedback system and how it regulates the female reproductive system.

3 Describe the rationale for the various treatments and cite dosages, side effects, cautions, contraindications, and drug interactions associated with estrogen and progestin therapy, selective estrogen receptor modulators, and drugs used in labour and delivery.

4 Develop a nursing care plan that includes all phases of the nursing process for the client receiving estrogens, progestins, oral contraceptives, and drugs used in labour and delivery.

5 Discuss combined oral contraceptives and selective estrogen receptor modulators.

6 List the expected therapeutic responses to the various women's health agents.

7 Describe the therapeutic responses to uterine stimulants and relaxants, as well as their mechanism of actions, side effects, contraindications, and drug interactions.

8 Discuss the concerns for hormonal replacement therapy (HRT) in women.

e-LEARNING ACTIVITIES

Student CD-ROM
- Review Questions: see questions 257–260
- Animations
- Medication Administration Checklists
- IV Therapy Checklists

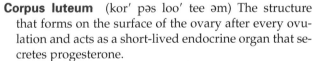 **Web site** (http://evolve.elsevier.com/Lilley/pharmacology/)
- Online Chapter Worksheet • Frequently Asked Questions
- Learning Tips and Content Updates • WebLinks • Online Appendices and Supplements • Mosby/Saunders ePharmacology Update • Access to *Mosby's Drug Consult*

DRUG PROFILES

GLOSSARY

Corpus luteum (kor' pəs loo' tee əm) The structure that forms on the surface of the ovary after every ovulation and acts as a short-lived endocrine organ that secretes progesterone.

Endocrine gland (en' doe krine) Part of a system of glands that secrete hormones into the blood.

Endometrium (en' doe mee' tree əm) The mucous membrane lining the uterus.

Estrogens The collective term for one of two major classes of female sex steroid hormones (the other being the *progestins*), with estradiol responsible for most estrogenic physiological activity.

Fallopian tube (fə loe' pee ən) The passage through which an ovum is carried from its ovary to the uterus.

Gonadotropin (gon' ə do troe' pin) The hormone that stimulates the testes and ovaries.

Implantation The attachment, penetration, and embedding of the fertilized ovum in the lining of the uterine wall; one of the first stages of pregnancy. (Also called *nidation,* from the Latin word *nidus* [nest]).

Menarche (mə nar' kee) The first menses in a young woman's life, and the beginning of cyclic menstrual function.

Menopause   The cessation of menses that marks the end of a woman's childbearing capability.

Menses   (men' seez) The normal flow of blood that occurs during menstruation.

Menstrual cycle   (men' strull) The recurring cycle of changes in the endometrium when the decidual layer is shed, regrows, proliferates, is maintained for several days, and is shed again at menstruation unless a pregnancy begins.

Nucleic acid   (noo klee' ik) A compound involved in energy storage and release and in the determination and transmission of genetic characteristics.

Osteoporosis   (os' tee oe pə roe' sis) A condition characterized by the progressive loss of bone density and thinning of bone tissue; associated with enhanced risk of fractures.

Ova   Female reproductive or germ cells (singular: ovum; also called *eggs*).

Ovarian follicle   The location of egg production and ovulation in the ovary; the precursor to corpus luteum.

Ovaries   (o' və reez) A pair of female gonads located on each side of the lower abdomen beside the uterus. They store and release ova during menstrual cycles.

Ovulation   The rupture of the ovarian follicle, resulting in the release of an unfertilized ovum into the peritoneal cavity.

Progestins   The collective term for the second major class of female hormones, with progesterone responsible for most progestational physiological activity.

Puberty   The period of life when the ability to reproduce begins.

Uterus   The hollow, pear-shaped female organ in which the fertilized ovum is implanted (see *implantation*) and the fetus develops.

Vagina   Part of the female genitalia that forms a canal from its external orifice through its vestibule to the uterine cervix.

OVERVIEW OF FEMALE REPRODUCTIVE FUNCTIONS

The female reproductive system consists of the **ovaries, fallopian tubes, uterus, vagina,** and the external structure known as the *vulva*. The development of these primary sex characteristics, their subsequent reproductive functions (starting at **puberty**), and their maintenance are controlled by pituitary **gonadotropin** hormones and the female sex steroid hormones—the **estrogens** and **progestins.** Pituitary gonadotropins include follicle stimulating hormone (FSH) and luteinizing hormone (LH). Both play a primary role in hormonal communication between the pituitary gland (Chapter 29) and the ovaries in the continuous regulation of the **menstrual cycle** from month to month.

Estrogens are also responsible for stimulating the development of secondary female sex characteristics, including characteristic breast, skin, and bone development and distribution of body fat and hair. Progestins promote optimal conditions for pregnancy in the **endometrium** just after **ovulation** and also promote the start of **menses** in the absence of a fertilized ovum.

The ovaries (female gonads) are paired glands located on each side of the uterus. They function both as **endocrine glands** and as reproductive glands. As reproductive glands, they produce mature **ova** within **ovarian follicles,** which are then ovulated, that is, released into the space in the peritoneal cavity between the ovary and the fallopian tube. Fingerlike projections known as *fimbriae* lie adjacent to each ovary and serve to "catch" the released ovum. Once inside the fallopian tube an ovum is moved through its lumen to the uterus. This occurs as a result of the muscular contractions of the tube walls and the actions of ciliated cells inside the lumen of the tube, which "beat" in a direction toward the uterus. Fertilization of the ovum, when it does occur, often takes place in the fallopian tube.

As endocrine glands, the ovaries are responsible for producing the two major classes of sex steroid hormones, estrogens and progestins. Chemically speaking, each of these two major classes includes several distinct hormones. However, only two of these hormones occur in significant amounts, and they have the greatest physiological activity. These are the estrogen *estradiol* and the progestin *progesterone.* Estradiol is the principle secretory product of the ovary and serves to promote several estrogenic effects. One of these effects is the regulation of gonadotropin (FSH, LH) secretion via negative feedback to the pituitary gland. Others include promotion of the development of women's secondary sex characteristics, monthly endometrial growth, thickening of vaginal mucosa, thinning of cervical mucus, and growth of the ductal system of the breasts. Progesterone is the principle secretory product of the **corpus luteum** and is responsible for progestational effects. These include tissue growth and secretory activity in the endometrium following the estrogen-driven proliferative phase of the menstrual cycle. This important secretory process is required for endometrial egg **implantation** and maintenance of pregnancy. Other progestational effects include induction of menstruation when fertilization has not occurred and, during pregnancy, inhibition of uterine contractions, increased viscosity of cervical mucus (protects fetus from external contamination), and growth of the alveolar glands of the breasts.

The uterus consists of three layers: the outer protective *perimetrium*, the muscular *myometrium*, and the inner mucosal layer, known as the *endometrium.* The myometrium provides the powerful smooth muscle contractions needed for childbirth, whereas the endometrium is the site of

- Implantation of a fertilized ovum and the subsequent development of the fetus
- Initiation of labour and birthing of the infant
- Menstruation

TABLE 33-1
PHASES OF THE MENSTRUAL CYCLE

Phase	Ovarian Follicle Activity	Endometrium Activity
Phase 1	Menstruation	Menstruation
Phase 2	Follicular phase (preovulatory)	Proliferative phase
Phase 3	Ovulation	Ovulation
Phase 4	Luteal phase (post-ovulatory)	Secretory phase

The vagina serves as a common passageway for birthing and menstrual flow. In addition, it is a receptacle for the penis during sexual intercourse and the sperm after male ejaculation.

The menstrual cycle usually takes roughly 1 month to complete. It commences during puberty with the first menses (**menarche**) and ceases with **menopause**, which in most women occurs between 45 and 55 years of age. The hormonally controlled menstrual cycle consists of four distinct but interrelated phases. These phases occur in overlapping sequence. Phase names correspond to activity in either the ovarian follicle or the endometrium (Table 33-1).

- **Phase 1:** The *menstruation phase*, which initiates the cycle and lasts from 5 to 7 days.
- **Phase 2:** The *follicular phase*, during which a mature ovum develops from an ovarian follicle. This phase is also called the *proliferative* or *preovulatory phase* and is characterized by rising estrogen secretion from the ovary and LH secretion from the pituitary gland. It terminates on or about day 14 of the cycle.
- **Phase 3:** The *ovulation phase* involves release of the unfertilized ovum from the ovary. This process occurs over a roughly 24- to 48-hour period starting at about day 14. Both estrogen and LH levels peak near this time.
- **Phase 4:** The final phase of the cycle is called the *luteal* or *post-ovulatory phase*. It is also called the *secretory phase*. It occurs when the corpus luteum forms from the ruptured ovarian follicle. The corpus luteum is a secretory mass of cells on the surface of the ovary. Its primary function is to produce progesterone, which helps to optimize the endometrial mucosa for implantation of a fertilized ovum. The corpus luteum also serves as an initial source of needed progesterone during early pregnancy. This function is later assumed by the developing placenta. If fertilization does not occur, the rising progesterone levels in the blood serve to initiate the start of menstruation. The corpus luteum then degenerates and the menstrual cycle begins again on or about day 28.

Figure 33-1 illustrates the sequence of hormone secretions and related events that take place during the menstrual cycle.

FEMALE SEX HORMONES

ESTROGENS

There are three major endogenous estrogens: estradiol, estrone, and estriol. All are synthesized from cholesterol in the ovarian follicles and have the basic chemical structure of a steroid, known as the steroid nucleus (Figure 33-2). For this reason they are sometimes referred to as steroid hormones. Estradiol is the principal and most active of the three and represents the end product of estrogen synthesis.

The exogenous estrogenic agents, those used as drug therapy, were developed because most of the endogenous estrogens are inactive when taken orally. These synthetic agents fall into two categories, steroidal and non-steroidal:

Steroidal
- conjugated estrogens
- synthetic conjugated estrogens
- esterified estrogens
- estradiol transdermal
- estradiol cypionate
- estradiol valerate
- ethinyl estradiol
- estradiol vaginal dosage forms
- estrone
- estropipate

Non-steroidal
- diethylstilbestrol
- diethylstilbestrol diphosphate

The most popular estrogen product in use today is an estrogen mixture known as conjugated estrogens. It contains a combination of natural estrogen compounds equivalent to the average estrogen composition of pregnant mare urine, hence its brand name of Premarin. There is also now a non-animal source for this conjugated estrogen product. A product called Estrace is composed of one estrogen, 17β-estradiol, which is structurally identical to estradiol produced by the female ovary but is obtained from soy beans. This product was developed in response to consumer demand from women who wanted an alternative to an animal-derived product. Ethinyl estradiol is one of the most potent of these estrogens and is used most commonly in oral contraceptive agents.

Non-steroidal estrogen agents do not have the basic steroid structure but can still act on estrogenic tissues throughout the body. There are two non-steroidal estrogen drug products on the Canadian market, diethylstilbestrol and diethylstilbestrol diphosphate. These are hormonal anticancer agents used for palliative treatment of prostatic carcinoma, particularly in advanced stages of prostate cancer (Chapter 46). An earlier form of diethylstilbestrol, more commonly known by its acronym DES, was originally given to pregnant women between 1940 and 1971 to prevent obstetric problems such as miscarriage and premature delivery. However, the drug was eventually associated with reproductive organ disease

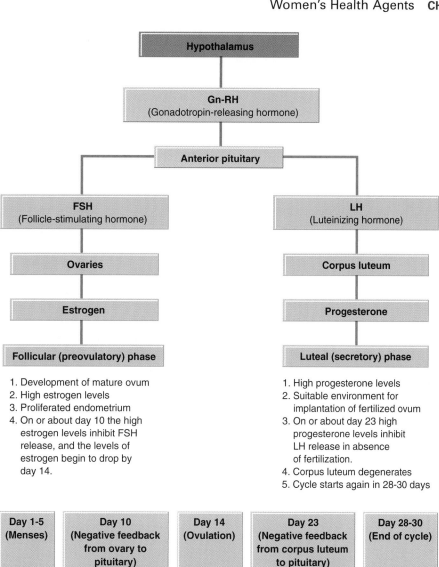

FIG. 33-1 Hormonal activity during monthly menstrual cycle. Gonadotropin-releasing hormone (Gn-RH) from the hypothalamus stimulates the pituitary gland, causing it to secrete follicle-stimulating hormone (FSH) early in the cycle (coinciding with menses) and later luteinizing hormone (LH). FSH stimulates the ovaries to produce estrogen (primarily estradiol). Later in the cycle the combined surges in the levels of estrogen, Gn-RH, FSH, and LH stimulate ovulation. The corpus luteum then secretes estrogen and progesterone, providing negative feedback to the hypothalamus and pituitary gland to reduce Gn-RH, FSH, and LH secretions. If the ovum (egg) is not fertilized by spermatozoa, levels of estrogen and progesterone then fall to their monthly lows, Gn-RH and FSH rise again, and the onset of menses begins a new cycle.

and malformations in both male and female offspring of mothers who received the drug during pregnancy. It is now contraindicated during pregnancy.

Mechanism of Action and Drug Effects

The binding of estrogen to estrogen receptors stimulates the synthesis of **nucleic acids** (deoxyribonucleic acid [DNA] and ribonucleic acid [RNA]) and proteins, which are the building blocks for all living tissue (see also Chapter 48). Estrogens are also required at puberty for the development and maintenance of the female reproductive system and the development of female secondary sex characteristics, a process known as *feminization*.

Estrogens produce their effects in estrogen-responsive tissues, which have a high content of estrogen receptors. These tissues include the female genital organs, the breasts, the pituitary gland, and the hypothalamus. At the time of puberty the production of estrogen increases greatly. This causes feminizing changes, such as the initiation of menses, the development of breasts, the redistribution of body fat, and softening of the skin. Estrogens play a role in the shaping of body contours and the skeleton. For

Indications for Estrogen Therapy

- Atrophic vaginitis (shrinkage of the vagina and/or urethra)
- Hypogonadism
- Oral contraception (in combination with a progestin)
- Ovarian failure or ovariectomy
- Uterine bleeding
- Kraurosis vulvae (atrophy and shrinkage of the skin of the vagina and vulva)
- Osteoporosis and prophylaxis
- Postpartum lactation (when a woman does not wish to lactate)
- Dysmenorrhea (painful or difficult menstruation)
- Vasomotor symptoms of menopause (e.g., hot flashes)

TABLE 33-2
ESTROGENS: COMMON ADVERSE EFFECTS

Body System	Side/Adverse Effects
Cardiovascular	Hypertension, thrombophlebitis, edema, palpitations
Central Nervous System	Headaches, depression, fatigue, irritability, dizziness
Gastrointestinal	Nausea, vomiting, abdominal cramps, pressure or pain, gallbladder disorder, asymptomatic liver dysfunction
Genitourinary	Amenorrhea, breakthrough uterine bleeding, dysmenorrhea, enlarged uterine fibromyomas, dyspareunia, reactivation of endometriosis, cystitis
Other	Tender breasts, fluid retention, decreased carbohydrate tolerance, visual disturbances

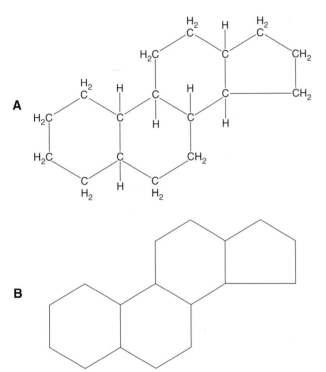

FIG. 33-2 Chemical structures for steroid nucleus. **A,** Detailed structure. **B,** Abbreviated structure.

Diethylstilbestrol

Between 1940 and 1971, an estimated 6 million mothers and their fetuses were exposed to diethylstilbestrol (DES). It was used to prevent reproductive problems such as miscarriage, premature delivery, intrauterine fetal death, and toxemia. This use resulted in significant complications of the reproductive system in both female and male offspring. In 2003, the Marketed Health Products Directorate and the Therapeutic Products Directorate of Health Canada issued a health professional advisory in a letter advising of the risk of genital and obstetrical complications in those exposed in utero, with recommended screening guidelines. Complications suspected to result from DES exposure are to be reported to the Canadian Adverse Drug Reaction Monitoring Program (CADRMP). D.E.S. Action Canada is a consumer organization that provides information that advocates on behalf of those exposed to DES.

instance, long bones are usually inhibited from growing, with the result that females are usually shorter than males.

Indications

Estrogens are used in the treatment or prevention of an assortment of disorders that primarily result from estrogen deficiency. These conditions are listed in Box 33-1.

Contraindications

Contraindications for estrogen administration include known drug allergy, active obstructive hepatic disease, any estrogen-dependent cancer, undiagnosed abnormal vaginal bleeding, pregnancy, classic migraine, thromboembolic disorder, and history of thromboembolic disorder such as stroke and thrombophlebitis. It should not be used during breastfeeding, as estrogen passes into the breast milk.

Side Effects and Adverse Effects

The most serious side and adverse effects of the estrogens are thromboembolic events. Rarely, they cause erythema multiforme, a rare skin disorder in which macules (red areas), papules (bumps), or subdermal vesicles (fluid-filled bumps) erupt on the hands and forearms. It can be recurrent or may run a severe course and fatally terminate in Stevens-Johnson syndrome, one of the most severe dermatological drug reactions. The most common undesirable effect of estrogens is nausea. Other undesirable effects are listed in Table 33-2. The use of DES in pregnancy (no longer allowed in Canada) is associated with serious adverse effects on the reproductive systems of both male and female children (Box 33-2).

DOSAGES Selected Estrogenic Agents

Agent	Pharmacological Class	Usual Dosage Range	Indications
conjugated estrogens	Estrogenic hormone mixture	PO: 0.3–1.25 mg daily	Atrophic vaginitis, kraurosis vulvae
		PO: 0.625–1.25 mg/day	Vasomotor symptoms of menopause
		PO: 10 mg tid × 3 mo	Breast cancer (palliative; male and female)
		PO: 1.25 mg/day cyclically, 3 wk on, 1 wk off or continuously	Ovariectomy, primary ovarian failure
		PO: 0.3–0.625 mg/day cyclically	Female hypogonadism
		PO: 1.25 mg q4h × 24 h, then 1.25 mg daily × 7–10 days	Abnormal uterine bleeding
estradiol	Estrogenic hormone	PO: 1 mg daily, adjusted to needs of client	Vasomotor symptoms of menopause, female castration, ovarian failure
		PO: 0.5 mg daily cyclically, can be titrated up or down	Osteoporosis prophylaxis
estradiol transdermal	Estrogenic hormone	Transdermal patch: 1 patch twice weekly for 50 μg/day, adapted to client needs	Vasomotor symptoms of menopause
NON-STEROIDAL diethylstilbestrol (DES) diphosphate	Synthetic non-steroidal estrogenic agent	PO: 1 mg tid IV: Induction: 500 mg/day 5–10 days, then 250 mg/day for 10–20 days Maintenance: 250–500 mg 3–4 times/week for 1–2 months then 250 mg weekly	Palliative treatment of inoperative prostate cancer

Interactions

Estrogens can decrease the activity of the oral anticoagulant, antidiabetic, and antihypertensive agents, and their concurrent use with rifampin, barbiturates, hydrantoins, carbamazepine, meprobamates, or phenylbutazone can decrease the estrogenic effect. Some herbal products such as St. John's wort, available over-the-counter, may affect the metabolism of estrogens. Smoking during estrogen therapy should be avoided because this too can diminish the estrogenic effect and add to the risk for thrombosis.

Dosages

See the table above for the recommended dosages of some of the many available estrogen products. See Appendix B for some of the common brands available in Canada.

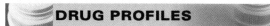

DRUG PROFILES

▸▸ estrogen

Estrogen replacement is indicated for the treatment of many clinical conditions, primarily those resulting from estrogen deficiency (see Box 33-1). Many of these conditions occur around menopause, when the endogenous estradiol level is declining. Any estrogen capable of binding to the estrogen receptors in target organs can alleviate these menopausal symptoms. As a general rule, however, the smallest dose of estrogen that alleviates the symptoms or prevents the condition is used for the shortest possible period.

Although estrogen and estrogen/progestin medication products are widely used for post-menopausal hormone replacement therapy (HRT), two recent studies demonstrated possible detriments to such therapy. The NIH-sponsored Women's Health Initiative (WHI) study found that research subjects who took a certain estrogen/progestin combination product had an increased risk of breast cancer, heart disease, stroke, and blood clots compared with the placebo group, but a reduced risk of hip fractures and colon cancer. Nonetheless, these preliminary results indicated that the risks outweighed the benefits associated with using combined HRT and the combined estrogen/progestin arm of the study was discontinued. A portion of the WHI study focusing on cognitive function, the WHI Memory Study (WHIMS), also demonstrated cognitive hazards in women receiving combination estrogen/progestin therapy. These clients showed an increased risk of developing dementia and reduced performance on tests of cognitive function. In March 2004 the estrogen-only arm HRT was also discontinued. The NIH concluded that there was no cardiovascular benefit to women and no increase in risk for breast or colorectal cancer. However, there was an increased risk of stroke and deep vein thrombosis and a reduction in risk for hip and other fractures in those women who have had a hysterectomy.

Estrogenic agents are contraindicated in the presence of hypersensitivity, thromboembolic disorders or a history of thromboembolic disorders (except in cases of cancer palliation), abnormal genital bleeding, estrogen-dependent neoplasms, and breast cancer. These agents are classified as pregnancy category X agents.

The principal pharmacological effects of all estrogens are similar because there are only slight differences in their chemical structure. These differences make for different potencies, which in turn make them useful for a variety of indications. They also allow the agents to be given by different routes of administration, and often at highly customized doses.

Many fixed estrogen/progestin combination products have emerged over the years. These are commonly referred to as *continuous-combined hormone replacement therapy* (CCHRT). The rationale for the development of these agents is that the use of estrogen alone has been associated with an increased risk of endometrial hyperplasia, a possible precursor of endometrial adenocarcinoma. The addition of continuous progestin reduces the incidence of endometrial hyperplasia. Examples of these fixed combinations are conjugated estrogens with medroxyprogesterone, norethindrone acetate with ethinyl estradiol, and estradiol with norethindrone.

PROGESTINS

Available progestational agents, or progestins, include both natural and synthetic agents. Progesterone is the principally active natural progestational hormone. It is produced by the corpus luteum after each ovulation and during pregnancy by the placenta. In addition, there are two other major natural progestins. One is 17-hydroxyprogesterone, an inactive metabolite of progesterone. The other is pregnenolone, a chemical precursor to all steroid hormones that is synthesized from cholesterol in the ovary. Because orally administered progesterone is relatively inactive and parenterally administered progesterone causes local reactions and pain, chemical derivatives were developed that are effective orally and also more potent. Their actions are also more specific and of longer duration. Some of the most commonly used progestins include

- medroxyprogesterone
- megestrol
- norethindrone
- norgestrel with ethinyl estradiol
- progesterone

Mechanism of Action and Drug Effects

All of these progestin products produce all of the same physiological responses as those produced by progesterone itself. These responses include inducing secretory changes in the endometrium, including diminished endometrial tissue proliferation; an increase in the basal body temperature; thickening of the vaginal mucosa; relaxation of uterine

TABLE 33-3	
PROGESTINS: COMMON ADVERSE EFFECTS	
Body System	**Side/Adverse Effects**
Central Nervous System	Headache, dizziness, nervousness, depression, insomnia, fatigue
Gastrointestinal	Nausea, vomiting, bloating, abdominal discomfort
Genitourinary	Amenorrhea, breakthrough uterine bleeding, spotting, changes in menstrual flow, changes in cervical erosion and secretions
Other	Edema, weight gain or loss, allergic rash, pyrexia (fever), somnolence or insomnia, mental depression, breast tenderness

smooth muscle; stimulation of mammary alveolar tissue growth; feedback inhibition (negative feedback) of release of pituitary gonadotropins (FSH, LH); and alterations in menstrual blood flow, especially in the presence of estrogen.

Indications

Progestins are useful in the treatment of functional uterine bleeding caused by a hormonal imbalance, fibroids, or uterine cancer; the treatment of primary and secondary amenorrhea; the adjunctive and palliative treatment of some cancers and endometriosis; and alone or in combination with estrogens for the prevention of conception. They may also be useful to prevent a threatened miscarriage and alleviate the symptoms of premenstrual syndrome (PMS). Specifically, medroxyprogesterone and progesterone have been used to treat hormone imbalance, primary or secondary amenorrhea, and functional bleeding of the uterus, although medroxyprogesterone is the one most commonly used for this. Norethindrone may be used to treat female hormone imbalance and endometriosis but is more commonly used alone or in combination with estrogens as a contraceptive. Megestrol is commonly used as adjunct therapy in the treatment of breast and endometrial cancers. When estrogen replacement therapy is used after menopause, progestins are often included to decrease endometrial proliferation.

Contraindications

Contraindications for progestins are similar to those for estrogens.

Side Effects and Adverse Effects

The most serious undesirable effects of progestins include liver dysfunction, commonly manifested as cholestatic jaundice; thrombophlebitis; and thromboembolic disorders such as pulmonary embolism. The more common of these effects are listed in Table 33-3.

Interactions

Possible decreases in glucose tolerance when progestins are taken with antidiabetic agents may require that the dose of the antidiabetic agent be adjusted. The concurrent

DOSAGES   Selected Progestational Agents

Agent	Pharmacological Class	Usual Dosage Range	Indications
▶▶ medroxyprogesterone acetate	Progestin	PO: 2.5–10 mg/day for set number of days or cyclically (smaller doses may be given on a continuous daily basis)	Amenorrhea, uterine bleeding
		PO: 2.5–10 mg daily on last 10–13 days of each mo to accompany estrogen dosing	Vasomotor symptoms of menopause
		PO: 200–400 mg/day for endometrial cancer IM: 400–1000 mg/wk	Metastatic endometrial or renal cancer
		PO: 400–800 mg/day divided IM: 500 mg/day × 28 days, maintenance 500 mg twice/wk	Breast cancer
		IM: 50 mg/wk or 100 mg q2wk × 6 mos	Endometriosis
megestrol acetate	Progestin	PO: 400–800 mg/day	Severe weight loss in male and female clients with HIV/AIDS
		PO: 160 mg/day in divided doses	Breast cancer
		PO: 80–320 mg/day divided	Endometrial cancer
		PO: 120 mg/day, single dose	Advanced hormone-responsive carcinoma of prostate
progesterone	Progestin	Intravaginal gel: 90 mg once to twice daily for up to 12 wk	Progesterone deficiency in infertility
		PO: 200 mg at bedtime or 300 mg bid for set number of days or cyclically	Hormone replacement therapy
		IM: 5–10 mg daily for 6–8 days	Amenorrhea or functional uterine bleeding

use of medroxyprogesterone or norethindrone with some anticonvulsants, barbiturates, or rifampin induces increased metabolism of the progestin. Caution is also indicated for use with some natural health products as they may affect the metabolism of the progestins.

Dosages

For recommended dosages of the progestins, see the table above. See Appendix B for some of the common brands available in Canada.

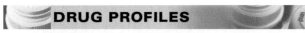

DRUG PROFILES

▶▶ *medroxyprogesterone*

Medroxyprogesterone inhibits the secretion of pituitary gonadotropins, which prevents follicular maturation and ovulation; stimulates the growth of mammary tissue; and has an antineoplastic action against endometrial cancer. It is used to treat uterine bleeding, secondary amenorrhea, endometrial cancer, endometriosis, and renal cancer, and is also used as a contraceptive. Its most common use is to prevent endometrial cancer caused by estrogen replacement. It is also sometimes used as adjunct therapy in certain types of cancer (Chapter 46). It is classified as a pregnancy category X agent and is contraindicated in clients with a history of thrombophlebitis, thromboembolic disorders, cerebral apoplexy, liver disease,

undiagnosed vaginal bleeding, pregnancy, suspected breast cancer, partial or complete loss of vision from ophthalmic vascular disorder, or drug hypersensitivity. Medroxyprogesterone is available in both oral (PO) and parenteral preparations. In oral form it is available as 2.5-, 5-, 10-, and 100-mg tablets. In parenteral form it is available as 50- and 150-mg/mL sterile suspensions for intramuscular (IM) injection. Recommended dosages are given in the table above.

PHARMACOKINETICS

Half-Life	Onset	Peak	Duration
14.5 hr	Unknown	IM: 3 weeks	IM: 3 mo

megestrol

Megestrol is a synthetic progestin that differs structurally from progesterone only in the addition of a methyl group on the steroid nucleus and a double bond. Although megestrol shares the actions of the progestins, it is primarily used in the palliative management of recurrent, inoperable, or metastatic endometrial or breast cancer. It is used for palliative treatment of hormone-responsive advanced prostate cancer. It has also been used for AIDS clients with anorexia, cachexia (wasting), or an unexplained, substantial weight loss. In addition, it may be used to stimulate appetite and promote weight gain in clients with cancer. It is available only in oral form as a 40-mg/mL oral suspension and as 40- and 160-mg tablets. It is also classified as a pregnancy category X

Emergency Post-coital Contraception

In Canada the use of emergency contraception (EC) is becoming better known. Commonly known as the "morning-after pill," levonorgestrel 0.75 mg has been available in Canada by prescription since 2000. Previously, EC had been used in specific settings, such as college and university health centres and family planning clinics, and for sexual assault victims in emergency rooms and other settings. EC has been controversial; although it is not usually considered an abortifacient, because one of its mechanisms of action is to prevent implantation of a fertilized egg, some people who consider fertilization to constitute conception do consider it a form of early abortion. On April 19, 2005, EC became available without a prescription, reclassified by Health Canada as a "behind the counter" drug, meaning that pharmacists are expected to provide counselling to clients requesting the drug. This decision provides equal access to women across Canada; previously legislation in British Columbia, Saskatchewan, and Quebec allowed pharmacists to dispense EC without a prescription.

Levonorgestrel (Plan B) pills are high-dose hormones. Levonorgestrel is considered to be more effective than the Yuzpe regimen (a combination of 100 μg of ethinyl estradiol and 500 μg of levonorgestrel, administered in two doses 12 hours apart). The mechanism of action of levonorgestrel may be through its inhibition of ovulation and disruption of the corpus luteum. In addition, it decreases the luteal phase and inhibits the secretion of pituitary hormones, while making the cervical mucus impossible to penetrate. EC pills also decrease the function of endometrial hormones and have an effect on the endometrium that makes implantation of the egg impossible. Contraindications include a history of thromboembolic disorders, stroke, and tumours of the liver and breast. Females who have a history of migraine headache, liver disease, and high BP are at a greater risk for complications with use of EC pills. Side effects include nausea, vomiting, abdominal pain, fatigue, and headache. If taken more than 72 hours after the sexual assault or unprotected intercourse, the rate of effectiveness declines to 85 percent.

Reference: Shibbald, B. (2005). News synopsis. Nonprescription status for emergency contraception. *Canadian Medical Association Journal, 172*(7), 861–2.

agent, and the contraindications to its use are the same as those of the other progestins. Recommended dosages are given in the table on p. 551.

PHARMACOKINETICS

Half-Life	Onset	Peak	Duration
34 hr	6–8 wk	1–3 hr	4–10 mo

CONTRACEPTIVE AGENTS

Contraceptive agents are medications used to prevent pregnancy. Contraceptive devices are non-drug methods of pregnancy prevention such as intrauterine devices (IUDs), male and female condoms, cervical diaphragms, and so forth. Clients must be informed that contraceptive drug therapy serves only to prevent pregnancy and does not prevent the transmission of sexually transmitted diseases, including HIV/AIDS. This even includes spermicidal agents such as the over-the-counter (OTC) foams for intravaginal use. These products most often contain the spermicide nonoxynol-9, which does kill sperm cells to prevent pregnancy but does not necessarily kill microbes capable of causing sexually transmitted diseases, including HIV.

Oral contraceptives are the most effective form of birth control currently available. Estrogen–progestin combinations, often referred to as "the pill," are oral contraceptives that contain both estrogenic and progestational steroids. The most common estrogenic component is ethinyl estradiol, a semi-synthetic steroidal estrogen. The most common progestin component is norethindrone.

Currently available oral contraceptives may be monophasic, biphasic, or triphasic. In monophasic agents, the estrogen and progestin doses are the same throughout the menstrual cycle. The biphasic agents contain a fixed estrogen dose but a low progestin dose for the first 10 days and a higher dose for the rest of the cycle, in 21- or 28-day dosage packages. The triphasic oral contraceptives contain three different estrogen–progestin dose ratios that are administered sequentially during the cycle in 21- or 28-day dosage packs. The triphasic products closely duplicate the normal hormonal levels of the female cycle. There are also progestin-only oral contraceptives.

Three other important contraceptive medications include a long-acting injectable form of medroxyprogesterone, a transdermal contraceptive patch, and most recently, an intravaginal contraceptive ring.

Mechanism of Action and Drug Effects

Oral contraceptives prevent ovulation by inhibiting the release of gonadotropins. They also increase uterine mucous viscosity, resulting in decreased sperm movement, so that even if an ovum were to be released, the sperm would be less likely to fertilize it. If an egg were to be somehow released and fertilized, the increased viscosity might inhibit implantation of the resulting zygote.

Oral contraceptives have many of the same effects as those normally produced by the endogenous estrogens and progesterone. The contraceptive effect mainly results from suppression of the hypothalamic–pituitary system, which in turn prevents ovulation. Other incidental benefits to their use are that they improve menstrual cycle regularity and decrease blood loss during menstruation. A decreased incidence of functional ovarian cysts and ectopic pregnancies has also been associated with

DOSAGES   Selected Contraceptive Medications

Agent	Pharmacological Class	Usual Dosage Range	Indications
ORAL CONTRACEPTIVES			
norethindrone and ethinyl estradiol	Biphasic: fixed estrogen–variable progestin 21- or 28-day products	For the most reliable contraceptive action, the client should take all preparations according to instructions from prescriber or client information product insert, at intervals not to exceed 24 h	Prevention of pregnancy
levonorgestrel/ ethinyl estradiol norethindrone and ethinyl estradiol	Monophasic: fixed estrogen-progestin combinations; 21- or 28-day products; 28-day products contain 7 inert tabs		
levonorgestrel/ ethinyl estradiol norethindrone and ethinyl estradiol	Triphasic: 3 or 4 monthly phases of variable estrogen and progestin combinations; 21- or 28-day products; 28-day products contain 7 inert tabs		
INJECTABLE CONTRACEPTIVES			
depot- ▸▸ medroxyprogesterone acetate	Progestin-only injectable contraceptive	IM: 150 mg q3mo	Prevention of pregnancy
TRANSDERMAL CONTRACEPTIVES			
norelgestromin and ethinyl estradiol	Fixed-combination estrogen-progestin transdermal contraceptive	Transdermal patch: 1 patch applied weekly × 3 each month, scheduled around menses in week 4	Prevention of pregnancy
INTRAVAGINAL CONTRACEPTIVES			
etonogestrel/ethinyl estradiol vaginal ring (NuvaRing)	Fixed-combination estrogen-progestin intravaginal contraceptive	One ring inserted into vagina by client and left in place for 3 weeks, followed by a 1-week removal. A new ring is then inserted 1 week later.	Prevention of pregnancy

their use. Drawbacks to their use include the risk of hypertension, thromboembolism, alterations in carbohydrate and lipid metabolism, increases in serum hormone concentrations, and alterations in serum metal and plasma protein levels. It is the estrogen component that appears to be the source of most of these metabolic effects.

Indications

Oral contraceptives are primarily used to prevent pregnancy. In addition, they are used to treat endometriosis and hypermenorrhea and to produce cyclic withdrawal bleeding. Occasionally combination oral contraceptives (COCs) are used to provide post-coital emergency contraception. Emergency contraception pills (ECPs) are not effective if the woman is pregnant and should be taken within 72 hours of unprotected intercourse with a follow-up dose 12 hours after the first dose. They are intended to prevent pregnancy after known or suspected contraceptive failure or unprotected intercourse. Triphasil, Min-Ovral, and Alesse are three ethinyl estradiol/levonorgestrel combination agents that are commonly used for this indication.

Contraindications

Contraindications to the use of oral contraceptives include known drug allergy to a specific product, pregnancy, and known high risk for or history of thromboembolic events such as myocardial infarction, venous thrombosis, pulmonary embolism, or stroke.

Side Effects and Adverse Effects

Common side effects and adverse effects associated with the use of oral contraceptives are listed in Table 33-4.

Interactions

Many drugs decrease the effectiveness of oral contraceptives. The drugs that have clinically relevant interactions with oral contraceptives are few and include the following:
- Antacids
- Anticonvulsants
- Antibiotics
- clofibrate
- griseofulvin
- isoniazid
- rifampin
- Sedatives and hypnotics

TABLE 33-4

ORAL CONTRACEPTIVES: COMMON ADVERSE EFFECTS

Body System	Side/Adverse Effects
Cardiovascular	Hypertension, thrombophlebitis, edema, thromboembolism, neuro-ocular lesions, pulmonary embolism, MI
Central nervous	Dizziness, headache, migraines, depression, stroke, mood changes
Gastrointestinal	Nausea, vomiting, diarrhea, anorexia, pancreatitis, cramps, bloating, constipation, increased appetite, increased weight, cholestatic jaundice, hepatic adenomas or benign liver tumours
Genitourinary	Amenorrhea, cervical neoplasia, breakthrough bleeding, dysmenorrhea, breast changes, breast cancer

Drugs that may have reduced effectiveness when taken with oral contraceptives include the following:
- Alcohol
- Anticoagulants
- Anticonvulsants
- Antidiabetic agents
- Antihypertensive agents
- Antipyretics
- aminocaproic acid
- caffeine
- clonidine
- guanethidine
- meperidine
- Sedatives and hypnotics
- theophylline
- TCAs
- Vitamin B$_{12}$

Dosages

For the recommended dosages of oral contraceptives, see the table on p. 553. See Appendix B for some of the common brands available in Canada.

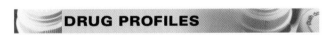

DRUG PROFILES

CONTRACEPTIVE AGENTS

Contraceptive agents are contraindicated in the following clinical situations: known or suspected breast cancer or any estrogen-dependent cancers, pregnancy, present or past thromboembolic disorders, undiagnosed abnormal genital bleeding, cerebrovascular and coronary artery disease, and benign or malignant liver tumours associated with estrogen use. Concurrent cigarette smoking increases the likelihood of these outcomes because of the effects of nicotine exposure on circulatory function. Oral contraceptives are classified as pregnancy category X agents. Examples of specific products appear in the table on p. 553.

CURRENT DRUG THERAPY FOR OSTEOPOROSIS

Approximately 16 percent of women aged 50 years or over in Canada currently are affected by **osteoporosis**; an additional 60 percent have decreased bone mineral density. Nearly 40 percent of Canadian white women over 50 years of age will develop an osteoporotic fracture, and the annual costs to society of treating osteoporosis and fractures was nearly $1.3 billion in 1993 and is expected to reach $32.5 billion by 2018. Supplemental calcium and vitamin D should be added to the diet if daily intake is inadequate. Risk factors for postmenopausal osteoporosis include Caucasian or Asian descent, slender body build, early estrogen deficiency, smoking, alcohol consumption, low-calcium diet, sedentary lifestyle, and family history of osteoporosis. Though osteoporosis primarily affects women, up to 20 percent of people with this disease are men.

Supplements of calcium and vitamin D are indicated for all women considered at risk for osteoporosis. These supplements play a major role in the prevention of this common bone disorder. Two major drug classes are currently the mainstays of treatment of active osteoporosis: the bisphosphonates and the selective estrogen receptor modifiers (SERMs). Currently available bisphosphonates used for osteoporosis treatment include alendronate, clodronate, etidronate, and risedronate. These agents have become the primary drugs of choice for this condition because they are the only drugs to date proven to reverse loss of bone mass. Raloxifene and tamoxifen are the currently available SERMs. Tamoxifen has been available for many years. It has primarily been used alone as an adjunct to surgery and radiation therapy for the treatment of breast cancer in women with negative axillary lymph nodes and in postmenopausal women with positive axillary lymph nodes. Adjuvant tamoxifen therapy reduces the occurrence of contralateral breast cancer in premenopausal or postmenopausal women with breast cancer. It has also been shown to be beneficial for primary prevention in women at a high risk for developing breast cancer, although this is not an approved use in Canada. Raloxifene, the newest SERM, has primarily been studied for prevention of osteoporosis, although many studies suggest that it may be beneficial in the treatment of osteoporosis as well. Other agents that have also shown beneficial results in the prevention and/or treatment of osteoporosis are calcium and vitamin D supplementation and the hormone calcitonin.

Mechanism of Action and Drug Effects

The mechanisms of action and drug effects of the bisphosphonates and SERMs are described in the drug profiles that follow.

Indications

Raloxifene is primarily used for the prevention of post-menopausal osteoporosis. Its use for the treatment of osteoporosis or the prevention of breast cancer is unknown at this point. Tamoxifen is used for the treatment and prevention of breast cancer. The bisphosphonates are used in both the prevention and treatment of osteoporosis.

Contraindications

Contraindications to the use of bisphosphonates include drug allergy, hypocalcemia, esophageal dysfunction, increased risk of aspiration, and the inability to sit or stand upright for at least 30 minutes after taking the medication. Contraindications to the use of SERMs include known drug allergy, elevated serum creatinine levels, overt osteomalacia (softening of the bones), pregnancy, and active thromboembolic disorder.

Side Effects and Adverse Effects

The primary side effects of SERMs are hot flashes and leg cramps. Like estrogens, they can increase the risk of venous thromboembolism and they are teratogenic (causing birth defects). Post-menopausal women taking raloxifene were no more likely to develop breast, uterine, or ovarian cancer than women taking a placebo. The most common side effects of bisphosphonates include headache, gastrointestinal (GI) upset, and joint pain. However, the bisphosphonates are usually well tolerated. There is a risk of esophageal burns with these medications if they become lodged in the esophagus before reaching the stomach. For this reason the client should take these medications with a full glass of water and remain sitting upright or standing for at least 30 minutes.

Interactions

Cholestyramine decreases the absorption of raloxifene, and raloxifene can decrease the effects of warfarin. Calcium supplements and antacids can interfere with the absorption of the bisphosphonates and therefore these drugs should be spaced 1 to 2 hours apart to avoid this interaction.

Dosages

For the recommended dosages of osteoporosis agents, see the table below. See Appendix B for some of the common brands available in Canada.

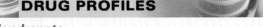

DRUG PROFILES

↠ alendronate

Alendronate is an oral bisphosphonate that is indicated for the prevention and treatment of osteoporosis in men and post-menopausal women to reduce the incidence of fractures. It is also indicated for the treatment of glucocorticoid-induced osteoporosis in men and women and for treatment of Paget's disease (a skeletal disease characterized by thickening and softening of bones). It works by inhibiting osteoclast-mediated bone resorption. Osteoclasts break down bone, causing calcium to be reabsorbed into the circulation, eventually leading to osteoporosis if not controlled. Alendronate was the first non-estrogen, non-hormonal option for preventing bone loss. Clodronate, etidronate, and risedronate are also available in Canada, while tiludronate is currently under investigation.

Data show that alendronate may reduce the risk of hip fracture by 51 percent, spinal fracture by 47 percent, and wrist fracture by 48 percent. It is contraindicated in women known to be hypersensitive to alendronate. Precaution should be taken in clients with dysphagia, esophagitis, esophageal ulcer, or gastric ulcer because it can be irritating. Case reports of esophageal erosions have been published. It is recommended that alendronate be given first thing in the morning upon rising with 200 to 250 mL of water and that the client not lie down for at least 30 minutes after taking it. When clients stabilized on alendronate are hospitalized and cannot adhere to these recommendations, the medication is often withheld. Alendronate has an extremely long terminal half-life, and going several days without taking a dose will do little if anything to the therapeutic efficacy of the drug.

Alendronate is available in 5-, 10-, 40-, and 70-mg tablets. Normal recommended dosages are 5 to 10 mg daily or 35 or 70 mg once weekly. The normal dose for prevention of osteoporosis in postmenopausal women is 5 mg daily and for treatment of osteoporosis is 10 mg daily or one 70-mg tablet once weekly. The normal dose for treatment of Paget's disease is 40 mg daily for six months. Pregnancy category C. Additional dosage information is provided in the table below.

DOSAGES   Selected Agents Used Specifically for Osteoporosis

Agent	Pharmacological Class	Usual Dosage Range	Indications
↠ alendronate	Bisphosphonate	PO: 5 mg daily or 35 mg/wk PO: 10 mg daily or 70 mg/wk	Osteoporosis prevention Osteoporosis treatment
calcitonin, salmon	Calcitonin hormonal substitute derived from salmon	IM/SC: 50–100 units daily or 50–100 units 3 times/wk Nasal spray: 200 units (1 spray) alternating nostrils daily	Osteoporosis treatment
raloxifene	Selective estrogen receptor modulator (SERM)	PO: 60 mg daily	Osteoporosis prevention and treatment
teriparatide	Parathyroid hormone derivative	SC: 250 μg once daily in thigh or abdomen	Osteoporosis treatment

PHARMACOKINETICS

Half-Life	Onset	Peak	Duration
10 yr	3 wk*	Unknown	Unknown

*Therapeutic effect.

raloxifene

Raloxifene is a SERM. It is used primarily for the prevention of post-menopausal osteoporosis. Raloxifene has beneficial effects on cholesterol, decreasing total and low-density lipoprotein (LDL) cholesterol without affecting high-density lipoprotein (HDL) or triglycerides. Raloxifene helps prevent osteoporosis by stimulating estrogen receptors on bone and increasing bone density. Raloxifene is contraindicated in women who are or may become pregnant and in women with active thromboembolic problems or history of venous thromboembolic events, including deep vein thrombosis (DVT), pulmonary embolism, and retinal vein thrombosis. It is also contraindicated in women known to be hypersensitive to raloxifene or other constituents of the tablets. It is available in 60-mg film-coated tablets. Pregnancy category X. Recommended dosages are listed in the table on p. 555.

PHARMACOKINETICS

Half-Life	Onset	Peak	Duration
27 hr	Unknown	Unknown	Unknown

teriparatide

Teriparatide is currently the only drug in the newest class of medications used against osteoporosis. It is a derivative of parathyroid hormone and works to treat osteoporosis by modulating the body's metabolism of calcium and phosphorus in a manner similar to natural parathyroid hormone. It is currently available only in injectable form in a 3-mL cartridge for pen use in a strength of 250 μg/mL. Pregnancy category C. Dosage information is provided in the table on p. 555.

DRUG THERAPY RELATED TO PREGNANCY, LABOUR, DELIVERY, AND THE POSTPARTUM PERIOD

Several drugs are available to increase the chances of conception for couples unable to conceive. A variety of medications are used to alter the dynamics of uterine contractions to either promote or prevent the start or progression of labour. In the immediate postpartum period, medications may also be used to promote rapid shrinkage of the uterus to reduce the risk of hemorrhage.

FERTILITY AGENTS

Infertility in women generally results from absence of ovulation (anovulation), which is usually due to various imbalances of female reproductive hormones. Such imbalances can occur at the level of the hypothalamus, the pituitary gland, the ovary, or any combination of these. Supplements of estrogens or progestins may be used to fortify the blood levels of these hormones when ovarian output is inadequate. The use of drug forms of these hormones was described earlier in this chapter.

Hormone deficiencies at the hypothalamic and pituitary levels are often treated with gonadotropin ovarian stimulants. These agents serve to stimulate increased secretion of gonadotropin-releasing hormone (Gn-RH) from the hypothalamus, which then results in increased secretion of FSH and LH from the pituitary gland. These hormones in turn stimulate the development of ovarian follicles and ovulation. They also stimulate ovarian secretion of the estrogens and progestins that are part of the normal ovulatory cycle. Proper selection and dosage adjustment of fertility agents often requires the expertise of a fertility specialist. The various medical techniques, including medications, used in the treatment of infertility are collectively now referred to as *assistive reproductive technology* (ART). One technique is *in vitro* fertilization, which involves fertilization of a woman's ovum with her partner's sperm in a laboratory setting, followed by medical implantation of the fertilized ovum into the woman's uterus. Infants born from the use of this technique are commonly referred to as "test tube babies." The success of such fertilization techniques may be further aided with medications such as those described earlier. Representative examples of ovulation stimulants include the drugs clomiphene, menotropins, and chorionic gonadotropin alfa.

Mechanism of Action and Drug Effects

Clomiphene is a non-steroidal ovulation stimulant that works by blocking estrogen receptors in the uterus and brain. This results in a false signal to the brain of low estrogen levels. The hypothalamus and pituitary gland in the brain then increase their production of Gn-RH (from the hypothalamus) and FSH and LH (from the pituitary), which stimulates the maturation of ovarian follicles. Ideally this leads to ovulation and increases the likelihood of conception in a previously infertile woman.

Menotropins is the drug name for a standardized mixture of FSH and LH that is derived from the urine of postmenopausal women. The FSH component stimulates the development of ovarian follicles leading to ovulation. The LH component stimulates the development of the corpus luteum, which supplies female sex hormones (estrogens and progestins) during the first trimester of pregnancy. Menotropins is also sometimes given to infertile male clients to stimulate spermatogenesis.

Chorionic gonadotropin alfa is a recombinant form (i.e., developed with recombinant DNA technology) of the hormone human chorionic gonadotropin. This hormone is naturally produced by the placenta during pregnancy and can be isolated from the urine of pregnant women. It is an analogue of LH and can provide a substitute for the natural LH surge that promotes ovulation. It does this by binding to LH receptors in the ovary and stimulating the rupture of mature ovarian follicles and subsequent development of the corpus luteum. Human chorionic gonadotropin (hCG) alfa also maintains the viability of the corpus luteum during early pregnancy. This is critical because the corpus luteum provides the supply of estrogens and progestins necessary to support the first trimester of pregnancy, until the placenta assumes this role. This drug is often given in a carefully timed fashion following therapy with menotropins or clomiphene, when client monitoring indicates sufficient maturation of ovarian follicles.

Indications

These agents are used primarily for the promotion of ovulation in anovulatory female clients. They may also be used to promote spermatogenesis in infertile men.

Contraindications

Contraindications for the ovarian stimulants include known drug allergy to any specific product and may also include primary ovarian failure, uncontrolled thyroid or adrenal dysfunction, liver disease, pituitary tumour, abnormal uterine bleeding, undiagnosed ovarian enlargement, sex hormone–dependent tumours, and pregnancy.

Side Effects and Adverse Effects

The most common adverse effects of the ovulation stimulants are listed in Table 33-5.

Interactions

Few drug interactions occur with fertility agents. The most notable are TCAs, butyrophenones (e.g., haloperidol), phenothiazines (e.g., promethazine), and the antihypertensive agent methyldopa. When any of these agents are used with the fertility agents, increased prolactin concentrations may occur, which may also impair fertility.

Dosages

For recommended dosages of the fertility agents, see the table below. See Appendix B for some of the common brands available in Canada.

DRUG PROFILES

choriogonadotropin alfa

Choriogonadotropin alfa is a synthetic recombinant analogue of natural hCG and has effects similar to this hormone. These include the rupture (and ovulation) of mature ovarian follicles and maintenance of the corpus luteum, which supplies estrogens and progestins during the first trimester of pregnancy until the placenta assumes this role. Natural forms of hCG, isolated from the urine of pregnant women, are also still available as the prescription drug products Profasi, Pregnyl, and various generic products. Contraindications for all of these medications are listed in the section on ovarian stimulants. Choriogonadotropin alfa is currently available only as 10,000 USP units/10 mL multi-dose vial for injection. Pregnancy category X. Commonly recommended dosages are given in the table below.

PHARMACOKINETICS

Half-Life	Onset	Peak	Duration
5.6 hr	2 hr	6 hr	36 hr

clomiphene

Clomiphene is primarily used to stimulate the production of pituitary gonadotropins, which in turn induces the maturation of the ovarian follicle and eventually ovulation. Contraindications are listed in the section on ovarian stimulants. It is currently available only in oral form as a 50-mg tablet. Pregnancy category X. Commonly recommended dosages are given in the table below.

PHARMACOKINETICS

Half-Life	Onset	Peak	Duration
5 days	4–12 days	Unknown	1 mo

TABLE 33-5
FERTILITY AGENTS: MOST COMMON ADVERSE EFFECTS

Body System	Side/Adverse Effects
Cardiovascular	Tachycardia, phlebitis, deep vein thrombosis, hypovolemia, stroke, pulmonary embolism, arterial occlusion
Central nervous	Dizziness, headache, flushing, depression, restlessness, anxiety, irritability, nervousness, fatigue, fever
Gastrointestinal	Nausea, bloating, constipation, abdominal pain, vomiting, anorexia
Other	Urticaria (hives), ovarian hyperstimulation, multiple pregnancies, blurred vision, diplopia (double vision), photophobia (intolerance of strong light), breast pain

DOSAGES   Selected Fertility Agents

Agent	Pharmacological Class	Usual Dosage Range	Indications
chorionic gonadotropin alfa	Ovulation stimulant, recombinant	SC/IM: 5000–10000 USP units given 1 day after last dose of follicle stimulant (e.g., menotropins)	Female infertility
clomiphene	Ovulation stimulant	PO: 50–100 mg daily for 5 days; cycle repeatable depending on response	Female infertility in selected clients
⯈⯈ **menotropins**	Gonadotropins (FSH/LH) ovulation stimulant	IM: 150 units daily for 5 days adjusted according to response, followed by chorionic gonadotropin	Female infertility, male infertility

»» *menotropins*

Menotropins is a purified preparation of the gonadotropins FSH and LH that is extracted from the urine of post-menopausal women. Other available medications with similar composition and functions include urofollitropin, follitropin alfa, and follitropin beta. Contraindications for all of these agents are listed in the section on ovarian stimulants. Menotropins is available only as a parenteral injection in the following potency: 75 units of FSH activity with 75 units of LH activity. Pregnancy category X. Commonly recommended dosages are given in the table on p. 557.

PHARMACOKINETICS

Half-Life	Onset	Peak	Duration
Unknown	Unknown	Unknown	Unknown

UTERINE STIMULANTS

The uterus undergoes several changes during normal gestation and childbirth that at different times make it either resistant or susceptible to various hormones and drugs. Three types of drugs are available in Canada to stimulate uterine contractions in order to promote the progression of labour: ergot derivatives, prostaglandins, and the hormone oxytocin. These agents all work on the uterus, a highly muscular organ that has a complex network of smooth muscle fibres and a large blood supply. These agents are often collectively referred to as *oxytocics*, named after the naturally occurring hormone oxytocin, whose action they mimic. It is one of the two hormones secreted by the posterior lobe of the pituitary gland. The other is vasopressin, which is also known as antidiuretic hormone (ADH).

Mechanism of Action and Drug Effects

The uterus of a woman who is not pregnant is relatively insensitive to oxytocin, but during pregnancy the uterus becomes more sensitive to oxytocin and is most sensitive at term (the end of gestation).

During childbirth, oxytocin stimulates uterine contraction, and during lactation it promotes the movement of milk from the mammary glands to the nipples. Oxytocin is available in a synthetic form called Pitocin. This agent is used to induce labour at or near full-term gestation and to enhance labour when uterine contractions are weak and ineffective. Oxytocic agents are also used to prevent or control uterine bleeding after delivery, to complete an incomplete abortion (including miscarriages), and to promote milk ejection during lactation.

Another class of oxytocic agents is the prostaglandins, natural hormones involved in regulating the network of smooth muscle fibres of the uterus. This network is known as the *myometrium*. The prostaglandins cause potent contractions of the myometrium and may also play a role in the natural induction of labour. When the prostaglandin concentrations increase during the final few weeks of pregnancy, mild myometrial contractions,

commonly known as Braxton-Hicks contractions, are stimulated. The prostaglandins may be used therapeutically to induce labour by softening the cervix (cervical ripening) and enhancing uterine muscle tone. Previously administered intravenously, prostaglandins were associated with significant side effects; however, the current use of intravaginal or intracervical local administration of prostaglandins is associated with fewer side effects, and smaller amounts have a significant softening effect on the cervix. Although not approved for this purpose in Canada, prostaglandins may also be used to stimulate the myometrium to induce abortion during the second trimester when the uterus is resistant to oxytocin. Examples of these drugs include dinoprostone and misoprostol. Misoprostol is a synthetic prostaglandin analogue used for clients taking NSAIDs for peptic ulcer prevention. It has been investigated as an agent for pre-induction cervical ripening; however, it has not been approved by Health Canada for this use. Carboprost tromethamine is another prostaglandin that is administered intramuscularly for the treatment of postpartum hemorrhage due to uterine atony.

The third major class of oxytocic agents is the ergot alkaloids, which are also potent simulators of uterine muscle. Ergot comes from a fungus, *Claviceps purpurea*, which grows on rye plants. The alkaloids are compounds derived from ergot. These agents increase the force and frequency of uterine contractions and are used after delivery of the infant and placenta to prevent postpartum uterine atony (lack of muscle tone) and hemorrhage.

One of the most politically charged prescription drugs ever approved by the FDA in the United States is the progesterone antagonist mifepristone, also known as RU-486 or the "abortion pill." This agent also stimulates uterine contractions to induce abortion and is often given with the synthetic prostaglandin agent misoprostol for this purpose. RU-486 is not available in Canada although another combination of drugs, methotrexate and misoprostol, may be used for early abortion.

Indications

The therapeutic uses of the oxytocic agents vary depending on the particular agent. Oxytocin is commonly used to induce labour in near-term or term pregnancies, to augment labour and promote contractions if labour is prolonged, to promote expulsion of the placenta and control uterine bleeding postpartum, to facilitate the completion of incomplete abortions after prostaglandin induction of the abortion, to promote milk ejection when the milk supply is inadequate, and to reduce postpartum breast engorgement. Prostaglandins such as dinoprostone are administered intravaginally or orally to induce abortion during the second trimester (beyond the twelfth week of gestation). Dinoprostone cervical gel may also be used to improve cervical inducibility (cervical "ripening") near or at term in women with a medical or obstetric need for labour induction. This agent prepares the cervix for the induction of labour and makes the process easier. Ergot alkaloids such as ergonovine are primarily used for the prevention and

DOSAGES **Selected Uterine Stimulants**

Agent	Pharmacological Class	Usual Dosage Range	Indications
▸▸dinoprostone	Prostaglandin E₂ abortifacient and cervical ripening agent	Vaginal insert (10 mg) placed transversely into posterior vaginal fornix (the space behind cervix)	Cervical ripening for induction of labour
		Cervical gel: 0.5 mg into cervical canal	Cervical ripening for induction of labour
		Tablets: 0.5 mg followed by 0.5 mg each hour, not to exceed 1.5 mg	Elective and indicated induction of labour
		Vaginal gel: 1 mg into posterior vaginal fornix, 1–2 mg repeated once 6 h later	Cervical ripening for induction of labour
▸▸ergonovine maleate	Oxytocic ergot alkaloid	IM/IV: 200 μg after delivery of placenta, repeatable at 2–4 h intervals, up to 5 doses	Postpartum or post-abortion uterine atony and hemorrhage
▸▸oxytocin	Oxytocic hypothalamic hormone	IV infusion: 10 units diluted in 1 L D5W at 1–20 microunits/min, titrated to effect	Labour induction
		IV infusion: 10–40 units in 1 L of D5W titrated to effect	Postpartum uterine atony and hemorrhage
		IV: 5–10 units by slow injection	
		IM: 5–10 units in a single dose after delivery of placenta	
misoprostol	Prostaglandin	PO: 400 μg 12 h before procedure
Intravaginally: 200 μg 9–10 h before procedure	Termination of pregnancy

treatment of postpartum and post-abortion hemorrhage caused by uterine atony or subinvolution. Although not approved by Health Canada, methotrexate, a folate agonist used for neoplastic diseases and as an antirheumatic drug, has been used in conjunction with the synthetic prostaglandin misoprostol to induce abortion through the first seven to eight weeks of pregnancy. The synthetic steroid mifepristone, a progesterone antagonist, may also be used in conjunction with misoprostol but it is also not approved by Health Canada.

Contraindications

Contraindications to the use of labour-inducing uterine stimulants include known drug allergy to a specific product and may include high-risk intrauterine fetal positions before delivery, placenta previa (improper placement of the placenta, blocking the opening), hypertonic uterus, uterine prolapse, or any condition in which vaginal delivery is contraindicated. Contraindications to the use of abortifacients also include known drug allergy, as well as the presence of an IUD, ectopic pregnancy, concurrent anticoagulant therapy or bleeding disorder, inadequate access to emergency health care, or the inability to understand or adhere with follow-up instructions.

Side Effects and Adverse Effects

The most common undesirable effects of oxytocic agents are listed in Table 33-6.

Interactions

There are few clinically significant drug interactions that occur with the oxytocic agents. The most common and important of these involve sympathomimetic drugs. The combination of drugs that produce vasoconstriction, such

TABLE 33-6
OXYTOCIC AGENTS: MOST COMMON ADVERSE EFFECTS

Body System	Side/Adverse Effects
Cardiovascular	Hypotension or hypertension, chest pain
Central nervous	Headache, dizziness, fainting
Gastrointestinal	Nausea, vomiting, diarrhea
Genitourinary	Vaginitis, vaginal pain, cramping
Other	Leg cramps, joint swelling, chills, fever, weakness, blurred vision

as sympathomimetics, with the oxytocic agents can result in severe hypertension.

Dosages

For the recommended dosages of selected oxytocic agents, see the table above. See Appendix B for some of the common brands available in Canada.

DRUG PROFILES

▸▸dinoprostone

Dinoprostone is a synthetic derivative of the naturally occurring hormone prostaglandin E₂. It is used for ripening of an unfavourable cervix in pregnant women at or near term with a medical or obstetric need for labour induction. The use of dinoprostone is contraindicated in hypersensitivity, uterine fibrosis, cervical stenosis, pelvic inflammatory disease, and respiratory disease. It is also contraindicated in clients who have undergone pelvic operations. It is available as a 10-mg vaginal insert, a 0.5-mg vaginal gel syringe and catheter, and oral 0.5 mg tablets. Pregnancy category C. Commonly recommended dosages are given in the table on p. 559.

PHARMACOKINETICS

Half-Life	Onset	Peak	Duration
Gel: N/A	Rapid	30–45 min	Unavailable
Tablet: 1 min	10 min	Unavailable	2–3 hr

⇥ *ergonovine maleate*

The ergot alkaloid ergonovine is primarily used in the immediate postpartum period to enhance myometrial tone and reduce the likelihood of postpartum uterine hemorrhage. Its use is contraindicated in clients with a known hypersensitivity to ergot medications and in those with pelvic inflammatory disease. It should also not be used to augment labour, before delivery of the placenta, or during a spontaneous abortion. Ergonovine is available in oral form as 200-μg tablets and as a 0.25-mg injection for intramuscular use. Intravenous (IV) administration is not recommended except in emergency situations. Pregnancy category C. Commonly recommended dosages are given in the table on p. 559.

PHARMACOKINETICS

Half-Life	Onset	Peak	Duration
<2 hr	PO: 5–15 min	30 min	3 hr
	IM: <5 min		

⇥ *oxytocin*

Oxytocin is the synthetic form of the endogenous hormone oxytocin and has all of its pharmacological properties. Oxytocin is contraindicated in clients with a history of hypersensitivity to the drug. Pregnancy category X, unless used to induce or augment labour. Commonly recommended dosages are given in the table on p. 559.

PHARMACOKINETICS

Half-Life	Onset	Peak	Duration
3–5 min	IV: Immediate	IV: Immediate	IV: 2–3 hr
	IM: <5 min	IM: Immediate	IM: 2–3 hr

UTERINE RELAXANTS

When contractions of the uterus begin before term it may be desirable to stop labour because premature birth, or labour before term, can have many detrimental effects, death of the neonate being the most serious consequence. Postponing delivery by relaxing the uterine smooth muscles and helping prevent contractions and the induction of labour increases the likelihood of the infant's survival. Only uterine contractions occurring between about 20 and 37 weeks of gestation are considered premature labour. Spontaneous labour occurring before the twentieth week is more commonly thought of as a spontaneous abortion, or miscarriage; it is commonly associated with a defective fetus and thus is usually not interrupted.

The non-pharmacological treatment of premature labour includes bed rest, sedation, and hydration. Drugs given to inhibit labour and maintain the pregnancy are called *tocolytics*. Tocolytics have generally been found useful only in the short term to delay labour long enough so that glucocorticoids (drug of choice is betamethasone) can be given to the mother to accelerate the maturity of fetal lung development. Generally, these agents can delay labour for approximately 48 hours. Although many different drugs can suppress pre-term labour, two commonly used tocolytic agents in the United States are ritodrine and terbutaline. Ritodrine was removed from the Canadian market because of side effects of maternal pulmonary edema. Terbutaline and ritodrine are classified as beta-adrenergic agents (see Chapter 17) and work by directly relaxing uterine smooth muscle. Calcium channel blockers such as nifedipine as well as non-steroidal anti-inflammatory drugs such as indomethacin have also been used to suppress labour. Concentrated solutions of the electrolyte magnesium sulphate may also be used intravenously for this purpose.

One common characteristic of tocolytics is that they relax uterine smooth muscle and stop the uterus from contracting. Magnesium sulphate works by directly relaxing uterine smooth muscle. It inhibits acetylcholine release at the neuromuscular junctions in the uterus. At therapeutic levels relaxation of the uterine muscle occurs.

NURSING PROCESS

■ Assessment

The client's baseline BP, weight, blood glucose levels, and liver and renal function studies should be documented before drug therapy is begun. It is also important for the nurse to assess the client's smoking history, including the number of packs per day and number of years. Drug allergies and any prescription and non-prescription drugs used should also be documented and noted. Before estrogen or progesterone agents are used the nurse should determine whether the client has any contraindications to their use, such as history of breast cancer, estrogen-dependent carcinomas, thromboembolic disorders, malignancies of the reproductive tract or abnormal vaginal bleeding, or pregnancy. These agents also should not be used in women who are breastfeeding; if the drug is needed, breastfeeding should be discontinued. Other contraindications include cerebral vascular disease, coronary artery disease, jaundice, hepatic lesions, and history of stroke. Cautions for the estrogens and progestins include smoking in a woman over the age of 35, uncontrolled hypertension, hyperlipidemia, migraines or other severe forms of headache, asthma, blood dyscrasias, diabetes, heart failure, depressive disorders, seizure disorders, and liver or renal disease. Drugs that interact with estrogens and progestins include anticoagulants, oral antidiabetic agents, TCAs, anticonvulsants, barbiturates, and steroids. Other drug interactions include any drug that is antagonized by hepatic enzyme-inducing drugs (e.g., rifampin, phenobarbital; see pharmacological principles). When COCs are used in emergency situations of post-coital conception they have the same cautions and contraindications as the other estrogens and progestins but are generally only one-time-use agents.

Dinoprostone, a new synthetic prostaglandin E_2 hormone, is indicated for the initiation and continuation of cervical ripening for women at or near term with a medical indication for the induction of labour. It is contraindicated with fibroids, pelvic inflammatory disease (PID), pelvic stenosis, respiratory disease, and pelvic operation. It is also contraindicated in women with a history of pelvic operations.

Before administering uterine stimulants such as oxytocin or prostaglandins, the nurse should determine and document the client's BP, pulse, and respiration. The fetal heart rate and contraction-related fetal heart rate should also be determined and recorded. The same considerations apply to ergot alkaloids, with assessment of the client particularly critical because these agents are most often used for the prevention and control of postpartum and post-abortion hemorrhage. The most notable drug interaction occurs with sympathomimetic drugs; the result is severe hypertension.

As mentioned previously in this chapter, uterine relaxants such as magnesium sulphate should be used only in women in premature labour who are in their twentieth to thirty-seventh week of gestation. Cautious administration is recommended in any client receiving them.

Before any of the fertility agents are administered, it is important for the nurse to determine whether there are any contraindications or cautions. Cautious use is recommended in clients with hypertension, seizure disorders, or diabetes mellitus. Contraindications include allergies, pregnancy, liver disease, and undiagnosed vaginal bleeding.

For the SERMs, such as alendronate and raloxifene, there are many contraindications and cautions. Cautions for these drugs include hepatic or renal dysfunction and use of estrogen. For alendronate, cautious use is recommended in clients with renal or hepatic impairment, mineral metabolism disorders, or upper GI disease. For raloxifene further cautions include leukopenia, thrombocytopenia, and the presence of cataracts. Contraindications include a history of or active venous thromboembolic events, pregnancy or the chance of pregnancy, lactation, DVT, pulmonary embolism, and retinal thrombosis. For alendronate, additional contraindications include the presence of esophageal abnormalities, delayed esophageal emptying, and the inability to remain upright (sitting or standing helps to prevent esophageal erosion and ulcers that result from reflux of the drug back into the esophagus). Drug interactions associated with alendronate include other drugs that cause GI distress, acetylsalicylic acid, and nonsteroidal anti-inflammatory drugs (NSAIDs). Drug interactions for raloxifene include warfarin, cholestyramine, and other highly protein-bound drugs (such as diazepam and diazoxide).

▌ Nursing Diagnoses

Nursing diagnoses pertinent to one or more drugs affecting women's health include the following:

- For SERM agents, risk of infection related to possible drop in white blood cell count.
- Disturbed body image related to physiological or pathological effects stemming from changes in female hormone levels, osteoporosis, or effects of breast cancer and its treatment.
- Deficient knowledge related to first-time drug therapy.

ETHNOCULTURAL IMPLICATIONS

Women's Health Issues and the Incidence of Ovarian Malignancies

The worldwide annual incidence of ovarian malignancy exceeds 140 000, and rates vary among countries. This variation may result from differences in the age of menarche, age of menopause, and rates of pregnancy, breastfeeding, or use of oral contraception. Rates of ovarian cancer are highest in Scandinavia, North America, and the United Kingdom. Approximately 2300 new cases and 1550 deaths occur each year in Canada as a result of ovarian cancer. Rates are lowest in Africa, India, China, and Japan. Risk factors include increasing age, family history of ovarian cancer, low fertility, use of fertility drugs, and low parity (number of births). Some case-control studies have found that using combined oral contraceptive pills for more than five years is associated with a 40 percent reduction in the risk of ovarian cancer.

Data from *Clinical Evidence Concise.* (Dec 2002). Available from http://www.clinicalevidence.com; http://www.unitedhealthfoundation.org; National Cancer Institute of Canada. (2004). Canadian cancer statistics (p. 18).

LEGAL and ETHICAL PRINCIPLES

Administration of Oxytocin

A client was admitted to labour and delivery for the delivery of her third child and was given oxytocin for induction of labour. The client eventually ended up having a hysterectomy because of a uterine tear, which resulted in uncontrolled heavy uterine bleeding that did not stop with repair of the tear. During the hysterectomy the client received several blood transfusions and subsequently developed hepatitis. The hospital, nurses, and physicians were sued for negligence and malpractice, and the court found in favour of the client. The healthcare professionals and the hospital were cited as failing to properly monitor and adhere to the standards of care for administration of oxytocin. What nursing actions could have easily been implemented to ensure client and fetal safety and to prevent harm or injury during drug administration? Would documentation of monitoring also be necessary?

- Acute pain related to the labour and delivery process and any associated abnormalities.
- Disturbed body image related to an abnormal pregnancy and/or associated complications.
- Anxiety related to possible fetal death or the complications of labour and pregnancy.
- Deficient knowledge related to first-time pregnancy and related unknown events or outcome of pregnancy.
- Disturbed body image related to inability to conceive.
- Anxiety related to unknown effects of treatment for infertility and success/failure rates.
- Deficient knowledge related to drug therapy for infertility.
- Deficient knowledge related to HRT in women.

■ Planning

Goals for clients receiving drugs for the treatment of various disorders and conditions of the female reproductive tract include the following:
- Client is free of body image disturbances.
- Client states the rationale for hormonal replacement, COCs, SERMs, uterine relaxants, or fertility drugs.
- Client states the side effects of specific medications.
- Client states the importance of adherence with hormonal therapy and other recommended pharmacological and non-pharmacological measures for the treatment of premature labour, pre-eclampsia, or fertility disorders.

■ *Outcome Criteria*

Outcome criteria for clients receiving agents used to treat various disorders and conditions of the female reproductive tract include the following:
- Client openly verbalizes her concerns, fears, and anxieties with staff about body image changes and the need for medication.
- Client is compliant with pharmacological and non-pharmacological therapy with successful management of osteoporosis, breast cancer, infertility, pre-eclampsia, or premature labour, or she experiences effective birth control.
- Client is free of complications and disturbing side effects associated with each group of drugs, such as chest pain, leg pain, blurred vision, thrombophlebitis, and leukopenia.
- Client returns for regular follow-up visits with physician to monitor therapeutic and adverse effects of treatment.

■ Implementation

Both estrogens and progestins should be administered in the lowest doses possible and then the doses titrated as needed. Intramuscular doses should be given deep in large muscle masses and the injection sites rotated. Oral forms should be taken with food or milk to minimize GI upset. Progestin-only oral contraceptive pills are taken daily. It is important for the client to take this oral contraceptive at the same time every day so that ef-

fective hormonal serum levels are maintained. Because the progestin-only pill leads to a higher incidence of ovulatory cycles, there is an associated increased rate of failure. This type of pill is usually used in women who cannot tolerate estrogens or for whom estrogens are contraindicated. Often it is more effective in women over 35 years of age. Combination estrogen/progestin pills are in low doses. The low-dose monophasic and multiphasic types have 21 days of pills followed by 7 days of placebo treatment, and the client needs to understand how this treatment regimen works. The nurse should emphasize to the client that the reduction of estrogen has been correlated to a decrease in side effects and a decrease in the risk for liver tumours, hypertension, and cardiovascular changes; however, more incidences of breakthrough bleeding will occur. The nurse should encourage clients taking these oral contraceptives do the following:
- Report weight gain (especially 2.25 kg or more in a week or 1 kg or more within a 24-hour period).
- Wear sunscreen or avoid sunlight because of increased susceptibility to sunburn.
- Double up on the medication if a dose is missed. Take the pills when the omission is remembered and then use another form of contraception for one complete cycle.

Clients should know that annual follow-up examinations, including a Papanicolaou (Pap) smear, pelvic examination, and a practitioner-performed breast examination, are necessary for the safe and effective use of oral contraceptives. The nurse should demonstrate breast self examination (BSE) and encourage clients to perform examinations monthly approximately 7 days after menstruation. Additional information on other forms of hormonal contraception is listed in Box 33-3.

Dinoprostone, the synthetic prostaglandin E_2, is available in gel, tablet, and vaginal insert forms. Client teaching tips and more information may be found on p. 564.

Oxytocin should be administered only as ordered and by following strictly any instructions or protocol. Clients should report strong contractions, edema, water intoxication (associated with headaches and nausea), palpitations, chest pain, and any perceived changes in fetal movement. Oxytocin should be administered only using an intravenous infusion pump and after dilution in D5W or 0.9 percent NS at a rate of 20 to 40 microunits/min or as ordered for completing an incomplete abortion; at no greater than 20 microunits/min for stimulating labour; and at 20 to 40 microunits/min for controlling postpartum bleeding. A crash cart should be kept on the unit, and magnesium sulphate should be kept at the client's bedside. Fetal heart rate and maternal vital signs should be monitored frequently and as needed during the infusion.

Fertility agents such as clomiphene are often self-administered. Specific instructions regarding their administration at home and the way to monitor drug effectiveness are important to enhancing the success of

New Category of Oral Contraceptives in Canada

Drospirenone/ethinyl estradiol, known by its trade name Yasmin, considered a breakthrough in modern oral contraceptives, has been on the market in the United States and Britain for more than five years and in January 2005 became available in Canada. It is the first in its category: a low-dose combination of ethinyl estradiol and a unique progestin called drospirenone. Drospirenone is similar to the natural form of the hormone progesterone. It possesses antimineralocorticoid activity, which, in birth control pills, is usually derived from the male hormone testosterone. The activity unique to drospirenone/ethinyl estradiol is the moderately increased excretion of sodium and water without the side effects usually found in birth control pills containing male hormone. Drospirenone/ethinyl estradiol provides effective oral contraception, excellent cycle control, and tolerability with a low rate of spotting and breakthrough bleeding.

Reference: Berlex Canada. (2005). First in new category of oral contraceptives approved. Yasmin arrives in Canada. Retrieved August 23, 2005, from http://www.berlex.ca/scripts/en/news/pr/pr011205.php.

CASE STUDY

Osteoporosis

T.L. is a relatively healthy 73-year-old female with newly diagnosed post-menopausal osteoporosis. She has been prescribed treatment with alendronate 10 mg orally every day. Approximately 5 days after initiating treatment, T.L. experiences dysphagia (difficulty swallowing) and odynophagia (pain with swallowing). She is scheduled for an endoscopy in the morning to rule out ulcerative esophagitis.
- What is alendronate and what are its indications?
- How could the adverse reaction to this medication administration have been prevented?
- What drug interactions are significant with alendronate?

For answers see http://evolve.elsevier.com/Lilley/pharmacology/.

treatment. Journal tracking of the medication regimen will be helpful to those involved in the care of the infertile client or couple.

COCs should be taken within 72 hours of unprotected intercourse and are *not* effective if the client is already pregnant.

The success of the SERMs is associated with thorough client teaching and ensuring that the client understands the drug therapy. With alendronate it is important for the nurse to emphasize the need to take the medication upon rising in the morning with a full glass

(200 to 250 mL) of plain water at least 30 minutes before the intake of any food, other fluids, or other medication. It is also important that the client not lie down for approximately 30 minutes to help prevent esophageal erosion or irritation. Any client taking raloxifene should be informed that this drug needs to be discontinued 72 hours before and during prolonged immobility. It can be resumed once the client becomes fully ambulatory.

HRT with estrogen and progestin pose new concerns for women. Recent research indicates that HRT may cause heart disease and breast cancer. The WHI study suggests that long-term HRT is *not* a good way to prevent osteoporosis and protect against coronary artery disease (CAD). Other forms of treatment are recommended, such as statins (for CAD) and bisphosphonates or raloxifene (for osteoporosis).

■ Evaluation

Therapeutic responses to estrogens include the disappearance of menopausal symptoms and the absence of breast engorgement. For men given estrogen for prostatic tumours, a therapeutic response is a decrease in the size of the tumour. The side effects of estrogens include thromboembolism, edema, jaundice, abnormal vaginal bleeding, hyperglycemia, nausea, vomiting, increased appetite, and weight gain. Therapeutic responses to progestins include a decrease in abnormal uterine bleeding and the disappearance of menstrual disorders such as amenorrhea. The side effects of progestins include edema, hypertension, cardiac symptoms, depression, changes in mood and affect, and jaundice.

Therapeutic effects of SERMs include increased bone density (with raloxifene) and improvement in or prevention of breast cancers (estrogen-receptor positive). Side effects include leukopenia, decreased platelets, risk for thrombophlebitis, hot flashes, and leg cramps.

Therapeutic effects of oxytocin and other uterine stimulants include stimulation of labour and control of postpartum bleeding. Adverse reactions include changes in vital signs with bradycardia, dysrhythmias, and premature ventricular contractions, severe abdominal pain and shock-like symptoms with a decrease in BP, and increased pulse. All of these indicate possible uterine rupture and fetal distress. The client should also be closely monitored for the occurrence of acceleration or deceleration and for the signs and symptoms of water intoxication. In addition, the physician should be notified if contractions last longer than 1 minute or do not occur.

The therapeutic effect of fertility agents is the successful fertilization of an ovum and resultant pregnancy. Adverse reactions for which the nurse should monitor include hot flashes, abdominal discomfort, blurred vision, GI upset, nervousness, depression, weight gain, and hair loss. Multiple births and birth defects are other possible consequences of therapy.

CLIENT TEACHING TIPS

Nurses should instruct clients as follows:

Oral Estrogens and Progestins

▲ Take this medication with food or milk to minimize upset stomach.

▲ Do a breast self examination, ideally 7 to 10 days after your period, and report any unusual lumps or bumps.

▲ Report chest pain, leg pain, blurred vision, headache, neck stiffness and pain, swelling, yellow discoloration of the skin or the white of the eye, clay-coloured stools, and vaginal bleeding.

▲ Do not breastfeed while taking this medication.

▲ Report any weight gain of more than 2 kg in a week or 1 kg or greater within a 24-hour period.

▲ Avoid sunlight or wear sunscreen because estrogens increase sensitivity to sunlight and ultraviolet light.

▲ (For clients on HRT) Hormone replacement is controversial. Current recommendations are that these hormones should not be taken to protect yourself against heart disease and osteoporosis.

Oral Contraceptives

▲ Take your medicine at the same time every day. If you miss a dose, take it as soon as you remember and use a backup form of contraception for one cycle. Do not double up on medication.

▲ Oral contraceptives will not protect you against sexually transmitted infections. For disease protection, you need to use condoms.

▲ Make follow-up appointments annually. If you have any problems, you will need to see the physician more frequently.

Emergency Contraception

▲ If you have unprotected intercourse and need emergency contraception, you can get it without prescription at a drug store. It should be taken within 72 hours of unprotected intercourse with a follow-up dose 12 hours later.

Fertility Agents

▲ Keep a daily journal of all medications, body changes and any other changes, your emotional and physical status, and any related signs and symptoms.

▲ Make sure to have regular follow-up visits to the physician.

▲ Make sure you understand all instructions about when and how to take your medication and about side effects to expect.

SERMs

▲ These drugs carry a risk of thrombophlebitis (blood clotting). Make sure you get your blood work done as the physician orders.

▲ Take this medication with meals to help decrease stomach upset.

POINTS to REMEMBER

▼ The first menses or menstrual cycle is called *menarche;* menstruation then typically occurs once a month until it ceases with menopause.

▼ The menstrual cycle consists of three phases: the menstrual phase, the follicular phase, and the luteal phase. The follicular phase is associated with high levels of estrogen. The luteal phase is associated with high levels of progesterone.

▼ Three major estrogens are synthesized in the ovaries: estradiol (principal estrogen), estrone, and estriol.

▼ Exogenous estrogens can be broken down into two main groups: steroidal estrogens (e.g., conjugated estrogens, esterified estrogens, estradiol) and the nonsteroidal estrogen diethylstilbestrol.

▼ Estrogens work by binding to and interacting with the estrogen receptors, increasing the synthesis of DNA and RNA.

▼ Ethinyl estradiol is a semisynthetic steroidal estrogen and the most orally active estrogenic drug.

▼ Progesterone is a hormone secreted by the corpus luteum.

▼ Progesterone is the principal natural progestational hormone.

▼ Chemical derivatives of progesterone are called *progestins.*

▼ Progestins have a variety of uses including treatment of uterine bleeding or amenorrhea and palliative treatment of some cancers.

▼ Oral contraceptives with a combination of estrogens and progestins are the most effective form of birth control currently available.

▼ Uterine stimulants (sometimes called *oxytocic agents*) include ergot derivatives, prostaglandins, and oxytocin.

▼ A thorough nursing assessment is necessary to ensure the safe and effective use of female reproductive agents. This should include information on the client's past medical problems, history of menses and problems with menstrual cycle, medications taken (prescribed and OTC), the number of pregnancies and miscarriages, the last menstrual period, and any related surgical or medical treatments.

▼ Client education should focus on the importance of the medication for managing the specific disease or disorder and also on the means to ensure a positive self-image and open communication.

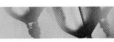

EXAMINATION REVIEW QUESTIONS

1 Which of the following are considered contraindications in Canada with the administration of dinoprostone?
  a. Termination of pregnancy after 20 weeks
  b. Gastrointestinal upset/ulcer disease
  c. Pelvic inflammatory disease
  d. Male clients with prostate cancer
2 Which of the following are side effects of oral contraceptives?
  a. Weight loss
  b. Benign liver tumours
  c. Diminished tanning of the skin
  d. Polyuria
3 Oxytocin is indicated for clients with which of the following?
  a. Severe acne with pregnancy
  b. Postpartum "blues"
  c. Suspicious skin lesions
  d. Labour at full term and not progressing
4 Which of the following is a side effect of an SERM?
  a. Hyperglycemia
  b. Polyuria
  c. Diabetes
  d. Esophageal abnormalities
5 The combination of oxytocin and sympathomimetics may be adverse to a client because of which of the following adverse effects?
  a. Dilation of veins
  b. Vasoconstriction
  c. Liver failure
  d. Multiple pregnancies

For answers see http://evolve.elsevier.com/Lilley/pharmacology/.

CRITICAL THINKING ACTIVITIES

1 K.T. has spent 14 hours in labour with her first pregnancy and has made little progress. She is becoming exhausted, and the uterine contractions have decreased in strength. Oxytocin is ordered to be given at a rate of 1 microunit/min. The normal concentration of oxytocin is 10 microunits/mL. What rate (in millilitres per hour) should the infusion be run at to deliver 1 microunit/min?

2 Why are oxytocics used to treat postpartum and postabortion bleeding caused by uterine relaxation and enlargement?
3 What is the primary mechanism by which oral contraceptives prevent pregnancy?

For answers see http://evolve.elsevier.com/Lilley/pharmacology/.

BIBLIOGRAPHY

Albanese, J., & Nutz, P. (2005). *Mosby's 2005 nursing drug cards.* St Louis, MO: Mosby.

American Psychiatric Association. (2000). *Diagnostic and statistical manual of mental disorders (DSM-IV-TR).* Arlington, VA: Author.

Anderson, P.O., Knoben, J.E., & Troutman, W.G. (2002). *Handbook of clinical drug data* (10th ed.). New York: McGraw-Hill/Appleton & Lange.

Berne, R., & Levy, M. (2002). *Principles of physiology* (3rd ed.). St Louis, MO: Mosby.

Black, D. (2003). What's new on contraception? *Canadian Journal of CME,* 65–72.

Boron, W.F., & Boulpaep, E.L. (2005). *Medical physiology.* Philadelphia: Saunders.

Briggs, G.G., Freeman, R.K., & Yaffe, S.J. (2003). *Drugs in pregnancy and lactation* (6th ed.). Philadelphia: Lippincott Williams & Wilkins.

Brown, J.P., Josse, R.G., & The Scientific Advisory Council of the Osteoporosis Society of Canada. (2002). 2002 clinical practice guidelines for the diagnosis and management of osteoporosis in Canada. Updated 2004. *Canadian Medical Association Journal, 167*(10 Suppl), S1–S34.

Canadian Pharmacists Association. (2003). *Therapeutic choices* (4th ed.). Ottawa, ON: Author.

Canadian Pharmacists Association. (2004). *Guide to drugs in Canada.* Toronto, ON: Dorling Kindersley.

Canadian Pharmacists Association. (2005). *Compendium of pharmaceuticals and specialties. The Canadian drug reference for health professionals.* Ottawa, ON: Author. [The subscription-based e-CPS is available at http://www.pharmacists.ca.]

Cheng, A., Williams, B.A., & Sivarajan, B.V. (Eds.). (2003). *The HSC handbook of pediatrics* (10th ed.). Toronto, ON: Elsevier.

Facts and Comparisons. (2004). *Drug facts and comparisons pocket version* (9th ed.). St Louis, MO: Wolters Kluwer Health.

Hardman, J.G, & Limbird, L.E. (2002). *Goodman and Gilman's the pharmacological basis of therapeutics* (10th ed.). New York: McGraw-Hill.

Health Canada. (2005). Drug product database (DPD). Retrieved August 23, 2005, from http://www.hc-sc.gc.ca/hpb/drugs-dpd/

Kasper, D.L., Braunwald, D., Faci, A., Hauser, S., Longo, D., & Jameson, J.L. (2005). *Harrison's principles of internal medicine* (16th ed.). New York: McGraw-Hill.

Katzung, B.G. (2004). *Basic and clinical pharmacology* (9th ed.). New York: McGraw-Hill.

Lacy, C.F., Armstrong, L.L., Goldman, M.P., & Lance, L.L. (2003). *Drug information handbook* (11th ed.). Hudson, OH: Lexi-Comp.

Larsen, P.R., Kronenberg, H.M., Melmod, S., & Polonsky, K.S. (2003). *Williams textbook of endocrinology* (10th ed.). Philadelphia: Saunders.

Lehne, R.A. (2004). *Pharmacology for nursing care* (5th ed.). St Louis, MO: Saunders.

Marketed Health Products and Therapeutic Products Directorates, Health Canada. (2003). Advisory on diethylstilbestrol (DES) and the risk of genital and obstetrical complications—health professional advisory. Retrieved August 22, 2005, from http://www.hc-sc.gc.ca/dhp-mps/medeff/advisories-avis/prof/2003/des_hpc-cps_e.html

McKenry, L.M., & Salerno, E. (2003). *Mosby's pharmacology in nursing—revised and updated* (21st ed.). St Louis, MO: Mosby.

Mosby. (2005). *Mosby's drug consult 2005: The comprehensive reference for generic and brand name drugs* (15th ed.). St Louis, MO: Mosby.

National Cancer Institute. (2005). Women's Health Initiative. The estrogen-alone study. Retrieved August 22, 2005, from http://www.nhlbi.nih.gov/whi/estro_alone.htm

Osteoporosis Society of Canada. (2004). New drug offers promise for patients with severe osteoporosis. Retrieved August 23, 2005, from http://www.osteoporosis.ca/english/News/forteo/default.asp?s=1

Shibbald, B. (2005). News synopsis. Nonprescription status for emergency contraception. *Canadian Medical Association Journal, 172*(7), 861–862.

Skidmore-Roth, L. (2006). *Mosby's 2006 nursing drug reference* (19th ed.). St Louis, MO: Mosby.

Men's Health Agents

After reading this chapter, the successful student will be able to do the following:

1 Discuss the normal anatomy, physiology, and functions of the male reproductive system.

2 Compare the indications for the various male reproductive agents.

3 Discuss the mechanisms of action, dosages, side effects, cautions, contraindications, dosage forms and routes, and drug interactions for the various men's health agents.

4 Develop a nursing care plan as related to the nursing process for the client receiving any of the men's health agents.

e-LEARNING ACTIVITIES

Student CD-ROM
- Review Questions: see questions 261–264
- Animations
- Medication Administration Checklists
- IV Therapy Checklists

 **Web site** (http://evolve.elsevier.com/Lilley/pharmacology/)
- Online Chapter Worksheet • Frequently Asked Questions
- Learning Tips and Content Updates • WebLinks • Online Appendices and Supplements • Mosby/Saunders ePharmacology Update • Access to *Mosby's Drug Consult*

DRUG PROFILES

danazol, p. 570	▶▶ sildenafil, p. 571
finasteride, p. 571	▶▶ testosterone, p. 572
fluoxymesterone, p. 572	

▶▶ Key drug.

GLOSSARY

Anabolic activity (an' ə bol' ik) Any metabolic activity that promotes the building up of body tissues, such as the activity produced by testosterone that causes the development of bone and muscle tissue. (Noun: anabolism.)

Androgenic activity (an' drə jen' ik) The activity produced by testosterone that causes the development and maintenance of the male reproductive system and other male secondary sex characteristics.

Androgens Male sex hormones responsible for mediating the development and maintenance of male sex characteristics. Chief among these are testosterone and various biochemical precursors.

Benign prostatic hypertrophy (BPH) Non-malignant (non-cancerous) enlargement of the prostate gland.

Catabolism The opposite of anabolism; any metabolic activity that results in the breaking down of body tissues. Examples of catabolic conditions include debilitating illnesses such as end-stage cancer and starvation (Noun: catabolism).

Erythropoietic effect (ə rith' ro poy et' ik) An effect that stimulates the production of red blood cells.

Prostate cancer A malignant tumour growth within the prostate gland.

Testosterone (tes tos' tə rone) The main androgenic hormone.

MALE REPRODUCTIVE SYSTEM

The male reproductive system consists of several structures, the testes and seminiferous tubules being the most important to this discussion. The testes are the male gonads, and they are a pair of oval glands located in the scrotal sac. They are the site of both reproductive (androgenic) and endocrine activity. The seminiferous tubules, which are channels in the testes, are the site of spermatogenesis, which is the process by which mature sperm cells are produced.

Androgens is the name for the group of male sex hormones (primarily testosterone) that function to mediate the normal development and maintenance of the primary male sex characteristics (normal male genital anatomy), as well as the secondary characteristics. Secondary male sex characteristics include growth and maturation of the prostate, seminal vesicles, penis, and scrotum; male hair distribution, such as facial, pubic, chest, and axillary hair; laryngeal enlargement and thickening of the vocal cords; and the defining of body musculature and fat distribution. Androgens must be secreted in adequate amounts for these characteristics to appear. Probably the most important androgen is **testosterone**, which is produced from clusters of interstitial cells located between the seminiferous tubules. Besides its **androgenic activity**, testosterone is also involved in the development of bone and muscle tissue, inhibition of protein **catabolism** (metabolic breakdown), and retention of nitrogen, phosphorus, potassium, and sodium. These contribute to its **anabolic activity**. The hormone initiates the synthesis of specific proteins needed for androgenic and anabolic activity by binding to chromatin in the nucleus of interstitial cells. In addition, testosterone appears to have an **erythropoietic effect**, in that it stimulates the production of red blood cells (Chapter 54).

ANDROGENS

Several synthetic derivatives of testosterone were developed with the intention of improving on the pharmacokinetic and pharmacodynamic characteristics of the naturally occurring hormone. One way that this was accomplished was by combining various esters with testosterone, resulting in a prolonged duration of action of the hormone. For example, testosterone propionate is formulated in an oily solution and its hormonal effects last for 2 to 3 days; the effects of testosterone cypionate and testosterone enanthate in oil last even longer. They can be administered once every 2 to 4 weeks. Orally administered testosterone has poor pharmacokinetic and pharmacodynamic characteristics because most of its dose is metabolized and destroyed by the liver before it can reach the circulation (first-pass effect). To circumvent this problem, researchers developed methyltestosterone and fluoxymesterone (both controlled substances in Canada). Newer transdermal dosage forms for testosterone, including skin patches and a gel, have provided another way to circumvent the first-pass effect.

There are other chemical derivatives of the naturally occurring testosterone known as *anabolic steroids*. These are synthetic agents that closely resemble the natural hormone, but possess high anabolic activity. One anabolic steroid drug product, nandrolone, is currently commercially available in Canada by prescription, as adjuvant treatment for certain types of anemia such as aplastic and sickle cell and with hereditary angioedema. An unlabelled use is for HIV wasting syndrome (debilitation related to disease-induced nutritional malabsorption). Anabolic steroids have a great potential for being misused by athletes, especially body builders and weight lifters, because of their muscle-building properties. Improper use of these substances can have many serious consequences, such as sterility, cardiovascular diseases, and even liver cancer. For this reason anabolic steroids are currently regulated under the Controlled Drugs and Substances Act applicable to Schedule IV. The trafficking, possession for the purpose of trafficking, possession for the purpose of exporting, and production, import, and export of anabolic steroids are illegal. This classification implies that misuse of the agent can lead to psychological or physical dependence, or both. Steroids can produce a variety of psychological effects that range from euphoria to hostility. They may be taken to feel powerful and energetic. However, steroids are also known to increase irritability, anxiety, and aggression, and to cause mood swings, manic symptoms, and paranoia, particularly when taken in high doses.

Another synthetic androgen is danazol. Its labelled uses include endometriosis and fibrocystic breast disease.

Mechanism of Action and Drug Effects

The drug forms of the natural and synthetic androgens and the synthetic anabolic steroids have effects similar to those of the endogenous androgens. These include stimulation of the normal growth and development of the male sex organs (primary sex characteristics) and development and maintenance of the secondary sex characteristics. One reason for the growth-promoting effects of androgens is that they stimulate the synthesis of ribonucleic acid (RNA) at the cellular level, thereby promoting cellular growth and reproduction. They also retard the breakdown of amino acids. These properties contribute to an increased synthesis of body proteins, which aids in the formation and maintenance of muscular and skeletal proteins. Another potent anabolic or tissue-building effect of androgens is the retention of nitrogen, also essential for protein synthesis. Nitrogen also promotes the storage in the body of inorganic phosphorus, sulphate, sodium, and potassium, all of which have important metabolic roles, including protein synthesis, nerve impulse conduction, and muscular contractions. All of these effects result in weight gain and an increase in muscular strength. Finally, androgens also stimulate the production of erythropoietin by the kidney, resulting in enhanced erythropoiesis (red blood cell synthesis). However, the administration of exogenous androgens causes the release of endogenous testosterone to be inhibited as the result of the feedback inhibition of pituitary luteinizing hormone (LH). Large doses of exogenous androgens may also suppress sperm production as the result of the feedback inhibition of pituitary follicle-stimulating hormone (FSH).

Androgen inhibitors are agents that block the effects of naturally occurring (endogenous) androgens in the body. This occurs via inhibition of a specific enzyme: 5-alpha-reductase. For this reason these agents are also called *5-alpha-reductase inhibitors*. One of the effects of endogenous androgens is the growth and maintenance of the prostate. When androgens are secreted in excessive amounts, the prostate enlarges, a condition known as **benign prostatic hypertrophy (BPH)**. BPH is amenable to treatment with a 5-alpha-reductase inhibitor. Currently, two such agents available are finasteride and dutasteride. They work by inhibiting the enzymatic process responsible for converting testosterone to 5-alpha-dihydrotestosterone (DHT), the androgen principally responsible for stimulating prostatic growth. Finasteride and dutasteride can dramatically lower the prostatic DHT concentrations, which helps to ease the passage of urine made difficult by the enlarged prostate. The drug effects of finasteride are limited primarily to the prostate, but this agent may also affect 5-alpha-reductase-dependent processes elsewhere in the body, such as hair follicles, skin, and the liver. For example, it has been noted that men taking finasteride experience increased hair growth as well. Therefore finasteride is also indicated for the treatment of male-pattern baldness. Results are encouraging. The inhibition of 5-alpha-reductase prevents the thinning of hair caused by increased levels of DHT. Finasteride is indicated for treating baldness only in men, and not in women. The long-term effects of dutasteride have not yet been determined as it only recently became available. However, established adverse effects are associated with the reproductive tract; for example, erectile dysfunction, decreased libido, and ejaculation disorders, as well as gynecomastia (breast development) have been noted. Finasteride and dutasteride can be teratogenic in pregnant women, and the manufacturers of these drugs do not recommend using them in women of any age (pregnant or not) or in children. However, another medication, minoxidil, can be used topically to treat baldness in both men and women. It is discussed in more detail in Chapter 55.

Another class of agents that may be used to help alleviate the symptoms of obstruction due to BPH are the alpha₁-adrenergic blockers (discussed in Chapter 17), most commonly terazosin, doxazosin, and tamsulosin. Tamsulosin appears to have a greater specificity for the alpha₁-receptors on the prostate and thus may cause less hypotension.

There are also two other classes of androgen inhibitors. The first are the androgen receptor blockers flutamide, nilutamide, and bicalutamide. These agents work by blocking the activity of androgen hormones at the level of the receptors in target tissues (e.g., prostate). For this reason these drugs are used in the treatment of **prostate cancer.** The second class is the gonadotropin-releasing hormone (Gn-RH) analogues, including leuprolide and goserelin. These agents work by inhibiting the secretion of pituitary gonadotropin, which eventually leads to a decrease in testosterone production. Both androgen receptor blockers and Gn-RH analogues are used most commonly to treat prostate cancer and are discussed in further detail in Chapter 46.

Sildenafil, better known as Viagra, is the first oral drug approved for the treatment of erectile dysfunction (ED). Two other drugs in the same class, vardenafil and taladafil, are now also available. Another agent, prostaglandin alprostadil, is also indicated for ED; however, this agent must be given by injection or pushed into the urethra. Sildenafil works by inhibiting the enzyme phosphodiesterase. This in turn allows buildup in the penis of the chemical cyclic guanosine monophosphate (cGMP), which causes relaxation of the smooth muscle in the corpora cavernosa (erectile tubes) of the penis, allowing the inflow of blood. Nitric oxide (NO) is also released inside the corpora cavernosa during sexual stimulation and contributes to the erectile effect.

A summary list of all of the men's health agents mentioned in the chapter appears in Box 34-1. More information on selected agents appears in the drug profile section of this chapter.

BOX 34-1
Currently Available Men's Health Agents

Alpha₁-Adrenergic Blockers
doxazosin
tamsulosin
terazosin

Anabolic Steroids
nandrolone

Androgens
danazol
fluoxymesterone
testosterone

Anti-Androgens
bicalutamide
flutamide
nilutamide

5-Alpha-Reductase Inhibitors
finasteride
dutasteride

Gn-RH Analogues
goserelin
leuprolide
triptorelin

Peripheral Vasodilator
minoxidil

Agents for Erectile Dysfunction
sildenafil
vardenafil
taladafil

Gn-RH, Gonadotropin-releasing hormone.

Indications

The primary use for androgens is replacement therapy. However, a variety of other uses for these agents are listed in Table 34-1.

Contraindications

Contraindications to the use of androgenic agents include known drug allergy and androgen-responsive tumours. Sildenafil is also contraindicated in men with major cardiovascular problems, especially if they use nitrate medications such as nitroglycerin.

Side Effects and Adverse Effects

Although rare, some of the most devastating effects of androgenic steroids occur in the liver, where they cause the formation of blood-filled cavities, a condition known as *peliosis of the liver*. This is a potential consequence of the long-term administration of androgenic anabolic steroids and can be life threatening. Other serious hepatic effects are hepatic neoplasms (liver cancer), cholestatic hepatitis, jaundice, and abnormal liver function. Fluid retention is another undesirable effect of androgens and may account for some of the weight gain seen. The serious adverse effects that can be caused by the androgens far outweigh the advantages to be gained from their use in those seeking improved athletic ability. Other less serious adverse effects of androgens are listed in Table 34-2.

Sildenafil has a relatively safe side effect profile. In clients with pre-existing cardiovascular disease, especially those taking nitrates (e.g., nitroglycerin, isosorbide mono- or dinitrate), sildenafil lowers blood pressure (BP) substantially and can lead to serious adverse events. Headache, flushing, and dyspepsia are the most common adverse effects reported. Priapism (prolonged erection) has been reported in clinical trials; however, in post-marketing surveillance, priapism has been reported infrequently.

Finasteride has been reported to cause loss of libido, loss of erection, ejaculatory dysfunction, hypersensitivity

reactions, gynecomastia, and severe myopathy. The drug has also caused a 50 percent decrease in prostatic specific antigen (PSA) concentrations. Pregnant women should not handle crushed or broken tablets regularly because of the possibility of topical absorption, which can lead to teratogenic effects.

Minoxidil can cause tachycardia, dizziness, angina pectoris, and marked fluid retention when taken orally. The topical formulation may also cause some of these adverse effects, but local irritation, itching, dryness, and erythema are more common, especially with the stronger 5 percent topical formulation. Allergic contact dermatitis has also been reported.

Interactions

All androgens, when used with oral anticoagulants, can significantly increase or decrease anticoagulant activity. They can also enhance the hypoglycemic effects of oral antihyperglycemic (antidiabetic) agents. Concurrent use with cyclosporine increases the risk of cyclosporine toxicity and is not recommended.

Dosages

For recommended dosages of the men's health agents, see the table on p. 571. See Appendix B for some of the common brands available in Canada.

DRUG PROFILES

danazol

Danazol is a synthetic derivative of ethisterone (which is derived from both progesterone and testosterone) that possesses weak androgenic activity. Its use is contraindicated in clients with significant cardiac, hepatic, or renal dysfunction, androgen-dependent tumour, any thromboembolic event, and those with porphyria; in women with undiagnosed abnormal vaginal bleeding;

TABLE 34-1

MEN'S HEALTH AGENTS: INDICATIONS

Androgen or Androgen Inhibitor	Indication(s)
danazol	Endometriosis
	Fibrocystic breast disease
danazol	Hereditary angioedema
finasteride	Benign prostatic hyperplasia (BPH)
	Male androgenetic alopecia
fluoxymesterone	Inoperable breast cancer
	Male hypogonadism
	Postpartum breast engorgement
minoxidil	Hypertension
	Male androgenetic alopecia
nandrolone	Senile and post-menopausal osteoporosis
sildenafil	Erectile dysfunction (ED)
testosterone	Primary or secondary hypogonadism

TABLE 34-2

ANDROGENS: COMMON ADVERSE EFFECTS

Body System	Side/Adverse Effects
Central nervous	Headache, anxiety, mental depression, generalized paraesthesia
Endocrine	Acne, gynecomastia in men
	In women, amenorrhea, menstrual irregularities, and virilization (deepening of voice, hirsutism, and clitoral enlargement)
Hematological	Polycythemia; suppression of clotting factors II, V, VII, X; increased serum cholesterol level
Other	Priapism or excessive sexual stimulation in males; male-pattern baldness; water retention, along with retention of sodium, chloride, potassium, and inorganic phosphates; stomatitis (inflammation of the mucous membrane of the mouth); hypercalcemia from osteolysis (breakdown of bone tissue)

and in pregnant or lactating women. It is currently available in 50-, 100-, and 200-mg strength capsules. Pregnancy category X. Refer to the table below for dosage information.

PHARMACOKINETICS

Half-Life	Onset	Peak	Duration
24 hr	4 wk	2 hr	Unknown

finasteride

Finasteride is contraindicated in clients who have shown a hypersensitivity to it and in pregnant women, and it is considered potentially dangerous for a pregnant woman to even handle crushed or broken tablets. It is currently available in two tablet forms of 1- and 5-mg strengths. The lower strength is indicated for androgenetic alopecia, which can occur in males. The higher strength is indicated for BPH. A similar but newer drug, dutasteride, is also indicated for BPH and

is currently available in 0.5-mg capsule form. Pregnancy category X (for both). Refer to the table below for dosage information.

PHARMACOKINETICS

Half-Life	Onset	Peak	Duration
4–15 hr*	3–12 mo†	8 hr‡	Unknown

*Varies with age.
†To reduce prostate size.
‡To lower DHT concentrations.

▸▸ sildenafil

Sildenafil is the first oral drug approved by Health Canada for treatment of ED. Another currently available agent for the treatment of ED is an injectable form of the prostaglandin alprostadil. Sildenafil potentiates the physiological sexual response, causing penile erection after sexual arousal by relaxing smooth muscle and increasing blood flow into the penis.

DOSAGES   Selected Men's Health Agents

Agent	Pharmacological Class	Usual Dosage Range	Indications
danazol	Pituitary gonadotropin inhibitor	**Adult** PO: 200–800 mg/day divided bid or qid for 3–6 mo	Endometriosis
		100–400 mg/day divided bid for up to 4–6 mo or regression of symptoms	Fibrocystic breast disease
finasteride	5-alpha-reductase inhibitor	**Adult** PO: 1 mg daily (Propecia)	Male androgenetic alopecia (baldness)—males only
		PO: 5 mg daily (Proscar)	BPH
vardenafil	Phosphodiesterase inhibitor	**Adult** PO: 5–20 mg 25–60 min before sexual activity; no more than once daily	ED
▸▸ sildenafil	Phosphodiesterase inhibitor	**Adult (males only)** PO: 25–100 mg 1 hr before sexual activity; no more than once daily	ED
dutasteride	5-alpha-reductase inhibitor	**Adult** PO: 0.5 mg daily	BPH
▸▸ testosterone cypionate	Androgenic hormone	**Adult** IM: 200–400 mg q3–4wk	Erectile dysfunction due to testicular deficiency, male climacteric
			Eunuchism, eunuchoidism (failure of the testes to develop)
		IM: 100–200 mg q3–6wk	Oligospermia (low sperm count)
		IM: 200–400 mg q3–4 wk	Anabolic effect, osteoporosis
testosterone, transdermal	Androgenic hormone	**Adult and adolescent** Androderm patch (applied to skin of back, abdomen, upper arms or thighs): 2.5–5 mg/day AndroGel (applied to shoulders, arms, or abdominal skin): 5 g daily (delivers 50 mg of testosterone) AndroGel pump: delivers 1.25 g of gel for each time pump is depressed (actuation)	Male hypogonadism

Sildenafil is contraindicated in clients with a known hypersensitivity to it. Sildenafil can potentiate the hypotensive effects of nitrates, and its administration to clients who are using organic nitrates, either regularly and/or intermittently, in any form is therefore contraindicated. It is available as 25-, 50-, and 100-mg tablets. It is classified as a pregnancy category B agent, though it is normally used only by males. A newer medication with similar dosage instructions and contraindications is vardenafil, which is available in tablet strengths of 5, 10, and 20 mg. Dosage information for both medications appears in the table on page 571.

PHARMACOKINETICS

Half-Life	Onset	Peak	Duration
4 hr	0.5–1 hr	1 hr	4 hr

GERIATRIC CONSIDERATIONS

Sildenafil: Use and Concerns

Over 10 million men in North America suffer from erectile disorder (ED). ED occurs with an increasing incidence as men age, with about 2 percent of clients being in their forties and 23 percent 65 years of age and older. Sildenafil is a prescription medication that is commonly ordered for ED, but not without concerns and cautions for the client. This is especially true for geriatric clients, who generally have other medical conditions (e.g., renal disorders, hypertension, diabetes) and are usually taking more than one other prescribed medication. Liver function declines with age; therefore drugs may not be as effectively metabolized in older adults as they are in younger adults. In addition, sildenafil is highly protein bound, causing it to stay in the body longer, thus creating more drug interactions. A decreased dosage of sildenafil, initially at 25 mg per day, is generally indicated for clients over 65 years of age and for those with liver or renal impairment. Side effects to be concerned about in all clients, particularly older clients, include headache, flushing, urinary tract infection, diarrhea, rash, and dizziness. Sildenafil should be used cautiously in clients who have cardiac disease and angina because these clients are at greater risk for complications, even more so if they are also on nitrates for their cardiovascular disease. This is especially problematic for the client over 65 years of age who is self-medicating.

Discussing topics of a sexual nature may be comfortable for some clients but anxiety producing for others. It is important for nurses to be aware of ethnocultural and gender differences with regard to how individuals perceive their own sexuality and how they generally deal with sexual performance issues. Nurses must be respectful of each person's beliefs and feelings not only about their sexuality, but about their whole self. This requires knowledge, sensitivity, and objectivity.

Source: Lacy, C.F., Armstrong, L.L., Goldman, M.P., & Lance, L.L. (2003). *Drug information handbook* (11th ed.). Hudson, OH: Lexi-Comp.

↦ *testosterone*

Testosterone is a naturally occurring anabolic steroid. It is used for primary and secondary hypogonadism but may also be used to treat oligospermia (low sperm count) and breast cancer. When used as replacement therapy a transdermal product is desirable. There is presently one transdermal patch and a nasal spray pump. They attempt to mimic the normal circadian variation in testosterone concentration seen in young healthy men where the maximum testosterone levels occur in the early morning hours and minimum concentrations in the evening. The transdermal delivery product Androderm is always applied to skin elsewhere on the body and never to the scrotal skin.

Testosterone is contraindicated for use in clients with severe renal, cardiac, or hepatic disease; hypersensitivity; pregnancy; lactation; and genital bleeding. Testosterone is considered a Schedule IV controlled substance under the Controlled Drugs and Substances Act. It is available as 100-mg/mL intramuscular injections; a 2.5- or 5.0-g transdermal gel in unit-dose packets or a 60 actuation metered-dose pump; 12.2- and 24.3-mg/day transdermal patches; and a 40-mg capsule. Pregnancy category X. Common dosages are listed in the table on p. 571.

PHARMACOKINETICS

Half-Life	Onset	Peak	Duration
10–100 min	1–2 hr	2–4 hr	2 hr–4 wk depending on dosage form

 NURSING PROCESS

■ Assessment

Androgenic agents are used for the treatment of a variety of disorders and diseases, including malignancies of the male reproductive system. Before any male reproductive agent is administered to a client, the purpose for its use and the client's urinary elimination patterns should be assessed and documented. Contraindications to the use of testosterone and related products include an allergy to the medication and renal, cardiac, and liver disease. Cautious use with careful monitoring is recommended in clients with diabetes and in those with a history of cardiovascular disease or myocardial infarction (MI). Because androgenic anabolic steroids such as testosterone and nandrolone increase weight and raise the potassium, chloride, nitrogen, and phosphorus levels, it is important for the nurse to determine and record the client's baseline weight, height, vital signs, and serum electrolyte levels. It is also important for the nurse to look at the results of laboratory tests that assess renal, cardiac, and liver functions, such as the blood urea nitrogen (BUN), creatinine, lactate dehydrogenase, creatine kinase, and bilirubin levels. PSA levels are often ordered before treatment with agents such as finasteride.

Specifically, danazol is contraindicated in clients with significant cardiac, hepatic, or renal dysfunction; in pregnant or lactating women; and in women with abnormal vaginal bleeding. Finasteride is contraindicated in clients with known allergies to the medication and in pregnant women because of its teratogenic effects. Nandrolone is contraindicated in clients with severe cardiac, liver, or renal disease; in pregnant women and those with abnormal vaginal bleeding; and in men with breast or prostate cancer. Sildenafil should be used cautiously in clients with cardiovascular disease, especially if they are also taking nitrates, because of related postural hypotensive effects and potential syncope. Drug interactions of androgenic agents include oral anticoagulants (warfarin sodium), steroids, insulin, and oral antihyperglycemic agents.

Nursing Diagnoses

Nursing diagnoses relevant to clients receiving androgenic agents include the following:
- Disturbed body image related to sexual dysfunction and/or diseases of the male reproductive tract.
- Fatigue related to side effects of medications.
- Excess fluid volume related to sodium retention caused by large dosages of androgenic agent.
- Disturbed body image related to sexual dysfunction associated with side effects (decreased libido, erectile dysfunction) of agents used to treat male reproductive malignancies.
- Risk for situational low self-esteem related to sexual dysfunction secondary to medications and/or disease states.
- Deficient knowledge related to misinterpretation of information about self-medication.

Planning

Goals for clients receiving androgenic agents include the following:
- Client maintains positive body image.
- Client maintains normal activity levels during androgenic therapy.
- Client maintains normal sodium and fluid volume levels.
- Client experiences minimal alterations in sexual integrity and function during androgenic therapy.
- Client remains adherent with androgenic therapy.
- Client verbalizes feelings and concerns about actual or perceived changes in sexual patterns.

Outcome Criteria

Outcome criteria related to the administration of androgenic agents include the following:
- Client verbalizes feelings, fears, and anxieties concerning potential for alteration in body image related to disease process or the side effects of androgenic therapy.
- Client maintains healthy activity level during androgenic therapy and suffers minimal fatigue with increased activities of daily living.
- Client states measures to be taken to minimize edema related to sodium retention stemming from the use of large dosages of androgens, such as dietary cautions.
- Client verbalizes feelings, anxieties, and fears of alteration in his or her sexual integrity or function during androgenic therapy and seeks counselling if needed.
- Client takes medications as prescribed.

Implementation

Intramuscular testosterone and related products should be injected deep and only after proper landmarking. Generally the lowest dose possible is prescribed to reduce side effects. Other dosage forms need to be given exactly as instructed. The metered-dose AndroGel pump requires priming prior to first use. It requires up to five depressions to remove the air, followed by gel discharge. The initial two gel discharges should be discarded so that an accurate gel dose is delivered. The gel should be discarded carefully to make sure other household members do not accidentally eat or touch it, especially pregnant or nursing women or children.

Finasteride may be given orally without regard to meals but should be protected from exposure to light and heat. When used for treatment of the urinary symptoms of BPH, finasteride should be administered orally for approximately 6 months, at which time the condition should be re-evaluated. Danazol should be given with milk or food to decrease GI upset. Clients taking sildenafil should be warned about potential side effects, such as flushing and headache. Minoxidil, in topical forms, may also lead to local reactions, and excessive rash or redness should be reported if they occur.

Nandrolone, an anabolic steroid, should be taken exactly as ordered and at the lowest possible dosage. If edema occurs, a low sodium diet may be recommended. It is only available in Canada for intramuscular use. See the Natural Health Therapies box for saw palmetto, an herbal supplement taken to relieve symptoms of enlarged prostate.

Teaching tips for clients receiving androgenic medications are presented in the box on p. 574.

NATURAL HEALTH THERAPIES

SAW PALMETTO *(Serenoa repens, Sabul serrulata)*

Overview
Saw palmetto is used as a diuretic, as a urinary antiseptic, and for its anabolic properties. It is most commonly used for the treatment of benign prostatic hypertrophy and is believed to inhibit dihydrotestosterone and 5-alpha-reductase.

Common Uses
Diuretic, urinary antiseptic, benign prostatic hypertrophy, alopecia

Adverse Effects
GI upset, headache, back pain, dysuria

Potential Drug Interactions
Anti-inflammatory agents, hormones such as estrogen replacement therapy and oral contraceptives, and immunostimulants

Contraindications
None

■ **Evaluation**

The therapeutic effect of androgenic agents is essentially the improvement of the condition and/or signs and symptoms for which the client is being treated. Some of the therapeutic effects may not be seen for 3 or 4 months. It is important for the nurse to observe and monitor the client for the side effects of these medications, such as hypercalcemia, hypoglycemia, hypertension, edema, changes in sexual functioning, and mood changes.

CLIENT TEACHING TIPS

The nurse should instruct the client on the following points, as relevant:

▲ Often it takes 3 to 4 months before therapeutic effects are seen with some of these medications.

▲ (For clients taking an androgen or a hormone-related drug) Never abruptly stop taking your medication. These medications should be discontinued only with a physician's order, and you will need to be monitored for several weeks while the dosage is tapered.

▲ If you are taking finasteride, you need to understand why you are taking it and know the side effects to report to your healthcare provider.

▲ (For a woman taking nandrolone) Notify your physician of any menstrual irregularities or of any decrease in the therapeutic effects.

POINTS to REMEMBER

▼ Androgens are the male sex hormones and are responsible for normal development and maintenance of male sex characteristics. The primary androgen is testosterone.

▼ Danazol and testosterone are exogenous agents.

▼ Testosterone is responsible for the development and maintenance of the male reproductive system and secondary sex characteristics. Since oral testosterone has poor pharmacokinetic and pharmacodynamic characteristics, testosterone is usually administered via injection, transdermal patch, or nasal metered-dose pump.

▼ The only anabolic steroids are chemical derivatives of testosterone responsible for bone and muscle development and decreased protein breakdown.

▼ Anabolic steroids are classified as controlled substances by the Canadian Controlled Drugs and Substances Act

(Schedule IV); the only one available by prescription in Canada is nandrolone.

▼ Anabolic inhibitors are used to block the effects of naturally occurring androgens and are also called *5-alpha-reductase inhibitors* because of the enzyme they block, which is needed to form testosterone.

▼ An example of an anabolic inhibitor is finasteride, which is usually indicated to stop growth of the prostate in men with BPH and to treat men with androgenic alopecia.

▼ Testosterone and related products, when administered intramuscularly, should be given deep in a large muscle mass.

▼ The therapeutic effects of androgenic agents often take 3 to 4 months to appear.

EXAMINATION REVIEW QUESTIONS

1 Which of the following is crucial to monitor in the client taking sildenafil?
   a. Daily weights, I&O, and weekly creatine
   b. I&O due to polyuria
   c. BP and drug interactions
   d. Nothing because this is a benign medication

2 An evening dose of sildenafil would be contraindicated in which of the following?
   a. 65 years of age
   b. Hypertension
   c. Hypervitaminosis
   d. Morning dose of antacids

3 Which of the following is an adverse effect of androgenic steroid use?
   a. Bradypnea
   b. Bradycardia

   c. Pyuria
   d. Polycythemia

4 Oral forms of minoxidil are associated with which of the following side effects?
   a. Gynecomastia
   b. Tachycardia
   c. Polyuria
   d. Severe myopathy

5 Drug interactions for saw palmetto include which of the following?
   a. Acetaminophen
   b. Vitamin C
   c. NSAIDs
   d. Estrogens

For answers see http://evolve.elsevier.com/Lilley/pharmacology/.

CRITICAL THINKING ACTIVITIES

1 How do finasteride and testosterone differ in their mechanisms of action?

2 Why might an androgen be prescribed in a client suffering from anemia?

3 Develop a teaching plan about the risks of anabolic steroids for an 18-year-old male football player and weightlifter.

For answers see http://evolve.elsevier.com/Lilley/pharmacology/.

BIBLIOGRAPHY

Albanese, J., & Nutz, P. (2005). *Mosby's 2005 nursing drug cards.* St Louis, MO: Mosby.

Avodart manufacturer's Web site. Retrieved August 24, 2005, from http://www.avodart.com

Canadian Pharmacists Association. (2003). *Therapeutic choices* (4th ed.). Ottawa, ON: Author.

Canadian Pharmacists Association. (2004). *Guide to drugs in Canada.* Toronto, ON: Dorling Kindersley.

Canadian Pharmacists Association. (2005). *Compendium of pharmaceuticals and specialties. The Canadian drug reference for health professionals.* Ottawa, ON: Author. [The subscription-based e-CPS is available at http://www.pharmacists.ca.]

Facts and Comparisons. (2004). *Drug facts and comparisons pocket version* (9th ed.). St Louis, MO: Wolters Kluwer Health.

Hardman, J.G., & Limbird, L.E. (2002). *Goodman and Gilman's the pharmacological basis of therapeutics* (10th ed.). New York: McGraw-Hill.

Health Canada. (2005). Drug product database (DPD). Retrieved August 24, 2005, from http://www.hc-sc.gc.ca/hpb/drugs-dpd/

Lacy, C.F., Armstrong, L.L., Goldman, M.P., & Lance, L.L. (2003). *Drug information handbook* (11th ed.). Hudson, OH: Lexi-Comp.

Larsen, P.R., Kronenberg, H.M., Melmod, S., & Polonsky, K.S. (2003). *Williams textbook of endocrinology* (10th ed.). Philadelphia: Saunders.

Lehne, R.A. (2004). *Pharmacology for nursing care* (5th ed.). St Louis, MO: Saunders.

Levitra manufacturer's Web site. Retrieved August 24, 2005, from http://www.levitra.com

Mosby. (2005). *Mosby's drug consult 2005: The comprehensive reference for generic and brand name drugs* (15th ed.). St Louis, MO: Mosby.

Skidmore-Roth, L. (2006). *Mosby's 2006 nursing drug reference* (19th ed.). St Louis, MO: Mosby.

PART SIX

Drugs Affecting the Respiratory System: Study Skills Tips

- STUDY ON THE RUN, PURR

STUDY ON THE RUN, PURR

The basic approach in applying Study on the Run (SOTR) is to make use of small blocks of time that are otherwise non-productive. Plan, Rehearse, and Review do not require that the entire chapter be covered in one study session. These steps produce their benefits by promoting repetition of learning.

Where Is the Time?

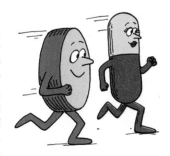

SOTR time is everywhere. In the course of a single day you might have an hour or more that can be used for SOTR actions. It is just a matter of becoming aware of little bits and pieces of your day that can ordinarily slip away without being productive. Small blocks of time are everywhere in your day; it just takes a little creativity on your part to become aware of them. Finishing an exam early, standing in the checkout line, waiting for the teakettle to boil, or even waiting for the washing machine to finish the last spin before you change loads can be time used for SOTR. Get creative and be flexible. Remember, every minute of time you use this way is a minute of time you will not have to find later.

SOTR and Plan

These sections have repeatedly stressed the importance of questioning as an essential component in Plan. Look at the chapter objectives for Chapter 36. There are five objectives presented for this chapter. Work on the questions for as many of these objectives as can be accomplished in the time you have. If you complete questions for only two objectives, do not look upon it as failing to complete something. Instead learn to view what you have done as that much less to do later. The time you spend now frees up that much more time during your large blocks of study time for intense study reading.

Will you forget the questions you generated in this session before you have the opportunity to read the chapter? If you make it a habit to ask questions as a continuing part of all study, you will find that you remember the focus questions well. If you have trouble remembering your own questions, use a pencil. Write questions in the margins of the text. Gradually you will find questioning becomes such an automatic procedure that you will be able to dispense with writing questions. You will remember them.

SOTR and Vocabulary

One of the most challenging aspects of a course like this is the almost overwhelming vocabulary load. As if the new vocabulary were not enough, you also need to keep reviewing previous parts and chapters because some term that was introduced three chapters ago has reappeared and you do not remember it clearly. Creating your own vocabulary cards is a perfect SOTR activity.

The basic card model is simple. The word, common form, prefix, or suffix appears on the card front. The back of the card may have just a little information, the minimum being a definition of what is on the front, or the back of the card may contain considerable information. Including part, chapter, and page number on the back helps you locate the term quickly if the need arises. In addition, you may want to add a specific example from the text or of your own creation to help clarify the term. Put as much information on the back as you find useful.

Creating Vocabulary Cards with SOTR

Use the time between classes to create several personal vocabulary cards. Grab your text and your blank note cards. Open to the next chapter you will be studying. Flip over to the glossary pages. Write the first word from the glossary on the front of a blank note card. Flip the card over. Write the part and chapter numbers and the page number for the glossary on the card. Pick a standard location for this. Put these numbers in a top corner or a bottom corner, but make sure you put them in the same corner every time. Eventually this becomes a habit and makes the preparation process faster. It also helps when you are making use of the cards because you will know exactly what information you put on the card and where you put it. Put this card aside and repeat the process with the next term in the glossary. In those few minutes before you go to class you can have completed the basic preparation for a full set of cards covering the 17 terms in the Chapter 36 glossary.

Notice that the paragraph above did not suggest copying the definition in the glossary at this time. The term may be much easier to understand when used in the context of a sentence and a paragraph. If, as you read the chapter, you feel that the glossary definition is also useful to have on this card, you can always flip back using the location information you put on the card.

SOTR and Vocabulary Review

Your vocabulary cards are ideal for SOTR action. Carry a deck of cards with you at all times. Whenever you have even a minute or two, you can pull out a stack of cards—cards from previous chapters or the current chapter. Use the oral ask-and-answer method discussed in the *Study Guide*. For instance, the first term in the glossary for Chapter 36 is *allergen*. Ask yourself aloud, "What is an allergen?" Then try to answer the question aloud. Answer: "An allergen is a substance that produces an allergic reaction." It is not necessary to recall the exact answer presented in the glossary and/or chapter. What is important is that you respond 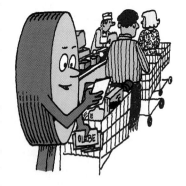 with a clear and meaningful answer. The answer given above is not exactly the same as that stated in the glossary, but the general concept is the same. Once you have stated

your answer, turn the card over and check to make sure that you were correct. Each time you do this with a term, you are strengthening your long-term memory and will find that it takes less and less time to recall the terms you need.

SOTR and Chapter Review

It can be overwhelming if you think that review means rereading the material and therefore you need large blocks of uninterrupted time. There is a much more efficient way to review, and it works well in short time blocks, which makes it a perfect technique for SOTR.

Look at the first page of Chapter 35. You should instantly see a number of visible structures that make it easy to review key terms and concepts without rereading the entire block of material. First, there is the chapter title: *Antihistamines, Decongestants, Antitussives, and Expectorants.* What are antihistamines? This is a question you would have generated when you were engaged in the Plan step of PURR. Now that you have read the chapter, repeat the question and answer it aloud. Answer aloud because you will hear what you say, and will either know the material or need to mark it to come back and reread. Now ask a more complex question: "What is the role of antihistamines? What do they do?" Now try to answer these questions. If you can, then you do not need to reread to find out what antihistamines are. Next, looking at p. 580 you will notice some things in **bold print**. Apply the same process. Using the bold face words and phrases as stimulus, ask questions and try to answer them to your own satisfaction. If you cannot develop a satisfactory answer, then you know that some rereading is needed. But it is very focused. You are not trying to reread everything on the page, only the material right there associated with the term.

Looking under the first major heading, Antihistamines, you will see a list. Look at the previous sentence: "This explains why the release of excessive amounts of histamine can lead to anaphylaxis and severe allergic symptoms and result in any or all of the following physiological changes." Ask questions. If you can answer, no reading is necessary. If you cannot answer, you know that the answers are found immediately after this sentence in the indented list. Use the structures in the chapter to accomplish focused review. Comprehension is improved, long-term memory is strengthened, and your test grades will reflect this.

The benefits of SOTR are enormous. There is no drawback. You are using time that otherwise would be "wasted." This time now becomes productive study time. The more active you become in looking for SOTR opportunities, the more you will find. The more SOTR time you spend, the better a student you will become.

Antihistamines, Decongestants, Antitussives, and Expectorants

OBJECTIVES

After reading this chapter, the successful student will be able to do the following:

1 Classify agents as antihistamines, decongestants, antitussives, and expectorants, and contrast these groups.

2 Discuss the mechanisms of action, indications, contraindications, cautions, adverse effects, dosage ranges, and various dosage forms for the use of antihistamines, decongestants, antitussives, and expectorants.

3 Develop a nursing care plan that includes all phases of the nursing process for clients taking any of the antihistamines, decongestants, antitussives, and expectorants.

e-LEARNING ACTIVITIES

Student CD-ROM
- Review Questions: see questions 265–270
- Animations
- Medication Administration Checklists
- IV Therapy Checklists

evolve Web site (http://evolve.elsevier.com/Lilley/pharmacology/)
- Online Chapter Worksheet • Frequently Asked Questions
- Learning Tips and Content Updates • WebLinks • Online Appendices and Supplements • Mosby/Saunders ePharmacology Update • Access to *Mosby's Drug Consult*

DRUG PROFILES

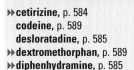

▶▶cetirizine, p. 584
codeine, p. 589
desloratadine, p. 585
▶▶dextromethorphan, p. 589
▶▶diphenhydramine, p. 585

fexofenadine, p. 585
▶▶guaifenesin, p. 590
▶▶loratadine, p. 583
oxymetazoline, p. 587

▶▶ Key drug.

GLOSSARY

Adrenergic (sympathomimetic) (a' drə ner' jik) Of or pertaining to sympathetic nerve fibres of the autonomic nervous system that use epinephrine or epinephrine-like substances as neurotransmitters.

Anticholinergic (parasympatholytic) (an' tee kol in er' jik) Of or pertaining to the blockade of acetylcholine receptors that results in the inhibition of the transmission of parasympathetic nerve impulses.

Antigen Any substance that is, upon entry into the body, capable of inducing a specific immune response and in turn reacting with the specific products of such a response, such as specific antibodies and specifically sensitized T-lymphocytes. Antigens can be soluble (e.g., foreign protein) or particulate (insoluble, e.g., a bacterial cell).

Antihistamine (an' tee his' tə meen) Any substance capable of reducing the physiological and pharmacological effects of histamine, including a wide variety of drugs that block histamine receptors.

Antitussive A drug substance that reduces coughing, often by inhibiting neural activity in the cough centre of the central nervous system (CNS).

Corticosteroids Any one of the hormones produced by the adrenal cortex, either in natural or synthetic form. They influence or control many key processes of the body, such as carbohydrate and protein metabolism, the maintenance of serum glucose levels, electrolyte and water balance, and the functions of the cardiovascular system, skeletal muscles, kidneys, and other organs.

Decongestant Any substance that reduces congestion or swelling, especially of the upper or lower respiratory tract.

Empirical therapy (em peer' ik əl) A method of treating disease based on observations and experience without

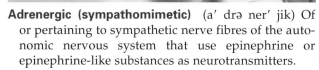

an understanding of the precise cause of or mechanism responsible for the disorder or the way in which the therapeutic agent or procedure effects improvement or cure.

Expectorant (ek spek′ tə rent) An agent that increases the flow of fluid in the respiratory tract, reducing the viscosity of bronchial and tracheal secretions and facilitating their removal by the cough reflex and ciliary action.

Histamine antagonist (his′ tə meen) A drug that competes with histamine for histamine receptors.

Influenza A highly contagious infection of the respiratory tract caused by a myxovirus and transmitted by airborne droplets.

Non-sedating antihistamines Newer medications that work peripherally to block the actions of histamine and therefore do not have the CNS effects that many of the older antihistamines have (also called *second-generation antihistamines*).

Peripherally acting antihistamines Another name for non-sedating antihistamines.

Reflex stimulation An irritation of the respiratory tract occurring in response to an irritation of the gastrointestinal tract.

Rhinovirus (ry′ no vy′ rəs) Any of about 100 serologically distinct ribonucleic acid (RNA) viruses that cause about 40 percent of acute respiratory illnesses.

Sympathomimetic drug A pharmacological agent that causes effects that mimic those resulting from the stimulation of organs and structures by the sympathetic nervous system. They do this by occupying adrenergic receptor sites and acting as an agonist or by increasing the release of norepinephrine at post-ganglionic nerve endings.

Upper respiratory tract infection (URTI) Any infectious disease of the upper respiratory tract, including the common cold, laryngitis, pharyngitis, rhinitis, sinusitis, and tonsillitis.

COLD MEDICATIONS

The agents used to treat the symptoms of the common cold are **antihistamines**, **decongestants**, **antitussives** (cough suppressants), and **expectorants**. Most common colds result from a viral infection, most often a **rhinovirus** or an **influenza** virus. These viruses typically invade the tissues (mucosa) of the upper respiratory tract (nose, pharynx, and larynx) to cause an **upper respiratory tract infection (URTI)**. The inflammatory response elicited by these invading viruses stimulates excessive mucus production. This fluid drips down the pharynx and into the esophagus and lower respiratory tract, which leads to symptoms typical of a cold: sore throat, coughing, and upset stomach. The irritation of the nasal mucosa often triggers the sneeze reflex and also causes the release of several inflammatory and vasoactive substances, which results in the dilation of the small blood vessels in the nasal sinuses and leads to nasal congestion. The treatment of the common symp-

toms of URTI involves the combined use of antihistamines, nasal decongestants, antitussives, and expectorants. However, they can only relieve the symptoms of a URTI. They can do nothing to eliminate the causative pathogen. Antivirals and antibiotics are currently the only agents that can do this, but treatment with these is often hampered by the fact that the viral or bacterial cause cannot be readily identified. Because of this the treatment rendered can only be determined on the basis of what is believed to be the most likely cause, based on presenting clinical symptoms. This is called **empirical therapy**. Some clients seem to gain benefit from the use of natural health products and other supplements, such as vitamin C, in terms of preventing the onset of cold signs and symptoms, or at least decreasing their severity. One herbal product commonly used for colds is echinacea (see box below). The practitioner should recognize, however, that there is limited controlled research data regarding the efficacy of herbal products and also that some of them can have significant drug–drug or drug–disease interactions.

NATURAL HEALTH THERAPIES

ECHINACEA (*ECHINACEA*)

Overview
The three kinds of echinacea are *Echinacea angustifolia, Echinacea pallida,* and *Echinacea purpurea.* Echinacea has been shown in clinical trials to reduce cold symptoms and recovery time when taken early in the illness. This is believed to be due to its immunostimulant effects. At this time there is no strong research evidence to warrant recommendations for urinary tract infections, wound healing, or prevention of colds; further study is needed to show evidence of its therapeutic effects and indications. The World Health Organization (WHO) has endorsed echinacea for the treatment of the common cold. However a new study released in 2005 (Sampson) disputes that extracts of echinacea alone or in combination have any significant outcome when taken for the common cold virus or any of the effects of the infection with the rhinovirus.

Common Uses
Stimulate immune system, antiseptic, antiviral, influenza-like respiratory infections, promote the healing of wounds, chronic ulcerations

Adverse Effects
Dermatitis, upset stomach or vomiting, dizziness, headache, unpleasant taste

Potential Drug Interactions
Amiodarone, cyclosporine, phenytoin, methotrexate, ketoconazole, barbiturates; tolerance likely to develop if used for more than 8 wk. Because some preparations have a high alcohol content, they may cause acetaldehyde syndrome in clients taking disulfiram to prevent alcohol abuse (Chapter 8).

Contraindications
Contraindicated for clients with AIDS, tuberculosis, connective tissue diseases, multiple sclerosis.

ANTIHISTAMINES

Histamine is a bodily substance that performs many functions. It is involved in central nervous system (CNS) transmission, dilation of capillaries, contraction of smooth muscles, stimulation of gastric secretion, and acceleration of the heart rate. There are two types of cellular receptors for histamine. Histamine$_1$ (H$_1$) receptors mediate smooth muscle contraction and dilation of capillaries, and histamine$_2$ (H$_2$) receptors mediate the acceleration of the heart rate and gastric acid secretion. This explains why the release of excessive amounts of histamine can lead to anaphylaxis and severe allergic symptoms and result in any or all of the following physiological changes:

- Constriction of smooth muscle, especially in the stomach and lungs
- Increase in body secretions
- Vasodilation and increased capillary permeability resulting in fluid movement out of the blood vessels and into the tissues, causing a drop in blood pressure (BP) and edema

Antihistamines are drugs that compete directly with histamine for specific receptor sites. For this reason they are also called **histamine antagonists**. Antihistamines that compete with histamine for the H$_2$ receptors are called *histamine$_2$* (H$_2$) antagonists or *H$_2$ blockers* and include such agents as cimetidine, ranitidine, famotidine, and nizatidine. Because they act on the gastrointestinal (GI) system, they are discussed in detail in Part Nine, which focuses on the agents that affect this system. The focus of this chapter is on the histamine$_1$ (H$_1$) antagonists (also called *H$_1$ blockers*); these are the agents more commonly known by the term *antihistamines*. They are useful agents because approximately 10 to 20 percent of the general population is sensitive to various environmental al-

lergens. Histamine is a major inflammatory mediator of many disorders, such as allergic rhinitis (e.g., hay fever, mould, and dust allergies), anaphylaxis, angioedema, drug fevers, insect bite reactions, and urticaria (itching).

H$_1$ antagonists include such drugs as diphenhydramine, chlorpheniramine, and fexofenadine. They are of greatest value in the treatment of nasal allergies, particularly seasonal hay fever. They are also given to relieve the symptoms of the common cold, such as sneezing and running nose. In this regard they are palliative, not curative; that is, they can help alleviate the symptoms of a cold but can do nothing to destroy the virus causing it.

The clinical efficacy of the more than one dozen different antihistamines is extremely similar, although they all have varying degrees of antihistaminic, anticholinergic, and sedating properties. The particular actions of, and hence indications for, a particular antihistamine are determined by its specific chemical makeup. All antihistamines compete with histamine for the H$_1$ receptors in areas such as the smooth muscle surrounding blood vessels and bronchioles. They also affect the secretions of the lacrimal, salivary, and respiratory mucosal glands, which are the primary anticholinergic actions of antihistamines. Because of their antihistaminic properties, they are indicated for the treatment of allergies. These agents also differ from each other in their potency and their adverse effects, especially in the degree of drowsiness they produce. The antihistaminic, anticholinergic, and sedative properties of some of the commonly used antihistamines are summarized in Fig. 35-1. These effects make them useful for the treatment of such problems as vertigo, motion sickness, insomnia, and cough. Some of the commonly used antihistamines are listed in Table 35-1, along with their various anticholinergic and sedative effects.

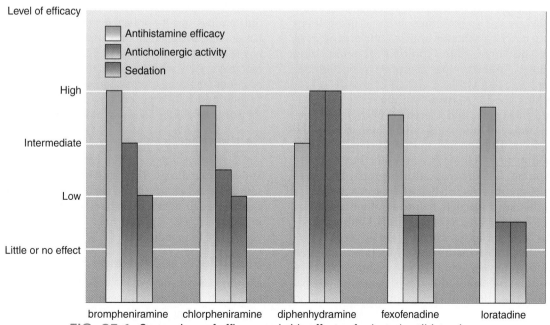

FIG. 35-1 Comparison of efficacy and side effects of selected antihistamines.

TABLE 35-1

EFFECTS OF VARIOUS ANTIHISTAMINES

Chemical Class	Anticholinergic Effects	Sedative Effects	Comments
ALKYLAMINES			
brompheniramine	Moderate	Low	Cause less drowsiness and more CNS stimulation; suitable for daytime
chlorpheniramine	Moderate	Low	use
ETHANOLAMINES			
clemastine	High	Moderate	Substantial anticholinergic effects; commonly cause sedation; with
diphenhydramine	High	High	usual doses drowsiness occurs in about 50% of clients; diphenhy-
dimenhydrinate	High	High	dramine and dimenhydrinate also used as anti-emetics
ETHYLENEDIAMINES			
pyrilamine	Low to none	Low	Weak sedative effects, but adverse GI effects are common
tripelennamine	Low to none	Moderate	
PHENOTHIAZINE			
promethazine	High	High	Principally used as antipsychotics; some are useful as antihistamines, antipruritics, and anti-emetics
PIPERIDINES			
azatadine	Moderate	Moderate	Commonly used in the treatment of motion sickness; hydroxyzine is
cyproheptadine	Moderate	Low	used as a tranquilizer, sedative, antipruritic, and anti-emetic
hydroxyzine	Moderate	Moderate	
MISCELLANEOUS			
fexofenadine	Low to none	Low to none	Minimal adverse effects from anticholinergic or sedative effects;
loratadine	Low to none	Low to none	almost exclusively antihistaminic effects, can be taken during the day because no sedative effects; in general they are longer acting and have fewer side effects

Mechanism of Action and Drug Effects

During allergic reactions, histamine and other substances are released from mast cells, basophils, and other cells in response to **antigens** circulating in the blood. The histamine molecules then bind to and activate other cells in the nose, eyes, respiratory tract, GI tract, and skin, producing the characteristic allergic signs and symptoms. For example, in the respiratory tract, histamine causes extravascular smooth muscle (e.g., in the bronchial tree) to contract, whereas antihistamines cause it to relax. Also, histamine causes pruritus by stimulating nerve endings. Antihistamines can prevent or alleviate this itching.

By blocking the H_1 receptors on the surfaces of basophils and mast cells, and thereby preventing the actions of histamine in these cells, antihistamines have the opposite effects. They do not push off histamine that is already bound to a cell surface receptor but compete with histamine for unoccupied receptors. Therefore these agents are most beneficial when given early in a histamine-mediated reaction, before all of the histamine binds to cell membrane receptors. This binding of H_1 blockers to these receptors prevents the adverse consequences of histamine binding: vasodilation; increased GI, respiratory, salivary, and lacrimal secretions; and increased capillary permeability with resultant edema. The various drug effects of antihistamines are listed in Table 35-2.

Indications

Antihistamines are more effective in preventing the actions of histamine than in reversing them once they have taken place. Because of their anticholinergic actions, they have a drying effect and reduce nasal, salivary, and lacrimal gland hypersecretion (runny nose and tearing and itching of eyes). In the skin they reduce capillary permeability, wheal-and-flare formation, and itching. Antihistamines are most beneficial in the management of nasal allergies, seasonal or perennial allergic rhinitis (e.g., hay fever), and some of the typical symptoms of the common cold. They are also useful in the treatment of allergic reactions, motion sickness, Parkinson's disease (PD; due to their anticholinergic effects), and vertigo. In addition, they are sometimes used as a sleep aid.

Contraindications

Antihistamines are generally contraindicated in cases of known drug allergy. They should also not be used as the sole drug therapy during acute asthmatic attacks. In such cases a rapidly acting bronchodilator such as albuterol, or in extreme cases epinephrine, is usually the most urgently needed medication.

Side Effects and Adverse Effects

Drowsiness is usually the chief complaint of people who take antihistamines, but these sedative effects vary from class to class (see Table 35-1). The anticholinergic (drying)

TABLE 35-2
ANTIHISTAMINES: DRUG EFFECTS

Body System	Histamine Effects	Antihistamine Effects
Cardiovascular (small blood vessels)	Dilation of blood vessels, increased blood vessel permeability (allows substances to leak into tissues)	Reduces dilation of blood vessels and increased permeability
Immune (release of various substances commonly associated with allergic reactions)	Mast cells release histamine and several other substances, resulting in allergic reactions	They do not stabilize mast cells, nor do they prevent the release of histamine and other substances, but they do bind to histamine receptors and prevent the actions of histamine
Smooth muscle (on exocrine glands)	Stimulates salivary, gastric, lacrimal, and bronchial secretions	Reduces salivary, gastric, lacrimal, and bronchial secretions

effects of antihistamines can cause such side effects as dry mouth, changes in vision, difficulty urinating, and constipation. Reported side effects and adverse effects of the antihistamines are listed in Table 35-3.

Interactions

Fexofenadine, when given with erythromycin or ketoconazole, can increase fexofenadine concentrations. This effect was demonstrated in animal studies but in healthy volunteers there was no significant increases in fexofenadine concentrations. The major difference between fexofenadine and terfenadine is that increased levels of fexofenadine do not result in severe cardiac rhythm disturbances. Terfenadine and a similar drug, astemizole, were pulled from the Canadian market in the 1990s because of significant numbers of fatal drug-induced cardiac dysrhythmias. Ketoconazole, cimetidine, and erythromycin may increase concentrations of loratadine. Alcohol, monoamine oxidase inhibitors (MAOIs), and CNS depressants may increase the CNS depressant effects of diphenhydramine and cetirizine.

Dosages

For the recommended dosages for selected antihistamines, see the dosages table on p. 584. See Appendix B for some of the common brands available in Canada.

DRUG PROFILES

Although some antihistamines are prescription drugs, most are available over the counter (OTC). Antihistamines are available in many dosage forms to be administered orally (PO), intramuscularly (IM), intravenously (IV), or topically.

NON-SEDATING ANTIHISTAMINES

A major advance in antihistamine therapy occurred with the development of the **non-sedating antihistamines** loratadine, cetirizine, and fexofenadine. These agents were developed in part to eliminate many of the unwanted side effects (mainly sedation) of the older antihistamines. These agents work peripherally to block the actions of histamine and therefore do not have the

TABLE 35-3
ANTIHISTAMINES: REPORTED ADVERSE EFFECTS

Body System	Side/Adverse Effects
Cardiovascular	Local anaesthetic (quinidine-like) effect on the cardiac conduction system resulting in dysrhythmias, arrest, hypotension, palpitations, syncope, dizziness, death (see Interactions section)
Central nervous	Sedation (mild drowsiness to deep sleep), dizziness, muscular weakness, paradoxical excitement, restlessness, insomnia, nervousness, seizures
Gastrointestinal	Anorexia, nausea, vomiting, diarrhea or constipation, hepatitis, jaundice
Other	Dryness of mouth, nose, and throat; urinary retention; erectile dysfunction; vertigo; visual disturbances; blurred vision; tinnitus; headache; rarely agranulocytosis, hemolytic anemia, leukopenia, thrombocytopenia, pancytopenia

CNS effects that many older antihistamines have. For this reason these agents are also called **peripherally acting antihistamines** because, unlike their traditional counterparts, they tend not to cross the blood–brain barrier. Another advantage is longer durations of action, which allows some of these agents to be taken only once a day, increasing adherence. These three drugs replace the two original non-sedating antihistamines terfenadine and astemizole, which were withdrawn from the U.S. and Canadian markets following several cases of fatal drug-induced cardiac dysrhythmias. Fexofenadine is actually the active metabolite of terfenadine but is not associated with such severe cardiac effects, nor are loratadine or cetirizine.

▸▸ loratadine

Loratadine is a non-sedating antihistamine. It needs to be taken only once a day. Structurally it is similar to cyproheptadine and azatadine, but unlike these agents it cannot distribute into the CNS, which alleviates the sedation effects associated with traditional antihistamines. Loratadine is used to relieve the symptoms of

DOSAGES **Selected Antihistamines**

Agent	Pharmacological Class	Usual Dosage Range	Indications
Non-Sedating Antihistamines			
⯈⯈ cetirizine	H₁ antihistamine	**Adult and pediatric ≥ 12 yr** 5–10 mg once daily, max 20 mg/day **Children 6–12 yr** 10 mL once daily or split bid **Pediatric 2–6 yr** 5 mg once daily or split bid	Allergic rhinitis, chronic urticaria
desloratadine	H₁ antihistamine	**Adult and pediatric ≥ 12 yr only** 5 mg once daily **Children 6–11 yr** 2.5 mg once daily **Pediatric 2–5 yr** 1.25 mg once daily	Allergic rhinitis, chronic urticaria
fexofenadine	H₁ antihistamine	**Adult and pediatric ≥ 12 yr** 60 mg bid or 120 mg once daily	Allergic rhinitis, chronic urticaria
⯈⯈ loratadine	H₁ antihistamine	**Adult and pediatric ≥ 12 yr** 10 mg once daily **Pediatric 2–9 yr** 5 mg once daily	Allergic rhinitis, chronic urticaria
Traditional Antihistamines (more commonly associated with sedation)			
chlorpheniramine (less sedating)	H₁ antihistamine	**Pediatric 2–6 yr** 1 mg (¼ of a 4-mg tab) **Pediatric 6–12 yr** 2 mg q4–6h, max 12 mg/24 hr **Adult** 4 mg q4–6h, max 24 mg/24 hr	Allergic rhinitis
⯈⯈ diphenhydramine (more sedating)	H₁ antihistamine	**Adult** IM/IV: 25–50 mg tid–qid **Pediatric ≥ 10 kg** IM/IV: 12.5–25 mg tid–qid **Adults and pediatric ≥ 12 yr** PO: capsules/caplets: 25–50 mg tid–qid; extra strength nighttime: 1 caplet at bedtime; junior strength chewable: 2–4 q4–6h to max 16/day; elixir: 10–20 mL q4–6h **Pediatric 6– <12 yr** Elixir: 5–10 mL q4–6h, max 4 doses/day; liquid: 10–20 mL q4–6h, max 4 doses/day **Pediatric 2–5 yr** Children's Liquid: 5 mL q4–6h **Pediatric <2 yr** Children's Liquid: 2.5 mL q4–6h	Allergic disorders, allergic reactions, anti-emetic, antihistamine, antispasmodic, motion sickness, post-operative nausea and vomiting
		Adult and pediatric ≥ 12 yr PO: 50 mg at bedtime	Nighttime sleep aid

seasonal allergic rhinitis (e.g., hay fever), as well as chronic urticaria. Loratadine has recently been converted to OTC status. However, its primary active metabolite, desloratidine, has recently come on the Canadian market and is also available OTC (see drug profile).

Drug allergy is its only contraindication. Loratadine is available in oral form as a 10-mg tablet, as a 1-mg/mL syrup, as a 10-mg rapidly disintegrating tablet, and in a combination tablet with the decongestant pseudoephedrine. Pregnancy category B. See the table above for dosage information.

PHARMACOKINETICS

Half-Life	Onset	Peak	Duration
7.8–24 hr	2 hr	8–12 hr	24 hr

⯈⯈ **cetirizine**

Cetirizine is the second non-sedating antihistamine added to the Canadian market. It is an active metabolite of the sedating antihistamine hydroxyzine, and it is also dosed once daily. It generally does not cause sedation, although sedation has been reported in up to 20 percent of clients receiving higher doses. It is used for symptoms of allergic rhinitis and chronic idiopathic urticaria and is available in 5-, 10-, and 20-mg tablets and in a 5-mg/5 mL oral syrup. Contraindications include drug allergies to either cetirizine or hydroxyzine. Pregnancy category B. See the table on p. 584 for dosing information.

PHARMACOKINETICS

Half-Life	Onset	Peak	Duration
8–11 hr	15–30 min	30–60 min	24 hr

desloratadine

Desloratadine is the primary active metabolite of loratadine and is a newer prescription drug that has taken the place of loratadine, which is now available OTC. Desloratadine is also a non-sedating antihistamine and needs to be taken only once a day. It is used to relieve the symptoms of seasonal allergic rhinitis and chronic urticaria. Although its parent compound loratadine has little if any clinically significant drug- or food-interaction activity, desloratadine is reported by its manufacturer to have even less. Drug allergy is its only contraindication. Desloratadine is currently available in oral form as a 5-mg tablet and a 0.5-mg/mL syrup. Pregnancy category B. See the table on p. 584 for dosage information.

PHARMACOKINETICS

Half-Life	Onset	Peak	Duration
27 hr	30 min	3 hr	24 hr

fexofenadine

Fexofenadine is the active metabolite of terfenadine. Terfenadine has numerous interactions with other drugs that are metabolized in the liver. These other drugs, such as erythromycin (an antibiotic) and ketoconazole (an antifungal drug), can lead to terfenadine buildup in the blood. There is a resulting potential for serious, sometimes fatal cardiac dysrhythmias. Terfenadine is the pro-drug precursor of fexofenadine, its active metabolite. Fexofenadine provides the same general therapeutic effects of terfenadine. It does not, however, block cardiac potassium channels or cause QT prolongation or ventricular dysrhythmias (notably torsades de pointes type ventricular tachycardia) as was sometimes observed to occur with terfenadine. For this reason terfenadine was voluntarily withdrawn from the market by its manufacturer in the 1990s and was replaced by fexofenadine.

Fexofenadine is indicated for the relief of symptoms associated with seasonal allergic rhinitis in adults and children 12 years of age and older. This drug is contraindicated in clients with known hypersensitivity to it or any of its ingredients. Fexofenadine is available in oral form in 60- and 120-mg tablets and in a combination tablet with the decongestant pseudoephedrine (Allegra-D). Pregnancy category C. See the table on p. 584 for dosage information.

PHARMACOKINETICS

Half-Life	Onset	Peak	Duration
14–16 hr	1–2 hr	2–3 hr	10–12 hr

TRADITIONAL ANTIHISTAMINES

The traditional antihistamines are the older agents that work both peripherally and centrally. They also have anticholinergic effects, which in some cases make them more effective than non-sedating antihistamines. Some of these commonly used older agents are diphenhydramine, brompheniramine, chlorpheniramine, dimenhydrinate, meclizine, and promethazine. These agents are used either alone or in combination with other drugs in the symptomatic relief of many disorders ranging from insomnia to motion sickness. Many clients respond to and tolerate the older agents quite well, and because many are generically available they are much less expensive. These agents are available both OTC and by prescription.

▶▶ diphenhydramine

Diphenhydramine is an older, traditional antihistamine that works both peripherally and centrally. It also has potent anticholinergic effects. It is one of the most commonly used antihistamines, in part because of its excellent safety profile and efficacy. It has the greatest range of therapeutic indications of any antihistamine available. It is used for the relief or prevention of histamine-mediated allergies and motion sickness, for post-operative nausea and vomiting, for the treatment of PD (due to its anticholinergic effects), and as a sleep aid. It is also used in conjunction with epinephrine in the management of anaphylaxis and in the treatment of acute dystonic reactions.

Diphenhydramine is classified as a pregnancy category B agent and is contraindicated in clients with a known hypersensitivity to it, nursing mothers, neonates, and clients with lower respiratory tract symptoms. It is available in oral, parenteral, and topical preparations. In oral form diphenhydramine is available as 25- and 50-mg caplets and 50-mg capsules, 12.5-mg chewable tablets, as a 12.5-mg/5 mL elixir, as a 6.25/5-mL liquid, and in several combination products that contain other cough and cold medications. In parenteral form diphenhydramine is available as a 50-mg/mL injection. In topical form diphenhydramine is available as a 2 percent cream. It also is available in combination with several other drugs that are commonly given topically, such as calamine, camphor, and zinc oxide. These combination preparations are available as creams and lotions. The recommended dosages for the oral and injectable forms are given in the dosages table on p. 584.

PHARMACOKINETICS

Half-Life	Onset	Peak	Duration
2–7 hr	15–30 min	1–2 hr	4 hr

OTHER ANTIHISTAMINES

Brompheniramine and chlorpheniramine are other antihistamines commonly used alone or in combination with other drugs as OTC cough and cold preparations. Dimenhydrinate is commonly used in the treatment of motion sickness, radiation sickness, post-operative vomiting, and drug-induced nausea and vomiting. It also has been used for the vertigo and nausea associated with Ménière's syndrome. It is available as a chewable tablet that can be quickly absorbed for rapid onset of action, which is helpful in sudden-onset vertigo or motion sickness. Meclizine is available OTC. One of the most commonly used anti-emetic agents, promethazine, is an antihistamine. It is available in oral preparations and as an injection. Following is a listing of many of the antihistamine products still available in Canada, including the commonly recommended dosages and other pertinent information:

- **azatadine** Available by prescription as 1-mg tablets. The recommended dosage is 1 to 2 mg twice daily. It is also available in combination with pseudoephedrine. Pregnancy category B.
- **brompheniramine** Available as 2-mg/5 mL and 4-mg/5 mL elixirs and 05-mg/mL drops in combination with other cold medicines. These dosage forms may be obtained OTC. The recommended oral dosage is 4 to 8 mg 3 to 4 times daily. Pregnancy category C.
- **chlorpheniramine** Available as 4-, 8-, and 12-mg tablets and a 2.5-mg/5 mL syrup. There are numerous cough and cold combinations available OTC. The recommended oral dosage is 4 mg every 4 to 6 hours. Pregnancy category B.
- **clemastine** Available by prescription or OTC as a 1-mg tablet. The recommended oral adult dosage is 1 mg 1 to 3 times daily. Pregnancy category B.
- **cyproheptadine** Available as a 2-mg/5 mL syrup and as a 4-mg tablet. The usual adult dosage is 4 mg 3 to 4 times daily. Available OTC. Pregnancy category B.
- **dimenhydrinate** An OTC drug available as a 15- and 50-mg tablet and 50-mg capsule; 100-mg combined release tablet; 25-, 50-, and 100-mg suppository; 3-mg/mL syrup; and 15-mg/5 mL liquid. It is also available in a parenteral form of 50 mg/mL. The recommended oral adult dosage is 50 to 100 mg every 4 to 6 hours, taken half an hour before travel. The recommended dosage for 6- to 12-year-old children is 25 to 50 mg every 6 to 8 hours, taken half an hour before travel. Pregnancy category B.
- **hydroxyzine** The hydrochloride salt of hydroxyzine is known as Atarax. Hydroxyzine is considered a weak anxiolytic. It has sedative and mild anti-anxiety activity similar to that of diphenhydramine. It is a prescription-only drug and is available as 10-, 25-, and 50-mg capsules; a 2-mg/mL and 10-mg/5 mL syrup; and a 50-mg/mL injection. Pregnancy category C.
- **meclizine** Available as a 25-mg chewable tablet OTC. The recommended adult oral dosage is 25 to 50 mg, repeated once every 24 hours as needed. Pregnancy category B.
- **promethazine** A prescription drug available as 25- and 28.2-mg/mL injections, 10-mg/5 mL syrup, and 25- and 50-mg tablets. The recommended adult dosage is up to 25 mg every 4 to 6 hours. Pregnancy category C.

DECONGESTANTS

Nasal congestion is due to excessive nasal secretions and inflamed and swollen nasal mucosa. The primary causes of nasal congestion are allergies and URTIs, especially the common cold. There are three separate groups of nasal decongestants: **adrenergics (sympathomimetics)**, which are the largest group; **anticholinergics (parasympatholytics)**, which are somewhat less commonly used; and selected topical **corticosteroids** (intranasal steroids).

Nasal decongestants can be taken orally to produce a systemic effect, inhaled, or administered topically to the nose. Each method of administration has its advantages and disadvantages. Decongestants administered by the oral route include pseudoephedrine, which is available OTC. A commonly used nasal decongestant spray is phenylephrine, which is also OTC.

Agents administered by the oral route produce prolonged decongestant effects, but the onset of activity is more delayed and the effect less potent than those of decongestants applied topically. However, the clinical problem of rebound congestion associated with topically administered agents is almost non-existent with oral doses. Inhalation decongestants used orally included desoxyephedrine and propylhexedrine. These formulations are not available on the Canadian market. The inhaler that is available in Canada contains oxymetazoline, a sympathomimetic that is associated with rebound congestion.

The topical administration of adrenergics into the nasal passages produces a potent decongestant effect with a prompt onset of action. However, sustained use of these agents for several days can cause rebound congestion, which only exacerbates the condition. Decongestants suitable for nasal inhalation include the following:
- ephedrine
- oxymetazoline
- phenylephrine

Inhaled intranasal steroids and anticholinergic agents are not generally associated with rebound congestion and are often used prophylactically to prevent nasal congestion in clients with chronic upper respiratory symptoms. Commonly used intranasal steroids include the following:
- beclomethasone dipropionate
- budesonide
- flunisolide
- fluticasone
- triamcinolone

The only commonly used intranasal anticholinergic at this time is ipratropium nasal spray.

Mechanism of Action and Drug Effects

Nasal decongestants are most commonly used for their ability to shrink engorged nasal mucous membranes and relieve nasal stuffiness. Adrenergic agents (e.g., ephedrine, oxymetazoline) accomplish this by constricting the small arterioles that supply the structures of the upper respiratory tract, primarily the blood vessels surrounding the nasal sinuses. When these blood vessels are stimulated by alpha-adrenergic drugs, they constrict. Because sympathetic nervous system (SNS) stimulation produces the same effect, these agents are sometimes referred to as *sympathomimetics*. Once these blood vessels shrink, the nasal secretions in the swollen mucous membranes are better able to drain, either externally through the nostrils or internally through reabsorption into the bloodstream or lymphatic circulation.

Nasal steroids are aimed at the inflammatory response elicited by the invading organisms (viruses and bacteria) or antigens. The body responds by producing inflammation in an effort to isolate or "wall off" the area, and by attracting various cells of the immune system to consume and destroy the offending antigen(s). Steroids exert their anti-inflammatory effect by causing these cells to be turned off or rendered unresponsive. Intranasal steroids are also discussed in Chapter 36.

Indications

Nasal decongestants reduce the nasal congestion associated with acute or chronic rhinitis, the common cold, sinusitis, and hay fever or other allergies. They may also be used to reduce swelling of the nasal passages and to facilitate visualization of the nasal and pharyngeal membranes before surgery or diagnostic procedures.

Contraindications

Contraindications to the use of decongestants include drug allergy and, in the case of adrenergic drugs, narrow-angle glaucoma, uncontrolled cardiovascular disease, diabetes, thyroid dysfunction, and prostatitis.

Side Effects and Adverse Effects

Adrenergic agents are usually well tolerated. Possible adverse effects of these agents include nervousness, insomnia, palpitations, and tremor. The most common side effects of intranasal steroids are localized and include mucosal irritation and dryness.

Although topically applied adrenergic nasal decongestant can be absorbed into the bloodstream, the amount is usually too small to cause systemic effects in normal doses. However, excessive doses of these medications are more likely to cause systemic effects elsewhere in the body. These may include cardiovascular effects such as hypertension and palpitations and CNS effects such as headache, nervousness, and dizziness. These systemic effects are the result of alpha-adrenergic stimulation of the heart, blood vessels, and CNS.

Interactions

There are few significant drug interactions with the nasal decongestants. Systemic **sympathomimetic drugs** and sympathomimetic nasal decongestants are more likely to cause drug toxicity when given together. MAOIs may result in additive pressor (i.e., raising of blood pressure) effects when given with sympathomimetic nasal decongestants.

Dosages

For the recommended dosages of oxymetazoline, the only nasal decongestant profiled, see the dosages table on p. 588.

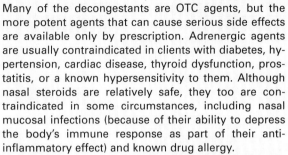

DRUG PROFILES

Many of the decongestants are OTC agents, but the more potent agents that can cause serious side effects are available only by prescription. Adrenergic agents are usually contraindicated in clients with diabetes, hypertension, cardiac disease, thyroid dysfunction, prostatitis, or a known hypersensitivity to them. Although nasal steroids are relatively safe, they too are contraindicated in some circumstances, including nasal mucosal infections (because of their ability to depress the body's immune response as part of their anti-inflammatory effect) and known drug allergy.

Steroids (e.g., beclomethasone, dexamethasone, and flunisolide) are discussed in greater detail in Chapter 36. The adrenergic agents such as oxymetazoline are discussed here. These are usually the first-line agents used in the treatment of nasal congestion because they are available OTC and are often intended for short-term symptom relief.

oxymetazoline

Oxymetazoline is chemically and pharmacologically similar to the other sympathomimetic agent xylometazoline. When these agents are administered intranasally, they cause dilated arterioles to constrict, thereby reducing nasal blood flow and congestion. During a cold, the blood vessels that surround the nasal sinus are usually dilated, swollen, and engorged with plasma, white blood cells, mast cells, histamines, and many other blood components that are involved in fighting infections of the respiratory tract. This swelling, or dilation, blocks the nasal passages, resulting in nasal congestion. Oxymetazoline and its chemically related cousins are classified as pregnancy category C agents and have the same contraindications as the other nasal decongestants. Nasally administered oxymetazoline is available as a 0.05 percent nasal solution and is meant to be instilled into each nostril. Common dosages for this agent are given in the dosages table on p. 588.

PHARMACOKINETICS

Half-Life	Onset	Peak	Duration
Unknown	5–10 min	Unknown	2–6 hr

ANTITUSSIVES

Coughing is a normal physiological function and serves the purpose of removing potentially harmful foreign substances and excessive secretions from the respiratory tract. The cough reflex is stimulated when receptors in the bronchi, alveoli, and pleura (lining of the lungs) are stretched. This causes a signal to be sent to the cough centre in the medulla of the brain, which in turn stimulates the cough. Although most of the time coughing is a beneficial response, there are times when it is not useful and may even be harmful (e.g., after a surgery such as hernia repair, or in cases of non-productive cough ["dry cough"]). In these situations, an antitussive agent may enhance client comfort and reduce respiratory distress.

DOSAGES **Selected Decongestant, Expectorant, and Antitussive Agents**

Agent	Pharmacological Class	Usual Dosage Range	Indication
codeine (as part of a combination product such as Dimetane-Expectorant-C, Dimetapp-C, CoActifed, Robitussin AC, others)	Opioid antitussive	*Adult and pediatric >12 yr* 20 mg q4h, max 120 mg/24 h *Pediatric 6– <12 yr* 10 mg q4h, max 60 mg/24 h *Pediatric 2–6 yr* 5 mg q4h, max 30 mg/24 h	Cough suppression
▸▸dextromethorphan (as part of a combination product such as Balminil DM, Benylin DM-E, Dimetapp DM, Robitussin-DM, others)	Non-opioid antitussive	*Adult and pediatric ≥12 yr* 30 mg q6h, max 120 mg/24 h *Pediatric 6–11 yr* 15 mg q6h, max 60 mg/24 h *Pediatric 2–6 yr* 7.5 mg q6h, max 30 mg/24 h	
▸▸guaifenesin [aka glyceryl guaiacolate] (Benylin E, Bismutal, Dimetane, Robitussin, others)	Expectorant	*Adult and pediatric ≥12 yr* 200 mg q6h *Pediatric 6– <12 yr* 100 mg q6h *Pediatric 2– <6 yr* 50 mg q6h	Relief of respiratory congestion, cough suppression
oxymetazoline	Alpha-adrenergic vasoconstrictor	*Adult and pediatric ≥6 yr* 0.05%, 2 or 3 sprays in each nostril q12h prn, usually for no more than 3–5 days; children 6–12: max 2 doses/24 h	Relief of nasal congestion

There are two main categories of antitussives: opioid and non-opioid.

Although all opioid agents have antitussive effects, only codeine and its semi-synthetic derivative hydrocodone are used as antitussives. Both agents are effective in suppressing the cough reflex and, if used in the prescribed manner, should not lead to dependency. The two drugs are usually incorporated into various combination dosage formulations with other respiratory drugs and are rarely used as single agents for the purpose of cough suppression.

Non-opioid antitussive drugs are less effective and are available either alone or in combination with other agents in an array of OTC cold and cough preparations. Dextromethorphan is the most widely used of these antitussive agents and is a derivative of the synthetic opioid levorphanol.

Mechanism of Action and Drug Effects

The opioid antitussives codeine and hydrocodone suppress the cough reflex through a direct action on the cough centre in the CNS (medulla). Opioid antitussives also provide analgesia and have a drying effect on the mucosa of the respiratory tract, which also increases the viscosity of respiratory secretions. This helps to reduce such symptoms as runny nose and post-nasal drip. The non-opioid cough suppressant dextromethorphan works in the same way. However, because it is not an opioid, it does not have analgesic properties, nor does it cause addiction or CNS depression. Another non-opioid antitussive is diphenhydramine.

Indications

Although they have other properties, such as the analgesic effect of opioid agents, antitussives are used primarily to stop the cough reflex when the cough is nonproductive and/or harmful.

Contraindications

The only absolute contraindication is drug allergy. Relative contraindications include use in opioid-dependent clients (for opioid antitussives) and use in clients at high risk for respiratory depression (e.g., frail geriatric clients). Such clients often are able to tolerate lower medication doses and still experience some symptom relief.

Side Effects and Adverse Effects

Following are the common side effects and adverse effects of selected antitussive agents:
• *codeine:* sedation, nausea, vomiting, lightheadedness, and constipation
• *dextromethorphan:* dizziness, drowsiness, and nausea
• *diphenhydramine:* sedation, dry mouth, and other anticholinergic effects
• *hydrocodone:* sedation, nausea, vomiting, lightheadedness, and constipation

Interactions

A few drug interactions are associated with opioid antitussives and dextromethorphan. Opioid antitussives (codeine and hydrocodone) may potentiate the effects of other opioids, general anaesthetics, tranquilizers, sedatives and hypnotics, tricyclic antidepressants (TCAs), MAOIs, alcohol, and other CNS depressants. Dextromethorphan may also potentiate the serotonergic effects of MAOIs and thus concurrent administration is contraindicated.

Dosages

For the recommended dosages of selected antitussive agents, see the dosages table on p. 588.

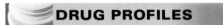
DRUG PROFILES

Antitussives come in many oral dosage forms and are available both with and without a prescription. Most of the narcotic antitussives are available only by prescription because of the associated abuse potential. Dextromethorphan is the most popular non-narcotic antitussive available OTC.

codeine

Codeine is a popular opioid antitussive agent. It is used in combination with many other respiratory medications to control coughs. Because it is an opioid it is potentially addictive and can depress respirations as part of its CNS depressant effects. For this reason codeine-containing cough suppressants are more tightly controlled (Controlled Drugs and Substances, Schedule I), but commonly available by prescription. These cough suppressants are available in many oral dosage forms: solutions, tablets, capsules, and suspensions. They are contraindicated in clients with a known hypersensitivity to opiates and in those suffering from respiratory depression, increased intracranial pressure, seizure disorders, or severe respiratory disorders. Pregnancy category C. Common dosages are listed in the table on p. 588.

PHARMACOKINETICS

Half-Life	Onset	Peak	Duration
2.9 hr (plasma)	30–60 min	1–2 hr	4–6 hr

▶▶ dextromethorphan

Dextromethorphan is a non-opioid antitussive that is available alone or in combination with many other cough and cold preparations. It is widely used because it is safe and non-addicting and does not cause respiratory or CNS depression. It is contraindicated in cases of drug allergy, asthma and emphysema, and persistent headache. Dextromethorphan is available as lozenges, a solution, liquid, suspension, liquid-filled capsules, freezer pops, granules, caplets, tablets (chewable, extended-release, and film-coated), and an extended-release syrup. Pregnancy category C. Common dosages are listed in the table on p. 588.

PHARMACOKINETICS

Half-Life	Onset	Peak	Duration
Unknown	15–30 min	Unknown	3–6 hr

EXPECTORANTS

Expectorants aid in the expectoration (i.e., coughing up and spitting out) of excessive mucus that has accumulated in the respiratory tract by disintegrating and thinning out the secretions. They are administered orally either as single agents or in combination with other drugs to facilitate the flow of respiratory secretions by reducing the viscosity of tenacious secretions. The actual clinical effectiveness of expectorants is highly questionable, however. Placebo-controlled clinical evaluations have failed to strongly confirm that expectorants reduce the viscosity of sputum. Despite this, expectorants are popular drugs and are contained in most OTC cold and cough preparations. The most common expectorant used in OTC products is guaifenesin (formerly known as *glyceryl guaiacolate*). Iodinated glycerol and potassium iodide are less commonly used and available only by prescription.

Mechanism of Action and Drug Effects

Expectorants work by one of two different mechanisms of action. The first is **reflex stimulation**: loosening and thinning of the respiratory tract secretions in response to a drug-induced irritation of the GI tract. The second is direct stimulation of the secretory glands in the respiratory tract. Iodine-containing products (iodinated glycerol and potassium iodide) are believed to work by this mechanism.

Indications

Expectorants are used for the relief of productive cough commonly associated with the common cold, bronchitis, laryngitis, pharyngitis, pertussis, influenza, and measles. They may also be used for the suppression of coughs caused by chronic paranasal sinusitis. By loosening and thinning sputum and the bronchial secretions, they may also indirectly diminish the tendency to cough.

Contraindications

Contraindications include drug allergy and possibly hyperkalemia (for potassium-containing expectorants).

Side Effects and Adverse Effects

The side effects and adverse effects of expectorants are minimal. The most common side effects of the individual expectorants are listed in Table 35-4.

Interactions

The drug interactions most commonly associated with expectorant use occur with the iodinated products. They may produce an additive or synergistic hypothyroid effect when used concurrently with lithium or antithyroid drugs. Their use with other potassium-containing drugs or potassium-sparing diuretics may

TABLE 35-4
EXPECTORANTS: REPORTED ADVERSE EFFECTS

Expectorant	Side/Adverse Effects
guaifenesin	Nausea, vomiting, gastric irritation
iodinated glycerol	GI irritation, rash, enlarged thyroid gland
potassium iodide	Iodism (iodine poisoning), nausea, vomiting, taste perversion

lead to the development of hyperkalemia, which can result in cardiac dysrhythmias or cardiac arrest.

Dosages

The recommended dosages of guaifenesin, the only expectorant profiled, are given in the dosages table on p. 588. See Appendix B for some of the common brands available in Canada.

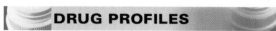

DRUG PROFILES

▶▶ *guaifenesin*

Guaifenesin is a commonly used expectorant that is available in several different oral dosage forms: capsules, tablets, solutions, and granules. It is used in the symptomatic management of coughs of varying origin. It is intended for the treatment of productive coughs by thinning difficult-to-cough-up mucus in the respiratory tract. There is little published pharmacokinetic data on guaifenesin, but its half-life is estimated at approximately 1 hour. Such a short half-life helps to explain why it is usually dosed several times throughout the day. Pregnancy category C. See the table on p. 588 for the common dosages.

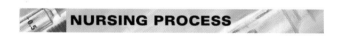

NURSING PROCESS

▌ Assessment

Assessment should begin with gathering data about the condition and/or allergic reaction for which the drug is indicated. For example, an allergic reaction to a drug, food, or substance may include signs and symptoms such as hives, wheezing or bronchospasm, tachycardia, or hypotension. The drug is selected based on the severity of the symptoms and the cause.

Before administering antihistamines the nurse must ensure that the client has no allergies to this group of medications, even though these drugs are used for allergic reaction. The antihistamines are contraindicated in clients suffering from an acute asthma attack and in those with lower respiratory tract disease. Cautious use, or close monitoring, should occur in clients with a history of increased intra-ocular pressure, cardiac or renal disease, hypertension, bronchial asthma, chronic obstructive pulmonary disease, peptic ulcer disease, convulsive disorders, or benign prostatic hypertrophy, and in pregnant women. Often these conditions may be exacerbated (worsened).

Most non-sedating antihistamines (e.g., fexofanadine, loratadine, desloratadine, and cetirizine) have the contraindication of hypersensitivity. However, there are specific contraindications to specific drugs. Fexofenadine is contraindicated in children under 12 years of age and in clients with renal impairment. Desloratadine is not recommended for children. Loratadine (OTC agent Claritin) should be avoided in children under 2 years of age. Cautious use of all these agents is called for in clients with impaired liver function or renal insufficiency and in breastfeeding women.

Before administering an antitussive agent, the nurse should assess the client for hypersensitivity to the agent and should also perform and document a respiratory and cough assessment. Decongestants may result in hypertension, palpitations, and CNS stimulation, and their use may be contraindicated in clients with disorders of these systems. Expectorants should be used with caution in geriatric and debilitated clients and in clients with asthma or respiratory insufficiency.

▌ Nursing Diagnoses

Nursing diagnoses appropriate for clients receiving any of the respiratory agents include the following:
- Impaired gas exchange related to the disorders affecting the respiratory system with increased congestion.
- Deficient knowledge related to the effective use of cold and other related products due to lack of information and client teaching.
- Risk for injury, falls, related to the sedating side effects of many of these respiratory agents (antihistamines, antitussives).

▌ Planning

Goals for clients receiving any of these respiratory agents include the following:
- Client states rationale for the use of antihistamine, expectorant, antitussive, or decongestant.
- Client states the side effects of medication.
- Client states the importance of adherence with therapy.
- Client identifies symptoms to report to the physician.
- Client states the importance of follow-up appointments with the physician.
- Client states relief of symptoms with treatment.

▌ *Outcome Criteria*

Outcome criteria pertaining to clients receiving any of these respiratory agents include the following:
- Client remains adherent with antihistamine therapy until symptoms are resolved or by physician's order.
- Client takes medications exactly as prescribed, no more and no less, to avoid complications of therapy and to experience maximal effectiveness.
- Client reports any of the following symptoms to the physician immediately: increase in cough, congestion, shortness of breath, chest pain, fever (oral temperature defined as >37°C; however, clinically a fever is usually 38°C), or any change in sputum production or colour (e.g., a change from clear to yellowish).
- Client reports resolution of symptoms and an improved health status.

▌ Implementation

Clients on antihistamines should take the medications as prescribed. Although taking antihistamines with meals slightly lowers absorption, it is generally advised because it minimizes GI upset. If clients complain of dry mouth they can suck on candy or chew gum, preferably sugarless, and perform frequent mouth care to ease the discomfort. OTC medications and other prescribed medications should not be taken with an antihistamine unless approved by the physician because of the serious drug interactions that can occur. Clients receiving any of the newer agents, such as non-sedating agents, should follow directions carefully for self-administration. A reduced dose at the initiation of therapy is recommended in clients with decreased renal functioning and in geriatric clients. Non-sedating H_1 receptor antagonist agents (antihistamines also) do not cross the blood–brain barrier as readily as do older antihistamines and are therefore less likely to cause sedation. They are generally well tolerated with minimal side effects. Clients taking any type of antihistamine should *always* be told to use caution while driving a car and participating in other activities that require mental alertness.

CASE STUDY

Asthma

A 13-year-old female, K.L., has had well-controlled asthma since 6 years of age. Her daily regimen consists of cromolyn sodium by nebulizer and inhaler. Loratadine has now been added to her treatment regimen. Since early spring she has been suffering from seasonal rhinitis. Her dose of loratadine is 10 mg once a day.
- What type of client education tips should you share with K.L. about loratadine?
- Why is it recommended that loratadine be given on an empty stomach?
- What directions should you give K.L. about taking loratadine in relation to mealtimes?

For answers see http://evolve.elsevier.com/Lilley/pharmacology/.

Clients taking expectorants should receive more fluids, unless contraindicated, to help loosen and liquefy secretions and to help with expectoration. Any cough or symptoms of fever should be reported to the physician.

Clients taking chewable or lozenge antitussive agents should avoid drinking fluids for 30 to 35 minutes after their use to prevent "washing away" their effect. Drowsiness or dizziness may occur with the use of antitussives; therefore clients should be cautioned against driving a car or participating in other activities that requires mental alertness until they feel back to normal.

Client teaching tips for these agents are presented in the box below.

■ Evaluation

A therapeutic response to respiratory agents would include a decrease in the symptoms of the condition for which they were prescribed. These include cough; congestion; nasal, salivary, and lacrimal gland hypersecretion; motion sickness; allergic rhinitis; PD (decrease in symptoms); and vertigo. Some of the antihistamines, such as diphenhydramine, are also helpful as a sleep aid, and a therapeutic response would be the successful induction of sleep. Non-sedating agents should result in a reduction of nasal congestion; sneezing; watery or red eyes; and itching of the nose, palate, and eyes. Adverse effects for which to monitor include excessive dry mouth, drowsiness, oversedation, dizziness (lightheadedness), paradoxical excitement, nervousness, dysrhythmias, palpitations, GI upset, urinary retention, fever, dyspnea, chest pain, palpitations, headache, or insomnia depending on the agent prescribed. (See Table 35-3 for other common side effects.)

CLIENT TEACHING TIPS

Clients should be educated thoroughly about the purpose of the medication, the expected side effects, and the drugs with which it interacts. Clients should be informed about the availability of newer, non-sedating antihistamines. The nurse should instruct clients on the following points:
- Report a fever (>38°C), cough, or other symptoms lasting longer than 1 week to your physician.
- Many drugs interact with other drugs, especially other cold products. Always check the package insert before taking any over-the-counter medication to make sure it doesn't interact with any other drug you're taking. Many over-the-counter products contain more than one active ingredient. You should be aware of all the drugs contained, and make sure none of them poses a problem for any conditions you may have or other drugs you may be taking.

Antihistamines
- Contact your healthcare provider if you become excessively sleepy, confused, or if you become dizzy and feel that you will faint.

Sedating Antihistamines, Antitussives
- Your medication may make you drowsy. If you find yourself becoming drowsy, do not drive a car, oper-

ate machinery, or do anything else requiring mental alertness.
- Do not drink alcohol or take other CNS depressants because this could increase the sedation.

Non-sedating Antihistamines
- Inform your physician and other healthcare providers (including dentists) that you are taking this medication.

Expectorants
- Drink plenty of fluids, unless you have been told otherwise; this will help get rid of secretions.

Decongestants
- For clients taking decongestants with cardiac and CNS stimulating effects: Don't drink coffee, tea, or cola, or use any other product containing caffeine while on this medication.

Antitussives
- Report to your physician a rash, a persistent headache or fever, or a cough that lasts longer than 1 week.
- If you are taking lozenges or chewable tablets, don't have anything to drink for 30 to 35 minutes after a dose to prevent "washing away" their effect.

POINTS to REMEMBER

▼ There are two types of histamine blockers: histamine₁ (H₁) blockers and histamine₂ (H₂) blockers:
- H₁ blockers are the agents most people are referring to when they use the term *antihistamine*. H₁ blockers prevent the harmful effects of histamine and are used to treat seasonal allergic rhinitis, anaphylaxis, reactions to insect bites, and so forth.
- H₂ blockers are used to treat gastric acid disorders, such as hyperacidity or ulcer disease.

▼ Non-sedating antihistamines are not associated with the sedating effect that most antihistamines have but have other bothersome (but not severe) side effects such as dry mouth.

▼ Decongestants consist of adrenergics and corticosteroids. Most of the drugs in this group are adrenergic drugs, such as pseudoephedrine and phenylephrine, and work by stimulating engorged and swollen blood vessels in the sinuses to constrict, which decreases pressure and allows mucous membranes to drain.

▼ Antitussives are used to stop or reduce coughing and may be either opioid (e.g., codeine, hydrocodone) or non-opioid (e.g., dextromethorphan) agents.

▼ Expectorants aid in the expectoration or removal of mucus and work by thinning and reducing the viscosity of secretions.

▼ Guaifenesin is believed to work by irritating the GI tract, causing reflex stimulation of the respiratory tract, resulting in expectoration of mucus.

▼ Clients should avoid consuming alcohol and taking other CNS depressants while they are taking antihistamines.

▼ A general warning for safe administration of antihistamines, decongestants, antitussives, and expectorants (especially the OTC and combination products): clients may not be aware of all ingredients in these products, including other drugs such as acetaminophen, acetylsalicylic acid, non-steroidal anti-inflammatory drugs (NSAIDs), and pseudoephedrine hydrochloride (a sympathomimetic).

EXAMINATION REVIEW QUESTIONS

1. H₁-blockers are indicated for which of the following?
   a. Tachycardia
   b. Urinary retention
   c. Ulcer disease
   d. Allergic rhinitis
2. Decongestants that have beta-stimulating effects may also result in which of the following side effects?
   a. Fever
   b. Bradycardia
   c. Hypertension
   d. CNS depression
3. Antihistamines have which of the following therapeutic effects?
   a. Prevention of the constriction of blood vessels in the nasal mucosa.
   b. Prevention of increased vascular permeability in the eyes.
   c. Stimulation of salivary, gastric, lacrimal, and bronchial secretions.
   d. Ability to bind to histamine receptors and prevent histamine release.
4. Which of the following actions are antitussives used for?
   a. Stopping or reducing coughing
   b. Constricting the blood vessels and relieving congestion
   c. Blocking the effects of histamine on the blood vessels
   d. Aiding in the removal of mucus by reducing the viscosity of respiratory secretions
5. The binding of H₁ blockers to the unoccupied receptors prevents which of the following?
   a. Vasodilation
   b. Leukopenic infiltration
   c. Decreased capillary permeability
   d. Diminished GI secretions

For answers see http://evolve.elsevier.com/Lilley/pharmacology/.

CRITICAL THINKING ACTIVITIES

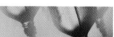

1. Why should antihistamines be used with caution in asthmatic clients?
2. Discuss the problem of rebound congestion when overusing nasal spray decongestants. Does this phenomenon also occur with oral decongestants? Explain your answer.
3. What additional nursing interventions would be helpful for an older client without major medical problems who is taking guaifenesin?

For answers see http://evolve.elsevier.com/Lilley/pharmacology/.

BIBLIOGRAPHY

Albanese, J., & Nutz, P. (2005). *Mosby's 2005 nursing drug cards.* St Louis, MO: Mosby.

Canadian Pharmacists Association. (2003). *Therapeutic choices* (4th ed.). Ottawa, ON: Author.

Canadian Pharmacists Association. (2004). *Guide to drugs in Canada.* Toronto, ON: Dorling Kindersley.

Canadian Pharmacists Association. (2005). *Compendium of pharmaceuticals and specialties. The Canadian drug reference for health professionals.* Ottawa, ON: Author. [The subscription-based e-CPS is available at http://www.pharmacists.ca.]

Cheng, A., Williams, B.A., & Sivarajan, B.V. (Eds.). (2003). *The HSC handbook of pediatrics* (10th ed.). Toronto, ON: Elsevier.

Facts and Comparisons. (2004). *Drug facts and comparisons pocket version* (9th ed.). St Louis, MO: Wolters Kluwer Health.

Hardman, J.G., & Limbird, L.E. (2002). *Goodman and Gilman's the pharmacological basis of therapeutics* (10th ed.). New York: McGraw-Hill.

Health Canada. (2005). Drug product database (DPD). Retrieved August 24, 2005, from http://www.hc-sc.gc.ca/hpb/drugs-dpd/

Fetrow, C.W., & Avila, J.R. (2000). *The complete guide to herbal remedies.*, Springhouse, PA: Springhouse.

Katzung, B.G. (2004). *Basic and clinical pharmacology* (9th ed.). New York: McGraw-Hill.

Lehne, R.A. (2004). *Pharmacology for nursing care* (5th ed.). St Louis, MO: Saunders.

Mosby. (2005). *Mosby's drug consult 2005: The comprehensive reference for generic and brand name drugs* (15th ed.). St Louis, MO: Mosby.

Sampson, W. (2005). Echinacea doesn't help children's colds. *The New England Journal of Medicine, 353,* 337–339.

Skidmore-Roth, L. (2006). *Mosby's 2006 nursing drug reference* (19th ed.). St Louis, MO: Mosby.

CHAPTER

36 Bronchodilators and Other Respiratory Agents

OBJECTIVES

After reading this chapter, the successful student will be able to do the following:

1 Describe the anatomy and physiology of the respiratory system.

2 Discuss the impact of respiratory agents on various lower and upper respiratory tract diseases.

3 List the various classifications of drugs, with specific examples, indicated for the treatment of lower and upper respiratory tract diseases as well as acute and chronic respiratory diseases.

4 Discuss the mechanisms of action, indications, contraindications, cautions, dosages, routes of administration, side effects, and toxic effects associated with the bronchodilators and other respiratory agents.

5 Explain the nursing process as it relates to a nursing care plan for the client receiving bronchodilators or other respiratory agents.

e-LEARNING ACTIVITIES

Student CD-ROM
- Review Questions: see questions 271–285
- Animations
- Medication Administration Checklists
- IV Therapy Checklists

evolve Web site (http://evolve.elsevier.com/Lilley/pharmacology/)
- Online Chapter Worksheet • Frequently Asked Questions
- Learning Tips and Content Updates • WebLinks • Online Appendices and Supplements • Mosby/Saunders ePharmacology Update • Access to *Mosby's Drug Consult*

DRUG PROFILES

▶▶**beclomethasone dipropionate**, p. 606
▶▶**epinephrine and ephedrine**, p. 601
    fluticasone, p. 607
    isoproterenol, p. 601
▶▶**montelukast**, p. 604

    nedocromil, p. 609
▶▶**salbutamol**, p. 601
    salmeterol, p. 602
    sodium cromoglygate, p. 608
▶▶**theophylline**, p. 599
    zafirlukast, p. 605

▶▶ Key drug.

GLOSSARY

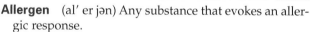

Allergen (al′ er jən) Any substance that evokes an allergic response.

Alveoli (al′ vee oe′ lee) Microscopic sacs in the lungs where oxygen is exchanged for carbon dioxide; also called *air sacs*.

Antibody (an′ tee bod ee) An immunoglobulin produced by lymphocytes in response to bacteria, viruses, or other antigenic substances.

Antigen (an′ ti jən) A substance (usually a protein) that causes the formation of an antibody and reacts specifically with that antibody.

Asthma (az′ muh) A chronic inflammatory disorder characterized by edema, mucus production, and airway inflammation.

Asthma attack The onset of wheezing together with difficulty breathing.

Bronchial asthma (brong′ kee əl) Recurrent and reversible shortness of breath resulting from narrowing of the bronchi and bronchioles.

Bronchodilators Medications that improve airflow by relaxing bronchial smooth muscle cells (e.g., xanthines, adrenergic agonists).

594

Chronic bronchitis (brong ky' tis) Chronic inflammation of the bronchi.

Emphysema (em' fə zee' muh) A condition of the lungs resulting from enlargement of the air spaces distal to the bronchioles.

Immunoglobulin (im' yoo no glob' yoo lin) Any of five structurally and antigenically distinct antibodies present in the serum and external secretions of the body.

Lower respiratory tract (LRT) The division of the respiratory system composed of organs located almost entirely within the chest.

Mast cell stabilizers Drugs such as sodium cromoglygate and nedocromil that stabilize the membranes of cells that normally release endogenous bronchoconstricting substances.

Status asthmaticus (sta' təs az mat' ik əs) A prolonged asthma attack.

Sympathomimetic bronchodilators A group of drugs with beta$_2$-receptor agonist activity in the lungs commonly used during the acute phase of an asthmatic attack to quickly reduce airway constriction and restore normal airflow; also called *beta-agonists* and *beta-adrenergic agonists*.

Upper respiratory tract (URT) The division of the respiratory system composed of organs located outside the chest cavity (thorax).

The main function of the respiratory system is to deliver oxygen to the cells that make up the body and then to remove carbon dioxide from these cells. To perform this deceptively simple task requires an intricate system of tissues, muscles, and organs called the *respiratory system*. It consists of two divisions, or tracts: the upper and lower respiratory tracts. The **upper respiratory tract (URT)** is composed of the structures that are located outside the chest cavity (thorax). These are the nose, nasopharynx, oropharynx, laryngopharynx, and larynx. The **lower respiratory tract (LRT)** is located almost entirely within the chest and is composed of the trachea, all segments of the bronchial tree, and the lungs. The URT and LRT have four main accessory structures that aid in their overall function. These are the oral cavity (mouth), the rib cage, the muscles of the rib cage (intercostal muscles), and the diaphragm. The URT and LRT together with the accessory structures make up the respiratory system, and they are in constant communication with each other as they perform the vital function of respiration and the exchange of oxygen for carbon dioxide.

The air we breathe is a mixture of many gases. During inhalation, oxygen molecules from the air diffuse across semi-permeable membranes of the **alveoli**, where they are exchanged for carbon dioxide molecules, which are exhaled. The lungs also filter, warm, and humidify the air we breathe. The oxygen is then delivered to the cells by the blood vessels that make up the circulatory system. It is here that the respiratory system "hands off" the oxygen it has extracted from inhaled air to the hemoglobin in red blood cells (RBCs). It is also here that the cellular metabolic waste product carbon dioxide is collected from the

tissues by the RBCs. This waste is then transported back to the lungs via the circulatory system, where it diffuses back across the alveolar membranes before being exhaled into the air. Other important functions of the respiratory system are speech, smell, and regulation of pH (acid–base balance).

DISEASES OF THE RESPIRATORY SYSTEM

Several diseases impair the function of the respiratory system. Those that affect the URT include colds, rhinitis, and hay fever. These and the agents used to treat them are discussed in Chapter 35. The major diseases that impair the function of the LRT include asthma, **emphysema,** and **chronic bronchitis**. The one feature these diseases have in common is that they all involve the obstruction of airflow through the airways. Chronic obstructive pulmonary disease (COPD) is the name applied collectively to emphysema and chronic bronchitis because the obstruction is relatively constant. Asthma that is persistent and present most of the time despite treatment is also considered a COPD. Cystic fibrosis and infant respiratory distress syndrome are other disorders that affect the LRT, but because their treatment is primarily non-pharmacological, they are not discussed here.

ASTHMA

Bronchial asthma is defined as a recurrent and reversible shortness of breath and occurs when the airways of the lung (bronchi and bronchioles) become narrow as a result of bronchospasm, inflammation and edema of the bronchial mucosa, and the production of viscid mucus. The alveolar ducts and alveoli distal to the bronchioles remain open, but the obstruction to the airflow in the airways prevents carbon dioxide from getting out of the air spaces and oxygen from getting into them. Wheezing, coughing, chest tightness, and difficulty breathing are the symptoms, and when an episode has a sudden and dramatic onset, it is referred to as an **asthma attack**. Most asthma attacks are short, and normal breathing is subsequently recovered. However, an asthma attack may be prolonged for several minutes to hours and not respond to typical drug therapy. This is a condition known as **status asthmaticus**. Hospitalization is often required. Among people with asthma, 50 percent have onset before the age of 10 and another 30 percent before the age of 40.

Asthma is not a disease but a symptom complex with many different etiologies and a number of predisposing, causal, and contributing risk factors. Asthma tends to run in families. Environmental triggers such as a viral infection, allergens, and pollutants are thought to interact with a hereditary predisposition to produce disease. Asthma occurs in approximately 10 percent of the Canadian pediatric population and 12.5 percent of the population older than 12 years of age. Asthma prevalence is increasing, especially among adult women.

Asthma is now considered a chronic inflammatory disorder characterized by edema, mucus production, and airway inflammation. An **allergen** is any substance that elicits an allergic reaction. The offending allergens are substances such as dust, mould, pollen, and animal dander, which are present in the environment throughout the year. Cigarette smoking or exposure to secondhand smoke is another common allergen. Exposure to the offending allergen causes an immediate reaction called the *early-phase response.* This is mediated by hypersensitive antibodies already present in the client's body that sense the allergen to be a foreign substance, or **antigen**. The **antibody** in asthma sufferers is usually **immunoglobulin** E (IgE), which is one of the five types of antibodies in the body (the others are IgG, IgA, IgM, and IgD). On exposure to the allergen, the client's body responds by mounting an immediate and potent antigen–antibody reaction. This reaction occurs on the surface of cells such as mast cells, which are rich in histamines, leukotrienes (LTs), and other mediators, and stimulates the release of inflammatory mediators. This in turn triggers the mucosal swelling and bronchoconstriction that are characteristic of an allergic asthma attack. The early-phase response lasts approximately one hour. The sequence of events in early-phase response is listed in Box 36-1.

Approximately 50 percent of clients with asthma experience a *late-phase response,* four to six hours after the initial response. It is thought that the mediators produced in the early-phase response attract additional inflammatory mediators, especially leukotrienes, which create a self-sustaining cycle of inflammation and obstruction. The clinical symptoms are the same as during the early phase. As a result of the inflammation, airways become sensitized or hyperresponsive such that subsequent episodes of asthma may be triggered not only by allergens but by respiratory stimuli such as strong odours, cold weather, and strenuous work or exercise. The risk factors that contribute to the etiology of asthma and their most likely causes are summarized in Table 36-1.

The National Asthma Task Force and the Canadian Asthma Consensus Group have established guidelines for the diagnosis and management of asthma, published in 2000 and 1999, respectively. The Global Initiative for Asthma (GINA) is an initiative between the U.S. National Heart, Lung, and Blood Institute, the NIH, and the World Health Organization (WHO) to reduce world asthma prevalence, morbidity, and mortality. Based on these guidelines, drugs are no longer classified as either anti-inflammatory or bronchodilator medications but as long-term control and quick-relief medications. The specific agents in each classification are listed in Box 36-2. The guidelines advocate a stepwise treatment approach (see Table 36-2 and Figure 36-1) and an individualized action plan.

CHRONIC BRONCHITIS

Chronic bronchitis is a continuous inflammation of the bronchi, although it is actually inflammation of the bronchioles that obstructs airflow. Manifestations must continue for at least three months of the year for two consecutive years to be defined as chronic bronchitis. Chronic bronchitis involves the excessive secretion of mucus and certain pathological changes in the bronchial structure. The disease can arise as the result of repeated

TABLE 36-1
ETIOLOGY OF ASTHMA

Factors	Most Likely Cause
Predisposing	Atopy (inherited allergic reaction), gender, genetics
Causal	Indoor allergens: dust, dander, cockroach, mould; outdoor allergens: pollens, fungi; occupational sensitizers
Contributing	Respiratory infections, air pollution, smoking, low income

BOX 36-1
Sequence of Events in Early-Phase Response of Asthma

- The offending allergen provokes the production of hypersensitive antibodies (most commonly IgE) that are specific to the allergen. This immunological response initiates client sensitivity.
- The IgE antibodies are homocytotrophic (that is, they have an affinity for similar cells) and collect on the surface of mast cells and basophils, thus sensitizing the client to the allergen.
- Subsequent allergen contact provokes the antigen–antibody reaction on the surface of mast cells.
- Mast cell integrity is then violated, and these cells release chemical mediators. They also synthesize and then release other chemical mediators. These mediators include bradykinin, eosinophil chemotactic factor of anaphylaxis (ECF-A), histamine, prostaglandins, and slow-reacting substance of anaphylaxis (SRS-A).
- The released chemical mediators, especially histamine and SRS-A, trigger the bronchial constriction and the asthma attack.

BOX 36-2
Classifications of Agents Used to Treat Asthma

Long-Term Control
antileukotriene agents
sodium cromoglycate
inhaled steroids
ipratropium
long-acting beta$_2$-agonists
nedocromil
theophylline

Quick-Relief
intravenous systemic corticosteroids
short-acting inhaled beta$_2$-agonists

episodes of acute bronchitis or in the context of chronic generalized diseases. It is usually precipitated by prolonged exposure to bronchial irritants. One of the most common is cigarette smoke. Some clients acquire the disease by other predisposing factors such as viral or bacterial pulmonary infections during childhood. Others may have mild impairment of the ability to inactivate proteolytic enzymes, which then damage the airway mucosal tissues. Unknown genetic characteristics may be responsible as well.

EMPHYSEMA

In emphysema, alveolar walls are destroyed and air spaces enlarged. This appears to stem from the effect of proteolytic enzymes released from leukocytes in the setting of alveolar inflammation. The partial destruction of alveolar walls reduces the surface area where oxygen and carbon dioxide are exchanged, thus impairing effective respiration. As with chronic bronchitis, smoking appears to be the primary precipitant of the underlying inflammation. There is also an associated genetic component in some people known as *alpha-antitrypsin deficiency*.

TABLE 36-2

STEPWISE APPROACH TO THE MANAGEMENT OF ASTHMA

Step	Drug Classification
Step 1: Mild intermittent	Short-acting inhaled beta$_2$-agonists prn
Step 2: Mild persistent	Sodium cromoglygate or nedocromil (particularly in children) and low-dose inhaled corticosteroids (preferred) plus short-acting inhaled beta$_2$-agonists prn Theophylline and antileukotriene agents considered second line
Step 3: Moderate persistent	Medium-dose inhaled corticosteroids Long-acting bronchodilator (salmeterol preferred) Short-acting inhaled beta$_2$-agonists prn
Step 4: Severe persistent	High-dose inhaled corticosteroids Long-acting bronchodilators Systemic corticosteroids Short-acting inhaled beta$_2$-agonists prn

TREATMENT OF DISEASES OF THE LOWER RESPIRATORY TRACT

In the past, the treatment of asthma and other COPDs focused primarily on drugs that cause airways to dilate. Now there is a greater understanding of the pathophysiology of asthma. The emphasis of research has shifted from the bronchoconstriction component of the disease to the inflammatory component. The role played by inflammatory cells and their mediators has become just as important as the bronchoconstriction component of the disease.

Classes of anti-asthmatic agents include beta-adrenergic agonists, selected anticholinergics, xanthine derivatives or theophyllines, corticosteroids, and indirect-acting anti-asthmatic drugs such as cromoglycate and nedocromil sodium. The antileukotriene agents include two LT receptor antagonists (LTRAs), zafirlukast and montelukast.

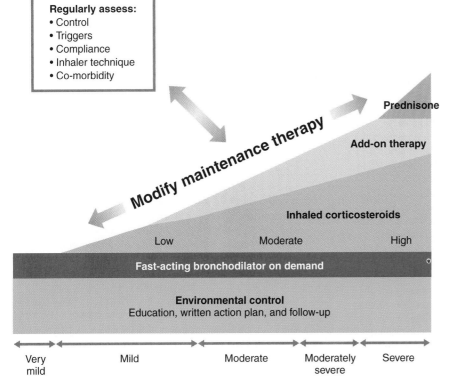

FIG. 36-1 Continuum of treatments for asthma management. (Reprinted with permission from A. Becker, W. Watson, A. Ferguson, H. Dimich-Ward, and M. Chan-Yeung (2004). The Canadian asthma primary prevention study: Outcomes at 2 years of age. *Journal of Allergy and Clinical Immunology, 113*, 650–656.)

A synopsis of how these agents work is provided in Table 36-3.

BRONCHODILATORS

Bronchodilator drugs are an important part of the pharmacotherapy for all COPDs. They are able to relax bronchial smooth muscle bands to dilate the bronchi and bronchioles that are narrowed as a result of the disease process. There are two classes of such agents: xanthine derivatives and beta-agonists.

XANTHINE DERIVATIVES (ALSO CALLED XANTHINES)

The natural xanthines consist of the plant alkaloids caffeine, theobromine, and theophylline, but only theophylline and its chemical derivatives are used as bronchodilators. Caffeine is primarily used as a central nervous system (CNS) stimulant (analeptic) and theobromine as a diuretic. Besides theophylline, which occurs in various salt forms, the other xanthine bronchodilators used clinically for the treatment of bronchoconstriction are aminophylline and oxtriphylline.

Because of their relatively slow onset of action, xanthines are used more for the prevention of asthmatic symptoms than for the relief of acute asthma attacks. They are also used as bronchodilators in the symptomatic treatment of the asthma and reversible bronchospasm that may occur in clients with chronic bronchitis or emphysema. Aminophylline is used in clients with status asthmaticus who have not responded to fast-acting beta-agonists such as epinephrine.

Mechanism of Action and Drug Effects

The mechanisms of action of theophylline and its chemical derivatives are similar. They all cause bronchodilation by increasing the levels of the energy-producing substance cyclic adenosine monophosphate (cAMP). They do this by competitively inhibiting phosphodiesterase (PDE), the enzyme responsible for breaking down cAMP. cAMP plays an integral role in the maintenance of open airways in clients with COPD because the level of its intracellular concentration determines smooth muscle relaxation and the inhibition of the IgE-induced release of the chemical mediators (histamine, slow-reacting substance of anaphylaxis [SRS-A], and others) that are responsible for causing an allergic reaction. An accumulation of cAMP therefore causes the constricted airways of the lung to dilate, relieving bronchospasm and allowing greater airflow into and out of the lungs. Xanthines also have other beneficial effects. They stimulate the CNS (though to a lesser degree than caffeine, another xanthine) thus directly stimulating the medullary respiratory centre. In large doses, theophylline and its derivatives may stimulate the cardiovascular system, resulting in both an increased force of contraction (positive inotrope) and an increased heart rate (positive chronotrope). The increased force of contraction increases cardiac output and hence blood flow to the kidneys. This, in combination with the ability of the xanthines

TABLE 36-3
MECHANISMS OF ANTI-ASTHMATIC DRUG ACTION

Anti-Asthmatic	Mechanism in Asthma Relief
Anticholinergics	Block cholinergic receptors, thus preventing the binding of cholinergic substances that cause constriction and increase secretions
Antileukotriene agents	Modify or inhibit the activity of leukotrienes, which decreases arachidonic-acid-induced inflammation and allergen-induced bronchoconstriction
Beta-agonists and xanthine derivatives	Raise intracellular levels of cyclic adenosine monophosphate (cAMP), which in turn produces smooth muscle relaxation and dilates the constricted bronchi and bronchioles
Corticosteroids	Prevent the inflammation commonly provoked by the substances released from mast cells
Mast cell stabilizers (sodium cromoglygate and nedocromil)	Stabilize the cell membranes in which the antigen–antibody reactions take place (the mast cell), thereby preventing the release of substances such as histamine that cause constriction

PEDIATRIC CONSIDERATIONS
Respiratory Agents

- Bronchodilators are often used in pediatric clients, but they should be used with *extreme caution*. The nurse must monitor for adverse effects such as tremors, restlessness, GI tract upset, hallucinations, dizziness, palpitations, and tachycardia.
- Xanthine derivatives should be used cautiously in pediatric clients, with extremely close monitoring of the blood levels and response to the medication; CNS- and cardiovascular-stimulating effects may be enhanced in children.
- Cromoglycate should be used for children only if the child and/or parent or caregiver can accurately demonstrate the correct use of the nebulizer and how to care for the equipment. Either child or parent must also be capable of monitoring for the adverse effects. Long-acting dosage forms are not recommended for children under the age of 6 years. Once-a-day dosage forms have not been established for children under the age of 12 years. Year-round therapy is important to adequately prevent asthma attacks. Nedocromil, another preventive agent (like sodium cromoglygate), is taken year-round. The safety and efficacy of nedocromil for children under the age of 3 years has not been established.
- A daily action plan should be kept documenting the date, time, drug used, signs and symptoms, and peak flow meter results. This will help determine the client's adherence with the regimen and the presence of therapeutic effects.

to dilate blood vessels in and around the kidney, increases the glomerular filtration rate, resulting in a diuretic effect.

Indications

Theophylline and the other xanthine derivatives are used to dilate the airways in clients with asthma, chronic bronchitis, or emphysema. They may be used in mild to moderate cases of acute asthma and as an adjunct agent in the management of COPD.

Contraindications

Contraindications to xanthine derivative therapy include drug allergy, uncontrolled cardiac dysrhythmias and seizure disorders, hyperthyroidism, and peptic ulcers.

Side Effects and Adverse Effects

The common side effects of the xanthine derivatives include nausea, vomiting, headache, and anorexia. In addition, gastroesophageal reflux has been observed during sleep. Cardiac side effects include sinus tachycardia, extrasystole, palpitations, and ventricular dysrhythmias but are usually associated with toxicity. Induced vomiting is not recommended for overdose and toxicity of xanthine derivatives because of the risk of sudden onset seizures. Activated charcoal should be administered as soon as possible.

Interactions

The use of xanthine derivatives with any of the following agents causes the serum level of the xanthine derivative to be increased: allopurinol, beta-blockers, calcium channel blockers, cimetidine, alpha interferon, erythromycin, mexiletine, propaferone, flu vaccine, and oral contraceptives. Their use with sympathomimetics, or even caffeine, can produce additive cardiac and CNS stimulation. St. John's wort (hypericum) is also reported to increase the rate of xanthine metabolism, presumably by enhancing the activity of liver enzymes. Thus higher doses of theophylline and other xanthine derivatives may be needed in clients using this popular herbal preparation. Cigarette smoking has a similar effect because of the enzyme-inducing effect of nicotine.

Dosages

For the recommended dosages of selected theophylline salts, see the table below. See Appendix B for some of the common brands available in Canada.

GERIATRIC CONSIDERATIONS

- Xanthine derivatives should be given cautiously with careful monitoring in geriatric clients because of their increased sensitivity to these drugs (due to decreased drug metabolism).
- With xanthines it is important to assess geriatric clients for signs of toxicity: restlessness, insomnia, irritability, tremors, nausea, and vomiting. Be careful to assess restlessness and its cause because it may be from hypoxia or from medication side effects.
- Inform geriatric clients not to chew or crush sustained-released forms; to be careful of drug interactions, especially with the use of other asthma-related drugs or bronchodilators; and to take their medication at the same time every day.
- Encourage geriatric clients to never omit or double up on doses. If they miss a dose they should contact their physician or healthcare provider for further instructions on dosing. Serum levels of the drug should be monitored to avoid possible toxicity and to make sure blood levels are therapeutic.
- Lower doses in the elderly may be necessary initially and possibly throughout therapy, with close monitoring for adverse effects and toxicity (cardiovascular and CNS stimulation).

DRUG PROFILES

▶▶ theophylline

Theophylline is one of the most commonly used of all the bronchodilators. It is used most commonly in the treatment of chronic respiratory disorders but may also be used for the relief of mild to moderate acute asthmatic attacks. Theophylline is available in oral, rectal, and parenteral dosage forms, but only with a prescription. These various preparations are listed in Table 36-4.

Theophylline is contraindicated in clients with a known hypersensitivity to xanthines and in clients with tachyarrhythmias. Its beneficial effects can be maximized by maintaining levels in the blood within a certain target range. If these levels become too high, many adverse effects can occur. If the levels become too low the client receives little therapeutic benefit. Although

DOSAGES Theophylline Salts

Agent	Pharmacological Class	Usual Dosage Range	Indications
aminophylline	Xanthine-derived bronchodilator	*Pediatric 6 mo–16 yr* IV: 0.2–0.9 mg/kg/h continuous infusion *Adult* IV: 0.7 mg/kg/h continuous infusion	Asthma
▶▶ theophylline	Xanthine-derived bronchodilator	*Adult & Pediatric <1yr** 16 mg/kg/day to max 400 mg/day in 3–4 divided doses	

*The dosage schedules and dosage forms used vary widely with age and clinical status.

the optimal level may vary from client to client, the common therapeutic range for theophylline in the blood is usually 55 to 110 μmol/L. The Canadian asthma consensus guidelines recommend that a serum concentration of 28 to 55 μmol/L will reduce side effects without loss of therapeutic benefit. Laboratory monitoring of drug blood levels is common to ensure adequate dosage, especially in the hospital setting. Aminophylline is simply a theophylline pro-drug that is 79 percent theophylline. It is often used for intravenous (IV) administration of xanthine derivative therapy in the hospital setting. Pregnancy category C. The commonly recommended dosages of both theophylline and aminophylline are given in the table on p. 599.

PHARMACOKINETICS

Half-Life	Onset	Peak	Duration
7–9 hr*	Unknown	1–2 hr	Varies with dosage form

*In healthy adults

BETA-ADRENERGIC AGONISTS

Beta-agonists are a large group of drugs that are commonly used during the acute phase of an asthmatic attack to quickly reduce airway constriction and restore airflow to normal. They are agonists or stimulators of the sympathetic nervous system (SNS) receptors (beta- and alpha-adrenergic receptors are discussed in depth in Part Three). These drugs imitate the effects of norepinephrine on these receptors. For this reason they are also called **sympathomimetic bronchodilators**. For a beta-agonist to dilate the airways it must stimulate the beta$_2$-adrenergic receptors located throughout the lungs. When these receptors are stimulated the constricted airways dilate; conversely, a non-specific beta-antagonist would cause the airways to constrict.

Beta-agonists, or sympathomimetic bronchodilators, are categorized according to the specific receptors they stimulate:

1 Non-selective adrenergic drugs, which stimulate the alpha, beta$_1$ (cardiac), and beta$_2$ (respiratory) receptors. Example: epinephrine.

2 Non-selective beta-adrenergic drugs, which stimulate both beta$_1$- and beta$_2$-receptors. Example: isoproterenol.

3 Selective beta$_2$ drugs, which primarily stimulate the beta$_2$-receptors. Example: salbutamol.

These drugs can also be categorized according to the route of administration as oral, parenteral, or inhalation agents. The various beta-agonist bronchodilators are listed in Table 36-5.

Mechanism of Action and Drug Effects

The bronchioles are surrounded by smooth muscle. If this smooth muscle contracts, the airways are narrowed and the amount of oxygen and carbon dioxide exchanged is reduced. The mechanism of action of beta-agonist bronchodilators begins at the specific receptor stimulated and ends with the dilation of the airways, but many reactions must take place at the cellular level for this bronchodilation to occur. When a beta$_2$-adrenergic receptor is stimulated by a beta-agonist, adenylate cyclase, an enzyme needed to make cAMP, is activated. The increased levels of cAMP made available by adenylate cyclase cause bronchial smooth muscles to relax, which results in bronchial dilation and increased airflow into and out of the lungs.

Non-selective adrenergic agonist drugs such as epinephrine also stimulate alpha-adrenergic receptors, causing vasoconstriction. This vasoconstriction reduces the amount of edema or swelling in the mucous membranes and limits the quantity of secretions normally secreted from these membranes. Such drugs also stimulate beta$_1$-receptors, resulting in cardiac side effects such as an increased heart rate and force of contraction. Thus adrenergic agonists with selectivity for the beta$_2$-receptors, such as salbutamol, are usually the best choice when only pulmonary effects are desired.

Drugs such as salbutamol that predominantly stimulate the beta$_2$-receptors have more specific drug effects. By predominantly stimulating the beta$_2$-adrenergic receptors of the bronchial, uterine, and vascular smooth muscles, they cause bronchodilation as one of the desirable effects. They may also have a dilating effect on the peripheral vasculature, resulting in a decrease in diastolic blood pressure (BP). Additionally, the beta$_2$-stimulants are thought to stimulate the Na^+/K^+-adenosinetriphosphatase (ATPase) cell membrane ion pump. This facilitates a temporary shift of potassium ions from the bloodstream into the cells, resulting in a

TABLE 36-4
AVAILABLE THEOPHYLLINE PREPARATIONS

Dosage Form	Strengths
ORAL	
Solution	80 mg/15 mL; 50 and 100 mg/5 mL; 10 mg/mL
Tablets	100, 200, and 300 mg
Extended-release tablets	100, 200, 225, 300, 350, 400, and 600 mg
PARENTERAL (AS AMINOPHYLLINE AND THEOPHYLLINE)*	
Injection	25 and 50 mg/mL (aminophylline) 0.8 and 0.16 mg/mL (theophylline)
RECTAL (AS AMINOPHYLLINE)*	
Suppository	250 and 500 mg

*Aminophylline = 79% theophylline.

TABLE 36-5
BETA-AGONIST BRONCHODILATORS

Drug	Type	Route of Administration
salbutamol	Beta$_2$	PO, inhalation
ephedrine	Alpha-beta	PO, IM, IV, SC
epinephrine	Alpha-beta	SC, IM, inhalation
isoproterenol	Beta$_1$-beta$_2$	IV, inhalation
fenoterol	Beta$_2$	Inhalation
formoterol	Beta$_2$	Inhalation
salmeterol	Beta$_2$	Inhalation
terbutaline	Beta$_2$	Inhalation

temporary decrease in serum potassium levels. This makes them useful in treating clients with acute hyperkalemia.

Some beta-agonist bronchodilators partially stimulate beta$_1$-receptors, causing CNS and cardiovascular system stimulation. This may result in nervousness, tremors, a fast heart rate, and elevated BP.

Other beta-agonist bronchodilators may stimulate both alpha- and beta-receptors. This stimulation of the alpha-adrenergic receptors mostly results in vasoconstriction, specifically of the arterioles in the skin, mucous membranes, and organs. However, it also results in the dilation of the arterioles in skeletal muscles. Some of this vasoconstriction can be beneficial in the management of certain respiratory disorders. For instance, a beta-agonist such as ephedrine that also stimulates alpha-receptors may also cause dilated blood vessels in the nasal mucosa to constrict, thereby reducing nasal congestion.

Indications

The therapeutic effects of the beta-agonists are mostly confined to the treatment of various pulmonary disorders. However, because they have effects outside the respiratory system they may also be used for the management of other disorders. The primary respiratory therapeutic effects are the relief of bronchospasm related to bronchial asthma, bronchitis, and other pulmonary diseases.

Contraindications

Contraindications include drug allergy and uncontrolled cardiac dysrhythmias.

Side Effects and Adverse Effects

Alpha-beta agonists produce the greatest array of undesirable effects. These include insomnia, restlessness, anorexia, cardiac stimulation, hyperglycemia, hypokalemia, tremor, and vascular headache. The side effects of the non-selective beta-agonists are limited to beta-adrenergic effects, including cardiac stimulation, tremor, anginal pain, and vascular headache. Beta$_2$ agents can cause both hypertension and hypotension, vascular headaches, and tremor. Overdose management may include careful administration of a beta-blocker while the client is under close observation. However, because the half-life of most adrenergic agonists is often relatively short, the client may just be observed while the body eliminates the medication.

Interactions

The use of beta-agonist bronchodilators with a non-selective beta-blocker antagonizes the bronchodilation. Their use with monoamine oxidase inhibitors (MAOIs) and other sympathomimetics is best avoided because of the enhanced risk for hypertension. Diabetics may require an adjustment in the dose of their hypoglycemic agent, especially clients receiving epinephrine, because of the increased blood glucose levels that can occur.

Dosages

For recommended dosages of selected beta-agonists, see the table on p. 602. See Appendix B for some of the common brands available in Canada.

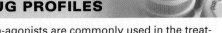

DRUG PROFILES

Although beta-agonists are commonly used in the treatment of an acute asthmatic attack, they are also used as decongestants and to treat hypotension and shock.

▶▶ *epinephrine and ephedrine*

Epinephrine and ephedrine are both beta-agonist bronchodilators that can also stimulate alpha$_1$-receptors. Their beta$_2$-stimulating properties result in bronchodilation. Their alpha$_1$-stimulating properties produce vascular effects elsewhere in the body. One of these is arteriolar constriction in the mucous membranes, making them useful as nasal decongestants.

Epinephrine is available intravenously for respiratory distress due to bronchospasm or anaphylactic shock. It is also used in sinusitis, hay fever, and rhinitis to relieve congestion. Ephedrine is available OTC in Canada at 8 mg and under. Both agents are available in several combination forms and are used to treat a variety of respiratory and non-respiratory disorders. However, those preparations used for the treatment of respiratory disorders are only given by the oral route. Because these drugs are available OTC, the Canadian medical community is concerned that individuals may be self-treating asthma and may fail to recognize early warning signs of a severe asthma attack, with dire consequences. Ephedrine and epinephrine administered via metered-dose inhaler are no longer drugs of choice in asthma treatment and are not available in Canada. Epinephrine is available as a 0.1- and 1.0-mg/mL solution for intravenous injection. Ephedrine is often abused as a stimulant and an anorexiant for weight loss. The availability of these drugs is also a contributing factor to the increase in methamphetamine abuse. Fatalities have been reported from abuse of this drug. Both drugs are classified as pregnancy category C. Commonly recommended dosages of epinephrine are given in the table on p. 602.

PHARMACOKINETICS

Half-Life	Onset	Duration	Peak
Unknown	Immediate	Rapid	Rapid (IV)

isoproterenol

Isoproterenol is available only with a prescription and is normally used in hospital. Its contraindications are the same as those for the beta$_2$-agonists such as salbutamol, but it is also contraindicated in clients with cardiac dysrhythmias or cardiac glycoside–induced tachycardia. Isoproterenol is currently available as a 0.2-mg/mL injection for intravenous use and a 0.5 percent solution for inhalation. Pregnancy category C. Common dosage recommendations are listed in the table on p. 602.

PHARMACOKINETICS

Half-Life	Onset	Peak	Duration
2.5–5 min	Immediate	1–2 hr	1–3 hr

▶▶ *salbutamol*

Salbutamol is one of the beta$_2$-specific bronchodilating beta-agonists. The others are fenterol, formoterol, salmeterol, and terbutaline. Salbutamol is most commonly used to treat acute attacks of bronchial asthma but may also be used to prevent them. If used too

DOSAGES Bronchodilators

Agent	Pharmacological Class	Usual Dosage Range	Indications
▸▸epinephrine	Alpha-beta–agonist	*Pediatric (all ages)* SC: 0.01–0.03 mg/kg q5min prn *Adult* SC/IM: 0.2–1.0 mg q15min–q4h IV: 0.1–0.25 mg Inhalation : 0.2.5–5 mg/inhalation prn	Asthma, bronchospasm
ipratropium	Anticholinergic	*Adult and pediatric ≥ 12 yr* MDI: 2 puffs tid–qid Nasal spray, 0.03%: 2 sprays bid–tid Nasal spray, 0.06%: 2 sprays bid–tid–qid Inhalation solution: 250–500 μg tid–qid *Pediatric 5–12 yr* Inhalation solution: 125–250 μg tid–qid	Asthma, bronchospasm
isoproterenol	Beta$_1$-beta$_2$–agonist	*Pediatric* IV: 0.05–1 μg/kg/min continuous infusion *Adult* IV: 10–20 μg/min continuous infusion	Asthma, bronchospasm, prevention of bradycardia following cardiac surgery
▸▸salbutamol	Beta$_2$-agonist	*Pediatric 2–6 yr* PO: 0.1 mg/kg tid–qid *Pediatric 6–12 yr* PO: 2 mg tid–qid *Adult and pediatric ≥ 12 yr* PO: 2–4 mg tid–qid Inhalation solution: 2.5–5 mg qid *Pediatric 5–12 yr* Inhalation solution: 0.25–0.5 mg qid *Adult and pediatric ≥ 4 yr* MDI: 1 puff q3–4/day Powder capsules: 100–200 μg via inhalation q4/day	Asthma, bronchospasm
salmeterol xinaforte	Beta$_2$-agonist	*Pediatric ≥ 4 yr* Inhalation aerosol: 2 × 25 μg inhalations twice daily Diskhaler disk: 1 blister (50 μg) twice daily	Long-term maintenance management of asthma, chronic bronchitis, emphysema

MDI, Metered-dose inhaler.

frequently, dose-related adverse effects may be seen as a result of salbutamol losing its beta$_2$-specificity, especially at larger doses. Thus the beta$_1$-receptors are stimulated, causing nausea, anxiety, palpitations, tremors, and an increased heart rate.

Salbutamol is contraindicated in clients with a hypersensitivity to sympathomimetics and in those who have tachyarrhythmias or severe cardiac disease. It is available only with a prescription. In oral form salbutamol is available as a 0.4-mg/mL syrup and 2- and 4-mg tablets. As an inhalation agent it is available in a metered-dose inhaler (MDI) that releases 100 μg per spray, a 100-, 200-, and 400-μg powder contained in a blister/disk formulation, a 0.05-, 1-, 2-, and 5-mg/mL solution, a plastic ampoule of 1 and 2 mg/mL and 2.5 and 5 mg/2.5 mL, and in nebules (Sterinebs) of 2.5 mg/mL for nebulization. Pregnancy category C. Commonly recommended dosages are listed in the table above.

PHARMACOKINETICS

Half-Life	Onset	Peak	Duration
2.7–5 hr	PO: 5–15 min	2–3 hr	3–6 hr

salmeterol

Salmeterol is a selective, long-acting beta-agonist (LABA), used as asthma maintenance therapy. Its unique 12-hour duration of action makes it an attractive alternative. Salmeterol is effective for both early-phase and late-phase response. Its full effect is apparent after the first or second dose. LABAs have been proven to improve lung functions, disease control, and quality of life for clients with asthma. Recently, salmeterol has come under scrutiny because of results of the Salmeterol Multi-center Asthma Research Trial (SMART), in which there was an increased risk of asthma- and respiratory-related deaths. In 2005, Health Canada issued safety information on the correct use of salmeterol and the salmeterol available in various combination products. LABAs should be used in the lowest possible dose.

PHARMACOKINETICS

Half-Life*	Onset	Peak*	Duration
Unknown	PO: 10–20 min	Unknown	12 hr

*Salmeterol acts locally in the lung; plasma levels do not predict therapeutic effect. The low therapeutic dose results in low or undetectable systemic levels.

Update on Metered Dose Inhalers

The global treaties curbing chlorofluorocarbons (CFCs), including the Montreal Protocol on Substances that Deplete the Ozone Layer, spurred Health Canada to phase out asthma inhalers that use CFCs as propellants. By 1996, Canada stopped producing and importing new CFCs. Amendments were made to the Ozone-depleting Substances Regulations, 1998, to allow for a phasing-out period, with production and importation of all products containing CFCs prohibited by January 1, 2005. Pharmaceutical companies have responded by developing alternative propellants, such as hydrofluoroalkane (HFA) and hydrofluorocarbon (HFC), as well as dry powder inhalers, which are activated by inspiration and thus do not require a propellant. Examples of both are listed below.

HFAs or HFCs
Proventil HFA

Dry Powder
Flovent Rotadisk
Pulmicort Turbuhaler
Serevent Diskus

OTHER RESPIRATORY AGENTS

Bronchodilators are just one type of agent used to treat asthma, chronic bronchitis, and emphysema. There are also other agents that are effective in suppressing various underlying causes of some of these respiratory illnesses. These drugs include anticholinergics (ipratropium), leukotriene receptor antagonist agents (montelukast and zafirlukast), corticosteroids (beclomethasone, budesonide, flunisolide and fluticasone), and **mast cell stabilizers** (sodium cromoglygate and nedocromil).

ANTICHOLINERGICS

Currently the only anticholinergic agent that is used in the treatment of COPD is ipratropium bromide. Many clients benefit from both a beta$_2$-agonist and an anticholinergic agent. Now there are two combination products containing either the beta$_2$-agonist salbutamol and ipratropium (Combivent), or fenoterol and ipratropium (Duovent UDV). Ipratropium is pharmacologically similar to atropine, and the salbutamol or fenoterol component produces local bronchodilation after inhalation. On the surface of the bronchial tree are receptors for acetylcholine (ACh), the neurotransmitter for the parasympathetic nervous system (PSNS). When the PSNS releases ACh from its nerve endings, the neurotransmitter binds to the ACh receptors on the surface of the bronchial tree, resulting in bronchial constriction and narrowing of the airways. An anticholinergic drug such as ipratropium bromide prevents this bronchoconstriction, thereby causing the airways to dilate. Because its actions are slow and prolonged, ipratropium is used for prevention of the bronchospasm associated with chronic bronchitis or emphysema and is not for the management of acute symptoms.

The most commonly reported adverse effects of ipratropium therapy are dry mouth or throat, GI distress, headache, coughing, and anxiety. It is classified as a pregnancy category B agent and is contraindicated in clients with a known hypersensitivity to it, atropine, or any of its derivatives. There are currently no drugs that are known to interact with ipratropium. The usual adolescent or adult dose is 1 or 2 inhalations 3 to 4 times daily.

PHARMACOKINETICS

Half-Life	Onset	Peak	Duration
1.6 hr	5–15 min	1–2 hr	4–5 hr

ANTILEUKOTRIENE AGENTS

The *leukotriene receptor antagonists (LTRAs)*, or antileukotriene agents, the earliest of which appeared in the 1990s, are the first new class of asthma medications to be introduced in Canada in more than 20 years

Before the use of antileukotriene agents, most asthma treatments focused on relaxing the squeeze of bronchial muscles with bronchodilators. In the last decade, researchers have begun to understand how asthma symptoms are caused by the immune system at the cellular level. A chain reaction starts when a trigger allergen, such as cat hair or dust, starts a series of chemical reactions in the body. This produces several substances, including a family of molecules known as *leukotrienes (LTs)*. In people with asthma these LTs cause inflammation, bronchoconstriction, and mucus production. This in turn leads to coughing, wheezing, and shortness of breath. Antileukotriene agents prevent LTs from attaching to receptors located on circulating cells and cells within the lungs. This blocks the inflammation in the lungs that leads to asthma symptoms. The research responsible for the discovery of these agents is the direct result of a Nobel Prize–winning discovery made by scientist Ben Samuelsson in 1979.

Currently there are three known subcategories of antileukotriene agents. Each subcategory modifies or inhibits the activity of LTs and thus relieves the inflammatory process underlying asthma. These subcategories are classified by the mechanisms by which they block the inflammatory process in asthma. The first class of antileukotriene agents inhibits the enzyme 5-lipoxygenase (zileuton and ICI-D2138, an investigational agent). Zileuton is the only one of this class of drugs available in the United States and it has not been approved for use in Canada. The second subcategory of antileukotriene agents inhibits 5-lipoxygenase-activating protein. Examples include MK-886, MK-591, and BAY-X-1005, all of which are still investigational compounds. The third subcategory of antileukotriene agents are the LTD4-receptor blockers (montelukast, pobilukast, pranlukast, tomelukast, verlukast, and zafirlukast). Montelukast, developed in Canada, and zafirlukast are the only members of this category currently available on the Canadian market.

Mechanism of Action and Drug Effects

Montelukast and zafirlukast work by blocking the action of leukotrienes on cells in the respiratory tract for these LTs, reducing inflammation.

The drug effects of antileukotriene agents are primarily limited to the lungs. Through their antagonist action on LT receptors, they prevent smooth muscle contraction of the bronchial airways, decrease mucus secretion, and reduce vascular permeability. Other LTs that these agents block prevent the mobilization and migration of such cells as neutrophils and leukocytes into the lungs. Decreased neutrophil and leukocyte infiltration to the lungs prevents inflammation in the lungs.

Indications

The antileukotriene agents montelukast and zafirlukast are used for the prophylaxis and chronic treatment of asthma in adults and children. Montelukast is considered safe in children 6 years of age and older and zafirlukast in children 12 years of age and older. These agents are not meant for the management of acute asthmatic attacks. Improvement is typically seen in about one week.

Contraindications

Drug allergy or other previous adverse drug reaction is the primary contraindication to use of antileukotriene agents.

TABLE 36-6
DRUG INTERACTIONS: ANTILEUKOTRIENE AGENTS

Drug	Mechanism	Result
MONTELUKAST		
phenobarbital	Increased metabolism	Decreased montelukast levels
ZAFIRLUKAST		
acetylsalicylic acid	Decreased clearance	Increased zafirlukast levels
erythromycin	Decreased bioavailability	Decreased zafirlukast levels
theophylline	Decreased bioavailability	Decreased zafirlukast levels
tolbutamide, phenytoin, carbamazepine	Inhibited metabolism	Increased tolbutamide, phenytoin, and carbamazepine levels
warfarin	Decreased clearance	Increased prothrombin (PT) time

Side Effects and Adverse Effects

The side effects of antileukotriene agents differ depending on the specific agent. Zafirlukast can cause headaches, nausea, and diarrhea. This agent may also lead to elevations in serum transaminases and liver dysfunction. For this reason, liver enzyme levels should be monitored regularly, especially early in the course of therapy.

Limited information exists regarding acute zafirlukast overdose and toxicity. Symptomatic and supportive measures are recommended.

There have been some case reports of Churg-Strauss syndrome in clients receiving montelukast. This consists of systemic necrotizing vasculitis (destruction of blood vessels) and is often manifested by tender subcutaneous nodules, large skin plaques, and markedly elevated eosinophil count in the blood (eosinophilia). It is usually treated with systemic (intravenous or oral) corticosteroid therapy.

Interactions

Montelukast has fewer drug interactions than zafirlukast. It does not interact with theophylline, warfarin, digoxin, prednisone, or either the estrogen or progestin components of combination oral contraceptives. Phenobarbital decreases montelukast concentrations. For information on the drugs that interact with zafirlukast see Table 36-6.

Dosages

For recommended dosages of selected antileukotriene agents, see the table below. See Appendix B for some of the common brands available in Canada.

DRUG PROFILES

Antileukotriene agents are a new class of asthma medications. Currently there are two antileukotriene agents available: zafirlukast and montelukast. They are primarily used for oral prophylaxis and treatment of chronic asthma. These agents are not recommended for treatment of acute asthma attacks.

▸▸ **montelukast**

Montelukast is the latest agent to become available in the antileukotriene class. It belongs to the same subcategory of antileukotriene agents as zafirlukast.

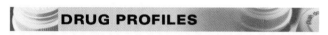

DOSAGES Selected Antileukotriene Agents

Agent	Pharmacological Class	Usual Dosage Range	Indications
▸▸montelukast	Leukotriene receptor antagonist	**Pediatric 2–5 yr** PO: 4 mg daily at bedtime **Pediatric 6–14 yr** PO: 5 mg daily at bedtime **Adult and pediatric ≥15 yr** PO: 10 mg daily at bedtime	Prophylaxis and maintenance treatment of asthma
zafirlukast	Leukotriene receptor antagonist	**Adult and pediatric ≥12 yr** PO: 20 mg bid	Prophylaxis and maintenance treatment of asthma

Montelukast and zafirlukast work by blocking LTD4-receptors to augment the inflammatory response. Montelukast offers the advantage of being Health Canada approved for use in children 2 years of age and older. It also has fewer side effects and drug interactions than zafirlukast. Montelukast is contraindicated in clients with a known hypersensitivity to it. It is available in 4- and 5-mg chewable tablets, a 10-mg film-coated tablet, and 4-mg packet of oral granules. Pregnancy category B. Common dosages are given in the table on p. 604.

PHARMACOKINETICS

Half-Life	Onset	Peak	Duration
2.7–5.5 hr	30 min	3–4 hr	24 hr
		2.5 hr (chewable)	

zafirlukast

Zafirlukast is an LTD4-receptor blocker. It is indicated for the prophylaxis and treatment of chronic asthma in adults and children 12 years of age and older. Zafirlukast is contraindicated in clients with a hypersensitivity to zafirlukast. It is available in oral form as a 20-mg tablet. Pregnancy category B. Common dosages are given in the table on p. 604.

PHARMACOKINETICS

Half-Life	Onset	Peak	Duration
10 hr	30 min	3–4 hr	12 hr

CORTICOSTEROIDS

Corticosteroids are used in the treatment of chronic asthma for their anti-inflammatory effects, which lead to decreased airway obstruction. Like ipratropium bromide, corticosteroids do not relieve the symptoms of acute asthmatic attacks but are used prophylactically to prevent an attack. Corticosteroids do this by preventing various non-specific inflammatory processes such as altered vascular permeability and the accumulation of inflammatory mediators such as polymorphonuclear leukocytes. They can be given by inhalation, orally, or even intravenously in severe cases of asthma when the agent cannot get to the airways because of the obstruction. Corticosteroids administered by inhalation have an advantage over orally administered corticosteroids in that their action is limited to the topical site of action—the lungs. This generally prevents systemic effects. The chemical structures of the corticosteroids given by inhalation have also been slightly altered to limit their systemic absorption from the respiratory tract. The corticosteroids administered by inhalation include beclomethasone dipropionate, budesonide, fluticasone, mometasone furoate monohydrate, and triamcinolone acetonide.

Mechanism of Action and Drug Effects

Although the exact mechanism of action of the corticosteroids has not been determined, it is conjectured that they have the dual effect of both reducing inflammation and enhancing the activity of beta-agonists.

The corticosteroids produce their anti-inflammatory effects through a complex sequence of actions. They stabilize the membranes of leukocytes (white blood cells, or WBCs) that normally release harmful bronchoconstricting substances (e.g., histamine, SRS-A). There are five different types of WBCs, each with its own specific characteristics, as summarized in Table 36-7.

Corticosteroids have also been shown to restore or increase the responsiveness of bronchial smooth muscle to beta-adrenergic receptor stimulation, which results in more pronounced stimulation of the beta$_2$-receptors by beta-agonist drugs such as salbutamol. It may take several weeks of continuous therapy before the full therapeutic effects of the corticosteroids are realized.

Most of the drug effects of inhaled corticosteroids are limited to their topical site of action in the lungs. Because of the chemical structure of these inhaled dosage forms, there is little systemic absorption of the agents when they are administered by inhalation at normal therapeutic doses. When there is significant systemic absorption, such as with high-dose intravenous or oral administration, corticosteroids can affect any of the organ systems in the body. Some of these systemic drug effects include adrenocortical insufficiency, increased susceptibility to infection, fluid and electrolyte disturbances, endocrine effects, dermatological effects, nervous system effects, bone loss, and osteoporosis.

Indications

Inhaled corticosteroids are now used for the primary treatment of bronchospastic disorders to control the inflammatory responses that are believed to be the cause of these disorders. They are often used concurrently with bronchodilators, primarily beta-adrenergic agonists. Xanthine bronchodilators are not as commonly used. They are not considered first-line agents for the management of acute asthmatic attacks or status asthmaticus.

Contraindications

Drug allergy is the primary contraindication. It should also be emphasized that these agents are not intended as sole therapy for acute asthma attacks.

Side Effects and Adverse Effects

The main undesirable local effects of corticosteroids on the respiratory system include pharyngeal irritation, coughing, dry mouth, and oral fungal infections. Systemic effects of inhaled dosage forms are rare because of the relatively low doses used for inhalation therapy. Caution is required in switching clients from systemic to inhaled corticosteroids, especially if they received high doses for an extended period. Deaths have been reported due to adrenal gland failure when the switch is made quickly. To prevent gland failure, systemic doses should be tapered slowly, with careful clinical monitoring. A client dependent on systemic corticosteroids may need up to one year of recovery time after discontinuation of systemic therapy.

TABLE 36-7

WHITE BLOOD CELLS (LEUKOCYTES)

Specific WBC*	Role in Inflammation	Corticosteroid Effect
GRANULOCYTES		
Neutrophils (65%)	Contain powerful lysosomes, which are digestive-like enzymes; release chemicals that destroy invading organisms and also attack other WBCs	Stabilize their cell membranes so that inflammation-causing substances are not released
Eosinophils (2%–5%)	Main function is in allergic reactions and in protecting against parasitic infections; ingest inflammatory chemicals and antigen–antibody complexes	Little if any effect
Basophils (0.5%–1%)	Contain histamine, an inflammation-causing substance, and heparin, an anticoagulant	Stabilize their cell membranes so that histamine is not released
AGRANULOCYTES		
Lymphocytes (25%)	2 types: T-lymphocytes and B-lymphocytes; T-cells attack infecting microbial or cancerous cells; B-cells produce antibodies against specific antigens	Decrease activity of the lymphocytes
Monocytes (3%–5%)	Produce macrophages, which can migrate out of the bloodstream to such places as mucous membranes, where they are capable of engulfing large bacteria or virus-infected cells	Inhibited macrophage accumulation in already inflamed areas, thus preventing more inflammation

*Percentage in parentheses is the proportion of the total number of leukocytes they constitute.

Interactions

Oral and intravenous corticosteroids can interact with many drugs. Drugs that can interact with oral or IV corticosteroids and therefore should be avoided include acetylsalicylic acid, alcohol, barbiturates, phenytoin, theophylline, anticoagulants, anticonvulsants, antidiabetic agents, antituberculin agents, antifungal agents, digitalis, diuretics, non-steroidal anti-inflammatory drugs (NSAIDs), oral contraceptives, estrogens, and macrolide antibiotics.

Inhaled corticosteroids generally cause few significant drug interactions because they are delivered directly to the site of action in the respiratory tract. Therefore they neither have systemic effects nor interact with systemically administered drugs. When a more pronounced anti-inflammatory effect is needed, as in an acute exacerbation of COPD or asthma, intravenous corticosteroids (e.g., methylprednisolone, hydrocortisone) are often used.

Dosages

For recommended dosages of selected corticosteroids, see the table on p. 607. See Appendix B for some of the common brands available in Canada.

DRUG PROFILES

Inhaled corticosteroids are contraindicated in clients who are hypersensitive to glucocorticoids, clients whose sputum is positive for *Candida* organisms, and clients with systemic fungal infection. All of the inhaled corticosteroids are classified as pregnancy category C agents and are available only with a prescription. Two new systems have become available in Canada that combine a steroid and a long-acting beta₂ receptor-agonist: budesonide and formoterol fumarate dihydrate (Symbicort Turbuhaler), and fluticasone propionate and salmeterol (Advair). These drugs with their different modes of action combine to have an additive effect and

COMMUNITY HEALTH POINTS

ADVAIR Diskus System

A newer drug for the treatment of asthma is fluticasone propionate (a corticosteroid) with the addition of a long-acting beta₂-receptor agonist (stimulant), salmeterol. This combination of drugs is found in the ADVAIR Diskus and is delivered via inhaler using a dry powder or through MDI. The circular double-foil pack contains "blisters" of the drug and a Diskhaler inhalation container/device. Following are important points to emphasize for client use at home:

* Various dosage forms are available, with 100/50, 250/50, and 500/50 dosages; the first number represents the fluticasone dose and the second number represents the salmeterol dose. The Advair aerosol is available in 125/25 and 250/25 fluticasone to salmeterol.
* This product is *not* for children.
* This product is *not* for acute attacks.
* *Never* exhale into the Diskus or MDI.
* Never take the device apart.
* Activate and use device only in a level and horizontal position.
* Keep the device dry.
* Always rinse the mouth with water without swallowing after treatment dosing to prevent oral candidiasis (fungal infection).

reduce asthma exacerbations. The systemic use of corticosteroids is discussed in detail in Chapter 43.

▶▶ *beclomethasone dipropionate*

Beclomethasone dipropionate is administered by oral inhalation for the treatment of bronchial asthma in clients who require corticosteroids on a long-term basis for the control of symptoms. It may also be used in clients who have not responded to an adequate trial of conventional therapy, usually xanthines and beta-agonists, as well as in the management of clients with COPD (such as

DOSAGES   Selected Corticosteroids

Agent	Pharmacological Class	Usual Dosage Range	Indications
▶▶ beclomethasone dipropionate	Synthetic glucocorticoid	**Adult and pediatric ≥6 yr** MDI: 1–2 puffs tid–qid	Asthma prophylaxis and maintenance treatment
		Nasal spray: 1–2 sprays in each nostril daily–qid depending on dosage form	Allergic rhinitis
budesonide	Synthetic glucocorticoid	**Adult and pediatric ≥6 yr** MDI: 1–2 puffs bid	Asthma prophylaxis and maintenance treatment
		Nasal spray: 2 sprays in each nostril bid or 4 sprays in each nostril once daily **Pediatric 12 mo–8 yr**	Allergic rhinitis
		Inhalation solution: 0.5–1 mg daily–bid	Asthma prophylaxis and maintenance treatment
flunisolide	Synthetic glucocorticoid	Nasal spray: 2 sprays bid	Allergic rhinitis
fluticasone propionate	Synthetic glucocorticoid	**Adult and pediatric ≥12 yr** Flovent, MDI, 3 strengths available: 50, 150, or 250 μg bid Flovent Diskus 5, inhalation powder, 3 strengths available: 50, 100, 500 μg/actuation **Pediatric 4–11 yr** 50–100 μg bid **Adult and pediatric ≥12 yr** 100–1000 μg bid	Asthma prophylaxis and maintenance treatment
triamcinolone acetonide	Synthetic glucocorticoid	**Adult and pediatric ≥12 yr** Nasal spray: 1–2 sprays each nostril once daily **Pediatric 4–12 yr** Nasal spray: 1–4 sprays each nostril once daily	Allergic rhinitis
mometasone furoate monohydrate	Synthetic glucocorticoid	**Adult and pediatric ≥12 yr** Nasal spray: 1–4 sprays each nostril once daily **Pediatric 3–11 yr** Nasal spray: 1 spray each nostril once daily **Adult and pediatric ≥12 yr** Nasal spray: 2–4 sprays each nostril bid	Allergic rhinitis Sinusitis

MDI, Metered-dose inhaler.

chronic bronchitis) whose disease has been stabilized with oral corticosteroid therapy.

When beclomethasone is administered by oral inhalation, the primary sites of action are the bronchi and the bronchioles. Little drug reaches the bloodstream through the respiratory tract because it is metabolically inactivated. Beclomethasone appears to have greater topical anti-inflammatory activity and to cause fewer adverse systemic effects. The use of an inhaled corticosteroid commonly allows for clients with chronic bronchial asthma to reduce or discontinue systemic corticosteroids. Beclomethasone is available as an aerosolized mist in an MDI that releases 42 mg per spray and is given by oral inhalation. Pregnancy category C. Commonly recommended dosages are listed in the table above.

PHARMACOKINETICS

42 μg/metered spray

Half-Life	Onset	Peak	Duration
3–15 hr	10 min	15–30 min	4–6 hr

fluticasone

Fluticasone is administered intranasally (Flonase; one inhalation in each nostril daily) and by oral inhalation (Flovent; usually one inhalation by mouth twice daily). It is used for the treatment of seasonal allergic rhinitis. Inhaled corticosteroids help to control symptoms of allergies through their anti-inflammatory activity. Recently fluticasone became available in combination with the long-acting bronchodilator salmeterol (Advair Diskus inhaler). This product has become popular with prescribers. Pregnancy category C.

MAST CELL STABILIZERS

The mast cell stabilizers sodium cromoglygate and nedocromil are additional agents that can be used in the treatment of asthma. Sodium cromoglygate and nedocromil are considered indirect-acting agents because they prevent the release of the various intracellular chemical mediators that cause bronchospasm, rather than blocking the receptors for these substances (e.g., histamine or LT receptors). They have no direct bronchodilator activity and are used only prophylactically. They are most effective in preventing the asthma caused by extrinsic factors such as allergens and exercise.

Mechanism of Action and Drug Effects

Mast cells function in a similar manner to the subset of lymphocytes in the blood known as *basophils* (Table 36-7). In fact, mast cells can be thought of as stationary basophils in various tissues, including those of the respiratory tract. As with basophils, when antibodies to a specific antigen bind to receptors on the surfaces of mast cells, inflammatory mediators such as histamine are released from inside the mast cells to take part in the body's inflammatory response. However, unlike basophils, which circulate as a component of the blood, mast cells are stationary. They are present in high concentrations in tissues more prone to injury, such as the nose, mouth, feet, internal body surfaces, and blood vessels.

As previously mentioned, these cells release the vasoconstrictive substances (e.g., histamine, SRS-A) responsible for causing bronchoconstrictive disorders such as asthma. Sodium cromoglygate and nedocromil exert their actions by stabilizing the membranes of the mast cells, thereby suppressing the release of the substances.

Nedocromil and sodium cromoglygate are alike in pharmacological effects, but nedocromil is more potent on a weight basis in inhibiting mediator release and the bronchoconstriction induced by various stimuli. Nedocromil also appears to affect a broader range of inflammatory cells (eosinophils, neutrophils, macrophages, mast cells, monocytes, and platelets). Nedocromil can inhibit both an acute bronchoconstrictor response and a delayed inflammatory response to inhaled antigens and irritants. It may also suppress cough by inhibiting the neuronal reflexes in airways.

The drug effects of sodium cromoglygate and nedocromil are primarily limited to the lungs, and when inhaled, little if any of the agent gets into the bloodstream to cause systemic effects. The primary drug effect of these agents is on the surface of cell membranes. Because these drugs can be administered by several different routes (orally, inhaled, and in the eye), they can get to all areas of the body where there are inflammatory cells (e.g., mast cells, monocytes, macrophages, neutrophils) and stabilize their cell membranes, thereby preventing the release of the harmful cellular contents that cause inflammation. Sodium cromoglygate and nedocromil may also inhibit the movement of some cells into and out of the tissues and blood vessels.

Indications

Sodium cromoglygate and nedocromil are used as adjuncts to the overall management of clients with asthma and are used solely for prophylaxis. These agents are of no value in the treatment of acute asthma attacks. They are used to prevent bronchospasm induced by exercise or by exposure to precipitating factors such as cold dry air, environmental pollutants, and allergens. They may also be used for the symptomatic prevention and treatment of seasonal or perennial allergic rhinitis. Sodium cromoglygate may be used to relieve allergic eye disorders that result in itching, tearing, redness, and discharge. It has also been administered orally for the prophylactic management of food allergies and for the treatment of chronic inflammatory bowel disease (Crohn's disease and ulcerative colitis). Nedocromil also has anti-inflammatory action.

Contraindications

Drug allergy is the primary contraindication. It should also be emphasized, as with inhaled corticosteroids, that mast cell stabilizers are a maintenance and prevention intervention and are not effective for treating acute asthma attacks.

Side Effects and Adverse Effects

Most of the side effects of sodium cromoglygate and nedocromil affect the respiratory system and include coughing, sore throat, rhinitis, and bronchospasm. Other effects include taste changes, dizziness, and headache.

Dosages

For the recommended dosages of sodium cromoglygate and nedocromil, see the table on p. 609. See Appendix B for some of the common brands available in Canada.

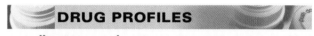

DRUG PROFILES

sodium cromoglygate

Sodium cromoglygate is a mast cell stabilizer that is indicated for the prevention of bronchospasms and bronchial asthmatic attacks. It seems to stabilize fewer cell types than nedocromil and is less potent. It was the first of the two agents in this drug class to be developed and used in clinical practice.

Sodium cromoglygate is contraindicated in clients who are hypersensitive to the drug or to its lactose filler, which may induce symptoms in lactose-intolerant clients. It is not intended for treating acute asthmatic symptoms. It is available for both oral and ophthalmic administration and for nasal and oral inhalation, and because of its many dosage formulations it may be used for the treatment of many disorders. The nasal spray is available in a 2 percent solution; the ophthalmic solution is also a 2 percent solution; the aerosolized oral inhalation agent delivers 800 mg per metered spray; the powder for oral inhalation is available as a 20-mg capsule; and the solution for nebulization has a concentration of 20 mg/2 mL. Pregnancy category B. Recommended dosages are given in the table on p. 609.

PHARMACOKINETICS

Half-Life	Onset	Peak	Duration
1.5 hr	Unknown	15 min	4–6 hr

DOSAGES   Mast Cell Stabilizers

Agent	Pharmacological Class	Usual Dosage Range	Indications
sodium cromoglygate	Mast cell stabilizer	**Adult and pediatric ≥2 yr** Nebulizer solution: 20 mg qid **Adult and pediatric ≥5 yr** MDI: 2 inhalations qid **Adult and pediatric ≥6 yr** Nasal spray: 1 spray each nostril 3–6 ×/day	Asthma Rhinitis
nedocromil	Mast cell stabilizer	**Adult and pediatric ≥ 12 yr** MDI: 2 inhalations qid **Adults & pediatric ≥3 yr** 1 drop each eye bid	Asthma Seasonal allergic conjunctivitis

nedocromil

Nedocromil is indicated for the prevention of bronchospasms and bronchial asthma attacks. Contraindications are the same as for sodium cromoglygate. Its particular mechanism of action has already been described. Nedocromil is available only as an aerosolized inhaler, and it is used only as an adjunct agent in the overall management of clients with mild to moderate bronchial asthma. It is available only with a prescription and comes in an MDI that delivers 2 mg per spray for oral inhalation. It also comes in a 2 percent ophthalmic solution. Pregnancy category B. Recommended dosages are given in the table above.

PHARMACOKINETICS

Half-Life	Onset	Peak	Duration
1.5 hr	Unknown	15 min	4–6 hr

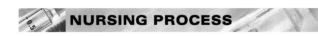

NURSING PROCESS

■ Assessment

The net drug effect of all the bronchodilators and other respiratory agents (beta-agonists, anticholinergics, xanthine derivatives, indirect-acting anti-asthmatics, antileukotrienes, mast cell inhibitors, and corticosteroids) is relaxation of the bronchial smooth muscle. There are as many indications as there are cautions and contraindications for the various respiratory agents. In a thorough assessment of clients receiving any of the respiratory agents, the client's skin colour, temperature, respirations (rate [<12 or >24 breaths/min] and rhythm), breath sounds, BP, and pulse should be monitored as needed. The nurse should also question whether the client is experiencing problems with cough, dyspnea, orthopnea, or respiratory distress; whether sternal retraction, cyanosis, restlessness, activity intolerance, or cardiac symptoms such as palpitations, hypertension, and tachycardia are occurring; and whether accessory muscles are being used to breathe. Clients should be asked to give a thorough history of their respiratory disease as well as of any allergens and allergic responses (especially sputum production), and to list any other medications and non-drug therapies. The type of asthma attack also needs to be assessed and documented because of the different indications for specific drugs.

Beta-agonists are contraindicated in clients with a history of cardiac disease, dysrhythmias, angina, hyperthyroidism, coronary artery disease, hypertension, diabetes, or convulsive disorders. Anticholinergic agents are contraindicated in clients with a history of benign prostatic hypertrophy or glaucoma. Xanthine derivatives such as theophylline are contraindicated in clients with a history of peptic ulcer disease, GI disorders, or hyperthyroidism, and cautious use (with close monitoring) is recommended in clients with a history of cardiac disorder. Corticosteroids are contraindicated in clients with an allergy to the drug and in those with a history of psychosis, fungal infections, acquired immunodeficiency syndrome (AIDS), tuberculosis, or idiopathic thrombocytopenia, as well as in children less than two years of age. Cautious use is recommended in clients with diabetes mellitus, glaucoma, osteoporosis, ulcer disease, renal disease, heart failure, edema, myasthenia gravis, seizure disorders, or esophagitis.

With antileukotrienes (e.g., montelukast and zafirlukast), it is important to assess for contraindications, such as clients who are allergic to the agent or have hepatic dysfunction (transaminase three times the normal level). There are also significant drug interactions with antileukotrienes.

Sodium cromoglygate and nedocromil are used for preventive management of asthma, not for the control of acute exacerbations of asthma. In fact, acute asthmatic attacks are considered contraindications to these two drugs. Use of the inhaled form of this medication in children younger than five years of age and in pregnant or lactating women is not recommended; however, preventive management may begin at an early age of six to eight years.

■ Nursing Diagnoses

Nursing diagnoses related to the administration of respiratory agents include the following:

- Impaired gas exchange related to pathophysiological changes caused by respiratory disease.
- Fatigue related to the disease process.
- Risk for injury related to the side effects of various respiratory medications.

- Anxiety related to uncertainty about respiratory disease and related drug therapy.
- Disturbed thought processes related to the CNS stimulation caused by bronchodilators.
- Deficient knowledge related to unfamiliarity with medication treatment regimen and the disease process.
- Non-adherence related to undesirable side effects of medication therapy.

Planning

Goals for the client receiving respiratory agents include the following:

- Client experiences minimal exacerbations of the disease while adherent with medication regimen.
- Client states the importance of rest to recovery.
- Client is free of self-injury related to either the disease or the side effects of the medication.
- Client remains adherent with the medication regimen and with the non-pharmacological therapies.
- Client follows up with healthcare providers as instructed by the physician.
- Client does not increase or decrease the dose or stop taking the medication without the approval of the physician.
- Client's respiratory status improves because of adherence with the medication therapy.

Outcome Criteria

Outcome criteria for clients receiving respiratory agents include the following:

- Client briefly describes the disease process, its signs and symptoms, and the precipitating factors.
- Client states measures to take to prevent self-injury resulting from the disease or the side effects of the medication, such as taking medications as prescribed.
- Client is well rested, with plans to rest during periods of exacerbation.
- Client states the expected side effects of the drug, such as palpitations, nervousness, mood changes, and insomnia.
- Client contacts the physician if increased dyspnea, shortness of breath, increased cough, or fever occur.
- Client states the importance of taking the medication as prescribed and the reasons for not stopping, increasing, or decreasing the dose.

Implementation

Nursing interventions that apply to clients with respiratory disease processes (e.g., COPD, asthma, upper and lower respiratory disorders) include client education and an emphasis on adherence and prevention. Measures to prevent, relieve, or decrease the manifestations of the disease should be emphasized to the client at all times during treatment, including increasing awareness of precipitating factors. Bronchodilators should be given exactly as prescribed and by the prescribed route (e.g., parenterally, orally, by intermittent positive pressure breathing, or by inhalation). The proper method for administering the inhaled forms of these agents should be demonstrated to the client with client return demonstrations. Clients should also be strongly discouraged from taking more than the prescribed dose of the

beta-agonists and xanthines because of their excessive cardiac demands and risk of hypertension and tachycardia with cardiac and CNS stimulation. The nurse should always identify the specific medication(s) clients are taking to make sure that there are no drug interactions. Combivent (salbutamol and ipratropium) is a combination product that contains a beta-agonist agent and an anticholinergic bronchodilator; both drugs require specific nursing actions. Community health care implications applicable to clients receiving inhalers are given in the box on p. 612.

Xanthine derivatives should also be given exactly as prescribed. If they are to be given parenterally, the nurse should always determine the correct diluent to be used, the amount of the agent, and the time to infuse medication, then use an infusion pump to ensure dosage accuracy and help prevent toxicity. To prevent sudden drug release with irritating effects on the gastric mucosa, timed-release preparations should not be crushed or chewed. Suppository forms of the drug should be refrigerated, and clients should be told to notify their physician if rectal burning, itching, or irritation occurs.

Corticosteroid inhalers should also be used exactly as prescribed, with cautions about overuse. All equipment (inhalers or nebulizers) should be kept clean, with filters cleaned and changed (nebulizers) and in good working condition. Clients should rinse their mouths after using the inhaler or nebulizer to help prevent thrush (oral candidiasis). Pediatric clients may need a physician's order to have these medications on hand at school and during athletic events or physical education. Peak flow meter use is also encouraged to help clients better regulate their disease.

Sodium cromoglygate, although not a bronchodilator, does have a role to play in the preventive treatment of asthma. It is available as a powder contained in a capsule (spincaps) that is administered by a specific type of inhaler, but in both adults and children it can also be administered by nebulizer. During a treatment session using either delivery system, the client may experience bronchospasms. If they continue, the client's condition should be stabilized, the session discontinued, and the physician notified. The proper technique for inhalant administration is presented in the Pediatric Considerations box on sodium cromoglygate therapy on p. 613. Other interventions such as forcing fluids and avoiding precipitating factors are also recommended.

The antileukotrienes montelukast and zafirlukast are given orally. Of most concern are the montelukast chewable tablets, which contain aspartame and approximately 0.842 mg of phenylamine per 5-mg tablet. Client education for the LT-receptor antagonists should emphasize that they are indicated for chronic, and not acute, asthma. These agents should be taken every night on a continuous schedule, even if symptoms improve.

Pediatric considerations relevant to treatment with the various respiratory agents are discussed in the box on p. 613. See the Case Study on p. 613 to evaluate understanding of the nursing process in a hospitalized client with a diagnosis of COPD. Client teaching tips for bronchodilators and other respiratory agents are presented in the box on p. 614.

NURSING CARE PLAN	Asthma

Thirteen-year-old Jennifer was recently diagnosed with asthma and is to begin nebulizer treatments with sodium cromoglygate bid. She has been adherent with her steroid inhaler and with other treatments for her asthma; therefore the physician believes that the sodium cromoglygate will help prevent some of her asthmatic attacks. Because you are the nurse on the "well" side of the pediatrician's office today you are to tell Jennifer about the medication, as well as how to best use two inhalers.

ASSESSMENT

Subjective Data
"I'm not sure that this stuff will work."

Objective Data
- 13-year-old newly diagnosed asthmatic
- Success with other therapies
- Listens and comprehends well
- States, "I want to get my asthma under control."
- Respiration rate 20
- Lungs clear
- BP 100/60
- Pulse 66

NURSING DIAGNOSIS

Deficient knowledge related to new diagnoses of asthma and its treatment

PLANNING

Goals
Client will remain adherent with new asthma treatment beginning with first dose forward

Outcome Criteria
Client will state the following about sodium cromoglygate therapy:
- Use
- Side effects
- Cautions
- Side effects to report to the physician

Client will state that she is having fewer to no asthmatic attacks.

IMPLEMENTATION

Client teaching should include the following:
- Remember that this medication is to be given by nebulizer for the time being and should be taken exactly as ordered (bid).
- Make sure that after you do the treatment you rinse your mouth out and gargle to prevent irritation of the mouth and throat.
- You may not see its full effects for about four weeks.
- Keep machinery clean as recommended by the manufacturer.
- Once we have discussed the medication, you will be all set to go because you already know how to use the machine.
- Side effects could include throat irritation, cough, nasal stuffiness, burning of the eyes, headache, nausea, dry mouth, bitter taste.
- Call the physician if you experience severe headaches, dizziness, rash, or joint pain or swelling.

EVALUATION

- Client will display a therapeutic response to sodium cromoglygate as evidenced by
  - Decrease in asthmatic symptoms
  - Decreased chest tightness and wheezing
  - Decrease in cough
  - Fewer asthma attacks
  - Regular respiratory rate and rhythm
  - No dyspnea
- Client will experience minimal side effects and report those indicated as a concern, such as
  - CNS excitation (tremors, seizures, irritability, hyperactivity)
  - Cardiovascular excitation (tachycardia, angina, hypertension, cardiac irregularities)

COMMUNITY HEALTH POINTS

Clients Receiving Salbutamol

- Instructions to clients regarding the proper use of inhaled forms of medications are crucial to ensuring their safe and effective use. Be sure to have clients demonstrate the technique for using an inhaler or nebulizer.
- Instructions regarding the care of the inhaler or nebulizer and associated equipment are also important. This involves washing the inhaler in warm water every day and drying it before reuse, or washing the tubing and other apparatus used with the nebulizer. A solution of white vinegar and water can be used to rinse out the tubing of the nebulizer. Always encourage clients to follow the manufacturer's recommendations regarding the use, storage, and cleaning of any equipment used.
- Children under the age of six are most prone to the CNS stimulation. Symptoms such as hyperactivity, excitement, nervousness, tachycardia, nausea, or vomiting should be reported immediately to the healthcare provider. The safety and efficacy of salbutamol by inhalation has not been established in children under six years of age.
- Tablet and syrup forms of the drug should be stored in light-resistant containers with a tight childproof lid, and out of the reach of children.
- If the client is receiving salbutamol and beclomethasone inhalation therapy, the salbutamol should be administered 20–30 min before the beclomethasone to allow deeper penetration of the beclomethasone (steroid) inhaled form, unless ordered differently by the healthcare provider.
- Warn clients that a potential side effect of salbutamol is dizziness.
- OTCs should be used only with the approval of the healthcare provider because of the many drug interactions with other cold and cough products.
- Clients must be warned not to allow the inhaler spray to get in their eyes.
- A therapeutic response to salbutamol inhaler use includes absence of wheezing and dyspnea.
- Clients must be instructed and reminded during home healthcare visits to use these medications *exactly* as prescribed; an overdose may precipitate palpitations, angina, hypertension, or dysrhythmias.
- If the therapeutic effects of this drug decrease, the client should contact the physician or healthcare provider. The client should not change the number of inhalations or doses on his or her own.
- Subjective improvement of symptoms with salbutamol should occur in about 15 min after the inhaled dosage is administered (60–90 min with oral liquid forms). If this does not occur, the client should contact their healthcare provider immediately for further instructions; immediate treatment with other drugs may be needed.

How to Check the Volume of Medication Left in an MDI Canister

MDIs may be checked for residual amounts of medication so that the client does not run out. First, obtain a container that is wider and longer than the inhaler and fill it ¾ full with water. Remove the mouthpiece and drop the inhaler into the container. If the canister drops to the bottom and lies on its side, then it is full. If it drops to the bottom and lands with the bottom of the inhaler pointing upward then it is about ¾ full. If it lands in the water with about ¼ of the bottom of the inhaler exposed, then it is approximately ½ full. If the canister leans to its side and is submerged except for about ¼ of the bottom of the inhaler, then it is most likely about ¼ full. If it floats on top of the water line it is most likely near empty. Be sure to tell clients that this method merely provides an estimate. They should refill prescriptions in plenty of time.

General Nursing Considerations for Clients Using an MDI and Spacer

The nurse must inform all clients who are using an MDI about how they help deliver medication directly to the lungs. Also explain that the pressurized canister contains measured doses of the medication. The Asthma Society of Canada recommends that spacers should always be used with MDIs that deliver inhaled corticosteroids or beta$_2$-receptor agonists. Instructions for the MDI should include the following:

- Shake the container thoroughly to activate drug and then breathe out fully through your mouth.
- Place the inhaler mouthpiece in front of your mouth with your lips around it or follow directions for using a spacer device, if provided. Breathe out through your nose, expelling as much air from the lungs as possible; close your lips and teeth around the open end of the mouthpiece, which should be placed well into your mouth, and aim the device toward the back of your throat.
- Activate the inhaler by pressing down on it at the same time that you are breathing in slowly and deeply.
- Count to five seconds while breathing in, then hold your breath for an additional ten seconds before exhaling slowly.
- If a second dose is recommended, wait two minutes then repeat directions.

To avoid any type of mouth infection from the use of an inhaled corticosteroid, clients should gargle with water and cleanse the mouth after the treatment. Instructions on inhalers may vary; therefore the nurse must demonstrate the technique to clients and clarify any other instructions with the healthcare provider. Children six years of age and even younger can usually be trained to use an MDI properly, but adult supervision is recommended. Return demonstration is effective.

Data from Asthma Society of Canada. (2005). Retrieved August 25, 2005, from http://www.asthma.ca/

▪ Evaluation

The therapeutic effects of any of the agents used to treat or prevent respiratory diseases include decreased dyspnea; decreased wheezing, restlessness, and anxiety; improved respiratory patterns with return to normal rate and quality; improved activity tolerance and arterial blood gas levels; increased quality of life; and decreased severity and incidence of respiratory symptoms. The therapeutic effects of bronchodilating agents such as xanthine derivatives or beta-agonists include decreased symptoms and increased ease of breathing. Peak flow meters are easy to use and serve as a monitor of treatment effectiveness. The respiratory rate, rhythm, depth, and lung fields should also return to normal. Other anti-asthmatic or bronchodilating agents should produce the same therapeutic effects.

Adverse effects for which to monitor in clients receiving beta-agonists include tachyarrhythmias, chest pain, restlessness, agitation, nervousness, and insomnia. Adverse effects of anticholinergic agents consist of dry mouth, constipation, headache, nervousness, nausea, and blurred vision. The xanthine derivatives may cause palpitations, tachyarrhythmias, chest pain, GI upset, agitation, headache, insomnia, and restlessness. Besides watching for the side effects of xanthine derivatives, the therapeutic blood levels should also be checked. (Theophylline is 55 to 110 μmol/L. Any level above this is considered toxic and may cause fatal reactions. The Canadian asthma consensus guidelines recommend that a serum concentration of 28 to 55 μmol/L will reduce side effects without loss of therapeutic benefit.) The adverse effects of sodium cromoglygate include hypotension, bitter taste, dizziness, nausea, vomiting, dysrhythmias, and restlessness.

Adverse effects for which to monitor in clients taking antileukotrienes include headache, dyspepsia, nausea, dizziness, and insomnia. Therapeutic effects include an improvement in the control of chronic asthma.

PEDIATRIC CONSIDERATIONS ◆▲▼■

Use of Sodium Cromoglygate and Nedocromil Sodium

- Children over six years of age who are being treated with sodium cromoglygate administered by nasal spray should be given only one spray in each nostril tid or qid, but only as ordered by the physician and not to exceed six doses in 24 h. This type of spray is usually indicated for the treatment of allergic rhinitis.
- Children over five years of age being treated for bronchospasms with inhaled forms of sodium cromoglygate are usually given 20 mg administered over <1 hour qid; those treated with nebulizer forms are usually given a dose of 20 mg qid. Nedocromil sodium should be dosed at two inhalations qid.
- Children over five years of age being treated for bronchial asthma are generally prescribed inhaler and nebulizer forms at a dose of 20 mg qid. Children are usually willing and eager to learn about ways to prevent respiratory difficulty; therefore it is important to show them and their family members or caregivers the proper inhalation technique, which is as follows: Have the child exhale, then put the inhaler in place. Have the child inhale deeply with the head tipped back to maximize the opening of the air passages. Sodium cromoglygate and nedocromil sodium should be administered during this deep inhalation. After inhaling, instruct the child to remove the inhaler while holding the breath, than exhale when needed and repeat as instructed.
- Children should be told that sodium cromoglygate capsules are not to be chewed.
- Nebulizer forms of sodium cromoglygate and nedocromil sodium should be administered as instructed and according to the physician's orders. All equipment, including the filter and tubing, should be kept clean. Filters need to be purchased well ahead of time; manufacturers' guidelines suggest changing them when they begin to appear grey. The tubing and mouthpieces should be cleaned according to the manufacturer's guidelines, using water and white vinegar. Specific instructions should be followed regarding proper breathing and use of the machine. Once the nebulizer session is over, the mouthpiece should be rinsed. The child should also rinse out his or her mouth with water.
- Acute bronchospasms may occur with either of these agents and should be reported to the physician or healthcare provider immediately. Use of the agents should be discontinued.
- Use of a spacer device may be indicated.
- Instructions on peak flow meters should be clear and concise, with an emphasis on their importance in prevention.

CASE STUDY ▶◀◀

Chronic Obstructive Pulmonary Disease

Ms. B. is a 73-year-old woman who worked in the local traffic tunnel for about 25 years. She has had COPD for ten years, caused by cigarette smoking and exposure to workplace environmental pollutants. She quit smoking about eight years ago and is now retired. She is frequently admitted to the hospital, and is now in hospital for treatment of an acute exacerbation of her COPD and an upper respiratory tract infection. The physician has ordered the following: aminophylline intravenously per respiratory therapy protocol, intravenous continuous infusion at a rate of 0.8 mg/kg/hr; chest physiotherapy bid and prn; cephalothin antibiotic therapy, 1 g intravenously in 30 mL NS q8h; I&O; daily weights; VS with breath sounds q2h and prn until stable; and salbutamol inhaler, 2 puffs q4h per respiratory therapy protocol.

- What nursing interventions would be most appropriate to help this client conserve energy while enhancing O_2 and CO_2 gas exchange?
- What is the rationale for the continuous intravenous infusion of aminophylline?
- What are the reasons for prescribing the salbutamol inhaler and the antibiotic? Be specific about the reasons for each.
- What would be the most important client education guidelines for Ms. B. about using oral aminophylline and the salbutamol inhaler at home?

For answers see http://evolve.elsevier.com/Lilley/pharmacology/.
VS, vital signs.

CLIENT TEACHING TIPS

The nurse should instruct the client as follows:
▲ You can help improve your breathing problems by maintaining a generally good state of health.
▲ As much as practical, avoid the things that worsen your symptoms, such as allergens, stress, smoking, and air pollutants.
▲ Drink plenty of fluids (at least 12 glasses a day, unless your physician has told you otherwise) to thin the mucus.
▲ Make sure you come in for follow-up visits.
▲ Eat a balanced diet.
▲ As much as practical, avoid excessive fatigue, heat, and cold.
▲ Don't drink coffee, tea, cola, or other caffeinated beverages because they may narrow your airways.
▲ Use your medications as ordered. Make sure you understand when to use it: Some medications are to be taken every day to keep your breathing clear; others should be used before participating in activities that may cause problems, such as aerobic exercise, or before exposure to cold.
▲ (Except for clients on xanthines) If you have a chronic respiratory disease, get flu and pneumonia vaccinations.
▲ If you get the flu or some other infection, especially anything in your throat or lungs, get it treated promptly.
▲ Always check with your physician before taking any other medication, even over-the-counter medications, because you may have side effects if you combine this medication with others.

Corticosteroids

Corticosteroid treatment in clients with a COPD requires much patience on the part of the nurse and much client education. Nurses should tell clients the following:
▲ Do not abruptly discontinue your medications. This could lead to serious consequences. If your physician decides you need to discontinue this medication for any reason, you will be weaned off gradually over one to two weeks under the physician's care.
▲ Wear a medical alert bracelet or tag and carry a card at all times that identifies you as a steroid user.
▲ Tell your physician immediately if you develop "moon face," acne, swelling, or new fat. These symptoms indicate excess steroid levels.
▲ Also tell the physician if you develop nausea, difficulty breathing, joint pain, weakness, and fatigue; this could indicate that you aren't getting enough steroid.
▲ Report chest pain or any weight gain of more than 2 kg in a week.
▲ Do not drink alcohol while on this medication.
▲ Tell any other healthcare provider, including a dentist, that you are on this medication. Many drugs interact with this medication, so the doctor will need to check carefully before prescribing.

▲ Do not take ASA (aspirin). Do not take any over-the-counter drugs without checking with your physician.

Beta-agonists

▲ Take the medication exactly as prescribed by the physician, with no omissions or double dosing.
▲ Notify your physician if you experience insomnia, jitteriness, restlessness, palpitations, chest pain, or any change in symptoms.

Xanthine Derivatives

▲ Take your medication exactly as ordered. It is important to take this medication at the same time every day. If you miss a dose by more than one hour, skip it. Never double up on doses.
▲ Notify your physician if you experience palpitations, nausea, vomiting, weakness, dizziness, chest pain, or convulsions.
▲ If you are taking sustained-released tablets, pills, or capsules, never crush or chew them.
▲ Check with your physician before getting an influenza vaccination or immunization.
▲ Tell any other healthcare providers, including your dentist, that you are on this medication. Check with your physician before taking any over-the-counter medications.
▲ Do not drink large amounts of coffee.

Mast Cell Stabilizers

▲ This drug needs to be administered consistently for the therapeutic effects to occur. Don't be discouraged if your symptoms don't improve at first; it may take up to four weeks before you see the benefits.
▲ You may experience throat irritation, cough, headache, a bitter or bad taste in the mouth, or dry mouth.

Inhaled Medication

▲ To use your inhaler, first exhale, then insert the inhaler, tip your head back, and breathe in deeply. Remove the inhaler and hold your breath for ten seconds (or as close to ten seconds as you can), then exhale.
▲ Gargle and rinse your mouth with water afterward to avoid irritations or infections of the mouth and throat.
▲ If you have a nebulizer, make sure you know how to use it properly. Change the filters when they become greyish. Clean the tubing and mouthpieces frequently with soap, water, and white vinegar. Disposable tubing and mouthpieces are available.
▲ If you are using an MDI, the first time you use it, discharge it at least once into the air before taking your dose. This will help ensure that you get the proper amount of medication. Do the same if the canister has been stored upright for a while.

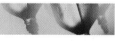

POINTS to REMEMBER

▼ Beta-agonists work by stimulating adenylate cyclase, which produces more cAMP and in turn causes relaxation of the smooth muscle that surrounds the airways.

▼ Beta-agonists may stimulate alpha- and beta-receptors, beta$_1$- and beta$_2$-receptors, or just beta$_2$-receptors.

▼ Beta$_2$-stimulants are the most specific for the lungs and have the fewest side effects.

▼ Xanthines include agents such as caffeine, theobromine, and theophylline and work by inhibiting phosphodiesterase.

▼ Phosphodiesterase breaks down cAMP, which is needed to relax smooth muscles.

▼ Theophylline is the most common xanthine; aminophylline is the parenteral form of theophylline.

▼ A major anticholinergic, ipratropium bromide (Atrovent), is the only agent in its category that is used for treatment of COPD.

▼ Anticholinergic agents are used for maintenance effects and not for relief of acute bronchospasms; they work by blocking the bronchoconstrictive effects of ACh.

▼ Corticosteroids are also used for treatment of the various respiratory disorders and have many indications. The most commonly used are beclomethasone, flunisolide, and triamcinolone. Corticosteroids work by stabilizing the membranes of cells that release harmful bronchoconstricting substances.

▼ Drugs such as sodium cromoglygate and nedocromil sodium are indicated only for prophylactic management of asthma and work by stabilizing the mast cell wall, helping to prevent potentially harmful vasoconstrictive substances from being released and exacerbating of asthma/bronchospasms.

▼ Nursing considerations vary depending on the drug. Contraindications to beta-agonist use include history of cardiac disease, dysrhythmias, angina, coronary artery disease, hypertension, and seizure disorders; anticholinergics are contraindicated in clients with benign prostatic hypertrophy or glaucoma; and xanthine derivatives are contraindicated in clients with a history of GI tract disorders or peptic ulcer disease.

▼ Sodium cromoglygate is used to prevent asthma, and treatment with this medication must be adhered to year-round. Client education is crucial to the success of this type of treatment.

▼ All respiratory agents should be given exactly as ordered and the diluent checked in terms of the proper amount and type of solution.

▼ The antileukotriene agents montelukast and zafirlukast are given orally. Side effects include headache, dizziness, insomnia, and dyspepsia.

EXAMINATION REVIEW QUESTIONS

1 The physician prescribes sodium cromoglygate to be given by nebulizer at home for an 11-year-old girl with a nine-year history of asthma. Which of the following is the rationale for the use of this medication? Sodium cromoglygate
   a. inhibits histamine release.
   b. inhibits mast cell degeneration.
   c. stimulates the release of bronchospastic agents.
   d. stimulates the substances that release acetylcholine.

2 Salbutamol's mechanism of action and related use include which of the following?
   a. Non-selective alpha-adrenergic receptor stimulation; used for bronchial secretion thickening
   b. Alpha- and beta-adrenergic receptor stimulation; used for bladder muscle contraction
   c. Beta$_2$-receptor stimulation; used for bronchospasms
   d. Beta$_1$-receptor stimulation; used for restriction of gaseous exchange

3 Which of the following is a side effect associated with xanthine derivatives?
   a. CNS depression
   b. Sinus tachycardia

   c. Increased appetite
   d. Temporary urinary retention

4 Indirect-acting agents (sodium cromoglygate and nedocromil), corticosteroids (e.g., triamcinolone), and anticholinergics (e.g., ipratropium bromide) are all used for clients with airway diseases (e.g., asthma, chronic bronchitis, emphysema):
   a. acutely.
   b. as needed.
   c. emergently.
   d. prophylactically.

5 Your client is changed from a xanthine to an antileukotriene (montelukast) for treatment of her asthma. Which of the following is a contraindication to its use?
   a. Polyuria
   b. Liver dysfunction
   c. Diabetes insipidus
   d. Transient urinary frequency

CRITICAL THINKING ACTIVITIES

1 Your client is taking a xanthine derivative and should not ingest xanthine-containing beverages. What are examples of these beverages, and why is it important to avoid consuming them while taking a xanthine derivative?

2 Discuss the necessary client education for the use of leukotriene modifiers, especially the rationale for the emphasis on taking the medication daily as ordered.

3 State the general guidelines for the use of an MDI, especially when it is new to the client.

For answers see http://evolve.elsevier.com/Lilley/pharmacology/.

BIBLIOGRAPHY

Albanese, J., & Nutz, P. (2005). *Mosby's 2005 nursing drug cards.* St Louis, MO: Mosby.

Asthma Society of Canada. (2005). Retrieved August 25, 2005, from http://www.asthma.ca/adults/

Asthma Guidelines Working Group of the Canadian Network For Asthma Care. (2005). Canadian pediatric asthma consensus guidelines, 2003 (updated to December 2004). *Canadian Medical Association Journal, 173*(6), S1–S56.

Becker, A., Watson, W., Ferguson, A., Dimich-Ward, H., Chan-Yeung, M. (2004). The Canadian asthma primary prevention study: Outcomes at 2 years of age. *Journal of Allergy and Clinical Immunology, 113*, 650–656.

Boulet, L.P., Becker, A., Bérebé, D., Beveridge, R., Ernst, P. and the Canadian Asthma Consensus Group. (1999). Canadian asthma consensus report. *Canadian Medical Association Journal, 161*(11 Suppl), S1–S62.

Canadian Pharmacists Association. (2003). *Therapeutic choices* (4th ed.). Ottawa, ON: Author.

Canadian Pharmacists Association. (2004). *Guide to drugs in Canada.* Toronto, ON: Dorling Kindersley.

Canadian Pharmacists Association. (2005). *Compendium of pharmaceuticals and specialties. The Canadian drug reference for health professionals.* Ottawa, ON: Author. [The subscription-based e-CPS is available at http://www.pharmacists.ca.]

Cheng, A., Williams, B.A., & Sivarajan, B.V. (Eds.). (2003). *The HSC handbook of pediatrics* (10th ed.). Toronto, ON: Elsevier.

Environment Canada. (2002). MDI information for health care professionals. Canada phases out CFC inhalers. Retrieved August 25, 2005, from http://www.ec.gc.ca/ozone/DOCS/SandS/mdi/EN/profession/article.cfm

Hardman, J.G., & Limbird, L.E. (2002). *Goodman and Gilman's the pharmacological basis of therapeutics* (10th ed.). New York: McGraw-Hill.

Health Canada. (2000). Risk of important drug interactions between St. John's Wort and prescription drugs. Retrieved August 25, 2005, from http://www.hc-sc.gc.ca/dhp-mps/medeff/advisories-avis/prof/2000/hypericum_perforatum_hpc-cps_e.html

Health Canada. (2005). Drug product database (DPD). Retrieved August 25, 2005, from http://www.hc-sc.gc.ca/hpb/drugs-dpd/

Health Canada. (2005). Health Canada endorsed important safety information on Serevent. Retrieved November 25, 2005 from http://www.hc-sc.gc.ca/dhp-mps/medeff/advisories-avis/prof/serevent_2_hpc-cps_e.html

Katzung, B.G. (2004). *Basic and clinical pharmacology* (9th ed.). New York: McGraw-Hill.

Lacy, C.F., Armstrong, L.L., Goldman, M.P., & Lance, L.L. (2003). *Drug information handbook* (11th ed.). Hudson, OH: Lexi-Comp.

Lehne, R.A. (2004). *Pharmacology for nursing care* (5th ed.). St Louis, MO: Saunders.

Lemière, C., Bai, T., Balter, M., Bayliff, C., Becker, A., Boulet, L-P., et al, on behalf of the Canadian Adult Consensus Group of the Canadian Thoracic Society. (2004). Adult asthma consensus guidelines update 2003. *Canadian Respiratory Journal, 11*(Suppl A), 9A–33A.

Mosby. (2005). *Mosby's drug consult 2005: The comprehensive reference for generic and brand name drugs* (15th ed.). St Louis, MO: Mosby.

The National Asthma Task Force. (2000). Prevention and management of asthma. Retrieved from http://www.phac-aspc.gc.ca/publicat/pma-pca00/pdf/asthma00e.pdf

Skidmore-Roth, L. (2006). *Mosby's 2006 nursing drug reference* (19th ed.). St Louis, MO: Mosby.

PART SEVEN

Anti-Infective and Anti-Inflammatory Agents: Study Skills Tips

- NURSING PROCESS
- ASSESSMENT
- NURSING DIAGNOSES
- EVALUATION

This study model focuses on the Nursing Process sections, using Chapter 37 as an example.

"The discussion of the nursing process will <u>focus</u> on each <u>major classification of antibiotics</u> to convey <u>general and specific information</u> about the various antibiotics."

The underlining in this paragraph is intended to point out the important information. The Nursing Process section focuses on major classifications. Another critical piece of this paragraph is the need to see both *general* and *specific* information about the classifications. Although the paragraph is only one sentence long, it clearly defines what you need to keep in mind as you study this section.

ASSESSMENT

What is the purpose of this section? Each time you begin to read the Nursing Process section of a chapter, you need to ask this question. What are you supposed to learn? What are you supposed to know? What are you supposed to be able to do? All these questions relate to your role as a nurse. Consider the following sentence from this section in Chapter 37.

"<u>Before administering</u> any antibiotic, it is <u>crucial to ensuring appropriate, effective treatment for the nurse to collect client data</u> on <u>age; hypersensitivity to drugs; hepatic (aspartate aminotransferase [AST] and alanine aminotransferase [ALT]), renal, and cardiac function (i.e., pertinent laboratory test results); culture and sensitivity results; and complete blood count (CBC), hemoglobin (Hgb), and hematocrit (Hct) values.</u>"

Assessment clearly has to do with client care. You are assessing clients in relation to the pharmacological interventions that this chapter discusses. I have done some underlining in this section to bring into sharper focus some of the things that you must be aware of as you study.

First, notice the use of the word *crucial* in the first line. Something is so important at this point that it cannot be ignored. Immediately the questioning process should be activated. What is crucial? The answer follows immediately in the sentence. You must have data collected on the client. The sentence goes on to identify the kind of data that should be available, and the sentence makes it clear that it has to be done "before administering." Each of the data factors is important, and each relates to other parts and chapters in this text.

The client's age should be known. Chapter 3 deals with pediatric and geriatric concerns. Children and elderly clients respond to drugs differently than adults. This would directly affect dosage and possibly even the choice of antibiotics to be administered. This also ties directly to the "effective treatment" referred to in this sentence.

The next data item is hypersensitivities. Some individuals are allergic to certain antibiotics. It would be dangerous and possibly fatal to administer an antibiotic to a client who is hypersensitive to it. This also connects with appropriate treatment. As you consider each of the underlined elements in this sentence, you must keep in mind its relationship to effectiveness and appropriateness.

Another data item specifies hepatic, renal, and cardiac functioning. As you read this you should instantly think what hepatic, renal, and cardiac mean. Then you should try to recall information from this chapter that related the specific antibiotics to these functions. Learning is cumulative. The Nursing Process section assumes you have read and understood what was presented earlier in the chapter.

One more aspect of this sentence is the use of standard medical abbreviations. In earlier Study Skills Tips it has been suggested that you prepare vocabulary cards for these abbreviations. You need to know what CBC, Hgb, and Hct mean, what they measure, and how they relate to appropriate administration of antibiotics. If these letters are not meaningful to you, then you will not be able to link what you know about the antibiotics with what you must know about administering them. Many test questions on nursing examinations use the standard abbreviations, and you must know them instantly and be able to relate them to the situation covered. What might a test question ask about these data elements as they apply to client care? This is what the nursing process is all about.

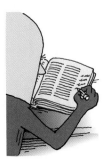

NURSING DIAGNOSES

The same first question applies here as in every other section. What am I supposed to learn? Since the focus is on administration of antibiotics, the expectation you should bring to this is an awareness of your role in diagnosis. What should you look for in working with clients that affects the administration of antibiotics?

This same procedure should be applied to the sections on Planning, Outcome Criteria, and Implementation. Consider what each of these headings suggests about the nursing process, and read and evaluate the information, relating it to what you have already learned. Also consider the implications of the information as possible test questions that may ask you to do more than recall specific facts. As an example, consider the following case:

Client A, age 23 years, has a fever of 38.2°C. She was admitted yesterday and delivered a healthy infant eight hours ago. She is breastfeeding the newborn. What antibiotics might be administered for the fever? What specific antibiotics should be used with caution or eliminated from consideration?

This case demonstrates the need to read and think critically. You need to not only remember the specific facts from the chapter, but also be able to take a case study example and apply those facts to that specific situation.

EVALUATION

This is the final section under Nursing Process. What are you supposed to evaluate?

"The therapeutic effects of antibiotics in general include a decrease in the signs and symptoms of the infection; a return to normal vital signs, including temperature; negative results of culture and sensitivity tests; a decrease to a normal CBC; and improved appetite, energy level, and sense of well-being." This sentence makes it clear that you are evaluating the client and his or her response to the antibiotics being administered. In evaluating the client, what should you look for? Given the focus in nursing process on contraindications, cautions, hypersensitivity, and reactions related to the administration of antibiotics, you should be evaluating two aspects of the client.

First you should look for the positive responses set forth in the above text sample that indicate the client is responding favourably to the treatment. But when you read the next sentence in this section, you see: "Common adverse reactions for which to monitor. . . " This says your role in evaluation is to monitor the client for negative responses and to be prepared to educate the client about these effects and possible steps to alleviate them.

The Nursing Process section in each chapter should be read carefully and thoughtfully because it is in this section that you begin to see how the complex pharmacological material presented earlier in the chapter fits into your role as a nurse. This material should be read with the same concern and care that you have given to the earlier part of the chapter, 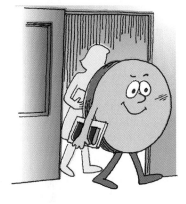 as this is the section in which you think about *applying* all you have learned. Apply the PURR model and be an active questioner and reader, and you will be successful in working with the Nursing Process in each chapter.

Antibiotics

OBJECTIVES

After reading this chapter, the successful student will be able to do the following:

1 Discuss the general principles of antibiotic therapy.

2 Explain how antibiotics work to rid the body of infection.

3 Discuss the pros and cons of antibiotic usage.

4 Describe concerns about the overuse of antibiotics.

5 Discuss the indications, cautions, contraindications, mechanisms of action, side effects, and toxicity associated with the various antibiotic groups.

6 List the classifications of antibiotics, with examples of specific drugs.

7 Develop a nursing care plan that includes all phases of the nursing process for the client receiving antibiotics.

e-LEARNING ACTIVITIES

Student CD-ROM
- Review Questions: see questions 286–300
- Animations
- Medication Administration Checklists
- IV Therapy Checklists

 **Web site** (http://evolve.elsevier.com/Lilley/pharmacology/)
- Online Chapter Worksheet • Frequently Asked Questions
- Learning Tips and Content Updates • WebLinks • Online Appendices and Supplements • Mosby/Saunders ePharmacology Update • Access to *Mosby's Drug Consult*

DRUG PROFILES

amikacin, p. 641
▶▶amoxicillin, p. 630
ampicillin, p. 630
▶▶azithromycin and clarithromycin, p. 636
▶▶cefazolin, p. 631
cefepime, p. 634
cefixime, p. 633
▶▶cefoxitin, p. 632
ceftazidime, p. 633
▶▶ceftriaxone, p. 633

cefuroxime, p. 633
▶▶cephalexin, p. 631
▶▶ciprofloxacin, p. 644
▶▶clindamycin, p. 644
cloxacillin, p. 630
dapsone, p. 645
demeclocycline, p. 639
▶▶doxycycline, p. 639
▶▶erythromycin, p. 636
▶▶gentamicin, p. 641
▶▶imipenem-cilastatin, p. 634

levofloxacin, p. 644
linezolid, p. 645
▶▶metronidazole, p. 645
nitrofurantoin, p. 645
▶▶penicillin G and penicillin V potassium, p. 629

quinupristin and dalfopristin, p. 646
sulfamethoxazole, p. 626
sulfisoxazole, p. 627
▶▶vancomycin, p. 646

 ▶▶ Key drug.

GLOSSARY

Aerobic Requiring oxygen for the maintenance of life.

Anaerobic Not requiring oxygen for the maintenance of life.

Antibiotic Of or pertaining to the ability to destroy or interfere with the development of a living organism. Term used most commonly to refer to antibacterial drugs.

Bactericidal antibiotic An antibiotic that kills bacteria.

Bacteriostatic antibiotic An antibiotic that does not actually kill but rather inhibits the growth of bacteria.

Beta-lactamase Any of a group of enzymes produced by bacteria that catalyze the chemical opening of the crucial beta-lactam ring structures in beta-lactam antibiotics.

Beta-lactamase inhibitor One of several medications added in combination with certain penicillin drugs to block the effect of beta-lactamase enzymes.

Beta-lactams The name for a broad, major class of antibiotics that includes four subclasses: penicillins, cephalosporins, carbapenems, and monobactams.

Empirical therapy Administration of antibiotics based on the most likely pathogens causing an apparent infection; involves the presumptive treatment of an infection to avoid treatment delay before specific culture information has been reported or obtained.

Glucose-6-phosphate dehydrogenase (G6PD) deficiency An inherited disorder in which the red blood cells are partially or completely deficient in glucose-6-phosphate dehydrogenase, a critical enzyme in the metabolism of glucose. Certain medications can cause hemolytic anemia in clients with this disorder. This is a type of *host factor* as related to drug therapy.

Host factors Factors that are unique to the body of a particular client that affect the client's susceptibility to infection and response to various antibiotic drugs.

Infection The invasion and multiplication of micro-organisms in body tissues.

Micro-organism A microscopic living organism (also called *microbe*).

Minimum inhibitory concentration (MIC) The lowest concentration of antibiotic required to inhibit the growth of a specific micro-organism; usually refers to blood concentrations.

Prophylactic antibiotic therapy Antibiotics taken before anticipated exposure to an infectious organism in an effort to prevent the development of infection.

Slow acetylator (a set' ə lay tər) A common genetic host factor that reduces the rate of metabolism of certain drugs.

Subtherapeutic Referring to antibiotic treatment that is ineffective for a given infection. Possible causes include inappropriate drug therapy, insufficient drug dosing, or bacterial drug resistance.

Superinfection (1) An infection occurring during antimicrobial treatment for another infection, resulting in overgrowth of a non-susceptible organism. (2) A secondary microbial infection that occurs in addition to an earlier primary infection, often due to weakening of the client's immune system function by the first infection.

Teratogen (ter' ə to jen) Any substance that can interfere with normal prenatal development and cause one or more developmental abnormalities in the fetus.

Therapeutic Of or relating to treatment that is considered beneficial. With regard to antibiotics, refers to drug therapy that results in sufficient concentrations of the drug in the blood or other tissues to render it effective against specific bacterial pathogens.

MICROBIAL INFECTION

A person is normally able to remain healthy and resistant to infectious **micro-organisms** because of the existence of certain host defences. These defences take various forms. They can be actual physical barriers such as intact

Bacterial Morphology
Shapes

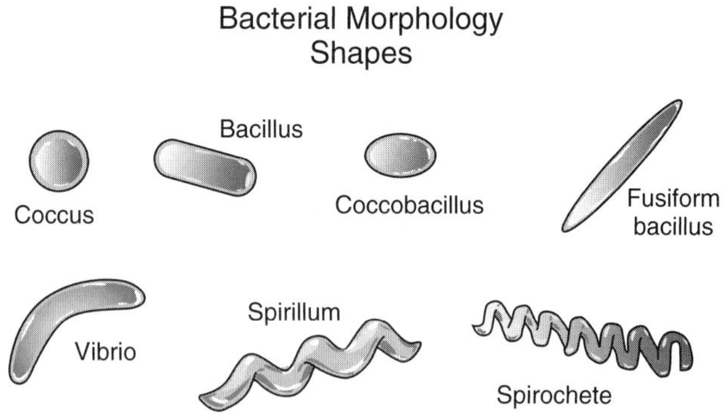

FIG. 37-1 Bacterial morphologies. (From Murray, P.R., Rosenthal, K.S., Kobayashi, G.S., & Pfaller, M.A. (2002). *Medical microbiology.* St Louis, MO: Mosby.)

skin or the ciliated respiratory mucosa. They can be physiological defences such as the gastric acid in the stomach and immune factors such as antibodies. They can also be the phagocytic cells (macrophages and polymorphonuclear neutrophils) that are part of the reticuloendothelial system.

Micro-organisms are everywhere, both in the external environment and in many parts of the internal environment of our bodies. They can be intrinsically harmful to humans, or they can be innocuous and even beneficial under normal circumstances but become harmful when these conditions are altered in some way. An example of an intrinsically harmful micro-organism is *Rickettsia rickettsii*, which causes Rocky Mountain spotted fever (RMSF). An example of a micro-organism that is only sometimes harmful is a certain species of *Streptococcus* that is normally present in the body. Streptococci usually do not cause harm, but under certain circumstances can cause endocarditis in clients whose heart valves have been damaged as a result of rheumatic fever. Every known major class of microbes has member organisms that can infect humans. This includes bacteria, viruses, fungi, and protozoans. The focus of this chapter is common bacterial **infections**.

Recall from microbiology that bacteria come in a number of different shapes. This property is called the *morphology* of a given type of bacteria (Figure 37-1). Bacteria may also group themselves into common recognizable patterns (Figure 37-2). One of the most important ways of categorizing different bacteria is on the basis of their response to the *Gram-stain* procedure (Figure 37-3). Bacterial species that stain purple using the Gram-stain dyes are classified as gram-positive organisms. Those bacteria that stain red are classified as gram-negative organisms. This seemingly simple difference proves to be significant in guiding the choice of **antibiotic** therapy.

Gram-positive organisms have cell walls with a much thicker component known as *peptidoglycan,* which refers to the protein (peptido-) and sugar (-glycan) chemistry of its structure. In addition, gram-positive organisms also have a thicker outer cell *capsule.* However, gram-negative

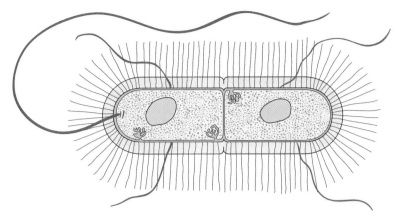

FIG. 37-2 A dividing bacterial cell with a single flagellum, four sex pili, numerous common fibriae, a cell wall, a cytoplasmic membrane, two nuclear bodies, three mesosomes, and numerous ribosomes. (From Greenwood, D., Slack, R., & Peutherer, J. (2002). *Medical microbiology* (16th ed.). Edinburgh, GB: Elsevier Science.)

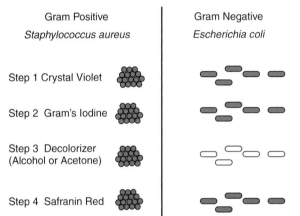

FIG. 37-3 Gram-stain morphology of bacteria. The crystal violet of Gram stain is precipitated by Gram iodine and is trapped in the thick peptidoglycan layer in gram-positive bacteria. The decolorizer disperses the gram-negative outer membrane and washes the crystal violet from the thin layer of peptidoglycan. Gram-negative bacteria are visualized by the red counterstain. (From Murray, P.R., Rosenthal, K.S., Kobayashi, G.S., & Pfaller, M.A. (2002). *Medical microbiology*. St Louis, MO: Mosby.)

organisms have a cell wall structure that is more complex, having a smaller outer capsule and peptidoglycan layer than gram-positive bacteria, but also having two cell membranes: an outer and inner membrane (Figures 37-4 and 37-5). These differences usually make gram-negative bacterial infections more difficult to treat because the drug molecules have a harder time penetrating the more complex gram-negative cell walls.

When a person's normal host defences are breached or somehow compromised, that person becomes susceptible to infection. The micro-organisms invade and multiply in the body tissues, and if the infective process overwhelms the body's own defence system, the infection becomes clinically apparent. The client then manifests the characteristic signs and symptoms of infection: fever, chills,

sweats, redness, pain and swelling, fatigue, weight loss, increased white blood cell (WBC) count, and the formation of pus. Not all clients will exhibit signs of infection. This is especially true in geriatric and immunocompromised clients.

Antibiotic therapy is often required to help the body and its normal host defences combat an infection. Antibiotics are most effective when their actions are combined with functioning bodily defence mechanisms. However, before considering specific types of drug therapy, we first review some general principles.

GENERAL PRINCIPLES OF ANTIBIOTIC THERAPY

Antibiotic drug therapy should begin with a clinical assessment of the client to determine whether the common signs and symptoms of infection are present. The client should also be assessed during and after antibiotic therapy to evaluate the effectiveness of the drug therapy, monitor for adverse drug effects, and make sure the infection is not recurring.

Often the signs and symptoms of an infection appear long before an organism can be identified. When this happens and the risk of life-threatening or severe complications is high, an antibiotic is given to the client immediately. The antibiotic selected is one that can best kill the micro-organisms known to be the most common causes of infection. This is defined as **empirical therapy**. Before the start of empirical antibiotic therapy, suspected areas of infection should be cultured in an attempt to identify a causative organism. It must be emphasized that culture specimens should be obtained *before* initiating drug therapy whenever possible. Otherwise the presence of antibiotics in the tissues may result in misleading culture results. If an organism is identified in the laboratory it is then tested for various antibiotic susceptibilities. The

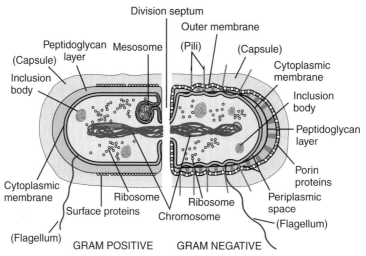

FIG. 37-4 Gram-positive and gram-negative bacteria. A gram-positive bacterium has a thick layer of peptidoglycan *(left)*. A gram-negative bacterium has a thin peptidoglycan layer and an outer membrane *(right)*. Structures in parentheses are not found in all bacteria. (From Murray, P.R., Rosenthal, K.S., Kobayashi, G.S., & Pfaller, M.A. (2002). *Medical microbiology*. St Louis, MO: Mosby.)

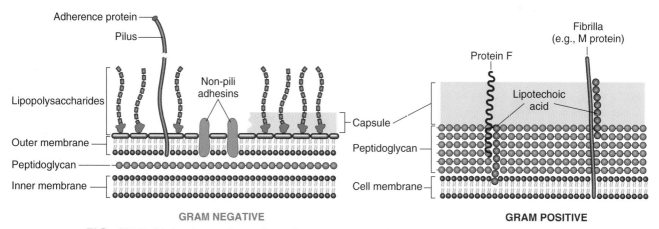

FIG. 37-5 Molecules on the surface of gram-negative and gram-positive bacteria involved in pathogenesis. Not shown is the type 3 secretory apparatus of gram-negative bacteria. (From Cotran, R.S., Kumar, V., & Collins, T. (1999). *Robbins pathologic basis of disease* (6th ed.). Philadelphia: Saunders.)

results of these tests can confirm whether the empirical therapy chosen is appropriate for eradicating the organism identified. If not, therapy can be adjusted to optimize its efficacy against the specific infectious organism(s).

Antibiotics are also given for prophylactic reasons. This is often the case when clients are scheduled to have a procedure in which the likelihood of dangerous microbial contamination is high. **Prophylactic antibiotic therapy** is used to prevent an infection. However, the risk of infection varies depending on the procedure being performed. For example, the risk of infection in a client undergoing coronary artery bypass surgery (with standard preoperative cleansing of the body) is relatively low compared with that in a person undergoing intra-abdominal surgery for the treatment of injuries suffered in a motor vehicle accident. In the latter case, bacterial contamination from the gastrointestinal (GI) tract is highly likely to be present in the abdominal cavity. This would constitute a contaminated or dirty surgical field, and therefore the likelihood of clinically serious infection would be high.

To optimize antibiotic therapy, the client should be monitored for both **therapeutic** efficacy and adverse drug effects. A therapeutic response to antibiotics is one in which there is a decrease in the specific signs and symptoms of infection compared with the baseline findings (e.g., fever, elevated WBC count, redness, inflammation, drainage, pain). Antibiotic therapy is said to be **subtherapeutic** when these signs and symptoms do not improve. This can result from using an incorrect route of administration, inadequate drainage of an abscess, poor antibiotic penetration to the infected area, subtherapeutic serum levels of the agent, or bacterial resistance to the antibiotic. Antibiotic therapy is considered toxic when the serum levels of the antibiotic are too high or when the client has an allergic or other major adverse reaction to the drug. These reactions include rash, itching, hives, fever, chills, joint pain, difficulty breathing, or wheezing. Relatively minor adverse drug reactions such as GI discomfort and diarrhea are quite common with antibiotic therapy and are usually not severe enough to require drug discontinuation.

Superinfections and antibiotic interactions with food and other drugs are other problems to be watched for in clients taking antibiotics. Superinfections occur when antibiotics reduce or completely eliminate the normal bacterial flora. This consists of certain bacteria and fungi that are needed to maintain normal function in various organs. When these bacteria or fungi are killed by antibiotics, other bacteria or fungi are permitted to take over and cause infection. An example of a **superinfection** caused by antibiotics is the development of vaginal yeast infections when the normal vaginal flora is reduced and yeast growth is no longer suppressed.

Another type of superinfection occurs when a second infection occurs closely following an initial primary infection, which may still be ongoing. A common example of this is when a client who has already developed a viral respiratory infection develops a secondary bacterial infection, probably because the virus weakened the immune system. Although the viral infection will not respond to antibiotic therapy, antibiotics may be needed to treat the secondary bacterial infection. This situation calls for some diagnostic finesse on the part of prescribers (e.g., nurse practitioners), who should avoid prescribing unnecessary antibiotics for a viral infection. The presence of coloured sputum (e.g., green or yellow) is one sign of a bacterial superinfection during a viral respiratory illness.

Clients will often expect to receive an antibiotic prescription even when they show no signs of a bacterial superinfection. From their perspective, they know they are sick and want some medicine to expedite their recovery from illness. This can create both diagnostic confusion and an emotional dilemma for the prescriber. Over the decades since antibiotics were first developed in the 1940s, many formerly treatable bacterial infections have become increasingly resistant to antibiotic therapy. This phenomenon is attributed partly to the overprescribing of antibiotics. Antibiotic resistance is now considered to be one of the world's most pressing public health problems. *Emerging infections,* such as those with drug-resistant bacteria, are a major culprit. Inappropriate antibiotic prescribing has had the effect of selecting out the most drug-resistant bacteria. Another factor that contributes to this problem is the tendency of many clients to not complete their antibiotic regimen. Clients should be counselled to take the entire course of prescribed antibiotic therapy, even if they feel that they are no longer ill. This increases the likelihood of a more complete bacterial kill for their infection, while reducing the likelihood of recurrent illness and survival of drug-resistant bacteria. The only usual exception to this is when culture results indicate that the chosen antibiotic therapy is not ideal for a particular type of bacterial infection. Clients should be educated as needed regarding such matters.

The chemical makeup of antibiotics can also cause the body to react in many ways. Food–drug and drug–drug interactions are common problems in clients taking antibiotics. One of the more common food–drug interactions is between milk or cheese and tetracycline, resulting in decreased absorption of tetracycline. An example of an antibiotic–drug interaction is between quinolone antibiotics and antacids, resulting in decreased absorption of quinolone antibiotics.

Other important factors essential to the appropriate use of antibiotics are host-specific factors, or **host factors.** These are the particular factors that pertain to the infected client and that can have an important bearing on the success or failure of antibiotic therapy. Some of these host factors are age, allergy history, organ function (kidneys and liver), pregnancy, genetic characteristics, site of infection, and host defences.

Age-related host factors apply to clients at either end of the age spectrum. For instance, infants and children may not be able to take certain antibiotics such as tetracyclines, because of their effects on developing teeth or bones; fluoroquinolones, which may also affect bone development in children; and sulphonamides, which may displace bilirubin from albumin and precipitate kernicterus (hyperbilirubinemia) in young clients. The aging process affects the function of various organ systems. As we age there is a gradual decline in the function of the kidneys and liver, the organs primarily responsible for metabolizing and eliminating antibiotics. Therefore, depending on the level of kidney or liver function for a given older adult, dosage adjustments may be necessary. Pharmacists often play a significant role in ensuring optimal dosing for a given client's level of organ function.

A history of allergic reactions must also be considered in selecting an antibiotic. Many people have allergic reactions to penicillins and sulphonamides. The most dangerous such reaction is anaphylactic shock, in which a client can suffocate from drug-induced respiratory arrest. This extreme outcome underscores the importance of assessing clients for drug allergies and documenting any known allergies clearly in the medical record. All reported drug allergies should be taken seriously and investigated further before making a final decision about whether to administer a given drug. Many clients will state that they are allergic to a medication when in fact they have had a common mild side effect such as stomach upset or nausea. Clients who report drug allergies should be asked to describe prior allergic reactions. The most common severe reactions, which need to be noted, include any difficulty breathing; significant rash, hives, or other skin reaction; and severe GI intolerance. Although some antibiotics are ideally taken on an empty stomach, eating a small amount of food with the medication may be sufficient to help the client tolerate it and realize its therapeutic benefits.

Pregnancy-related host factors are also important because several antibiotics can pass through the placenta to the fetus and harm the developing fetus. Such drugs are called **teratogens**. Their use in pregnant women can result in birth defects.

Many drugs, including certain antibiotics, depend on specific enzyme systems to chemically break them down (metabolize) so that they can be eliminated. However, some clients have certain genetic abnormalities that may result in deficiencies of the enzymes needed by these systems. This can result in toxic levels of the drug in the body. Two of the most common examples of such genetic host factors are **glucose-6-phosphate dehydrogenase (G6PD) deficiency** and **slow acetylator** metabolic status. The administration of such antibiotics as sulphonamides, nitrofurantoin, and dapsone to a person with G6PD deficiency may result in the hemolysis, or destruction, of red blood cells (RBCs). Slow acetylators metabolize certain drugs more slowly than usual, specifically with regard to a chemical step known as *acetylation*. This can lead to toxicity from drug accumulation. The most common example is the development of a peripheral neuropathy in a slow acetylator who is given typical adult doses of the antituberculosis drug isoniazid (Chapter 39).

The anatomic site of the infection is another important host factor to consider when determining not only which antibiotic to use but also the dose, route of administration, and duration of therapy.

Consideration of these host factors helps ensure that the most appropriate antibiotic is selected for a particular client. Additional client assessment and routine monitoring of antibiotic therapy increase the likelihood that it will be safe and effective.

ANTIBIOTICS

Antibiotics are classified into many broad categories based on their chemical structure. Some of the more common of these categories are sulphonamides, penicillins, cephalosporins, macrolides, fluoroquinolones, aminoglycosides, and tetracyclines. In addition to chemical structure, the characteristics that distinguish one class of agents from the next include antibacterial spectrum, mechanism of action, potency, toxicity, and pharmacokinetic properties. The four most common mechanisms of antibiotic action include interfering with bacterial cell wall synthesis, interfering with protein synthesis, interfering with deoxyribonucleic acid (DNA) replication, and acting as an antimetabolite to disrupt other critical metabolic reactions inside the bacterial cell. Figure 37-6 lists the mechanisms of action of several major antibiotic classes. Perhaps the greatest challenge in understanding antimicrobial therapy is remembering which types and species of micro-organisms a given drug can act against. The list of individual micro-organisms that a given drug acts against can be quite extensive and seem daunting to the inexperienced practitioner. Most antimicrobials have activity against only one *type* of microbe (e.g., bacteria, viruses, fungi, protozoans). However, a few drugs do have activity against more than one class of organisms. Understanding of antimicrobial therapy will deepen with

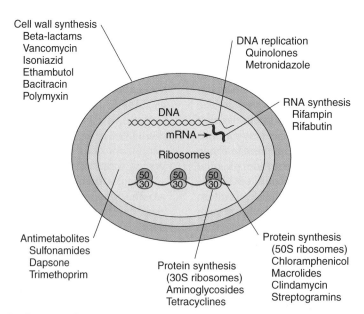

FIG. 37-6 Basic sites of antibiotic activity. (From Murray, P.R., Rosenthal, K.S., Kobayashi, G.S., & Pfaller, M.A. (2002). *Medical microbiology.* St Louis, MO: Mosby.)

clinical experience. It is always appropriate to check reference materials or consult with colleagues (e.g., nurses, pharmacists, physicians) when questions remain.

SULPHONAMIDES

Sulphonamides are a chemically related group of antibiotics that are synthetic derivatives of sulphanilamide. They were one of the first groups of drugs used as antibiotics, and some of the more commonly prescribed agents are sulfadiazine, sulfamethoxazole, and sulfisoxazole. Sulfasalazine, another sulphonamide, is used for ulcerative colitis and rheumatoid arthritis and not as an antibiotic. The antibiotic activity of sulphonamides is the result of their ability to antagonize or inhibit an enzyme that is essential for the growth and proliferation of certain bacteria, and they are effective against a wide range of organisms. These antibiotics achieve high concentrations in the kidneys, through which they are eliminated. Therefore they are primarily used in the treatment of urinary tract infections (UTI), but they are sometimes also used for respiratory tract infections. In addition they are routinely combined with other antibiotics for a synergistic drug effect.

Mechanism of Action and Drug Effects

Sulphonamides do not actually destroy bacteria but instead they inhibit their growth. For this reason they are considered **bacteriostatic antibiotics**. They inhibit the growth of susceptible bacteria by preventing the synthesis of folic acid, a B-complex vitamin that is required for the proper synthesis of purines and nucleic acid. Folic acid is composed of a molecule of para-aminobenzoic acid (PABA), pteridine, and glutamic acid. Sulphonamides compete with the PABA for the enzyme that incorporates the PABA into the folic acid molecule during biosynthesis. Because sulphonamides block a specific step in a biosynthetic pathway, they are also considered antimetabolites. However, micro-organisms that can use preformed folic acid are not affected by the sulphonamides.

A common combination is the sulphonamide agent sulfamethoxazole with trimethoprim (a non-sulphonamide). Commonly available in combination tablet form or as an oral suspension, together these two antibiotics block two successive steps in the bacterial folic acid pathway. Unfortunately, however, many organisms once susceptible to the sulphonamides are now resistant to them.

Only micro-organisms that synthesize their own folic acid are inhibited by sulphonamides. Animals and bacteria that are capable of using exogenous folic acid precursors or preformed folic acid are not affected by them. Human cells can use preformed folic acid and are therefore not affected by sulphonamides.

Indications

The sulphonamides are used for the treatment of UTIs caused by susceptible strains of *Enterobacter* spp., *Escherichia coli*, *Klebsiella* spp., *Proteus mirabilis*, *Proteus vul-*

garis, and *Staphylococcus aureus*. In addition, sulphonamides are the drugs of choice for the treatment of nocardiosis, *Pneumocystis carinii* pneumonia (PCP), and infections secondary to the bacteria *Stenotrophomonas maltophilia*. They are also excellent drugs for the treatment of upper respiratory tract infections. Sulphonamides are used as adjuncts in the treatment of malaria and toxoplasmosis and as alternative agents for the management of chlamydial infections. Specifically, sulfapyridine is used for the second-line treatment of a herpes-like skin infection known as *dermatitis herpetiformis*; sulfadiazine, sulfisoxazole, and sulfamethoxazole are all used for the treatment of nocardiosis (infection by the bacterium *Nocardia*, which starts in the lungs and can spread to the brain); and sulfasalazine is used to treat ulcerative colitis.

Contraindications

Sulphonamides are contraindicated in cases of known drug allergy to sulphonamides or chemically related drugs such as sulphonylureas (used for diabetes), thiazide and loop diuretics, and carbonic anhydrase inhibitors (Chapter 25).

Side Effects and Adverse Effects

Sulphonamide drugs are a common cause of allergic reactions. These agents are included in several drug classes, including antimicrobials, diuretics, oral hypoglycemics, and carbonic anhydrase inhibitors. Although immediate reactions can occur, sulphonamides typically cause delayed cutaneous reactions. These reactions often begin with fever followed by a rash (morbilliform eruptions, erythema multiforme, or toxic epidermal necrolysis). Other reactions to sulphonamides include mucocutaneous, GI, hepatic, renal, or hematological complications, all of which may be fatal. It is believed that sulphonamide reactions are immune mediated and involve the production of reactive metabolites. It is important to differentiate between sulphites and sulphonamides. Sulphites are commonly used as preservatives in everything from wine to food to injectable drugs. Reported side effects of sulphonamide drugs are listed in Table 37-1.

TABLE 37-1
SULPHONAMIDES: REPORTED ADVERSE EFFECTS

Body System	Side/Adverse Effects
Blood	Agranulocytosis, aplastic anemia, hemolytic anemia, thrombocytopenia
Gastrointestinal	Nausea, vomiting, diarrhea, pancreatitis
Integumentary	Epidermal necrolysis, exfoliative dermatitis, Stevens-Johnson syndrome, photosensitivity
Other	Convulsions, crystalluria, toxic nephrosis, headache, peripheral neuritis, urticaria

Interactions

Sulphonamides can have clinically significant interactions with a number of other medications. Sulphonamides can potentiate the hypoglycemic effects of sulphonylureas in diabetes; the toxic effects of phenytoin; and the anticoagulant effects of warfarin, which can lead to hemorrhage. Sulphonamides can inhibit the immunosuppressant effects of cyclosporine for transplant clients but can also increase the likelihood of cyclosporine-induced nephrotoxicity. Clients receiving any of these combinations may require more frequent monitoring to ensure optimal drug effects.

Laboratory Test Interactions

Sulphonamides can increase the serum levels of aspartate aminotransferase, acetyltransferase, and alkaline phosphatase.

Dosages

For recommended dosages of selected sulphonamides, see the table below. See Appendix B for some of the common brands available in Canada.

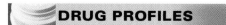

DRUG PROFILES

Sulphonamides are classified as pregnancy category C agents. They are contraindicated in clients with a known hypersensitivity to sulphonamides, in pregnant women at term, and in infants under two months of age.

sulfamethoxazole

Sulfamethoxazole is a sulphonamide antibiotic. Because it is eliminated by means of the kidneys and reaches high concentrations there, it is commonly used to treat UTIs caused by susceptible organisms. The drug is currently available only in combination with antimetabolite trimethoprim in a fixed combination containing a 5:1 ratio of sulfamethoxazole to trimethoprim. As explained earlier, this combination of agents sequentially inhibits two steps in the folic acid pathway, giving it antibacterial synergism. It is commonly used in the treatment of UTIs caused by susceptible bacteria, PCP, ear infections (otitis media), bronchitis, gonorrhea, and many other infectious conditions. It is also used for prophylaxis in human immunodeficiency virus (HIV)-infected clients, especially against PCP (Chapter 38). This fixed combination is available as an oral suspension containing 40 mg/5 mL of trimethoprim and 200 mg/5 mL of sulfamethoxazole, as well as three strengths of oral tablets containing 20, 80, and 400 mg and 100, 160, and 800 mg of trimethoprim and sulfamethoxazole respectively. It is also available in a fixed-combination agent containing 16 mg/mL of trimethoprim and 80 mg/mL of sulfamethoxazole to be given as an intravenous (IV) injection. Pregnancy category C. Recommended dosages of the sulfamethoxazole products are listed in the table below.

PHARMACOKINETICS

Half-Life	Onset	Peak	Duration
7–12 hr	Variable	2–4 hr (plasma)	Up to 12 hr

DOSAGES — Selected Sulphonamides and Combination Drug Products

Agent	Pharmacological Class	Usual Dosage Range	Indications
sulfamethoxazole/ trimethoprim	Sulphonamide/folate antimetabolite	**Adult and pediatric** IV: 5–20 mL/kg/day divided bid–qid **Pediatric <12 yr** PO:* 20 mg trimethoprim/kg/day and 100 mg sulfamethoxazole/kg/day in 4 divided doses **Adult** PO: 3 tablets or 1.5 DS tablets twice daily **Adult** PO:* 80–160 mg trimethoprim/800 mg sulfamethoxazole once daily **Pediatric <12 yr** PO: 6 mg trimethoprim/kg/day, plus 30 mg sulfamethoxazole/kg/day divided bid	GI infections, UTIs, upper and lower respiratory tract infections, uncomplicated gonococcal urethritis, shigellosis enteritis, PCP in infants and children PCP prophylaxis, chronic chest infection prophylaxis
▸▸ erythromycin/ sulfisoxazole	Macrolide/ sulphonamide	**Pediatric >2 mo only** PO: 50 mg/kg/day erythromycin and 150 mg/kg/day sulfisoxazole (max 6 g/day) equally divided doses tid–qid × 10 days	*Haemophilus influenzae, Streptococcus pneumoniae, Staphylococcus pyrogenes, Branhamella catarrhalis* otitis media
sulfisoxazole	Sulphonamide	**Adult** PO: 2–4 g load, then 4–8 g/day divided q4–6h **Pediatric ≥2 mo** PO: 75 mg/kg load, then 150 mg/kg/day divided q4–6h	Otitis media, UTIs, *Haemophilus influenzae* meningitis, nocardiosis, toxoplasmosis

*Each tablet contains 80 mg trimethoprim and 400 mg sulfamethoxazole; double strength (DS): 160 mg trimethoprim and 800 mg sulfamethoxazole; 5-mL ampoule contains 80 mg trimethoprim and 400 mg sulfamethoxazole; 5-mL oral suspension contains 40 mg trimethoprim and 200 mg sulfamethoxazole.
UTI, Urinary tract infection; *PCP*, *Pneumocystis carinii* pneumonia.

sulfisoxazole

Sulfisoxazole is a short-acting sulphonamide antibiotic that is primarily used alone for its ability to effectively inhibit bacterial organisms in the urinary tract. It is more commonly used in combination with erythromycin in pediatric clients. This particular combination acts synergistically so that less of each drug can be used. This drug combination has good activity against those organisms that commonly cause ear infections (otitis media) in small children and so is available in a pediatric-strength oral suspension for this purpose. Unlike sulfamethoxazole, it is not available as a parenteral agent. It is available as a 500-mg tablet and a fixed-combination product containing 600 mg of sulfisoxazole and 200 mg of erythromycin per 5 mL. Pregnancy category C. Recommended dosages are given in the table on p. 626.

PHARMACOKINETICS

Half-Life	Onset	Peak	Duration
4.6–7.8 hr	Variable	1–4 hr (plasma)	4–6 hr

BETA-LACTAM ANTIBIOTICS

The **beta-lactam** antibiotics are commonly used agents, so named because of the beta-lactam ring that is part of the chemical structure (Figure 37-7). This broad group of drugs includes four major subclasses: penicillins, cephalosporins, carbapenems, and monobactams. Some bacterial strains produce the enzyme **beta-lactamase**. This enzyme provides a mechanism for bacterial resistance to infection. The enzyme can break the chemical bond between the carbon (C) and nitrogen (N) atoms in

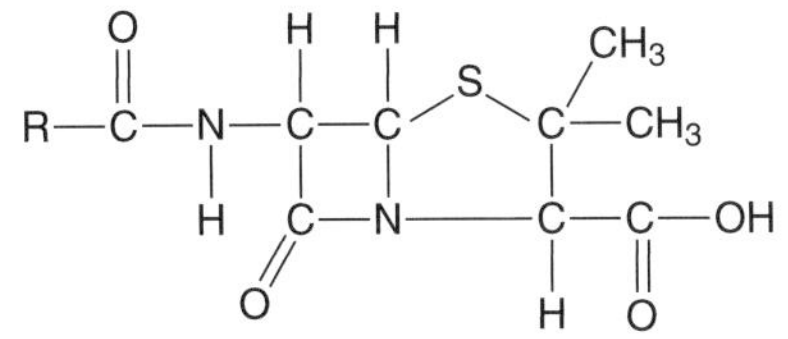

FIG. 37-7 Chemical structure of penicillins. *R*, Variable portion of drug chemical structure.

the structure of the beta-lactam ring. When this happens, all beta-lactam drugs lose their antibacterial efficacy. Because of this, additional drugs known as **beta-lactamase inhibitors** are added to the dosage forms of several different penicillin beta-lactam antibiotics to make the drug more powerful against beta-lactamase–producing bacterial strains. All four classes of beta-lactam antibiotics are now examined individually in more detail.

PENICILLINS

The penicillins are a large group of chemically related antibiotics that are derived from a mould fungus often seen on bread or fruit. The penicillins can be divided into four subgroups based on their structure and the spectrum of bacteria that they can kill: natural penicillins, penicillinase-resistant penicillins, aminopenicillins, and extended-spectrum penicillins. Examples of antibiotics in each subgroup and a brief description of their characteristics are given in Table 37-2.

Natural penicillins were first introduced in the early 1940s during World War II, and to this day they have remained effective and safe antibiotics. They are **bactericidal antibiotics** and can kill a wide variety of gram-positive and some gram-negative bacteria. Penicillins work by inhibiting bacterial cell wall synthesis. However, some bacteria have acquired the capacity to produce enzymes capable of destroying penicillins. These enzymes are called *beta-lactamases,* and they can inactivate the penicillin molecules by opening the beta-lactam ring. Beta-lactamases that specifically inactivate penicillins are called *penicillinases.* Bacterial strains that produce these drug-inactivating enzymes were a therapeutic obstacle until drugs were synthesized that inhibit these enzymes. Two of these beta-lactamase inhibitors are clavulanic acid (also called *clavulanate*) and tazobactam. By binding with the beta-lactamase enzyme itself, they prevent the enzyme from breaking down the penicillin. Examples of currently available penicillin–beta-lactamase inhibitor combinations are as follows:

- amoxicillin + clavulanic acid = Clavulin
- ticarcillin + clavulanic acid = Timentin
- piperacillin + tazobactam = Tazocin

TABLE 37-2
PENICILLIN CLASSIFICATION

Subclass	Generic Drug Names	Description
Extended-spectrum penicillins (aminopenicillins)	amoxicillin, ampicillin, pivampicillin, pivmecillinam	Have an amino group attached to their penicillin nucleus structure that enhances their activity against gram-negative bacteria compared with natural penicillins. Have wider spectra of activity than any other penicillins.
Natural penicillins	penicillin G, penicillin G benzathine, penicillin V	Although many modifications of the original natural (mould-produced) structure have been made, these are the only ones in current clinical use. Penicillin G is the injectable form for IV or IM use; penicillin V is a PO dosage form (tablet and liquid).
Penicillinase-resistant agents	cloxacillin	Stable against hydrolysis by most staphylococcal penicillinases (enzymes that normally break down the natural penicillins).
Anti-pseudomonal penicillins	piperacillin sodium	Piperacillin is not absorbed when given orally.

Mechanism of Action and Drug Effects

The mechanism of action of penicillins involves several steps that together result in the inhibition of bacterial cell wall synthesis. In the first step, penicillin molecules slide through the bacterial cell walls to get to their site of action. However, some penicillins are too large to pass through these openings in the cell walls, and because they cannot get to their site of action they cannot kill the bacteria. On the other hand, some bacteria can make the openings in their cell walls smaller so that the penicillin cannot get through to kill them. The penicillin molecules that do gain entry into the bacteria must then find the appropriate binding sites. These are known as penicillin-binding proteins (PBPs). By binding to this protein, the penicillin interferes with the normal cell wall synthesis, causing the formation of defective cell walls that are unstable and easily broken down (Figure 37-6). Bacterial death usually results from lysis (rupture) of the bacterial cells due to drug-induced disruption of cell wall structure.

Penicillins inhibit the cell wall synthesis of bacteria only, not of other cells in the body. Therefore the drug effects of penicillins are limited to the killing of bacteria. In humans this has the therapeutic effect of destroying invading bacteria that are responsible for infections without damage to human cells.

Indications

Penicillins are indicated for the prevention and treatment of infections caused by susceptible bacteria. The micro-organisms most commonly destroyed by penicillins are gram-positive bacteria, including the *Streptococcus* spp., *Enterococcus* spp., and *Staphylococcus* spp. Most penicillins have little if any ability to kill gram-negative bacteria, although some of the extended-spectrum penicillins can do so.

TABLE 37-3

PENICILLINS: REPORTED ADVERSE EFFECTS

Body System	Side/Adverse Effects
Central nervous	Lethargy, hallucinations, confusion, anxiety, depression, twitching, coma, convulsions
Gastrointestinal	Nausea, vomiting, diarrhea, black hairy tongue, increased AST and ALT levels, abdominal pain, colitis
Hematological	Anemia, increased bleeding time, bone marrow depression, eosinophilia, neutropenia, leukopenia, granulocytopenia
Metabolic	Hyperkalemia, hypokalemia, alkalosis
Other	Taste alterations; sore mouth; dark, discoloured, or sore tongue; hives; rash; Jarisch-Herxheimer reaction (an inflammatory reaction in syphilitic tissue caused by a rapid release of toxins from the bacteria under attack)

AST, Aspartate aminotransferase; *ALT,* alanine aminotransferase.

Contraindications

Penicillins are usually safe and well-tolerated. The only usual contraindication is known drug allergy.

Side Effects and Adverse Effects

Allergic reactions to penicillin occur in 0.7 to 8 percent of treatment courses. The most common reactions to penicillin include urticaria, pruritus, and angioedema. About 10 percent of allergic reactions are life threatening, and 10 percent of these are fatal. A wide variety of idiosyncratic (unpredictable) drug reactions can occur, such as maculopapular eruptions, eosinophilia, Stevens-Johnson syndrome (a potentially fatal skin disorder), and exfoliative dermatitis. Maculopapular rash occurs in about 2 percent of treatment courses with penicillin and 5.2 percent to 9.5 percent with ampicillin. Clients who are allergic to penicillins may also be sensitive to other beta-lactam antibiotics such as cephalosporins. Prescribers often consider cephalosporins for clients reporting a penicillin allergy. The exact incidence of cross-reactivity between cephalosporins and penicillins is not known; however, it is believed to be low. Clients reporting penicillin allergy should be asked to describe their prior allergic reaction. The decision to continue with cephalosporin therapy in such cases is often a matter of clinical judgement, based on the severity of reported prior reactions to penicillin drugs, the nature of the infection and its drug susceptibility if known, and the availability and client tolerance of other alternative antibiotics. Macrolide antibiotics, discussed later in this chapter, are a commonly used alternative class of medications for clients reporting allergy to penicillins or cephalosporins.

Allergies aside, penicillins are generally well tolerated and associated with few adverse effects. As with many drugs, the most common adverse are GI in nature. The most common side effects and adverse effects are listed in Table 37-3.

Interactions

There are many drugs that interact with penicillins; some have beneficial effects, and others have harmful effects. The most common and clinically significant interactions are listed in Table 37-4.

Dosages

For dosage information on selected penicillins, see the table on p. 629. See Appendix B for some of the common brands available in Canada.

DRUG PROFILES

Penicillins are classified as pregnancy category B agents. They are safe antibiotics and are contraindicated only in clients with a hypersensitivity to them. Because of their relatively safe side effect profile, there are otherwise few contraindications to their use.

NATURAL PENICILLINS

▸▸ penicillin G and penicillin V potassium

Penicillin G has three salt forms: benzathine, potassium, and sodium. All of these forms are given by injection, either intravenously or intramuscularly (IM). The benzathine salt is used as a longer-acting intramuscular injection. It is available only through Health Canada's Special Access Programme, to be used for treating the sexually transmitted infection syphilis because often only one injection is needed and therefore it can be given once at a clinic that treats sexually transmitted infections (STIs).

Penicillin V potassium is available only in oral (PO) preparations. It is contraindicated in clients who are hypertensive to it. It is available as a 125- and 250-mg/5-mL oral solution and 300- and 500-mg tablets. Pregnancy category B. Commonly recommended dosages are given in the table below.

PHARMACOKINETICS

Half-Life	Onset	Peak	Duration
30 min	Variable	30–60 min (plasma)	4–6 hr

TABLE 37-4

PENICILLINS: DRUG INTERACTIONS

Drug	Mechanism	Result
Aminoglycosides and clavulanic acid	Additive	More effective killing of bacteria
NSAIDs	Compete for protein binding	More free and active penicillin (may be beneficial)
Oral contraceptives	Decrease effectiveness	May decrease efficacy of the contraceptive (controversial)
probenecid	Competes for elimination	Prolongs the effects of penicillins
rifampin	Inhibition	May inhibit the killing activity of penicillins
warfarin	Increases metabolism	Penicillins may increase metabolism of warfarin, decreasing its effect

DOSAGES   Selected Penicillins

Agent	Pharmacological Class	Usual Dosage Range	Indications
▸▸ amoxicillin	Extended-spectrum penicillin (aminopenicillin)	**Adult and pediatric >20 kg** PO: 250–500 mg q8h **Pediatric <20 kg** PO: 20–40 mg/kg/day divided q8h	Various susceptible gram-negative and gram-positive infections
ampicillin	Extended-spectrum penicillin (aminopenicillin)	**Adult** PO/IV/IM: 1–14 g/day divided q4–6h **Pediatric** 25–200 mg/kg/day divided q4–6h	Primarily gram-negative infections such as *Shigella, Salmonella, Escherichia, Haemophilus, Proteus,* and *Neisseria* spp.; some gram-positive infections
cloxacillin	Penicillinase-resistant penicillin	**Adult** PO/IM/IV: 250–500 mg q4–6h **Pediatric** PO/IM/IV: 50–200 mg/kg/day divided q6–12h	Penicillinase-producing staphylococcal infections
▸▸ penicillin V potassium	Natural penicillin	**Adult and pediatric >12 yr** PO: 300 mg q6–8 h IM: 1–20 million units/day IV: 20 million units/day q4–6h divided **Pediatric 1 mo – <12 yr** PO: 150–500 mg 3–6 divided doses IV: 25 000–400 000 units/day q4–6h divided PO: 250 mg bid continuous	Primarily gram-positive infections such as *Streptococcus* (including pneumococcus) and *Staphylococcus* spp. Rheumatic fever prophylaxis
piperacillin sodium	Anti-pseudomonal penicillin	**Adult >12 yr** IM/IV: 3–4 g q4–6h, max 2 g per IM site	Primarily gram-negative infections such as *Pseudomonas, Escherichia, Proteus,* and *Enterobacter* spp., but also *Streptococcus faecalis* (aka *Enterococcus*), which is gram-positive

PENICILLINASE-RESISTANT PENICILLINS

cloxacillin

Cloxacillin is the only available penicillinase-resistant penicillin. It is available in oral and injectable forms. Cloxacillin is able to resist the breakdown of the penicillin-destroying enzyme (penicillinase) commonly produced by bacteria such as staphylococci. For this reason it may also be referred to as an antistaphylococcal penicillin. The chemical structure of cloxacillin features a large, bulky side-chain near the beta-lactam ring. This side-chain serves as a barrier to the penicillinase enzyme, preventing it from breaking the beta-lactam ring, which would inactivate the drug. There are, however, certain strains of staphylococci, specifically *Staphylococcus aureus,* that are resistant to cloxacillin. Such bacteria often require more powerful antibiotic regimens. The only usual contraindication is drug allergy. Cloxacillin is available in oral form as 250- and 500-mg capsules and a 125-mg/5-mL solution, and in parenteral form as 250- and 500-mg and 1- and 2-g injections. Commonly recommended dosages are given in the table on p. 629.

PHARMACOKINETICS

Half-Life	Onset	Peak	Duration
20–30 min	Variable	30–60 min	6 hr (IV)

AMINOPENICILLINS

There are three aminopenicillins: amoxicillin, ampicillin, and pivampicillin. Because of the presence of a free amino group (–NH$_2$ in their chemical structure), aminopenicillins have enhanced activity against gram-negative bacteria, against which the natural and penicillinase-resistant penicillins are relatively ineffective. Amoxicillin is an analogue of ampicillin, and pivampicillin is a pro-drug of ampicillin. Pivampicillin has no antibacterial activity until hydrolyzed to ampicillin in the body. Contraindications include drug allergy. Pregnancy category B.

▶▶ amoxicillin

Amoxicillin is a commonly prescribed aminopenicillin. Amoxicillin is used to treat infections caused by susceptible organisms in the ears, nose, throat, genitourinary (GU) tract, skin, and skin structures. It is available as 100-mg tablets; 250- and 500-mg capsules; and a 125- and 250-mg/5-mL powder for oral suspension. Commonly recommended dosages are given in the table on p. 629.

PHARMACOKINETICS

Half-Life	Onset	Peak	Duration
1–1.3 hr	0.5–1 hr	1–2 hr	6–8 hr

ampicillin

Ampicillin trihydrate is the prototypical aminopenicillin, and it differs from penicillin G only in that it has the amino group on its molecular structure. It is available in two different salt forms: trihydrate and sodium. Like penicillin G, each salt form allows it to be administered by a different route. Ampicillin trihydrate is administered orally and ampicillin sodium is given parenterally. Trihydrate ampicillin is available as 250- and 500-mg

capsules; a 125-mg tablet; and 125-, 250-, and a 500-mg/5-mL oral suspension. Ampicillin sodium is available as 250-, 500-, 1000-, and 2000-mg vials for injection. Commonly recommended dosages are given in the table on p. 629.

PHARMACOKINETICS

Half-Life	Onset	Peak	Duration
PO: 0.7–1.4 hr	Variable	1–2 hr (serum)	4–6 hr

EXTENDED-SPECTRUM PENICILLINS

By making a few changes in the basic penicillin structure, another generation of penicillins was produced with a wider spectrum of activity than either of the other two classes of semi-synthetic penicillins (penicillinase-resistant penicillins and aminopenicillins) or by the natural penicillins. Two of these extended-spectrum penicillins are currently available: piperacillin and pivmecillinam. Ticarcillin, also an extended-spectrum antibiotic, is available only in a newer combination drug product described later.

These extended-spectrum drugs have activity against some bacteria that the other classes of penicillins cannot kill, such as the *Pseudomonas* spp. They also have stability against the beta-lactamase enzymes produced by *Proteus* spp. Both of these bacterial genera are among the more difficult infections to treat.

Piperacillin is given only intravenously, whereas pivmecillinam is given only orally. The only usual contraindication is drug allergy. Ticarcillin and piperacillin are available in fixed-combination products that include beta-lactamase inhibitors. The ticarcillin fixed-combination product (Timentin) includes clavulanate potassium. Piperacillin is combined with tazobactam in a product called Tazocin. Common dosage recommendations for piperacillin are listed in the table on p. 629.

PHARMACOKINETICS

pivmecillinam HCL: 185-mg tablets

Half-Life	Onset	Peak	Duration
0.8–1 hr	Variable	0.5–2 hr (serum)	6 hr

piperacillin sodium: 2-, 3-, and 4-g vials for injection

Half-Life	Onset	Peak	Duration
0.9–1.3 hr	Variable	IV: 5 min (serum)	Variable

CEPHALOSPORINS

Cephalosporins are semi-synthetic antibiotic derivatives of cephalosporin C, a substance produced by a fungus but synthetically altered to produce an antibiotic. The cephalosporins are structurally and pharmacologically related to penicillins. Like penicillins, they are bactericidal and work by interfering with bacterial cell wall synthesis. They also bind to the same *penicillin-binding proteins* (PBPs) inside bacteria.

Cephalosporins can destroy a broad spectrum of bacteria because of the chemical changes that have been made to their basic structure. Modifications to this chemical structure by pharmaceutical scientists have given rise to four generations of cephalosporins. Depending on the generation, these drugs may be active against gram-positive, gram-negative, or **anaerobic** bacteria. They are not active against fungi and viruses. The different drugs of each generation have certain chemical similarities and thus can kill similar spectra of bacteria. In general, first-generation cephalosporins have the best gram-positive coverage but poor gram-negative coverage; third-generation cephalosporins have the best gram-negative coverage but poor gram-positive coverage; and second-generation agents have intermediate coverage. Over the past several years, cephalosporins with a broader spectrum of antibacterial activity than even the third-generation cephalosporins have emerged. These agents are classified by some references as *fourth-generation* cephalosporins. They typically have more activity against gram-positive bacteria than third-generation cephalosporins, but they still maintain strong gram-negative coverage as well. Cefepime is the only fourth-generation cephalosporin available in Canada. The currently available parenteral and oral cephalosporin antibiotics are listed in Table 37-5.

The safety profiles, contraindications, and pregnancy ratings of the cephalosporins are similar to those of the penicillins. The most commonly reported side effects include mild diarrhea, abdominal cramps or distress, rash, pruritus, redness, and edema. Because cephalosporins are chemically similar to penicillins, a person who has had an allergic reaction to penicillin may also have an allergic reaction to a cephalosporin. This is referred to as *cross-sensitivity*. Various investigators have observed that the incidence of cross-sensitivity between penicillins and cephalosporins is between 1 and 18 percent. However, only those clients who have had a serious anaphylactic reaction to penicillin should definitely not be given cephalosporins. As a class the cephalosporins are safe and effective antibiotics, and they should not be unnecessarily avoided out of excessive concern about possible cross-sensitivity.

Penicillins and cephalosporins are practically identical in their mechanism of action, drug effects, therapeutic effects, side effects and adverse effects, and drug interactions. For that reason this information is not repeated for the cephalosporins and the reader is referred to the pertinent discussion in the section on the penicillin agents. Cephalosporins of all generations are safe agents that are categorized as pregnancy category B drugs. They are contraindicated in clients who have shown a hypersensitiv-

ity to them and in infants younger than one month of age. The prototypical first-, second-, third-, and fourth-generation cephalosporins are described in the following drug profiles section.

Dosages

For the recommended dosages of selected cephalosporin agents, see the table on p. 632. See Appendix B for some of the common brands available in Canada.

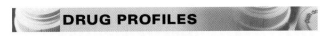

DRUG PROFILES

FIRST-GENERATION CEPHALOSPORINS

First-generation cephalosporins are usually active against gram-positive bacteria and have limited activity against gram-negative bacteria. They are available both in parenteral and oral forms. There are three first-generation cephalosporins currently available: cefadroxil, cefazolin, and cephalexin.

▸▸ cefazolin sodium

Cefazolin is a prototypical first-generation cephalosporin. As with all first-generation cephalosporins, it has excellent coverage against gram-positive bacteria but limited coverage against gram-negative bacteria. It is available only in a parenteral formulation as 500-1000-, and 10 000-mg vials for intramuscular or intravenous injection. Commonly recommended dosages are given in the table on p. 632.

PHARMACOKINETICS

Half-Life	Onset	Peak	Duration
1.2–2.2 hr	Variable	1–2 hr	Variable

▸▸ cephalexin

Cephalexin is a prototypical oral first-generation cephalosporin. It also has excellent coverage against gram-positive bacteria but limited coverage against gram-negative bacteria. It is available only in oral formulations of 250- and 500-mg capsules and tablets and a 125- and 250-mg/5-mL oral suspension. Commonly recommended dosages can be found in the table on p. 632.

PHARMACOKINETICS

Half-Life	Onset	Peak	Duration
0.5–1.2 hr	Variable	1 hr	6–12 hr

TABLE 37-5

CEPHALOSPORINS: PARENTERAL AND ORAL PREPARATIONS

First Generation		Second Generation		Third Generation		Fourth Generation	
IV	PO	IV	PO	IV	PO	IV	PO
cefazolin	cefadroxil		cefaclor		cefixime	cefepime	
	cephalexin	cefoxitin	cefuroxime axetil	cefotaxime			
		cefuroxime	cefprozil	ceftazidime			
		cefotetan		ceftriaxone			

DOSAGES — Selected Cephalosporins

Agent	Pharmacological Class	Usual Dosage Range	Indications
▸▸ cefazolin sodium	First-generation cephalosporin	**Adult** IV/IM: 500–1000 mg q6–8h **Pediatric** IV/IM: 25–50 mg/kg/day divided q6–8h	Comparable to cephalexin plus some penicillinase-producing and more gram-negative organisms; pre-op and post-op prophylaxis
cefepime	Fourth-generation cephalosporin	**Adult and pediatric >40 kg** IV/IM: 500–2000 mg once to twice daily **Pediatric 2 mo – ≤40 kg** IV/IM: 50 mg/kg q12h	Has extensive gram-negative coverage, including intra-abdominal infections
cefixime	Third-generation cephalosporin	**Adult** PO: 400 mg/day **Pediatric <50 kg** PO: 8 mg/kg/day divided	Primarily gram-negative infections of urinary, respiratory, and GU tracts and otitis media; some *Streptococcus* (gram-positive) spp. infections
▸▸ cefoxitin sodium	Second-generation cephalosporin	**Adult** IV/IM: 3–12 g/day divided q4–6h **Pediatric** IV/IM: 80–160 mg/kg/day divided q4–6h, not to exceed 12 g/day	Comparable to cephalexin plus more gram-negative coverage
ceftazidime	Third-generation cephalosporin	**Adult** IV/IM: 250–2000 mg q8–12h **Pediatric >1 mo** IV/IM: 10–33 mg/kg/day divided q8–12h	More extensive gram-negative coverage, including *Pseudomonas* spp.
▸▸ ceftriaxone	Third-generation cephalosporin	**Adult** IV/IM: 1–2 g divided once to twice daily **Pediatric** IV/IM: 50–100 mg/kg/day divided once to twice daily	Comparable to ceftazidime, plus used for pre-op surgical prophylaxis
cefuroxime*	Second-generation cephalosporin	**Adult ≥12 yr** PO (tabs): 125–500 mg bid **Pediatric >3 mo** PO oral suspension: 20–30 mg/kg/day divided bid **Adult** IV/IM: 750–1500 mg q8h **Pediatric >1 mo – 12 yr** IV/IM: 30–100 mg/kg/day, divided q6–8h	Comparable to cephalexin, plus more gram-negative coverage
▸▸ cephalexin	First-generation cephalosporin	**Adult** PO: 1–4 g/day divided bid–qid **Pediatric** PO: 30 mg/kg/day bid, max 2 g	Various susceptible gram-positive and gram-negative bacterial infections of respiratory and GU tracts; skin; bone; and otitis media

*Cefuroxime is a pro-drug for PO use that is hydrolyzed into the active ingredient in the fluids of the GI tract.

SECOND-GENERATION CEPHALOSPORINS

Second-generation cephalosporins have coverage against gram-positive organisms similar to the first-generation cephalosporins but enhanced gram-negative coverage. They include both parenteral and oral formulations. Like first-generation agents, second-generation cephalosporins are also excellent prophylactic antibiotics because of their favourable safety profile, broad range of organisms they can kill, and relatively low cost. There are three parenteral second-generation cephalosporins currently available: cefoxitin, cefuroxime, and cefotetan. These agents differ slightly with regard to their antibacterial coverage. Cefoxitin and cefotetan, known collectively as cephamycins, may have better coverage against various anaerobic bacteria such as *Bacteroides fragilis*, *Peptostreptococcus* spp.,

and *Clostridium* spp. than the other agents in this class. This is because they differ structurally from the other agents in the class by having a methoxy group rather than a hydrogen group on the beta-lactam ring of the cephalosporin nucleus.

▸▸ cefoxitin

Cefoxitin is a parenteral second-generation cephalosporin. It has excellent gram-positive coverage and better gram-negative coverage than the first-generation agents. Because it is a cephamycin it can kill anaerobic bacteria. Cefoxitin has been used extensively as a prophylactic antibiotic in clients undergoing such surgical procedures as abdominal or colorectal operations because it can kill the bacteria that usually reside in these areas (gram-positive and gram-negative bacteria and anaerobes). Its contraindications are the same as those of the other cephalosporins, namely known drug allergy or prior severe allergic reaction to a penicillin agent. Cefoxitin is available only in parenteral preparations as 1-, 2-, and 10-g vials for injection. Pregnancy category B. Commonly recommended dosages can be found in the table on p. 632.

PHARMACOKINETICS

Half-Life	Onset	Peak	Duration
30–60 min	Variable	20–30 min	Variable

cefuroxime

Cefuroxime sodium is the parenteral form of this second-generation cephalosporin. The oral form is a different salt of cefuroxime, cefuroxime axetil. Cefuroxime is a versatile second-generation cephalosporin. It is also widely used as a prophylactic antibiotic for various surgical procedures. It has more activity against gram-negative bacteria than first-generation cephalosporins but a narrower spectrum of activity against gram-negative bacteria than third-generation cephalosporins. Unlike the cephamycins, it does not kill anaerobic bacteria. Cefuroxime axetil is a pro-drug. It has little antibacterial activity until it is hydrolyzed in the liver to its active cefuroxime form. It is available as 250- and 500-mg film-coated tablets and as a 125-mg/5-mL oral suspension. Cefuroxime sodium is available as 750-mg, 1.5-g, and 7.5-g vials for injection. Commonly recommended dosages can be found in the table on p. 632.

PHARMACOKINETICS

Half-Life	Onset	Peak	Duration
1.2 hr	Variable	2.2–3 hr	6–8 hr

THIRD-GENERATION CEPHALOSPORINS

The currently available third-generation cephalosporins include cefixime, ceftazidime, and ceftriaxone. These are the most potent of the three generations of cephalosporins in fighting gram-negative bacteria, but they generally have less activity than first- and second-generation agents when it comes to destroying gram-positive bacteria. As with all of the different classes of both penicillins and cephalosporins, slight modifications in the chemical structure have endowed specific agents with certain advantages over the others.

Because of specific changes in its basic cephalosporin structure, ceftazidime has significant activity against *Pseudomonas* spp. In fact, this third-generation agent has the best activity of all the cephalosporins against this difficult-to-treat gram-negative bacterium. Ceftriaxone is an extremely long-acting third-generation agent that can be given only once a day in the treatment of most infections. It also has the unique characteristic of being able to pass easily through the blood–brain barrier. For this reason it is one of the few cephalosporins indicated for the treatment of meningitis, an infection of the meninges of the brain. Cefixime is currently the only third-generation cephalosporin available for oral use. All the other third-generation agents are only available in parenteral forms.

cefixime

Structurally, cefixime is similar to cefotaxime and ceftriaxone, but one aspect of its structure allows for better GI absorption. It has better activity against gram-negative bacteria than other oral cephalosporins such as cefaclor, cefuroxime axetil, or cefprozil. However its gram-negative activity is less than that of many of the other parenterally administered third-generation cephalosporins, especially against Enterobacteriaceae such as *Enterobacter* and *Pseudomonas* spp. Cefixime is a prescription-only drug that has the same pregnancy rating and contraindications as the other cephalosporins. Cefixime is available as a 100-mg/5-mL oral suspension and as 400-mg film-coated tablets. Commonly recommended dosages can be found in the table on p. 632.

PHARMACOKINETICS

Half-Life	Onset	Peak	Duration
3–4 hr	Variable	4 hr	12–24 hr

▶▶ ceftriaxone

Ceftriaxone is a parenterally administered third-generation cephalosporin that has a long half-life and can be given once a day. Structurally it resembles other third-generation agents such as cefotaxime, but it has an acidic enol group believed to be responsible for its long half-life. The spectrum of activity for ceftriaxone is similar to that of the other third-generation agents. It can be given both intravenously and intramuscularly. In some cases of infections, one intramuscular injection can eradicate the infection. Ceftriaxone is 93 to 96 percent bound to plasma protein, a proportion higher than that of many of the other cephalosporins. It can also easily pass through the meninges and diffuse into the cerebrospinal fluid (CSF), making it an excellent agent for the treatment of central nervous system (CNS) infections. Ceftriaxone is available as an injection that can be given either intramuscularly or intravenously. It is available as 250-mg, 1-g, 2-g, and 10-g vials. Commonly recommended dosages can be found in the table on p. 632.

PHARMACOKINETICS

Half-Life	Onset	Peak	Duration
4.3–8.7 hr	Variable	IM: 2–4 hr	24 hr

ceftazidime

Ceftazidime is a parenterally administered third-generation cephalosporin with excellent coverage against difficult-to-treat gram-negative bacteria such as *Pseudomonas* spp. It is the third-generation cephalosporin of choice for many indications because of its excellent spectrum of activity and safety profile. It can be given either intramuscularly or intravenously and to children as well as adults. It is available as 1-g, 2-g, and 6-g vials for injection. One idiosyncrasy of this particular drug is the buildup of gas in the medication vial when its powder is reconstituted with diluent—sometimes so much that it expels the needle right out of the vial. Commonly recommended dosages are given in the table on p. 632.

PHARMACOKINETICS

Half-Life	Onset	Peak	Duration
2 hr	Variable	IM: 1 hr	8–12 hr

FOURTH-GENERATION CEPHALOSPORINS

cefepime

Cefepime is the prototypical fourth-generation cephalosporin. It is currently the only fourth-generation cephalosporin available in Canada. Cefepime is a broad-spectrum cephalosporin that most closely resembles ceftazidime in its spectrum of activity but has increased activity against many *Enterobacter* spp. and gram-positive organisms. This characteristic defines it as a fourth-generation cephalosporin. It has a broader spectrum of antibacterial activity, especially against gram-positive bacteria, than the third-generation agents. It may also be more resistant to beta-lactamases, the enzymes capable of inactivating beta-lactam antibiotics such as cephalosporins. Cefepime is indicated for the treatment of uncomplicated and complicated UTIs, uncomplicated skin and skin-structure infections, and pneumonia. It is used as monotherapy for the empirical treatment of fever in clients with neutropenia. Its only usual contraindication is known drug allergy. Cefepime is available only in parenteral preparations of 1-g and 2-g vials for injection. Pregnancy category B. Commonly recommended dosages can be found in the table on p. 632.

PHARMACOKINETICS

Half-Life	Onset	Peak	Duration
2 hr	0.5 hr	0.5–1.5 hr	8–12 hr

CARBAPENEMS

Carbapenems have among the broadest antibacterial spectra of any antibiotics to date. Because of this they are often reserved for complicated body cavity and connective tissue infections in acutely ill hospitalized clients. One relatively rare but serious hazard of carbapenem use is drug-induced seizure activity. This is one reason that carbapenem therapy is chosen carefully and often used only as a last resort in the seriously ill.

▶▶ imipenem-cilastatin

Imipenem-cilastatin is a fixed combination of imipenem, which is a semi-synthetic carbapenem antibiotic similar to beta-lactam antibiotics, and cilastatin, an inhibitor of an enzyme that breaks down imipenem. Imipenem has a wide spectrum of activity against gram-positive and gram-negative aerobic and anaerobic bacteria. Cilastatin is unique in inhibiting an enzyme in the kidneys called *dihydropeptidase*, which would otherwise break down the imipenem. Cilastatin also blocks the renal tubular secretion of imipenem, which prevents imipenem from being metabolized by the kidneys, the primary route of excretion of the agent. Meropenem (Merrem) is the second agent in this class of antibiotics called carbapenems. Meropenem appears to be somewhat less active than imipenem-cilastatin against gram-positive organisms, more active against Enterobacteriaceae, and equally active against *Pseudomonas aeruginosa*. However, meropenem is the only carbapenem currently indicated for treatment of bacterial meningitis. The newest carbapenem is ertapenem, which has a spectrum of activity comparable to imipenem-cilastatin. Note that only imipenem is combined with the dihydropeptidase inhibitor cilastatin. Neither meropenem nor ertapenem is susceptible to this enzyme, which gives them one advantage over imipenem-cilastatin.

Imipenem-cilastatin exerts its antibacterial effect by binding to penicillin-binding proteins inside bacteria, which in turn inhibits bacterial cell wall synthesis. It also kills bacteria and is therefore bactericidal. Unlike many of the penicillins and cephalosporins, imipenem-cilastatin is resistant to the antibiotic-inhibiting actions of beta-lactamases. Potential drug interactions include cyclosporine, ganciclovir, and probenecid. All three of these agents are known to potentiate the CNS side effects (including seizures) of imipenem and should not be used concurrently with it. The most serious adverse effect associated with imipenem-cilastatin therapy is seizures, which have been reported to occur in up to 1.5 percent of clients receiving more than 500 mg every six hours. However, in clients receiving high doses of the agent (>500 mg q6h) there is about a 10 percent incidence of seizures. Seizures are more likely in geriatric and renally impaired clients. Seizures have also been associated with both meropenem and ertapenem, but data to date suggest a lower incidence.

Imipenem-cilastatin is indicated for the treatment of bone, joint, skin, and soft tissue infections; bacterial endocarditis caused by *S. aureus*; intra-abdominal bacterial infections; pneumonia; UTIs and pelvic infections; and bacterial septicemia caused by susceptible bacterial organisms. Imipenem-cilastatin is contraindicated in clients with a known hypersensitivity to it or to local anaesthetics of the amide type (dibucaine or lidocaine). Imipenem-cilastatin is available only in parenteral form as 250- and 500-mg vials for intravenous injection. All dosage forms contain the same number of milligrams of both imipenem and cilastatin. Pregnancy category C. Common dosages are given in the table on p. 646.

PHARMACOKINETICS

Half-Life	Onset	Peak	Duration
2–3 hr	Variable	2 hr	6–8 hr

MONOBACTAMS

Monobactams are synthetic beta-lactam antibiotics that are primarily active against aerobic gram-negative bacteria, including *E. coli*, *Klebsiella* spp., and *Pseudomonas* spp. Currently there are no monobactam antibiotics marketed in Canada.

MACROLIDES

The macrolides are a large group of antibiotics that first became available in the early 1950s with the introduction of erythromycin. Macrolides are considered bacteriostatic; however, in high enough concentrations they may be bactericidal to some susceptible bacteria. There are three main macrolide antibiotics: azithromycin, clarithromycin, and erythromycin. Azithromycin and clarithromycin are two of the newer agents in the class, and together with the original agent, erythromycin, are widely used. Although the spectra of antibacterial activity of both azithromycin and clarithromycin are similar to that of erythromycin, the former have longer durations of action, which allows them to be given less often. They produce fewer and milder GI tract side effects than erythromycin, and they need to be given for shorter lengths of time than many of the erythromycin products. They also exhibit better efficacy in eradicating various bacteria and are capable of better tissue penetration. Erythromycin has a bitter taste and is quickly degraded by the acidity of the stomach. Several salt forms and many dosage formulations have been developed to circumvent these problems (see Table 37-6).

Mechanism of Action and Drug Effects

The mechanism of action of macrolide antibiotics is similar to that of other antibiotics. They bind to the 50S ribosomal subunit inside the cells of bacteria and by so doing prevent the bacteria from producing the protein they need to grow, with the result that the bacteria eventually die (Figure 37-6). This action can immediately kill some susceptible strains of bacteria if the concentration of the macrolide is high enough.

Macrolides are effective against a wide range of infections. These include various infections of the upper and lower respiratory tract, skin, and soft tissue caused by some strains of *Streptococcus* and *Haemophilus;* spirochetal infections such as syphilis and Lyme disease; gonorrhea; *Chlamydia* and *Mycoplasma* infections; and *Listeria monocytogenes* and *Corynebacterium* infections. Because of its GI tract–irritating properties, erythromycin affects the motility of the GI tract. This property has been studied experimentally and may prove to be of benefit in increasing GI motility in conditions such as diabetic gastroparesis (delayed gastric emptying in diabetics).

Macrolides are also unusually effective against several bacterial species that often reproduce *inside* host cells instead of just in the bloodstream or interstitial spaces. Common examples include *Listeria, Chlamydia, Legionella* (e.g., Legionnaire's disease), *Neisseria* (e.g., gonorrhea), and *Campylobacter.*

Indications

Infections caused by *Streptococcus pyogenes* (group A beta-hemolytic streptococci) are inhibited by macrolides, as are mild to moderate upper and lower respiratory tract infections caused by *Haemophilus influenzae.* Spirochetal infections that are treated with erythromycins and other macrolides are syphilis and Lyme disease. Various forms of gonorrhea and *Chlamydia* and *Mycoplasma* infections are also susceptible to the effects of macrolides.

Erythromycin's ability to irritate the GI tract, stimulating smooth muscle and GI motility, may be of benefit to clients with decreased GI motility. It is also of some benefit in facilitating the passage of feeding tubes from the stomach into the small bowel.

Azithromycin and clarithromycin are used for the treatment of *Mycobacterium avium* complex (MAC) infections, a common *opportunistic infection* (OI) often associated with HIV/AIDS (acquired immunodeficiency syndrome; Chapter 38). Clarithromycin is also approved for use in triple therapy in combination with omeprazole (used for acid suppression) and the antibiotic amoxicillin for the treatment of active ulcer associated with *Helicobacter pylori.*

Contraindications

The only usual contraindication to macrolide use is known drug allergy. In fact, as indicated earlier, macrolides are often used as alternative drugs for clients with allergies to beta-lactam antibiotics.

Side Effects and Adverse Effects

Many of the older macrolide products, primarily erythromycin derivatives, have many side effects. Most affect the GI tract, although the incidence seems to be lower with azithromycin and clarithromycin. Reported adverse effects are listed in Table 37-7.

TABLE 37-6

ERYTHROMYCIN FORMULATIONS

Formulation	Benefit
SALT FORMS	
Stearate salt	Developed to overcome bitter
Estolate	taste of erythromycin
Ethylsuccinate ester	
DOSAGE FORMULATION	
Film coated	Developed to overcome bitter
Enteric coated (pellets and particles)	taste and to protect erythromycin from acid degradation in the stomach
STRUCTURAL CHANGES **Semi-Synthetic Macrolides**	
Azide group (azithromycin) Methylation of hydroxyl group (clarithromycin)	Developed to improve resistance to acid degradation in the stomach and increase tissue penetration to improve antibiotic efficacy

TABLE 37-7

MACROLIDES: REPORTED ADVERSE EFFECTS

Body System	Side/Adverse Effects
Cardiovascular	Palpitations, chest pain
Central nervous	Headache, dizziness, vertigo, somnolence
Gastrointestinal	Nausea, hepatotoxicity, heartburn, vomiting, diarrhea, stomatitis, flatulence, cholestatic jaundice, anorexia
Integumentary	Rash, pruritus, urticaria, thrombophlebitis (IV site)
Other	Hearing loss, tinnitus

Agent	Pharmacological Class	Usual Dosage Range	Indications
▶▶azithromycin	Semi-synthetic macrolide	**Adult** PO: 500 mg × 1 dose, then 250 mg/day × 4 days **Pediatric** 30 mg/kg × 1 dose or 10 mg/kg/day × 3 days or 10 mg/kg × 1 dose, then 5 mg/kg/day × 4 days	Comparable to erythromycin, but focusing on GU and respiratory tracts, including MAC
▶▶clarithromycin	Semi-synthetic macrolide	**Adult** PO: 250–500 mg q12h **Pediatric** PO: 7.5 mg/kg bid (max 500 mg/dose)	Comparable to erythromycin, but focusing on GI and respiratory tracts, including MAC
▶▶erythromycin	Natural macrolide	**Adult*** PO: 250 mg q6h; 333 mg q8h; 500 mg q12h **Pediatric*** 30–100 mg/kg/day divided qid	Various gram-positive, gram-negative, and miscellaneous organisms causing infections in respiratory and GI tracts and skin

*There are many types of dosage forms and dosages may vary from those listed.
MAC, *Mycobacterium avium* complex

Interactions

There are a number of potential drug interactions with the macrolides. Carbamazepine, cyclosporine, digoxin, theophylline, and warfarin compete with the macrolides for hepatic metabolism, resulting in enhanced effects of the second drug. Sometimes this is done intentionally so that smaller doses of the interacting drugs can be given, possibly decreasing the incidence of side effects. Other times it is unintentional and can result in toxicity. Such drug combinations should be avoided when possible. When they are used, the client should be observed for signs of drug toxicity and appropriate lab measurements (e.g., blood drug levels) should be taken. Two properties of macrolides that are the source of many of these interactions are that they are highly protein bound and they are metabolized in the liver. Drugs that are bound to protein are usually bound to albumin in the blood, making them inactive. When they are displaced from these binding sites on albumin and are then free and unbound, they become active. Therefore when a client is given two or more drugs that compete for the same binding sites on albumin in the blood, one will not successfully bind, with the result that it is free in the blood and active. That drug will then have a greater action or effect in the body. In the liver, drug interactions commonly arise from competition between different drugs for metabolic enzymes, specifically an enzyme complex known as the *cytochrome P450 complex*. The result is a delay in the metabolic clearance of one or more interacting drugs and thus a prolonged and possibly toxic drug effect.

Dosages

For dosage information on selected macrolide antibiotics, see the table above. See Appendix B for some of the common brands available in Canada.

DRUG PROFILES

Macrolide antibiotics are used to treat a variety of infections ranging from Lyme disease to Legionnaire's disease. Of the three macrolide agents currently available, erythromycin has been around the longest and has been the mainstay of treatment for various infections for more than four decades. Azithromycin and clarithromycin have fewer side effects and a better pharmacokinetics profile than older agents.

Macrolides are contraindicated in clients with known drug allergy. As previously noted, because these agents are highly protein bound and metabolized in the liver, they may interfere with other drugs that are also highly protein bound or hepatically metabolized.

▶▶ *erythromycin*

Erythromycin, which goes by many product names, is the most commonly prescribed macrolide antibiotic. It is available in several different salt and dosage forms for oral use that were developed to circumvent some of the drawbacks it has chemically. (These benefits are summarized in Table 37-8.) An IV form is also available, as well as topical forms for dermatological use (Chapter 55) and ophthalmic dosage forms (Chapter 56).

The absorption of oral erythromycin is enhanced if it is taken on an empty stomach, but because of the high incidence of stomach irritation, many of these agents are taken after a meal or snack. Pregnancy category B. The various salt forms and dosage formulations, their strengths, and product names are listed in Table 37-8.

▶▶ *azithromycin and clarithromycin*

Azithromycin and clarithromycin are semi-synthetic macrolide antibiotics that differ structurally from erythromycin and as a result have better side effect profiles and pharmacokinetic properties. They also cause less

TABLE 37-8
ERYTHROMYCIN DOSAGE FORMS AND PRODUCT NAMES

Dosage Form Name	Strength	Product Name
ERYTHROMYCIN BASE (PO)		
Capsules		
Delayed-release (enteric coated)	250 mg	Apo-Erythro E-C
Tablets	250, 333, 500, and 600 mg	Nu-Erythromycin-S, PCE Tab, Erythro-Base Tab, Erythro-ES, E.E.S. 600, Erythromycine, Erybid
Capsules		
Delayed-release (enteric-coated pellets)	250 and 333 mg	Eryc
ERYTHROMYCIN ESTOLATE (PO)		
Oral suspension	250 mg/5 mL	Novo-Rythro
ERYTHROMYCIN ETHYLSUCCINATE (PO)		
Tablets		
Film-coated	600 mg	Apo Erythro E.S. tab
Powder for oral suspension	40 mg/mL and 200 and 400 mg/5 mL	Novo-Rythro, EryPed 200, E.E.S. 200 Granules, EryPed 400
ERYTHROMYCIN STEARATE (PO)		
Tablets		
Film-coated	250 and 500 mg	Nu-Erythromycin-S, Erythro-500
Oral suspension	50 mg/mL	Erythrocin
Erythromycin lactobionate (IV)	500 mg and 1 g	erythromycin lactobionate (generic only)

GI tract irritation. Both have similar spectrums of activity that differ only slightly from that of erythromycin, and the two agents are used for the treatment of both upper and lower respiratory tract and skin structure infections.

Azithromycin is capable of excellent tissue penetration, allowing it to reach high concentrations in infected tissues. It also has a long duration of action, allowing it to be dosed once daily. Azithromycin is available in oral form as 250- and 600-mg tablets; as 100-mg/5-mL and 200-mg/5-mL suspensions, and 1-g powder for single dose pack oral suspension; and as a 500-mg vial for parenteral administration. Azithromycin is recommended for use in adults and children. Food decreases both the rate and extent of GI absorption. Pregnancy category B. Commonly recommended dosages can be found in the table on p. 636.

Clarithromycin can be given only twice daily and is recommended for use in adults and children 12 years of age and older. Its safety and efficacy in younger clients has not been established. It is also available in oral form as 250- and 500-mg tablets, a 500-mg extended-release tablet, and as a 125-mg/5-mL and 250-mg/5-mL oral suspension. Pregnancy category C. Common dosages are found in the table on p. 636.

PHARMACOKINETICS
azithromycin (oral)

Half-Life	Onset	Peak	Duration
6–8 hr	Variable	2.5 hr	Up to 24 hr

clarithromycin

Half-Life	Onset	Peak	Duration
3–7 hr	Variable	2 hr	Up to 12 hr

TETRACYCLINES

The tetracyclines are a small chemically related group of five antibiotics, three of which are naturally occurring and two of which are semi-synthetic. They are derivatives of *Streptomyces* organisms. Although the tetracyclines are bacteriostatic, the body's own host defence mechanisms are helping to kill bacteria as well. Demeclocycline, oxytetracycline, and tetracycline occur naturally. Doxycycline and minocycline are semi-synthetic (see Table 37-9).

Tetracyclines are chemically and pharmacologically similar to one another. The most significant chemical characteristic of these agents is their ability to bind (chelate) to divalent (Ca^2, Mg^2) and trivalent metallic (Al^3) ions to form insoluble complexes. If they are given with milk, antacids, or iron salts, oral absorption is considerably reduced. In addition, their strong affinity for calcium usually precludes their use in pediatric clients younger than eight years of age because they can result in significant tooth discoloration. They should also be avoided in pregnant women and nursing mothers. The drugs do pass into breast milk and can discolour the teeth of nursing children.

TABLE 37-9

AVAILABLE TETRACYCLINE ANTIBIOTICS

Generic Name	Description
NATURAL TETRACYCLINES	
demeclocycline	Derived from *Streptomyces* spp. by a fer-
oxytetracycline	mentation process
tetracycline	
SEMI-SYNTHETIC TETRACYCLINES	
doxycycline	Chemical derivative of oxytetracycline
minocycline	Chemical derivative of tetracycline

Tetracyclines primarily differ from one another in the following ways:

- *Oral absorption rates:* All are adequately absorbed, but doxycycline and minocycline are absorbed the most.
- *Body tissue penetration:* Doxycycline and minocycline possess the best penetration potential (brain and CSF).
- *Half-life and resulting dosage schedule:* See the table on p. 639 and Pharmacokinetics information in the Drug Profiles section.

Mechanism of Action and Drug Effects

Tetracyclines work by inhibiting protein synthesis in susceptible bacteria. For this synthesis to occur, transfer ribonucleic acid (RNA) must bind to the messenger RNA ribosome. The tetracyclines obstruct this synthesis by binding to that portion of the ribosome called the *30S subunit* (Figure 37-6). This in turn shuts down many of the bacterium's essential functions, such as growth and repair, so that eventually the bacterium stops growing and dies.

Tetracyclines are used primarily for their antibiotic effects. They inhibit the growth of and kill a wide range of *Rickettsia, Chlamydia,* and *Mycoplasma* organisms, as well as a variety of gram-negative and gram-positive bacteria. They are also useful in the treatment of spirochetal infections such as syphilis and Lyme disease. Demeclocycline possesses a unique drug effect in that it inhibits the action of antidiuretic hormone (ADH), making it useful in the treatment of the syndrome of inappropriate antidiuretic hormone (SIADH). Another drug effect of tetracyclines is their ability to cause inflammation that results in fibrosis in the lungs. This is a useful property in clients with pleural or pericardial effusions caused by metastatic tumours, thoracentesis, or thoracostomy tubes because when instilled into the pleural space of the lungs they cause scar tissue to form, thereby reducing the fluid accumulation.

Indications

Tetracyclines have a wide range of activity and all drugs in this class have essentially the same antimicrobial spectrum. They inhibit the growth of many gram-negative and gram-positive organisms and even some protozoa. Traditionally used to treat acne in adolescents and adults, they are also considered the drugs of choice for the treat-

ment of the following infections caused by susceptible organisms:

- *Chlamydia:* Lymphogranuloma venereum; psittacosis; and non-specific endocervical, rectal, and urethral infections.
- *Mycoplasma:* Mycoplasma pneumonia.
- *Rickettsia:* Q fever, rickettsial pox, RMSF, scrub typhus, typhus.
- *Other bacteria:* Acne control, brucellosis, chancroid, cholera, granuloma inguinale, shigellosis, and spirochetal relapsing fever. In addition, it is used for the treatment of Lyme disease and as part of the treatment regimen for *Helicobacter pylori* infections associated with peptic ulcer disease. It is also used as an alternative agent in penicillin-allergic clients for treatment of gonorrhea and syphilis.
- *Protozoa:* Balantidiasis.

Contraindications

The only usual contraindication is known drug allergy. However, tetracyclines should also be avoided by pregnant and nursing women and should not be given to children under the age of eight years.

Side Effects and Adverse Effects

All tetracyclines cause similar side effects and adverse effects. They can cause discoloration of the permanent teeth and tooth enamel hypoplasia in both fetuses and children and possibly retard fetal skeletal development if taken during pregnancy. Other clinically significant undesirable effects include photosensitivity, with the highest incidence with demeclocycline, and alteration of the intestinal flora, resulting in diarrhea, pseudomembranous colitis, and overgrowth of non-susceptible organisms (superinfection), especially *Candida* and pediatric staphylococcal enteritis.

They can also alter the vaginal flora, resulting in moniliasis; cause reversible bulging fontanelles in neonates; precipitate thrombocytopenia, possible coagulation irregularities, and hemolytic anemia; and exacerbate systemic lupus erythematosus. Other effects include gastric upset, enterocolitis, and maculopapular rash.

Interactions

Several significant drug interactions are associated with tetracyclines. When taken with antacids, antidiarrheal agents, dairy products, or iron preparations, the oral absorption of the tetracycline is reduced. They can potentiate the effects of oral anticoagulants, necessitating more frequent monitoring of anticoagulant effect and possible dose adjustment. They can also antagonize the effects of bactericidal antibiotics. In addition, depending on the dose, they can cause the blood urea nitrogen (BUN) levels to be increased.

Dosages

For dosage information for selected tetracyclines, see the table on p. 639. See Appendix B for some of the common brands available in Canada.

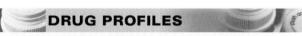

DOSAGES   Selected Tetracyclines

Agent	Pharmacological Class	Usual Dosage Range	Indications
demeclocycline	Tetracycline	**Adult** PO: 150 mg qid or 300 mg bid **Pediatric >8 yr*** 6–12 mg/kg divided bid–qid	Broad antibacterial coverage, including infections of skin, respiratory, GI, and GU tracts
▸▸ doxycycline	Tetracycline	**Adult** PO: 200 mg first day, then 100 mg qd thereafter **Pediatric >8 yr*** PO: 4.4 mg/kg first day followed by 2.2 mg/kg/day thereafter	Comparable to demeclocycline

*Tetracyclines are contraindicated in children >8 yr and in pregnant women because of risk of significant tooth discoloration in children.

DRUG PROFILES

Tetracyclines were one of the first classes of antibiotics capable of a wide range of antibiotic coverage. They are also unique in treating conditions other than bacterial infections. They are used for the treatment of SIADH and as sclerosing (tissue-hardening) agents in the treatment of pleural effusions. They are prescription-only drugs that are potentially harmful to children younger than eight years of age and should not be given to pregnant women because by binding to calcium they can prevent normal bone growth and cause tooth enamel hypoplasia in the child or the fetus. They are also contraindicated in clients who have had hypersensitivity reactions to them in the past and in lactating women. Resistance to one tetracycline implies resistance to all tetracyclines. They are classified as pregnancy category D agents.

demeclocycline

Demeclocycline is a naturally occurring tetracycline antibiotic that is derived from strains of *Streptomyces*. It is used both for its antibacterial action and for its ability to inhibit SIADH. Demeclocycline has all the characteristics of this class of tetracyclines. It is available only in oral form as 150- and 300-mg film-coated tablets. Pregnancy category D. Commonly recommended dosages can be found in the table above.

PHARMACOKINETICS

Half-Life	Onset	Peak	Duration
10–17 hr	Variable	3–4 hr	6–12 hr

▸▸ doxycycline

Doxycycline is a semi-synthetic tetracycline antibiotic that was made by altering the naturally occurring tetracycline oxytetracycline. Doxycycline is available in Canada in the salt form hyclate. It is useful in the treatment of rickettsial infections such as Rocky Mountain Spotted Fever (RMSF), chlamydial and mycoplasmal infections, gonorrhea, spirochetal infections, and many gram-negative infections. Doxycycline may also be used as a sclerosing agent in the treatment of pleural effusions. It is available in oral form as a 44 mg/unit subgingival controlled-release gel, 20- and 100-mg tablets, and 100-mg capsules. Pregnancy category D. Commonly recommended dosages can be found in the table above.

PHARMACOKINETICS

Half-Life	Onset	Peak	Duration
14–24 hr	Variable	1.5–4 hr	Up to 12 hr

AMINOGLYCOSIDES

The aminoglycosides are a group of natural and semi-synthetic bactericidal antibiotics; that is, they destroy bacteria rather than inhibit their growth. Like the tetracyclines, they are derived from *Streptomyces* organisms. The aminoglycoside antibiotics available for clinical use are listed in Table 37-10. These agents can be given by several different routes, but they are not given orally because of their poor oral absorption. An exception is neomycin, which is administered orally to decontaminate the GI tract prior to surgical procedures. It is also commonly used as a rectal enema for this same purpose.

The three aminoglycosides most commonly used for the treatment of systemic infections are amikacin, gentamicin, and tobramycin. The serious toxicities of the aminoglycosides are renal failure and hearing loss (ototoxicity). Certain optimal drug blood levels are strived for to prevent these toxicities from occurring and to optimize the antibiotic killing power. Following are the levels for a few of these agents:

	Peak	Trough
amikacin	20–35 μg/mL	<10 μg/mL
gentamicin and tobramycin	5–12 mg/mL	<2 mg/mL

The ototoxicity associated with aminoglycoside use involves both auditory impairment and vestibular damage and is thought to be due in part to damage to the eighth cranial nerve inflicted by the agents proper. Symptoms include dizziness, tinnitus, and hearing loss. Aminoglycosides are excreted solely in the urine and are directly toxic to proximal tubular cells. The nephrotoxicity, or

TABLE 37-10
AVAILABLE AMINOGLYCOSIDE ANTIBIOTICS

Origin	Aminoglycoside Product	Description
Natural	Gentamicin neomycin paromomycin streptomycin tobramycin	All derived from *Streptomyces* spp. by a fermentation process
Semi-synthetic	amikacin	Chemical derivative of kanamycin

renal failure, is manifested by urinary casts, proteinuria, and increased BUN and serum creatinine levels. In light of these potentially serious toxicities, clients receiving aminoglycosides should be monitored for the signs and symptoms of renal failure (rising BUN and creatinine levels) and hearing loss (fullness in ears, ringing in ears, and dizziness). The risk of these toxicities is greatest in clients with pre-existing renal impairment, clients already receiving other renally toxic drugs, and clients on high doses of or prolonged aminoglycoside therapy.

Although originally given in three daily intravenous doses, the current predominant practice is *once daily aminoglycoside dosing*, especially for clients with normal renal function. The **minimum inhibitory concentration (MIC)** is the lowest concentration in tissue of a drug needed to inhibit bacterial growth. This is usually measured as the serum or plasma drug concentration taken from an arterial or venous blood sample. It has been shown that other classes of antibiotics, such as beta-lactams, work on *time-dependent killing,* that is, the amount of time above MIC that is crucial for maximal bacterial kill. However, aminoglycosides work primarily based on *concentration-dependent killing,* where achieving an increase in plasma concentration above MIC, but for no particular length of time, enhances the bacterial kill by the drug. Several clinical studies have shown that once daily aminoglycoside dosing provides a sufficient plasma drug concentration for bacterial kill, along with equal or less risk of toxicity. The most important goal is a trough concentration (the serum level at its low point, just before the next dose) at or below 2 mg/mL for gentamicin and tobramycin, the most commonly used agents, and below 10 μg/mL for amikacin. Trough concentrations above 2 mg/mL are associated with greater risk of both ototoxicity and nephrotoxicity. Standard once daily doses range from 2 to 5 mg/kg/dose adjusted for the client's level of renal function. A once daily regimen, rather than the traditional three times daily regimen, also reduces the required nursing care time and often allows for outpatient or even home-based aminoglycoside drug therapy. Another advantage is that peak concentrations are expected to be high and thus need not be measured. Only the serum trough concentration needs to be obtained every four to five days of therapy. If therapy is continued for only four days or less, then the trough concentration need not be measured at all. However, three times a day at 1 mg/kg every eight hours is still used and is recommended for more serious infections or for those with impaired renal function.

Aminoglycosides should be administered with caution in premature and full-term neonates because the immaturity of their kidneys can result in prolonged action and a greater risk of toxicities. Aminoglycosides have been shown to cross the placenta and cause fetal harm when administered to pregnant women. There have been several reports of total, irreversible bilateral congenital deafness in the children of women taking aminoglycosides during pregnancy. Therefore aminoglycosides should be used in pregnant women only in the event of life-threatening situations or severe infections when safer drugs either cannot be used or are ineffective. The pregnancy categories of the various aminoglycosides are as follows: gentamicin, C; tobramycin, D; amikacin, D; kanamycin, D; neomycin, C; netilmicin, D; and streptomycin, B. These antibiotics are also distributed in breast milk; therefore their use should be avoided in lactating women. Aminoglycosides are contraindicated in clients with a known hypersensitivity or a history of a serious toxic reaction to them.

Mechanism of Action and Drug Effects

Aminoglycosides, like tetracyclines, bind to ribosomes and thereby prevent protein synthesis in bacteria (Figure 37-6). Specifically, they bind to the 30S ribosomal subunit, a structure that needs to be functioning for protein synthesis to occur. When this process is disrupted the bacterial cell eventually dies.

Aminoglycosides can kill both gram-positive and gram-negative bacteria but are customarily used to kill gram-negative bacteria such as *Pseudomonas* spp., *E. coli, Proteus* spp., *Klebsiella* spp., *Serratia* spp., and others because there are less toxic antibiotics that are effective against the gram-positive bacteria. Often they are used in combination with other antibiotics such as cephalosporins, penicillins, or vancomycin because they have a *synergistic effect;* that is, the combined effect of the two antibiotics is greater than that of either agent alone. Aminoglycosides are relatively inactive against fungi, viruses, and most anaerobic bacteria. Some aminoglycosides (e.g., streptomycin) are active against *Mycobacterium* spp. Other agents, such as paromomycin, are active against protozoal infections (Chapter 41).

Indications

The toxicity associated with aminoglycosides restricts their use to the treatment of serious gram-negative infections and specific conditions involving gram-positive cocci, in which case gentamicin is usually given in combination with a penicillin. Paromomycin is used to treat amoebic dysentery, a protozoal intestinal disease (Chapter 41).

TABLE 37-11
AMINOGLYCOSIDES: COMPARATIVE SPECTRA OF ANTIMICROBIAL ACTIVITY

Aminoglycoside	Spectrum
amikacin sulphate	*Acinetobacter* spp., *Citrobacter* spp., *Enterobacter aerogenes*, *Escherichia coli*, *Klebsiella pneumoniae*, *Proteus* spp., *Providencia* spp., *Pseudomonas* spp., *Salmonella* spp., *Serratia* spp., *Staphylococcus* infections
gentamicin sulphate	*E. aerogenes*, *E. coli*, *K. pneumoniae*, *Proteus* spp., *Pseudomonas* spp., *Salmonella* spp., *Serratia* spp. (non-pigmented), *Shigella* spp.
neomycin sulphate	Toxicity limits use to GI tract (hepatic coma, *E. coli* diarrhea, and antisepsis) and as a topical antibacterial
paromomycin sulphate	Amoebic dysentery
streptomycin sulphate	Granuloma inguinale, plague, brucellosis, tularemia, TB, non-hemolytic *Streptococcus* endocarditis, MAC
tobramycin sulphate	*Citrobacter* spp., *Enterobacter* spp., *E. coli*, *Klebsiella* spp., *Proteus* spp., *Providencia* spp., *P. aeruginosa*, *Serratia* spp.

MAC, Mycobacterium avium complex.

The selection of an aminoglycoside is based on the susceptibility of the causative organism. Serious *Pseudomonas* infections are treated with a suitable aminoglycoside and an extended-spectrum penicillin. Refer to Table 37-11 for the antibacterial spectra of specific aminoglycosides.

Contraindications

The only usual contraindication is known drug allergy. However, aminoglycosides are generally not favoured for long-term use because of the risks of oto- and nephrotoxicity. All are rated pregnancy category D.

Side Effects and Adverse Effects

Aminoglycosides are potent antibiotics and are capable of potentially serious toxicities, especially to the kidneys and to hearing. As a result they are generally reserved for the treatment of more serious or life-threatening infections. Other undesirable effects include headache, paraesthesia, neuromuscular blockade, dizziness, vertigo, skin rash, fever, and overgrowth of non-susceptible organisms.

Interactions

Several significant drug interactions are associated with aminoglycosides. They should not be used with neurotoxic or nephrotoxic drugs such as colistimethate, ethacrynic acid, furosemide, and polymyxin B. The concurrent administration of dimenhydrinate can mask aminoglycoside toxicity, and the co-administration of a neuromuscular blocking agent can increase their activity. Calcium salts can be administered to reverse the blockade. In addition, their use with oral anticoagulants can increase the anticoagulant activity because they decrease intestinal vitamin K synthesis, which normally balances the effect of oral anticoagulant drugs such as warfarin.

Dosages

For recommended dosages of selected aminoglycosides, see the table on p. 642. See Appendix B for some of the common brands available in Canada.

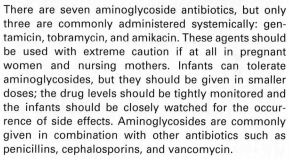

DRUG PROFILES

There are seven aminoglycoside antibiotics, but only three are commonly administered systemically: gentamicin, tobramycin, and amikacin. These agents should be used with extreme caution if at all in pregnant women and nursing mothers. Infants can tolerate aminoglycosides, but they should be given in smaller doses; the drug levels should be tightly monitored and the infants should be closely watched for the occurrence of side effects. Aminoglycosides are commonly given in combination with other antibiotics such as penicillins, cephalosporins, and vancomycin.

amikacin

Amikacin is a semi-synthetic aminoglycoside antibiotic derived by chemically altering kanamycin, a naturally occurring aminoglycoside. Its therapeutic drug levels are much higher than those of the other two agents. The peak levels should be between 20 and 35 μg/mL, and the trough level should be less than 10 μg/mL. Aiming for blood drug levels in this range ensures sufficient antibiotic to destroy the maximum amount of bacteria while preventing nephrotoxicity and ototoxicity. Amikacin is available as 250-mg/mL IV injections. Pregnancy category D. Commonly recommended dosages can be found in the table on p. 642.

PHARMACOKINETICS

Half-Life	Onset	Peak	Duration
2–3 hr	Variable	1 hr	8–12 hr

▸▸ gentamicin

Gentamicin is a naturally occurring aminoglycoside obtained from cultures of *Micromonospora purpurea*. It is one of the most commonly used aminoglycosides. It can be given either intravenously or intramuscularly, with the dosage the same for both routes. It is indicated for the treatment of several susceptible gram-positive and gram-negative bacteria. The common therapeutic drug levels for gentamicin and tobramycin are lower than those for amikacin. Gentamicin is available in several dosage forms. It is available as 1-, 1.2-, 1.6-, and 40-mg/mL injections for intramuscular or

DOSAGES | Selected Aminoglycosides

Agent	Pharmacological Class	Usual Dosage Range	Indications
amikacin	Aminoglycoside	**Adult** IV: 15 mg/kg/day divided q12h **Pediatric** IV: 15–30 mg/kg/day divided q8h **Neonatal** IV: 15–20 mg/kg/day divided q12h × 7 days, then 20–30 mg/kg/day q8h	
▸▸gentamicin sulphate	Aminoglycoside	**Adult** IV/IM: 3–5 mg/kg/day divided once daily–qid **Pediatric** IV/IM: 7.5 mg/kg/day divided q8h **Neonatal** IV: 2.5–3 mg/kg/dose q8h	Primarily gram-negative infections along with severe staphylococcal infections
tobramycin	Aminoglycoside	**Adult** IV/IM: 300 mg bid × 28 days **Pediatric** IV/IM: 7.5 mg/kg/day divided q8h **Neonatal** IV/IM: 3 mg/kg q24h or 2.5 mg/kg q12h	

intravenous use. For intravenous use it is also combined with sodium chloride at 1.4 mg/mL. It is also available as a 0.3 percent, 3 mg/mL solution for ophthalmic use (Chapter 56). Gentamicin also is available as a 1 percent ointment for topical application on superficial skin infections, burns, and skin ulcers (Chapter 55). Commonly recommended dosages can be found in the table above.

PHARMACOKINETICS

Half-Life	Onset	Peak	Duration
2 hr	Variable	0.5–2 hr	8–12 hr

FLUOROQUINOLONES

Fluoroquinolones are potent broad-spectrum antibiotics. They kill bacteria rather than inhibit their growth and are therefore bactericidal. The first agents of this type to become available were the original quinolones cinoxacin (no longer available in Canada) and nalidixic acid. These two agents have narrower spectra of antibacterial activity than the newer, more potent, and less toxic fluoroquinolones and are therefore seldom used anymore. A fluorine atom was added onto the basic quinolone structure to create these newer agents, and this increased their antibacterial potency and made them able to kill a broader range of bacteria. However, both generations of drugs are commonly referred to as "quinolones" for brevity. There are currently six fluoroquinolone antibiotics, including norfloxacin, ciprofloxacin, ofloxacin, levofloxacin, moxifloxacin, and gatifloxacin.

Fluoroquinolones are active against a wide variety of gram-negative and selected gram-positive bacteria. Ciprofloxacin, norfloxacin, and ofloxacin are effective against an extensive spectrum of gram-negative bacteria. Levofloxacin is a newer fluoroquinolone antimicrobial that is somewhat more active than older fluoroquinolones against gram-positive organisms such as *Streptococcus pneumoniae,* including strains highly resistant to penicillin. Other gram-positive organisms such as *Enterococcus* and *S. aureus* are also susceptible. The characteristics of fluoroquinolone antibiotics and their therapeutic effects are summarized in Table 37-12.

Gatifloxacin and moxifloxacin have similar *in vitro* (laboratory) activity. Gatifloxacin is two to four times and moxifloxacin is four to eight times more active than levofloxacin against *S. pneumoniae,* including strains highly resistant to penicillin. It is uncertain whether these *in vitro* differences will mean anything clinically. Both gatifloxacin and moxifloxacin are active against some strains of *S. aureus* and enterococci, but multi-drug-resistant *S. aureus* (MRSA) and vancomycin-resistant enterococci are generally also resistant to gatifloxacin and moxifloxacin. The activity of gatifloxacin and moxifloxacin against many enteric gram-negative bacteria and *P. aeruginosa* is similar to that of levofloxacin and less than that of ciprofloxacin. Gatifloxacin and moxifloxacin have some *in vitro* activity against anaerobic bacteria. With the exception of norfloxacin, these antibiotics have excellent oral absorption. In many cases oral absorption is as fast as intravenous. However, taking antacids with fluoroquinolones greatly reduces their oral absorption. Fluoroquinolones are primarily excreted by the kidneys, which contain a high percentage of unchanged drug. Together with the fact that they have extensive gram-negative coverage, this makes them suitable for treating UTIs. Their use in children is not currently recommended

TABLE 37-12
FLUOROQUINOLONE ANTIBIOTIC CHARACTERISTICS

Generic Drug Name	Antibacterial Spectrum	Common Indications
norfloxacin	Extensive gram-negative and selected gram-positive coverage	Urinary tract infections, prostatitis, STIs
ciprofloxacin	Comparable to norfloxacin	Anthrax (inhalational, post-exposure); respiratory, skin, urinary tract, prostate, intra-abdominal, GI, bone and joint infections; typhoid fever; STIs; selected nosocomial pneumonias (i.e., acquired in hospital)
ofloxacin	Comparable to norfloxacin	Lower respiratory, skin, urinary tract, and prostate infections; STIs
levofloxacin	Comparable to norfloxacin	Respiratory, skin, and urinary tract infections
moxifloxacin		Respiratory and skin infections; CAP caused by PRSP
gatifloxacin		Respiratory and urinary tract infections

STI, Sexually transmitted infection; *CAP,* community-acquired pneumonia; *PRSP,* penicillin-resistant *Streptococcus pneumoniae.*

because they have been shown to affect cartilage development in laboratory animals.

Mechanism of Action and Drug Effects

Quinolone antibiotics destroy bacteria by altering their DNA (Figure 37-6). They accomplish this by interfering with DNA gyrase, the enzyme necessary for the synthesis of bacterial DNA. If bacteria cannot produce DNA, they die. Quinolones do not seem to affect the mammalian enzyme and therefore do not inhibit the production of human DNA.

The drug effects of quinolone antibiotics are mostly limited to their effects on bacteria. They kill susceptible strains of gram-negative and some gram-positive organisms. Some quinolones are also believed to diffuse into and concentrate themselves in human neutrophils, killing such bacteria as *S. aureus, Serratia marcescens,* and *Mycobacterium fortuitum* that sometimes accumulate in these cells.

Indications

Quinolone antibiotics are used in the treatment of various bacterial infections. The particular bacteria and the body site infected determine which quinolone is selected. Table 37-12 lists the available fluoroquinolone antibiotics, the broad range of bacteria they kill, and the indications for their use according to body site.

Contraindications

The most common contraindication is known drug allergy. However, quinolones also have some unique contraindications related to cardiac function. Dangerous cardiac dysrhythmias are more likely to occur when quinolones are taken by clients receiving class IA and class III antiarrhythmic agents such as disopyramide and amiodarone. For this reason, such drug combinations should be avoided.

Side Effects and Adverse Effects

Fluoroquinolones are capable of causing both serious and bothersome adverse effects, the most common of which are listed in Table 37-13. Bacterial overgrowth is another

TABLE 37-13
FLUOROQUINOLONES: REPORTED ADVERSE EFFECTS

Body System	Side/Adverse Effects
Central nervous	Headache, dizziness, fatigue, insomnia, depression, restlessness, convulsions, increased intracranial pressure, toxic psychosis
Gastrointestinal	Nausea, constipation, increased AST and ALT levels, flatulence, heartburn, vomiting, diarrhea, oral candidiasis, dysphagia, pseudomembranous colitis
Integumentary	Rash, pruritus, urticaria, flushing
Other	Fever, chills, blurred vision, tinnitus, crystalluria, hypoglycemia

AST, Aspartate aminotransferase; *ALT,* alanine aminotransferase.

possible complication of quinolone therapy, but this is more commonly associated with long-term use.

Interactions

There are several drugs that interact with fluoroquinolones with significant consequences. Antacids, iron or zinc preparations, and sucralfate greatly reduce the oral absorption of the fluoroquinolone. Probenecid can reduce the renal excretion of the fluoroquinolone, and the use of some fluoroquinolones with theophylline may increase the toxicity of the bronchodilator. Nitrofurantoin, discussed later in this chapter, can antagonize the antibacterial activity of the fluoroquinolones, and oral anticoagulants should be used with caution in clients receiving fluoroquinolones because of the antibiotic-induced alteration of the intestinal flora, which affects vitamin K synthesis.

Dosages

For recommended dosages of selected fluoroquinolones, see the table on p. 644. See Appendix B for some of the common brands available in Canada.

DOSAGES **Selected Fluoroquinolones ("Quinolones")**

Agent	Pharmacological Class	Usual Dosage Range	Indications
▸▸ciprofloxacin	Fluoroquinolone	**Adult*** IV: 400–1200 mg/day, q8–12h PO: 500–1000 mg q12h	Broad gram-positive and gram-negative coverage for infections throughout the body
levofloxacin	Fluoroquinolone	**Adult only** IV/PO: 250–500 mg once daily	Various susceptible bacterial infections

*Not normally recommended for children <18 yr because of adverse musculoskeletal effects shown in studies of immature animals.

DRUG PROFILES

Quinolones are broad-spectrum synthetic antibiotics with bactericidal activity. They are effective in both oral and parenteral forms and are used to treat a variety of infections, including urinary tract, lower respiratory tract, bone and joint, and skin and skin structure infections, as well as STIs. Because of their excellent oral bioavailability, the oral forms of many of these quinolones are just as effective as their parenteral counterparts when given to clients with a functioning GI tract. Quinolones are prescription-only agents that are classified as pregnancy category C. They are contraindicated in clients with a known hypersensitivity to them.

▸▸ ciprofloxacin

Ciprofloxacin was one of the first of the newer broad-coverage, potent fluoroquinolones to become available. It has the advantage and convenience of an oral medication and because of its excellent bioavailability, it can work as well as many intravenous antibiotics. It is also capable of killing a wide range of gram-negative bacteria and is even effective against traditionally difficult to kill gram-negative bacteria such as *Pseudomonas*. Some anaerobic bacteria as well as atypical organisms such as *Chlamydia*, *Mycoplasma*, and *Mycobacterium* can also be killed by ciprofloxacin. It is available in both oral and parenteral forms. In oral form it is available as 250-, 500-, and 750-mg tablets and 500- and 1000-mg film-coated extended-release tablets. In parenteral form it is available in doses of 2 mg/mL contained in premixed bags of 100 and 200 mL for intravenous infusion or in a 10-g/100-mL oral suspension. Ciprofloxacin is also available as a 0.3 percent ophthalmic solution and a 0.3 percent ophthalmic ointment (Chapter 56), as well as a 2-mg/mL otic suspension in combination with hydrocortisone 10 mg/mL (Chapter 57). Pregnancy category C.

PHARMACOKINETICS

Half-Life	Onset	Peak	Duration
3–4.8 hr	Variable	1–2.3 hr	Up to 12 hr

levofloxacin

Levofloxacin is one of the newer quinolones. It has a broad spectrum of activity similar to ciprofloxacin, but it has the advantage of once-daily dosing, as does gatifloxacin. Levofloxacin is available in 250-, 500-, and 750-mg tablets and in premixed intravenous minibags

of 50, 100, and 150 mg to provide 5-mg/mL strength. Pregnancy category C.

PHARMACOKINETICS

Half-Life	Onset	Peak	Duration
6–8 hrs	Variable	1–2 hr	Up to 24 hr

MISCELLANEOUS ANTIBIOTICS

There are a number of antibiotics that do not fit into any of the previously described broad categories. Most have somewhat unique indications or are especially preferred for a particular type of infection. Although they may not be used as often as drugs from the major classes, they are still of clinical importance. Several of these agents are described individually. See the table on p. 646 for dosing information.

▸▸ clindamycin

Clindamycin is a semi-synthetic derivative of lincomycin, an older antibiotic. Like many semi-synthetic derivatives, it was improved over its predecessor agents through the addition of certain chemical groups to the basic structure, with the result that it is more effective and causes fewer adverse effects than its parent compound.

Clindamycin can be either bactericidal or bacteriostatic, depending on the concentration of the drug at the site of infection and on the infecting bacteria. It inhibits protein synthesis in bacteria by binding to the 50S ribosomal subunit, the same site as erythromycin (Figure 37-6). It is indicated for the treatment of bone infections such as osteomyelitis and septic arthritis, PCP, GU tract infections, intra-abdominal infections, anaerobic pneumonia, septicemia caused by streptococci and staphylococci, and serious skin and soft tissue infections caused by susceptible bacteria. Most aerobic gram-positive bacteria, including staphylococci, streptococci, and pneumococci, are susceptible to clindamycin's actions. It also has the special advantage of being active against several anaerobic organisms and is most often used for this purpose.

Clindamycin is classified as a pregnancy category B agent and is contraindicated in clients with a known hypersensitivity to it, those with ulcerative colitis or enteritis, and infants younger than one month. GI tract side effects are the most common and include nausea, vomiting, abdominal pain, diarrhea, pseudomembranous colitis, and anorexia. Clindamycin is available in both oral and parenteral form. In oral form it is available as 150- and 300-mg capsules and as a 75-mg/5-mL oral suspension. In parenteral form it is available in 150-mg/mL vials for injection. It is also available in various topical forms (Chapter 55). Common dosages are found in the table on p. 646.

PHARMACOKINETICS

Half-Life	Onset	Peak	Duration
3.5–4.5 hr	Variable	45 min	6 hr

dapsone

Dapsone is an antibiotic of the *sulphone* class, which is structurally different from the sulphonamides described earlier. It has been used clinically for several decades. Its official indications include leprosy and another skin condition known as *dermatitis herpetiformis*. This is an *idiopathic* (cause unknown) recurring inflammatory skin condition with lesions that can resemble herpes blisters but that is not caused by a herpes virus. Leprosy is an infectious skin condition also known as *Hansen's disease*. It is characterized by disfiguring nodular skin lesions and is caused by *Mycobacterium leprae,* a bacterium of the same genus that causes tuberculosis *(Mycobacterium tuberculosis).* Unlabelled (non–Health Canada approved) uses include PCP and toxoplasmosis (associated with HIV/AIDS) and some rheumatic disorders. Drug resistance has become an increasing problem with dapsone, and liver toxicity and pancreatitis have been reported. Dapsone is contraindicated in cases of drug allergy. It is currently available only in 100-mg tablets. Pregnancy category C. Dosage information appears in the table on p. 646.

PHARMACOKINETICS

Half-Life	Onset	Peak	Duration
10–50 hr	Unknown	4–8 hr	>3 wk

linezolid

Linezolid is the first antibacterial drug in a new class of antibiotics known as oxazolidinones. Linezolid has received approval for treatment of community-acquired and hospital-acquired pneumonia, uncomplicated and complicated skin and skin structure infections, intraabdominal infections, and gram-positive infections in infants and children. Linezolid is particularly useful in treating infections resistant to other antibiotics. One such infection is vancomycin-resistant *Enterococcus faecium* (VREF or VRE), which is notoriously difficult to treat and is often *nosocomial* (acquired while hospitalized). Another virulent nosocomial infection is commonly known as *methicillin-resistant Staphylococcus aureus* (MRSA), although methicillin, a penicillinase-resistant penicillin, has recently been removed from the Canadian market, largely because of bacterial resistance to it. MRSA, which can cause serious infections in hospital, is resistant not only to penicillinase-resistant penicillins but to many other types of antibiotics, and is

thus also called multi-drug-resistant *Staphylococcus aureus*.

The most commonly reported side effects attributed to linezolid are headache, nausea, and diarrhea. Other reported side effects are oral and vagina moniliasis, hypertension, dyspepsia, pruritus, and tongue discoloration. It has also been shown to cause myelosuppression including leukopenia, thrombocytopenia, anemia, and pancytopenia. It is contraindicated in clients with a known hypersensitivity to it. It is available in various injectable forms for intravenous use, and in 400- and 600-mg tablets for oral use. Pregnancy category C. Common dosages are listed in the table on p. 646.

PHARMACOKINETICS

Half-Life	Onset	Peak	Duration
5 hr	1–2 hr	1–2 hr	12 hr

▶▶ metronidazole

Metronidazole is an antimicrobial, trichomonacidal, and bactericidal agent of the class *nitroimidazole*. It has especially good activity against anaerobic organisms and is widely used for intra-abdominal and gynecological infections that are caused by such organisms. Examples of the *anaerobes* include *Peptostreptococcus* spp., *Eubacterium* spp., *Bacteroides* spp., and *Clostridium* spp. The drug is also indicated for treatment of protozoal infections such as amoebiasis and trichomoniasis (Chapter 41). Like the quinolones, it works by interfering with microbial DNA synthesis (Figure 37-6). Metronidazole is contraindicated in cases of drug allergy. It is available in 250- and 500-mg tablets, a 750-mg extended-release tablet, a 500-mg capsule, and a premixed 100 mL bag of 5-mg/mL solution for intravenous infusion. It is also available as a vaginal cream, gel, and inserts and a topical gel or cream. It is classified as a pregnancy category B drug, though it is not recommended for use during the first trimester of pregnancy. Common dosages are listed in the table on p. 646.

PHARMACOKINETICS

Half-Life	Onset	Peak	Duration
6–12 hr	Unknown	1–2 hr	Unknown

nitrofurantoin

Nitrofurantoin is an antibiotic agent of the class *nitrofuran*. It is indicated primarily for uncomplicated UTIs caused by bacterial species *E. coli* and *S. saprophyticus*. The drug is believed to work by interfering with the activity of enzymes that regulate bacterial carbohydrate metabolism and also by disrupting bacterial cell wall formation. It is contraindicated in cases of drug allergy and also in cases of significant renal function impairment because the drug concentrates in the urine. Clinical side effects most often reported are nausea, headache, and flatulence. A more severe adverse effect is an acute, subacute, or chronic pulmonary reaction. Changes in liver function may also occur. The drug is available in 50- and 100-mg capsules and tablets. Pregnancy category B. Dosage information appears in the table on p. 646.

Selected Miscellaneous Antibiotics

Agent	Pharmacological Class	Usual Dosage Range	Common Indications
▸▸clindamycin	Lincosamide	**Adult** IV/IM: 1200– 2700 mg divided PO: 150–300 mg q6h **Pediatric >1 mo** IV/IM: 20–40 mg/kg/day divided tid–qid PO: 8–20 mg/kg/day tid–qid **Pediatric <1 mo** IV/IM: 10–20 mg/kg/day tid–qid	Anaerobes; streptococcal and staphylococcal infections of bone, skin, respiratory, and GU tract
dapsone	Sulphone	**Adult and pediatric** PO: 50–300 mg once daily	Leprosy (Mycobacterium leprae); dermatitis herpetiformis
▸▸imipenem-cilastatin	Antibiotic combination	**Adult** IV: 250 mg–1 g q6–8h	Anti-infective
linezolid	Oxazolidinone	**Adults only** IV/PO: 400–600 mg q12h	VRE; skin and respiratory infections caused by various Staphylococcus and Streptococcus spp.
▸▸metronidazole	Nitroimidazole	**Adult*** IV: 500 mg q8h PO: 500 mg q8h	Primarily anaerobic and gram-negative infections of abdominal cavity, skin, bone, and respiratory and GU tracts
nitrofurantoin	Nitrofuran	**Adult and pediatric >12 yr** PO: 100 mg bid **Pediatric** PO: 12.5–50 mg/ qid	Primarily UTIs caused by gram-negative organisms and Staphylococcus aureus
quinupristin/dalfopristin	Streptogramins	**Adult and pediatric** IV: 7.5 mg/kg q8–12h	VRE; skin infections caused by streptococcal and staphylococcal infections
▸▸vancomycin	Tricyclic glycopeptide	**Adult** IV/PO: 500–2000 mg q12–24h **Pediatric** IV/PO: 10 mg/kg q6h **Infants and neonates** IV/PO: 10–15 mg/kg q8–12h	Severe staphylococcal infections, including MRSA; other serious gram-positive infections, including Streptococcus spp.

*Not normally used in children, except for cases of amoebiasis.
GU, Genitourinary; VRE, vancomycin-resistant Enterococcus; UTI, urinary tract infection; MRSA, multi-drug-resistant Staphylococcus aureus.

PHARMACOKINETICS

Half-Life	Onset	Peak	Duration
20–60 min*	Unknown	Unknown	Unknown

*This is the plasma half-life, depending on renal function. The primary site of drug action is in the lumen of the urinary tract, including the bladder.

quinupristin and dalfopristin

Quinupristin and dalfopristin are two streptogramin antibacterials marketed in a 30:70 combination. They are approved for intravenous treatment of bacteremia and life-threatening infection caused by vancomycin-resistant Enterococcus (VRE) and for treatment of complicated skin and skin structure infections caused by S. aureus and S. pyogenes. These two streptogramin antibacterials work synergistically on the bacterial ribosome to disrupt protein synthesis (Figure 37-6).

Common side effects are arthralgias and myalgias, which may become severe. Adverse effects related to the infusion site, including pain, inflammation, edema, and thrombophlebitis, have developed in about 75 percent of clients treated through a peripheral intravenous line. The drug is contraindicated in clients with a known hypersensitivity to it. It is available as a 500-mg powder for injection containing 350 mg of dalfopristin and 150 mg of quinupristin. Pregnancy category B. Common dosages are listed in the table above.

PHARMACOKINETICS

Half-Life	Onset	Peak	Duration
1–3 hr	1–2 hr	3–4 hr	8–12 hr

▸▸ vancomycin

Vancomycin is a natural bactericidal antibiotic structurally unrelated to any other commercially available antibiotics. It destroys bacteria by binding to the bacterial cell wall, producing immediate inhibition of cell wall synthesis, leading to bacterial death (Figure 37-6). This mechanism differs from that of beta-lactam antibiotics.

It is the antibiotic of choice for the treatment of MRSA infection and infections caused by many other gram-positive bacteria. It is not active against gram-negative bacteria, fungi, or yeast. Oral vancomycin is indicated for the treatment of antibiotic-induced pseudomembranous colitis *(Clostridium difficile)* and for the treatment of staphylococcal enterocolitis. Because the oral formulation is poorly absorbed from the GI tract, it is used for its local effects on the surface of the GI tract. The parenteral form is indicated for the treatment of bone and joint infections and bacterial bloodstream infections caused by *Staphylococcus* spp. It is also used to treat susceptible strains of endocarditis. Resistance to vancomycin has been noted with increasing frequency in clients with *Enterococcus* infections. Resistant strains have been isolated most often from GI tract infections but have also been isolated from skin, soft tissue, and bloodstream infections.

Vancomycin is contraindicated in clients with a known hypersensitivity to it. It should be used with caution in those with pre-existing renal dysfunction or hearing loss, as well as in geriatric clients and neonates. Vancomycin is similar to the aminoglycosides in that there are specific drug levels in the blood that are safe. If the levels are too low (<5 mg/mL), the dosage may be subtherapeutic. If the blood levels are too high (>40 mg/mL), the drug may cause toxicity, most seriously ototoxicity (hearing loss) and nephrotoxicity (kidney damage). Optimal blood levels of vancomycin should be a peak level of 30 to 40 mg/mL and a trough level of 5 to 10 mg/mL. If these levels are achieved, then the antibacterial effect of the vancomycin will usually be optimal and the side effects minimal. It should be noted that there are no consistent peak and trough concentrations with efficacy and toxicity in the literature. It is advised that you refer to your local laboratory services for recommended values. Vancomycin is available in both oral and parenteral forms. In oral form it is available as 125- and 250-mg capsules and 1- and 10-g solutions. In parenteral form it is available in 500-mg and 1-g vials for intravenous infusions. Pregnancy category C (injectable forms) and B (oral forms). Common dosages are given in the table on p. 646.

PHARMACOKINETICS

Half-Life	Onset	Peak	Duration
4–6 hr	Variable	1 hr	Up to 12 hr

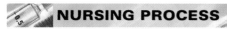

NURSING PROCESS

The discussion of the nursing process will focus on each major classification of antibiotics to convey general and specific information about the various antibiotics.

■ Assessment

Before administering any antibiotic, it is crucial to ensuring appropriate treatment for the nurse to collect client data on age; hypersensitivity to drugs; hepatic (aspartate aminotransferase [AST] and alanine aminotransferase [ALT]), renal, and cardiac function (i.e., pertinent laboratory test results); culture and sensitivity results; and complete blood count (CBC), hemoglobin (Hgb), and hematocrit (Hct) values. It may also be necessary to monitor bowel status and patterns. Assessing for bleeding, such as for ecchymosis (bleeding gums), may also be necessary. With any antibiotic therapy it is important for the nurse to assess for overgrowth of infection as evidenced by fever, lethargy, perineal itching, or other relevant manifestations. The status of the client's immune system and overall condition is also important because if the immune system is deficient in some way, the client's ability to physically resist infection will be diminished. It is also important for the nurse to obtain and document a list of all prescribed and over-the-counter (OTC) medications the client is taking so that drug interactions can be averted. A culture and sensitivity should be obtained before beginning therapy.

■ *Penicillins*

Contraindications to the use of penicillins include a known hypersensitivity to them. Cautious use is generally recommended in neonates and in pregnant or lactating women. The client must also be assessed for a history of asthma, a sensitivity to multiple allergens, or a sensitivity to cephalosporins, because a client with any of these conditions may also be allergic to penicillin agents. The drugs that interact with these agents are listed in Table 37-4.

■ *Cephalosporins*

Before receiving any of the cephalosporins, the client should be assessed thoroughly for the existence of any hypersensitivity, including a hypersensitivity to penicillins. Cautious use is recommended in clients who have a history of any type of drug allergy or who have impaired renal or liver function. In addition, cautious use, with careful and frequent monitoring of the client's vital signs and any complaints of dyspnea, hives, and so on, is recommended for clients who are also taking furosemide, ethacrynic acid, colistin, or aminoglycosides. (See Table 37-4, which gives information on the drug interactions associated with the penicillins; these are comparable for the cephalosporins.)

■ *Sulphonamides*

Any client who is to receive a sulphonamide agent should first be assessed for any drug allergies. Other contraindications include pregnancy, lactation, severe hepatitis, glomerular nephritis, and uremia. Cautious use is recommended in clients with impaired liver or renal function, severe allergies, or bronchial asthma, and in clients also taking anticoagulants or oral antidiabetic agents of the sulphonylurea group. There are many drug–drug interactions that need to be assessed for with this particular class of antibiotics, and they vary from drug to drug.

■ *Tetracyclines*

Contraindications to the use of tetracyclines include pregnancy and hypersensitivity. They also should not be given to children under eight years of age. Cautious use is recommended in lactating women and in clients with renal or hepatic disease. Drugs and substances that interact with tetracyclines include antacids, dairy products, penicillins, and oral anticoagulants. Doxycyclines also have many drug–drug interactions that need to be assessed for before use, such as antacids, iron, phenytoin, anticoagulants, barbiturates, and oral contraceptives.

■ *Aminoglycosides*

Aminoglycosides should be used with caution in clients with impaired renal function. There are also many medications that interact with aminoglycosides and that should not be given in conjunction with this antibiotic group. These agents include oral anticoagulants, diuretics, cephalothins, skeletal muscle relaxants, and general anaesthetic agents. The aminoglycosides are also ototoxic and nephrotoxic; therefore, baseline hearing tests and renal function studies (BUN and serum and urine creatinine levels) should be performed and the results documented. Nephrotoxic effects are manifested by decreased urine creatinine clearance and increased serum creatinine levels.

■ *Clindamycin*

Hypersensitivity to either clindamycin or to its parent agent lincomycin is a contraindication to its use. It is also contraindicated in clients with ulcerative colitis or enteritis and in infants younger than one month. Cautious use of clindamycin is recommended in clients with renal disease, liver disease, or GI disorders; in geriatric clients; and in pregnant or lactating women. Drugs that interact with it include muscle relaxants, chloramphenicol, and erythromycin.

■ *Quinolones*

Quinolones (or fluoroquinolones) are used most commonly to treat urinary, GI, and upper respiratory infections. They should not be used in clients who are allergic to any of the agents. Cautious use is recommended in clients who have seizure disorders or renal disease, in geriatric clients, and in children. They should also be used cautiously in pregnant or lactating women. There are many drug–drug interactions for which to assess before use; a few include antacids, anticoagulants, antineoplastics, and theophylline.

■ *Macrolides*

Macrolides are contraindicated in clients with a known allergy to these drugs. They should be used cautiously in clients with impaired liver function. There are also many drug–drug interactions: a few examples include clindamycin, theophylline, antihistamines, penicillins, and oral anticoagulants.

■ *Vancomycin*

Vancomycin, a tricyclic glycopeptide, is contraindicated in clients with hearing loss and those who are allergic to the medication. Cautious use is recommended in geriatric clients, neonates, pregnant or lactating women, and clients with compromised renal function. Drugs that interact or are incompatible with vancomycin include the aminoglycosides, cephalosporins, polymyxin, cisplatin, and amphotericin B. The combined use of these agents with vancomycin may precipitate nephrotoxicity or ototoxicity.

■ Nursing Diagnoses

Nursing diagnoses appropriate for clients receiving antibiotics include the following:
- Risk for infection related to the client's compromised immune system status before treatment.
- Risk for injury to self (compromised organ function) related to side effects of medications (e.g., ototoxicity and nephrotoxicity) and from a weakened physical state.
- Acute pain related to infection and adverse reaction to medications.
- Deficient knowledge related to lack of information and experience with the medication regimen.
- Ineffective therapeutic regimen management related to lack of information about the proper use of antibiotics and the need for client education.

■ Planning

Goals of nursing care in clients receiving antibiotics include the following:
- Client is free of the signs and symptoms of infection once therapy is completed.
- Client experiences minimal side effects of antibiotic therapy.
- Client remains adherent with therapy.
- Client returns for follow-up visits as recommended.
- Client completes medical regimen of entire course of antibiotics as ordered.

■ *Outcome Criteria*

Goals related to the administration of all antibiotics are as follows:
- Client experiences increased sense of well-being related to resolving infection.
- Client states the signs and symptoms of an infection (e.g., fever, pain, malaise) and reports them if they occur after a few days on antibiotics.
- Client is able to identify the side effects of antibiotic therapy such as GI upset, nausea, and diarrhea (specific to each class).
- Client experiences increased periods of comfort and improved energy levels related to a resolving infectious process and minimal side effects of therapy.
- Client states the reasons for adherence with therapy (i.e., to adequately eradicate bacteria).

- Client states the measures to take to minimize the GI distress associated with antibiotic therapy, such as taking with yogourt or other foods, as appropriate.
- Client keeps follow-up appointments with the physician or other healthcare provider to be evaluated for therapeutic effects or complications of therapy.

Implementation

Some common nursing interventions apply to the antibiotics as a whole; different interventions also apply to specific classes or agents.

Penicillins

Any client taking a penicillin should be carefully monitored for at least 30 minutes after its administration so that an allergic reaction will not go undetected. Penicillin G binds to food and is poorly absorbed in an acidic medium; therefore it should be given one hour before or two hours after meals. In addition, the effectiveness of oral penicillins is decreased when they are taken concurrently with caffeine, citrus fruit, cola beverages, fruit juices, or tomato juice. The intramuscular administration of a penicillin such as penicillin G sodium may cause irritation to localized tissue; therefore it should be administered into a large muscle mass. Intramuscular medications should be diluted well in the diluent recommended by the manufacturer and the sites rotated. When administering intravenous ampicillin, it should be diluted according to the manufacturer's guidelines and infused over the recommended time. The intravenous infusion sites should be assessed frequently and changed every 48 hours, or as dictated by institutional policy. Intravenous administration is to be avoided, except for ampicillin. The nurse should always double-check to make sure that, if the medication has been ordered to be given intravenously, it indeed can be given by this route. Intramuscularly administered imipenem-cilastin is often reconstituted with lidocaine without epinephrine and is given in a deep, large muscle mass. Intravenous imipenem-cilastin must be mixed with appropriate diluents (0.9 percent NaCl, 50 percent dextrose [D50], 0.45 NaCl) and administered over 20 to 30 minutes (250 to 500 mg dose).

Should the client experience an anaphylactic reaction to a penicillin, management often includes the intravenous or subcutaneous (SC) administration of epinephrine; maintenance of the client's airway; and other supportive treatment such as the administration of steroids, vasopressors, or oxygen, or implementation of cardiopulmonary resuscitation.

Cephalosporins

Orally administered cephalosporins should be given with food to decrease GI upset, even though this will delay absorption. Intramuscular injections may be irritating and so should be given deep in a large muscle mass. If accidental subcutaneous injection occurs, sterile abscesses may form. Intravenous infusion sites should be assessed frequently for redness, swelling, and heat and should be changed every 48 hours, or as dictated by institutional policy. Alcohol, when used with some of the cephalosporins, may result in Antabuse-like reactions (flushing, palpitations, severe vomiting, and sometimes respiratory depression); therefore, always check for this contraindication before giving the medication. To ensure safety with the newer cephalosporins, the nurse must check drug names carefully because there are many agents that sound alike or are spelled alike.

Sulphonamides

Sulphonamides should always be given with plenty of fluids (at least 2000 to 2400 mL per day) to prevent the crystalluria that can occur with the oral forms. Oral forms will cause less GI upset if taken with milk or food.

Tetracyclines

Tetracyclines should not be given with dairy products, antacids, sodium bicarbonate, kaolin-pectin, or iron because these chelate or bind with the tetracycline, resulting in a decreased antibiotic effect. These foods and drugs can be given two hours before or three hours after the tetracycline. Oral forms should be given with at least 240 mL of fluid. Intravenous tetracycline should be given per physician's orders and manufacturer's guidelines regarding diluents. Intravenously administered doxycycline is irritating to the veins; therefore, the intravenous infusion site should be checked daily and changed every 72 hours or per policy. Diluents include 0.9 percent NaCl, Ringer's, lactated Ringer's (LR), and D5/LR.

Quinolones

Quinolones should be taken exactly as prescribed and for the full course of treatment. The client should limit the intake of alkaline foods and drugs such as antacids, dairy products, peanuts, vegetables, and sodium bicarbonate. Any of the quinolone agents should be administered only after culture and sensitivity testing has been done on a fresh urine sample from the client. Fluid intake of up to 3 L/day should be encouraged, unless contraindicated.

Oral fluoroquinolones are tolerated more easily with food. These agents are often phototoxic. If an intravenous infusion of lincomycin is ordered, 1 g of the medication should be diluted in 100 mL or more of 5 percent dextrose in water (D5W) or normal saline (NS), but not to the extent that a rate of infusion of 100 mL/hr would be exceeded. Intramuscular injections should be given deep in the muscle and the sites rotated. Oral forms should be given with at least 240 mL of fluid and on an empty stomach.

Miscellaneous Antibiotics

Vancomycin should be reconstituted for intravenous administration according to the manufacturer's guidelines and should be infused over at least 60 minutes. Extravasation may cause local skin irritation and damage; therefore, frequent monitoring of the intravenous tube and site is needed. Sterile water for reconstitution is recommended, and if further intravenous dilution is needed, D5W or NS may be used. If Redman's syndrome occurs (decreased blood pressure, flushing of neck and face), an antihistamine may need to be ordered. Adequate hydration (at least 2 L of fluids/24 h unless contraindicated) is also important with vancomycin to prevent nephrotoxicity.

Clindamycin should be administered as ordered and if given intravenously should be given by infusion, not by an intravenous push. No more than 1200 mg should be infused in a single one-hour infusion, and the usually recommended dilution and dosage is 300 mg/50 mL of com-

patible fluids delivered over more than ten minutes. Intramuscular injections of the agent should be given deep in a large muscle mass and the sites rotated. Oral forms should be given with at least 240 mL of fluids.

Teaching guidelines for clients receiving antibiotics are listed in the box below.

■ Evaluation

The therapeutic effects of antibiotics in general include a decrease in the signs and symptoms of the infection; a return to normal vital signs, including temperature; negative results of culture and sensitivity tests; a decrease to a normal CBC; and improved appetite, energy level, and sense of well-being.

Common adverse reactions for which to monitor in clients taking penicillins include rash, dermatitis, fever, joint pain, and itching. Clients taking cephalosporins should be watched for the occurrence of diarrhea, abdominal pain, colitis symptoms, headache, fever, chills, nausea, vomiting, rash, or dyspnea. Adverse reactions to the sulphonamides for which to monitor include leukopenia, nausea, vomiting, abdominal pain, hepatitis syndrome, renal failure, nephrosis, and Stevens-Johnson syndrome. Tetracyclines may cause diarrhea, hepatotoxicity, nausea, stomatitis, pericarditis, rash, fever, headache, and oral candidiasis or other superinfections. Quinolones may cause lethargy, dizziness, or confusion. Vancomycin may cause hearing loss and ringing or roaring in the ears, and its use should be discontinued if these symptoms appear. The physician should be notified if any unusual side effects occur or if fever, sore throat, restlessness, wheezing, or tightness in the chest arises. Treatment with clindamycin, although an agent in a different class of antibiotics, requires similar nursing interventions, and the client education guidelines are also similar.

CASE STUDY

Antibiotic Therapy

Mr. G. is a resident of an assisted care facility who had a left-sided stroke five years ago. Presently his cardiovascular status and cerebrovascular status are stable. However, he has had a productive cough for two days and a low-grade fever. On physical assessment and chest X-ray examination, the physician diagnoses him with LLL pneumonia. The physician orders oral ciprofloxacin 200 mg q12h and oral theophylline 300 mg q12h. Maalox has been ordered prn for GI upset.

- What drug interactions or other potential problems should the nurse be concerned about with the use of ciprofloxacin and the other medications ordered for Mr. G.?
- What parameters should be assessed and monitored with ciprofloxacin to determine whether the drug is working? Explain your answer.
- If Mr. G.'s signs and symptoms improve, could it mean that he just had a viral infection?

For answers see http://evolve.elsevier.com/Lilley/pharmacology/.

CLIENT TEACHING TIPS

The nurse should instruct the client as follows:
- ▲ Take any antibiotic exactly as prescribed and for the time specified.
- ▲ Take your medication with at least 180 to 240 mL of water; it will be absorbed better.
- ▲ If you have a drug allergy, you should wear a medical alert tag, bracelet, or necklace.

Penicillins
- ▲ Take your medication with 180 to 240 mL of water and on an empty stomach.
- ▲ Report any new symptoms of sore throat, fever, muscle weakness, or joint pain to the physician immediately.

Cephalosporins
- ▲ Take your medication with meals to minimize stomach problems.
- ▲ Do not drink alcohol or use products that contain alcohol (such as some cough syrups and mouth-

washes). You could have an extremely unpleasant reaction.
- ▲ You can eat yogourt or drink buttermilk to prevent or decrease the diarrhea that this drug sometimes causes.
- ▲ Take this medication exactly as prescribed and for the specified time.
- ▲ If you develop a newly sore throat, or have any bruising, bleeding, or joint pain, notify the physician immediately.

Sulphonamides
- ▲ Drink at least ten glasses of fluid per day, unless your physician has told you otherwise.
- ▲ Avoid sunlight and tanning beds while on this medication, because it makes you more sensitive to sunlight.
- ▲ Do not take any over-the-counter medications while on this medication, especially vitamin C and ASA (Aspirin), because they interact with your medication.

▲ If you are taking oral contraceptives, use a backup form of contraception while you are taking this medication and for the rest of the cycle, because this medication decreases the contraceptive effect.

▲ Notify your physician if you develop a new symptom of fever or sore throat, or if mouth sores, easy bruising, or skin rash occurs.

Tetracyclines

▲ Avoid sun exposure and tanning beds while on this medication, because it makes you more sensitive to sunlight.

▲ While you are taking this medication, avoid milk and other dairy products, iron preparations, and antacids. These products make the medication less effective.

▲ Take this medication with at least a three-quarters-full glass of fluid, preferably water (but never milk).

Quinolones

▲ Drink at least 12 glasses of fluids per day, unless your physician has told you not to.

▲ Some people get dizzy while taking this drug; if you do, get whatever help you need to do everyday activities.

▲ Notify your physician if you develop a new fever, sore throat, or headache, or if you develop a rash or become agitated or confused.

▲ Some of the agents are phototoxic.

Lincomycin and vancomycin

▲ If you are taking oral medication, take with food to minimize stomach problems, and drink plenty of fluids.

▲ Take this medication at the times ordered; it is important to keep the right levels of medication in your body.

▲ Report to your doctor if you develop a new sore throat, fever, rash, or excessive fatigue.

POINTS to REMEMBER

▼ There are seven main classes of antibiotic agents: sulphonamides, penicillins, cephalosporins, macrolides, quinolones, aminoglycosides, and tetracyclines. These classes of antibiotics differ in the way in which they destroy bacteria.

▼ Antibiotics are either bacteriostatic or bactericidal. Bacteriostatic means that the antibiotic inhibits the growth of the bacterium but does not directly kill it. Bactericidal means that the antibiotic directly kills the bacterium.

▼ Most antibiotics work by inhibiting bacterial cell wall synthesis in some way. Bacteria survive for years because they can adapt to their surroundings. If a bacterium's surroundings include an antibiotic, over time it can mutate in such a way that it can survive an attack by an antibiotic. The production of beta-lactamases is one way in which bacteria can fend off the effects of antibiotics.

▼ The most common side effects of antibiotics are nausea, vomiting, and diarrhea.

▼ Antibiotics should always be taken for the length of time prescribed.

▼ A therapeutic response to antibiotic treatment includes disappearance of fever, lethargy, drainage, and redness.

▼ Each class of antibiotics has specific side effects and drugs that the agents interact with and must be carefully assessed and monitored.

▼ Because normal bacteria are killed off during antibiotic therapy, superinfections may occur during therapy and may be identified by the following signs and symptoms: a new fever, perineal itching, oral and/or vaginal candidiasis, a new cough, and lethargy.

EXAMINATION REVIEW QUESTIONS

1 Your client is scheduled for colorectal surgery tomorrow. He is not septic, his WBC count is normal, he has no fever, and he is otherwise in good health. The GI surgeon asks you to recommend a cephalosporin for prophylaxis. What generation of cephalosporin would you recommend, and why?
   a. A third-generation cephalosporin because it is the most potent
   b. A second-generation cephalosporin because it is the least toxic
   c. A first-generation cephalosporin because it kills the bacteria that are most common in this surgical field
   d. A second-generation cephalosporin because it kills the bacteria that are most common in this surgical field

2 Therapeutic effects associated with antibiotics include which of the following?
   a. Decrease in Hgb
   b. Elevated WBC count
   c. Increase in Hgb
   d. Decreased WBC count

3 The quinolone antibiotics, such as ciprofloxacin and ofloxacin, are unique in their mechanism of action in that they
   a. interfere with DNA gyrase.
   b. prevent the synthesis of folic acid.
   c. bind to penicillin-binding proteins.
   d. bind to 30S and 50S ribosomal subunits.

4 Macrolide antibiotics, such as azithromycin and clarith-romycin, differ from the prototype macrolide (erythromy-cin) in that they have which of the following characteristics?
   a. Complete action against all bacteria
   b. Antifungal properties
   c. Better efficacy and longer duration of action
   d. Shorter onset of action and no side effects

5 Which of the following is an expected side effect of aminoglycoside agents?
   a. Glaucoma
   b. Palpitations
   c. Nephrotoxicity
   d. Diabetes mellitus

For answers see http://evolve.elsevier.com/Lilley/pharmacology/.

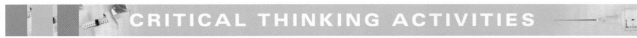

CRITICAL THINKING ACTIVITIES

1 Explain the rationale for not taking dairy products, iron, or calcium with tetracycline. What would be recom-mended if these products are not taken out of the diet?

2 Ms. S. is taking an aminoglycoside for the treatment of a recurrent UTI. What conditions should be assessed for or laboratory studies performed before the initiation of therapy?

3 What symptoms would alert the nurse to the fact that a client is suffering from a superinfection or overgrowth of normal flora stemming from the use of tetracycline?

For answers see http://evolve.elsevier.com/Lilley/pharmacology/.

BIBLIOGRAPHY

Albanese, J., & Nutz, P. (2005). *Mosby's 2005 nursing drug cards.*, St Louis, MO: Mosby.

Anderson, P.O., Knoben, J.E., & Troutman, W.G. (2002). *Handbook of clinical drug data* (10th ed.). New York: McGraw-Hill/Appleton & Lange.

Canadian Committee on Antibiotic Resistance (CCAR). (2004). Canadian committee on antibiotic resistance report. *The Canadian Journal of Infectious Diseases and Medical Microbiology*, *15*(5).

Canadian Pharmacists Association. (2003). *Therapeutic choices* (4th ed.). Ottawa, ON: Author.

Canadian Pharmacists Association. (2004). *Guide to drugs in Canada.* Toronto, ON: Dorling Kindersley.

Canadian Pharmacists Association. (2005). *Compendium of pharmaceuticals and specialties. The Canadian drug reference for health professionals.* Ottawa, ON: Author. [The subscription-based e-CPS is available at http://www.pharmacists.ca.]

Centers for Disease Control and Prevention (CDC). (2005). *Background on antibiotic resistance.* Retrieved August 27, 2005, from http://www.cdc.gov/drugresistance/community/

Cheng, A., Williams, B.A., & Sivarajan, B.V. (Eds.). (2003). *The HSC handbook of pediatrics* (10th ed.). Toronto, ON: Elsevier.

Facts and Comparisons. (2004). *Drug facts and comparisons pocket version* (9th ed.). St Louis, MO: Wolters Kluwer Health.

Greenwood, D., Slack, R., & Peutherer, J. (2002). *Medical microbiology* (16th ed.). Edinburgh, GB: Elsevier Science.

Hardman, J.G., & Limbird, L.E. (2002). *Goodman and Gilman's the pharmacological basis of therapeutics* (10th ed.). New York: McGraw-Hill.

Health Canada. (2005). Drug product database (DPD). Retrieved August 27, 2005, from http://www.hc-sc.gc.ca/hpb/drugs-dpd/

Kasper, D.L., Braunwald, D., Faci, A., Hauser, S., Longo, D., & Jameson, J.L. (2005). *Harrison's principles of internal medicine* (16th ed.). New York: McGraw-Hill.

Katzung, B.G. (2004). *Basic and clinical pharmacology* (9th ed.). New York: McGraw-Hill.

Lacy, C.F., Armstrong, L.L., Goldman, M.P., & Lance, L.L. (2003). *Drug information handbook* (11th ed.). Hudson, OH: Lexi-Comp.

Lehne, R.A. (2004). *Pharmacology for nursing care* (5th ed.). St Louis, MO: Saunders.

Mandell, G.L., Bennett, J.E., & Dolin, R. (2005). *Principles and practice of infectious diseases* (6th ed.). Philadelphia: Elsevier Churchill Livingstone.

Mosby. (2005). *Mosby's drug consult 2005: The comprehensive reference for generic and brand name drugs* (15th ed.). St Louis, MO: Mosby.

Murray, P.R., Greenwood, D., Slack, R., & Peutherer, J. (2002). *Medical microbiology* (16th ed.). St. Louis, MO: Mosby.

Skidmore-Roth, L. (2006). *Mosby's 2006 nursing drug reference* (19th ed.). St Louis, MO: Mosby.

Steinhauer, R. (2002). The emergency management plan. *RN*, *65*(6), 40–45.

DRUG PROFILES

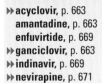

▸▸acyclovir, p. 663
amantadine, p. 663
enfuvirtide, p. 669
▸▸ganciclovir, p. 663
▸▸indinavir, p. 669
▸▸nevirapine, p. 671

oseltamivir and zanamivir, p. 664
ribavirin, p. 664
tenofovir, p. 671
▸▸zidovudine, p. 672

▸▸ Key drug.

GLOSSARY

Antibody (an' tee bod' ee) Immunoglobulin molecule that has an antigen-specific amino acid sequence and is synthesized by the humoral immune system (antibodies produced from B-cells) in response to exposure to a specific antigen, the purpose of which is to attack and destroy molecules of this antigen.

Antigen (an' ti jen) A substance, usually a protein, that is foreign to a host (e.g., human) and that causes the formation of an antibody and reacts specifically with that antibody. Examples of antigens include bacterial exotoxins and viruses. An allergen (e.g., dust, pollen, mold) is a specific type of antigen that causes allergic reactions (Chapter 36).

Antiretroviral agent A more specific term for antiviral drugs that work against retroviruses such as HIV (see *retrovirus*).

Antiviral agent A general term for any drug that destroys viruses either directly or indirectly by suppressing their replication.

Cell-mediated immunity The cell-mediated immune system is one of two major parts of the immune system. It is mediated primarily by T-lymphocytes (T-cells) and other immune system cells (e.g., monocytes, macrophages, neutrophils) other than B-cells. T-cells mount their immune response through such activities as release of cytokines (chemicals that stimulate other protective immune functions), as well as more direct action such as phagocytosis (eating) of antigens. Cell-mediated immunity is also referred to as the *non-specific immune response* because it does not involve antibodies that are specific for a given antigen (see *humoral immune system*).

Deoxyribonucleic acid (DNA) (dee ok' si ry' boe noo klay' ik) A nucleic acid composed of *nucleotide* units that contain molecules of the sugar deoxyribose, phosphate groups, and purine and pyrimidine bases. DNA molecules transmit genetic information and are found primarily in the nuclei of cells. (Compare with *ribonucleic acid [RNA].*)

Fusion   The process by which viruses attach themselves to, or fuse with, the cell membranes of host cells, in preparation for infecting the cell for purposes of viral replication (see *replication*).

Fusion inhibitors (FIs)   The newest class of anti-HIV drugs. There is currently only one FI, which acts by disrupting the viral fusion process.

Genome   The complete set of genetic material of any organism; may be multiple chromosomes (groups of DNA or RNA molecules) in higher organisms; a single chromosome as in bacteria; or a one- or two- DNA or RNA molecule, as in viruses.

Herpesvirus   Any virus of the family Herpesviridae; includes many types, including herpes simplex type 1 (HSV-1, which causes mucocutaneous herpes—usually with perioral blisters); herpes simplex type 2 (HSV-2, which causes genital herpes); varicella-zoster (also called *herpes zoster, herpes simplex type 3,* or *HSV-3*) which causes both chicken pox and shingles; herpesvirus type 4 (also called *Epstein-Barr virus* [EBV]); and herpes virus type 8, which is believed by some to cause *Kaposi's sarcoma,* a cancer associated with AIDS.

Host   Any organism (human, animal, or plant) that is infected with a micro-organism, such as bacteria or viruses.

Human immunodeficiency virus (HIV)   The retrovirus that causes AIDS.

Humoral immune system   The second of two major parts of the immune system that consists of B-lymphocytes (B-cells) and their functions. Their chief function is to differentiate (change) into plasma cells, which can produce antibodies directed against specific antigens. For this reason, humoral immunity is also referred to as the *specific immune response.*

Immunoglobulin   (im' yoo noe glob' yoo lin) (Synonymous with immune globulin.) A glycoprotein synthesized and used by the humoral immune system to attack and kill any substance that is foreign to the body. An immunoglobulin with an antigen-specific amino acid sequence is called an *antibody* and is able to recognize and inactivate molecules of a specific antigen (see *antibody* and *antigen*).

Influenza virus   The virus that causes influenza, an acute viral infection of the respiratory tract. There are three types of influenza virus: A, B, and C. Currently there are medications to treat only types A and B.

Nucleic acids   A general term referring to DNA and RNA. These complex biomolecules contain the genetic material of all living organisms, which is passed to future generations during reproduction.

Nucleoside   A structural component of nucleic acid molecules (DNA or RNA), which consists of a purine or pyrimidine base attached to a sugar molecule.

Nucleotide   A nucleoside that is attached to a phosphate unit, which makes up the side chain "backbone" of a DNA or an RNA molecule.

Protease   An enzyme that breaks down the amino acid structure of protein molecules by chemically cleaving the peptide bonds that link together the individual amino acids.

Protease inhibitors (PIs)   A major class of anti-HIV drugs that work to prevent HIV replication by inhibition of the enzyme protease.

Replication   Any process of duplication or reproduction, such as that involved in the duplication of nucleic acid molecules (DNA or RNA) during the reproduction processes of all living organisms. This is also the term used most often to describe the entire process of viral reproduction, which occurs only inside the cells of an infected host organism.

Retrovirus   Any virus belonging to the family Retroviridae. These viruses contain RNA (as opposed to DNA) as their genome and replicate using the enzyme reverse transcriptase. The most clinically significant retrovirus is currently HIV (see *HIV*).

Reverse transcriptase   An RNA-directed DNA-polymerase enzyme. Such an enzyme promotes the synthesis of a DNA molecule from an RNA molecule, which is the "reverse" of the usual process. HIV replicates in this manner.

Reverse transcriptase inhibitors (RTIs)   A major class of anti-HIV drugs that work to prevent HIV replication by inhibition of the reverse transcriptase enzyme.

Ribonucleic acid   (RNA) A nucleic acid composed of nucleotide units (see *nucleotide*) that contain molecules of the sugar ribose, phosphate groups, and purine and pyrimidine bases. RNA molecules transmit genetic information and are found in both the nuclei and cytoplasm of cells. (Compare with *DNA*.)

Virion   A mature virus particle.

Virus   The smallest class of micro-organisms; can replicate only inside host cells.

GENERAL PRINCIPLES OF VIROLOGY

Viruses are tiny micro-organisms, usually many times smaller than bacteria. For this reason they are usually seen only with the strongest microscopes, such as an electron microscope. All viruses are *obligate intracellular parasites.* This means that, unlike bacteria, viruses can only reproduce, or replicate, inside the cells of their **host,** which can be human, animal, plant, or even other types of micro-organisms (e.g., bacteria, protozoans). It must be emphasized that viruses are not cells, per se, but instead are particles that infect and replicate inside cells. A virus particle is known as a **virion.** Compared with other organisms, virions have a relatively simple structure that consists of the following parts: the genome, the capsid, and the envelope. The **genome** is the inner core of the virion, which consists of single- or double-stranded **deoxyribonucleic acid (DNA)** or **ribonucleic acid (RNA)** molecules, but not both. Viruses have the simplest genome of all organisms because the cells of more complex organisms have either much larger nucleic acid strands or multiple strands, which make up chromosomes. The latter is the case with higher organisms, including humans. The viral capsid is a protein coat that serves to surround and protect the genome. It also plays a role in the fusion process between the virions and the host cells. The envelope is the outermost layer of the virion and occurs in some, but not all, viruses. It has a lipoprotein (lipid and protein) structure containing viral **antigens** that are often chemically specific for various proteins on the surface of the host cell membranes (cell surface proteins). This biochemical specificity, when present, also facilitates the fusion (viral attachment) process. The **human immunodeficiency virus (HIV)** functions in this manner.

Viruses can enter the body through at least four routes: inhalation through the respiratory tract, ingestion via the gastrointestinal (GI) tract, transplacentally via mother to infant, and inoculation via skin or mucous membranes. The inoculation route can take several forms, including sexual contact, blood transfusions, sharing of syringes or needles (as in injection drug use [IDU]), organ transplants, and animal bites (including human, animal, insect, spider, and others). Once inside the body the virus particles, or virions, begin to attach themselves to the outer membranes of host cells (cell membranes or plasma membranes). The viral genome then passes through the plasma membrane into the cytoplasm of the host cell. It later enters the cell nucleus, where the **replication** process begins. The virion may use its own or host enzymes (or both) to direct the replication process. In the host cell nucleus, the viral genome uses the cell's own genetic material (ribonucleic acid [RNA] and deoxyribonucleic acid [DNA]) to synthesize viral **nucleic acids** and proteins. These are then used to construct complete new virions, including genome, capsid, and envelope (if applicable). These new virions then exit the infected host cell by budding through the plasma membrane and go on to infect other host cells, where the replication process continues. This process is called the *cytopathic effect* and usually results in the destruction of the host cell. Repeated over time, cumulative host cell destruction gives rise to the pathological effects of the virus, which can eventually impair or even kill the host organism. Although this cytopathic effect is the most common outcome, there are other possible outcomes of viral infection. Viral transformation involves mutation of the host cell DNA or RNA, which can result in malignant (cancerous) host cells. Viruses that can induce cancer in this way are known as *oncogenic* viruses. More common than viral transformation is latent, or dormant, infection, in which the virions remain inside host cells but do not actively replicate to any significant degree. For example, HIV infection may have a lengthy dormant phase of ten years or more before developing into AIDS in an infected person. HIV infection is discussed in greater detail later in this chapter in the section on retroviruses.

Viruses are said to be ubiquitous (widespread) in the environment, and most viral infections may not even be noticed before they are eliminated by the host's immune system. These are referred to as "silent" viral infections. Although the host's immune system does act to neutralize viral infection, it can become overwhelmed depending on the strength, or virulence, of the virus and how rapidly it replicates inside host cells. However, in most cases a person's immune system is able to arrest and eliminate the virus. Host immune responses to viral infections are classified as non-specific or specific. Non-specific immune responses include phagocytosis (eating) of viral particles by leukocytes (white blood cells [WBCs]) such as neutrophils, macrophages, monocytes, and T-lymphocytes (T-cells). These immune system cells may also kill virally infected host cells to curb the growth and spread of infection. These types of immune responses are collectively referred to as **cell-mediated immunity**. Specific immune responses include the production from B-lymphocytes (B-cells) of antibodies. These are immune system proteins (**immunoglobulins**) that are chemically specific for viral antigens. This type of immune response is also called *humoral immunity*. Immune system function is discussed in further detail in Chapters 44 and 47.

OVERVIEW OF THE VIRAL ILLNESSES AND THEIR TREATMENT

At least six classes of DNA viruses and at least 14 classes of RNA viruses are known to infect humans. Some of the more prominent viral illnesses include smallpox (poxviruses), sore throat and conjunctivitis (adenoviruses), warts (papovaviruses), influenza (orthomyxoviruses), respiratory infections (coronaviruses, rhinoviruses), gastroenteritis (rotavirus, Norwalk-like viruses), HIV/AIDS (**retroviruses**), herpes (**herpesviruses**), and hepatitis (hepadnaviruses). It is currently feared that smallpox, once thought eradicated through vaccine programs, may reemerge as a weapon of bioterrorism. Effective drug therapy is currently available only for a relatively small number of active viral infections. The drug therapy for hepatitis is discussed further in Chapter 47 on immunomodulating agents. HIV belongs to the unusual viral class known as *retroviruses* and is discussed in greater detail in a separate section of this chapter.

Fortunately, many viral illnesses are survivable (e.g., chicken pox), even if bothersome and uncomfortable. The incidence of some of these illnesses has been reduced by the development of effective vaccines (e.g., polio, smallpox, measles, chicken pox). Vaccines are discussed in more detail in Chapter 45. However, many other viral illnesses are either fatal or have much more severe long-term outcomes (e.g., hepatitis, HIV).

Antiviral agents are chemicals that kill or suppress viruses either by destroying virions or by inhibiting their ability to replicate. Even the best medications currently available probably never fully eradicate a virus completely from its host. However, the body's immune system has a better chance of controlling or eliminating a viral infection when the ability of the virus to replicate itself is suppressed. Agents that actually destroy virions include various disinfectants and immunoglobulins. Disinfectants such at povidone iodine are *virucides* that are commonly used to disinfect medical equipment, as well as various parts of the body during invasive procedures. Such agents are discussed further in Chapter 42.

Immunoglobulins are concentrated antibodies that can attack and destroy viruses. They are isolated and pooled from human or animal blood. They may be non-specific (e.g., human gamma globulin) or specific (e.g., rabies immunoglobulin, varicella-zoster immunoglobulin). Although such substances can technically be thought of as antiviral drugs, they are more commonly thought of as immunizing agents and are therefore also discussed in further detail in Chapter 45. A few antiviral agents, such as the interferons, stimulate the body's immune system to kill the virions directly. These agents are discussed in Chapter 47.

In contrast to the various types of antiviral agents listed, the medications that are generally thought of as antiviral drugs per se are currently all synthetic compounds that work by inhibiting viral replication as opposed to directly destroying mature virions themselves. As mentioned earlier, relatively few of the numerous known viruses can be controlled to varying degrees by the currently available antiviral agents. Some of these viruses are as follows:

- Cytomegalovirus (CMV)
- Hepatitis viruses
- Herpes viruses
- HIV
- H5N1 strain of avian influenza ("bird flu")
- **Influenza viruses** ("the flu")
- Respiratory syncytial virus (RSV)

Active viral infections are usually much more difficult to eradicate than those of other microbes such as bacteria. One reason is that viruses can replicate only inside host cells rather than independently replicating in the bloodstream or other tissues. Antiviral drugs therefore must usually enter these cells to disrupt viral replication. The need to develop antiviral drugs that are not overly toxic to host cells is one reason that relatively few effective antiviral medications have been brought to the market. However, the HIV/AIDS pandemic that began in the early 1990s strongly boosted antiviral drug research. This has resulted in more available antiviral drugs than ever before for HIV and other viral infections, such as influenza, CMV, and varicella-zoster virus (VZV).

Another major reason viral illnesses are difficult to treat is that the virus has often replicated itself many thousands or even millions of times before symptoms of illness appear. This amplifies the difficulty of eradicating the virus, even with potent medications. Therefore one goal in the field of infectious disease treatment is to be able to diagnose viral illnesses before an infecting virus has undergone widespread replication in a human host. This would theoretically allow the dual benefit of both early drug therapy and easier elimination of the virus by the host's immune system.

Recall that for a virus to replicate, virions must first attach themselves to host cell membranes in a process known as **fusion**. Once inside the cell the viral genome makes use of cellular genetic processes to generate viral nucleic acids and proteins, which are then used to build new viral particles, or virions (Figure 38-1). All mature virions contain a genome that consists of DNA or RNA, but not both. However, both molecules may temporarily occur simultaneously during the viral replication process. Antiviral drugs inhibit this replication process in various

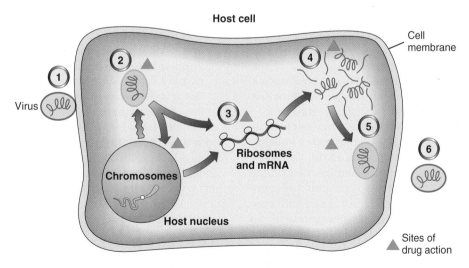

1. Attachment to host cell
2. Uncoating of virus, and entry of viral nucleic acid into host cell nucleus
3. Control of DNA, RNA, and/or protein production
4. Production of viral subunits
5. Assembly of virions
6. Release of virions

FIG. 38-1 Virus replication. Some viruses integrate into host chromosomes with development of latency. (Modified from Brody, T.M., Larner, J., & Minneman, K.P. (1998). *Human pharmacology: molecular to clinical* (3rd ed.). St Louis, MO: Mosby.)

TABLE 38-1
DNA AND RNA CHARACTERISTICS

Characteristic	DNA	RNA
Type of sugar	Deoxyribose	Ribose
Nucleoside pairing	cytosine with guanine	cytosine with guanine
	adenine with thymine	adenine with uracil

Purines: adenine and guanine; pyrimidine: cytosine, thymine, and uracil.
DNA, Deoxyribonucleic acid; *RNA,* ribonucleic acid.

TABLE 38-2
CHARACTERISTICS OF NUCLEOSIDE ANALOGUES

Antiviral Agent	Nucleoside Analogue of	Antiviral Activity
PURINE NUCLEOSIDES (GUANINE [G] AND ADENOSINE [A])		
acyclovir, valacyclovir	guanine	HSV-1 and -2, VZV
didanosine (ddI)	adenosine	HIV
Famciclovir	guanine	HSV-1 and -2, VSV
Ganciclovir, valganciclovir	guanine	CMV retinitis and systemic CMV infection
ribavirin	guanine	RSV
PYRIMIDINE NUCLEOSIDES (CYTOSINE [C], THYMINE [T], AND URACIL [U])		
idoxuridine (IDU)	thymine	HSV
lamivudine (3TC)	cytosine	HIV
stavudine (d4T)	thymine	HIV
trifluridine	thymine	HSV
zalcitabine (ddC)	cytosine	HIV
zidovudine (AZT)	thymine	HIV

HSV, Herpes simplex virus (types 1 and 2); *VZV,* varicella-zoster virus; *HIV,* human immunodeficiency virus; *CMV,* cytomegalovirus; *RSV,* respiratory syncytial virus.

ways. Most antiviral drugs enter the same cells that the viruses enter. Once inside, the antiviral drugs interfere with viral nucleic acid synthesis. Other antiviral drugs work by preventing the fusion process itself. If a virion cannot fuse with and enter a host cell, it cannot replicate, and it dies.

The best responses to antiviral drug therapy are usually seen in clients with a competent immune system. Such an immune system can work synergistically with the drug to eliminate or effectively suppress viral activity. Clients who are already immunocompromised because of various illnesses are at greater risk for opportunistic viral infections that would not normally harm an immunocompetent person. The most common examples of such clients include cancer clients with leukemia or lymphoma, organ transplant recipients, and clients with AIDS. These clients are prone to frequent and often severe opportunistic infections (OIs) of many types, including other viruses, bacteria, fungi, and protozoans. Such OIs often require long-term prophylactic anti-infective drug therapy to control the infection and prevent recurrence.

Most of the antiviral drugs are synthetic purine or pyrimidine nucleoside analogues, which means that they are chemically patterned after adenine, guanine, thymine, cytosine, or uracil. These are the five organic bases that are the major structural components of nucleic acids. Recall that there are two types of nucleic acid. The first is DNA, which consists of long chains of deoxyribose sugar molecules, phosphate groups, and purine (adenine or guanine), together with pyrimidine (cytosine or thymine) bases. The second type of nucleic acid is RNA, which consists of long chains of ribose sugar molecules linked to phosphate groups and purine (adenine or guanine), together with pyrimidine (cytosine or uracil) bases. A **nucleoside** is a single unit consisting of a base and its attached sugar molecule; a **nucleotide** is a nucleoside plus its attached phosphate molecule. The differences between DNA and RNA are listed in Table 38-1. Selected currently available antiviral agents along with their nucleoside type (purine vs. pyrimidine) and their antiviral activity are summarized in Table 38-2.

Antiviral agents are used to treat a variety of viral infections ranging from herpes to AIDS, but the effectiveness of these drugs varies widely among clients and even over time for the same client. The specific antiviral activities for several of the currently available antiviral agents are summarized for the different agents in Table 38-3.

Antiviral medications are broadly subdivided into the following two major categories:

1 *Antiviral agents,* which is now commonly used as a general term for those medications used to treat infections of viruses other than HIV.
2 **Antiretroviral agents,** which are used primarily in the treatment of infections caused by HIV, the virus that causes AIDS. Although antiretroviral drugs also fall under the broader category of antiviral agents in general, their mechanisms of action are unique to the AIDS virus and so they are more commonly referred to by their subclassification.

Both classes of drugs are discussed in separate sections of this chapter. However, the indications, adverse effects, and interactions for several common antiviral agents of both types are summarized in Table 38-3, Table 38-4, and Box 38-1, respectively. Before examining these two major drug classes in detail we first examine, as an example, one common viral illness.

VARICELLA-ZOSTER VIRUS (CHICKEN POX, SHINGLES)

The latency period associated with HIV infection was mentioned earlier. Another important and common example of latent viral infection involves the VZV. This is a type of herpesvirus (human herpesvirus type 3) that most commonly causes chicken pox (varicella) in childhood, remains dormant for many years, and then re-emerges in later adulthood as painful herpes zoster lesions, or shingles.

TABLE 38-3

ANTIVIRAL THERAPEUTIC EFFECTS

Antiviral	Viral Activity	Therapeutic Effect
acyclovir, famciclovir, valacyclovir	HSV-1 and -2, VZV	Acyclovir is used topically, PO, and IV, for treatment of herpes simplex, encephalitis, and most other significant herpes infections. Administration as soon as possible produces the best results. These agents reduce viral shedding, decrease local symptoms, and decrease severity and duration of illness.
amantadine	Influenza A	Used for the treatment and prophylaxis of influenza A, but ineffective against influenza B. Most effective if given before exposure or within 48 h of development of symptoms. Reduces fever and palliates symptoms of influenza.
ganciclovir, foscarnet	CMV	Ganciclovir is the older and more studied of these agents. Now available in a variety of formulations (PO, parenteral, and an ocular implant). Has been shown to be effective not only for CMV retinitis but also for other CMV infections such as GI infection and pneumonitis and for prevention of CMV in recipients of solid organ transplants and in clients with HIV infection. Primary dose-limiting toxicity of ganciclovir is bone marrow toxicity. Foscarnet is less toxic to the bone marrow but can cause renal failure. It is available only through Health Canada's Special Access Programme.
delavirdine, efavirenz, nevirapine	HIV	In combination with nucleoside analogues, these two NNRTI are used to treat HIV-infected clients, including newly infected asymptomatic clients.
didanosine, lamivudine, stavudine, zalcitabine, zidovudine	HIV	Approved for the treatment of HIV-related infections. Produce a significant reduction in mortality and incidence of opportunistic infections, improve physical performance, and significantly improve T-cell counts.
idoxuridine, trifluridine	HSV	Used to treat herpes simplex keratitis. Used only topically because of significant liver and bone marrow toxicity.
indinavir, ritonavir, saquinavir, nelfinavir, amprenavir, atazanavir, lopinavir-ritonavir	HIV	Newer class of drugs for the treatment of HIV infection when antiretroviral therapy is warranted. Used in combination with nucleoside analogues. All are potent inhibitors of the HIV protease enzyme, which is critical to replication of the virus that causes AIDS.
ribavirin, RSV immunoglobulin	Influenza A and B, RSV, Lassa virus, Hantavirus	Severe RSV bronchopneumonia can be treated using an aerosol (ribavirin) or an IV infusion (RSV immunoglobulin). These products have been shown to improve oxygenation, decrease viral shedding, and alleviate pneumonia symptoms. Inhalation treatment with ribavirin has also been shown to be effective in influenza A and B infections. PO and parenteral treatment are effective for Lassa fever virus and Hantavirus.

HSV, Herpes simplex virus; *VZV,* varicella zoster virus; *CMV,* cytomegalovirus; *NNRTI,* non-nucleoside reverse transcriptase inhibitors; *RSV,* respiratory syncytial virus.

TABLE 38-4

SELECTED ANTIVIRALS: ADVERSE EFFECTS

Antiviral Agent	Side/Adverse Effects
acyclovir	Most common: nausea, vomiting, diarrhea, headache, rash, paraesthesia, asthenia (weakness), transient burning when topically applied
amantadine	CNS: insomnia, nervousness, lightheadedness; GI: anorexia, nausea, anticholinergic effects
didanosine	CNS: peripheral neuropathies, seizures; GI: pancreatitis, lactic acidosis, severe hepatomegaly
foscarnet	CNS: headache, fatigue, seizures; Metabolic: hypocalcemia, hypophosphatemia, hypokalemia; GU: acute renal failure; Hematological: bone marrow suppression; GI: nausea, vomiting, diarrhea
ganciclovir	Hematological: bone marrow toxicity; GI: diarrhea, nausea, anorexia, vomiting; CNS: headache, seizures; Other: pyrexia, cough
idoxuridine	Nothing significant
indinavir	Nausea, abdominal pain, headache, diarrhea, vomiting, weakness or fatigue, insomnia, flank pain, taste changes, acid regurgitation, back pain, indirect hyperbilirubinemia, nephrolithiasis/urolithiasis
nevirapine	Rash, fever, nausea, headache, fatigue, increases in liver function tests
ribavirin	Rash, conjunctivitis, anemia, mild bronchospasm
trifluridine	Burning, swelling, stinging, photophobia, pain, epithelial keratopathy
zalcitabine	Peripheral neuropathy, nausea, ulcerative stomatitis, rash, ulcers
zidovudine	Asthenia, bone marrow suppression, fever, nausea, headache, GI pain

BOX 38-1

Antiviral Drugs: Interactions

Acyclovir with the Following
- interferon: additive antiviral effects
- probenecid and cimetidine: increased acyclovir levels by decreasing renal clearance

Amantadine with the Following
- anticholinergic drugs: increased adverse anticholinergic effects
- CNS stimulants: additive CNS stimulant effects

Didanosine with the Following
- allopurinol: increased risk of dose-related toxicities
- antacids: increased absorption of didanosine, which is beneficial
- dapsone: may interfere with GI absorption of dapsone
- ganciclovir: administration of didanosine concurrently or two hours before ganciclovir may increase toxicity of didanosine
- itraconazole and ketoconazole: didanosine decreases their absorption; give two hours apart
- methadone: decreased total drug exposure levels of didanosine (as measured by "area under the curve" [AUC], or summed serum levels over a period of time including peaks and troughs)
- quinolones: didanosine decreases absorption of some quinolone antibiotics
- retrovirals: decreased AUCs of delavirdine and indinavir when co-administered with didanosine
- ribavirin: may increase the risk of adverse reactions of didanosine
- tetracyclines: decreased absorption of tetracyclines; give two hours before tetracyclines
- zalcitabine: additive toxicity (peripheral neuropathies); avoid giving together
- zidovudine: additive and synergistic effect against HIV

Ganciclovir with the Following
- foscarnet: additive or synergistic effect against CMV and HSV-2
- didanosine: didanosine levels increased significantly
- imipenem-cilastatin: increased risk of seizures
- probenecid: compete for renal tubule secretion, increased risk of ganciclovir toxicity
- zidovudine: increased risk of hematological toxicity, (i.e., bone marrow suppression)

Indinavir with the Following
- didanosine: alters the optimal pH of the stomach for indinavir to be maximally absorbed

- drugs metabolized by the CYP3A4 hepatic microsomal enzyme system (terfenadine, astemizole, cisapride, ergot derivatives, triazolam, pimozide, and midazolam): competition for metabolism resulting in elevated blood levels and potential toxicity
- HMG-CoA Reductase Inhibitors: increased risk of myopathy and rhabdomyolysis (breakdown of muscle fibres)
- itraconazole: increased plasma concentrations of indinavir
- rifampin: markedly diminished plasma concentrations of indinavir
- St. John's Wort: decreases indinavir concentrations sufficiently that virologic response may be lost with possible resistance to indinavir or to the class of protease inhibitors
- sildenafil: increase sildenafil concentrations and may increase sildenafil-associated adverse effects (hypotension, visual changes, priapism)

Nevirapine with the Following
- drugs metabolized by the CYP3A4 hepatic microsomal enzyme system: increased metabolism of these drugs
- ketoconazole: significant reduction of ketoconazole levels
- oral contraceptives: decreased plasma concentrations of oral contraceptives
- methadone: decreased plasma concentrations of methadone
- protease inhibitors: decreased plasma concentrations of protease inhibitors

Zalcitabine with the Following
- antacids: reduced zalcitabine absorption
- cimetidine: decreased zalcitabine renal elimination
- drugs associated with pancreatic, peripheral neuropathy, and renal toxicities: should be avoided because of additive toxicities
- zidovudine: additive or synergistic effect against HIV

Zidovudine with the Following
- beta-interferon: increased serum levels of zidovudine
- cytotoxic agents: increased risk for hematological toxicity
- didanosine and zalcitabine: additive or synergistic effect against HIV
- ganciclovir and ribavirin: antagonize the antiviral action of zidovudine
- probenecid: increased serum levels of zidovudine

Chicken pox is usually an uncomfortable but self-limiting disease of childhood. However, it is highly contagious and easily spread by either direct contact with weeping lesions or via droplet inhalation. It may also lead to significant scarring. The serious condition known as Reye's syndrome (fatty liver damage with encephalopathy), as well as other viral infections such as influenza, may also complicate varicella. Herpes zoster, more commonly known as *shingles*, is caused by the reactivation of VZV from its dormant state, often decades af-

ter a case of childhood chicken pox. It is also referred to more simply as *zoster*. Its most common manifestation is skin lesions known as *dermatomes* that follow nerve tracts along the skin surface. The most common site of these lesions is around the side of the trunk, though they can appear in other areas (e.g., dermatomes along the trigeminal nerves of the face). Zoster lesions are often quite painful and some clients require narcotics for pain control. In addition, post-herpetic neuralgias (long-term nerve pain) remain following shingles outbreaks in up to 50 percent of geriatric clients. Early administration of antiviral drugs such as acyclovir may speed recovery, but this effect is usually not dramatic. The best results are usually seen when the antiviral agent is started within 72 hours of symptom onset. Active childhood varicella (chicken pox) infections, as mentioned earlier, are usually self-limiting and are not normally treated with antiviral drugs, except in high-risk (e.g., immunocompromised) pediatric clients. However, varicella virus vaccine was Health Canada approved in 1998 and is now routinely recommended for healthy children between 12 and 18 months of age who have not had chicken pox, susceptible older children and adolescents, children and adolescents on chronic salicylate acid therapy or with cystic fibrosis, and susceptible household contacts of immunocompromised persons. It has even been shown effective for producing VZV immunity in HIV-positive children who are reasonably healthy. As this newly vaccinated pediatric population ages it will become known whether the VZV vaccine also protects against shingles. There is currently no specific vaccine for shingles.

In a small percentage of shingles cases, skin lesions may progress beyond the usual dermatome regions and the virus can cause solid organ infections such as pneumonitis, hepatitis, encephalitis, and optic neuritis (infection of the optic nerve). Such infections are uncommon, but geriatric and immunocompromised clients (e.g., those with HIV/AIDS, organ transplants, or cancer) are the most vulnerable to these more serious VZV exacerbations. These infections can also be due to first time exposure to varicella (chicken pox). In general these more serious infections require intravenous (IV) antiviral agents, especially in high-risk clients. Intravenous acyclovir is the most commonly used drug. Acyclovir can sometimes prevent fatalities or disability in the most serious infections. Less serious infections are usually treated orally with acyclovir, valacyclovir, or famciclovir. These drugs are discussed further in Chapter 55. Though VZV reactivation is comparable in pathology to that caused by herpes simplex virus (HSV; e.g., oral or genital herpes lesions), VZV reactivation occurs much less regularly than does HSV because of a lack of reactivation genes. Because secondary bacterial infections (e.g., group A streptococcus skin infection) are common with VZV exacerbations, antibiotics may also be needed. This is especially true in cases of ophthalmic involvement.

Approximately 95 percent of pregnant women have VZV antibodies, which protect the fetus from viral infection. However, first time exposure to VZV infection can pose a teratogenic risk in pregnant women, especially during the first trimester. If the infection manifests in a pregnant woman within five days of delivery, a dose of varicella-zoster immunoglobulin (VZIG) is recommended for the infant. It may also be beneficial to both mother and infant when given to the mother during pregnancy, preferably as soon as possible after diagnosis of infection. Both varicella virus vaccine and VZIG are discussed further in Chapter 45.

ANTIVIRAL AGENTS (NON-RETROVIRAL)

These agents are used to treat non-HIV viral infections such as those caused by influenza viruses, HSV, VZV, CMV, and hepatitis A, B, and C viruses (HAV, HBV, and HCV). Hepatitis treatment is discussed in further detail in Chapter 47 because it involves unique drug therapy.

Mechanism of Action and Drug Effects

Most of the current antiviral drugs work by blocking the activity of a polymerase enzyme, which normally catalyzes the synthesis of new viral genomes. The result is impaired viral replication, which ideally results in viral concentrations small enough to be eliminated by the client's immune system. If this does not occur, the virus may either enter a dormant state or remain at a low level of replication with continuous drug therapy. For some of the more serious viral infections, such as HIV or HCV, long-term drug therapy is often necessary.

Indications

Indications for several commonly used antiviral agents, including antiretroviral agents, are summarized in Table 38-3.

Contraindications

Most of the non-retroviral antiviral agents are surprisingly well tolerated. The only usual contraindication for a given agent is known severe drug allergy, keeping in mind that the seriousness of a given client's illness may leave few treatment options.

Side Effects and Adverse Effects

The side effects and adverse effects of the antiviral agents are as different as the agents themselves. Each has its own specific side effect profile. Because viruses reproduce in human cells and therefore have many of the same features as these cells, it is hard to target a unique enzyme or other feature of the virus. Selective killing is difficult, and as a result many healthy human cells, in addition to virally infected cells, may be killed in the process, resulting in more serious toxicities. However, this effect is usually not as pronounced as in cancer chemotherapy, which often kills many more healthy cells. The more serious adverse effects are listed by agent in Table 38-4.

Interactions

Significant drug interactions occur most often when antiviral agents are administered via systemic routes, such as intravenously and orally. Topical application to the eye or body involves few drug interactions (see Box 38-1).

Dosages

See the dosages table on p. 662 for doses of the commonly used non-retroviral antiviral drugs. See Appendix B for some of the common brands available in Canada.

DOSAGES Antiviral Drugs (Non-Retroviral)

Agent	Pharmacological Class	Usual Dosage Range	Indications
▸▸acyclovir	Anti-herpesvirus	**Pediatric** IV: 15–45 mg/kg/day divided q8h × 7–10 days **Pediatric 12 yr–adult** IV: 5–10 mg/kg q8h × 7–10 days PO: 200–800 mg q4h 5×/day × 7–10 days, or 400 mg bid up to 12 mo **Pediatric and Adult** PO: 20 mg/kg (max 800 mg/dose) qid × 5 days	HSV-1 and HSV-2, including genital herpes, mucocutaneous herpes, and herpes encephalitis; herpes zoster (shingles); higher dose therapy for acute episodes; lower dose therapy for viral suppression Chicken pox (varicella)
amantadine	Anti-influenza	**Pediatric 1–9 yr** PO: 4.5–9 mg/kg/day divided bid or tid, max 150 mg/day **Pediatric 9–12 yr** PO: 100 mg bid **Adolescent and Adult 13–64 yr** PO: 200 mg divided once or twice daily **Adult >65 yr** 100 mg daily	Influenza virus type A
famciclovir	Anti-herpesvirus	**Adult** PO: 125 mg bid–500 mg tid × 5–7 days	Herpes zoster (shingles); recurrent genital herpes
foscarnet	Anti-CMV, anti-HSV	**Adult** IV induction: 60 mg/kg q8h × 14 days; maintenance: 90–100 mg/kg daily over 2 h by infusion pump after initial induction	CMV retinitis; HSV infections that are resistant to standard drug therapy
▸▸ganciclovir	Anti-CMV	**Adult** IV: 5 mg/kg q12h × 2–3 wk, followed by 5 mg/kg/day 7 days/wk or 6 mg/kg/day 5 days/wk PO: 1000 mg tid with food	CMV retinitis; prevention (in high-risk clients) or treatment of extra-ocular CMV infection (e.g., in CNS or GI tract)
oseltamivir	Anti-influenza	**Pediatric 1–12 yr <15 kg*** PO: 30 mg bid **15–23 kg** PO: 45 mg bid **23–40 kg** PO: 60 mg bid **>40 kg or 13 yr–adult** PO: 75 mg bid × 5 days	Influenza A or B infection
ribavirin	Anti-RSV	**Pediatric** Aerosol: 6 g reconstituted to 20 mg/mL via continuous aerosol × 12 hr/day × 3–7 days	Severe RSV infection in hospitalized infants and toddlers
valacyclovir	Anti-herpesvirus	**Adult** PO: 500–1000 mg bid–tid × 3–10 days	Herpes zoster (shingles); genital herpes
valganciclovir	Anti-CMV	**Adult** PO: 900 mg bid × 3 wk with food	CMV retinitis
zanamivir	Anti-influenza	**Pediatric ≥7 yr–adult** Inhalation†: 10 mg (2 × 5–mg powder doses) bid; first day's doses must be at least 2 h apart and q12h thereafter.	Influenza A or B infection

*Use liquid oral suspension for doses <75 mg
†Use bronchodilator inhaler first if applicable.
Note: Where pediatric doses are not provided, dosing guidelines for pediatric clients are not firmly established for the drug in question and should be based on the careful clinical judgement of a qualified prescriber.
HSV, Herpes simplex virus (types 1 and 2); CMV, cytomegalovirus; RSV, respiratory syncytial virus.

DRUG PROFILES

NON-RETROVIRAL ANTIVIRAL AGENTS

Antiviral agents are now commonly used to treat active infection with several viruses, including influenza viruses, HSV, VZV, CMV, and RSV. More effective methods of drug development have resulted in many new antiviral drugs over the past two decades.

amantadine

One of the earliest antiviral drugs, amantadine is active only against influenza A viruses. It is used both prophylactically and therapeutically. It has been shown to be effective, if not life-saving, when used prophylactically in geriatric, chronically ill, or immunocompromised clients in whom influenza A infection can be particularly devastating. It may also be used prophylactically when influenza vaccine is either not available or is contraindicated for a given client. Criteria for its use as an early vaccination are outlined by the National Advisory Committee on Immunization. When used therapeutically to treat active influenza A infections it can reduce recovery time.

Amantadine is contraindicated in clients with a known hypersensitivity to it, lactating women, children under 12 months of age, and clients with an eczematic rash. Amantadine is available only in oral (PO) form as a 50-mg/5-mL solution and 100-mg capsules or tablets. Commonly recommended dosages can be found in the table on p. 662.

PHARMACOKINETICS

Half-Life	Onset	Peak	Duration
15 hr	Unknown	1–4 hr	12–24 hr

NEURAMINIDASE INHIBITORS

▶▶ acyclovir

Acyclovir is a synthetic nucleoside analogue of guanine that is mainly used to suppress the replication of HSV-1 and -2 and VZV, which causes chicken pox and shingles. Acyclovir is considered the drug of choice for the treatment of both initial and recurrent episodes of both of these viral infections.

Acyclovir is available in oral, topical, and parenteral formulations. It is available in oral form as a 200-mg/5-mL suspension and 200-, 400-, and 800-mg tablets. In parenteral form it is available as a 25-mg/mL solution and as a 500-mg and 1-g powder for reconstitution and intravenous infusion. Other similar antiviral drugs include valacyclovir and famciclovir. (Note the slight inconsistencies in the spelling of these drug names.) These latter two drugs are currently available only for oral use and are indicated for the treatment of shingles and the suppression of genital herpes in immunosuppressed clients. Valacyclovir is a pro-drug that is metabolized to acyclovir in the body. It has the advantage of greater oral bioavailability and less frequent dosing (three times daily versus five times daily for acyclovir). It may also provide more effective relief of pain from zoster lesions.

Acyclovir is the only agent of the three that is currently available in intravenous form. It is also available in topical form as a 5 percent ointment (see Chapter 55). Acyclovir is contraindicated in clients hypersensitive to it. Pregnancy category C. Commonly recommended dosages can be found in the table on p. 662.

PHARMACOKINETICS

Half-Life	Onset	Peak	Duration
2.1–5 hr	Unknown	PO: 1.5–2 hr	4–5 hr

▶▶ ganciclovir

Like acyclovir, ganciclovir is a synthetic analogue of guanine, but it has a very different spectrum of antiviral activity. CMV is carried by up to 50 percent of the adult population and normally causes no harm. However, in immunocompromised clients (including premature infants) it can cause life-threatening or disabling opportunistic infections. Ganciclovir is the antiviral agent most often used in the treatment of CMV infection. Ganciclovir also has activity against HSV-1 and -2, Epstein-Barr virus (HSV-4), and VZV but is not normally used for the treatment of infection caused by these other viruses because there are other less toxic antiviral agents that are just as effective in inhibiting them. Foscarnet, available only through Health Canada's Special Access Programme, may be used for the treatment of CMV or for acyclovir resistant HSV/VZV.

A common site of CMV infections in the immunocompromised client involves the eye, and the result is CMV retinitis, a devastating viral infection that can lead to blindness. Ganciclovir is most commonly administered intravenously or orally. However, there is also an ophthalmic form for treating active CMV retinitis, which must be surgically inserted (see Chapter 56). Ganciclovir is also administered to prevent CMV disease in high-risk clients, such as those receiving organ transplants.

A dose-limiting toxicity of ganciclovir treatment is bone marrow suppression, including granulocytopenia, anemia, and thrombocytopenia. Dose adjustments may need to be made for someone with renal failure, as ganciclovir is excreted by the kidneys. Ganciclovir also causes temporary or permanent inhibition of spermatogenesis whereas foscarnet can cause renal toxicity. These toxicities should be kept in mind when deciding which agent is more appropriate in a particular patient. For example, a heart transplant recipient who contracts CMV retinitis is immunocompromised because of immunosuppressant drug therapy and is most likely taking cyclosporine, which is nephrotoxic. Therefore using foscarnet in this patient may be more dangerous than using ganciclovir. On the other hand, a patient who contracts a CMV infection and is immunocompromised because of a bone marrow transplant might be better treated using foscarnet.

Ganciclovir is available in oral form as 250- and 500-mg capsules, as an ocular implant, and in parenteral form as a 500-mg injection for intravenous infusion. Ganciclovir is contraindicated in clients with a hypersensitivity to either it or acyclovir. Pregnancy category C. Commonly recommended dosages can be found in the table on p. 662.

PHARMACOKINETICS

Half-Life	Onset	Peak	Duration
2.5–3.6 hr	Unknown	Variable	Variable

oseltamivir and zanamivir

Oseltamivir and zanamivir both belong to one of the newest classes of antiviral agents, known as neuraminidase inhibitors. These agents are active against influenza virus types A and B. They are indicated for the treatment of uncomplicated acute illness caused by influenza infection in adults. They have been shown to reduce the duration of influenza infection by several days. The neuraminidase enzyme enables budding virions to escape from infected cells and spread throughout the body. Neuraminidase inhibitors are designed to stop this process in the body, speeding recovery from infection.

The most commonly reported adverse events with oseltamivir are nausea and vomiting, and those with zanamivir are diarrhea, nausea, and sinusitis. Oseltamivir is now available as a 75-mg capsule and a 12-mg/mL oral suspension. It is indicated for both prophylaxis and treatment of influenza infection. Zanamivir is available in blister packets of 5 mg of dry powder for inhalation. It is currently indicated only for treatment of active influenza illness. Treatment with oseltamivir or zanamivir ideally should begin within two days of influenza symptom onset. Oseltamivir and zanamivir are contraindicated in clients with known hypersensitivity to them, and both are classified as pregnancy category C agents. Commonly recommended dosages can be found in the table on p. 662.

ribavirin

Ribavirin is a unique antiviral agent in that it is given only by oral or nasal inhalation. It is a synthetic nucleoside analogue of guanosine, as are many of the other antiviral agents, but it has a spectrum of antiviral activity that is broader than that of other currently available antiviral agents. It interferes with both RNA and DNA synthesis and as a result inhibits both protein synthesis and viral replication overall.

The inhalational form has been available for close to a decade. It is used primarily in hospitalized infants for treatment of severe lower respiratory tract infections caused by RSV. Because ribavirin may cause fetal toxicity when administered to pregnant women, it is a pregnancy category X agent and contraindicated in pregnant women; the risk of teratogenic or embryocidal effects far outweighs any benefits to be gained in the treatment of the generally self-limiting RSV infections. More recently, 200-mg capsules and tablets for oral use have become available for use in the treatment of hepatitis C in combination with interferon alfa-2b. Commonly recommended dosages can be found in the table on p. 662.

PHARMACOKINETICS

Inhalational form

Half-Life	Onset	Peak	Duration
1.4–2.5 hr*	Unknown	End of inhalation period	Variable

*In respiratory secretions.

OVERVIEW OF HUMAN IMMUNODEFICIENCY VIRUS INFECTION AND THE ACQUIRED IMMUNODEFICIENCY SYNDROME PANDEMIC

The first cases of AIDS were recognized in 1981 in 31 previously healthy homosexual men in Los Angeles and New York City. The first case in Canada was reported in 1982. These first clients mysteriously developed *Pneumocystis carinii* pneumonia (PCP) or Kaposi's sarcoma, both normally extremely rare illnesses. Within months similar disease patterns were recognized in injected drug users and in hemophiliac clients who had been transfused with blood-derived clotting factors. Other cases began to occur in hospitalized clients transfused with a variety of blood-derived products. In 1983, the human T-cell lymphotropic virus type 3 (HTLV-3) was isolated from a client with lymphadenopathy (swollen lymph nodes) and in 1984 was demonstrated to be the cause of AIDS. This virus was later renamed human immunodeficiency virus (HIV), a member of the retrovirus family. There are two recognized types of HIV: HIV-1 and HIV-2. Both cause AIDS, but HIV-2 is primarily localized in western Africa, with HIV-1 causing the majority of the HIV pandemic in the rest of the world. By 1985, a laboratory technique known as an *enzyme-linked immunosorbent assay* (ELISA) was developed. This technique allowed for detection of HIV exposure based on the presence of human antibodies to the virus in blood samples. This diagnostic breakthrough led to an appreciation of the enormity of HIV prevalence both in high-risk groups in the United States and Canada and as an emerging world pandemic, especially in developing countries. This laboratory screening technique also helped to restore the safety of the transfusion blood supply, though it is not 100 percent reliable. In addition to HIV-1 and HIV-2, there are two other retroviruses known to infect humans: HTLV-1 and -2. HTLV-1 is an oncogenic virus capable of causing certain types of leukemia, whereas HTLV-2 is not associated with any specific disease.

The retrovirus family got its name upon discovery of a unique feature of its replication process. Retroviruses are all RNA viruses and are unique in their use of the enzyme **reverse transcriptase** during their replication process. This enzyme promotes the synthesis of complementary ("mirror image") DNA molecules from the viral RNA genome. A second enzyme, integrase, promotes the integration of this viral DNA into the host cell DNA. This hybrid DNA complex is known as a *pro-virus*. It produces new viral RNA genomes and proteins, which in turn combine to make mature HIV virions that infect other host cells. Another important enzyme is **protease**, which serves to chemically separate the new viral RNA from viral protein molecules. These components are initially synthesized into one large macromolecular strand, and the protease enzyme breaks up this strand into its key components. Figure 38-2 illustrates the major structural features of the HIV virion, and Figure 38-3 illustrates the steps in its replication process. Non-retroviruses, on the other hand, primarily use host cell enzymes (DNA or RNA polymerases) to synthesize viral nucleic acids. Reverse transcriptase itself is actually an RNA-dependent DNA polymerase and is sometimes also referred to by this name. However, reverse transcriptase is not normally found in host cells—both reverse transcriptase and integrase are carried by the virus itself. This "reversal" of the usual replication processes leads to the enzyme name

reverse transcriptase, and also to the *retrovirus* name for this family of viruses. Reverse transcriptase also differs from host cell nucleic acid polymerases in another significant way. It has a higher rate of errors when stringing together the purine and pyrimidine bases (A, T, G, C) during transcription of the viral RNA genome into a DNA molecule during the replication process. This allows for more frequent genetic mutations among HIV virions and often results in viral strains that are resistant both to medications and to the client's immune system. Such mutations also hamper the development of an effective vaccine against the virus. However, clinical vaccine trials are currently underway in both Thailand and the United States, using two different vaccine strains that are specific to each geographic area.

The most common routes of transmission for HIV are sexual activity, IDU, and perinatally from mother to child. Heterosexual transmission is most common in Africa. In Canada, according to the latest statistics, unprotected sex among male homosexuals remains the most common cause of new cases (40 percent), with heterosexual vaginal or anal intercourse (25 percent) and IDU (30 percent) as additional causes. Young people aged 15 to 29 years make up 27.4 percent of cases. Aboriginal peoples in Canada have significantly higher rates of HIV than the general population.

In heterosexual transmission, male-to-female transmission is more common. However, there are documented cases of female-to-male sexual transmission that demonstrate the infectiousness of both vaginal secretions

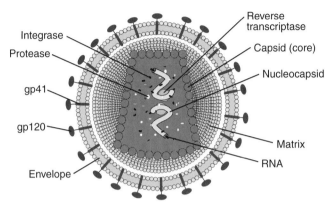

FIG. 38-2 Human immunodeficiency virus (HIV). Within the core capsid, the diploid, single-stranded, positive-sense RNA is complexed to nucleoprotein. (From Newman, W.A. (2003). *Dorland's illustrated medical dictionary* (30th ed.). Philadelphia: Saunders.)

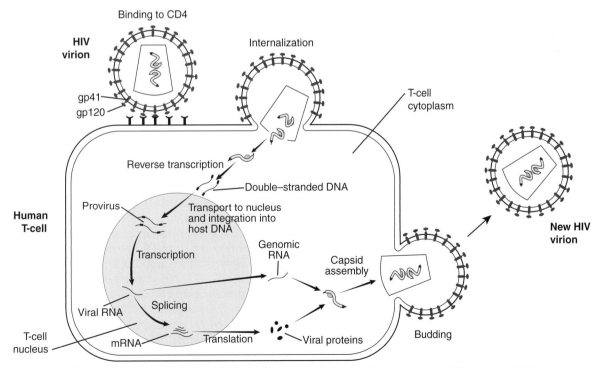

FIG. 38-3 Life cycle of the HIV virus. The extracellular envelope protein gp120 binds to CD4 on the surface of T-lymphocytes or mononuclear phagocytes, while the transmembrane protein glycoprotein 41 (gp41) mediates the fusion of the viral envelope with the cell membrane. (From Newman, W.A. (2003). *Dorland's illustrated medical dictionary* (30th ed.). Philadelphia: Saunders.)

Recommendations for Occupational HIV Exposure Chemoprophylaxis

Type of Exposure	Source	Prophylaxis	Therapy
Percutaneous	Blood	Recommended	Zidovudine + lamivudine +/– indinavir
	Fluid containing visible blood or other potentially infectious fluid or tissue	Offer	Zidovudine + lamivudine
Mucous membrane	Blood	Offer	Zidovudine + lamivudine +/– indinavir
	Fluid containing visible blood or other potentially infectious fluid or tissue	Offer	Zidovudine +/– lamivudine
Skin (i.e., prolonged contact, extensive area, area without skin integrity)	Blood	Offer	Zidovudine + lamivudine +/– indinavir

and menstrual blood. Cases of sexual transmission via oral mucosa are also documented, though uncommon. However, it should be emphasized that no solid evidence to date confirms transmission of HIV by more casual contact, including hugging, kissing, coughing, sneezing, swimming in pools,, and sharing of food, water, eating utensils, or toilet facilities. It is also not transmitted by insect bites, unlike some viral illnesses. Although HIV can be isolated from almost any body fluid, including tears, sweat, saliva, and urine, its concentrations in these fluids are much lower than those in blood and genital secretions. In approximately 6 percent of cases, specific risk factors cannot be determined.

The risk of transmission to healthcare workers resulting from percutaneous (needle stick) injuries is currently calculated at 0.32 percent. The observance of Standard Precautions in avoiding contact with all body fluids during client care dramatically reduces the risk of caregiver infection (see Box 9-1).

The rate of new infections is rising more rapidly in minority populations, especially among Blacks and Aboriginal people. Worldwide there are now more than 30 million cases of HIV/AIDS, with more than 80 percent occurring in developing countries. People in these countries often lack access to adequate drug therapy, resulting in millions of orphaned children each year.

An untreated pregnant woman with HIV has a 15 to 30 percent likelihood of transmitting the virus to her infant. This can occur transplacentally, causing infection *in utero*, or during birth. When the first antiretroviral drugs were developed in the 1980s, it was feared that they would be too toxic and even teratogenic if given to pregnant women. However, prophylactic antiretroviral treatment of infected mothers has been shown to reduce infant infection by at least two-thirds and is not normally harmful to either mother or infant. Medication may also be given prophylactically to the newborn infant, typically for the first six weeks of life. Of course infants and children with established HIV infection must continue on medication indefinitely. Breast milk can transmit the virus to the infant in 10 to 20 percent of cases, and therefore breastfeeding is contraindicated in more developed countries. In developing countries, however, breastfeeding may be the

only available source of nutrition for the infant and therefore worth the risk. This is especially true if medications and other health services are lacking, as is often the case. Box 38-2 summarizes key epidemiological concepts related to HIV/AIDS.

HIV infection that is untreated or treatment resistant eventually leads to immune system failure. The clinical spectrum of the disease often progresses over a period of several years, and the typical course proceeds through a recognized natural history of HIV infection:

1. Primary acute infection
2. Asymptomatic infection
3. Early symptomatic infection
4. Advanced immunodeficiency with opportunistic complications

Primary acute infection refers to the acute viral illness associated with the host response to the virus during the first few weeks after initial exposure to the virus. During this time clients may be asymptomatic, but 25 to 65 percent will show signs of a mild illness that is comparable to an infectious mononucleosis-like illness called the acute retroviral syndrome. This occurs approximately one to six weeks (with a peak occurring at three weeks) after exposure to the virus. Presenting symptoms are generally non-specific and variable and include fever, rash, pharyngitis, night sweats, malaise, myalgia, lymphadenopathy ("swollen glands"), anorexia, and diarrhea. These symptoms are usually mild and resolve spontaneously about the time of seroconversion, which is when the client's own antibodies to the virus (HIV antibodies) begin to appear in blood samples. At this point the client is said to be HIV positive.

The asymptomatic infectious stage occurs next and can last from one to ten years. During this time the virus is present in the blood at low levels and has a low rate of replication. CD4 positive (CD4$^+$) cell counts are usually still within normal limits. CD4 refers to the protein on the cell surface of helper T-lymphocytes, to which HIV attaches itself. These helper T-cells function by releasing cytokines. These are chemicals that activate and modulate *cellular immune function*, which is a general term for all immune system actions other than those of antibodies. (**Antibody**-related immune system activity is also

BOX 38-2

Epidemiology of HIV Infection

Disease Viral Factors
- Developed virus is easily inactivated and must be transmitted in body fluids
- Disease has a long prodromal or incubation period
- Virus can be shed before development of identifiable symptoms

Transmission
- Virus is present in blood, semen, and vaginal secretions

Who Is At Risk?
- Intravenous drug users; sexually active people with many partners (homosexual and heterosexual); prostitutes; newborns of HIV-positive mothers
- Blood and organ transplant recipients and hemophiliacs who received transfusions before 1985 (pre-screening programs)

Geographic Factors
- There is a continuously expanding epidemic worldwide
- No particular seasonal pattern of infection (unlike, e.g., influenza)

Modes of Control
- Antiviral drugs limit progression of disease
- Vaccines for prevention and treatment are in trials
- Safer, monogamous sex helps limit spread
- Sterile injection needles should be used
- Large-scale screening programs have been developed for blood for transfusions, organs for transplants, and clotting factors used by hemophiliacs

From Murray, P.R., Greenwood, D., Slack, R., & Peutherer, J. (2002). *Medical microbiology* (16th ed.). St Louis, MO: Mosby.

referred to as **humoral immune system** function.) Helper T-lymphocytes circulate in the blood and are the primary target cells for HIV. HIV may also infect macrophages, which are usually stationary (non-circulating) CD4-positive (CD4$^+$) cells that remain in various tissues (e.g., lungs, skin, brain) to prevent infection, but it is ultimately through widespread destruction of the helper T-cells in the blood that HIV infection eventually weakens the client's immune system. Characteristic of infection with HIV is persistent generalized lymphadenopathy, defined as the infection of the lymph nodes with CD4$^+$ cells in at least two sites outside the inguinal (groin) area that lasts for a minimum of three to six months.

Once the CD4$^+$ cell count reaches $200\mu/L$ to $500\mu/L$ the infection progresses to a highly symptomatic state. Viral replication increases dramatically, resulting in increasing destruction of helper T-cells and a corresponding decrease in CD4$^+$ counts. At this point there is a major decline in immune system function, and the effects of the illness begin to seriously affect the entire body. Fever, night sweats, and malaise resume and are now accompanied by localized infections, lymphadenopathy, and nervous system manifestations. *Candida* or thrush, shingles,

herpes, and Kaposi's sarcoma are common infections. Oral hairy leukoplakia, characterized by white lesions at the edge of the tongue, is an Epstein-Barr virus often typical of this phase and is an indicator that the disease is progressing.

Generally a diagnosis of AIDS is made once the client meets specific criteria determined by the Centers for Disease Control and Prevention (CDC). AIDS is diagnosed when one of the following develops: the CD4$^+$ count drops to a level below $200/\mu L$ (in Canada and Europe the CD4$^+$ count is not included in the definition of AIDS); certain opportunistic infections (OIs) or opportunistic cancers appear; and wasting syndrome or dementia occurs. HIV wasting syndrome involves major weight loss, chronic diarrhea, frequent or even constant fever, and chronic fatigue.

OIs are so named because the destruction by HIV of the client's immune system gives the "opportunity" for normally harmless micro-organisms in the body to proliferate into serious infections. They may become life threatening or produce significant disability. CMV retinitis, for example, can cause blindness. OIs often begin with atypical bacterial infections such as *Mycobacterium avium* complex (MAC) and *pneumocystic carinii* pneumonia (the species name *carinii* is pronounced kar-ee-nee). Other common OIs include parasitic infections such as cryptosporidial diarrhea and toxoplasmosis encephalitis; viral infections such as HSV mouth ulcers, esophagitis, pneumonitis, CMV pneumonia, and retinitis; and fungal infections such as candidiasis of the GI and respiratory tracts.

Tuberculosis (TB) is usually more severe in persons with AIDS and is currently the leading cause of death worldwide for HIV-infected clients. Dually infected clients are 100 times more likely to develop active TB and become infectious than clients infected with TB alone. About 40 percent of HIV-infected clients in Canada are believed to be co-infected with HCV, which also tends to be more severe in HIV clients. The most common route of transmission is through needle sharing, with sexual and perinatal routes much less common. HCV is the most important cause of chronic liver disease in Canada. HCV-induced liver failure is the most common reason for liver transplantation, and liver cancer may also occur secondary to HCV infection. Many other OIs may also occur, as indicated in Box 38-3.

A similar opportunistic situation occurs with HIV-associated neoplasms. The most common of these include Kaposi's sarcoma, non-Hodgkins lymphoma, and invasive cancer of the cervix. In addition to its attack on helper T-cells and macrophages, the virus itself can also cause additional pathology in such organs as the brain (HIV-induced encephalopathy and dementia), bone marrow, lungs (recurrent pneumonia), and skin. All of these manifestations are said to be the defining conditions of HIV/AIDS.

The viral load, which is measured as the number of viral RNA copies per millilitre of blood, also continues to rise uncontrollably. If this condition continues, death often ensues. Figure 38-4 illustrates events that roughly correlate with the progress of HIV infection.

Indicator Diseases of AIDS*

Opportunistic Infections
Protozoal
Toxoplasmosis of the brain
Extrapulmonary cryptosporidiosis with diarrhea
Isosporiasis with diarrhea
Disseminated or extrapulmonary coccidomycosis

Fungal
Candidiasis of the esophagus, trachea, bronchi, and
   lungs
PCP
Histoplasmosis (disseminated or extrapulmonary)

Viral
CMV disease
CMV retinitis
HSV infection (persistent or disseminated)
Progressive multifocal leukoencephalopathy
Extrapulmonary cryptococcosis

Bacterial
Mycobacterium avium complex (MAC) (disseminated)
Any "atypical" mycobacterial disease
Mycobacterium tuberculosis
Salmonella septicemia (recurrent)
Pyogenic bacterial infections (multiple or recurrent)

Opportunistic Neoplasias
Kaposi's sarcoma
Burkitt's lymphoma
Immunoblastic lymphoma
Primary lymphoma of the brain
Invasive cervical cancer

Others
HIV wasting syndrome
HIV encephalopathy
Lymphoid interstitial pneumonia

Modified from Mandell, G.L., Bennett, J.E., & Dolin, R. (2005). *Principles and practice of infectious diseases* (6th ed.). Philadelphia: Elsevier Churchill Livingstone.
*Manifestations of HIV-infection–defining AIDS according to criteria of the CDC.

Advances in antiretroviral drug therapy have given rise to increasingly greater numbers of long-term survivors of HIV infection. Long-term survival is defined as living with the illness for at least 10 to 15 years after infection. Some particularly remarkable clients have lived for several years with CD4 counts remaining at the often fatal levels of $200/\mu L$ or less. Improved drug therapy against both HIV and OIs is still believed to play an important role in these unusual cases. Other remarkable clients are the long-term non-progressors. These are long-term survivors who have maintained normal CD4 counts and low HIV viral loads, despite not receiving *any* anti-HIV drug treatment. These clients are usually able to mount especially strong cell-mediated and humoral immune responses that prevent progression of the viral infection. They are also the subject of much research aimed at identifying the mechanisms of their survival and hopefully finding ways to share these advantages with other clients.

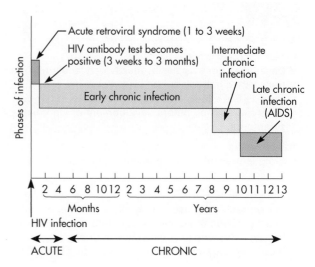

FIG. 38-4 Time course and stages of HIV disease. A long clinical latency period follows the initial mononucleosis-like symptoms. The progressive decrease in the number of CD4 T-cells, even during the latency period, allows opportunistic infections to occur. The stages (World Health Organization and Centers for Disease Control and Prevention) in HIV disease are defined by the CD4 T-cell levels and occurrence of opportunistic disease. (From Lewis, S., Heitkemper, M., & Dirksen, S. (Eds.) (2004). *Medical-surgical nursing: Assessment and management of clinical problems* (6th ed.) p. 627. St Louis, MO: Mosby.)

ANTIRETROVIRAL AGENTS

Much has happened in medical science since the AIDS virus was first identified in the early 1980s. The increasing urgency and public awareness of the HIV epidemic has stimulated much research into the fields of immunology and pharmacology. This has resulted in the development of several increasingly effective antiretroviral agents, as well as antiviral agents in general. Although new drug combinations have definitely prolonged lives and offered hope to many people, these medications are often not without significant toxicities. Furthermore, HIV/AIDS is still not normally considered to be a curable disease, though there have been some remarkable recoveries and apparent cures in a small number of individuals. There are now five classes of antiretroviral agents, including three distinct classes of **reverse transcriptase inhibitors (RTIs)**; the **protease inhibitors** (PIs); and the newest class, the **fusion inhibitors**, which currently includes only one medication.

Mechanism of Action and Drug Effects

Although HIV/AIDS is a complex illness, the mechanisms of action of the various drug classes are, fortunately, straightforward and distinct. The name of each class of medication provides a reminder of its role in suppressing the viral replication process. RTIs work by blocking activity of the enzyme reverse transcriptase, which promotes the synthesis of new viral DNA molecules from the RNA genome of the parent virion. There are currently three subclasses of RTIs: nucleoside RTIs, or NRTIs (six drugs); non-nucleoside RTIs, or NNRTIs (three drugs); and nucleotide RTIs, or NTRTIs (one drug).

There are currently eight protease inhibitors (PIs), including one combination drug product, which consists of two PIs. These agents work by inhibiting the protease retroviral enzyme. This enzyme promotes the breakup of chains of protein molecules at designated points, a process necessary for viral replication. There is currently only one fusion inhibitor. This compound is named enfuvirtide and works by inhibiting viral fusion. This is the process by which an HIV virion attaches to (fuses with) the membrane of a host cell (T-lymphocyte) before infecting it in preparation for viral replication.

Single-drug therapy was most common in the early years of the HIV epidemic, partly due to a lack of treatment options. However, both the development of multiple antiretroviral drugs and the emergence of resistant viral strains have given rise to combination drug therapy as the current standard of care. This is the most effective treatment to date and is referred to as *highly active antiretroviral therapy* (HAART). HAART usually includes at least three medications. The most commonly recommended drug combinations include two or three NRTIs, two NRTIs plus one or two PIs, and an NRTI plus an NNRTI plus one or two PIs.

All antiretroviral agents have, to varying degrees, similar therapeutic effects. They reduce the viral load, which is the number of viral RNA copies per millilitre of blood. A viral load of less than 50 copies/mL is considered to be undetectable and is a primary goal of antiretroviral therapy. HIV-infected clients should ideally be followed by practitioners with extensive training in drug therapy for infectious diseases. These practitioners must often make careful choices and changes in drug therapy over time, based on a given client's clinical response and severity of any drug-related toxicities.

Indications

As indicated in Table 38-3, the only usual indication for all of the current antiretroviral agents is active HIV infection. Prophylactic therapy is also given to individuals (e.g., healthcare workers) with known potential exposure to HIV (e.g., via needle stick injuries in hospitals—see Research box on p. 666).

Contraindications

Keeping in mind the potentially fatal outcome of HIV infection, the only usual contraindication to a given medication is known severe drug allergy or other intolerable toxicity. Fortunately, the two decades that saw the rise of the HIV pandemic were also marked by the development of several categories of antiretroviral medications. Most of the current antiretroviral drug classes now have several alternative drugs to choose from should a client be especially intolerant of a given agent.

Side Effects and Adverse Effects

Common adverse effects of selected antiretroviral agents are listed in Table 38-4. It is not uncommon to need to modify drug therapy because of side effects. The goal is to find the regimen that will best control a given client's infection, with as tolerable a side effect profile as possible. Different clients can vary widely in their drug tolerance, and a given client's drug tolerance may change over time. Thus medication regimens must often be strategically individualized and evolve with the course of the client's illness.

Interactions

Common drug interactions involving selected antiretroviral agents are listed in Box 38-1.

Dosages

Dosage information for all of the currently available antiretroviral medications is listed in the dosages table on p. 670–671. Profiles of selected drugs follow. See Appendix B for some of the common brands available in Canada.

DRUG PROFILES

enfuvirtide

Enfuvirtide is the newest medication in the newest class of antiretroviral drugs. It received approval by Health Canada in 2004 and is classified as a fusion inhibitor. It works by suppressing the fusion process whereby a virion is attached to the outer membrane of a host T-cell before entry into the cell and subsequent viral replication. This mechanism of action serves as yet another example of how antiretroviral drugs are strategically designed to interfere with specific steps of the viral replication process. As mentioned previously, the use of combinations of drugs that work by different mechanisms improves a client's chances for continued survival by reducing the likelihood of viral resistance to the drug therapy regimen. Enfuvirtide is indicated for treatment of HIV infection in combination with other antiretroviral drugs. Its only current contraindication is known severe drug allergy. Adult and pediatric clients have shown comparable tolerance of the drug in clinical trials thus far. The drug is currently available only in injectable form as a 90-mg vial of powdered drug for reconstitution and subcutaneous (SC) injection. Pregnancy category has yet to be classified. Dosing information appears in the table on p. 670.

PHARMACOKINETICS

Half-Life	Onset	Peak	Duration
4 hr	Unknown	6 hr	Unknown

▸▸ *indinavir*

Indinavir belongs to the PI class of antiretroviral agents. Others include ritonavir, saquinavir, nelfinavir, atazanavir, amprenavir, and the combination product lopinavir/ritonavir. Indinavir can be taken in combination with other anti-HIV therapies or alone. Indinavir therapy produces increases in CD4+ cell counts, an important measure of immune system function. It also produces

DOSAGES Antiretroviral Agents

Agent	Pharmacological Class	Usual Dosage Range	Indications
abacavir	Nucleotide reverse transcriptase inhibitor (NRTI)	*Pediatric 3 mo–12 yr* PO: 8 mg/kg bid (max 300 mg/dose) *12 yr–adult* PO: 300 mg bid	
amprenavir	Protease inhibitor (PI)	*Pediatric 4–12 yr* PO: 20 mg/kg bid or 15 mg/kg tid *Adult >12 yr* PO: 1200 mg bid	
delavirdine	Non-nucleoside reverse transcriptase inhibitor (NNRTI)	*16 yr–adult* PO: 400 mg tid	
didanosine	Nucleotide reverse transcriptase inhibitor (NRTI)	*Pediatric 2 weeks to <8 mo* PO: 100 mg/m² divided q12h *Pediatric >8 mo* PO: 120 mg/m² divided q12h *Adult (depending on weight)* PO: 250–400 mg/day or 125–250 mg bid	
efavirenz	Non-nucleoside reverse transcriptase inhibitor (NNRTI)	*Pediatric 3 yr–adult* PO: 200–600 mg once daily based on weight table	
enfuvirtide	Fusion inhibitor	*Pediatric 6–16 yr* SC: 2 mg/kg bid (max 90 mg/dose) *17 yr–adult* SC: 90 mg bid	
≫ indinavir	Protease inhibitor (PI)	*Adult* PO: 800 mg q8h *Pediatric >3 yr* PO: 500 mg/m² q8h	
lamivudine	Nucleotide reverse transcriptase inhibitor (NRTI)	*Pediatric 3 mo–15 yr* PO: 4 mg/kg bid (max 150 mg/dose) *16 yr–adult* PO: 100 mg daily	HIV infection
nelfinavir	Protease inhibitor (PI)	*Pediatric 2–13 yr* PO: 25–30 mg/kg tid *14 yr–adult* PO: 625–750 mg bid–tid	
≫ nevirapine	Non-nucleoside reverse transcriptase inhibitor (NNRTI)	*Pediatric 2 mo–8 yr* PO: 120 mg/m² daily × 14 days, then 200 mg/m² bid *>8–15 yr* PO: 120 mg/m² daily × 14 days, then 120 mg/m² bid *Adult* PO: 200 mg qd × 14 days, then bid	
ritonavir	Protease inhibitor (PI)	*Pediatric 2–12 yr* PO: 400 mg/m² bid *Adult* PO: 600 mg bid (max 1200 mg)	
saquinavir	Protease inhibitor (PI)	*16 yr–adult* PO (Invirase): 600 mg tid	
stavudine	Nucleotide reverse transcriptase inhibitor (NRTI)	*Pediatric (specific ages not listed)* PO: 1 mg/kg q12h *Adult <60 kg* PO: 30 mg q12h *≥60 kg* PO: 40 mg q12h	
tenofovir	Nucleotide reverse transcriptase inhibitor (NTRTI)	*Adult* PO: 300 mg once daily	
zalcitabine	Nucleotide reverse transcriptase inhibitor (NRTI)	*13 yr–adult* PO: 0.75 mg q8h	

Continued

DOSAGES   Antiretroviral Agents—cont'd

Agent	Pharmacologic Class	Usual Dosage Range	Indications
▸▸zidovudine	Nucleotide reverse transcriptase inhibitor (NTRTI)	**Pediatric infants 0–6 wks*** PO: 2 mg/kg q6h starting within 12 h after birth IV: 1.5 mg/kg q6h **3 mo–12 yr** PO: 180 mg/m² q6h IV: 120 mg/m² q6h (max 160 mg/dose) **Adult** PO: 200 mg q12h or 300 mg q8h IV: 1–2 mg/kg q4h **Pregnant women** PO: 100 mg 5×/day during pregnancy until start of labour, then give IV bolus dose of 2 mg/kg over 1 h followed by an IV infusion of 1 mg/kg/h until the umbilical cord is clamped	
Combination Drug Products			HIV infection
abacavir/ lamivudine/ zidovudine	Triple-drug combination nucleoside reverse transcriptase inhibitor	**Adolescent or adult ≥40 kg** PO: 1 tab bid (1 tab = 300 mg abacavir + 150 mg lamivudine + 300 mg zidovudine)	
lamivudine/ zidovudine	Double-drug combination nucleoside reverse transcriptase inhibitor	**12 yr–adult** PO: 1 tab bid (1 tab = 150 mg lamivudine + 300 mg zidovudine)	
lopinavir/ ritonavir	Double-drug combination protease-inhibitor	**Pediatric 7–14 kg** PO: 12 mg/kg bid **Pediatric 15–40 kg** PO: 10 mg/kg bid **Pediatric >40 kg or adult** PO: 3 caps or 5 mL bid (1 cap = 133.3 mg lopinavir + 33.3 mg ritonavir; for the oral solution 5 mL contains 80 mg lopinavir + 20 mg ritonavir)	

*Drug should be continued either IV or PO through at least six weeks of age.
Note: Where pediatric doses are not provided, dosing guidelines for pediatric clients are not firmly established for the drug in question and should be based on the careful clinical judgement of a qualified prescriber.

significant reductions in viral load, or levels of HIV in the bloodstream. PIs are commonly given in combination with two RTIs to maximize efficacy and decrease the likelihood of viral drug resistance. Indinavir is relatively well tolerated in most clients. Nephrolithiasis (kidney stones) can occur in approximately 9.8 percent of clients. Clients who take indinavir are encouraged to drink at least 1.5 L of liquids every day to maintain hydration and help avoid nephrolithiasis. Indinavir is contraindicated in clients with clinically significant hypersensitivity to any of its components. Indinavir is available only in oral form as 200- and 400-mg capsules. Pregnancy category C. The commonly recommended dosage can be found in the table on p. 670.

PHARMACOKINETICS

Half-Life	Onset	Peak	Duration
1.5–2.5 hr	2 wk*	0.5–1 hr	6 mo

*Therapeutic effects.

▸▸ nevirapine

Nevirapine is an NNRTI. This is the second class of antiviral agents indicated for the treatment of HIV infection. Other currently available NNRTIs include delavir-

dine and efavirenz. These agents are often used in combination with NRTIs such as zidovudine.

Nevirapine is well tolerated when compared with other therapies for HIV. The most common adverse events associated with nevirapine therapy are rash, fever, nausea, headache, and abnormal liver function tests. The greatest risk of severe adverse skin reactions and hepatic toxicity occurs during the first 18 weeks of therapy; close monitoring is recommended. Nevirapine is contraindicated in clients with clinically significant hypersensitivity to any of its components. Nevirapine is available in oral form as a 200-mg tablet. Pregnancy category C. Commonly recommended dosage can be found in the table on p. 670.

PHARMACOKINETICS

Half-Life	Onset	Peak	Duration
25–30 hr	2 hr*	2–4 hr	24 hr

*Therapeutic effects.

tenofovir

Tenofovir is the first NTRTI. It was approved in Canada in March 2004 with conditions. It is an analogue of adenine but has an attached phosphate group, which distinguishes this drug class from the nucleoside RTIs. It is indicated for use against HIV infection in combination with other antiretroviral drugs. It is reserved for clients who have not had success with other antiretroviral regimes. It is contraindicated in cases of known drug allergy and is currently available only as a 300-mg tablet. It is currently classified as a pregnancy category B drug, though it is still quite new. Dosage information appears in the table on p. 670.

PHARMACOKINETICS

Half-Life	Onset	Peak	Duration
Unknown	Unknown	1 hr	Unknown

▸▸ *zidovudine*

Zidovudine is a synthetic nucleoside analogue of thymidine that has had an enormous impact on the treatment and quality of life of clients infected with HIV who have AIDS. It was the first, and for a long time the only, anti-HIV medication that offered clients with AIDS any hope in the early years of the epidemic. HIV requires reverse transcriptase for viral replication. This enzyme is inhibited by zidovudine, as well as the other NRTIs: lamivudine, zalcitabine, didanosine, stavudine, and abacavir. Although there have been many new therapies approved recently, none currently available can eradicate the infection completely. They are effective in that they decrease the viral load and delay immunological decline. However, HIV over time can become resistant to the effects of RTIs. For this reason it is common practice to now use multiple agents in the treatment of HIV infection. Zidovudine, along with various other antiretroviral agents, is given to HIV-infected pregnant women and even to newborn babies to prevent maternal transmission of the virus to the infant. These six antiretroviral agents are all approved for the treatment of HIV/AIDS. When effective, treatment leads to a significant reduction in mortality and the incidence of opportunistic infections, the improvement of a client's physical condition, and a significant improvement in T-cell counts.

The major dose-limiting adverse effect of zidovudine is bone marrow suppression, and this is often the reason a client with an HIV infection has to be switched to another anti-HIV agent such as zalcitabine or didanosine. Some clients may be taking a combination of two of these agents, in lower doses, to maximize their combined actions. This strategy may decrease the likelihood of toxicity. The combination of various nucleoside analogues is so common that pharmaceutical companies have begun to make combination products. An example is Combivir, which is a single tablet that combines 150 mg of lamivudine and 300 mg of zidovudine.

Zidovudine is contraindicated in clients with a known hypersensitivity to it. It is available in both oral and parenteral formulations. In parenteral form it is available as a 10-mg/mL injection for intravenous infusion. In oral form it is available as a 100-mg capsule and a 50-mg/5-mL solution. Pregnancy category C. Commonly recommended dosages can be found in the table on p. 671.

PHARMACOKINETICS

Half-Life	Onset	Peak	Duration
1.1 hr	Unknown	0.5–1.5 hr	3–5 hr

OTHER SIGNIFICANT VIRAL ILLNESSES OF RECENT CONCERN

There are numerous other viral infections that could be discussed in this chapter. However, four of recent special significance are briefly discussed here: hantavirus, West Nile virus (WNV), and sudden acute respiratory syndrome (SARS). All three of these viral infections have resulted in significant morbidity and mortality and often require aggressive supportive care in an intensive care unit (ICU) setting.

Hantaviruses

Hantaviruses are members of the bunyavirus family. There are several known hantavirus serotypes. An outbreak of a serious respiratory illness known as hantavirus pulmonary syndrome occurred in northeastern Arizona in 1993. It resulted in several deaths and it was determined that a specific serotype of hantavirus, known as the Sin Nombre virus (Spanish for "without name"), was the causative organism. This virus is carried by rodents (e.g., the deer mouse) and spread by contact with rodent feces, especially by inhalation of fecal particles. Treatment often requires intensive supportive care with ventilator support of respiratory function. No definitive viral drug therapy currently exists for hantavirus infection, though the drug ribavirin has been used in some cases without marked success. Prevention involves keeping homes free of rodents and rodent feces and avoiding contact with rodents in rural areas. Canada's first case occurred in 1994 in British Columbia. There have been a total of 57 cases in Canada with 19 deaths from hantavirus.

West Nile Virus

In 1999 the first North American cases of WNV occurred in New York City. WNV is a member of the arbovirus family and is transmitted to humans by mosquitoes. It also infects animals, primarily birds, and has been detected in horses and cows. In humans it can lead to meningitis and encephalitis. In 2001 an epidemic occurred with over 4000 documented human cases, including 284 deaths. Organ transplant clients were one of the key groups infected. The first human documented cases of WNV in Canada occurred in 2001. In 2003, 14 deaths occurred from WNV and there have been 12 reported deaths in 2005. The virus can also be transmitted through blood transfusions and has been detected in breast milk. There is new evidence that healthcare workers can get WNV via needle sticks or cuts. It is currently being investigated for maternal–fetal transmission during pregnancy. In June 2003, Health Canada began screening blood donations for WNV using a test developed by the Canadian Blood Services. There is currently no specific antiviral medication available. In cases of encephalitis, aggressive supportive measures such as monitoring and control of intracranial pressure (ICP) can be crucial. Mannitol diuresis is one method of reducing ICP. Prevention focuses on reducing mosquito reproduction by eliminating unneeded pools of water near residential environments.

SARS

November 2002 was marked by the emergence of a new, serious viral infectious disease known as sudden acute respiratory syndrome, or SARS. A large outbreak later occurred in Singapore in March of 2003. This outbreak was eventually traced to a traveller returning from Hong Kong. Cases later appeared in Europe and North America, with the first case reported in Canada on February 23, 2003. As of August 2003, there had been 438 probable and suspect SARS cases in Canada, including 44 deaths. The cause of SARS is still being determined but it is thought to be caused by a member of the coronavirus family. Coronaviruses commonly cause mild to moderate upper respiratory illnesses in humans, including the common cold. The U.S. Centers for Disease Control and Prevention (CDC), along with a Canadian laboratory, recently sequenced the genome of the coronavirus that has since been named SARS-CoV.

SARS can range from a mild to life-threatening respiratory syndrome. The illness usually resolves on its own within three to four weeks. However, 10 to 20 percent of clients thus far have required mechanical ventilation and intensive care support, with a 3 percent overall fatality rate. Although clients have been given empirical drug therapy, including various antibiotics, the antiviral agents ribavirin and oseltamivir, and corticosteroids, no drug therapy to date has been definitively proven helpful. The illness appears to be easily spread via inhalational and contact routes, and healthcare workers are at especially high risk. Several nurses and physicians caring for SARS clients have become infected themselves. Face masks that meet the N-95 standard for respiratory pathogens are recommended, along with gloves and gowns, when delivering client care, and clients should be placed in appropriate isolation. Eye protection is also recommended until all routes of transmission are further clarified. These are currently the only preventive measures recommended. Much remains to be learned about this emerging illness, including its causes and effective treatments, if any.

Avian Flu

An emerging public health issue is the H5N1 strain of avian influenza, which is creating worldwide concern about a pandemic. Three types of influenza viruses can affect humans: types A, B, and C. However, only the influenza A virus naturally infects birds. Because influenza viruses mutate frequently, there is fear that this virus may undergo an abrupt major change, creating a new pathogenic form of influenza A that can infect humans. Although human-to-human transmission of the virus is considered to be rare, there have been reported cases of strains of avian influenza in humans. These have been found primarily in Asia and are associated with close direct contact with infected poultry or contaminated surfaces. In an effort to contain the virus, the entire poultry population in Hong Kong was destroyed. This same strategy has been used in Canada when low pathogenic strains of the virus were found in farms in British Columbia. The Public Health Agency of Canada is main-

taining close surveillance of the virus. There is no vaccine ready for commercial production, although one is under development. Health Canada has stockpiled 23 million doses of oseltamivir as a preventative strategy.

NURSING PROCESS

■ Assessment

Before administering an antiviral agent the nurse should perform a thorough assessment to find out what underlying diseases the client may have and his or her medical history. This is important to ensure safe medication use. The nurse should also find out whether the client has any known allergies to the medication or whether he or she has suffered any side effects of the medication in the past. It is also important to assess the client's nutritional status and baseline vital signs because of the profound effects viral illnesses can have on them, especially if the client is also immunosuppressed. Contraindications to the use of most of the antiviral agents include herpes zoster infection in immunosuppressed clients. Cautious use, with careful monitoring, is recommended in clients who have renal or hepatic disease, who are dehydrated or in electrolyte imbalance, who are pregnant or lactating, or who have seizure disorders.

Amantadine is contraindicated in children under one year of age and should be used cautiously in clients suffering from heart failure (because of its cardiovascular side effects) or orthostatic hypotension. A reduction of the amantadine dosage may be needed for clients who have a history of seizures, uncontrollable psychoses, or renal impairment. Laboratory results that should be obtained before the start of therapy include white blood cell (WBC) count, red blood cell (RBC) count, blood urea nitrogen (BUN), creatinine clearance, and liver function studies. Culture and sensitivity testing should also be done before initiation of therapy. Drug interactions include anticholinergics (such as atropine and atropine-like drugs), CNS stimulants, and alcohol.

Zidovudine has been used in clients with HIV infections but is associated with many side effects and is capable of significant drug interactions that may increase the risk of toxicity. Vital signs, complete blood counts (CBCs) and liver function tests need to be assessed and documented before therapy is initiated. It is also crucial for the nurse to assess and document symptoms such as fever, night sweats, lymph node swelling, diarrhea, cough, anorexia, and yeast infections. Drug interactions include any bone marrow suppressing drugs such as dapsone, vincristine, adriamycin, vinblastine, and interferon alfa. Clarithromycin may reduce peak levels of zidovudine.

Most antivirals should be administered with caution in those clients who have renal or hepatic dysfunction. Because zidovudine suppresses bone marrow functioning, it should not be used in conjunction with other agents that do the same because of the resulting additive adverse effects. Other drugs that interact with zidovudine include ganciclovir, probenecid, phenytoin, methadone, and fluconazole.

Other antiviral agents have their own important parameter-related assessments. With ribavirin, assessment of the respiratory system, including breath sounds, cough, and sputum production, is required because of the potential for pulmonary problems. Indinavir and nevirapine are contraindicated in clients who are allergic to their chemical properties. Renal studies should be assessed before the use of indinavir, and hepatic function studies should be assessed before the use of nevirapine.

Acyclovir, used for herpes and varicella-zoster (within 24 hours of appearance of the typical rash of chicken pox), should be used cautiously in clients with decreased renal functioning because of associated nephrotoxicity; laboratory data for renal function should be collected. Vital signs and the characteristics of any visible lesions should be assessed and documented. Drug interactions include any other type of nephrotoxic drugs (e.g., aminoglycoside antibiotics).

Ganciclovir is contraindicated in clients with an absolute neutrophil count (ANC) of less than 0.5×10^9 cells/L because there is a greater risk of infection. Clients with decreased renal function usually receive a decreased dose. For CMV retinitis there may be alterations in vision and formation of exudative (weeping) lesions. Liver function tests, BUN, serum creatinine, CBCs, and platelet counts should be assessed and documented.

Tenofovir is contraindicated in cases of known drug allergy. It is a pregnancy category B drug. Tenofovir is relatively new (approved by Health Canada in 2004 with conditions) and should be administered only after careful assessment.

When drugs are used in combination, lower doses of each drug are required, and this may help to decrease toxicity. The combination of various nucleoside analogues is so common that pharmaceutical companies have begun to make combination products. An example is Combivir, which is a single tablet that combines 150 mg of lamivudine and 300 mg of zidovudine. Because of the potentially fatal outcome of HIV infection, the only usual contraindication to a given medication is known severe drug allergy or other intolerable toxicity.

The PIs are to be given with caution to those with a history of renal disorders or decreased functioning. Renal function studies should be assessed and documented. They are pregnancy category C drugs.

SARS is a viral infection that Canada and the international population must confront now and in the future. The symptoms of SARS may range from mild to life threatening and may resolve on their own within three to four weeks; however, some 10 to 20 percent of afflicted clients have required mechanical ventilation and intensive care support, and there is a 3 percent overall mortality rate. Although clients have been given empirical drug therapy, including antiviral agents (e.g., ribavirin and oseltamivir) and corticosteroids, no drug to date has definitively proved helpful although there are several in testing. The illness appears to be easily spread via inhalation and contact; therefore nurses and other healthcare workers are at especially high risk for exposure and/or contracting the illness. It is important for the nurse to take proper precautions when assessing a client with possible or diagnosed SARS virus and to ensure that they and all other healthcare workers in contact with the client are aware of the nature of the client's illness to prevent the spread of the virus. Standard precautions should be taken automatically.

Nursing Diagnoses

Nursing diagnoses appropriate for clients receiving antiviral agents include the following:
- Acute pain related to the signs and symptoms associated with viral infections.
- Risk for injury related to falls due to the side effects of antiviral medications.
- Deficient knowledge related to the lack of information about viral infections, their transmission, and treatment.
- Activity intolerance related to weakness secondary to decreased energy from pathology of viral infections.
- Risk for infection related to viral and/or antiviral medication-induced compromised physical status.

Planning

Goals pertaining to clients receiving antiviral agents include the following:
- Client is free of symptoms of viral infection once therapy is completed.
- Client remains adherent with therapy.
- Client experiences improved energy and appetite and improved ability to engage in activities of daily living.
- (for genital herpes) Client states the rationale for therapy for active sexual partners.
- Client experiences minimal side effects of antiviral agent.

Outcome Criteria

Outcome criteria for clients receiving antiviral agents include the following:
- Client experiences increased periods of comfort as a result of successful treatment of viral infection.
- Client states the effect of a viral infection on health (e.g., compromised immune system) and need for appropriate treatment.
- Client states the rationale for treatment.
- (for genital herpes) Client states the rationale for treatment of any partners with whom the client has been sexually active to prevent worsening of symptoms and to decrease severity of episodes related to genital herpes.
- Client identifies the possible side effects of the antiviral agent, such as diarrhea, headache, nausea, and insomnia.

Implementation

Nursing interventions pertinent to clients receiving antiviral agents include use of the appropriate technique of application or administration of ointment, aerosol powders, or intravenous or oral forms of medication (see Box 9-1). Hands should be washed before and after administering the medication to prevent contamination of the site and spread of infection to others. In addition, strict adherence to Standard Precautions is important to the safety of both the client and the nurse.

Amantadine must be taken as ordered, and syrup forms are available. The full course of treatment should be taken, and if a dose is missed it is important for the client to take the dose as soon as it is remembered or contact the healthcare provider for further instructions. Should dry mouth occur, sugarless candy and gum might be helpful. Daily mouth care, including the use of dental floss, and regular dental preventive visits are encouraged. Saliva substitutes may be needed for amantadine and other drugs. If dryness of the mouth continues for more than two weeks, the healthcare provider should be contacted. Livedo reticularis (red–blue network mottling of skin caused by congestion of the superficial capillaries) may occur, and client education about this is important. Discontinuation of the drug will reverse this effect.

Topical antiviral agents such as acyclovir should be applied in accordance with the manufacturer's guidelines or physician's orders, and gloves must be used to prevent the spread of infection to others. Intravenously administered acyclovir should be diluted in recommended solutions such as sterile water for injection or in the solutions recommended by the manufacturer. Intravenous administration is usually done over one hour, but all sources of drug information should be consulted first to determine the correct timing.

Acyclovir and many of the other antiviral agents interact with several drugs, listed earlier. Fluid intake of at least 2400 mL/day should be encouraged in clients receiving acyclovir by any route, unless contraindicated. This is to prevent crystalluria. Intravenous infusions should be administered slowly over at least one hour and the intravenous infusion sites watched closely for the development of redness, swelling, or heat. Acyclovir sodium should not be administered subcutaneously, intramuscularly (IM), orally, or ophthalmically. Many intravenous agents and solutions are incompatible with intravenous acyclovir, and the nurse should check and recheck compatibilities before co-administering other agents or solutions.

COMMUNITY HEALTH POINTS

Alternative Approaches to Treatment

Many alternative approaches (such as homeopathic therapy, naturopathic therapy, and use of herbal products) exist to treat various disease processes, including AIDS and HIV. Even if healthcare providers do not support these alternative approaches, they should give clients the resources to make the best informed decision.

The following are a few online resources for clients:
- http://www.cdnaids.ca/
- http://www.patients.uptodate.com/
- http://www.hc-sc.gc.ca/dc-ma/aids-sida/index_e.html
- http://www.nih.gov

Other sources include journals, such as *AIDS Patient Care* and *Alternative Therapy in Health and Medicine.*

Zanamivir is to be used, if indicated, within two days of the onset of flu symptoms. It comes in a powder for inhalant use.

Clients taking ribavirin for RSV treatment via the Viratex Small Particle Aerosol Generator (SPAG) device should be taught how to properly mix and administer the drug. The powder should be reconstituted according to the manufacturer's guidelines. Residues in the equipment should be discarded before adding fresh medication. (Note: Drugs administered via Viratex SPAG equipment should be administered 12 to 18 hours daily for up to seven days, beginning within three days of the onset of symptoms. Generally the dose of ribavirin is 20 mg/mL.)

Indinavir and nevirapine are administered orally. With indinavir, clients should drink at least 1.5 L of fluids every day to maintain adequate hydration and help prevent nephrolithiasis. Orally administered didanosine should be given every 12 hours, or as ordered, and on an empty stomach one hour before meals or two hours after meals. Antifungals are incompatible with didanosine. Buffered powder solutions for oral administration should be mixed in at least 115 mL of water—not fruit juice or acid-containing juices—and the solution should be drunk immediately after mixing.

PIs should be administered with forcing of fluids to help minimize nephrolithiasis; 3000 mL/day is recommended unless contraindicated. Client teaching tips are presented in the box on p. 676.

■ Evaluation

The therapeutic effects of antiviral agents depend on the type of viral infection and the immune and general status of the client. This could range from delayed progression of AIDS to a decrease in flu-like symptoms and the frequency of herpetic flare-ups and OIs. Herpetic lesions should crust over, and the frequency of recurrence should decrease. Adverse reactions to specific antiviral agents should be monitored for. These specific reactions are listed in Table 38-4.

CASE STUDY

Antiviral Therapy

One of your clients, Z.K., a 33-year-old biology professor, has just begun therapy with zidovudine for an opportunistic infection. She is to be dosed with 200 mg PO q4h and will be taking the medication at home. She is inquiring about the new medication regimen, drug interactions, side effects, and any other important information and how this medication differs from other antivirals.
- Develop a client teaching guide for Z.K., emphasizing any specific cautions and symptoms to report to the healthcare provider.
- Compare and contrast the various antiviral agents.
- At what level of platelets and white blood cells would the zidovudine likely be discontinued or the dose changed?

For answers see http://evolve.elsevier.com/Lilley/pharmacology/.

CLIENT TEACHING TIPS

The nurse should instruct the client as follows:

▲ Take these medications exactly as prescribed and for the full course of therapy.

▲ Some antiviral agents may cause dizziness; be careful about driving or other activities requiring alertness until you find out how this medication affects you.

▲ Practise good hygiene. Be careful about washing hands, especially before contact with food or other people.

▲ Be aware that antiviral agents are not cures but do help to manage the related symptoms.

Acyclovir Ointment

▲ Do not use any other additional creams or ointments on the site. Wear a glove or finger cot when applying topical solutions to affected areas, and keep these areas clean and dry.

Antiretrovirals

▲ Check with your physician before taking any other prescribed or over-the-counter medications or natural health medications.

▲ It is especially important to check with your physician if you are taking St. John's wort. It will decrease the effectiveness of indinavir and some other drugs and increase viral resistance. If you are currently taking St. John's wort, consult your physician about potential interactions.

▲ Avoid crowds and people with infections.

▲ Practise safer sex.

▲ Take zidovudine on an empty stomach.

▲ Zidovudine may, rarely, cause hair loss. If this occurs, you may want to consider a wig or hairpiece.

POINTS to REMEMBER

▼ Currently those viruses that are killed by antivirals include the following: CMV, HSV, HIV, influenza A, and RSV.

▼ Viruses are difficult to kill and to treat because they live inside human cells.

▼ Most antiviral drugs work by inhibiting replication of the viral cell.

▼ Antiviral drugs include synthetic purine and pyrimidine nucleoside analogues.

▼ Antiviral drugs "trick" the virus into thinking that the drugs are either a purine (a human amino acid [adenine or guanine]) or a pyrimidine (another amino acid [cytosine or thymine]). These drugs are then taken up by the virus, and the virus uses this "trick" substance to try to replicate itself. The virion ends up dying because this substance is not the "real" substance.

▼ Antivirals must be able to enter cells infected with virus, interfere with ability of virus to bind to cells, and stimulate the body's immune system.

▼ Purine analogue antivirals are synthetic analogues of purine nucleosides such as adenine and guanine. They include acyclovir, didanosine, and ganciclovir.

▼ Pyrimidine analogues are synthetic analogues of pyrimidine nucleoside such as cytosine and thymine. They include zalcitabine and zidovudine.

▼ An important nursing consideration is that these drugs should be administered only after reading and understanding all physician orders and after a thorough nursing assessment, including the client's nutritional status and baseline vital signs.

▼ Contraindications to the use of antiviral agents include herpes zoster in immunosuppressed clients.

▼ Antivirals are *not* recommended for clients with renal, hepatic, or seizure disorders; pregnant or lactating women; and clients who are dehydrated or in electrolyte imbalance.

▼ Many drugs interact with the antiviral agents; therefore the nurse should always check to make sure the client is taking none of these agents before administering the antiviral agent.

EXAMINATION REVIEW QUESTIONS

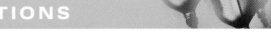

1 Which if the following may result from treatment with zidovudine?
   a. Erythematous scrotal areas
   b. Bleeding hematoma in lungs
   c. Livedo reticularis
   d. Bone marrow suppression

2 Recommendations for occupational HIV exposure may include the use of which of the following?
   a. zidovudine, methotrexate, and amines
   b. lamivudine and thiamine

   c. zidovudine, lamivudine, and indinavir
   d. lamivudine, tyramine, and acyclovir

3 Which of the following is a caution for antiviral use?
   a. Use of normal dosages of acetaminophen
   b. Use of fat- or water-soluble vitamins
   c. HIV infection
   d. Seizure disorders

4 Which of the following would be reported to the physician?
a. Mild vomiting for eight hours
b. Bone marrow suppression
c. One to two nights of insomnia
d. Hematocrit of 0.40 and hemoglobin of 160 g/L

5 Which of the following is a contraindication to the use of amantadine?
a. Polycythemia
b. Heart failure
c. Polyuria
d. Photophobia

For answers see http://evolve.elsevier.com/Lilley/pharmacology/.

CRITICAL THINKING ACTIVITIES

1 A 19-year-old male university student from Hong Kong was diagnosed with HIV approximately seven months ago. He has been going through several treatment regimens but the infectious disease physician is going to change his medication. He has been on several anti-HIV agents and is now being treated with didanosine. He has experienced some bone marrow depression off and on during the last few months. Which condition(s) and/or health concern(s) would most likely lead to a change to didanosine? Discuss your answer. Also, what side effects may compound the problem of altered RBCs and even platelets with this drug?

2 A young adult female client underwent a bone marrow transplant and, less than a year afterward, contracted CMV. Would antiviral agents be problematic if this client were pregnant? Tell why or why not and explain your answer.

3 Discuss the drugs that are being used to treat opportunistic infections prophylactically. What information should you include in your health teaching?

For answers see http://evolve.elsevier.com/Lilley/pharmacology/.

BIBLIOGRAPHY

Albanese, J., & Nutz, P. (2005). *Mosby's 2005 nursing drug cards.* St Louis, MO: Mosby.

Canadian Blood Services. (2003). Canadian Blood Services launches early test for West Nile Virus. Retrieved August 27 from http://www.bloodservices.ca/

Canadian Pharmacists Association. (2003). *Therapeutic choices* (4th ed.). Ottawa, ON: Author.

Canadian Pharmacists Association. (2004). *Guide to drugs in Canada.* Toronto, ON: Dorling Kindersley.

Canadian Pharmacists Association. (2005). *Compendium of pharmaceuticals and specialties. The Canadian drug reference for health professionals.* Ottawa, ON: Author. [The subscription-based e-CPS is available at http://www.pharmacists.ca.]

Cheng, A., Williams, B.A., & Sivarajan, B.V. (Eds.). (2003). *The HSC handbook of pediatrics* (10th ed.). Toronto, ON: Elsevier.

Facts and Comparisons. (2004). *Drug facts and comparisons pocket version* (9th ed.). St Louis, MO: Wolters Kluwer Health.

Genome Canada. (2003). Lab decodes genes of virus tied to SARS. Retrieved August 28, 2005 from http://www.genome-canada.ca/GCmedia/articlesTranscriptions/indexDetails.asp?id=96&l=e

Greenwood, D., Slack, R., & Peutherer, J. (2002). *Medical microbiology.* (16th ed.). Edinburgh, GB: Elsevier Science.

Gutfreund, K.S., & Bain, V.G. (2000). Chronic viral hepatitis C: Management update. *Canadian Medical Association Journal, 162*(6), 827–833.

Hardman, J.G., & Limbird, L.E. (2002). *Goodman and Gilman's the pharmacological basis of therapeutics* (10th ed.). New York: McGraw-Hill.

Health Canada. (2000). Potentially harmful drug interaction between St. John's wort and prescription drugs. Retrieved November 25, 2005, from http://www.hc-sc.gc.ca/ahc-asc/media/advisories-avis/2000/2000_36_e.html.

Health Canada. (2004). Approval of Viread with conditions. Retrieved August 27, 2005, from http://www.hc-sc.gc.ca/dhp-mps/medeff/advisories-avis/prof/2004/viread_dhcpl_e.html

Health Canada. (2005). Drug product database (DPD). Retrieved August 28, 2005, from http://www.hc-sc.gc.ca/hpb/drugs-dpd/

Health Canada. (2005). West Nile virus. Retrieved August 27, 2005, from http://www.hc-sc.gc.ca/dc-ma/wnv-vno/index_e.html

Kasper, D.L., Braunwald, D., Faci, A., Hauser, S., Longo, D., & Jameson, J.L. (2005). *Harrison's principles of internal medicine* (16th ed.). New York: McGraw-Hill.

Katzung, B.G. (2004). *Basic and clinical pharmacology* (9th ed.). New York: McGraw-Hill.

Lacy, C.F., Armstrong, L.L., Goldman, M.P., & Lance, L.L. (2003). *Drug information handbook* (11th ed.). Hudson, OH: Lexi-Comp.

Lehne, R.A. (2004). *Pharmacology for nursing care* (5th ed.). St Louis, MO: Saunders.

Lewis, S.M., Heitkemper, M.M., & Dirksen, S.R. (Eds.). (2004). *Medical-surgical nursing. Assessment and management of clinical problems* (6th ed.). St Louis, MO: Mosby.

Mandell, G.L., Bennett, J.E., & Dolin, R. (2005). *Principles and practice of infectious diseases* (6th ed.). Philadelphia: Elsevier Churchill Livingstone.

Mosby. (2005). *Mosby's drug consult 2005: The comprehensive reference for generic and brand name drugs* (15th ed.). St Louis, MO: Mosby.

Murray, P.R., Greenwood, D., Slack, R., & Peutherer, J. (2002). *Medical microbiology.,* St Louis, MO: Mosby.

Public Health Agency of Canada. (2004). HIV/AIDS Epi Update. Retrieved August 27, 2005, from http://www.hc-sc.gc.ca/dc-ma/aids-sida/index_e.html

Public Health Agency of Canada. (2004). Learning from SARS—Renewal of Public Health in Canada—executive summary. Retrieved August 27, 2005, from http://www.phac-aspc.gc.ca/publicat/sars-sras/naylor/exec_e.html

Public Health Agency of Canada. (2004). SARS: Severe acute respiratory distress syndrome. Retrieved August 28, 2005, from http://www.phac-aspc.gc.ca/sars-sras/

Public Health Agency of Canada. (2005). Avian influenza. Retrieved November 25, 2005 from http://www.phac-aspc.gc.ca/influenza/avian_e.html

RocheCanada. (2005). Information for the patient. "Fuzeon" Enfuvirtide for injection. Retrieved August 28, 2005, from http://www.rochecanada.com/pdf/fuzeonpiE.pdf

Skidmore-Roth, L. (2006). *Mosby's 2006 nursing drug reference* (19th ed.). St Louis, MO: Mosby.

Weir, E., & Shapiro, H. (2004). West Nile virus: Round five. *Canadian Medical Association Journal, 170*(11), 1669–70.

CHAPTER
39 Antituberculous Agents

OBJECTIVES

After reading this chapter, the successful student will be able to do the following:

1 Identify the various first-line and second-line agents used for the treatment of tuberculosis.

2 Discuss the mechanisms of action, dosages, side effects, indications for treatment, cautions, contraindications, and drug interactions associated with the various antituberculous agents.

3 Develop a nursing care plan that includes all phases of the nursing process for clients receiving antituberculous drugs.

4 Develop a teaching guide for clients receiving an antituberculous agent.

e-LEARNING ACTIVITIES

Student CD-ROM
- Review Questions: see questions 307–311
- Animations
- Medication Administration Checklists
- IV Therapy Checklists

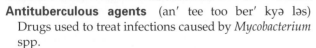 **Web site** (http://evolve.elsevier.com/Lilley/pharmacology/)
- Online Chapter Worksheet • Frequently Asked Questions
- Learning Tips and Content Updates • WebLinks • Online Appendices and Supplements • Mosby/Saunders ePharmacology Update • Access to *Mosby's Drug Consult*

DRUG PROFILES

ethambutol, p. 683
▶▶isoniazid, p. 683
pyrazinamide, p. 684
rifabutin, p. 684

rifampin, p. 684
rifapentine, p. 684
streptomycin, p. 684

▶▶ Key drug.

GLOSSARY

Antituberculous agents (an′ tee too ber′ kyə ləs) Drugs used to treat infections caused by *Mycobacterium* spp.

Bacillus (bə sil′ əs) Rod-shaped bacteria.

Multi-drug-resistant tuberculosis (MDR-TB) Tuberculosis (TB) that demonstrates resistance to two or more drugs.

Primary (first-line) agents First-choice drugs.

Primary TB infection A client's first TB infection.

Rapid acetylator An individual heterozygous or homozygous for the *fast* allelic variant of the acetylation enzyme, causing isoniazid to be metabolized rapidly in the liver.

Reinfection The most chronic form of TB.

Secondary (second-line) agents Second-choice drugs.

Slow acetylator An individual homozygous for the *slow* allelic variant of the acetylation enzyme, causing isoniazid to be metabolized slowly in the liver.

Tubercle bacilli (too′ ber kəl) Rod-shaped TB bacteria.

TUBERCULOSIS

Mycobacterium tuberculosis is the bacterium that causes tuberculosis (TB). It is an **aerobic bacillus,** which means that it is a rod-shaped micro-organism (bacillus) that requires a large supply of oxygen for it to grow and flourish (aerobic). This bacterium's need for a highly oxygenated body site explains why *Mycobacterium* infections most commonly affect the lungs, the growing ends of bones, and the brain (cerebral cortex), with the kidney, liver, and genitourinary tract all being less common sites of infection.

These **tubercle** (tuberculous) **bacilli** are transmitted from one of three sources: humans, cows (bovine), or birds (avian), although bovine and avian transmissions are much less common than human transmission. Tubercle bacilli are conveyed in droplets expelled by infected people or animals during coughing or sneezing and then inhaled by the new host. After these infectious droplets are inhaled, the infection spreads to the susceptible organ sites by means of the blood and lymphatic system. However, TB does not develop in all people who inhale these infectious droplets. Instead, the bacteria become dormant and walled off by calcified or fibrous tissues. This makes TB difficult to treat, as does its slow growth rate. Most bactericidal (bacteria-killing) drugs work by disrupting critical cellular metabolic processes in the organism. Slow-growing micro-organisms are less metabolically active, and thus less susceptible to drugs. Many of the antibiotics used to treat TB work by inhibiting growth rather than directly killing the organism.

TB can inflict devastating and irreversible damage in persons whose host defences have been broken down as a result of immunosuppressive drug therapy, chemotherapy for cancer, or an immunosuppressive disease such as AIDS. The first infectious episode is considered the **primary TB infection; reinfection** represents the more chronic form of the disease.

Canada has one of the lowest reported incidence rates of TB in the world. After a steady decline up to 1987, due in part to improved public health education and treatment, the Canadian incidence has levelled off, with 1634 new cases reported to the Canadian Tuberculosis Reporting System (CTBRS) in 2002. TB is much more prevalent elsewhere, and the worldwide incidence continues to grow. Many millions of people worldwide have some form of tuberculous infection.

Several factors have contributed to this global health-care crisis, but one important source of the problem is the increasing number of people who are particularly susceptible to the infection—homeless and undernourished or malnourished people; people with HIV/AIDS; people taking immunosuppressant drugs; drug abusers; and people suffering from cancer. Those at high risk of contracting the disease also tend to live in crowded and poorly sanitized facilities.

In Canada, TB incidence is highest among the foreign-born population. In 2002, foreign-born citizens made up 19 percent of the Canadian population, but 67 percent of the new cases reported to the CTBRS. Of as much concern as the increasing number of TB cases is the appearance of drug-resistant TB. For instance, the CTBRS observed that from 1992 to 2002, 34 percent of Canadian clients with TB were resistant to at least one antituberculous drug. Disease resistance to two or more antituberculous drugs is called **multi-drug-resistant TB (MDR-TB)**. MDR-TB is responsible for 1.6 percent of all cases in Canada and is six times as likely to be found in recent immigrants. Primary drug resistance was found in eight percent of people infected with both HIV and TB.

ANTITUBERCULOUS AGENTS

The agents used to treat infections caused by all forms of *Mycobacterium* are called antituberculous agents, and these agents fall into two categories: **primary (first-line)** and **secondary (second-line) agents**. The antimycobacterial activity, efficacy, and potential adverse and toxic effects of the various agents determine the class to which they belong. Isoniazid (INH) is the most commonly used antituberculous agent. It can be used either as the sole agent in the prophylaxis of TB or in combination with other antituberculous agents. The various first- and second-line antibiotic agents are listed in Box 39-1.

An important consideration during drug selection is the relative likelihood of drug-resistant organisms and drug toxicity. Following are other key elements important to the planning and implementation of effective therapy:

1 Drug-susceptibility tests should be performed on the first *Mycobacterium* sp. that is isolated from a client specimen (to prevent the development of MDR-TB).
2 Before the results of the susceptibility tests are known, the client should be started on a drug regimen. Effective treatment regimens are divided into two short-course regimens. The initial short-course is the intensive or induction phase, where a combination of drugs are used to kill rapidly growing TB and to prevent the possibility of the organism becoming drug resistant. This is followed by an intermittent continuation phase, where sterilizing drugs are used to kill the intermittently growing TB organisms. For example, first-line drugs consisting of isoniazid, rifampin, pyrazinamide (PZA), and ethambutol or streptomycin, used in combination, are 95 percent effective in combatting the infection.
3 Once drug susceptibility results are available, the regimen should be adjusted accordingly.
4 Client adherence with, and the adverse effects of, the prescribed drug therapy should be monitored closely because the incidence of both client non-adherence and adverse effects is high.

BOX 39-1
First- and Second-Line Antituberculous Agents

First-Line Agents
ethambutol
isoniazid
pyrazinamide (PZA)
rifabutin
rifampin
rifapentine
streptomycin

Second-Line Agents
amikacin
cycloserine
levofloxacin
ofloxacin

Mechanism of Action and Drug Effects

The mechanisms of action of the various antituberculous drugs vary. Some inhibit protein synthesis or cell wall synthesis of *M. tuberculosis*. The **antituberculous agents** are listed in Table 39-1 by their mechanism of action.

Indications

The drug effects of the antituberculous agents are primarily limited to their ability to kill *M. tuberculosis*, but other strains of *Mycobacterium* may also be susceptible to

---

RESEARCH

Tuberculosis: What Is DOT, and How Is Tuberculosis Tracked?

TB is a disease caused by the bacterium *Mycobacterium tuberculosis*. *M. tuberculosis* can attack any part of the body, but it specifically attacks the lungs. At one time it was the leading cause of death in Canada. Antibiotic treatment for TB began to appear in the 1940s, and although there has been a steady decline in the incidence in Canada, the increase in number of multidrug resistant cases is a clear indication of the need for increased research and a need to track cases.

In Canada, the target groups for screening and management of TB are those with the highest incidence: new immigrants, those seeking refugee status, and First Nations and Inuit groups. Guidelines for the investigation and follow-up of individuals under medical surveillance for tuberculosis were prepared by the *Immigration Subcommittee of the Canadian Tuberculosis Committee* in 2003 and approved by the Canadian Tuberculosis Committee and the Canadian Thoracic Society. In addition, Health Canada's First Nations and Inuit Health Branch (FNIHB) has developed a TB elimination strategy intended to reduce the incidence of TB in those groups to less than 1 per 100 000. The Canadian Tuberculosis Standards provide the national guidelines for the treatment of TB with an interim elimination goal of a five percent reduction in the number of TB cases. Within the new guidelines, published in 2002, are specific criteria for the diagnosis and management of TB in children.

Health Canada-approved drugs for treating TB include isoniazid, rifampin, ethambutol, and pyrazinamide (PZA). These are considered first-line drugs and the core of initial treatment regimens. Streptomycin is a first-line drug and is still used as initial treatment, but resistance to it continues to form.

Direct Observation of Therapy (DOT)

DOT involves providing antituberculous drugs directly to the client and watching as the client takes the medication. It is the recommended and preferred strategy for managing the treatment regimen for all clients with TB.

Data from Long, R. (Ed.). (2000). *Canadian tuberculosis standards* (5th ed.). Canadian Lung Association, Canadian Thoracic Society, Health Canada. Retrieved August 28, 2005, from http://www.hc-sc.gc.ca/hpb/lcdc/publicat/cts-ncla00

---

the killing actions of these drugs. They are used as the initial treatment for clients with uncomplicated pulmonary TB and for most children and adults with extrapulmonary TB. Antituberculous drug effects have not been fully tested in pregnant women, but the combination of isoniazid and ethambutol has been used to treat pregnant women with clinically apparent TB without teratogenic complications.

Besides being used for the initial treatment of TB, antituberculous agents have also proved effective in the management of treatment failures and relapses. Infection with species of *Mycobacterium* other than *M. tuberculosis* (MOTT) and atypical mycobacterial infections have also been successfully treated with these agents. Non-tuberculous mycobacteria (NTM) may also be susceptible to antituberculous drugs. However, in general, antituberculous agents are not as effective against other species of *Mycobacterium* as they are against *M. tuberculosis*. Some of these other species that may be of particular concern in immunocompromised clients such as AIDS clients are *Mycobacterium avium-intracellulare*, *Mycobacterium flavescens*, *Mycobacterium marinum*, and *Mycobacterium kansasii*. Additional *Mycobacterium* infections that may respond to antituberculous agents are those caused by *Mycobacterium fortuitum*, *Mycobacterium chelonae*, *Mycobacterium smegmatis*, *Mycobacterium xenopi*, and *Mycobacterium scrofulaceum*. Treatment regimens for these non-TB mycobacterial infections often include the macrolide antibiotics clarithromycin or azithromycin (Chapter 37), either alone or in combination with one or more antituberculous agents.

In summary, antituberculous drugs are primarily used for the prophylaxis or treatment of TB. The effectiveness of these agents depends on the type of infection, adequate dosing, sufficient duration of treatment, drug adherence, and the selection of an effective drug combination. The indications of the different antituberculous drugs are listed in Table 39-2.

Contraindications

Contraindications to the use of various antituberculous agents include severe drug allergy and major renal or liver dysfunction. However, contraindications must be balanced against the urgency of treating a potentially fatal infection. In extreme cases clients are sometimes given a drug to which they have some degree of allergy with supportive care to help them tolerate the medication. Examples of such supportive care might include antipyretic (e.g., acetaminophen), antihistamine (e.g., diphenhydramine), or even corticosteroid (e.g., prednisone or methylprednisolone) therapy.

Reported contraindications that are specific to cycloserine include epilepsy and significant mental illness. One relative contraindication to ethambutol is optic neuritis. Chronic alcohol use, especially when associated with major liver damage, may also be a contraindication to any antituberculous drug therapy, keeping in mind the caveats mentioned earlier.

TABLE 39-1

ANTITUBERCULOUS AGENTS: MECHANISMS OF ACTION

Drugs	Description
INHIBIT PROTEIN SYNTHESIS	
Amikacin, rifabutin, rifampin, rifapentine, streptomycin	Streptomycin works by interfering with normal protein synthesis and production of faulty proteins. Rifampin acts at a different point in the protein synthesis pathway: it inhibits RNA synthesis and may also inhibit DNA synthesis. Human cells are not as sensitive as the mycobacterial cells and are not affected by rifampin except at high drug concentrations.
INHIBIT CELL WALL SYNTHESIS	
Cycloserine, isoniazid	Cycloserine acts by inhibiting the amino acid (D Alanine) involved in the synthesis of cell walls. Isoniazid also acts at least partly to inhibit the synthesis of wall components, but the mechanisms of this agent are still not clearly understood.
OTHER MECHANISMS	
ethambutol, isoniazid, PZA	Other proposed mechanisms of action for isoniazid exist. Isoniazid is taken up by mycobacteria cells and undergoes hydrolysis to isonicotinic acid, which reacts with cofactor nicotinamide adenine dinucleotide (NAD) to form a defective NAD that is no longer active as a co-enzyme for certain life-sustaining reactions in the *Mycobacterium tuberculosis* organism. Ethambutol affects lipid synthesis, resulting in the inhibition of mycolic acid incorporation into the cell wall, thus inhibiting protein synthesis. The mechanism of action of PZA in the inhibition of TB is unknown. It can be either bacteriostatic or bactericidal, depending on the susceptibility of the particular *Mycobacterium* organism and the concentration of the drug attained at the site of infection.

TABLE 39-2

ANTITUBERCULOUS AGENTS: INDICATIONS

Drug	Indications
amikacin	Used in combination with other antituberculous agents in treatment of clinical TB. Not intended for long-term use.
cycloserine	Used with other antituberculous agents for treatment of active pulmonary and extrapulmonary TB after failure of first-line agents.
ethambutol	First-line agent for treatment of TB.
isoniazid	Used alone or in combination with other antituberculous agents in treatment and prevention of clinical TB.
PZA	Used with other antituberculous agents in treatment of clinical TB.
rifabutin	Used to prevent or delay development of *Mycobacterium avium-intracellulare* bacteremia and disseminated infections in clients with advanced HIV infection.
rifampin	Used with other antituberculous agents in treatment of clinical TB.
	Used in treatment of diseases caused by mycobacteria other than *M. tuberculosis*.
	Used for preventive therapy in clients exposed to isoniazid-resistant *M. tuberculosis*.
	Used to eliminate meningococci from the nasopharynx of asymptomatic *Neisseria meningitidis* carriers when risk of meningococcal meningitis is high.
	Used for chemoprophylaxis in contacts of clients with *Haemophilus influenzae* type B (Hib) infection.
	Used with at least one other anti-infective agent in treatment of leprosy.
	Used in treatment of endocarditis caused by methicillin-resistant staphylococci, chronic staphylococcal prostatitis, and multiple-anti-infective–resistant pneumococci.
rifapentine	Used with other antituberculous agents in treatment of clinical TB.
streptomycin	Used in combination with other antituberculous agents in treatment of clinical TB and other mycobacterial diseases.

TABLE 39-3

ANTITUBERCULOUS AGENTS: COMMON ADVERSE EFFECTS

Drug	Side/Adverse Effects
amikacin	Ototoxicity, nephrotoxicity
cycloserine	Psychotic behaviour, seizures
ethambutol	Retrobulbar neuritis (inflammation of the optic nerve, impairing vision), blindness
isoniazid	Peripheral neuritis, hepatotoxicity
levofloxacin, ofloxacin	Dizziness, headache, GI disturbances, visual disturbances, insomnia
PZA	Hepatotoxicity, hyperuricemia
rifabutin	GI tract disturbances, rash, neutropenia, brown-orange discoloration of urine, feces, saliva, sputum, sweat, tears, skin
rifampin	Hepatitis; hematological disorders; reddish discoloration of urine, tears, sweat, sputum
rifapentine	GI upset, red-orange discoloration of tears, sweat, skin, teeth, tongue, sputum, saliva, urine, feces, cerebrospinal fluid
streptomycin	Ototoxicity, nephrotoxicity, blood dyscrasias

Side Effects and Adverse Effects

Antituberculous agents are fairly well tolerated. Isoniazid, one of the mainstays of treatment, is noted for causing pyridoxine deficiency and liver toxicity. For this reason supplements of pyridoxine (vitamin B_6; see Chapter 52) are often given concurrently with isoniazid, with a common oral dose of 50 mg daily. The most problematic drugs and their associated adverse effects are listed in Table 39-3.

Interactions

Drugs that interact with antituberculous agents can cause significant effects. See Table 39-4 for a summary of these interactions. Besides these drug interactions, isoniazid can cause false-positive urine glucose test (e.g., Clinitest) readings and an increase in the serum levels of the liver function enzymes alanine aminotransferase (ALT) and aspartate aminotransferase (AST).

Dosages

For the recommended dosages of selected antituberculous agents, see the dosages table on p. 683. See Appendix B for some of the common brands available in Canada.

TABLE 39-4

ANTITUBERCULOUS AGENTS: DRUG INTERACTIONS

Drug	Mechanism	Results
AMINOSALICYLATE		
probenecid	Reduce excretion	Increased aminosalicylate levels
salicylates	Additive effects	Aminosalicylate toxicity
ISONIAZID		
antacids	Reduce absorption	Decreased isoniazid levels
cycloserine, rifampin	Additive effects	Increased CNS and hepatic toxicity
disulfiram	Additive effects	Coordination difficulties and psychotic episodes
phenytoin, carbamazepine, valproic acid	Decrease metabolism	Increased phenytoin, carbamazepine, and valproic acid effects
Warfarin	Inhibits metabolic metabolism	Increases in international normalized ratio
STREPTOMYCIN		
Nephrotoxic and neurotoxic drugs	Additive	Increased toxicity
Oral anticoagulants	Alter intestinal flora	Increased bleeding tendencies
RIFAMPIN		
Beta-blockers Benzodiazepines Calcium channel blockers amiodarone, buspirone, chloramphenicol, clarithromycin, oral anticoagulants, oral antidiabetics, oral contraceptives, clofibrate	Increase metabolism	Decreased therapeutic effects of these drugs
clarithromycin, delavirdine	Decrease metabolism	Increased plasma levels of rifampin
aminosalicylic acid, antacids, ketoconazole	Decrease metabolism	Decreased serum levels of rifampin

DRUG PROFILES

Antituberculous drugs can only be obtained by prescription and are indicated for the treatment of many different *Mycobacterium* infections, including *M. tuberculosis,* the organism that causes TB. They are available in many different dosage forms, including orally (PO), intravenously (IV), and intramuscularly (IM) administered agents.

ethambutol

Ethambutol is a first-line bacteriostatic agent used in the treatment of TB that is believed to work by diffusing into the mycobacteria and suppressing ribonucleic acid (RNA) synthesis, thereby inhibiting protein synthesis. Ethambutol is included with isoniazid, streptomycin, and rifampin in many TB combination-drug therapies because resistance develops quickly if used as a single agent. It may also be used to treat other mycobacterial

diseases. It is contraindicated in clients with a hypersensitivity to it and those with optic neuritis. It is available only in oral form as 100-mg and 400-mg tablets. Pregnancy category B. The usual recommended dosages are given in the dosages table below.

PHARMACOKINETICS

Half-Life	Onset	Peak	Duration
3–4 hr	Variable	2–4 hr	Up to 24 hr

▸▸ isoniazid

Isoniazid is the most widely used antituberculous agent and the mainstay of TB treatment. It may be given either as a single agent for prophylaxis or in combination with other antituberculous drugs for the treatment of active TB. It is a bactericidal agent that kills the mycobacteria by disrupting cell wall synthesis and essential

DOSAGES   Selected Antituberculous Agents

Agent	Pharmacological Class	Usual Dosage Range	Indications
ethambutol	Synthetic first-line antimycobacterial	**Adult and pediatric** PO: 15–25 mg/kg/day; may also be divided in 2×/wk and 3×/wk dosage regimens with higher doses; pediatric max 1 g/day or 2.5 g twice weekly	
▸▸ isoniazid	Synthetic first-line antimycobacterial	**Adult** PO: 5–10 mg/kg daily (max 300 mg) or 15 mg/kg 1–3×/wk (max 900 mg/dose) **Pediatric** PO: 10–20 mg/kg/day (max 300 mg) or 20–40 mg/kg 2–3×/wk (max 900 mg/dose)	Active TB
pyrazinamide (PZA)	Synthetic first-line antimycobacterial	**Adult and adolescent** PO: 15–30 mg/kg/day (max 2 g) or 50–70 mg/kg 2–3×/wk (max 3–4 g/dose) **Pediatric** PO: 30 mg/kg/day (max 2 g) or 2–3×/wk (max 3–4 g/dose)	
rifabutin	Semi-synthetic first-line antimycobacterial antibiotic	**Adult only** PO: 300 mg once to twice daily	
rifampin	Semi-synthetic first-line antimycobacterial antibiotic	**Adult** PO: 600 mg q24h × 2 days **Pediatric >1 mo** PO: 10 mg/kg q12h × 2 days (max 600 g) **Neonates <1 mo** PO: 5 mg/kg q12h × 2 days **Adult** PO: 600 mg qd × 4 days **Pediatric >1 mo** PO: 20 mg/kg qd × 4 days (max 600 g) **Neonates <1 mo** PO: 5 mg/kg/day × 4 days	*N. meningitis* prophylaxis *H. influenza* type b
streptomycin	Antimycobacterial aminoglycoside antibiotic	**Adult** IM: 15–25 mg/kg 2–3×/wk (max 1 g/dose) **Pediatric** IV: 20–40 mg 1–2×/wk (max 1 g)	Active TB

cellular functions. Isoniazid is metabolized in the liver through a process called *acetylation,* which requires a certain enzymatic pathway to break down the drug. Most individuals are either intermediate or **rapid acetylators**, meaning their liver enzymes can metabolize the isoniazid fairly quickly in the liver. However, some people are homozygous for the *slow* allelic variant of the liver enzyme. Such individuals are called **slow acetylators** and their enzyme variant metabolizes isoniazid much more slowly than the intermediate or rapid acetylators, resulting in accumulation and longer half-life of the drug in the body. Slow acetylators may therefore have more adverse events brought on by drug accumulation. The dosages of isoniazid may need to be adjusted upward or downward respectively in rapid and slow acetylator clients depending on the specific severity of their enzyme metabolic rate. Approximately 50 to 60 percent of Blacks and those of European and South Indian descent are slow acetylators; 90 percent of people of Inuit, Japanese, and Chinese descent are rapid acetylators.

Isoniazid is currently available only in oral formulations as a 50-mg/5-mL solution and as 50-, 100-, and 300-mg tablets. A combination product contains 120 mg of rifampin, 50 mg isoniazid, and 300 mg of PZA in tablet form. Isoniazid is contraindicated in clients with a hypersensitivity to it and in those with previous isoniazid-associated hepatic injury or acute liver disease. Pregnancy category C. The usual recommended dosages of isoniazid are given in the table on p. 683.

PHARMACOKINETICS

Half-Life	Onset	Peak	Duration
1–4 hr	Variable	1–2 hr	Up to 24 hr

pyrazinamide

Pyrazinamide (PZA) is an antituberculous drug that can be either bacteriostatic or bactericidal, depending on its concentration at the site of infection and the particular susceptibility of the mycobacteria. It is commonly used in combination with other antituberculous drugs for the treatment of TB. Its mechanism of action is unknown, but it is believed to work by inhibiting lipid and nucleic acid synthesis in the mycobacteria. PZA is available in oral form in a 500-mg tablet. It is contraindicated in clients who have had a hypersensitivity reaction to it. Pregnancy category C. The usually recommended dosages are given in the table on p. 683.

PHARMACOKINETICS

Half-Life	Onset	Peak	Duration
9–10 hr	Variable	2 hr	Up to 24 hr

rifabutin

Rifabutin is the second of two currently available rifamycin antibiotics, following rifampin. It is commonly used to prevent infections caused by *Mycobacterium avium* complex (MAC) in clients with advanced HIV. It is not administered to clients with active TB as a single agent as it can lead to the development of TB resistant to rifabutin and rifampin. A notable side effect of

rifabutin is that it can turn urine, feces, saliva, skin, sputum, sweat, and tears a red-orange to red-brown color. It is also associated with neutropenia and occasionally thrombocytopenia. Rifabutin is currently available only as a 150-mg capsule and is contraindicated in cases of known drug allergy. Pregnancy category B. Dosage information appears in the table on p. 683.

rifampin

Rifampin is the first of the rifamycin class of synthetic macrocyclic antibiotics, which also includes rifabutin and rifapentine. The term *macrocyclic* connotes the large and complex hydrocarbon ring structure included in all the rifamycin compounds. Rifampin has activity against many *Mycobacterium* spp., as well as against meningococcus, *Haemophilus influenzae* type B, and leprosy. It is a broad-spectrum bactericidal agent that kills the offending organism by inhibiting protein synthesis. Rifampin is used in combination with other antituberculous agents in its treatment of TB. Rifampin is available in both oral and parenteral formulations and, as previously mentioned, in combination with isoniazid. As an oral agent it is available as 150- and 300-mg capsules.

Rifampin is contraindicated in clients with a known hypersensitivity to it. Pregnancy category C. The usual recommended dosages are given in the dosages table on p. 683.

PHARMACOKINETICS

Half-Life	Onset	Peak	Duration
3 hr	Variable	2–4 hr	Up to 24 hr

rifapentine

Rifapentine is a derivative of rifampin. It is currently being used only in clinical trials in Canada. Rifapentine has a much longer duration of action than rifampin and possibly better efficacy. It has been shown to have greater antimycobacterial efficacy and macrophage penetration. Its accumulation in tissue macrophages allows it to work synergistically against bacterial cells that are ingested by the macrophage during phagocytosis ("cell eating"). Rifapentine is indicated for pulmonary TB and comes as a 150-mg tablet. It is contraindicated in patients with a hypersensitivity to it. Pregnancy category C.

streptomycin

Streptomycin is an aminoglycoside antibiotic currently available only in generic form. Introduced in 1944, it was the first drug that could effectively treat TB. Because of its toxicities it is used most commonly today in combination-drug regimens for the treatment of MDR-TB infections. Streptomycin is currently available only in a 1-g parenteral formulation. It is contraindicated in clients hypersensitive to it. Pregnancy category D. The usual recommended dosages are given in the table on p. 683.

PHARMACOKINETICS

Half-Life	Onset	Peak	Duration
2–3 hr	Variable	1–2 hr	Up to 24 hr

NURSING PROCESS

Assessment

Before administering any of the first-line and second-line antituberculous agents, the nurse should obtain a thorough medical history on the client and perform a complete assessment. Liver function studies should be performed in clients who used to receive isoniazid or rifampin because of the hepatic impairment these agents can cause. This is especially important in geriatric clients and in clients who consume alcohol daily because of the greater likelihood of liver disorders in such clients. A thorough neurological assessment is also called for because of the increased incidence of peripheral neuropathies of the feet and hands in clients taking isoniazid. It is also important for the nurse to check the client's complete blood count (CBC), hemoglobin (Hgb) level, and hematocrit (Hct) value before administering isoniazid because of the hematological disorders that this drug may precipitate. Renal studies, such as the creatinine and blood urea nitrogen (BUN) levels, and urinalysis should also be performed both at the start of isoniazid or rifampin therapy and during therapy. Assess colour of skin and any excrement for a baseline characteristic colour. Contraindications to the use of rifampin, rifabutin, and rifapentine include hypersensitivity. Contraindications to the use of isoniazid include allergy to the drug, liver or renal disease, pregnancy, and lactation. The drugs that interact with these agents are listed in Table 39-4. Sputum cultures are routinely done as part of the workup in clients; therefore the nurse should always check these results before administering the specific antituberculous drugs to confirm that the appropriate agent is being given.

PZA, ethambutol, and streptomycin are the other first-line agents used in the treatment of TB. Baseline liver function tests should be performed in clients who are to be given PZA because of the hepatotoxicity it can cause. It can also cause hyperuricemia; therefore gout or flare-ups of gout may occur in susceptible clients. The Hgb levels and Hct values should also be checked. Contraindications to the use of any of these three agents include hypersensitivity.

Ethambutol may cause a decrease in visual acuity resulting from optic neuritis; therefore a thorough eye examination with each eye tested separately may be called for before starting therapy. In addition, the client's baseline liver function status, Hgb levels, and Hct values should be determined. Contraindications include hypersensitivity and optic neuritis. Cautious use is called for in clients with liver or renal disease, hematological disorders, or diabetes.

Streptomycin is contraindicated in clients with renal disease and in those with a hypersensitivity to the agent. The client's BUN and creatinine levels should be measured and urinalysis performed before the start of therapy. It should be used carefully in geriatric clients and in clients with hearing disorders because of the ototoxicity it can cause.

The assessment aspect of the nursing care in clients being given any of the other second-line agents (see Table 39-2) is similar.

Nursing Diagnoses

Nursing diagnoses for clients receiving antituberculous agents include the following:
- Risk for injury related to non-adherence to drug therapy and to an overall status of poor health.
- Ineffective therapeutic regimen management of TB related to poor adherence to therapy.
- Ineffective family therapeutic regimen management related to poor adherence and poor housing and living conditions.
- Deficient knowledge related to the disease process and treatment protocol.

Planning

Goals for clients receiving antituberculous agents are focused on client safety and adherence with therapy:
- Client experiences minimal side effects of the treatment for TB.
- Client takes medication regularly and for the length of time prescribed.
- Client remains free of injury related to drug interactions.
- Client remains free of toxic effects or reports them to the physician immediately.

Outcome Criteria

The outcome criteria for clients receiving antituberculous agents are also focused on client safety and adherence.
- Client states the therapeutic effects of the treatment (improved signs and symptoms and killing of mycobacterium) and possible side effects (neuropathies, GI upset).
- Client states the importance of taking the medication regularly and for the length of time prescribed to prevent complications, relapses, or recurrences.
- Client states the drugs that interact with antituberculous agent such as salicylates, antacids, and anticoagulants.
- Client reports toxic effects, such as renal or liver dysfunction, hearing loss, and blindness, to the physician should they occur.
- Client shows improvement of disease state with a decreased cough and fever and normal laboratory values.

Implementation

Because drug therapy is the mainstay of the treatment for TB and often lasts for up to 24 months, client education is critical, with a special emphasis on adherence. Simple, clear, and concise instructions should be given to the client. This should include the fact that multiple drugs are generally used and that 90 percent cure rates can be achieved with combination therapy consisting of isoniazid and rifampin (if the client is strictly adherent with therapy). All antituberculous agents should be given exactly as ordered and at the same time every day. Consistent use and dosing are critical to maintaining steady blood levels and minimizing the chances of resistance to the drug therapy.

Generally speaking, oral preparations should be given with meals to diminish GI tract upset, even though it is often recommended that they be given either one hour before or two hours after meals. An anti-emetic may be necessary in some clients. Intramuscularly administered agents such as streptomycin should be given deep in a large muscle mass and the sites rotated. Pyridoxine in doses of 200 to 300 mg/day may be ordered in clients taking cycloserine or isoniazid to prevent the associated neurotoxicity.

Client teaching tips are presented in the box below.

■ Evaluation

The nurse should always document clients' response, or lack of response, to therapy. The therapeutic response to antituberculous therapy is reflected by a decrease in the symptoms of TB, such as cough and fever, and by weight gain. The results of laboratory studies (culture and sensitivity tests) and the chest X-ray findings should confirm the clinical findings. Clients with drug-resistant disease do not show a clinical response to the therapy, and laboratory findings confirm this.

Clients also need to be monitored for adverse reactions, including fatigue, nausea, vomiting, numbness and tingling of the extremities, fever, loss of appetite, depression, and jaundice. For other adverse effects of rifampin, rifabutin, and rifapentine, see the client teaching tips below. The physician should be notified if any of these occur, and the incident should be documented accordingly.

CASE STUDY

Tuberculosis

For a project that received new funding, you and five of your community health nursing peers have been asked to give some mini-presentations to various large work settings in the community. One place is in your health department with the nurses who work in the adult clinic.
- What are some key Internet resources you can share with staff regarding TB infections, control guidelines, and Canadian recommendations?
- What information could then be used or shared with clients in the adult clinic?
- What conditions in the community are considered high-risk for transmission of diseases such as TB?

For answers see http://evolve.elsevier.com/Lilley/pharmacology/.

CLIENT TEACHING TIPS

The nurse should instruct the client as follows:
▲ Take all medications exactly as ordered by the physician.
▲ To achieve a cure, you must keep taking the medication as ordered and for the ordered length of time, and keep follow-up appointments with your physician.
▲ Do not consume alcohol while you are receiving this medication.
▲ Always check with your physician before taking any other type of medication, whether prescribed by another doctor or over-the-counter.
▲ See your healthcare provider at least monthly during treatment.
▲ Your disease is contagious, and will be for a while. Take some precautions to make sure you don't infect your family or others. Make sure to wash your hands and cover your mouth when you cough or sneeze. Don't leave tissues you have coughed or spat into lying around. It's best to flush them down the toilet.
▲ Take good care of yourself. Eat a balanced diet, and get enough rest and relaxation.
▲ Keep all medications away from children.
▲ Always wear a medical alert tag or bracelet naming the medications you are taking.

Isoniazid

▲ (For diabetic clients) Monitor your blood glucose levels using a glucometer because this medication can affect blood sugar.
▲ If you are prescribed pyridoxine by your physician, take it regularly; it can prevent some of the side ef-

fects of this medication, such as numbness and tingling.

Isoniazid or Rifampin

▲ Report any of the following side effects to the physician immediately: fever, nausea, vomiting, loss of appetite, unusual bleeding, numbness and tingling in your hands and feet, and reddish discoloration to urine, sweat, tears, and mucus in your mouth. The discoloration will go away when you stop taking the drug; however, contact lenses may be permanently stained. (Contact lens discoloration may also occur with rifabutin and rifapentine.)

Rifampin

▲ (For women taking oral contraceptives) You will need to switch to another form of birth control, because oral contraceptives become ineffective when given with this medication.

Rifabutin

▲ You may notice a brown-orange discoloration of your skin, sweat, tears, urine, feces, mucus in your mouth, and saliva.

Rifapentine

▲ This drug may result in a red-orange discoloration of the skin, teeth, tears, saliva, mucus in your mouth, urine, feces, and tongue.

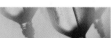

POINTS to REMEMBER

▼ Primary (first-line) antituberculous agents include ethambutol, isoniazid, PZA, rifampin, and streptomycin.

▼ These drugs are used to treat pulmonary and extrapulmonary *M. tuberculosis* infections. Depending on the agent used, these may also be used for disseminated infections in clients with advanced HIV infections and endocarditis.

▼ Side effects of the PAS regimen include GI tract disturbances and hepatotoxicity. Side effects of other agents include the following:
  • ethambutol: retrobulbar neuritis and blindness
  • isoniazid: peripheral neuritis and hepatotoxicity
  • rifabutin: GI tract disturbances, rash, and neutropenia

• rifampin: hepatitis
• streptomycin: hepatotoxicity, ototoxicity, nephrotoxicity, and blood dyscrasias

▼ Nursing considerations include the following:
  • Client education should include the importance of strict adherence to the treatment regimen for improvement of condition or cure.
  • Education that clients should not consume alcohol while taking any of these medications.

▼ Vitamin B₆ is needed to combat peripheral neuritis associated with isoniazid.

▼ Women taking oral contraceptive therapy who are prescribed rifampin should be counselled on other forms of birth control because of the ineffectiveness of oral contraception while on rifampin.

EXAMINATION REVIEW QUESTIONS

1 Which of the following side effects are expected with the use of either isoniazid or rifampin?
   a. Headache and neck pain
   b. Glaucoma and gynecomastia
   c. Reddish-brown urine and emesis
   d. Numbness or tingling of extremities

2 Why would a client need pyridoxine when taking isoniazid?
   a. To improve energy
   b. To reduce GI side effects
   c. To combat cardiac abnormalities
   d. To prevent neurological side effects

3 Which of the following should women taking oral contraceptives with rifampin expect?
   a. Have an annual Pap smear
   b. Have reddish-brown vaginal discharge
   c. Switch to an alternate form of birth control
   d. Experience increased energy level and breast discharge

4 When are TB clients considered contagious?
   a. During any phase of the illness
   b. Any time up to 18 months after therapy
   c. During the post-ictal phase of TB
   d. During the initial period of the illness and its diagnosis

5 Which of the following would be a therapeutic response to antituberculous drugs?
   a. The client states that he or she is feeling much better.
   b. There is no fever, white blood cell (WBC) count is 21 × 10⁹/L, and cough has subsided.
   c. The client reports a decrease in cough and night sweats and few side effects.
   d. There is a decrease in symptoms supported by improved chest X-ray results, sputum culture, and sensitivity tests.

For answers see http://evolve.elsevier.com/Lilley/pharmacology/.

CRITICAL THINKING ACTIVITIES

1 What is considered a therapeutic response to antituberculous drugs?

2 Is there any concern for the female taking oral contraceptives while taking rifampin? Explain your answer.

3 What parameters should be assessed while a client is taking antituberculous drugs and why?

For answers see http://evolve.elsevier.com/Lilley/pharmacology/.

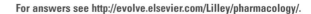

BIBLIOGRAPHY

Albanese, J., & Nutz, P. (2005). *Mosby's 2005 nursing drug cards.* St Louis, MO: Mosby.

Anderson, P.O., Knoben, J.E., & Troutman, W.G. (2002). *Handbook of clinical drug data* (10th ed.). New York: McGraw-Hill/Appleton & Lange.

Canadian Pharmacists Association. (2003). *Therapeutic choices* (4th ed.). Ottawa, ON: Author.

Canadian Pharmacists Association. (2004). *Guide to drugs in Canada.* Toronto, ON: Dorling Kindersley.

Canadian Pharmacists Association. (2005). *Compendium of pharmaceuticals and specialties. The Canadian drug reference for health professionals.* Ottawa, ON: Author. [The subscription-based e-CPS is available at http://www.pharmacists.ca.]

Cheng, A., Williams, B.A., & Sivarajan, B.V. (Eds.). (2003). *The HSC handbook of pediatrics* (10th ed.). Toronto, ON: Elsevier.

Facts and Comparisons. (2004). *Drug facts and comparisons pocket version* (9th ed.). St Louis, MO: Wolters Kluwer Health.

Health Canada. (2005). Drug product database (DPD). Retrieved August 28, 2005, from http://www.hc-sc.gc.ca/hpb/drugs-dpd/

Heywood, N., Kawa, B., Long, R., Njoo, H., Panaro, L., & Wobeser, W. on behalf of the Immigration subcommittee of the Canadian Tuberculosis Committee. Guidelines for the investigation and follow-up of individuals under medical surveillance for tuberculosis after arriving in Canada: A summary. *Canadian Medical Association Journal, 168*(12), 1563–1565.

Katzung, B.G. (2004). *Basic and clinical pharmacology* (9th ed.). New York: McGraw-Hill.

Lacy, C.F., Armstrong, L.L., Goldman, M.P., & Lance, L.L. (2003). *Drug information handbook* (11th ed.). Hudson, OH: Lexi-Comp.

Lehne, R.A. (2004). *Pharmacology for nursing care* (5th ed.). St Louis, MO: Saunders.

Long, R. (Ed.). (2000). *Canadian tuberculosis standards* (5th ed.). Canadian Lung Association, Canadian Thoracic Society, Health Canada. Retrieved August 28, 2005, from www.hc-sc.gc.ca/hpb/lcdc/publicat/cts-ncla00

Mandell, G.L., Bennett, J.E., & Dolin, R. (2005). *Principles and practice of infectious diseases* (6th ed.). Philadelphia: Elsevier Churchill Livingstone.

Mosby. (2005). *Mosby's drug consult 2005: The comprehensive reference for generic and brand name drugs* (15th ed.). St Louis, MO: Mosby.

Skidmore-Roth, L. (2006). Mosby's *2006 nursing drug reference* (19th ed.). St Louis, MO: Mosby.

Antifungal Agents

OBJECTIVES

After reading this chapter, the successful student will be able to do the following:

1 Identify the various antifungal medications.

2 Describe the mechanisms of action, indications, contraindications, routes of administration, side and toxic effects, and drug interactions associated with the use of antifungal agents.

3 Develop a nursing care plan that includes all phases of the nursing process for clients receiving antifungal medications.

4 Develop teaching guidelines for clients receiving antifungal medications.

e-LEARNING ACTIVITIES

Student CD-ROM
- Review Questions: see questions 312–315
- Animations
- Medication Administration Checklists
- IV Therapy Checklists

evolve Web site (http://evolve.elsevier.com/Lilley/pharmacology/)
- Online Chapter Worksheet • Frequently Asked Questions
- Learning Tips and Content Updates • WebLinks • Online Appendices and Supplements • Mosby/Saunders ePharmacology Update • Access to *Mosby's Drug Consult*

DRUG PROFILES

▸▸**amphotericin B,** p. 692   **nystatin,** p. 694
   caspofungin, p. 694   **terbinafine HCl,** p. 694
▸▸**fluconazole,** p. 694   **voriconazole,** p. 696

▸▸ Key drug.

GLOSSARY

Allylamine antifungal   One of the newer of the five major classes of antifungal agents, currently containing a single drug, terbinafine HCl.

Azoles   One of the most common of the five major classes of antifungal agents. This class of drugs includes both the imidazoles and the triazoles.

Echinocandin   The newest of the five major classes of antifungal agents, currently containing a single drug, caspofungin.

Ergosterol   (er gos' tə rol) An unsaturated hydrocarbon of the vitamin D group isolated from yeast, mushrooms, ergot, and other fungi; the main sterol in fungal membranes.

Fungi   (fun'guy *or* fun' jy) A large, diverse group of eukaryotic, thallus-forming micro-organisms that require an external carbon source. Fungi include yeasts and moulds, as well as mushrooms.

Imidazoles   (im' id a zolz) A subclass of the azoles, which are a major class of antifungal agents. The drugs in this class are ketoconazole, miconazole, clotrimazole, econazole, and butoconazole. All work by inhibiting a needed enzyme in susceptible fungi.

Moulds   Multicellular fungi characterized by long, branching filaments called *hyphae,* which entwine to form a mycelium.

Mycosis   (my koe' sis) The general term for any fungal infection.

Oral candidiasis   (kan' də die' ə sis) Overgrowth of the yeast known as *Candida albicans* occurring in the tissues of the mouth (also called *thrush*).

Pathological fungi   Fungi that cause mycoses.

Polyenes   (pol e' enz) One of the five major classes of antifungal agents. This class includes amphotericin B and nystatin. Polyenes work by binding to sterols in fungal membranes, allowing potassium and magnesium ions to leak out of the cell and altering fungal cellular metabolism, which leads to the death of the organism.

Sterol The substance in the cell membranes of fungi to which polyenes bind.

Triazoles A subclass of the azoles, which are a major class of antifungal agents. Included in this class are butoconazole, clotrimazole, econazole, miconazole, terconazole, fluconazole, itraconazole, and voriconazole.

Yeast infection An infection caused by *Candida* (single-celled fungi) that most commonly infects the mouth (thrush), esophagus, and genitourinary tract (e.g., vaginal candidiasis).

Yeasts Single-celled fungi that reproduce by budding.

FUNGAL INFECTIONS

Fungi are a large and diverse group of micro-organisms that include all yeasts and **moulds.** Yeasts are single-celled fungi that reproduce by budding and are actually very useful organisms. They are used for baking and in alcoholic beverages. Moulds are multicellular and are characterized by long, branching filaments called *hyphae*, which entwine to form a "mat" called a *mycelium*. Some fungi are part of the normal flora of the skin, mouth, intestines, and vagina.

The infection caused by a fungus is called a **mycosis**. Fungi that can cause clinically significant infections are called **pathological fungi**, and the infections range from mild and superficial to severe and life threatening. These infections can be contracted by several different routes: they can be ingested orally; they can become implanted under the skin after injury; and, if the fungal spores are airborne, they can be inhaled. There are four general types of mycotic infections: systemic, cutaneous, subcutaneous, and superficial. Many fungal infections are superficial and the symptoms primarily annoying; others are systemic and can be life threatening. The most severe systemic fungal infections generally afflict people whose host immune defences are compromised. Commonly these are clients who have received organ transplants and are on immunosuppressive drug therapy, cancer clients immunocompromised as the result of chemotherapy, and clients with AIDS. In addition, the use of antibiotics, antineoplastics, or immunosuppressants such as corticosteroids may result in colonization of *Candida albicans*, followed by the development of a systemic infection. When this affects the mouth, it is referred to as **oral candidiasis**, or *thrush*. It is common in newborns and immunocompromised clients. Vaginal candidiasis, commonly called a **yeast infection**, often afflicts pregnant women, women with diabetes mellitus, women taking antibiotics, and women taking oral contraceptives. The characteristics of some of the systemic, cutaneous, and superficial mycotic infections are summarized in Table 40-1.

ANTIFUNGAL AGENTS

The drugs used to treat fungal infections are called antifungal agents. Systemic mycotic infections and some cutaneous or subcutaneous mycoses are treated with oral or parenteral agents, but these constitute a fairly small group of agents, only three or four of which are commonly used. There are few such agents because the fungi that cause these infections have proved to be difficult to kill, and research into new and improved agents has occurred at a slow pace, with relatively few important advances yielded so far. One difficulty is that often the chemical concentrations required for these experimental agents to be effective cannot be tolerated by human beings. Those agents that have met with success in the treatment of systemic and severe cutaneous or subcutaneous mycoses are amphotericin B, fluconazole, griseofulvin, itraconazole, ketoconazole, miconazole, nystatin, terbinafine HCl, and voriconazole.

Topical antifungal agents are by far the most commonly used drugs in this class and are most often used without prescription for the treatment of cutaneous or subcutaneous mycoses. A few are available in special formulations for use in the eye. These drugs are discussed in more detail in chapters 55 and 56.

Topical antifungals approved for clinical use are butoconazole, butenafine, ciclopirox, clioquinol, clotrimazole, econazole, ketoconazole, miconazole, nystatin, terbinafine HCl, and terconazole. Topical antifungals are most commonly used in the treatment of oral, dermatological, and vaginal candidiasis, although occasionally a systemic antifungal is used in the management of severe cases.

Antifungal agents can be broken down into five major groups based on their chemical structures, which in turn determine their mechanisms of action: griseofulvin, allylamine (terbinafine HCl), **polyenes** (amphotericin B and nystatin), **echinocandins** (anidulafungin, caspofungin, and micafungin), and the **azoles**, which include both the **imidazoles** and the **triazoles** (ketoconazole, butoconazole, miconazole, clotrimazole, econazole, terconazole, fluconazole, itraconazole, and voriconazole).

Mechanism of Action and Drug Effects

The different classes of agents have different mechanisms of action. Griseofulvin, one of the older types, works by preventing susceptible fungi from reproducing. It enters the fungal cell through an energy-dependent transport system and inhibits fungal mitosis (cell division) by binding to key structures known as *microtubules*. This in turn disrupts the mitotic spindle structure, which arrests the metaphase of cell division. It has also been proposed that griseofulvin causes the production of defective DNA, which is then unable to replicate. Although griseofulvin is still currently available on the Canadian market, its clinical use has largely been supplanted by newer antifungal drug classes.

The polyenes act by binding to **sterols** in the cell membranes of fungi, the main sterol in fungal membranes being **ergosterol**. Human cell membranes have cholesterol instead of ergosterol. Because polyene antifungals have a strong chemical affinity for ergosterol instead of cholesterol, they do not bind to human cell membranes and therefore do not kill human cells. Once the polyene drug

TABLE 40-1
MYCOTIC INFECTIONS

Mycosis	Fungus	Endemic Location	Reservoir	Transmission	Primary Tissue Affected
SYSTEMIC INFECTION					
Aspergillosis	*Aspergillus* spp.	Universal	Soil	Inhalation	Lungs
Blastomycosis	*Blastomyces dermatitidis*	North America	Soil, animal droppings	Inhalation	Lungs
Coccidioidomycosis	*Coccidioides immitis*	Southwestern United States	Soil, dust	Inhalation	Lungs
Cryptococcosis	*Cryptococcus neoformans*	Universal	Soil, pigeon droppings	Inhalation	Lungs/meninges of brain
Histoplasmosis	*Histoplasma capsulatum*	Universal	Soil, droppings of chickens and other birds	Inhalation	Lungs
CUTANEOUS INFECTION					
Candidiasis	*Candida albicans*	Universal	Humans	Direct contact, non-susceptible antibiotic overgrowth	Mucous membrane/skin disseminated (may be systemic)
Dermatophytes, tinea	*Epidermophyton* spp., *Microsporum* spp., *Trichophyton* spp.	Universal	Humans	Direct and indirect contact with infected persons	Scalp, skin
SUPERFICIAL INFECTION					
Tinea versicolor	*Malassezia furfur*	Universal	Humans	Unknown*	Skin

*Malassezia spp. are a usual part of the normal human flora and appear to cause infection only in certain individuals.

molecule binds to the ergosterol, a channel forms in the fungal cell membrane that allows potassium and magnesium ions to leak out of the cell. This loss of ions causes fungal cellular metabolism to be altered, leading to death of the cell.

The azoles act as either fungistatic or fungicidal agents, depending on their concentration in the fungus. They are most effective in combating rapidly growing fungi and work by inhibiting fungal cell cytochrome P-450 enzymes. These enzymes are needed to produce ergosterol. When the production of ergosterol is inhibited, other sterols, called *methylsterols*, are produced instead. This results in a problem similar to that caused by the polyene antifungals, namely a leaky cell membrane that allows needed electrolytes to escape. The fungal cells die because they cannot carry on cellular metabolism. Pathological fungi susceptible to these agents are listed in Box 40-1.

Indications

Indications are specific to both the antifungal agent and the type of infection being treated. The side effects of the newer antifungals are fewer and less serious than those of the older agents. However, the agent of choice for the treatment of many severe systemic fungal infections remains one of the oldest antifungals, amphotericin B, which often does have major side effects. Amphotericin B

is effective against a wide range of fungi. It is effective for treating aspergillosis, disseminated candidiasis, blastomycosis, candidiasis, coccidioidomycosis, cryptococcosis, fungal endocarditis, histoplasmosis, fungal septicemia, and many other systemic fungal infections. The activity of nystatin is similar to that of amphotericin B, but its usefulness is limited because of its toxic effects when given in the doses required to accomplish the same antifungal actions as those of amphotericin B. It is also not available in a parenteral form.

Fluconazole and itraconazole are synthetic azole antifungals, as are all of the drugs with an "-azole" suffix. Fluconazole can pass into the cerebrospinal fluid (CSF) and inhibit cryptococcal fungi. This makes it effective in the treatment of cryptococcal meningitis. Both drugs are active against oropharyngeal and esophageal *Candida* infections. Itraconazole, on the other hand, is capable of only poor CSF penetration but can be widely distributed throughout other areas of the body. It is indicated for the treatment of fungal infections in immunocompromised and non-immunocompromised clients with oral and/or esophageal candidiasis. The other systemic imidazole, ketoconazole, also has poor CNS penetration, but it inhibits many dermatophytes and fungi that cause systemic mycoses; however it is not active against *Aspergillus* organisms or phycomycetes such as *Mucor* spp. Fortunately, the newest imidazole antifungal agent, voriconazole, is particularly effective against the tenacious invasive *Aspergillus* organism.

Fluconazole is the most effective for combatting infections with *Candida* and *Cryptococcus.* Its approved use is for the more serious candidal infections of the urinary tract, peritonitis, pneumonia, cryptococcal meningitis, and oropharyngeal and esophageal candidiasis.

Griseofulvin inhibits dermatophytes of *Microsporum, Trichophyton,* and *Epidermophyton* spp. It has no effect on filamentous fungi such as *Aspergillus,* yeasts such as *Candida* spp., or dimorphic species such as *Histoplasma.*

Terbinafine HCl is a synthetic allylamine derivative used primarily to treat topical fungal infections such as tinea cruris, tinea corporis, and tinea pedis. It is also used in a systemic oral form for treatment of onychomycoses—fungally infected fingernails or toenails. The azole itraconazole is also sometimes used for this purpose.

The echinocandins, licensed in Canada in 2002, are fungicidal and less toxic to the host. They have a novel mechanism of action. These drugs target a major enzyme, glucan synthase, an integral component in the fungal cell membrane. Caspofungin, indicated for the treatment of invasive candidiasis, is the sole drug currently available in this class. Micafungin and anidulafungin are in clinical trials.

Contraindications

The most common contraindications for antifungal agents are drug allergy, liver failure, and, for griseofulvin, porphyria (a disorder involving the production of heme, which can manifest in cutaneous or CNS symptoms). Itraconazole should not be used for treating onychomycoses in clients with severe cardiac problems.

Side Effects and Adverse Effects

Drug interactions and hepatotoxicity are the primary concerns with most antifungal agents, but intravenous amphotericin B is associated with a multitude of adverse effects. The most common and problematic side effects are listed in Table 40-2.

Interactions

Many important drug interactions, some life threatening, are associated with antifungal agents. A common underlying source of the problem is that many of the antifungal drugs, as well as other agents, are metabolized by an enzyme system in the liver, called the cytochrome P-450 system, that is under heavy demand. When two agents that are both broken down by this system are given together, they compete for the limited number of enzymes, and one of the drugs ends up accumulating. Interactions are summarized in Table 40-3.

Dosages

For the recommended dosages of selected antifungal agents, see the table on p. 695. See Appendix B for some of the common brands available in Canada.

DRUG PROFILES

▸▸ *amphotericin B*

Amphotericin B remains the agent of choice for the treatment of severe systemic mycoses. Its main drawback is its many adverse effects. Almost all clients given the agent intravenously experience fever, chills, hypotension, tachycardia, malaise, muscle and joint pain, anorexia, nausea and vomiting, and headache. For this reason pre-treatment with an antipyretic (acetaminophen), antihistamines, and anti-emetics may be given to decrease the severity of this reaction.

Lipid formulations of amphotericin B have been developed in an attempt to decrease the side effects and increase efficacy. There are currently three lipid preparations of amphotericin B: amphotericin B lipid complex, amphotericin B cholesteryl complex, and liposomal amphotericin B. These forms are much more expensive than conventional amphotericin B and therefore are often used only when clients are intolerant of or refractory to non-lipid amphotericin B.

Amphotericin B is a prescription-only drug that is available in parenteral, topical, and oral dosage forms. It is contraindicated in clients who have shown hypersensitivity reactions to it and in those suffering from severe bone marrow suppression. It is available as a 50-mg vial for injection. The lipid preparations of amphotericin B are administered parenterally and are available as a 5-mg/mL single-use vial, a 100-mg/20-mL vial, and 50-mg vials of powdered drug for injection. Often a 1-mg test dose is given over 20 to 30 minutes to see if the client will tolerate the amphotericin. It has been used as a local irrigant (bladder irrigation) for the treatment of candidal cystitis and has been used intrapleurally and intraperitoneally for the treatment of fungal infections in

TABLE 40-2
ANTIFUNGALS: COMMON ADVERSE EFFECTS AND CAUTIONS

Body System	Side/Adverse Effects	Caution
AMPHOTERICIN B		Recheck dosage and type of amphotericin B being administered
Cardiovascular	Cardiac dysrhythmias, hypotension, shock	
Central nervous	Neurotoxicity; visual disturbances; convulsions; numbness, tingling, or pain in hands or feet	
Kidneys	Renal toxicity, potassium loss	
Pulmonary	Pulmonary infiltrates, other respiratory difficulties	
Other (infusion-related)	Fever, chills, headache, malaise, nausea, dyspepsia, cramping epigastric pain, occasionally hypotension, rash, hepatotoxicity	
FLUCONAZOLE		Use with caution in clients with renal or hepatic dysfunction
Gastrointestinal	Nausea, vomiting, diarrhea, stomach pain	
Other	Increased AST and ALT levels, headache, skin rash	
GRISEOFULVIN		Avoid during pregnancy
Central nervous	Headache, peripheral neuritis, paraesthesia, confusion, dizziness, fatigue, insomnia, psychosis	
Ears, eyes, nose, and throat	Blurred vision, oral candidiasis, furry tongue, transient hearing loss	
Gastrointestinal	Nausea, vomiting, anorexia, diarrhea, dyspepsia, cramps, dry mouth, flatulence, increased thirst, dysgeusia (impaired or distorted sense of taste)	
Genitourinary	Proteinuria, precipitate porphyria	
Hematological	Leukopenia, granulocytopenia, neutropenia, monocytosis	
Integumentary	Rash, urticaria, photosensitivity, angioedema, systemic lupus erythematosus	
ITRACONAZOLE		Can trigger rare episodes of serious cardiovascular adverse effects
Central nervous	Headache, dizziness, insomnia, somnolence, depression	
Gastrointestinal	Nausea, vomiting, anorexia, diarrhea, cramps, abdominal pain, flatulence, hepatotoxicity	
Genitourinary	Gynecomastia (breast development in men), erectile dysfunction, decreased libido	
Integumentary	Pruritus, fever, rash	
Other	Edema, fatigue, malaise, hypertension, hypokalemia, tinnitus, hypertriglyceridemia, adrenal insufficiency	
KETOCONAZOLE		Avoid contact with eyes
Central nervous	Headache, dizziness, somnolence	
Gastrointestinal	Nausea, vomiting, anorexia, diarrhea, abdominal pain, dyspepsia, hepatotoxicity, GI bleeding	
Genitourinary	Gynecomastia, erectile dysfunction, menstrual irregularities	
Hematological	Thrombocytopenia, eosinophilia leukopenia, hemolytic anemia	
Integumentary	Pruritus, fever, chills, photophobia, rash, dermatitis, purpura, urticaria	
Other	Hypoadrenalism, hyperuricemia, hypothyroidism	
MICONAZOLE		Local irritation may occur; avoid contact with eyes
Central nervous	Headache	
Gastrointestinal	Nausea, vomiting, anorexia, diarrhea, cramps	
Genitourinary	Vulvovaginal burning, itching, edema, pelvic cramps	
Integumentary	Pruritus, flushing, anaphylaxis, hives	
NYSTATIN		Local irritation may occur
Gastrointestinal	Nausea, vomiting, anorexia, diarrhea, cramps	
Integumentary	Rash, urticaria	
TERBINAFINE HCL		Rarely causes irritation
Central nervous	Headache, dizziness, difficulties with concentration	
Gastrointestinal	Nausea, vomiting, diarrhea, cramps, GI irritation, dyspepsia, gastritis	
Integumentary	Rash, eczema, urticaria, pruritus	
Other	Alopecia (hair loss), fatigue	

TABLE 40-3
ANTIFUNGAL DRUGS: DRUG INTERACTIONS

Drug	Possible Effects
AMPHOTERICIN B	
Digitalis glycosides	Amphotericin B–induced hypokalemia may increase the potential for digitalis toxicity
Antineoplastic agents	Additive nephrotoxicity, bronchospasm, hypotension
Thiazide diuretics	Severe hypokalemia or decreased adrenal cortex response to corticotropin
FLUCONAZOLE, ITRACONAZOLE, AND MICONAZOLE	
cyclosporine, phenytoin	Increased plasma concentrations of both agents
Oral anticoagulants	Increased effects of anticoagulants seen as increases in prothrombin time
Oral hypoglycemics	Reduced metabolism of hypoglycemic agents
GRISEOFULVIN	
Oral anticoagulants	Decreased effects of anticoagulants seen as decreases in prothrombin time
Oral contraceptives, estrogen-containing products	Decreased effectiveness of these agents
KETOCONAZOLE AND MICONAZOLE	
Alcohol and other hepatotoxic drugs	Increased risk of hepatotoxicity
Antacids, anticholinergics, H_2 blockers, omeprazole	Increased GI tract pH, which can reduce absorption of ketoconazole
cyclosporine	Increased cyclosporine levels and potential for nephrotoxicity
isoniazid, rifampin	Decreased serum levels of ketoconazole

those body cavities. Pregnancy category B. The recommended dosages are given in the table on p. 695.

PHARMACOKINETICS*

Half-Life	Onset	Peak	Duration
1–15 days	Variable	1 hr	18–24 hr

*For conventional (non-lipid) injection; lipid formulations have shorter half-lives.

caspofungin

Caspofungin is the second-newest antifungal agent, approved in 2003. It is used for treating severe *Aspergillus* infection (invasive and esophageal aspergillosis) in clients who are intolerant of or refractory to other drugs. Its only currently listed contraindication is drug allergy. It is available only in injectable forms as 50- and 70-mg vials of powder for intravenous infusion. Pregnancy category C. Dosage information appears in the table on p. 695.

PHARMACOKINETICS

Half-Life	Onset	Peak	Duration
9–50 hr	Unknown	Unknown	Unknown

▸▸ fluconazole

Fluconazole has proved to represent a significant improvement in the area of antifungal treatment. It has a much better side effect profile than that of amphotericin B, and it also has excellent coverage against many fungi. Oral fluconazole has excellent bioavailability, which means that almost the entire dose administered is absorbed into the circulation. Fluconazole is a prescription-only antifungal agent that is available in both an oral (PO) and a parenteral formulation. The oral and intravenous doses are identical. It is contraindicated in

clients hypersensitive to it. It is available as 50- and 100-mg tablets; a powdered dosage form to make a 10-mg/mL oral suspension; and as a 200-mg intravenous injection. Pregnancy category C. The recommended dosages are given in the table on p. 695.

PHARMACOKINETICS

Half-Life	Onset	Peak	Duration
22–50 hr	PO: <1 hr	PO: 1–2 hr	Variable

nystatin

Nystatin is a polyene antifungal agent that is often applied topically for the treatment of candidal diaper rash, taken orally as prophylaxis against candidal infections during periods of neutropenia in clients receiving immunosuppressive therapy, and used for the treatment of oral and vaginal candidiasis. It is not available in a parenteral form but does come in several oral and topical formulations. It is currently available as 100 000-unit/mL oral drops and oral suspension, a 500 000-unit oral tablet for systemic use; as a topical cream, ointment, and powder in concentrations of 100 000 units/g; a 100 000-unit vaginal tablet; and a 500-mg vaginal suppository. Nystatin is contraindicated in clients with a known hypersensitivity to it. Pregnancy category C. The recommended dosages are given in the table on p. 695.

PHARMACOKINETICS

Half-Life	Onset	Peak	Duration
Unknown	2 hr	Unknown	Unknown

terbinafine HCl

Terbinafine HCl is classified as an **allylamine antifungal** agent and is currently the only drug in its class. It is available in a topical cream and spray for treating

DOSAGES   Selected Antifungal Agents

Agent	Pharmacological Class	Usual Dosage Range	Indications
▸▸amphotericin B	Polyene antifungal	IV: Initial daily dose, 0.25 mg/kg; titrate up to 1–1.5 mg/kg/day (max 1.5 mg/kg/day) Topical: apply cream or lotion bid–qid	Broad spectrum of systemic fungal infections Topical candidiasis
amphotericin B lipid complex (ABLC); doses vary with product as follows: Abelcet Amphotec AmBisome	Polyene antifungal	*Adult and pediatric* IV: 5 mg/kg once daily, infused at 2.5 mg/kg/h IV: 3–4 mg/kg/day, infused at 1 mg/kg/h IV: 3–6 mg/kg/day, infused over 1–2 h	Systemic fungal infections
caspofungin	Echinocandin antifungal	*Adult only* IV: 70 mg loading dose on day 1, followed by 50 mg/day thereafter; infuse doses over 1 h	Esophageal candidiasis, invasive candidiasis, invasive aspergillosis in clients intolerant of or refractory to other drugs
▸▸fluconazole	Synthetic triazole antifungal	*Adult* PO: 200 mg qd *Pediatric* PO: 6 mg/kg/day *Adult* IV/PO: 100–400 mg/day × 2–5 wk (dose and duration depending on severity of infection) *Pediatric* IV/PO: 3–12 mg/kg, same guidelines as for adult *Adult* IV/PO: 200–400 mg/day × 10–12 wk after negative CSF cultures *Pediatric* Titrate pediatric doses as for adult	Prevention of recurrence of cryptococcal meningitis Oropharyngeal and esophageal candidiasis, systemic candidiasis Cryptococcal meningitis
nystatin	Polyene antifungal	*Infant* PO: 100 000 units (2 mL) oral suspension in oral cavity tid–qid *Adult and pediatric* PO: 400 000–600 000 units (4–6 mL) oral suspension in oral cavity qid *Adult only* PO (tab): 500 000–1 000 000 units (1–2 tabs) tid Topical (cream, lotion, or powder): apply bid–tid Vaginal: Insert one vaginal tablet once to twice daily × 2 wk	Oral candidiasis Intestinal candidiasis Topical candidiasis Vaginal candidiasis
terbinafine HCl	Synthetic allylamine antifungal	*Adult only* PO: 250 mg/day × 6 wk (fingernail); × 12 wk (toenail) Topical cream or solution: apply bid to affected area × 2–6 wk	Onychomycosis (fungal infection of finger- or toenails) Athlete's foot (tinea pedis), jock itch (tinea cruris), or ringworm (tinea corporis)
voriconazole	Synthetic triazole antifungal	*Adult ≥40 kg* PO: loading dose of 400 mg × 2 doses q12h, then 200 mg bid maintenance *<40 kg* PO: loading dose of 200 mg × 2 doses q12h, then 100 mg bid maintenance IV: loading dose of 6 mg/kg/ mL × 2 doses q12h, then 4 mg/kg bid	Invasive aspergillosis; other major fungal infections in clients who do not tolerate or respond to other antifungal agents

superficial dermatological infections, including tinea pedis (athlete's foot), tinea cruris (jock itch), and tinea corporis (ringworm). A 250-mg oral tablet is also available for systemic use and is used primarily to treat onychomycoses of the fingernails or toenails. Terbinafine HCl is contraindicated in cases of known drug allergy or severe kidney or liver disease. Pregnancy category B. Dosing information appears in the table on p. 695.

PHARMACOKINETICS

Half-Life	Onset	Peak	Duration
22–26 hr	Unknown	2 hr	Unknown

voriconazole

Voriconazole is currently the newest antifungal agent on the Canadian market, approved by Health Canada in 2004. It is used for treating severe fungal infections caused by *Aspergillus* spp. (invasive aspergillosis). Voriconazole is contraindicated in clients with a known drug allergy to it. It should not be co-administered with certain other drugs metabolized by the cytochrome P-450 enzyme CYP3A4 (e.g., quinidine) because of the risk of serious cardiac dysrhythmias. The drug is available in oral form as 50- and 200-mg tablets and in parenteral form as a 200-mg vial of lyophilized voriconazole for injection. Pregnancy category D. Dosage information appears in the table on p. 695.

PHARMACOKINETICS

Half-Life	Onset	Peak	Duration
Unknown due to non-linear kinetics	Unknown	1–2 hr	Unknown

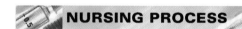

NURSING PROCESS

■ Assessment

Before administering amphotericin B or any of the other antifungal agents it is important for the nurse to identify any contraindications to the medication, such as hypersensitivity. Cautious use of these agents is recommended in pregnant or lactating women. Griseofulvin is contraindicated in clients with a hypersensitivity to it or with porphyria, hepatic disease, or lupus. Cautious use is recommended in clients known to be hypersensitive to penicillin and in pregnant women. The contraindications to ketoconazole use are hypersensitivity, pregnancy, lactation, and meningitis, with cautious use recommended in clients who have renal or hepatic disease. Miconazole is contraindicated in clients with a known hypersensitivity to it and should be used cautiously in pregnant women or clients with renal or hepatic disease.

Before administering any of the systemic antifungal agents the nurse should assess the client's vital signs and weight and check the baseline complete blood count (CBC), hemoglobin (Hgb) level, hematocrit (Hct) value, and red blood cells (RBCs). Baseline renal and liver function studies should also be obtained and documented. Clients who are to receive ketoconazole should have their liver function assessed because of the hepatotoxicity it can cause. Miconazole use is associated with adverse cardiovascular effects; therefore pulse, blood pressure, and electrocardiogram (ECG) should be checked and any history of cardiac disease documented. Griseofulvin may precipitate severe blood dyscrasias and therefore it is important to assess CBCs with this drug. Clients taking the newer antifungals caspofungin or fluconazole should be assessed for drug allergies. Terbinafine HCl is contraindicated in those clients with known allergy to antifungals and in those with severe renal or liver disease. Voriconazole is contraindicated if the client is taking drugs such as quinidine and other drugs metabolized by the cytochrome P-450 enzyme CYP3A4; interactions could induce serious cardiac dysrhythmias.

■ Nursing Diagnoses

Nursing diagnoses appropriate for clients receiving antifungals include the following:
- Acute pain related to symptoms of the infectious process.
- Deficient knowledge related to lack of information and experience with the antifungal drug therapy.
- Risk for injury related to side effects of the medication treatment regimen.

■ Planning

Goals for clients receiving antifungals include the following:
- Client states the rationale for adherence with medication therapy.
- Client states the common side effects of the specific antifungal medication.
- Client experiences minimal side effects and signs and symptoms of the infection.
- Client exhibits relief of the symptoms of the fungal infection.
- Client states the importance of follow-up appointments.

■ *Outcome Criteria*

Outcome criteria relevant to clients receiving systemic antifungal agents include the following:
- Client is free of the complications or suffers minimal side effects of the antifungal agents, such as nausea, vomiting, and gastrointestinal (GI) upset.
- Client remains adherent with the medication regimen and experiences relief of infection, including normal cultures and no fever.
- Client experiences improved appetite and energy levels after taking the antifungal agents for the prescribed period.
- Client returns to the physician regularly as recommended by the healthcare provider for CBC with differential.

■ Implementation

The nursing interventions appropriate to clients receiving antifungal agents vary depending on the agent. Amphotericin B given intravenously must be diluted properly according to the manufacturer's guidelines. Sterile water or normal saline (NS) is recommended for its reconstitution, and 5 percent dextrose in water (D5W) may be used for infusion, with a test dose of 1 mg/20 mL of D5W infused over 30 minutes. Infusion usually requires an IV access line or lumen dedicated solely to this drug. The main-line IV solution must be D5W, and no other medications or solutions may be co-infused into the amphotericin B line. Intravenous infusion pumps are recommended. The amphotericin B solution should be protected from light and should not be filtered. Caspofungin, a newer agent, is also given intravenously but should be used cautiously.

Fluconazole is administered either orally or intravenously, and when administered intravenously it should be diluted exactly according to the manufacturer's instructions. There are two different formulations of amphotericin B. One formulation (Fungizone) contains the detergent deoxycholate. A newer formulation (Amphotec, Abelcet) is associated with less toxicity. However, the dosages differ, with much higher dosages used with the newer formulation than with the deoxycholate-containing formulation. Therefore the nurse must use caution by checking and rechecking that the dose is appropriate to the formulation used. Because of the necrosis that results from extravasation of the agent at the intravenous infusion site, the nurse should check the site hourly.

Griseofulvin must be given carefully and the client frequently checked during infusions. Oral forms should be given with meals to decrease GI upset.

Voriconazole should be administered cautiously and with constant monitoring of cardiac function.

Clients receiving ketoconazole should not take alkaline products or antacids for at least two hours before or after dosing, and it should not be taken with coffee, tea, or acidic fruit juices. As with any other orally administered antifungal agents, taking ketoconazole with food helps minimize GI upset. Miconazole often causes nausea and vomiting; therefore the use of an anti-emetic may be helpful. Often a physician will order a test dose to be given to the client so that any untoward reactions can be identified.

It is often necessary for the nurse to check the vital signs of clients receiving any of the antifungals by IV every 15 to 30 minutes during infusion. It is important for the nurse to monitor the intake and output amounts, urinalysis findings, and specific gravity of the urine in clients receiving these medications to identify any deleterious drug effects on the kidneys. It is also important for the nurse to weigh clients weekly and to document these weights because a gain of more than 1 kg in a week may indicate medication-induced renal damage. The nurse must always be aware of newer drugs on the market. For example, voriconazole has severe cautions that could lead to serious health complications if it is administered in the wrong situation and with other drugs with which it interacts negatively.

Client teaching tips for antifungal agents are presented in the box below.

■ Evaluation

The therapeutic effects of antifungals include an easing of the symptoms of the infection, with complete resolution seen in clients who are fully adherent with the therapy. In systemic infections, improved energy levels and normal temperature and other vital signs also indicate a therapeutic response. Side effects for which to monitor in clients receiving these agents are listed in Table 40-2.

CLIENT TEACHING TIPS

Amphotericin B

Some clients receiving amphotericin B may need long-term treatment (i.e., weeks to months). If so, nurses should instruct clients as follows:

▲ Side effects may include ringing in the ears, blurred vision, burning and itching at the infusion site, headache, rash, fever, chills, and upset stomach. Notify a healthcare provider if these occur.

▲ Weigh yourself weekly and notify the physician if you gain more than 1 kg in a week.

Vaginal Infection

▲ Abstain from sexual intercourse until the treatment is completed and the infection is resolved.

▲ Continue to take the medication even if actively menstruating.

▲ Notify physician if symptoms persist after treatment is completed.

POINTS to REMEMBER

▼ Fungi are a large and diverse group of micro-organisms and consist of yeast and moulds.

▼ Yeast are single-celled fungi that may be harmful (causing infections) or helpful (e.g., when baking or brewing beer).

▼ Moulds are multicellular and characterized by long, branching filaments called *hyphae.*

▼ Candidiasis is an opportunistic fungal infection caused by *Candida albicans* and occurs in clients taking broad-spectrum antibiotics, antineoplastics, or immunosuppressants and in immunocompromised persons. When candidiasis occurs in the mouth, it is commonly termed *oral candidiasis* or *thrush.* It is more commonly seen in newborns or immunocompromised persons.

▼ Vaginal candidiasis is a yeast infection and occurs mostly in clients with diabetes mellitus, women taking oral contraceptives, and pregnant women.

▼ Antifungals may be administered either systemically or topically.

▼ Some of the most common systemic antifungals are amphotericin B, fluconazole, itraconazole, and ketoconazole; some of the most common topical antifungals are clotrimazole, miconazole, and nystatin.

▼ Several chemical categories of antifungals include both the topical and systemic agents, each with its own unique way of killing fungi.

▼ Nursing considerations for systemic antifungals include the following:

• Before administering these drugs, the nurse must thoroughly assess clients to find out whether they have a known hypersensitivity to the medication, what other drugs (prescribed and OTC) are being taken, and renal and liver function status.

• Amphotericin B must be properly diluted according to the manufacturer's guidelines and administered using an intravenous infusion pump. Tissue extravasation of fluconazole at the intravenous infusion site leads to tissue necrosis; therefore the site should be checked hourly and the assessment documented.

• Therapeutic effects include improved energy levels, normal temperature, and normal vital signs.

EXAMINATION REVIEW QUESTIONS

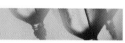

1 Which of the following poses a contraindication to the use of griseofulvin?
   a. Endocrine disease
   b. Hepatic disease
   c. Cardiac disease
   d. Pulmonary disease

2 The nurse should monitor which of the following laboratory parameters in clients receiving amphotericin?
   a. Chloride
   b. Potassium
   c. Hematocrit
   d. Serum creatine

3 Which of the following is a common underlying source of many of the drug interactions with antifungals?
   a. Polyuria
   b. Gallbladder metabolism
   c. Bone distribution
   d. Cytochrome P-450 enzyme system

4 Which of the following statements is most accurate regarding the use of antifungal agents in candidiasis infections?
   a. Amphotericin B is marketable because of its lack of side effects, its ease of use in home settings, and its ease of use in the transbuccal or sublingual dosage form.

   b. The mechanism of action of amphotericin B against bacterial, candidiasis, and tuberculin infections exceeds that of any other antifungal agent.

   c. Amphotericin B and other antifungals have minimal side effects and little chance of toxicity when used parenterally.

   d. Fluconazole, oral dosage, may not be the drug of choice in some clients, but for treating vaginal yeast infections it has shown to be convenient and more bioavailable.

5 Antifungals may lead to significant drug interactions if given with which of the following drugs that are also metabolized by cytochrome P-450?
   a. quinidine
   b. vitamins
   c. acetaminophen
   d. insulin

For answers see http://evolve.elsevier.com/Lilley/pharmacology/.

CRITICAL THINKING ACTIVITIES

1 What laboratory data and other assessment data should be considered before administering any of the systemic antifungals? Specify the data and identify the reason for their importance.

2 One of your clients is to receive amphotericin B. However, the client's liver and renal function is somewhat impaired.

What laboratory studies are important to monitor, and why is the administration of amphotericin B problematic in this type of client?

3 What instructions should accompany a prescription of ketoconazole?

For answers see http://evolve.elsevier.com/Lilley/pharmacology/.

BIBLIOGRAPHY

Albanese J., & Nutz, P. (2005). *Mosby's 2005 nursing drug cards.* St Louis, MO: Mosby.

Canadian Paediatric Society. (2000). Antifungal agents for common paediatric infections. Reaffirmed 2005. *Paediatrics & Child Health, 5*(8), 477–482.

Canadian Pharmacists Association. (2003). *Therapeutic choices* (4th ed.). Ottawa, ON: Author.

Canadian Pharmacists Association. (2004). *Guide to drugs in Canada.* Toronto, ON: Dorling Kindersley.

Canadian Pharmacists Association. (2005). *Compendium of pharmaceuticals and specialties. The Canadian drug reference for health professionals.* Ottawa, ON: Author. [The subscription-based e-CPS is available at http://www.pharmacists.ca.]

Cheng, A., Williams, B.A., & Sivarajan, B.V. (Eds.). (2003). *The HSC handbook of pediatrics* (10th ed.). Toronto, ON: Elsevier.

Facts and Comparisons. (2004). *Drug facts and comparisons pocket version* (9th ed.). St Louis, MO: Wolters Kluwer Health.

Hardman, J.G., & Limbird, L.E. (2002). *Goodman and Gilman's the pharmacological basis of therapeutics* (10th ed.). New York: McGraw-Hill.

Health Canada. (2005). Drug product database (DPD). Retrieved August 28, 2005, from http://www.hc-sc.gc.ca/hpb/drugs-dpd/

Huang, C.C., & Nunley, J.R. (2003). Dermatologic look-alikes. *Clinical Advisor, 6*(3), 95–98.

Katzung, B.G. (2004). *Basic and clinical pharmacology* (9th ed.). New York: McGraw-Hill.

Kumar, A. (2004). Update on antifungal therapy. *Infectious Diseases and Microbiology Rounds, 3*(9). Retrieved August 28, 2005, from http://www.idrounds.ca/crus/idmbeng_1104.pdf

Lacy, C.F., Armstrong, L.L., Goldman, M.P., & Lance, L.L. (2003). *Drug information handbook* (11th ed.). Hudson, OH: Lexi-Comp.

Mandell, G.L., Bennett, J.E., & Dolin, R. (2005). *Principles and practice of infectious diseases* (6th ed.). Philadelphia: Elsevier Churchill Livingstone.

Mosby. (2005). *Mosby's drug consult 2005: The comprehensive reference for generic and brand name drugs* (15th ed.). St Louis, MO: Mosby.

Skidmore-Roth, L. (2006). *Mosby's 2006 nursing drug reference* (19th ed.). St Louis, MO: Mosby.

CHAPTER

41 Antimalarial, Antiprotozoal, and Anthelmintic Agents

OBJECTIVES

After reading this chapter, the successful student will be able to do the following:

1 Identify the various antimalarial, antiprotozoal, and anthelmintic agents.

2 Contrast the signs and symptoms associated with these infectious processes.

3 Discuss the infections that are labelled malarial, protozoal, and/or helminthic in origin.

4 Discuss the mechanisms of action, indications, cautions, contraindications, side effects, dosages, and routes of administration associated with each antimalarial, antiprotozoal, and anthelmintic agent.

5 Develop a nursing care plan that includes all phases of the nursing process for clients receiving antimalarial, antiprotozoal, or anthelmintic agents.

e-LEARNING ACTIVITIES

Student CD-ROM
- Review Questions: see questions 316–318
- Animations
- Medication Administration Checklists
- IV Therapy Checklists

evolve Web site (http://evolve.elsevier.com/Lilley/pharmacology/)
- Online Chapter Worksheet • Frequently Asked Questions
- Learning Tips and Content Updates • WebLinks • Online Appendices and Supplements • Mosby/Saunders ePharmacology Update • Access to *Mosby's Drug Consult*

DRUG PROFILES

atovaquone, p. 707
▶▶chloroquine and hydroxychloroquine, p. 705
▶▶mebendazole, p. 711
mefloquine, p. 705
▶▶metronidazole, p. 707

paromomycin, p. 709
pentamidine, p. 709
praziquantel, p. 711
▶▶primaquine, p. 705
pyrimethamine, p. 706

▶▶ Key drug.

GLOSSARY

4-Aminoquinoline derivatives (uh mee' noe kwin' o leen) A major class of antimalarial agents that includes the drugs chloroquine and hydroxychloroquine. They work by binding to key enzymes in the cells of the malaria parasite. This results in inhibition of deoxyribonucleic acid (DNA), ribonucleic acid (RNA), and protein synthesis, as well as impaired utilization of host (human) hemoglobin during the erythrocytic stages of infection.

Anthelmintic (ant' hel min' tik) A drug that destroys or prevents the development of parasitic worm (helminthic) infections. Also called *antihelmintic* or *vermicide*. Notice that the terms for the drug categories are usually spelled with only one "h," in the second syllable, whereas the term for worm infection (*helminthic*) is spelled with two "h's," appearing in both the second and third syllables of the term.

Antimalarial A drug that destroys or prevents the development of the malaria parasite (*Plasmodium* sp.) in human hosts. Antimalarial agents are a subset of the antiprotozoal agents.

Antiprotozoal (an' tee proe' tə zoe' əl) A drug that destroys or prevents the development of protozoa in human hosts.

Erythrocytic phase   (e rith′ roe si′ tik) The phase of the asexual cycle of the malaria parasite that occurs inside the erythrocyte. Also called the *blood phase*.

Exoerythrocytic phase   (ek′ soe e rith′ roe si′ tik) The phase of the asexual cycle of the malaria parasite that occurs outside the erythrocyte, primarily in liver tissues. Also called the *tissue phase*.

Helminthic infection   (hel min′ thik) A parasitic worm infection.

Malaria   A protozoal infectious disease caused by four species of the genus *Plasmodium*. Malaria is the most significant infectious disease worldwide in terms of human morbidity and mortality.

Parasite   Any organism that feeds on another living organism in a way that results in harm to that organism.

Parasitic protozoa   Harmful protozoa that live on or in human beings or animals and cause disease in the process.

Plasmodium   (plaz moe′ dee əm) The genus of protozoa that causes malaria.

Protozoa   Single-celled organisms, such as amoebas. They form a sub-kingdom of the kingdom Protista, which also includes bacteria and fungi.

There are more than 28 000 known types of **protozoa**. Those that live on or in humans are termed **parasitic protozoa**. Billions of people worldwide are infected with these organisms, constituting a serious health problem. Some of the more common protozoal infections are malaria, leishmaniasis, trypanosomiasis, amoebiasis, giardiasis, and trichomoniasis. They are relatively uncommon in Canada but are becoming increasingly prevalent among immunocompromised persons, including those with AIDS. Protozoal diseases are especially prevalent among people living in tropical climates because it is easier for protozoa to survive and be transmitted in these year-round warm and humid environments. Even though the population of Canada is relatively free of many of these protozoal infections, international travel and the immigration of people from other countries where such infections are endemic are providing opportunities for increased exposure. Approximately 1.7 million Canadians travel annually to tropical countries that are potentially malaria-endemic. As many as 400 to 1000 cases a year of imported malaria are reported to Health Canada. Some of these cases are severe and can result in death.

MALARIA

The most significant protozoal disease in terms of morbidity and mortality is **malaria**. In Africa alone it accounts for more than one million infant deaths a year. Symptoms include fever and influenza-like symptoms, such as chills, headache, sweating, muscle aches, fatigue, and malaise; these symptoms may be intermittent. If untreated, the spleen and the liver become enlarged, anemia develops, and jaundice appears. Symptoms of severe untreated in-

fection can include coma (cerebral malaria), anemia, gastroenteritis, renal failure, and difficulty breathing. Death may occur from general debility, anemia, or clogging of the vessels of cerebral tissues by affected red blood cells.

Malaria is caused by a genus of protozoa called ***Plasmodium***, which includes four species, each with its own characteristics and resistance to **antimalarials**: *Plasmodium vivax, Plasmodium falciparum, Plasmodium malariae*, and *Plasmodium ovale*. Although *P. vivax* is the most widespread, *P. falciparum* is nearly as widespread and more drug resistant. The two remaining species are much less common and geographically limited, but can still cause serious malarial infections. Most commonly malaria is transmitted by the bite of an infected female *anopheles* mosquito. This type of mosquito is endemic to many tropical regions of the earth. Rarely, malaria can also be transmitted by blood transfusions, congenitally from mother to infant via an infected placenta, or through the use of shared contaminated needles. Despite the combined efforts of many countries to eradicate malaria, it remains the most devastating infectious disease in the world. Many lives are lost, and the cost of treating and preventing the disease imposes a tremendous economic burden on the often poor countries where the disease is prevalent.

The life cycle of the *Plasmodium* is quite diverse and involves many stages. It has two interdependent life cycles: the sexual cycle, which takes place inside the mosquito, and the asexual cycle, which occurs in the human host. In addition, the asexual cycle of the **parasite** consists of a phase outside the erythrocyte (primarily in liver tissues) called the **exoerythrocytic phase** (also called the *tissue phase*) and a phase inside the erythrocyte called the **erythrocytic phase** (also called the *blood phase*). The malarial parasite undergoes many changes during these two phases (Figure 41-1).

ANTIMALARIAL AGENTS

Antimalarial agents administered to humans cannot affect the parasite during its sexual cycle when it resides in the mosquito. Instead, these agents work against the parasite during its asexual cycle, which takes place within the human body. Chloroquine, hydroxychloroquine, quinine, quinidine, halofantrine, and mefloquine are all antimalarial drugs that kill the malarial parasite during the blood phase. Primaquine is able to kill the parasite during both the tissue and blood phases. Often these drugs are given in various combinations to achieve an additive or synergistic antimalarial effect. The management of malaria is changing as the prevalence of drug-resistant malaria increases. For example, in Canada, doxycycline is used to treat cases of drug-resistant malaria.

Mechanism of Action and Drug Effects

The mechanisms of action of the chemical families of antimalarial agents differ. The **4-aminoquinoline derivatives** (chloroquine and hydroxychloroquine) work by inhibiting deoxyribonucleic acid (DNA) and ribonucleic

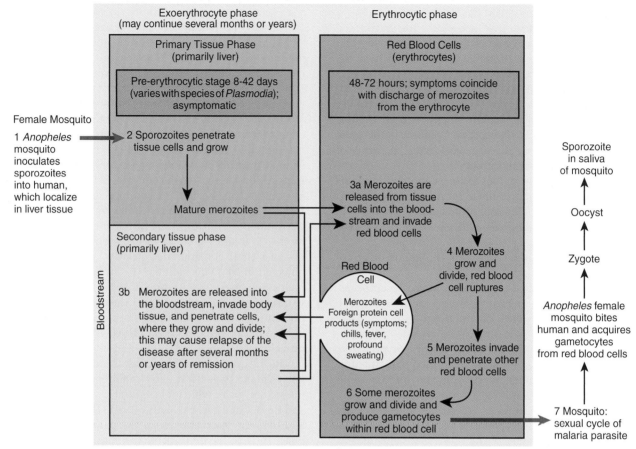

FIG. 41-1 Life cycle of the malarial parasite. (From McKenry, L.M., & Salerno, E. (2003). *Mosby's pharmacology in nursing—revised and updated* (21st ed.). St Louis, MO: Mosby.)

acid (RNA) polymerase, an enzyme essential to DNA and RNA synthesis by the parasite cells. Parasite protein synthesis is also disrupted because protein synthesis is dependent on proper nucleic acid (DNA and RNA) function. These drugs are also believed to raise the pH within the parasite, which has the effect of interfering with the parasite's ability to metabolize and utilize erythrocyte hemoglobin and is one reason the drugs are ineffective during the exoerythrocytic phase (tissue phase) of infection. All of these actions contribute to the destruction of the parasite. Quinine, quinidine, and mefloquine are also thought to raise the pH within the parasite.

The diaminopyrimidines (pyrimethamine and trimethoprim) work by inhibiting dihydrofolate reductase, an enzyme that is needed for the production of certain vital substances in malarial parasites. Specifically, inhibiting this enzyme blocks the synthesis of tetrahydrofolate, a precursor of purines and pyrimidines (nucleic acid components), and certain amino acids (protein components) essential for the growth and survival of plasmodia parasites. These two agents are also effective only during the erythrocytic phase and are often used with a sulphonamide or sulphone for synergistic effects. Tetracyclines (e.g., doxycycline) and clindamycin may

also be used in combination with some of the other antimalarial agents described earlier.

Primaquine has the ability to bind to and alter parasitic DNA and is one of the few agents effective in the exoerythrocytic phase.

The drug effects of the antimalarial agents are mostly limited to their ability to kill parasitic organisms, most of which are *Plasmodium* spp. Some of these agents do, however, have other drug effects. Chloroquine and hydroxychloroquine also have anti-inflammatory effects and are sometimes used in the treatment of rheumatoid arthritis and systemic lupus erythematosus. Quinine and quinidine, two plant alkaloids from the bark of the South American cinchona tree, can also decrease the excitability of both cardiac and skeletal muscles. Quinidine is still used to treat certain types of cardiac dysrhythmias (Chapter 22). A compound with a similar name and comparable chemical structure, quinacrine, is also effective against malaria and giardiasis, but it is no longer available in Canada.

Indications

Antimalarial agents are used to kill *Plasmodium* organisms, the parasites that cause malaria. Chloroquine and related compounds (the 4-aminoquinolines) remain the drugs of choice for the prevention and treatment of susceptible strains of malarial parasites. They are highly toxic to all *Plasmodium* spp., except in resistant cases of *P. falciparum*, which occur in many areas of the world, including Asia, Africa, and South America.

Chloroquine is taken once weekly, beginning one week before entering a chloroquine-sensitive malarial region, during the period of exposure, and for four weeks after leaving the malarial region. According to the Canadian Recommendations for the Prevention and Treatment of Malaria Among International Travellers, individuals who are unable to tolerate chloroquine should use atovaquone/proguanil, doxycycline, or mefloquine.

Atovaquone/proguanil is a fixed drug combination of atovaquone 250 mg and proguanil 100 mg. Atovaquone (ATQ) is a novel antimalarial belonging to the hydroxynapthaquinone class. It is an analogue of ubiquinone and, in combination with proguanil, is now considered in Canada to be first-line chemoprophylaxis for chloroquine- and mefloquine-resistant areas and uncomplicated multi-drug-resistant *P. falciparum* malaria. Atovaquone/proguanil is taken daily, beginning one day before entering the malarial region, during the period of exposure, and for one week after leaving the malarial region.

Mefloquine is a newer antimalarial agent that may also be used for first-line chemoprophylaxis of malaria in chloroquine-resistant areas. Mefloquine is taken weekly, beginning one week before entering the malarial region, during the period of exposure, and for four weeks after leaving the malarial region.

Primaquine is still considered an effective antimalarial agent for eradicating the parasite during the exoerythrocytic phase (tissue phase). Primaquine is used in Canada as an alternative chemoprophylactic agent when other regimes are inappropriate or contraindicated. Primaquine is taken daily, beginning one day before entry into the malarial region, during the period of exposure, and for four weeks after leaving the malarial region.

Doxycycline is also an alternative agent, taken daily, beginning one day before entering the malarial region, during the period of exposure, and for four weeks after leaving the malarial region. It may also be used in the treatment of chloroquine-resistant *P. falciparum*.

Pyrimethamine is another antimalarial antibiotic that was commonly used in combination with another antibiotic, sulfadoxine. However, resistance to this combination is now common.

Quinine is used for treatment of malaria. Although not considered the optimum, quinidine gluconate, administered parenterally, is indicated for the treatment of *P. falciparum malaria*. Quinidine should not be used alone but is more commonly used in combination with pyrimethamine or a tetracycline (such as doxycycline).

Contraindications

Contraindications to various antimalarial agents include drug allergy, glucose-6-phosphate dehydrogenase (G6PD) enzyme deficiency, optic neuritis, visual field changes, tinnitus (ringing in the ears), certain inflammatory diseases

TABLE 41-1
ANTIMALARIAL DRUGS: COMMON ADVERSE EFFECTS

Body System	Side/Adverse Effects
CHLOROQUINE	
Gastrointestinal	Diarrhea, anorexia, nausea, vomiting
Other	Alopecia (hair loss), dizziness, personality changes, stomatitis (inflammation of the mouth), blurred vision, retinopathy, hair bleaching, exacerbation of psoriasis
MEFLOQUINE	
Central nervous	Headache, dizziness, insomnia, mood changes, strange vivid dreams, dizziness, convulsions, depression, psychosis, anxiety, mood change
Gastrointestinal	Nausea, diarrhea
PRIMAQUINE	
Gastrointestinal	Nausea, vomiting, abdominal pain
Other	Headaches, pruritus, dark discoloration of urine, hemolytic anemia due to G6PD deficiency
PYRIMETHAMINE	
Gastrointestinal	Anorexia; nausea; colic; taste disturbances; soreness, redness, swelling, or burning of tongue; diarrhea; throat pain; swallowing difficulties; sore throat
Other	Fever, increased weakness, rash, leukopenia, anemia, thrombocytopenia, severe hypersensitivity reactions, insomnia
QUININE	
Central nervous	Visual disturbances, dizziness, severe headaches, tinnitus, hearing loss
Cardiovascular	Conduction disturbances, ventricular tachycardia, angina
Gastrointestinal	Diarrhea, nausea, vomiting, abdominal pain or discomfort
Other	Rash, pruritus, hives, respiratory difficulties, wheezing, hypoglycemia

(primaquine), megaloblastic anemia secondary to folic acid deficiency (pyrimethamine), and pregnancy (quinine). Severe renal, hepatic, or hematological dysfunction may also be a relative contraindication to the use of antimalarial agents.

Side Effects and Adverse Effects

Antimalarial agents cause diverse side effects and adverse effects, listed in Table 41-1.

Interactions

Some common drug interactions associated with antimalarial drugs are listed in Table 41-2 on p. 705.

Dosages

For the recommended dosages for selected antimalarial agents, see the dosages table on p. 704. See Appendix B for some of the common brands available in Canada.

DOSAGES Selected Antimalarial Agents

Agent	Pharmacological Class	Usual Dosage Range	Indications
atovaquone/ proguanil	Antimalarial	**Adult** PO: 1 tab daily × 7 days **Pediatric** PO: 11–20 kg: ¼ tablet daily 21–30 kg: ½ tablet daily 31–40 kg: ¾ tablet daily >40 kg: 1 tablet daily × 7 days	Malaria prophylaxis
		Adult PO: 4 tabs daily × 3 days **Pediatric** PO: 11–20 kg: 1 tab daily 21–30 kg: 2 tabs daily 31–40 kg: 3 tabs daily >41 kg: 4 tabs daily × 7 days	Malaria treatment
⟩⟩chloroquine	Synthetic antimalarial and anti-amoebic	**Adult** PO: 300 mg base weekly, beginning 1 wk before and continuing for 4 wk after visiting endemic area **Pediatric** PO: 5 mg/kg base weekly; max 300 mg	Malaria prophylaxis
		PO: 600 mg base day 1, followed by 300 mg 6 h later and daily for days 2 and 3 **Pediatric** PO: 25 mg base/kg total over 3 days	Malaria treatment
⟩⟩hydroxychloroquine	Synthetic antimalarial	**Adult*** PO: 310 mg base weekly, beginning 2 wk before and continuing through 8 wk after visiting endemic area	Malaria prophylaxis
		PO: 620 mg base day 1, followed by 310 mg 6–8 h later and daily for days 2 and 3	Malaria treatment
mefloquine	Synthetic antimalarial	**Adult** PO: 250 mg weekly beginning 1 wk before travel and continuing until 4 wk after visiting endemic area **Pediatric** PO: Weekly dosing as above based on weight as follows: 10–19 kg: ¼ tab 20–29 kg: ½ tab 30–45 kg: ¾ tab >46 kg: 1 tab (250 mg)	Malaria prophylaxis
		Adult PO: 1250 mg (5 tabs) as single dose **Pediatric** PO: 15–25 mg/kg in a single dose, not to exceed 1250 mg	Malaria treatment (not routinely recommended)
⟩⟩primaquine	Synthetic antimalarial	**Adult** PO: 35 mg base daily × 14 days **Pediatric** 0.5 mg base/kg/day daily × 14 days	For cure or relapse prevention of malaria infection with *Plasmodium vivax*; may also be used for *P. vivax* prophylaxis in clients intolerant of chloroquine or if chloroquine is not available
pyrimethamine	Folic acid antagonist, antimalarial, anti-toxoplasmotic agent	**Adult and pediatric >10 yr** PO: 50 mg daily × 2 days **Pediatric 4–10 yr** PO: 25 mg daily × 2 days	Malaria treatment

*Only adult doses are given. Pediatric doses range from 5–10 mg/kg but should not exceed adult doses.

TABLE 41-2
ANTIMALARIAL AGENTS: DRUG INTERACTIONS

Drug	Mechanism	Result
CHLOROQUINE		
cimetidine	Decreased metabolism of chloroquine	Increased serum chloroquine levels
Hepatotoxic drugs, alcohol	Increased chloroquine levels in liver	Increased hepatotoxicity
MEFLOQUINE		
Beta-blockers, calcium channel blockers, phenothiazines, nonsedating antihistamines, tricyclic antidepressants, quinidine, quinine	Unknown	Increased risk of dysrhythmia, cardiac arrest, seizures
PRIMAQUINE		
Other hemolytic agents	Unknown	Increased risk for myelotoxic effects (monitor for muscle weakness)

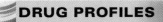

DRUG PROFILES

ANTIMALARIAL AGENTS

The dosing instructions for several of the antimalarial agents can be confusing because tablet strengths on the medication packaging often indicate the strength of the tablet in terms of the entire salt form of the drug, not just the active ingredient itself, which is referred to as the *base ingredient*. However, dosing guidelines often list recommended dosages in terms of the base ingredient and not the entire salt. For example, as described later in the drug profile for chloroquine, the tablets come in 250-mg strengths of the salt form of the drug, but these tablets actually only have 150 mg of the active ingredient or base. Nurses must be mindful of these distinctions.

▸▸ chloroquine and hydroxychloroquine

Chloroquine is a synthetic antimalarial agent that is chemically classified as a 4-aminoquinoline derivative. It is also indicated for treatment of other parasitic infections, such as amoebiasis. Hydroxychloroquine is another synthetic 4-aminoquinoline derivative that differs from chloroquine by only one hydroxyl group (–OH). Its efficacy in treating malaria is comparable to that of quinine. Both medications also possess anti-inflammatory actions and have been used to treat rheumatoid arthritis and systemic lupus erythematosus since the 1950s. However, hydroxychloroquine is preferred for inflammatory illnesses because of its reduced risk of causing ocular toxicity at the high doses required.

Contraindications include known drug allergy, visual field changes, and psoriasis, keeping in mind that sound clinical judgement may still warrant the use of the medication in urgent clinical situations.

Chloroquine is available in both a parenteral and an oral (PO) formulation. Chloroquine hydrochloride is used in the parenteral form in a strength of 40 mg/mL for injection. Chloroquine phosphate is used in the oral form as 250-mg (150-mg chloroquine base) tablets. Hydroxychloroquine is available only as a sulphate salt for oral use in 200-mg tablets (150-mg base). Both drugs are classified as pregnancy category C agents but should be used for pregnant women only in truly urgent situations. These drugs are also distributed into breast milk, with one study demonstrating about one-third the level of chloroquine in breast milk as in the mother's bloodstream. Commonly recommended dosages are listed in the dosages table on p. 704.

PHARMACOKINETICS
chloroquine

Half-Life	Onset	Peak	Duration
3–5 days	8–10 hr	2 hr	Variable

chloroquine hydroxychloroquine

Half-Life	Onset	Peak	Duration
32–50 days	several hr* 4–6 wk†	few hr* several mo†	Variable

*For malaria.
†For rheumatic diseases.

mefloquine

Mefloquine is an analogue of quinine that is indicated for the management of mild to moderate acute malaria and for the prevention and treatment of chloroquine-resistant malaria and multi-drug-resistant strains of *P. falciparum*. The drug is commonly used prophylactically by travellers to malaria-endemic areas. The tetracycline antibiotic doxycycline (Chapter 37) is also commonly used for this purpose. Mefloquine is contraindicated in clients with known drug allergy to it. It is available in 250-mg tablets, taken orally. Pregnancy category C. Commonly recommended dosages are listed in the dosages table on p. 704.

PHARMACOKINETICS

Half-Life	Onset	Peak	Duration
Days to weeks	<24	7–24 hr	Variable

▸▸ *primaquine*

Primaquine is similar in chemical structure and antimalarial activity to the 4-aminoquinolines, but it is classified as an 8-aminoquinoline. It is one of the few agents that can destroy malarial parasites in their exoerythrocytic phase (tissue phase).

Primaquine is contraindicated in clients with a known hypersensitivity to it, as well as in those with anemia, lupus erythematosus, methemoglobinemia, porphyria, rheumatoid arthritis, methemoglobin reductase deficiency, and G6PD deficiency. It is available as a 15-mg oral tablet. Pregnancy category C. Commonly recommended dosages are listed in the dosages table on p. 704.

PHARMACOKINETICS

Half-Life	Onset	Peak	Duration
4–10 hr	<2 hr	1–3 hr	24 hr

pyrimethamine

Pyrimethamine is a synthetic antimalarial agent that is structurally related to trimethoprim (Chapter 37). These two agents are sometimes referred to as *diaminopyrimidines*. Pyrimethamine is contraindicated in clients with known drug allergy to it or with megaloblastic anemia caused by folate deficiency. It is available only in an oral formulation as a 25-mg tablet. Pyrimethamine and trimethoprim are both classified as pregnancy category C agents. Commonly recommended dosages are listed in the dosages table on p. 704.

PHARMACOKINETICS

Half-Life	Onset	Peak	Duration
4 days	<6 hr	2–6 hr	Up to 2 wk

PROTOZOAL INFECTIONS

Although malaria is the most common, other common protozoal infections include amoebiasis, giardiasis, pneumocystosis, toxoplasmosis, and trichomoniasis. Like malaria, these are more prevalent in tropical regions. The protozoal parasites that most often cause these infections are, respectively, *Entamoeba histolytica*, *Giardia lamblia*, *Toxoplasma gondii*, and *Trichomonas vaginalis*.

These protozoal infections can be transmitted in a number of ways: from person to person (e.g., via sexual contact), through the ingestion of contaminated water or food, through direct contact with the parasite, or by the bite of an insect (mosquito or tick). Parasitic infections are often classified according to where they occur in the body. They can be systemic and occur throughout the body or be localized to a specific region. For example, amoebiasis most commonly affects the gastrointestinal (GI) tract (e.g., amoebic dysentery),

whereas pneumocystosis is predominantly a pulmonary infection.

The more common protozoal infections are listed in Table 41-3, along with a brief description of the infection and the **antiprotozoal** agents commonly used in their treatment. Clients whose immune system is compromised, such as those with leukemia, those with transplanted organs who are on immunosuppressive drugs, and those with AIDS, are at particular risk for acquiring a protozoal infection. Often such infections are fatal in these clients.

ANTIPROTOZOAL AGENTS

The most commonly used antiprotozoal agents are as follows:

- metronidazole and paromomycin: used for the treatment of intestinal amoebiasis
- chloroquine and metronidazole: used for the treatment of extraintestinal amoebiasis
- atovaquone, pentamidine, and pyrimethamine: used for the treatment of other protozoal infections

Mechanism of Action and Drug Effects

The mechanisms of action of the antiprotozoal agents are as different as the agents themselves. The most commonly used of these agents together with a brief description of their mechanisms of action are given in Table 41-4. Pyrimethamine is discussed earlier in this chapter in the section on malaria.

The drug effects of these antiprotozoal agents are primarily limited to their ability to kill various forms of protozoal parasites, but these differ from agent to agent. The drug effects of the antiprotozoal agents that have not yet been mentioned are summarized in Table 41-5.

Indications

Antiprotozoal agents are used to treat protozoal infections ranging from intestinal amoebiasis to pneumocystosis.

TABLE 41-3

TYPES OF PROTOZOAL INFECTIONS

Protozoal Infection	Description	Antiprotozoal Agent
Amoebiasis	Infection that mainly resides in the large intestine but can also migrate to other parts of the body, such as the liver. Produced by the protozoal parasite *Entamoeba histolytica*. Usually transmitted in contaminated food or water.	metronidazole, paromomycin
Giardiasis	Caused by *Giardia lamblia*. The most common intestinal protozoal infection, usually residing in the intestinal mucosa (most commonly the duodenum). May cause diarrhea, bloating, and foul-smelling stools. Transmitted by contaminated food or water or by contact with stool from infected persons. In Canada is referred to as "beaver fever."	metronidazole
Pneumocystosis	Pneumonias caused by *Pneumocystis carinii* that occur almost exclusively in immunocompromised people. Always fatal if left untreated.	dapsone, atovaquone, primaquine pentamidine, clindamycin, trimetrexate
Toxoplasmosis	Caused by *Toxoplasma gondii*. Can produce systemic infection in both immunocompetent and immunocompromised hosts. Domesticated animals, usually cats, serve as intermediate host for parasites, passing infective oocysts in their feces.	sulphonamides with pyrimethamine, clindamycin, metronidazole
Trichomoniasis	Sexually transmitted disease caused by *Trichomonas vaginalis*.	metronidazole

Atovaquone and pentamidine are used for the treatment of *P. carinii* infection. Paromomycin is used to treat intestinal amoebiasis, the usual causative organism being *Entamoeba histolytica*. Metronidazole is effective against several forms of bacteria, including anaerobic bacteria (Chapter 37), as well as against protozoa and helminths (parasitic worms). Worm infection (helminthiasis) is discussed later in this chapter.

Contraindications

Contraindications to the use of antiprotozoal drugs include known drug allergy. Additional contraindications may include serious renal, liver, or other illnesses, weighing the seriousness of the infection against the client's overall condition.

Side Effects and Adverse Effects

The side effects and adverse effects of antiprotozoal agents vary greatly depending on the agent, and those specific to various common antiprotozoal agents are listed in Table 41-6.

Interactions

The common drug and laboratory test interactions associated with the use of antiprotozoal agents are listed in Table 41-7. Some of these interactions can result in severe toxicities, and it is therefore important to know of them and to understand the mechanism involved.

Dosages

For dosage information on selected antiprotozoal agents, see the dosages table on p. 709. See Appendix B for some of the common brands available in Canada.

DRUG PROFILES

Antiprotozoal agents are used for a number of infectious diseases, including infections with *Pneumocystis carinii* and *Trichomonas vaginalis,* amoebic dysentery (*Entamoeba histolytica*), toxoplasmosis, and giardiasis, among many others. All require a prescription, and are available in a number of dosage forms including oral, injectable, and inhalation aerosol.

atovaquone

Atovaquone is a synthetic antiprotozoal agent indicated for the treatment of mild to moderate *P. carinii* pneumonia in clients who cannot tolerate trimethoprim/sulfamethoxazole (Chapter 37). The mechanism of atovaquone is unclear, but it appears to kill protozoa by inhibiting protozoal production of vital substances such as nucleic acids and ATP. Atovaquone is contraindicated in clients with known drug allergy. It is available only orally as a 750-mg/5-mL suspension. Pregnancy category C. Commonly recommended dosages are given in the dosages table on p. 709.

PHARMACOKINETICS

Half-Life	Onset	Peak	Duration
2–3 days	8–24 hr	24–96 hr	Unknown

▸▸ metronidazole

Metronidazole is an antiprotozoal agent that also has fairly broad antibacterial activity as well as **anthelmintic** activity. The therapeutic uses of metronidazole are many and varied; it is used for trichomoniasis, amoebiasis, giardiasis, anaerobic bacterial infections, and antibiotic-induced pseudomembranous colitis (Chapter 37). It can directly kill protozoa by causing free-radical reactions that damage their DNA and other vital biomolecules.

Contraindications to metronidazole use include known drug allergy and first trimester of pregnancy. It is available as an oral preparation in the form of

TABLE 41-4

ANTIPROTOZOAL AGENTS: MECHANISMS OF ACTION

Antiprotozoal Agent	Mechanism of Action
atovaquone	Protozoal energy is generated in mitochondria. Atovaquone selectively inhibits mitochondrial electron transport, resulting in no energy, and cell death. Also inhibits pyrimidine synthesis, causing the protozoa to be unable to make life-sustaining substances.
metronidazole	Bactericidal, amoebicidal, and trichomonacidal. Can also kill anaerobic bacteria, which it accomplishes by disrupting the synthesis of DNA and other nucleic acids needed for the survival of many organisms.
paromomycin	A luminal or contact amoebicide that can also kill susceptible bacteria. A direct-acting agent, it kills by inhibiting protein synthesis in susceptible bacteria by binding to the 30S ribosomal subunit.
pentamidine	Inhibits production of much-needed substances such as DNA and RNA. Can bind to and aggregate ribosomes. Is directly lethal to *Pneumocystis carinii* by inhibiting glucose metabolism, protein and RNA synthesis, and intracellular amino acid transport.

TABLE 41-5

ANTIPROTOZOAL AGENTS: DRUG EFFECTS

Antiprotozoal Agent	Drug Effects
atovaquone	Used for treatment of acute mild to moderately severe *Pneumocystis carinii* pneumonia (PCP)
metronidazole	An antibacterial (including anaerobes), antiprotozoal, and anthelmintic agent
paromomycin	Indicated for treatment of acute and chronic intestinal amoebiasis
pentamidine	Used for prevention and treatment of *P. carinii* pneumonia

TABLE 41-6
ANTIPROTOZOAL AGENTS: ADVERSE EFFECTS

Body System	Side/Adverse Effects
ATOVAQUONE	
Cardiovascular	Hypotension
Hematological	Anemia, neutropenia
Integumentary	Rash, oral candidiasis
Gastrointestinal	Anorexia, increased AST and ALT levels, elevated amylase and alkaline phosphatase, nausea, vomiting, diarrhea, constipation, abdominal pain, dyspepsia
Central nervous	Dizziness, headache, anxiety, insomnia
Respiratory	Sinusitis, rhinitis, cough
Metabolic	Hypoglycemia
Other	Sweating, fever
METRONIDAZOLE	
Central nervous	Headache, dizziness, confusion, fatigue, convulsions, peripheral neuropathy, transient ataxia, insomnia, confusion, hallucinations
Eyes, ears, nose, and throat	Blurred vision, sore throat, dry mouth, metallic taste, glossitis (inflammation of the tongue)
Gastrointestinal	Abdominal cramps, pseudomembranous colitis, nausea, vomiting, diarrhea, anorexia, dyspepsia, constipation
Genitourinary	Darkened urine, dysuria, vaginal *C. albicans*
Hematological	Leukopenia, bone marrow depression
Integumentary	Rash, pruritus, urticaria, flushing
PAROMOMYCIN	
Gastrointestinal	Stomach cramps, nausea, vomiting, diarrhea
PENTAMIDINE	
Cardiovascular	Hypotension, dysrhythmias
Hematological	Anemia, leukopenia, thrombocytopenia
Integumentary	Pain at injection site, pruritus, urticaria, rash
Genitourinary	Acute renal failure
Gastrointestinal	Increased AST and ALT levels, acute pancreatitis, metallic taste, nausea, vomiting, diarrhea
Central nervous	Disorientation, hallucinations, dizziness, confusion
Respiratory	Cough, shortness of breath, bronchospasm
Metabolic	Hyperkalemia, hypocalcemia, hypoglycemia followed by hyperglycemia
Other	Fatigue, chills, night sweats

TABLE 41-7
ANTIPROTOZOAL AGENTS: DRUG AND LABORATORY TEST INTERACTIONS

Antiprotozoal Agent	Interacting Drug or Substance	Mechanism	Result
atovaquone	Highly protein-bound drugs	Compete for binding on protein, resulting in free, active atovaquone	May increase drug concentrations and drug effects
metronidazole	Alcohol	Increased plasma acetaldehyde concentration after ingestion of alcohol by decreasing the absorption of vitamin K from the intestines due to the elimination of the bacteria needed to absorb vitamin K	"Disulfiram (Antabuse) reaction": flushing, palpitations, severe vomiting, possible respiratory depression
	warfarin		May increase action of warfarin
Paromomycin pentamidine	aminoglycoside, amphotericin B, colistin, cisplatin, methoxyflurane, polymyxin B, or vancomycin	Additive nephrotoxic effects	Nephrotoxicity

DOSAGES   Selected Antiprotozoal Agents

Agent	Pharmacological Class	Usual Dosage Range	Indications
atovaquone*	Synthetic antipneumo-cystis agent	*Adult and adolescents 13–16 yr* PO: 750 mg bid with meal × 21 days	Treatment of active PCP
▸▸ metronidazole	Amoebicide, antibacterial, trichomonacide	*Adult* PO: 500–750 mg tid 3 × 5–10 days *Pediatric* PO: 35–50 mg/kg (max 750 mg/dose) tid × 5–7 days	Amoebiasis, including amoebic liver abscess
		Adult PO: 250 mg bid × 5–7 days *Pediatric* PO: 25–35 mg/kg/day bid × 5–7 days	Giardiasis
		Adult only 1-day treatment PO: 2 g × 1 dose after a meal *Adult 10-day treatment* PO: 250 mg tid × 10 days	Trichomoniasis
paromomycin	Anti-amoebic aminoglycoside antibiotic (also has antibacterial properties, but is not normally used for this purpose)	*Adult and pediatric* PO: 25–35 mg/kg/day divided tid with meals × 5–10 days	Acute and chronic intestinal amoebiasis
pentamidine	Synthetic antipneumo-cystis agent	*Adult and pediatric* Inhalation aerosol: 300 mg q4wk IV/IM: 4 mg/kg/day × 14 days	Prophylaxis of PCP Treatment of active PCP

*A combination product containing atovaquone and proguanil is also used against malaria.
PCP, Pneumocystis carinii pneumonia.

250- and 500-mg capsules, a 250-mg tablet, and a 750-mg extended-release tablet, and parenterally in the form of a 5-mg/mL solution for intravenous (IV) infusion. It is also available in topical cream, lotion, and gel, and a vaginal gel. Pregnancy category X (first trimester) and B (second and third trimesters). Commonly recommended dosages are given in the dosages table above.

PHARMACOKINETICS

Half-Life	Onset	Peak	Duration
8–12 hr	>1.5 hr	PO: 1–2 hr	Variable

paromomycin

Paromomycin is an aminoglycoside antibiotic that is used for the treatment of intestinal amoebiasis. It directly kills intestinal protozoa when it comes in contact with them. Its bactericidal activity appears to be related to its ability to inhibit protein synthesis in susceptible organisms by binding to the 30S ribosomal subunit.

Contraindications include known drug allergy, renal failure, and gastrointestinal obstruction. It is only available in oral form as a 250-mg capsule. Pregnancy category C. Commonly recommended dosages are given in the dosages table above.

PHARMACOKINETICS

Half-Life	Onset	Peak	Duration
Unknown	Unknown	Unknown	Unknown

pentamidine

Pentamidine is an antiprotozoal agent that is used mainly for the management of *P. carinii* pneumonia, though it is sometimes used for treating various other protozoal infections. It works by inhibiting protein and nucleic acid synthesis. It is used both to treat active pneumocystosis and as prophylaxis in clients at high risk for initial or recurrent *Pneumocystis carinii* pneumonia (PCP), such as those with HIV/AIDS.

Hypersensitivity to the agent is the sole contraindication to its use. However, even if a given client does not tolerate inhaled forms of the drug, intramuscular (IM) or intravenous injection may still be necessary given the seriousness of PCP infection, and there are no absolute contraindications to the injectable routes of administration. The drug should also be used with caution in clients with blood dyscrasias, hepatic or renal disease, diabetes mellitus, cardiac disease, hypocalcemia, or hypertension. Pentamidine is available as a 300-mg vial of powdered drug for intravenous or intramuscular administration. Pregnancy category C. Commonly recommended dosages are given in the dosages table above.

PHARMACOKINETICS

Half-Life	Onset	Peak	Duration
6–9 hr	0.5–1 hr	<1 hr	Variable

HELMINTHIC INFECTIONS

Parasitic **helminthic infections** (worm infections) are a worldwide problem. No country is spared. It has been estimated that one-third of the world's population is infected with these parasites, but people in developing countries where sanitary conditions are often poor are by far the most common victims. The incidence of worm infections in the inhabitants of developed countries where sewage treatment is adequate is much lower, and usually only a few select helminthic diseases are the source of the problem. The most prevalent helminthic infection in Canada is enterobiasis, caused by one genus of roundworm, *Enterobius*.

Helminths that are parasitic in humans are classified in the following way:
- Platyhelminthes (flatworms)
- Cestodes (tapeworms)
- Trematodes (flukes)
- Nematoda (roundworms)

The characteristics of a few of the most common of the many helminthic infections are summarized in Table 41-8. These usually reside in the intestines of their host but can also reside in other tissues.

ANTHELMINTIC AGENTS

Unlike the single-celled protozoa, helminths are larger, have complex multicellular structures, and are members of the animal kingdom. Anthelmintic agents (also spelled *anthelminthic*) work to destroy these organisms by disrupting their structures. The currently available anthelmintic drugs in Canada are quite specific in the worms that they can kill. For this reason the causative worm in an infected host should be accurately identified before the start of treatment. This can usually be done by analyzing samples of feces, urine, blood, sputum, or tissue from the infected host for the presence of the particular parasite ova or larvae. However, sometimes the "suspected" worm will be treated.

The only anthelmintics commonly used in Canada are mebendazole and praziquantel.

Mebendazole is considered a broad spectrum anthelmintic and is used for single and mixed infestations. It is effective in the treatment of nematodes (pinworm, roundworm, whipworm, hookworm) and cestodes (large tapeworms) but not trematodes. Praziquantel is an agent that can kill trematodes (flukes, including schistosoma) but not nematodes and cestodes.

Mechanism of Action and Drug Effects

Mebendazole selectively and irreversibly inhibits the uptake of glucose and other nutrients. This results in the depletion of endogenous glycogen stores, eventual autolysis of the parasitic worm, and death. Praziquantel works by increasing the permeability of the cell membrane of susceptible worms to calcium. Calcium loss leads to contraction and paralysis of the worms' musculature, immobilizing their suckers so that they can no longer grip the wall of the mesenteric vein where they usually reside. They are then dislodged by normal blood flow and end up in the liver, where they are killed by host tissue reactions.

The anthelmintic agents have no drug effects other than the ability to kill various forms of worms and flukes.

Indications

Anthelmintic agents are used to treat roundworm, tapeworm, and fluke infection. Mebendazole is indicated specifically for trichuriasis (whipworm), enterobiasis, ascariasis, *Ancylostoma* infection (common hookworm), *Necator americanus* infection (American hookworm), *Strongyloides stercoralis*, and *Talenia solium* (large tapeworms). Praziquantel is indicated for schistosomiasis and opisthorchiasis (liver fluke).

Contraindications

The only usual contraindication to a specific anthelmintic drug product is known drug allergy. Praziquantel is also contraindicated in clients with *ocular cysticercosis* (tapeworm infection of the eye).

TABLE 41-8
HELMINTHIC INFECTIONS

Infection	Organism	Source	Site	Treatment
NEMATODA (ROUNDWORMS)				
Ascariasis	*Ascaris lumbricoides* (giant roundworm)		small intestine	mebendazole
Enterobiasis	*Enterobius vermicularis* (pinworm)		large intestine	mebendazole
PLATYHELMINTHES (INTESTINAL TAPEWORM OR FLATWORMS)				
Diphyllobothriasis	*Diphyllobothrium latum* (fishworm)	fish		niclosamide,* paromomycin, or praziquantel
Hymenolepiasis	*Hymenolepis nana* (dwarf tapeworm)			niclosamide,* paromomycin, or praziquantel
Taeniasis	*Taenia saginata* (beef tapeworm)	beef		niclosamide,* paromomycin, or praziquantel
	Taenia solium	pork		niclosamide,* paromomycin, or praziquantel

*Niclosamide is not available in Canada.

Side Effects and Adverse Effects

The adverse effects of mebendazole are limited to diarrhea, abdominal pain, and myelosuppression. Adverse effects of praziquantel include dizziness, headache, malaise, drowsiness, abdominal pain, and nausea.

Interactions

Praziquantel should be used with caution in clients with hepatic impairment or cardiac disease. It should not be used in pregnant women and breastfeeding should be stopped during treatment.

Dosages

For dosage information for selected anthelmintic agents, see the table below. See Appendix B for some of the common brands available in Canada.

DRUG PROFILES

Anthelmintics are available only as oral preparations and require a prescription. Different drugs are selected for different helminthic species.

▸▸ *mebendazole*

Mebendazole is a synthetic anthelmintic agent that may be used in the treatment of many types of roundworm and a few types of tapeworm infections. It is classified as a pregnancy category C agent, but it should be used in pregnant women only when the potential benefits justify the possible risks to the fetus. It is contraindicated in clients hypersensitive to it and is available only in an oral formulation as a 100-mg tablet. Commonly recommended dosages are listed in the dosages table below.

PHARMACOKINETICS

Half-Life	Onset	Peak	Duration
6–12 hr	<2 hr	2–4 hr	Variable

praziquantel

Praziquantel is one of the primary anthelmintic agents used for the treatment of various fluke infections. It is also useful against many species of tapeworm. It is contraindicated in clients who are hypersensitive to it and in clients with ocular worm infestation (ocular cysticercosis). It is available only in an oral formulation as a

600-mg film-coated tablet. Pregnancy category B. Commonly recommended dosages are listed in the dosages table below.

PHARMACOKINETICS

Half-Life	Onset	Peak	Duration
0.8–1.5 hr	<1 hr	1–3 hr	Variable

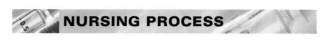

NURSING PROCESS

■ Assessment

Before beginning treatment with an antimalarial agent the nurse should obtain a thorough assessment and document the findings. Contraindications include pregnancy, porphyria, G6PD deficiency, and a history of drug allergy to these medications. Baseline vital signs should be checked, and any malaria-related symptoms (e.g., chills, profound sweating, headache, nausea, joint aching, and fatigue to exhaustion) documented. Other signs and symptoms include periodic diaphoresis (seating) and a remittent fever as high as 40° to 40.5°C. Baseline visual acuity and electrocardiogram (ECG) are also important to assess and document.

Antiprotozoal agents are contraindicated in clients with a history of hypersensitivity to the medication and in those with renal, cardiac, thyroid, or liver disease. Pregnancy is also a contraindication. The client's baseline visual acuity should be determined and documented. With any of the anthelmintic agents contraindications include pregnancy and a history of hypersensitivity. With these agents and other drugs discussed it is important for the nurse to assess and document the client's energy level, activities of daily living, weight, appetite, and symptoms. Along with contraindications and cautions, the nurse should assess for possible drug interactions (see Tables 41-2 and 41-7).

■ Nursing Diagnoses

Nursing diagnoses applicable to clients receiving any of the antimalarials, antiprotozoals, or anthelmintics include the following:
- Risk for injury related to medication side effects.
- Imbalanced nutrition, less than body requirements, related to the disease process and side effects of medication.

DOSAGES Selected Anthelmintic Agents

Agent	Pharmacological Class	Usual Dosage Range	Indications
▸▸ mebendazole	General anthelmintic	**Adult and pediatric >2 yr** PO: 100 mg single dose, repeat in 2–4 wks PO: 100 mg bid × 3 days	Enterobiasis Trichuriasis, ascariasis, ankylostomiasis, strongyloidiasis, taeniasis, mixed infections
praziquantel	Trematode anthelmintic	**Adult and pediatric >4 yr** PO: approx 25 mg/kg tid × 1 day PO: 20 mg/kg tid × 1 day	Fluke infections Schistosomiasis

- Deficient knowledge related to the infection and its treatment.
- Ineffective therapeutic regimen management related to poor adherence to treatment and lack of knowledge about the infection and its treatment.

■ Planning

Goals for clients being treated with any of the antiparasitic medications include the following:
- Client is free of self-injury related to the side effects of medication.
- Client maintains normal body weight during drug therapy.
- Client remains adherent with drug therapy for prescribed length of time.
- (when used for malaria prophylaxis) Client remains free of malarial symptoms.
- Client experiences minimal body image changes related to disease.
- Client states side effects of medication, as well as symptoms or adverse reactions to report to the physician.

■ *Outcome Criteria*

Outcome criteria for clients receiving any of the antiparasitic medications include the following:
- Client states measures to minimize self-injury related to the side effects of medication, such as dosing, time of day, and drug interactions.
- Client lists foods to be included in his or her diet, according to Canada's Food Guide, to improve overall health.
- Client states the symptoms of the infection, such as fever, lethargy, and loss of appetite.
- Client understands the rationale for treatment for prescribed length of time.
- Client states the symptoms to report to the physician, such as worsening of infection, anorexia, and fever.
- Client verbalizes feelings about altered body image openly with healthcare professional.
- Client states the importance of adhering with therapy and returning for follow-up visits to the physician to monitor progress and for adverse reactions.

■ Implementation

Chloroquine and hydroxychloroquine are administered orally and should be given exactly as prescribed. At the start of the treatment for malaria the client is given a loading dose, followed by half the dose on the next two days. For prophylaxis of malaria, treatment with these agents is usually started one to two weeks before the person is exposed to the region with malaria and for four weeks after the person has left the region; the medication is taken once weekly on the same day of the week during this time span. Mefloquine should be administered once weekly as ordered with at least 240 mL of water.

Any syrup forms of these agents should be stored in tight and closed containers to prevent chemical changes in the drug. Quinine sulphate, an antiprotozoal, must be administered intact because it is irritating to the GI mucosa. Most of the antiprotozoal agents (e.g., atovaquone, paromomycin) should be given with food when taken orally.

It is important when administering metronidazole or pentamidine by intramuscular or intravenous routes to follow drug company recommendations about dilution and intravenous infusion rates.

Anthelmintic agents should be administered as ordered and for a prescribed length of time.

See the box on p. 713 for teaching tips for clients receiving these agents.

■ Evaluation

The nurse should monitor the client for the therapeutic effects of the antimalarials, antiprotozoals, and anthelmintic agents, such as the decrease and/or resolution of all symptoms. If prolonged therapy is necessary with antimalarials, complete blood count (CBC) and urinalysis should be performed regularly and the client observed for the signs and symptoms of hemolysis. An ECG may be desirable before and during treatment if the client has or has had a cardiac disease. An eye examination should be done if the client experiences visual disturbances. Side effects to watch for are visual changes, possible irreversible retinal damage, cardiac dysrhythmias, and thrombocytopenia.

Antimalarial medications may precipitate hemolysis in clients with G6PD deficiency (mostly black clients and those of Mediterranean ancestry); therefore such clients should be closely monitored for hemolysis occurrence.

With antiprotozoal agents the client should be monitored for visual disturbances, GI distress, blurred vision, and altered hearing.

Clients taking anthelmintics should be monitored for fever, pallor, anorexia, and sudden decrease in red blood cells (RBCs), white blood cells (WBCs), and hemoglobin (Hgb).

CLIENT TEACHING TIPS

The nurse should instruct the client as follows:
▲ Keep all medications out of the reach of children.
▲ Take this medication exactly as prescribed, for the full prescribed period.
▲ (for most of these agents) Take with food to reduce the chance of upset stomach.

Antimalarials

▲ This medication often causes stomach upset; however, this may be decreased if the medication is taken with food. Contact your healthcare provider if you experience nausea, vomiting, profuse diarrhea, or abdominal pain.
▲ (for atovaquone) Take with food, preferably fatty foods.
▲ Quinidine products may cause dizziness, visual blurring, or yellow discoloration of the skin.
▲ Preventive treatment reduces the risk of malaria but does not eliminate it. Malaria can be effectively treated early on, but delay may result in a serious and even fatal outcome. Watch for symptoms of malaria, such as fever, chills, sweating, abdominal pain, muscle aches, and fatigue. These may occur as early as one week after first exposure and as late as several years after you have left the malarial region, but typically within three months.

▲ If you have had malaria, seek immediate treatment if your symptoms recur, such as high fever, chills, abdominal pain, and fatigue.
▲ Take your entire course of medication, as prescribed. Most antimalarials must be taken for four weeks after returning from a malaria-endemic area. (Atovaquone/proguanil, is taken for one week after returning.)
▲ Report any side effects to your physician, such as blurred vision or other visual disturbances, dizziness, headache, ringing in your ears, hearing problems, and upset stomach.

Metronidazole

▲ Be aware that this drug may leave a metallic taste in you mouth and your urine may turn dark.
▲ Do not consume alcohol in any form while taking this medication. A very unpleasant and even dangerous reaction can occur.

Anthelmintics

▲ Notify your physician immediately if you experience fatigue, fever, pallor, loss of appetite, darkened urine; or abdominal, leg, or back pain.

POINTS to REMEMBER

▼ Malaria is caused by *Plasmodium*, a particular genus of protozoa, and is transmitted by the bite of an infected female mosquito.
▼ Atovaquone 250 mg/proguanil HCl 100 mg is first-line chemoprophylaxis for chloroquine- and mefloquine-resistant malaria areas. Primaquine is an alternative chemoprophylactic agent when other regimens are contraindicated.
▼ Other common protozoal infections are amoebiasis, giardiasis, pneumocystosis, toxoplasmosis, and trichomoniasis. The most toxic protozoal infections are those caused by *Cryptosporidium* spp., *Isospora belli*, *P. carinii*, and *Toxoplasma gondii*.
▼ Protozoa are parasites that may be transmitted by person-to-person contact, contaminated water or food, direct contact with the parasite, or the bite of an insect (mosquito or tick).
▼ Antiprotozoals include atovaquone and pentamidine and are commonly used to treat *P. carinii* infections.
▼ Metronidazole is an antibacterial, antiprotozoal, and anthelmintic.

▼ Paromomycin directly kills protozoa such as *Entamoeba histolytica*.
▼ Anthelmintics are drugs used to treat parasitic worm infections caused by platyhelminthes (flatworms), cestodes (tapeworms), nematodes (roundworms), and trematodes (flukes).
▼ Nursing considerations include the following:
• Contraindications to the use of antimalarial agents include pregnancy, psoriasis, porphyria, G6PD deficiency, and a history of drug allergy.
• Baseline vital signs should be monitored and documented.
• Contraindications to the use of antiprotozoals include hypersensitivity; underlying renal, cardiac, thyroid, or liver disease; and pregnancy.
• Contraindications to the use of anthelmintics include a history of hypertension, hypersensitivity, visual difficulty, intestinal obstruction, inflammatory bowel disease, malaria, pregnancy, and severe hepatic, renal, or cardiac disease.

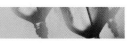

EXAMINATION REVIEW QUESTIONS

1 Which of the following would be appropriate to include in teaching clients about the side effects of antimalarials?
 a. Skin may turn "blotchy" while the client is on these medications.
 b. They may leave a metallic taste in the client's mouth and cause a loss of appetite.
 c. These drugs are not associated with GI upset and can be taken on an empty stomach.
 d. These agents may cause fever, anorexia, and alopecia.

2 Which of the following are drug interactions with antimalarials?
 a. Acetaminophen
 b. Ibuprofen
 c. Beta-blockers
 d. Vitamins

3 With use of antimalaria drugs, baseline assessment must include which of the following?
 a. ECG
 b. Ammonia levels
 c. Magnesium levels
 d. CT scan

4 Antimalarial drugs are used to treat clients with infections caused by which genus and species of protozoa?
 a. *Plasmodium* spp.
 b. *Candida albicans*
 c. *Pneumocystis carinii*
 d. *Mycobacterium tuberculosis*

For answers see http://evolve.elsevier.com/Lilley/pharmacology/.

CRITICAL THINKING ACTIVITIES

1 One of your clients has been taking the antiprotozoal agent atovaquone for *P. carinii* infection. What life-threatening reaction is related to the use of this drug? What should the nurse monitor for? Why is it also recommended that clients take atovaquone with meals (especially fatty foods)?

2 Your roommate is travelling to a country where there is high risk for malaria infection. She asks you what you

think the physician will order for her, if anything at all. After researching this, what would you most likely tell her?

3 What should be the emphasis of client teaching to a 21-year-old female who is travelling to a country with high risk of malaria exposure? Explain your answer.

For answers see http://evolve.elsevier.com/Lilley/pharmacology/.

BIBLIOGRAPHY

Albanese, J., & Nutz, P. (2005). *Mosby's 2005 nursing drug cards.* St Louis, MO: Mosby.

Canadian Pharmacists Association. (2003). *Therapeutic choices* (4th ed.). Ottawa, ON: Author.

Canadian Pharmacists Association. (2004). *Guide to drugs in Canada.* Toronto, ON: Dorling Kindersley.

Canadian Pharmacists Association. (2005). *Compendium of pharmaceuticals and specialties. The Canadian drug reference for health professionals.* Ottawa, ON: Author. [The subscription-based e-CPS is available at http://www.pharmacists.ca.]

Cheng, A., Williams, B.A., & Sivarajan, B.V. (Eds.). (2003). *The HSC handbook of pediatrics* (10th ed.). Toronto, ON: Elsevier.

Facts and Comparisons. (2004). *Drug facts and comparisons pocket version* (9th ed.). St Louis, MO: Wolters Kluwer Health.

Hardman, J.G., & Limbird, L.E. (2002). *Goodman and Gilman's the pharmacological basis of therapeutics* (10th ed.). New York: McGraw-Hill.

Health Canada. (2005). Drug product database (DPD). Retrieved August 29, 2005, from http://www.hc-sc.gc.ca/hpb/drugs-dpd/

Kasper, D.L., Braunwald, D., Faci, A., Hauser, S., Longo, D., & Jameson, J.L. (2005). *Harrison's principles of internal medicine* (16th ed.). New York: McGraw-Hill.

Katzung, B.G. (2004). *Basic and clinical pharmacology* (9th ed.). New York: McGraw-Hill.

Lacy, C.F., Armstrong, L.L., Goldman, M.P., & Lance, L.L. (2003). *Drug information handbook* (11th ed.). Hudson, OH: Lexi-Comp.

Lehne, R.A. (2004). *Pharmacology for nursing care* (5th ed.). St Louis, MO: Saunders.

Mandell, G.L., Bennett, J. E., & Dolin, R. (2005). *Principles and practice of infectious diseases* (6th ed.). Philadelphia: Elsevier Churchill Livingstone.

Mosby. (2005). *Mosby's drug consult 2005: The comprehensive reference for generic and brand name drugs* (15th ed.). St Louis, MO: Mosby.

Public Health Agency of Canada. (2004). Canadian recommendations for the prevention and treatment of malaria among international travellers. Retrieved August 29, 2005, from http://www.phac-aspc.gc.ca/publicat/ccdr-rmtc/04vol30/30s1/page9_e.html

Skidmore-Roth, L. (2006). *Mosby's 2006 nursing drug reference* (19th ed.). St Louis, MO: Mosby.

Antiseptic and Disinfectant Agents

CHAPTER
42

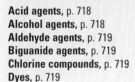

GLOSSARY

Acid A compound that yields hydrogen ions when dissociated in solution.

Aldehyde (al′ də hide) Any of a large category of organic compounds derived from a corresponding alcohol by the removal of two hydrogen atoms, as in the conversion of ethyl alcohol to acetaldehyde.

Antiseptic A chemical that can be applied to the surfaces of both living tissue and non-living objects that inhibits the growth and reproduction of micro-organisms without necessarily killing them. Antiseptics are also called static agents.

Community-acquired infection An infection acquired from the environment, including infections acquired indirectly through the use of medications.

Disinfectant A chemical applied to non-living objects to kill micro-organisms. Also called *cidal agents*.

Nosocomial infection (nos′ o koe′ mee əl) An infection acquired at least 72 hours after hospitalization, often caused by *Candida albicans*, *Escherichia coli*, hepatitis viruses, herpes zoster virus, *Pseudomonas* organisms, or *Staphylococcus* spp.; also called *hospital-acquired infection*.

Spore (1) A fastidious (hard to kill), dormant structure formed by certain bacterial species (e.g., *Bacillus* spp.). (2) The reproductive structure of certain lower micro-organisms, including protozoa and fungi.

Topical antimicrobial (an′ tee my kroe′ bee əl) A substance applied to any surface that either kills micro-organisms or inhibits their growth or replication.

COMMUNITY-ACQUIRED AND NOSOCOMIAL INFECTIONS

Infectious organisms—bacteria, fungi, and viruses—can be acquired from a number of different sources, such as hospitals, workplaces, nursing homes, and home. These can, however, be categorized into two main sites of origin: the community and the hospital. **Community-acquired infections** are defined as infections contracted either in the

TABLE 42-1

CHANGING PREVALENCE OF NOSOCOMIAL PATHOGENS

Period	Cause for Change	Pathogen
Before 1940	No antibiotics	Group A streptococci
Mid-1950s	Antibiotic era	Coagulase-positive *Staphylococcus aureus*
Today	New antibiotics	Gram-negative bacilli (*Pseudomonas* spp.), fungi or yeast *(Candida albicans),* herpesvirus, MRSA, VRE spp., *Clostridium difficile (C. difficile)*

MRSA, Multi-drug-resistant *Staphylococcus aureus; VRE,* vancomycin-resistant *Enterococcus.*

TABLE 42-2

ANTISEPTICS VERSUS DISINFECTANTS

	Antiseptics	Disinfectants
Where used	Living tissue	Non-living tissue
Toxic?	No	Yes
Potency	Less	More
Activity against organisms	Primarily inhibits growth (bacteriostatic)	Kills (bactericidal)

home or any place in the community outside of a healthcare facility. Hospital-acquired infections, more commonly known as **nosocomial infections**, are defined as those contracted in a hospital or institutional setting, such as a nursing home, that were not present or incubating in the client on admission to the hospital. In other words, they are acquired during the hospital stay and from the hospital. A newer, more general term is *healthcare-acquired infections,* recognizing that other types of healthcare facilities (e.g., clinics, dialysis centres) can also be sources of infection.

Nosocomial infections are much more difficult to treat, for several reasons. First, the causative micro-organisms have been exposed to many strong antibiotics in the past, and those that are left alive are the most drug resistant and the most virulent. The particular organisms that cause these infections have changed over time. These various pathogens and the reasons for their prevalence are summarized in Table 42-1.

Nosocomial infections develop in 5 to 10 percent of hospitalized clients, and the cost of treating them because of the extra hospitalization required amounts to nearly $3.9 million annually in Canada. Most of these infections (70 percent or more) are either urinary tract infections (UTIs) or post-operative wound infections. Often they are acquired from various devices, such as mechanical ventilators, intravenous (IV) infusion lines, catheters, and dialysis equipment. The risk of acquiring a nosocomial infection is particularly high in critical care, dialysis, oncology, transplant, and burn units. This is because the host defences of clients in these areas are typically compromised, making them more vulnerable to infection. Nurses need to be aware of both types of infections and the methods used to reduce their incidence.

TOPICAL ANTIMICROBIALS

Topical antimicrobials are agents that can be used to reduce the risk of nosocomial infections. They are substances that are applied to any surface for the purpose of

either inhibiting or killing as many micro-organisms as possible in a given pathogen population. There are two categories of these agents: antiseptics and disinfectants. **Disinfectants** are able to kill organisms and are used only on non-living objects to destroy organisms that may be present on them. They are sometimes called *cidal agents.* **Antiseptics** generally only inhibit the growth of micro-organisms but do not necessarily kill them. and are applied exclusively to living tissue. They are also called *static agents.* Often the terms *disinfectant* and *antiseptic* are used interchangeably and their actions and uses confused. However, it is important to keep the distinction in mind because using the wrong agent for the purpose can be harmful. The differences between disinfectants and antiseptics in a clinical sense are summarized in Table 42-2. Some antiseptic agents differ from disinfectants in their chemical makeup; others may simply be a diluted version of a disinfectant. Table 42-3 contains a list of these agents classified according to their chemical structure.

Mechanism of Action and Effects

Antimicrobial agents either inhibit the growth of micro-organisms or destroy them, but the extent to which they do this depends on the number and type of micro-organisms present, the concentration of the agent, the client's temperature, and the time of exposure to the agent. The mechanisms of action of the various antiseptics and disinfectants vary greatly. Some are strong oxidizing or alkylating agents; others work by damaging microbial cell walls. The various mechanisms are discussed by drug class in the drug profiles, but for the purpose of clarity the mechanisms by which the various agents either kill or inhibit the growth of micro-organisms are summarized in Table 42-4.

Indications

Living tissue such as skin and mucous membranes cannot be sterilized. However, the risk of infection can be minimized by reducing the number of micro-organisms on such tissues. Antiseptics are applied to these living tissues to inhibit the growth of the micro-organisms that typically reside on the tissue surfaces (normal flora) and that can do harm if they get into the body through an incision in the skin or by means of an injection. For example, these agents

TABLE 42-3

DISINFECTANTS AND ANTISEPTICS: CHEMICAL CATEGORIES

Agent	Antiseptic	Disinfectant
ACIDS		
Acetic	X	X
Benzoic	X	
Boric	X	
Lactic	X	
ALCOHOLS		
Ethanol	X	X
Isopropanol	X	X
ALDEHYDES		
Formaldehyde		X
Glutaraldehyde		X
BIGUANIDES		
Chlorhexidine gluconate	X	
DYES		
Gentian violet	X	
Carbol-fuchsin	X	
HALOGENS		
Chlorine Compounds		
Sodium hypochlorite	X	X
Halazone		X
Iodine Compounds		
Iodine (tincture and solution)	X	X
Iodophors (povidone)	X	
Mercurials		
Merbromin	X	
Thimerosal	X	
Yellow mercuric oxide	X	
Silver		
Silver nitrate	X	
NITROFURAZONE	X	
OXIDIZING AGENTS		
Benzoyl peroxide	X	
Hydrogen peroxide	X	X
Potassium permanganate	X	
PHENOLIC COMPOUNDS		
Hexachlorophene	X	
Hexylresorcinol	X	
Resorcinol	X	
SURFACE-ACTIVE AGENTS		
Benzalkonium chloride	X	
Cetylpyridinium chloride	X	

are contained in the presurgical scrubs (soaps) used by members of surgical teams to wash their hands in preparation for surgery. They are also applied to the client's skin before the incision is made. The removal of germs is only temporary, and is limited to the skin surface. However, during emergency surgical operations, antiseptic solutions may be quickly poured or splashed onto the skin surface or used to irrigate the open surgical field when the urgency of the situation does not permit sufficient time for the usual pre-operative skin cleansing.

Systemic agents (e.g., cefazolin, 1 g intravenously preop) are often administered to surgical clients as prophylaxis against infection caused by micro-organisms living in the internal body environment (see Chapter 37). Antimicrobial agents, including antiseptics, are also commonly used to irrigate body cavities either directly during surgery or through specially designed transdermal catheter devices. Besides these surgical soaps and topical solutions, antiseptics are also contained in salves, ointments, mouthwashes, and douches.

Inanimate objects such as tabletops and surgical equipment may be treated with disinfectants, as well as by autoclaving, radiation, heat, and so on. Disinfectants are also used on instruments and other inanimate objects (fomites) that may harbour pathogens and introduce them into a new host. Instruments acquire microbes by being placed on or inserted into anatomic sites in clients where many organisms naturally dwell (e.g., thermometers, which are placed orally, rectally, or under the axilla; and colonoscopes, which are used in examinations of the lower GI tract [colonoscopy]). Before their use in other clients, the bacteria, fungi, viruses, and **spores** that may have been acquired from the previous client's tissues must be removed from the instrument surfaces.

The therapeutic effects of the antiseptics and disinfectants vary from class to class. Some agents are potent and effective against many types of micro-organisms. Others are less potent and have limited activity against only a few micro-organisms. The range of micro-organisms against which these agents are effective is indicated for the various chemical classes of antimicrobial agents in Table 42-5.

Contraindications

The only usual contraindication to the use of a particular antiseptic agent is known client allergy to a specific product.

Side Effects and Adverse Effects

Antiseptics and disinfectants are safe agents, relatively speaking, and when used in the appropriate manner they are effective. However, some of them are capable of causing some side effects and adverse effects, mostly topical skin irritations. The others have no known adverse effects but at most may cause some skin irritation if used in exceedingly high concentrations. The agents and their side effects and adverse effects are summarized in Table 42-6.

Interactions

Few drugs interact with the antiseptics, although other topical agents that also irritate the skin may produce an additive effect when given in combination. In addition, a

TABLE 42-4

ANTISEPTICS AND DISINFECTANTS: MECHANISMS OF ACTION

Agent	Mechanism of Action	Comments
Alcohols	Denature or essentially destroy the micro-organism's protein; some may directly lyse the micro-organism.	60–70% concentration, most effective; >90% or <60% concentration, ↓ bactericidal activity.
Aldehydes	Act via alkylation, inhibiting the formation of the essential amino acid methionine.	Bacteriostatic or bactericidal depending on concentration.
Biguanides	Disrupt bacterial cytoplasmic membranes and inhibit membrane-bound ATPase (inhibit cell wall synthesis).	Chlorhexidine.
Halogens	Precipitate protein and oxidize essential enzymes by binding to and changing structure of proteins.	Iodine compounds: bactericidal; mercurials: bacteriostatic; chlorine compounds: bactericidal.
Oxidizing agents	Attack membrane lipids, DNA, and other essential components of the cell.	3–6% concentration: bactericidal and virucidal; 10–25% concentration: sporicidal.
Phenolic compounds	Interrupt bacterial electron transport (cellular respiration of micro-organisms) and inhibit other membrane-bound enzymes; high concentrations rupture bacterial membranes.	Bacteriostatic or bactericidal depending on concentration.
Surface-active agents	Denature or essentially destroy the micro-organism's protein, cell membrane, and cytoplasm components.	↓ Concentrations: bacteriostatic; ↑ concentrations: bactericidal and fungicidal.

ATPase, Adenosinetriphosphatase.

TABLE 42-5

ANTISEPTICS AND DISINFECTANTS: THERAPEUTIC EFFECTS

	Therapeutic Effects				
Agent	Bacteria	Tubercle Bacilli	Fungi	Viruses	Spores
Alcohols	X	X	X	X	
Aldehydes	X	X	X	X	X
Chlorhexidine	X		X		
Chlorine compounds	X	X	X	X	
Dyes	X				
Iodine compounds	X	X	X	X	x
Mercurial compounds	x				
Oxidizing agents	X			X	x
Phenolic compounds	X	X	X	X	
Silver compounds	X				
Surface-active agents	X		X	x	

X, Static or cidal activity; *x,* some activity if high concentrations of agent and lengthy exposure.

topical agent that augments the systemic absorption of an antiseptic may increase the likelihood of systemic toxicity from that agent. However, because most of these agents are used for short periods there is little opportunity for them to interact with other agents. Because disinfectants are not used for direct topical application to clients there is of course no opportunity for drug interactions to occur.

Dosages

For information on the recommended dosages and concentrations for selected antimicrobial agents, see the dosages table on p. 720. See Appendix B for some of the common brands available in Canada.

DRUG PROFILES

Following are descriptions of the various chemical categories of antimicrobials.

ACID AGENTS

Acetic acid (vinegar), benzoic acid, boric acid, and lactic acid are all members of the **acid** family of antiseptic and disinfectant agents. They are commonly used because of their practicality, availability, and low cost. All of these acid agents either kill micro-organisms or inhibit their growth by creating an acidic environment for organisms that require a neutral or alkaline medium to live and grow. Acetic acid in a 5 percent solution kills many organisms. In this concentration it is used as a vaginal douche for antisepsis and as a mild antiseptic deodorant for the collection containers of indwelling urinary drainage catheters, for bladder irrigation, and for diaper soaks. Acetic acid is also used as a buffer in hemodialysis solution. See the dosages table on p. 720 for dosage and concentration information.

ALCOHOL AGENTS

Isopropanol (isopropyl alcohol) and ethanol are both members of the alcohol category of antiseptics. The alcohol solutions are most effective at a concentration of 60 to 70 percent; at a concentration of more than 95 percent or less than 60 percent their "cidal" activity dramatically decreases.

TABLE 42-6

ANTISEPTIC AND DISINFECTANT AGENTS: ADVERSE EFFECTS

Body System	Side/Adverse Effects
ALCOHOLS	
Integumentary	Excessive dryness of the skin.
ALDEHYDES	
Integumentary	Burns to skin or mucous membranes.
CHLORHEXIDINE GLUCONATE	
Central nervous	Use as a pre-operative scrub or as a wash for neonates and burn clients has been stopped because absorption from the skin into systemic circulation has resulted in serious CNS toxicity.
HEXYLRESORCINOL	
Hepatic	Toxicity resulting from systemic absorption from the skin.
Cardiovascular	Myocardial toxicity resulting from systemic absorption from the skin.
Integumentary	May produce burns on skin or mucous membranes.
IODINE COMPOUNDS	
Integumentary	Iodine at concentrations >3% may produce skin blistering. Burns may appear with *tincture of iodine* when the treated area is covered with an occlusive dressing. It may stain skin and cause irritation and pain at wound sites.
SURFACE-ACTIVE AGENTS	
Integumentary	Chemical burns if left in contact with skin for too long, as in wet packs for occlusive dressings.

These agents kill micro-organisms by either denaturing their cellular proteins or directly lysing their cell membranes. Both isopropyl and ethyl alcohol are able to kill bacteria, tubercle bacilli, fungi, and viruses. See the dosages table on p. 720 for the concentration information on isopropanol.

ALDEHYDE AGENTS

Formaldehyde and glutaraldehyde are members of the **aldehyde** category of agents. These disinfectants act by means of alkylation, inhibiting the formation of the essential amino acid methionine. This either kills organisms or inhibits their growth, depending on the concentration of the solution. The aldehydes, such as formaldehyde and glutaraldehyde, are active against all types of micro-organisms, including bacteria, tubercle bacilli, fungi, viruses, and spores. Because these agents are somewhat caustic, they can cause burns to the skin or mucous membranes if used as antiseptics. For this reason they are used mostly as disinfectants. Formaldehyde comes in a 23-percent concentration and glutaraldehyde in a 2-percent solution. Both agents are commonly used as disinfectants for instruments, with glutaraldehyde preferred for disinfecting and sterilizing surgical equipment. See the dosages table on p. 720 for the concentration information for formaldehyde.

BIGUANIDE AGENTS

Chlorhexidine gluconate is a biguanide agent with antiseptic activity. Biguanides act by disrupting bacterial cytoplasmic membranes and inhibiting membrane-bound adenosinetriphosphatase (ATPase), which results in the inhibition of cell wall synthesis. Chlorhexidine is active against both gram-positive and gram-negative bacteria.

It is used as a bactericidal skin cleansing solution and is useful as a surgical scrub, a handwashing agent for healthcare personnel, and a skin wound cleanser. It may also be used to treat aphthous ulcers of the mouth and for the prevention of dental caries. When used as directed it causes few side effects. See the dosages table on p. 720 for concentration information.

DYES

Gentian violet, crystal violet, methyl violet, brilliant green, and fuchsin are all rosaniline dyes. These are basic dyes that are currently used only occasionally as antiseptic or antiprotozoal agents. Gentian violet is used topically as a 1- to 2-percent preparation, and it has both antibacterial and antifungal activity. See the dosages table on p. 720 for dosage information.

CHLORINE COMPOUNDS

Chlorine compounds actively kill bacteria, tubercle bacilli, and viruses but are only partially active against fungi. They have no activity against spores. Dilute sodium hypochlorite is commonly used as an antiseptic irrigation. Its antibacterial action is due to the hypochlorous acid that forms when chlorine reacts with water. Hypochlorous acid is rapidly antibacterial.

Sodium hypochlorite in a 10.8-percent solution is commonly used to disinfect utensils, walls, furniture, floors, and swimming pools; in a 0.5 percent solution it is used on skin surfaces for the treatment of fungous infections such as athlete's foot (tinea pedis). The strength of most household bleach solutions such as Javex or Clorox is 5.25 percent sodium hypochlorite. Public health outreach programs are giving small bottles of bleach to intravenous drug users, who frequently share needles and are

DOSAGES **Selected Antiseptic and Disinfectant Agents**

Agent	Pharmacological Class	Usual Concentration or Dosage Range	Indications
acetic acid	Antibacterial, antifungal acid, microbial	Solution: 2%, 4–5% (vinegar)	Antibacterial, antifungal
benzalkonium chloride	Broad-spectrum cationic detergent, surface-active antimicrobial	Solution 0.08% dilutions Antiseptic towel/wipe: 0.4% Topical spray Otic solution/powder	Skin cleanser, instrument storage, surface cleaner
carbolic acid	Phenolic antiseptic	Spray: 0.5% Gargle: 1.4%	Oral antiseptic Topical anaesthetic
chlorhexidine gluconate	Broad-spectrum biguanide antimicrobial	Liquid: 20% Soap: 2% Sponge: 0.05%	Cleanser, surgical scrub
formaldehyde	Broad-spectrum aldehyde antimicrobial	Solution: 0.23% Topical lotion: 2%	General disinfectant Skin-drying agent
gentian violet	Antibacterial/antifungal dye	Solution: 1%, 2%; apply qd–bid	Topical anti-infective
hydrogen peroxide	Oxidizing agent	Solution: 3%, 6%, 35%	Wound cleansing, antiseptic
iodine	Broad-spectrum iodine antimicrobial	Solution/tincture: 2.5%, apply once to twice daily	Topical antiseptic
isopropanol	General alcohol antiseptic/disinfectant/astringent	Solution: 62%, 70%, 75%, 99%	Skin astringent, cleansing agent, utensil disinfectant
povidone-iodine	Broad-spectrum iodine antimicrobial	Aerosol: 5% Topical stick: 0.75%, 10% Topical ointment: 10% Topical liquid: 21% Solution: 10% Mouthwash: 1.0% Surgical scrub: 7.5% Prep pad: 1% Vaginal douche: 10% Vaginal suppository: 200 mg	Topical antiseptic
sodium hypochlorite	Broad-spectrum antimicrobial/disinfective	Solution: Numerous strengths/concentrations available	Topical antiseptic
thimerosal	Organomercurial antiseptic	Solution: 0.2%, 0.3%, 0.375%, 0.4%; apply once to three times daily	Topical antiseptic

at increased risk for HIV, in the hope that if they do share injection equipment they will at least disinfect it, thus reducing the spread of HIV and other dangerous microbes. See the dosages table above for dosage information.

Halazone is a chloramine compound. Chloramines are chlorine-related compounds but are more stable, less irritating, and slower and more prolonged in their action than their chlorine cousins. Halazone is the only chloramine product used in Canada. It is available in tablet form for sanitizing drinking water. Adding 1 or 2 tablets to a litre of water can kill water-borne pathogens within 30 to 60 minutes.

MERCURIAL AGENTS

Topical mercurial antiseptics are relatively weak in their actions. They are primarily bacteriostatic agents whose effectiveness is enhanced by the vehicle in which they

are contained. Inorganic mercury compounds such as ammoniated mercury ointment owe their effectiveness primarily to these vehicles, which sustain the bacteriostatic action of the agent. Organic mercurial agents such as thimerosal are more bacteriostatic, less irritating, and less toxic than inorganic mercurials. Other mercury compounds used as topical anti-infectives include merbromin, yellow mercuric oxide, and triclosan. Mercurial antiseptics probably act by inhibiting bacterial sulphhydryl enzymes, but they may also inhibit tissue enzymes as well, which reduces their usefulness. Ammoniated mercury is used for the treatment of psoriasis, impetigo, dermatomycoses, pediculosis pubis (crabs), seborrheic dermatitis, and superficial pyodermas (pus-producing skin infections). Skin irritations, as well as hypersensitivity to the agents, have been reported as side effects of these compounds. See the

TABLE 42-7

IODINE FORMULATIONS

Iodine Formulation	Composition	Uses
Aqueous solution	5% iodine and 5% potassium iodide	These forms of iodine are used preoperatively to disinfect the skin. They are applied topically for their antimicrobial effects against bacteria, fungi, viruses, protozoa, and yeasts.
Iodine topical solution	2.5% iodine	
Iodine tincture	2% iodine in alcohol solution	
Strong iodine solution	5% iodine in alcohol	
Povidone-iodine	Iodine with polyvinylpyrrolidone	Used as a 10% applicator solution or as a 2% scrub, spray, foam, vaginal gel, ointment, mouthwash, perineal wash, or whirlpool concentrate.
Tincture of iodine	2% iodine and 2.5% potassium iodide in 83.7% ethyl alcohol	For cutaneous infections caused by bacteria and fungi. Even a 1% tincture will kill almost an entire bacterial population in 1.5 min. Three drops in 1 L of drinking water will reduce amoeba and bacteria counts in 15 min without impairing palatability.
Iodophors	Iodine compounds with a carrier that acts as a sustained-release pool of iodine	Widely used as antiseptics.

dosages table on p. 720 for the dosage information for thimerosal.

IODINE COMPOUNDS

Iodine (tincture and solution) is a non-metallic element that readily forms salts when combined with many other elements. Although it is a non-metallic element, it has a bluish black metallic lustre and a characteristic odour. It is only slightly soluble in water but is completely soluble in alcohol and in aqueous solutions of sodium iodide and potassium iodide. Iodine tincture and solution are both active against and kill all forms of micro-organisms: bacteria, tubercle bacilli, fungi, viruses, and spores. Their activity against spores depends on the concentration and the timing of administration. There are actually many forms of iodine, some of which are listed in Table 42-7. See the dosages table on p. 720 for the recommended dosages and concentrations of a few of them.

OXIDIZING AGENTS

Hydrogen peroxide is one of three members of the oxidizing family of antiseptic agents, the other agents being benzoyl peroxide and potassium permanganate. Oxidizing agents work by attacking membrane lipids, DNA, and other essential components of the micro-organism's cell. In concentrations of 3 to 6 percent they are bactericidal and virucidal; at 10 to 35 percent they are sporicidal.

The use of hydrogen peroxide as a solution to irrigate wounds is controversial. It can destroy newly forming cells as well as bacteria.

PHENOLIC COMPOUNDS

Carbolic acid (phenol) and Lysol are phenolic compounds used primarily as disinfectants. Because these agents cause burning and possibly blistering, they should not be allowed to come in contact with the skin in concentrations stronger than 2 percent and never in contact with areas where the skin is broken.

Phenolic compounds work by interrupting bacterial electron transport (cellular respiration of micro-organisms) and inhibiting other membrane-bound enzymes. At high concentrations they rupture bacterial membranes. Depending on the concentration of the phenolic compound they can be either static or cidal in their actions. The phenolic compounds are active against bacteria, tubercle bacilli, fungi, and viruses, but not spores. See the dosages table on p. 720 for concentration information on carbolic acid.

Hexachlorophene and resorcinol are two other phenolic compounds. Hexachlorophene is available by prescription only and is used as a surgical scrub as well as a bacteriostatic skin cleanser. Its use should be avoided in infants because they are particularly susceptible to transdermal absorption of this agent, with the risk of such serious neurotoxic effects as seizures. Resorcinol is bactericidal and fungicidal and is about one-third as effective as carbolic acid. It is used to treat acne, ringworm, eczema, psoriasis, seborrheic dermatitis, and similar skin lesions.

SURFACE-ACTIVE AGENTS

Benzalkonium chloride and cetylpyridinium chloride are surface-active agents. They work by denaturing the micro-organism or essentially destroying its protein, cell membrane, and cytoplasm components. At low concentrations they are bacteriostatic and at high concentrations they are bactericidal and fungicidal. These agents are used to treat bacteria, fungi, and some viral topical infections.

Substances such as organic matter, soaps, anionic detergents, and tap water that contain metallic ions will absorb the active ingredient and thereby weaken the surface-acting agent. See the dosages table on p. 720 for concentration information on benzalkonium chloride.

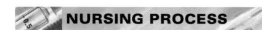

NURSING PROCESS

Assessment

When any type of topical medication such as an antiseptic is to be administered, the concentration of the medication, length of exposure to the skin, condition of the skin, size of area affected, and hydration status of the skin must be taken into consideration. Before applying any topical medication, it is important for the nurse to find out whether the client has any drug allergies or has shown any previous sensitivity to antiseptics or other topical agents. If an iodine-based agent such as povidone-iodine is being applied, the nurse should question the client about allergies to iodine or seafood, which are contraindications. Clients being treated with peroxide agents should be asked about previous allergies and local reactions to the medication.

The risk of reactions to the antibacterial topical agents is greater because of the sensitivity of clients to antibiotics in different dosage forms. Should a client have an allergy to a particular type of antibacterial agent, that specific agent should not be used topically, regardless of the dosage form. Culture and sensitivity reports will identify appropriate antibacterial therapy.

Nursing Diagnoses

Nursing diagnoses appropriate for the use of antiseptics include the following:

- Risk for infection related to compromised skin integrity.
- Risk for infection related to skin trauma or injury resulting from adverse reactions to the topical agent.
- Deficient knowledge related to topical agents and their proper use.

Planning

Goals related to the administration of antiseptics include the following:

- Client remains free of adverse reactions to the agent when used for the treatment of skin injury or infection.
- Client shows evidence of resolution of infection.
- Client is adherent with the medication regimen.
- Client experiences minimal to no adverse reactions to medication.
- Client returns for follow-up visits with physician if recommended.

Outcome Criteria

Outcome criteria in clients treated with antiseptics include the following:

- Client experiences minimal discomfort (such as stinging, itching, burning) from the use of the agent.
- Client experiences maximal therapeutic effects of medication once therapy is complete, with intact skin and no redness or drainage.

- Client demonstrates proper technique for applying topical antiseptic with applicator, tongue blade, gloved hand, and proper handwashing technique.
- Client states those situations (adverse reactions to medication or worsening of symptoms of infection) when the physician should be notified immediately.

Implementation

Before applying any topical agent, the nurse should check the physician's order, gather the needed supplies, and wash his or her hands. Standard Precautions should be followed (see Box 9-1). Non-sterile gloves are adequate if the skin is intact and there are no indications of additional risk factors; if the skin is not intact or the nurse judges it appropriate, sterile gloves and technique should be used. The nurse should follow any specific application directions (e.g., the order may specify that the agent be applied with a tongue depressor or that an occlusive dressing be placed). As with any procedure, the nurse should always ensure the client's privacy and comfort level. The skin site should be thoroughly cleansed. In general, before additional doses of a topical medication are applied, the site should be cleansed not only of any debris but also of any residual medication, using soap and water or normal saline (NS).

When using a lotion, the nurse should store it under the conditions recommended by the manufacturer and shake it well before using. Creams and ointments are often applied with a sterile cotton-tipped applicator or tongue blade. Any dressings should be applied as ordered and special attention paid to the directions for the application of occlusive, wet, or wet-to-dry dressings. Client education about the medication and dressings is important to the safe and effective use of these agents. The nurse should make sure to document the site of application and any drainage from the site, whether there is any swelling, the temperature and colour of the site, and any pain or other sensations.

After administering the medication, the nurse should wash his or her hands, dispose of contaminated dressings, record the nature of the procedure and findings, and maintain asepsis (surgical asepsis if the wound is open in any way or if the skin is not intact). The nurse should always make sure that the client is in no danger of causing harm to the site.

Client teaching tips for antiseptic agents are presented on p. 723.

Evaluation

When antiseptics are used, the client's therapeutic response may be manifested by improved healing of the affected area or decreased symptoms of inflammation or infection. When the agent is used prophylactically, such as preoperatively, the therapeutic response is prevention of infection. When using disinfectants on inanimate objects the nurse must ensure that clients are not exposed to the agent. It is also important for the nurse to evaluate clients for any side effects or adverse reactions (see Table 42-6).

CLIENT TEACHING TIPS

Nurses should teach clients how to properly apply the medication, dressings, and bandage and how to change any dressings so that they can do these things at home after discharge. The nurse should make sure the client or caregiver can do these tasks adequately. Clients should also be given written instructions, pamphlets, or other aids that clarify the procedure and reinforce the importance of doing it correctly.

The nurse should instruct clients as follows:

▲ Wash your hands before and after applying any topical medication. Handwashing is extremely important because it avoids contaminating the wound and helps to prevent the spread of infection.

▲ Make sure you have all the supplies you need at home (e.g., tape, gauze dressings and pads, tongue blades, cotton-tipped applicators, and gloves).

▲ Follow the instructions you have been given on applying medication and changing dressings. Shake lotions well before use and apply gently but firmly by tapping the skin surface area. Use a tongue blade or cotton-tipped applicator to apply creams and ointments.

▲ Note any unusual odour, drainage, or colour of the skin.

POINTS to REMEMBER

▼ Topical antimicrobials (antiseptics and disinfectants) are used to reduce the risk of nosocomial infections and are applied to topical surfaces to inhibit or kill as many micro-organisms as possible.

▼ Disinfectants are antimicrobials that are used only on non-living objects and that kill any organisms on these objects. They are *not* the same as antiseptics.

▼ Antiseptics are antimicrobials that are used only on living tissues and primarily inhibit growth and reproduction of micro-organisms.

▼ Antiseptics and disinfectants are categorized by their chemical makeup and include such agents as alcohols, aldehydes, phenolic compounds, biguanides, surface-active agents, acid agents, dyes, oxidizing agents, chlorine and iodine compounds, and mercurial agents.

▼ Nursing considerations include the following:
• Always observe Standard Precautions whenever applying topical agents.
• Always apply these agents to clean, dry skin unless otherwise ordered or specified.
• Be sure to instruct clients concerning the proper application technique before their discharge home.

EXAMINATION REVIEW QUESTIONS

1 Which of the following statements best describes the purpose of antimicrobials?
a. Bactericidal function and use in all open wounds
b. Reduction of all viral risks to the client
c. Disinfectant purpose to reduce all levels of bacteria
d. Reduction in risk of some nosocomial infections

2 Which of the following is considered to be a property of an antiseptic agent?
a. Useful on non-living tissues
b. More potent than a disinfectant
c. Bacteriostatic
d. Bactericidal

3 Which of the following is a commonly identifiable pathogen found in newly prevalent nosocomial infections?
a. *Neisseria*
b. *Haemophilus influenzae*

c. Hepatitis C
d. Gram-negative bacilli

4 Which of the following most correctly describes topical disinfectants?
a. Are bactericidal to non-living tissue
b. Sterilize all surfaces
c. Prevent spread of herpes and HIV
d. Kill all living tissue in the organism

5 Which of the following substances would be most effective to kill bacteria on an operating room floor?
a. A vaccine
b. An antiseptic
c. An antibiotic
d. A disinfectant

For answers see http://evolve.elsevier.com/Lilley/pharmacology/.

CRITICAL THINKING ACTIVITIES

1 What is the main purpose of using antiseptics and disinfectants?

2 Can disinfectants and antiseptics be used interchangeably? Why or why not?

3 How would you know that a client is having a therapeutic response to an antiseptic?

For answers see http://evolve.elsevier.com/Lilley/pharmacology/.

BIBLIOGRAPHY

Albanese, J., & Nutz, P. (2005). *Mosby's 2005 nursing drug cards.* St Louis, MO: Mosby.

Canadian Pharmacists Association. (2003). *Therapeutic choices* (4th ed.). Ottawa, ON: Author.

Canadian Pharmacists Association. (2004). *Guide to drugs in Canada.* Toronto, ON: Dorling Kindersley.

Canadian Pharmacists Association. (2005). *Compendium of pharmaceuticals and specialties. The Canadian drug reference for health professionals.* Ottawa, ON: Author. [The subscription-based e-CPS is available at http://www.pharmacists.ca.]

Cheng, A., Williams, B.A., & Sivarajan, B.V. (Eds.). (2003). *The HSC handbook of pediatrics* (10th ed.). Toronto, ON: Elsevier.

Health Canada. (2005). Drug product database (DPD). Retrieved August 30, 2005, from http://www.hc-sc.gc.ca/hpb/drugs-dpd/

Facts and Comparisons. (2004). *Drug facts and comparisons pocket version* (9th ed.). St Louis, MO: Wolters Kluwer Health.

Lacy, C.F., Armstrong, L.L., Goldman, M.P., & Lance, L.L. (2003). *Drug information handbook* (11th ed.). Hudson, OH: Lexi-Comp.

Lehne, R. A. (2004). *Pharmacology for nursing care* (5th ed.). St Louis, MO: Saunders.

Mosby. (2005). *Mosby's drug consult 2005: The comprehensive reference for generic and brand name drugs* (15th ed.). St Louis, MO: Mosby.

Skidmore-Roth, L. (2006). *Mosby's 2006 nursing drug reference* (19th ed.). St Louis, MO: Mosby.

Thibodeau, G.A., & Patton, K.T. (2003). *Anatomy and physiology* (5th ed.). St Louis, MO: Mosby.

Anti-Inflammatory, Antirheumatic, and Related Agents

OBJECTIVES

After reading this chapter, the successful student will be able to do the following:

1 Discuss the inflammatory response and the part it plays in the generation of pain.

2 Compare the various disease processes that are often identified as inflammatory in nature, such as rheumatoid arthritis, osteoarthritis, degenerative joint disorders, and gout.

3 Contrast the various non-steroidal anti-inflammatory drugs (NSAIDs), anti-gout agents, and antirheumatic agents in relation to their mechanisms of action, indications, side effects, dosage ranges, cautions, contraindications, drug interactions, and toxicities.

4 Develop a nursing care plan that includes all phases of the nursing process for the client receiving NSAIDs, anti-gout agents, antirheumatic agents, and other anti-inflammatory agents.

e-LEARNING ACTIVITIES

Student CD-ROM
- Review Questions: see questions 322–331
- Animations
- Medication Administration Checklists
- IV Therapy Checklists

evolve **Web site** (http://evolve.elsevier.com/Lilley/pharmacology/)
- Online Chapter Worksheet • Frequently Asked Questions
- Learning Tips and Content Updates • WebLinks • Online Appendices and Supplements • Mosby/Saunders ePharmacology Update • Access to *Mosby's Drug Consult*

DRUG PROFILES
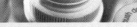

▶▶ allopurinol, p. 735
▶▶ acetylsalicylic acid, p. 732
auranofin, p. 737
gold sodium thiomalate, p. 737
▶▶ celecoxib, p. 734
colchicine, p. 736

etanercept, p. 737
▶▶ ibuprofen, p. 734
indomethacin, p. 733
▶▶ ketorolac, p. 734
leflunomide, p. 737
probenecid, p. 736
sulfinpyrazone, p. 736

▶▶ Key drug.

GLOSSARY

Acute salicylate overdose (sal i′ sil′ ate) Produces signs and symptoms similar to those of chronic intoxication, but the effects are often more pronounced and occur more quickly.

Chronic salicylate intoxication A toxic condition caused by the ingestion of salicylate, most often in ASA or oil of wintergreen.

Disease-modifying antirheumatic drugs (DMARDs) Medications used in the treatment of rheumatic diseases that have the potential to arrest or slow the actual disease process as opposed to, like the non-steroidal anti-inflammatory drugs (NSAIDs), providing only anti-inflammatory and analgesic effects.

Done nomogram (nom′ ə gram) A standard plot of graphic data, originally published in 1960 in the journal *Pediatrics*, for rating the severity of acetylsalicylate toxicity following overdose. Serum salicylate levels are plotted against time elapsed after ingestion.

Non-steroidal anti-inflammatory drugs (NSAIDs) A large and chemically diverse group of drugs that possess analgesic, anti-inflammatory, antirheumatic, and antipyretic (fever-reducing) activity.

Salicylism (sal′ i sil′ iz əm) The syndrome of salicylate toxicity, including such symptoms as tinnitus (ringing in the ears), nausea, and vomiting.

725

NON-STEROIDAL ANTI-INFLAMMATORY DRUGS

Non-steroidal anti-inflammatory drugs (NSAIDs) are among the most commonly prescribed drugs. Every year approximately ten million prescriptions are written for these agents in Canada. This represents over 5 percent of all prescriptions. There are currently more than 15 different NSAIDs available in Canada. Some are used much more commonly than others, and a given client may respond better to some NSAIDs than others, both in terms of symptom relief and side effect profile. NSAIDs comprise a large and chemically diverse group of drugs that possess analgesic, anti-inflammatory, antirheumatic, and antipyretic activity. The list of uses for these versatile drugs is as lengthy as the list of agents. They are used for the relief of mild to moderate headaches, myalgia, neuralgia, and arthralgia; alleviation of postoperative pain; inhibition of platelet aggregation; relief of the pain associated with arthritic disorders such as rheumatoid arthritis, juvenile arthritis, ankylosing spondylitis, and osteoarthritis; and treatment of gout and hyperuricemia.

The use of plants containing salicylates as medicinal agents goes back more than 1000 years. North American Aboriginal people used willow bark juice as an antipyretic, and South African Hottentots used a similar mixture as an antirheumatic. Willow and poplar were used as sources of medicinal compounds by both Greek and Roman physicians. Such notable physicians as Hippocrates, Pliny the Elder, and Celsus all chronicled the beneficial effects of these salicylate-containing agents in the treatment of such diverse ailments as gout, fever, sciatica, and earache.

The most common and first drug in this class was salicylic acid, and it was Hermann Kolbe who devised an economical procedure for the manufacture of a synthetic form of salicylic acid, which made its mass production, and hence availability, possible. Subsequently, in 1899 the most famous descendent of salicylic acid, acetylsalicylic acid (ASA, aspirin), was marketed and rapidly became the most widely used drug in the world. The success of ASA established the importance of drugs with antipyretic, analgesic, anti-inflammatory, and antirheumatic properties—the properties that all NSAIDs share.

However, along with its widespread use came evidence of its potential for causing major toxicological effects. Gastrointestinal intolerance, bleeding, and renal impairment became major factors limiting its long-term administration. As a result, efforts were mounted to develop agents that did not have the side effects of aspirin. This led to the discovery of other NSAIDs, which in general are associated with a lower incidence of toxicity and less serious toxicities, and are also better tolerated than ASA in clients with chronic diseases.

As a point of drug therapy clarification, special emphasis must be given to the widely used drug known as acetaminophen. This medication is available both with and without prescription in many single-drug and combination-drug products that are available for all ages. In clinical practice the drug name acetaminophen is commonly abbreviated as "APAP," which is an acronym for its chemical name, acetyl-para-aminophenol. As discussed in Chapter 10, acetaminophen primarily has only analgesic and antipyretic effects and lacks any significant anti-inflammatory or antirheumatic effects. For these reasons it is normally used only for control of fever and mild to moderate pain and not as the primary drug therapy for inflammatory or rheumatic conditions. However, it is sometimes used as an adjunct or secondary medication for these conditions.

Before getting into the in-depth discussion of the NSAID agents, it is important to explain the body's arachidonic acid metabolic pathway. The beneficial effects of NSAIDs are thought to result primarily from their inhibition of this pathway.

ARACHIDONIC ACID PATHWAY

Arachidonic acid is released from phospholipids in cell membranes in response to a triggering event (e.g., an injury). It is metabolized by either the prostaglandin (PG) pathway or the leukotriene (LT) pathway, both of which are "branches" of the arachidonic acid pathway, as shown in Figure 43-1. Both of these pathways result in inflammation and pain characteristic of the body's response to injury or inflammatory illnesses such as arthritis.

In the PG pathway, arachidonic acid is converted by cyclo-oxygenase (COX) into various PGs such as prostacyclin (PGI_2), as well as into thromboxane A_2 (TXA_2). PGs indirectly mediate and perpetuate inflammation by inducing vasodilation and enhancing vasopermeability. These effects in turn potentiate the action of pro-inflammatory substances, such as histamine and bradykinin, in the production of edema and pain. The LT pathway utilizes lipoxygenases to metabolize the arachidonic acid and convert it into various LTs. Although the actions of these compounds are not as well understood as those of PGs, they also appear to be mediators of inflammation. Some LTs promote vasoconstriction, bronchospasms, and vascular permeability.

Pain, headache, fever, and inflammation are all consequences (symptoms) of the activation of the arachidonic acid pathway.

When PGs are injected into research subjects, they experience skeletal pain and headache. Stimuli that would normally not be painful, such as simply moving a joint through its natural range of motion, become painful because of the inflammatory process at work. These symptoms arise as a result of PG-induced hyperalgesia (excessive motor sensitivity). Fever results when PGE_2 is synthesized in the pre-optic hypothalamic region, the area of the brain that regulates temperature.

The inflammatory response is mediated by a host of endogenous compounds, including proteins of the complement system, histamine, serotonin, bradykinin, LTs,

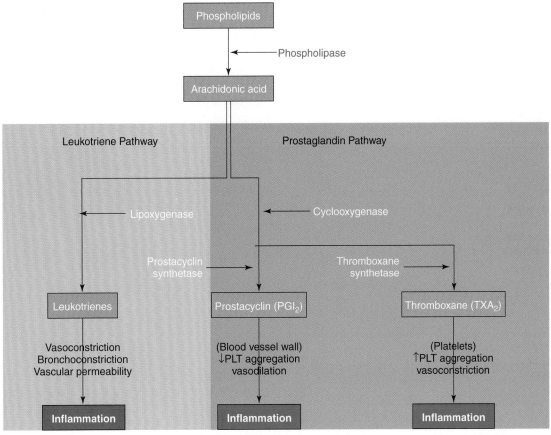

FIG. 43-1 Arachidonic acid pathway.

and PGs, the latter two being major contributors to the symptoms of inflammation.

NON-STEROIDAL ANTI-INFLAMMATORY DRUGS

Many NSAIDs are on the market and new agents are constantly becoming available; yet they can all be placed into one of seven structurally and historically related groups (see Box 43-1). The carboxylic acid agents are more commonly called *salicylates* and, as previously noted, were the first NSAIDs to be isolated and used therapeutically.

Currently at least one NSAID has been approved for each of the therapeutic indications listed in Box 43-2, and an NSAID is considered the drug of choice for the treatment of most of these conditions. This list of indications will continue to grow as more is learned about the mechanisms by which pain and inflammation are modified. Almost all NSAIDs are used for the treatment of rheumatoid arthritis and degenerative joint disease.

More NSAIDs are becoming available in long-acting sustained-release formulations. Some recent examples are naproxen sodium and diclofenac sodium. Medication adherence is enhanced with once-a-day medications. This

may increase the efficacy of these agents for the treatment of chronic disease states such as osteoarthritis.

Mechanism of Action and Drug Effects

NSAIDs work through inhibition of the LT pathway, the PG pathway, or both. More specifically, NSAIDs relieve pain, headache, and inflammation by blocking the chemical activity of either or both of the enzymes COX (PG pathway) and lipoxygenase (LT pathway). This limits inflammatory effects (see Figure 43-1). Both of these mechanisms differ from that of the opioids, which relieve pain by interfering with its recognition in the brain. Furthermore it is now recognized that there are at least two types or *isoforms* of COX. COX-1 is the isoform of the enzyme that promotes the synthesis of homeostatic PGs, which have primarily beneficial effects on various body functions. One example is their role in maintaining an intact GI mucosa. In contrast, the COX-2 isoform promotes the synthesis of PGs that are involved in inflammatory processes. In 1999 the newest class of NSAIDs, the COX-2 inhibitors, appeared on the Canadian market. These NSAIDs work by specifically inhibiting the COX-2 isoform of cyclo-oxygenase and have limited or no COX-1 effects. Previous NSAID groups inhibited both COX-1

BOX 43-1

Chemical Categories of NSAIDs

Acetic Acids
diclofenac sodium
diclofenac potassium
indomethacin
sulindac

Carboxylic Acids
Acetylated
ASA
etodolac
diflunisal

Non-acetylated
ketorolac
magnesium salicylate
sodium salicylate

COX-2 Inhibitors
celecoxib

Fenamic Acids
mefenamic acid

Napthylalkanones (non-acidic)
nabumetone

Oxicams
meloxicam
piroxicam

Propionic Acids
flurbiprofen
ibuprofen
ketoprofen
naproxen
oxaprozin

BOX 43-2

NSAIDs: Health Canada–Approved Indications

- Acute gout
- Acute gouty arthritis
- Acute painful shoulder
- Ankylosing spondylitis
- Bursitis
- Fever
- Juvenile rheumatoid arthritis
- Mild-to-moderate pain
- Osteoarthritis
- Primary dysmenorrhea
- Rheumatoid arthritis
- Tendinitis
- Various ophthalmic uses

The drug effects of NSAIDs are wide and varied. The main drug effects of NSAIDs are analgesic, anti-inflammatory, and antipyretic. NSAIDs are used principally in the symptomatic treatment of mild to moderate pain, fever, inflammatory diseases, and rheumatic fever.

One notable effect of the salicylates, especially ASA, is its inhibition of platelet aggregation, also known as its *antiplatelet activity*. Although all NSAIDs can be ulcerogenic and induce GI bleeding, as mentioned earlier, most of these effects are due to drug activity against tissue COX-1. ASA has the unique property of being an irreversible inhibitor of COX-1 in the platelets themselves. For this reason it is often used both prophylactically and following myocardial infarction (MI) to aid in the prevention of platelet aggregation and reinfarction from a resulting fibrin clot. This property of ASA and its related clinical uses serve to distinguish ASA from the other NSAIDs.

Indications

Some of the more noted therapeutic uses of this broad class of agents are listed in Table 43-1, but they are primarily used for their analgesic, anti-gout, anti-inflammatory, and antipyretic effects; for the relief of vascular headaches; and for platelet inhibition.

NSAIDs are also widely used for the treatment of rheumatoid arthritis and osteoarthritis, as well as other inflammatory conditions. They also have proved beneficial as adjunctive pain relief medications in clients with chronic pain syndromes, such as pain from bone cancer and chronic back pain. For the relief of pain they are sometimes combined with an opioid. This can provide pain relief mediated by a mechanism of action different from that of opioids. They also do not cause many of the

and COX-2 activity. The greater enzyme specificity of the COX-2 inhibitors allows for the beneficial anti-inflammatory effects associated with all other NSAIDs while reducing the prevalence of side effects, such as GI ulceration, associated with the anti–COX-1 activity of the more non-specific NSAIDs.

The LT pathway is inhibited by some antirheumatic agents but not by salicylates. Several anti-inflammatory drugs block both the PG pathway and the LT pathway, whereas others only weakly inhibit COX but primarily inhibit lipoxygenase.

NSAIDs reduce fever by inhibiting PGE_2, specifically by inhibiting its biosynthesis within the pre-optic hypothalamic region of the brain, which regulates body temperature.

TABLE 43-1
SUGGESTED NSAIDS FOR CLIENTS WITH VARIOUS MEDICAL CONDITIONS

Medical Condition	Recommended NSAID
Ankylosing spondylitis	indomethacin, naproxen, flurbiprofen
Diabetic neuropathy	sulindac
Dysmenorrhea	Fenamates, naproxen, ibuprofen
Gout	indomethacin, naproxen, sulindac
Headaches	ASA, ibuprofen
Hepatotoxicity	ibuprofen, piroxicam, fenamates
History of ASA or NSAID allergy	Avoid if possible; if deemed necessary consider a non-acetylated salicylate
Hypertension	sulindac, non-acetylated salicylate, ibuprofen, etodolac
Osteoarthritis	diclofenac, oxaprozin, indomethacin
Risk for gastrointestinal toxicity	COX-2 inhibitor celecoxib, non-acetylated salicylate, enteric-coated ASA, diclofenac, nabumetone, etodolac, ibuprofen, oxaprozin
Risk for nephrotoxicity	sulindac, non-acetylated salicylate, nabumetone, etodolac, diclofenac, oxaprozin
Warfarin therapy	sulindac, naproxen, ibuprofen, oxaprozin

undesirable effects of opioids, mainly respiratory depression. However, unlike opioids, their effectiveness is limited by a ceiling effect: beyond a certain level, increased doses increase the risk of adverse effects without a corresponding increase in the therapeutic effect. In contrast, opioid doses may be titrated almost indefinitely to increasingly higher levels, especially for terminally ill clients with severe pain.

Salicylates have an additional beneficial property: potent effects on the aggregation properties of platelets. For this reason they are commonly used for both prophylaxis and treatment of arterial, and possibly venous, thrombosis. Other NSAIDs generally lack these antiplatelet effects. However, they can be ulcerogenic, with possible blood loss, by inhibition of the synthesis of protective PGs, which normally function to protect the GI mucosa. Other NSAIDs are commonly used in the treatment of gout, which is caused by the overproduction of uric acid, decreased uric acid excretion, or both processes. This can often result in hyperuricemia (too much uric acid in the blood), a condition that causes joint pain as a result of the deposition of needlelike crystals of urate precipitate in tissues and the joints.

The appropriate selection of an NSAID calls for a consideration of the client's history, including any prior medical conditions, the intended use of the agent, the client's previous experience with NSAIDs, the client's preference, and the cost. The NSAIDs recommended for use with certain underlying medical conditions are listed in Table 43-1.

Contraindications

Contraindications to NSAIDs include known drug allergy and conditions that place the client at risk for bleeding. These conditions include rhinitis (risk of epistaxis [nosebleed]) and peptic ulcer disease. NSAIDs are also not advised during pregnancy, especially during the last trimester, because of the risk for maternal bleeding and possible miscarriage.

TABLE 43-2
NSAIDS: SIDE EFFECTS AND ADVERSE EFFECTS

Body System	Side/Adverse Effects
Cardiovascular	Moderate to severe non-cardiogenic pulmonary edema
Gastrointestinal	Most frequent: dyspepsia, heartburn, epigastric distress, nausea
	Less frequent: vomiting, anorexia, abdominal pain, GI bleeding, mucosal lesions (erosions or ulcerations)
Hematological	Altered hemostasis through effects on platelet function
Hepatic	Acute reversible hepatotoxicity
Renal	Reduction in creatinine clearance, acute tubular necrosis with renal failure
Other	Skin eruption, sensitivity reactions, tinnitus, hearing loss

Side Effects and Adverse Effects

The potential adverse effects of NSAIDs listed in Table 43-2 do not apply to all agents, but they do apply to many of them. One of the more common complaints and potentially serious adverse effects of the NSAIDs is GI distress. This can range from mild symptoms such as heartburn to GI bleeding. In fact, the adverse effects of salicylates mainly involve the GI tract and, besides bleeding, include symptomatic GI disturbances and mucosal lesions (e.g., erosive gastritis, gastric ulcer). These problems apparently are more commonly associated with ASA use than with the use of other NSAIDs.

Many of the side effects and adverse effects of NSAIDs are secondary to their inactivation of protective PGs that help maintain the normal integrity of the stomach lining. When the formation of these beneficial PGs is inhibited, this protective barrier is eliminated. This sets up a perfect environment for ulceration and GI bleeding. To further complicate matters, NSAIDs also prolong bleeding by inhibiting production by the platelets of TXA_2. This can exacerbate GI bleeding because TXA_2 is a potent promoter of platelet aggregation, a necessary step in the body's anti-bleeding mechanism. However, an agent called misoprostol has proved successful in preventing the gastric ulcers and hence GI bleeding that can occur in clients receiving NSAIDs. It is a synthetic PGE_1 analogue that potently inhibits gastric acid secretion, which it does by directly inhibiting the function of parietal cells. It also has a cyto-protective component, although the mechanism responsible for this action is unclear. It may prevent disruption of the gastric mucosal barrier, stimulate mucus secretion, stimulate alkaline (bicarbonate) secretion, or enhance mucosal blood flow. It also causes uterine contractions. Because of this, although not Health Canada approved, it is sometimes used with other drugs to induce abortion (Chapter 33). It should thus be avoided in pregnant women who do not intend to terminate their pregnancies.

The kidneys are also dependent to some extent on PGs, especially in renally compromised clients, because these organs rely on PGs to stimulate vasodilation and increase renal blood flow. If NSAIDs inhibit this compensatory mechanism, it may be enough to precipitate acute or chronic renal failure, depending on the client's current level of renal function. Geriatric clients are at greater risk for this adverse drug reaction.

Toxicity and Management of Overdose

There are both chronic and acute manifestations of salicylate toxicity. **Chronic salicylate intoxication** is known as **salicylism** and results from either short-term high doses or prolonged therapy. The most common signs and symptoms of acute or chronic salicylate intoxication are listed in Table 43-3.

The most common manifestations of chronic intoxication in adults are tinnitus and hearing loss. Those in children are hyperventilation and central nervous system (CNS) effects such as dizziness, drowsiness, and behavioural changes. These effects usually arise when serum salicylate concentrations exceed 2.89 to 4.3 mmol/L. Metabolic complications such as metabolic acidosis and respiratory alkalosis often occur to varying degrees in cases of chronic salicylate intoxication. Metabolic acidosis can also occur with acute intoxication, but it is usually less severe. Hypoglycemia is also likely to occur and can be life threatening.

The treatment of chronic intoxication is based on the presenting symptoms. Serum salicylate concentrations may be determined but are not as useful in estimating the severity because symptoms of severe intoxication tend to have slower onset and appear less severe than those of acute onset intoxication. The suggested treatment for chronic salicylate intoxication is summarized in Table 43-4.

The signs and symptoms of **acute salicylate overdose** are similar to those of chronic intoxication, but the effects are often more pronounced and occur more quickly. Acute salicylate overdose usually results from the ingestion of a single toxic dose, and its severity can be estimated based on the estimated amount (in mg/kg of body weight) ingested, as follows:

- Little or no toxicity: <150 mg/kg
- Mild to moderate toxicity: 150–300 mg/kg
- Severe toxicity: 300–500 mg/kg
- Life-threatening toxicity: >500 mg/kg

It should be noted, however, that even doses lower than 150 mg/kg have resulted in fatal toxicity, whereas some clients have survived ASA overdoses as high as 130 g. A serum salicylate concentration measured six hours or more after the ingestion may be used in conjunction with the **Done nomogram** to estimate the severity of intoxication and help guide treatment. The Done nomogram is a graphic plot of serum salicylate levels (in milligrams per decilitre [mg/dL] and millimoles per litre [mmol/L]) as a function of elapsed time following salicylate ingestion. It was first published in a 1960 issue of the journal *Pediatrics* and may still be used today for gauging acute salicylate toxicity. Although it has historical significance, it should not be used in isolation to determine toxicity or to guide therapy. This nomogram is intended only for estimating the severity of acute intoxications in pediatric clients if the time of ingestion is known, and is not considered useful for chronic salicylate intoxication or for enteric-coated or sustained release products.

The pathophysiological mechanism of salicylate overdose is complex because of the variety of toxic effects

TABLE 43-3

ACUTE OR CHRONIC SALICYLATE INTOXICATION: SIGNS AND SYMPTOMS

Body System	Signs and Symptoms
Cardiovascular	Increased heart rate
Central nervous	Tinnitus, hearing loss, dim vision, headache, dizziness, mental confusion, lassitude, drowsiness
Gastrointestinal	Nausea, vomiting, diarrhea
Metabolic	Sweating, thirst, hyperventilation

TABLE 43-4

ACUTE SALICYLATE INTOXICATION: TREATMENT

Severity	Treatment
Mild	1. Dosage reduction or discontinuation of salicylates 2. Symptomatic and supportive therapy
Severe	1. Discontinuation of salicylates 2. Intensive symptomatic and supportive therapy 3. Dialysis if: high salicylate levels (>7.3 mmol/L after acute ingestion and >4.4–5.1 mmol/L for chronic salicylism), unresponsive acidosis (pH <7.1), impaired renal function or renal failure, pulmonary edema, persistent CNS symptoms (e.g., seizures, coma), progressive deterioration despite appropriate therapy

produced by salicylates, although the principal effects are extensions of the agents' pharmacological actions:

- Local GI tract irritation
- Direct CNS stimulation of respiration
- Altered glucose metabolism (stimulation of gluconeogenesis and lipid metabolism)
- Increased tissue glycolysis
- Interference with hemostatic mechanisms

The treatment of acute toxicity stemming from a salicylate overdose involves intensive symptomatic and supportive therapy. The treatment goals should consist of removing salicylate from the GI tract and/or preventing its further absorption; correcting fluid, electrolyte, and acid-base disturbances; and implementing measures to enhance salicylate elimination. The measures to be taken to achieve these treatment goals are listed in Table 43-5.

An acute overdose of non-salicylate NSAIDs (e.g., ibuprofen) causes effects similar to those of salicylate overdose, but they are generally not as extensive or as dangerous. These symptoms include CNS toxicities such as drowsiness, lethargy, mental confusion, paraesthesias (abnormal touch sensations), numbness, aggressive behaviour, disorientation, seizures, and GI toxicities such as nausea, vomiting, and GI bleeding. Intense headache, dizziness, cerebral edema, cardiac arrest, and death have also been known to occur in extreme cases. For suspected overdose, consultation with a Poison Control Centre is recommended. Treatment should consist of the immediate removal of the ingested agent, first by gastric lavage and then by the administration of activated charcoal, with supportive and symptomatic treatment initiated thereafter. N-acetylcysteine is the antidote of choice for acetaminophen toxicity. Hemodialysis appears to be of no value in enhancing the elimination of NSAIDs.

Interactions

Drug interactions with salicylates and other NSAIDs can result in significant complications and morbidity. Some of the more common of these are listed in Table 43-6.

TABLE 43-5
ACUTE SALICYLATE INTOXICATION: TREATMENT GOALS

Treatment Goal	Measure
Reduce salicylate absorption	Gastric lavage* Activated charcoal
Treat fluid and electrolyte imbalance	Appropriate fluid replacement and electrolyte therapy should be implemented promptly, based on fluid, acid–base, and electrolyte status. Therefore, arterial pH and blood gases and electrolytes, serum creatine, BUN, and blood glucose should be determined.
Enhance salicylate elimination	Alkaline diuresis: intravenous administration of sodium bicarbonate to alkalinize the urine to a pH of ≥7.5 with sufficient urine flow. Hemodialysis: the same considerations as those that apply to chronic intoxication.
Provide symptomatic and supportive measures	Hypotension and/or hemorrhagic complications: fluids and transfusions, along with possible vitamin K injections. Respiratory depression: may require assisted pulmonary ventilation and oxygen. Seizures: intravenous administration of a benzodiazepine or short-acting barbiturate.

*Effective up to 3–4 h after acute ingestion and maybe up to 10 h after ingestion in the event of massive overdose.

TABLE 43-6
SALICYLATES AND OTHER NSAIDS: DRUG INTERACTIONS

Drug	Mechanism	Result
Alcohol	Additive effect	Increased GI bleeding
Anticoagulants	Platelet inhibition, hypoprothrombinemia	Increased bleeding tendencies
Antihyperglycemic agents	Increased antihyperglycemic response to sulphonureas	Reduced blood glucose
ASA and other salicylates with NSAIDs	Reduce NSAID absorption, additive GI toxicities	Increased GI toxicity with no therapeutic advantage
Corticosteroids and other ulcerogenic agents	Additive toxicities	Increased ulcerogenic effects
cyclosporine	Inhibits renal prostaglandin synthesis	May increase the nephrotoxic effects of cyclosporine
Hypotensive agents and diuretics	Inhibit prostaglandin synthesis	Reduced hypotensive and diuretic effects
phenytoin	Inhibit phenytoin metabolism	Increase phenytoin serum levels
Protein-bound drugs	Compete for binding	More pronounced drug actions
Uricosurics	Antagonism	Decreased uric acid excretion

These agents can also interfere with laboratory test results. Specifically, salicylates can cause the serum levels of alanine aminotransferase (ALT), aspartate aminotransferase (AST), and alkaline phosphatase to be increased. This is indicative of liver enzyme elevation. However, such elevations are usually minor and transient, and only rarely has severe hepatic toxicity been reported secondary to NSAID therapy or even overdosage. The hematocrit (Hct) values, hemoglobin levels (Hgb), and red blood cell (RBC) counts can all be decreased in clients suffering from GI bleeding stemming from the use of salicylates or other NSAIDs. NSAID use can also cause the serum levels of potassium to be elevated (hyperkalemia) and the serum levels of sodium to be lowered (hyponatremia).

Dosages

For the recommended dosages of various NSAIDs, see the dosages table on p. 733. See Appendix B for some of the common brands available in Canada.

DRUG PROFILES

Chemically speaking, the broad drug category of NSAIDs includes four major categories of carboxylic acids (acetic acids, propionic acids, pyranocarboxylic acids, and pyrrolizine carboxylic acids) along with the newest class of NSAIDs, the COX-2 inhibitors.

ACETIC ACIDS

Salicylates are chemically classified as carboxylic acids. Although ASA is the most commonly used of all these agents, the others have many of the same beneficial effects. ASA is available without prescription, but many of the other salicylate drugs do require a prescription. In Canada this includes diflunisal. Magnesium salicylate comes only as a non-prescription product (e.g., Herbogesic, Kneerelief Tablets). Salicylates are primarily available in oral (PO) preparations in capsule or tablet form. Other available dosage forms include an ASA chewing gum tablet (Aspergum) and 150- and 650-mg ASA rectal suppositories.

Indomethacin is one of the commonly used acetic acid or acetylated NSAIDs, the others being ASA, diflunisal, diclofenac, etodolac, and sulindac. Acetylation refers to the presence of an acetyl or –CH$_2$COOH functional group in the chemical structure of a given drug. This occurs when an acetic acid molecule (CH$_3$COOH) attaches to the ring structure of the drug, losing a hydrogen ion (H$_1$) in the process. There is conflicting evidence in the literature as to whether non-acetylated NSAIDs are as effective as the acetylated ones. The difference if any appears to be slight, but it is known that non-acetylated salicylates, with the exception of diflunisal, are weaker inhibitors of the COX enzyme than are the acetylated NSAIDs. However, all NSAIDs are still related in terms of their chemical structure and pharmacological action.

All NSAIDs are generally rated as pregnancy category B or C agents for use during the first two trimesters of pregnancy. However, all are rated pregnancy category D during the third trimester. The reasons for this are that some NSAIDs, such as ASA, have been shown to be both teratogenic and embryocidal in animals. NSAIDs use has also been associated with both excessive maternal bleeding and neonatal NSAID toxicity during the perinatal period. Neonatal NSAID exposure can also result in the reduction of needed PG synthesis by the infant's body; therefore NSAIDs are generally not recommended for use by nursing mothers because these medications can be excreted into human milk.

▶▶ ASA

Acetylsalicylic acid (ASA) is the prototype salicylate and NSAID and is the most widely used drug in the world. First introduced in the late 1800s, it remains a mainstay of many drug treatment regimens. ASA is capable of many beneficial therapeutic effects, including analgesic, anti-inflammatory, and antipyretic effects. It also has been shown to have an antithrombotic effect, which is the result of its ability to inhibit platelet aggregation by blocking platelet COX. This in turn results in reduced formation by the platelets of TXA$_2$, a substance that normally promotes platelet aggregation. This antiplatelet action has made ASA, along with thrombolytic drugs (Chapter 27), a primary drug in the treatment of acute MI and many other thromboembolic disorders. In fact, a daily ASA tablet (81 mg or 325 mg) is now routinely recommended as prophylactic therapy for adults who have strong risk factors for developing coronary artery disease or stroke, even if they have no prior history of such an event. The 81-mg (which is traditionally thought of as "children's" ASA) and the 325-mg strengths appear to be equally beneficial for the prevention of thrombotic events. For this reason the lower strength is often chosen for clients who have any elevated risk of bleeding, such as those with prior stroke history or history of peptic ulcer disease and those taking the anticoagulant warfarin. ASA is also often used to treat the pain associated with headache, neuralgia, myalgia, and arthralgia, as well as other pain syndromes resulting from inflammation. These include arthritis, pleurisy, and pericarditis. Clients with systemic lupus erythematosus may also benefit from ASA therapy because of its antirheumatic effects.

ASA is available in many dosage forms: chewing gum, tablets, delayed released enteric-coated tablets, capsules, and rectal suppositories. It is also contained in many combination products; some of the more popular of these are ASA, butalbital, and caffeine combinations (Fiorinal) and ASA combined with various antacids (Bufferin). ASA also is available in special enteric-coated dosage forms to decrease GI toxicities.

ASA use is contraindicated in clients with a known hypersensitivity to salicylates; those with GI bleeding, bleeding disorders, vitamin K deficiency, or a peptic ulcer; in children younger than 12 years of age; and in children with flu-like symptoms. Its use should also be avoided in nursing mothers because salicylates are known to be excreted in breast milk and could pose a toxicity risk to the nursing infant. Pregnancy category C (category D during the third trimester). Commonly recommended dosages are listed in the dosages table on p. 733.

DOSAGES   Most Commonly Used NSAIDs

Agent	Pharmacological Class	Usual Dosage Range	Indications
▸▸acetylsalicylic acid (ASA)	Salicylate	**Adult** PO/PR: 325–650 mg q4h (max 4 g/day) PO/PR: 975 mg 4–6 ×/day (max 3.2 g/day) PO/PR: 650 mg bid (× 14 days; 80–325 mg/day based on client needs **Pediatric <12 yr** PO/PR: 10–15 mg/kg q6h (max 2.4 g) PO/PR: 60–125 mg/kg divided q4–6h	Fever, pain Anti-inflammatory Thromboprevention, post-MI Fever, pain Anti-inflammatory
▸▸celecoxib	COX-2 inhibitor	**Adult** PO: 100–200 mg once daily PO: 400 mg bid	Arthritis, acute pain, primary dysmenorrhea Reduction of number of hereditary colon polyps in familial adenomatous polyposis
▸▸ibuprofen	Propionic acid	**Adult and pediatric >12 yr** 200–400 mg q4d (max 1200 mg/day) **Pediatric >2 yr** 100–300 mg q6–8h (max 400–1200 mg/day)	Arthritis, fever, pain, dysmenorrhea
▸▸indomethacin	Acetic acid	**Adult** PO: 25–50 mg bid–tid (max 200 mg/day) **Pediatric** PO: 2–4 mg/kg/day divided bid–qid (max 200 mg/day)	Arthritis, including acute gouty arthritis, acute painful shoulder due to bursitis or tendinitis
▸▸ketorolac	Pyrrolizine carboxylic acid	**Adult*** PO: 10 mg q4–6h (max 40 mg/day) IV/IM: 15–60 mg q6–12h (max 120 mg/day if <65 yr; max 60 mg/day if >65 yr)	Acute painful conditions that would otherwise require opioid level analgesia; PO form is recommended only in transition from injectable form to oral form

*Pediatric dosing guidelines are not as well established but the recommended range for IV, IM, or PO use is 0.4–1 mg/kg as a single dose for acute conditions (e.g., sports injury).

PHARMACOKINETICS

Half-Life	Onset	Peak	Duration
2–30 hr	15–30 min	1–2 hr	4–6 hr

▸▸ indomethacin

Like the other NSAIDs, indomethacin has analgesic, anti-inflammatory, antirheumatic, and antipyretic properties. Its therapeutic actions are of particular use in the treatment of rheumatoid arthritis, osteoarthritis, acute bursitis or tendinitis, ankylosing spondylitis (spinal arthritis), and acute gouty arthritis. An injectable form of the drug is also used intravenously to promote closure of patent ductus arteriosus (PDA) in premature infants. This is one of the structures in the neonatal heart that normally closes on its own shortly after delivery in infants who are carried to term. In premature infants, however, the ductus arteriosus sometimes remains open ("patent"), allowing oxygenated and non-oxygenated blood to mix in the baby's heart, impairing tissue oxygenation. Both indomethacin and the PGE_1 (alprostadil) can hasten PDA closure and improve neonatal circulation.

Indomethacin should not be used with agents that are ulcerogenic, corticosteroids, anticoagulants, and ASA products.

Because of its potent actions, indomethacin is available only by prescription. It can be administered orally, rectally, and by IV. The oral dosage forms are 25- and 50-mg capsules. The rectal suppositories contain 50 and 100 mg of the agent. In parenteral form indomethacin is available as a 1-mg intravenous injection. Hypersensitivity to it, asthma, severe renal and hepatic disease, and ulcer disease are all contraindications to its use. Indomethacin is considered as a pregnancy category B agent for women in the first or second trimester of pregnancy, but its use during the last trimester is not recommended (pregnancy category D) because it may inhibit PG synthesis in the fetus. For the same reason it is also not recommended for use in nursing women. Commonly recommended dosages are listed in the dosages table above.

PHARMACOKINETICS

Half-Life	Onset	Peak	Duration
1.5–2 hr	<30 min	0.5–3 hr	4–6 hr

PROPIONIC ACIDS

▶▶ ibuprofen

Ibuprofen is the prototype NSAID in the propionic acid category, which also includes flurbiprofen, ketoprofen, naproxen, and oxaprozin. Ibuprofen is the most commonly used of the propionic acid agents because of its numerous indications and relatively safe side effect and adverse effect profiles. Ibuprofen is also available OTC, either alone or in many combinations with other agents. To reduce toxicity and prevent some of the dose-related side effects, the maximum strength of the OTC ibuprofen preparations is 400 mg per tablet. Ibuprofen and other drugs in this category interact adversely with anticoagulants and ASA.

Ibuprofen is an excellent drug for the treatment of rheumatoid arthritis, osteoarthritis, primary dysmenorrhea, gout, dental pain, and musculoskeletal disorders. Ibuprofen is available as a 40-mg/mL infant oral drop solution; a 100-mg/5-mL pediatric oral suspension; 100-, 200-, 400-, and 600-mg regular tablets; 50- and 100-mg chewable tablets; and 200-mg liquid gel capsules.

It is not recommended for nursing women because it can inhibit PG synthesis in the infant. Its only absolute contraindication is drug allergy. Pregnancy category B (category D during the third trimester). Commonly recommended dosages are listed in the dosages table on p. 733.

PHARMACOKINETICS

Half-Life	Onset	Peak	Duration
2 hr	<30 min	1–2 hr	4–6 hr

▶▶ ketorolac tromethamine

Ketorolac is classified as a pyrrolizine carboxylic acid and is currently the only drug in this category, having a unique chemical structure. Although it does have some anti-inflammatory activity, it is used primarily for its powerful analgesic effects, which are comparable to those of narcotic agents such as morphine. It is indicated for the treatment of moderate to severe acute pain such as that resulting from orthopedic injuries. The opioid-level analgesic potential of the drug can make it a particularly desirable choice for opiate-addicted clients who have acute pain control needs, because ketorolac lacks the addictive properties of the true opioids. Ketorolac is the only NSAID that can be given by oral, injectable, and ophthalmic routes. It is available as a 10-mg tablet; a 10- and 30-mg injection; and a 0.4 percent and 0.5 percent ophthalmic solution (Chapter 56).

Ketorolac is available only by prescription. It is indicated for short-term (up to five days) management of moderate to severe acute pain. It is not indicated for minor or chronic painful conditions. Ketorolac is a potent NSAID with many contraindications. Pregnancy category C (category D during the third trimester). Commonly recommended dosages are listed in the dosages table on p. 733.

PHARMACOKINETICS

Half-Life	Onset	Peak	Duration
5–7 hr	0.5–1 hr	1.5–3 hr	6 hr

COX-2 INHIBITORS

This class of drugs inhibit cyclo-oxygenase 2. The only COX-2 inhibitor currently available is celecoxib. In the fall of 2004, another COX-2 inhibitor, rofecoxib, was voluntarily removed from the Canadian market because of post-market findings of an increased risk of cardiovascular disease, especially myocardial infarction and stroke. In the spring of 2005, valdecoxib was also removed voluntarily from the Canadian market because of serious, potentially life-threatening skin reactions. As of September 2005, despite an expert panel's recommendations that rofecoxib be reintroduced, Health Canada had not taken a position on its reintroduction.

Drug interactions with COX-2 inhibitors include ACE inhibitors, diuretics, salicylates, corticosteroids, warfarin, lithium, and anticoagulants.

▶▶ celecoxib

Celecoxib is indicated for the treatment of osteoarthritis and rheumatoid arthritis and the reduction of adenomatous colorectal polyps in clients with familial adenomatous polyposis (FAP). It is believed to work by inhibiting PG synthesis via inhibition of COX-2 but not COX-1.

COX-2 selective agents decrease the production of the inflammatory PGs that result from the activity of the COX-2 enzyme without decreasing the production of the beneficial PGs produced by COX-1, which are important in regulating other body functions, thus avoiding some of the toxicity associated with NSAID therapy.

The COX-2 selective inhibitor has little effect on platelet function. This agent was designed primarily to cause fewer GI adverse effects relative to other NSAIDs. However, it is not totally devoid of GI toxicity. Gastritis and upper GI bleeding have been reported, though much less frequently than with older NSAIDs. The most common adverse effects include fatigue, dizziness, headache, lower extremity edema, hypertension, diarrhea, dyspepsia, flatulence, nausea, heartburn, and epigastric discomfort. Potential drug interactions include angiotensin converting enzyme (ACE) inhibitors, ASA, methotrexate, and warfarin.

Celecoxib is contraindicated in individuals with known drug allergy. It is available as a 200-mg capsule. Pregnancy category C. Commonly recommended dosages are given in the dosages table on p. 733.

PHARMACOKINETICS

Half-Life	Onset	Peak	Duration
11 hr	0.75–1 hr	3 hr	4–8 hr

ENOLIC ACIDS, FENAMIC ACIDS, AND NON-ACIDIC COMPOUNDS

The last three chemical categories of NSAIDs consist of the smallest number of agents, and the indications for their use are limited. Both piroxicam and meloxicam belong to the enolic acid family of NSAIDs. Today these compounds are more commonly called *oxicams*. They are potent agents that can produce severe GI toxicities. Oxicams are commonly used in the treatment of painful osteoarthritis (arthrosis, degenerative joint disease), rheumatoid arthritis, mild to severe acute pain, and gouty arthritis. Both are available only in oral dosage formulations and have contraindications similar to those of the other NSAIDs. Pregnancy category C (category D during the third trimester).

Enolic agents enhance the effects of oral anticoagulants, insulin and oral antidiabetic agents, corticosteroids, and male or female hormones.

Mefenamic acid belongs to the category of fenamic acids. It is an older agent and not used as commonly as the other NSAIDs. It is indicated for the treatment of mild to moderate pain, osteoarthritis, and rheumatoid arthritis. Pregnancy category C (category D during the third trimester of pregnancy).

Nabumetone is a relatively new NSAID that is better tolerated by people who cannot tolerate the GI effects of other NSAIDs. It is classified as a naphthylalkanone and is currently the only drug in its class. It is relatively nonacidic compared with most of the other NSAIDs, which probably accounts for its improved GI tolerance. Currently it is indicated only for the treatment of osteoarthritis and rheumatoid arthritis. It has contraindications similar to those of the other NSAIDs. Pregnancy category C (category D during the third trimester).

ANTIRHEUMATIC AGENTS

As previously emphasized in this chapter, all NSAIDs have some antirheumatic activity. However, certain other types of medications are recognized primarily for their antirheumatic properties, as opposed to the analgesic, anti-inflammatory, and antipyretic properties that are associated with NSAIDs. These agents are referred to here as antirheumatic agents, and they are further subdivided into the anti-gout and anti-arthritic agents. Although some of these agents have additional medical uses, they are commonly used to treat the prevalent rheumatic conditions known as gout and arthritis. These drugs have characteristics that make them different from NSAIDs and for this reason are discussed separately. Additional antirheumatic agents are discussed in Chapter 47 because of their distinct mechanisms of action.

GOUT AND ANTI-GOUT AGENTS

Gout is a condition that results from inappropriate uric acid metabolism. People with gout either overproduce or underexcrete uric acid, an end product of purine metabolism. Purines are part of the normal dietary intake and are used to make the essential nucleoside and nucleotide structural units of DNA and RNA. During their metabolism they are converted from hypoxanthine to xanthine and eventually to uric acid. (The normal pathway for the purine metabolism is depicted in Figure 43-2.) When the body contains too much uric acid, deposits of uric acid crystals collect in tissues and joints. These crystals are like small needles that jab and stick into sensitive tissues and joints, causing the pain of gout.

Anti-gout agents are targeted at the underlying defect in uric acid metabolism, which causes either overproduction or underexcretion of uric acid. Both of these pathological processes lead to tissue accumulations of uric acid crystalline deposits (gouty deposits) and symptoms of gout. Although not all gouty deposits occur within joints, gouty arthritis is the condition of one or more inflamed joints resulting from gouty deposits that collect inside the joint anatomy. This is also called *articular gout*, whereas gout that occurs in tissues outside of the joints is called *abarticular gout*.

DRUG PROFILES

Anti-gout agents include such drugs as allopurinol, colchicine, probenecid, and sulfinpyrazone.

▶▶ *allopurinol*

Allopurinol relieves gout by inhibiting the enzyme xanthine oxidase, which thereby prevents uric acid production. Allopurinol is indicated for clients whose gout is caused by the excess production of uric acid (hyperuricemia). Oxypurinol, a metabolite of allopurinol, also prevents uric acid production. Oxypurinol is available as an orphan drug for clients with hyperuricemia who are intolerant to allopurinol therapy.

Allopurinol is contraindicated in clients with a hypersensitivity to it. Significant adverse effects to the

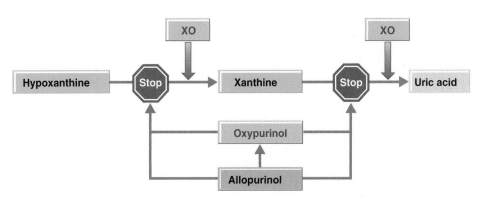

FIG. 43-2 Uric acid production. *XO*, Xanthine oxidase.

agent include agranulocytosis, aplastic anemia, and serious and potentially fatal skin conditions such as exfoliative dermatitis, Stevens-Johnson syndrome, and toxic epidermal necrolysis. Azathioprine and mercaptopurine both interact with allopurinol, and because of the important interactions that can result, their doses may have to be adjusted. Allopurinol is available only in oral preparations as 100-, 200-, and 300-mg tablets. The recommended adult dosage is 100 to 800 mg/day divided into one to three doses. A single dose should not exceed 300 mg. Pregnancy category C.

colchicine

Colchicine is an anti-gout medication that has weak anti-inflammatory activity, no effect on the urinary excretion of uric acid, and no analgesic activity. It appears to be effective in the treatment of gout by reducing the inflammatory response to the deposits of urate crystals in joint tissue. There are many possible explanations for its ability to do this, but the one most favoured is that it inhibits polymorphonuclear leukocyte metabolism, mobility, and chemotaxis.

Colchicine is a powerful inhibitor of cell mitosis and can cause short-term leukopenia. For this reason it is generally used for the treatment of acute attacks of gout. Its more severe side effects can include nausea, vomiting, abdominal pain, and diarrhea, which can lead to more problems if peptic ulcer or spastic colon are present; the drug should be stopped should such toxic effects appear. Colchicine can also cause bone marrow depression and agranulocytosis, thrombocytopenia, or aplastic anemia if used for long periods of time. It can also cause renal damage and hematuria. Hypersensitivity is the only contraindication to its use. The drug is available in 0.6- and 1-mg tablets. The usual adult dosage is an initial dose of 1 to 1.2 mg initially, then 0.5 or 0.6 mg every two hours until the gout pain disappears or until nausea, vomiting, or diarrhea develops. Doses for prophylaxis of recurrent gout range from 0.5 mg one to four times weekly to 1.8 mg daily, depending on how frequently attacks occur. Pregnancy category D.

probenecid

The beneficial effect of probenecid in the treatment of gout is the increased excretion of uric acid in the urine by inhibiting its reabsorption by the kidney. Drugs that promote uric acid excretion are known as *uricosurics*. In clients whose gout is due to the underexcretion of uric acid, urate crystals form because uric acid is not being excreted in the urine in sufficient quantities. Instead, most of the uric acid is being reabsorbed from the renal tubules back into the bloodstream and then conveyed throughout the body. Probenecid works by preferentially binding to the special transporter protein in the proximal convoluted renal tubule that takes uric acid from the urine and places it back into the blood. The probenecid is then reabsorbed back into the bloodstream while the uric acid remains in the urine and is excreted. Probenecid also delays the renal excretion of penicillin, thus increasing the serum levels of penicillin and prolonging its effect (Chapter 37). Probenecid is available as a 500-mg oral tablet. The usual adult dosage is 250 mg twice a day with food, milk, or

antacids for one week, followed by 500 mg twice daily thereafter. This dose may be adjusted as needed to maintain desirable serum uric acid levels. Pregnancy category B.

sulfinpyrazone

Sulfinpyrazone works similarly to probenecid. It is also a uricosuric agent. It is chemically related to phenylbutazone, an early NSAID, which is still available on the Canadian market in 100-mg tablet form. Like other NSAIDs, however, sulfinpyrazone can be ulcerogenic and is therefore contraindicated in clients with peptic ulcer disease. Sulfinpyrazone is available in 100- and 200-mg tablets. The usual adult dosage is 100 to 200 mg twice a day for one week. The subsequent adjusted maintenance dosage can range from 200 to 800 mg daily. Pregnancy category C (category D during the third trimester).

ANTI-ARTHRITIC AGENTS

Anti-arthritic agents suppress arthritic inflammation and are therefore used in the treatment of rheumatoid arthritis. These drugs are considered to be more powerful than the NSAIDs in that they do not merely provide anti-inflammatory and analgesic effects but can actually arrest or slow the degenerative disease processes associated with arthritis. For these reasons this class of medications is also referred to as the **disease-modifying antirheumatic drugs (DMARDs)**. DMARDs often have a slow onset of action of several weeks, versus minutes to hours for NSAIDs. For this reason DMARDs are sometimes also referred to as *slow-acting antirheumatic drugs (SAARDs)*. They are also commonly thought of as second-line agents for the treatment of arthritis because they can have much more toxic side effects than the NSAIDs. However, the use of the term *second-line agents* can be misleading because DMARDs may be appropriately used as first-line drug therapy, in spite of their greater toxicity, for more severe cases of arthritis as diagnosed by a rheumatologist.

Grading of the severity of a given case of arthritis often depends on careful evaluation by the prescriber of such factors as radiographic (X-ray) evidence and various laboratory indicators such as serum rheumatoid factor and antinuclear antibody. Less severe cases of arthritis are the more common clinical picture, however, and in such cases DMARDs are in fact used as second-line therapy, usually only after a client has failed at least a three-month trial of NSAID therapy.

DMARDs exhibit anti-inflammatory, anti-arthritic, and immunomodulating effects and work by inhibiting the movement of various cells into an inflamed, damaged area, such as a joint. These cells (neutrophils, monocytes, and macrophages) are responsible for causing many of the deleterious effects of chronic rheumatoid arthritis. By preventing the accumulation of these inflammatory cells in the area of the diseased joint, anti-arthritic agents prevent progression of the disease.

A newer type of agent, referred to as a *biological response modifier*, can be used for clients who do not respond to DMARDs. A drug in this category, etanercept, works by binding to and neutralizing tumour necrosis factor (TNF). TNF is a known pro-inflammatory cytokine, a non-antibody protein that is released by the body as part of the inflammatory process.

Another approach to active rheumatoid arthritis is represented by the new agent leflunomide, which modulates or alters the response of the immune system to rheumatoid arthritis. It has antiproliferative, anti-inflammatory, and immunosuppressive activity.

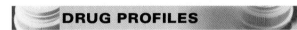

DRUG PROFILES

auranofin

Auranofin is an orally active anti-arthritic agent. Twenty-nine percent of it is gold, and like all anti-arthritic agents it has anti-inflammatory, anti-arthritic, and immunomodulating effects. It is poorly absorbed orally—only about 25 percent of the medication is absorbed from the GI tract into the blood. Auranofin is contraindicated in clients with a history of gold-induced necrotizing enterocolitis, pulmonary fibrosis, exfoliative dermatitis, bone marrow aplasia, or other types of blood dyscrasia. It is available in 3-mg capsules for oral use. The normal recommended adult dosage is 6 mg once per day or 3 mg twice per day. The dosage can be increased to 9 mg after six months of therapy if the response is inadequate. Pregnancy category C.

gold sodium thiomalate

Gold sodium thiomalate is a parenterally administered anti-arthritic agent. It is roughly 50 percent gold, and currently available only in an injectable form of 10-, 25-, and 50-mg/mL. It is made by complexing gold with thiomalate via a sulphur linkage. Like other anti-arthritic agents, it has anti-inflammatory, anti-arthritic, and immunomodulating effects. It is administered by the intramuscular (IM) route only, with weekly injections ranging from 10 to 100 mg. It requires regular monitoring, with either dose reduction or discontinuation if symptoms of toxicity appear, as detected by complete blood count (CBC), urinalysis, and kidney and liver function tests.

etanercept

Etanercept is the newest agent indicated for the treatment of moderately to severely active rheumatoid arthritis in clients who have not responded to one or more of the DMARDs, such as gold compounds or methotrexate. It is more commonly referred to as a biological response modifier. It was approved by Health Canada in 2001. It can be used in combination with methotrexate in clients who do not respond adequately to methotrexate alone. Methotrexate (see Chapter 46) is most commonly used as an anticancer drug. However, it is also used both orally and by injection for treating more severe cases of rheumatoid arthritis. Etanercept reduces inflammation by binding to and neutralizing tumour necrosis factor (TNF), a known pro-inflammatory cytokine. Etanercept has been shown to decrease joint swelling, tenderness, and morning stiffness. It has an extremely long half-life (92 hours), which allows it to be dosed just twice a week. The recommended dose of etanercept is 25 mg subcutaneously (SC) twice weekly. The most common side effect is a mild injection site reaction that typically subsides in three to five days. Malignancies are the most common severe adverse effect. Other adverse reactions include mild upper respiratory tract symptoms such as cough, rhinitis, sinusitis, upper respiratory tract infections, and pharyngitis. Etanercept is available as a 25-mg vial of powdered drug for injection. Pregnancy category B.

leflunomide

Leflunomide is a new agent indicated for the treatment of active rheumatoid arthritis. It modulates or alters the response of the immune system to rheumatoid arthritis. It has antiproliferative, anti-inflammatory, and immunosuppressive activity. Its most common side effects are diarrhea, respiratory tract infection, alopecia, elevated liver function tests, hypertension, and rash. It is contraindicated in women who are or may become pregnant and should not be used by nursing mothers or those with a hypersensitivity to it. Leflunomide is most commonly given by a loading dose of 100 mg daily for three days, then a maintenance dose of 20 mg daily. ASA, NSAIDs, and/or low-dose corticosteroids may be continued during leflunomide therapy. It is available as 10-, 20-, and 100-mg tablets. Pregnancy category X.

NURSING PROCESS

■ Assessment

Before administering NSAIDs, the nurse must assess the client for the following contraindications to their use: allergies to any of the classes of NSAIDs, GI lesions, gastric ulcerations, peptic ulcer disease, bleeding disorders, third trimester of pregnancy, and lactation. Cautious use with careful monitoring of the client for the occurrence of side effects or toxicity is recommended in pregnant women in the first or second trimester; clients with renal, cardiac, or hepatic disease; clients taking glaucoma agents (especially with enolic agents such as phenylbutazone); geriatric clients; and clients taking agents for psychiatric illness (especially with indomethacin or sulindac). Hypersensitivity is a contraindication to the use of salicylates, and if the client has a history of asthma there is a higher risk for allergic reactions to salicylates (or ASA products). Salicylates are also not to be given to children under 12 years of age because of the risk of Reye's syndrome (see the Pediatric Considerations box on p. 739). Salicylates have the same cautions as NSAIDs.

A thorough medication history is needed to determine if the client is taking any drugs (including prescription drugs, OTC drugs, and natural health products) that may interact with NSAIDs. Drug interactions for NSAIDs and salicylates include alcohol, heparin, phenytoin, anticoagulants, corticosteroids, and sulpha antibiotics. Other specific drug interactions for NSAIDs are as follows:

- Indole agents (e.g., indomethacin, sulindac): avoid agents that are ulcerogenic, corticosteroids, anticoagulants, and ASA products
- Enolic agents (e.g., phenylbutazone): enhance the effects of oral anticoagulants, insulin and oral antidiabetic agents, corticosteroids, and male or female hormones
- Phenylpropionic agents (e.g., ibuprofen, naproxen): interact adversely with anticoagulants and ASA
- ibuprofen and naproxen: anticoagulants, ASA, steroids, phenylbutazone
- indomethacin: corticosteroids, phenylbutazone, salicylates, anticoagulants
- phenylbutazone: oral anticoagulants, oral antidiabetic agents, insulin, penicillin, sulphonamides, barbiturates, sex hormones, steroids
- sulindac: ASA

The COX-2 inhibitor celecoxib has the same contraindications as other NSAIDs, but in some situations it has been found to have less severe side effects. Contraindications include allergy to ASA or sulphonamides and third trimester of pregnancy. Cautious use is recommended in geriatric clients and in those with renal or hepatic dysfunction (often a reduction of dose by 50 percent may be necessary), history of GI ulcers, fluid retention, heart failure, and hypertension. Drug interactions include ACE inhibitors, diuretics, salicylates, corticosteroids, warfarin, lithium, and anticoagulants.

Ketorolac is indicated only for short-term use (no more than five days) and for clients experiencing severe acute pain. It is contraindicated in clients with active or past peptic ulcer disease, a history of a confirmed stroke, recent GI bleeding, or gastritis, and during the preoperative period. Cautious use includes the careful self-administration of OTCs, ASA, and other forms of NSAIDs (e.g., prescription and non-prescription drugs). Drug interactions include OTC preparations such as ASA, ASA-containing drugs, NSAIDs (e.g., ibuprofen), alcohol, corticosteroids, lithium, anticoagulants, ACE inhibitors, diuretics, and antiepileptic drugs. The nurse must assess the length of time the drug needs to be used before administering it because Ketorolac is only recommended for use for up to five days, whether used alone or in combination of dosage forms (e.g., injectable plus tablets).

Laboratory tests reflecting the functioning level of the cardiac, renal, and liver systems; levels of RBCs; and Hgb, Hct, and platelet counts should be determined and the results documented before NSAIDs or DMARDs are used. In addition, laboratory studies that assess the status of other diseases (inflammatory-type diseases) may be ordered, such as an evaluation of rheumatoid factors, sedimentation rate values, and immunoglobulins.

Before and during the administration of anti-arthritic drugs (also called *antirheumatic drugs* or *DMARDs*), which include NSAIDs, penicillamine, gold products, immunosuppressants, antimalarials, and cytotoxic agents, it is important for the nurse to assess the client's respiratory function, such as dyspnea, wheezing, or history of any other respiratory problems, because the drug may need to be discontinued in these situations. Renal status and hepatic function must also be assessed because decreased function of these organs may necessitate a decrease in dosage. Contraindications to their use include hypersensitivity, lupus erythematosus, uncontrolled diabetes mellitus, heart failure, renal and liver disease, and hypertension. Anti-arthritic agents should be used cautiously with geriatric clients, children, pregnant women, and clients with blood dyscrasias. Drug interactions for which to assess include penicillamine, phenylbutazone, immunosuppressants, antimalarials, and cytotoxic agents, which may all lead to increased occurrence of blood dyscrasias. The newer antirheumatics, or DMARDs (e.g., leflunomide and etanercept), carry a high risk of liver toxicity if given with methotrexate or with other agents that are hepatotoxic.

Before administering colchicine (an anti-gout drug), it is important for the nurse to assess the client for any contraindications, such as allergies, severe GI disorders, blood dyscrasias, renal or hepatic disease, and cardiac diseases. Cautious use is recommended in geriatric clients and in clients with GI disorders. Drug interactions for colchicine include CNS depressants and sympathomimetics; simultaneous use of these medications (with colchicines) may lead to enhanced effects of the CNS depressants and the sympathomimetics.

Allopurinol is contraindicated in clients with known allergies to the medication. It should be administered cautiously in clients with renal or hepatic disease. Drug interactions include mercaptopurine and azathioprine (increased bone marrow depression when used with allopurinol) and cyclophosphamide (increased action of the allopurinol).

Nursing Diagnoses

Nursing diagnoses relevant to the use of NSAIDs and other anti-inflammatory agents should always take into consideration the specific indication for the agents and the client's medical diagnosis. The following nursing diagnoses may be appropriate:

- Acute pain related to disease process or injury.
- Activity intolerance related to the disorder, condition, or disease process causing the pain.
- Risk for injury to self related to the influence of the disease or treatment.
- Ineffective health maintenance related to lack of knowledge about pharmacological and non-pharmacological measures of treatment.
- Deficient knowledge related to first-time drug therapy for pain or disease process.

Planning

Goals pertinent to clients receiving NSAIDs and other anti-inflammatory agents include the following:

- Client is able to describe the use of the medication as it relates to the relief of inflammation and pain.

- Client experiences pain relief or relief of symptoms within expected period.
- Client uses non-pharmacological measures along with drug therapy to decrease inflammation so that he or she can increase activities of living (ADLs), including walking.
- Client reports adverse effects to the physician as indicated.
- Client remains adherent with medication therapy.

▨ *Outcome Criteria*

Outcome criteria for clients receiving NSAIDs and other anti-inflammatory agents include the following:

- Client states that pain is characteristic of inflammation, injury, or related disease and will decrease with therapy.
- Client identifies factors that aggravate or alleviate pain, such as movement, activity, noises, and so on.
- Client states non-pharmacological measures to use to promote comfort (e.g., hot or cold packs, physical therapy, relaxation therapy) and to increase ADLs, including walking.
- Client states side effects of NSAIDs, such as GI upset, heartburn, nausea and vomiting, and anorexia.
- Client discusses symptoms to report to the physician immediately, such as epigastric distress, nausea and vomiting, abdominal pain, dyspnea, and bleeding or easy bruising.
- Client states the importance of correct dosing and consistency in self-administering medication.
- Client returns for follow-up visits with the physician.

▨ Implementation

The client should be educated about the various side effects of NSAIDs, including the acetic acids and the propionic, pyranocarboxylic, and pyrrolizine acids (see Table 43-2 for those of the most commonly used agents). Should side effects become severe or intolerable or GI bleeding or abdominal pain occur, the physician must be contacted immediately. It is important for the nurse to prevent or decrease GI irritation by encouraging clients to take NSAIDs with food, milk, or an antacid. However, clients should still be watched closely for any unusual bleeding (such as in the stool) because of the increased risk for GI ulcerations. In addition, it is important for the nurse to explain to the client the difference between the medication's onset of action for the relief of acute pain as opposed to its more delayed effect when used for the relief of arthritis pain; in the latter case the therapeutic effects may not be realized for three to four weeks. Enteric-coated tablets should not be crushed or chewed. Treatment of salicylate overdose is usually by lavage, activated charcoal, and supportive treatment.

Clients on COX-2 inhibitors should not consume alcohol, ASA, or any OTC agents.

Ketorolac (IM, IV, or tablets) is for short-term use only (five days or less). It is critical that dosing orders be

---

PEDIATRIC CONSIDERATIONS ◆▲◣◆▮

Reye's Syndrome

Reye's syndrome occurs primarily in children, with peak incidence between six months and 15 years of age. This syndrome may be a life-threatening illness characterized by encephalopathy, liver damage, and other serious complications. It is associated with the administration of ASA. Reye's syndrome usually occurs after a viral infection, such as chicken pox or influenza B, during which time ASA is often given for fever.

Signs and Symptoms
- Altered liver function
- Encephalopathy
- Fatty degeneration of the viscera
- Changes in level of consciousness
- Coma, flaccid paralysis, loss of deep tendon reflexes
- Hypoglycemia
- Seizures
- Vomiting

Medical Management
- Supportive treatment in ICU
- Maintain life functions, regain metabolic balance, and control cerebral edema
- IV glucose (10 percent or higher) for treatment of hypoglycemia
- Monitor blood sugars; insulin may be needed
- Vitamin K for clotting problems
- Fresh-frozen plasma may be needed if there is significant bleeding
- Prophylactic anti-epileptic drugs
- Monitor intracranial pressure
- Cautious fluid administration
- Osmotic diuretics may be needed with steroids for cerebral edema

Nursing Management
- Critical care setting
- Assess neurological status, vital signs, and arterial and central venous pressures
- Monitor blood gases and intracranial pressure
- Control temperature to prevent elevations and increased O_2 demands
- Elevate head of bed
- Record intake and output
- Hyperventilation may be needed with intubation to reduce intracranial pressure by lowering CO_2 levels and increasing O_2 levels
- Quiet environment
- Handle gently
- Monitor O_2 for seizure activity
- Family support
- Physical and emotional support for child and family with recovery
- Spiritual care

Educate the public about Reye's Syndrome to help prevent this severe and potentially life-threatening reaction.

checked carefully and that maximum doses do not exceed the manufacturer's guidelines or physician's orders. The ophthalmic solution of ketorolac should be given carefully and as ordered. This drug may delay eye wound healing and lead to corneal epithelial breakdown.

Anti-arthritic agents, such as gold sodium thiomalate, should never be given intravenously and when indicated to be given intramuscularly should be given in deep muscle. It is important for the client to remain recumbent for at least ten minutes and to remain under medical observation for 30 minutes after the injection because of the potential for an anaphylactic response.

The DMARDs (e.g., leflunomide) may be used with NSAIDs or low-dose corticosteroids and should be continued only if ALT levels are watched closely. These drugs are to be given exactly as ordered.

The anti-gout drugs are somewhat different from the NSAIDs and have different nursing considerations. Colchicine should be taken on an empty stomach for more complete absorption, which means one hour before meals or two hours after meals. Clients should be instructed to increase their fluid intake (unless contraindicated) to 3 to 4 L in 24 hours. Clients must also be instructed to not consume alcohol or OTC cold relief products that contain alcohol while taking this medication. In addition, clients with gout must be instructed that adherence with the entire medical regimen is critical to the success of the treatment.

Allopurinol should be given with meals to decrease the likelihood of GI symptoms (nausea, vomiting, anorexia). If the allopurinol is being administered in conjunction with chemotherapy (to decrease hyperuricemia associated with the malignancy and treatment), it should be given a few days before. Clients taking allopurinol should be informed to increase fluid intake to 3 to 4 L per day, to avoid hazardous activities if dizziness or drowsiness occurs with the medication, and to avoid the use of alcohol and caffeine because these drugs will increase uric acid levels and decrease the levels of allopurinol.

See the box on p. 741 for client teaching tips for the use of NSAIDs.

Evaluation

NSAIDs—whether acetic, propionic, pyranocarboxylic, or pyrrolizine acid—may vary in their potency and anti-inflammatory effects. Therapeutic responses to NSAIDs include the following: decrease in acute pain; decrease in swelling, pain, stiffness, and tenderness of a joint or muscle area; return to normal laboratory values (CBC, RBC, Hgb level, Hct, and sedimentation rates); and return to a less inflamed state as evidenced by X-ray examination, computed tomography (CT) scan, or magnetic resonance imaging (MRI). The COX-2 inhibitor should also result in improved joint function and fewer inflammation-based signs and symptoms. Clients should begin to show improvement in ADLs and mobility. Monitoring for the occurrence of side effects and monitoring of liver function studies is essential to the safe and effective use of the COX-2 inhibitor (see Table 43-2).

Evaluating therapeutic responses to all other anti-arthritic agents and DMARDs includes monitoring for the increased ability to move joints with less discomfort and an overall increased sense of improvement in the condition.

Toxicity to gold products is evident by a decreased Hgb level, a white blood cell (WBC) count of less than 4.0 $\times 10^9$/L, platelets less than 150 $\times 10^9$/L, hematuria, severe diarrhea, itching, and proteinuria. Toxicity to DMARDs is evident by an elevation of ALT level.

A therapeutic response to anti-gout drugs (e.g., colchicines) includes decreased pain in joints and increased sense of well-being. The client should be monitored closely for or should report to the physician increased pain, blood in the urine, excessive fatigue and lethargy, and chills or fever. A therapeutic response to allopurinol, an anti-gout drug, includes a decrease in pain in the joints, a decrease in uric acid levels, and a decrease of stone formation in the kidneys.

CASE STUDY

Post-operative Pain

One of your post-operative abdominal surgery clients is complaining of abdominal pain, nausea, and breakthrough pain after receiving the pain protocol for Dilaudid PCA and ketorolac intramuscularly. She has received ketorolac for 15 days and in multiple doses. A GI ulcer is now diagnosed and has been attributed to the ketorolac; however, the client has a past history of gastritis and reflux disease and a five-year history of ulcer disease.

- What is the action of ketorolac?
- What could have been done to prevent the GI bleeding and ulcer formation with the ketorolac?
- What concerns would you have regarding the past history of GI disorders and how could you have handled this potential risk to the client? Was there any problem with the number of days ordered? Is ketorolac available orally, or only in injectable forms?

For answers see http://evolve.elsevier.com/Lilley/pharmacology/.

CLIENT TEACHING TIPS

NSAIDS

▲ Clients should understand that NSAIDs are used for the treatment of pain, an injury, or a disease process and that they work by decreasing the inflammation that leads to pain.

▲ Clients should know the most common side effects of the NSAIDs, which are as follows:
  - *ibuprofen:* heartburn, GI upset, ulcers, nausea
  - *indomethacin:* headache, nausea, vomiting, GI upset, ulcers, hemorrhage, hemolytic anemias, epistaxis, blurred vision, rash, leucopenia
  - *naproxen:* vomiting, blurred vision, decreased Hgb level and Hct value
  - *piroxicam:* GI upset, elevated blood urea nitrogen (BUN) level, dizziness, vertigo, edema, tinnitus, GI ulcer
  - *sulindac:* GI upset, GI discomfort, ulcers, rash, tinnitus, diarrhea, nausea

The nurse should instruct the client as follows:

▲ Take this medication with food, milk, or an antacid.

▲ Check your stools from time to time, and report to the physician if you notice blood in the stools.

▲ These drugs interact with many other drugs. Make sure your physician is aware of any drugs you are taking.

▲ Tell any other healthcare providers, including your dentist, that you are taking this drug.

▲ Check with your doctor before taking over-the-counter medications.

▲ Do not take ASA (aspirin) unless it is prescribed for you.

COX-2 Inhibitor

▲ Take only the prescribed dose.

▲ Avoid alcohol, ASA, and over-the-counter medications.

▲ Report to the physician immediately any stomach pain or other stomach problems, unusual bleeding, blood in vomit or stool, chest pain, or palpitations.

Anti-Arthritic Agents

▲ Take the medication exactly as prescribed.

▲ Get lab work done monthly as ordered.

▲ Report any skin conditions, fatigue, or sores in the mouth.

▲ Report to the physician any blood in your stools or urine, bleeding gums, or easy bruising.

▲ Unless the doctor has told you otherwise, drink eight to twelve glasses of fluid a day.

▲ It may take up to three to four months for the drug to reach the levels in your blood where it becomes really effective.

▲ Use sunscreen. This drug may make you more sensitive to sunlight.

▲ (For women of childbearing age who may be sexually active) Use contraception while taking this medication.

▲ Do not consume alcohol while taking this medication. This includes over-the-counter cold relief products that contain alcohol.

▲ (For clients with gout) To be successful in treating your gout, you must follow the whole treatment plan, not just medication.

Allopurinol

▲ Drink 3 to 3.5 L of fluids a day.

▲ If you become dizzy or drowsy, avoid hazardous activities.

▲ Do not drink alcohol, or use any over-the-counter medicine containing alcohol. Do not drink coffee, tea, cola drinks or any other product containing caffeine. Alcohol and caffeine will make your condition worse and your medication less effective.

POINTS to REMEMBER

▼ NSAIDs are one of the most commonly prescribed categories of drugs.

▼ The first drug in this category to be synthesized was salicylic acid.

▼ There are now many different NSAIDs, but only a few are commonly used.

▼ NSAIDs act by working in the arachidonic acid pathway.

▼ NSAIDs have analgesic, anti-inflammatory, and antipyretic activity; ASA also has antiplatelet activity.

▼ NSAIDs are often used in the treatment of gout, osteoarthritis, juvenile arthritis, rheumatoid arthritis, dysmenorrhea, and musculoskeletal injuries such as strains and sprains.

▼ The three main side effects of NSAIDs are GI intolerance, bleeding (often GI bleeding), and renal impairment.

▼ Misoprostol may be given to prevent GI intolerance and ulcers resulting from NSAIDs. It is classified as a PG analogue.

▼ There are many contraindications to the use of NSAIDs, such as allergies to them, GI tract lesions, peptic ulcers, and bleeding disorders.

▼ Most oral NSAIDs are better tolerated if taken with food to minimize GI upset.

▼ Clients on NSAIDs should be closely monitored for the occurrence of bleeding, such as blood in the stools or vomit.

▼ When NSAIDs are used to decrease inflammation in the joints of arthritis clients, therapeutic effects usually take up to three to four weeks.

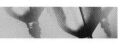

EXAMINATION REVIEW QUESTIONS

1 Which of the following drugs may be given to prevent the GI side effects of NSAIDs?
a. misoprostol
b. metoprolol
c. metoclopramide
d. magnesium sulphate

2 Which of the following manifestations indicates that your client is suffering from NSAID toxicity?
a. Nausea
b. Anorexia
c. Severe abdominal pain
d. Cerebral edema

3 Anti-gout drugs work by which of the following mechanisms?
a. Increasing blood oxygen levels
b. Decreasing leukocytes and platelets
c. Increasing protein and rheumatoid factors
d. Decreasing serum uric acid levels

4 Which of the following statements is most accurate about many of the anti-gout drugs?
a. Drink only limited amounts of fluid with the drug.
b. Limited movements of joints and oliguria are common side effects.
c. Cancer cell death and related by-product levels, such as uric acid, may be controlled through use of allopurinol.
d. When given with NSAIDs and colchicine, there are few adverse effects.

5 Which of the following is the only NSAID available in oral, ophthalmic, and parenteral dosage forms?
a. ketorolac
b. ibuprofen
c. colchicine
d. sulfinpyrazone

For answers see http://evolve.elsevier.com/Lilley/pharmacology/.

CRITICAL THINKING ACTIVITIES

1 Is the following statement true or false? Acetaminophen is an NSAID and exerts anti-inflammatory, antipyretic, analgesic, and antiplatelet effects. Explain your answer.

2 What are the drug interactions for NSAIDs? What problems may occur if these drugs are used with NSAIDs?

3 Describe the protocol for treating salicylate intoxication of a chronic nature.

For answers see http://evolve.elsevier.com/Lilley/pharmacology/.

BIBLIOGRAPHY

Albanese, J., & Nutz, P. (2005). *Mosby's 2005 nursing drug cards.*, St Louis, MO: Mosby.

Boron, W.F., & Boulpaep, E.L. (2005). *Medical physiology.* St Louis, MO: Elsevier Saunders.

Canadian Pharmacists Association. (2003). *Therapeutic choices* (4th ed.). Ottawa, ON: Author.

Canadian Pharmacists Association. (2004). *Guide to drugs in Canada.* Toronto, ON: Dorling Kindersley.

Canadian Pharmacists Association. (2005). *Compendium of pharmaceuticals and specialties. The Canadian drug reference for health professionals.* Ottawa, ON: Author. [The subscription-based e-CPS is available at http://www.pharmacists.ca.]

Cheng, A., Williams, B.A., & Sivarajan, B.V. (Eds.). (2003). *The HSC handbook of pediatrics* (10th ed.). Toronto, ON: Elsevier.

Drummond, R., Kadri, N., & St-Cyr, J. (2001). Delayed salicylate toxicity following enteric-coated acetylsalicylic acid overdose: a case report and review of the literature. *Canadian Journal of Emergency Medicine, 3.* Retrieved March 17, 2006, from http://www.caep.ca/004.cjem-jcmu/004-00.cjem/vol-3.2001/v31-044.htm

Facts and Comparisons. (2004). *Drug facts and comparisons pocket version* (9th ed.). St Louis, MO: Wolters Kluwer Health.

Hardman, J.G., & Limbird, L.E. (2002). *Goodman and Gilman's the pharmacological basis of therapeutics* (10th ed.). New York: McGraw-Hill.

Health Canada. (2005). Drug product database (DPD). Retrieved September 1, 2005, from http://www.hc-sc.gc.ca/hpb/drugs-dpd/

Health Canada. (2004). Advisory. Health Canada informs Canadians of Vioxx withdrawal by Merck & Co. Retrieved September 1, 2005, from http://www.hc-sc.gc.ca/ahc-asc/media/advisories-avis/2004/2004_50_e.htm

Kasper, D.L., Braunwald, D., Faci, A., Hauser, S., Longo, D., & Jameson, J.L. (2005). *Harrison's principles of internal medicine* (16th ed.). New York: McGraw-Hill.

Katzung, B.G. (2004). *Basic and clinical pharmacology* (9th ed.). New York: McGraw-Hill.

Lacy, C.F., Armstrong, L.L., Goldman, M.P., & Lance, L.L. (2003). *Drug information handbook* (11th ed.). Hudson, OH: LexiComp.

Lehne, R.A. (2004). *Pharmacology for nursing care* (5th ed.). St Louis, MO: Saunders.

Mosby. (2005). *Mosby's drug consult 2005: The comprehensive reference for generic and brand name drugs* (15th ed.). St Louis, MO: Mosby.

Murray, S. (2005). Drug regulation. Health Canada lukewarm on Vioxx panel findings. *Canadian Medical Association Journal, 173*(4), 350.

Pfizer. (2005). Pfizer Canada to suspend sales of Bextra in compliance with Health Canada concerns over skin reactions. Retrieved November 25, 2005, from http://www.pfizer.ca/english/newsroom/press

Skidmore-Roth, L. (2006). *Mosby's 2006 nursing drug reference* (19th ed.). St Louis, MO: Mosby.

Immune and Biological Modifiers and Chemotherapeutic Agents: Study Skills Tips

- TIME MANAGEMENT
- EVALUATE PRIOR PERFORMANCE
- ANTICIPATE THE TEST
- PLAN FOR DISTRIBUTED STUDY

TIME MANAGEMENT

The first step in preparing for a chapter or part exam is to plan for the time needed. Let us begin by assuming that the next test you have will cover the chapters in Part Eight. First examine the material to determine just how much there is to cover. Look at the objectives, the glossary, and the number of pages of text in each chapter. This will help you determine just how big a task you face. As you are doing this, also consider how much study time you have been devoting to these chapters in the days before the exam. If you have been doing regular study with frequent review sessions, then the demand on your time in the day or two just before the exam will be less than if you have to do a major cram session to try to catch up on study that has been put off. The basic question to answer here is a simple one. "How much time do I need to schedule for exam preparation?" The answer varies with each student. Some will need six, eight, or more hours of preparation time in the two to three days before the exam. Others will find that three, four, or five hours will be adequate. You must assess your own learning and prior success to determine what time is necessary for you, but you must set time aside and use it effectively.

One thing should play a major role in determining the time you will need to set aside. Evaluate your performance on prior exams. How have you been doing? How much time have you been spending to achieve that level? If you are not achieving according to your capabilities, then you should certainly consider spending more time preparing for the next exam. If you are achieving at a sat-

isfactory level, then plan on devoting about the same amount of time to test preparation.

The next step in preparing for an exam is to organize the time. Write down what you are going to study and when and how much time you will spend. Consider the following example based on the material in Chapters 46 and 47:

1 Review Chapter 46 objectives. Monday, 4:00 to 4:30 P.M. Note objectives that are unclear for further review.
2 Question and Answer review, Monday, 4:30 to 5:15 P.M.
3 Self-test, Chapter 46 glossary. Monday, 6:30 to 7:00 P.M. Note terms that need further review for mastery.
4 Review Chapter 47 objectives. Monday, 7:00 to 7:30 P.M.
5 Question and Answer review, Monday, 7:30 to 8:00 P.M.
6 Self-test, Chapter 47 glossary. Monday, 8:00 to 8:30 P.M.

The advantage to this test preparation model is that you now know where you must focus in the days before the exam.

EVALUATE PRIOR PERFORMANCE

As you begin preparing to review for any exam, take some time to look back at previous exams. Evaluate your performance, and use that evaluation to improve on subsequent tests. As you look at prior tests consider the following factors:

What Type of Errors Did I Make?

Students often find that they miss certain question types or forms. Assess your errors and try to pinpoint any recurring patterns in your mistakes. Did you miss questions that contained an exemption in the multiple choice stem? Questions that state "all of the following except" or ask "Which of the following would not be. . . " are exemption questions. Students often choose one of the apparently correct responses. Read the question carefully to see whether you are looking for a correct or an incorrect answer. An exemption stem is asking for the response choice that is "wrong."

Did I Have Trouble With Questions That Required Mastery of Terminology?

Look at questions that demanded mastery of the terms from the chapters. If you missed more than one or two questions of that type, then you know you need to spend more time reviewing terminology.

Did I Miss Concept Questions?

If the question asked you to apply a principle, evaluate a drug response, or in some other way apply knowledge from the course, you are dealing with concepts rather than facts. If you missed a number of concept questions, then you should spend more of your review time studying applications and principles than memorizing facts and terms.

Did I Make Errors Because I Did Not Know the Material?

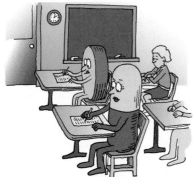

This question focuses on the quality of your learning. If you miss one or two questions on an exam because you did not learn (or did not remember) the material, it is not a major problem.

There will almost always be one or two questions that you do not remember. But if you had to guess on several questions because you did not recall any information that seemed relevant, you may need to put more time into review. It is essential that you acknowledge to yourself that you have missed questions because you did not know the material. Once you have acknowledged the problem, take steps to correct it. You may need to do more oral rehearsal so that the material is stored in long-term memory.

ANTICIPATE THE TEST

Do not wait until exam time to find out what you should know. As you do your review try to think like the instructor. Generate questions that you think might be a part of the test. This does not mean you need to try to write multiple choice stems and choices, but you should be trying to focus your review in a way that will facilitate learning and long-term memory.

Here are some examples of questioning that you might use based on material found in Chapter 47.

1 What are immunomodulators (IMs)?
2 What is the role of IMs in the care of clients with cancer?
3 What is the role of the immune system in treating cancer?

The sample questions were drawn from just the first few pages of the chapter. The first question focuses on literal comprehension. This type of question is easy to generate. Being able to answer such questions is important, but if all of your questions are literal, it may be difficult to answer questions that require application of principles and concepts. For that reason it is 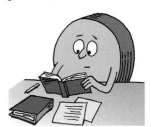 essential that some questions require analysis, synthesis, and/or evaluation of the material. Question 3 is an example of this type of question. Answers to these questions require the learner to put together the literal information and relate the terms to the concepts being explained.

PLAN FOR DISTRIBUTED STUDY

Many students wait too long to begin the review for a test. This forces them into a pattern of long hours of intensive study all packed into the last day or two before the exam. Although cramming does work to some degree, it is not the most effective way to learn. A better model is to distribute the review over a period of several days with short, 30-minute to 1-hour study sessions several times each day. Distributing practice in this way allows time for you to think about what you have been learning, and it fosters long-term memory.

Spend more of your review time doing oral rehearsal (asking and answering questions) than simply rereading material. Oral rehearsal encourages active learning, which enhances your ability to concentrate, improves comprehension and memory, and thus improves test performance.

Immunosuppressant Agents

CHAPTER

44

OBJECTIVES

After reading this chapter, the successful student will be able to do the following:

1 Discuss the role of immunosuppressive therapy in organ transplant recipients and in the treatment of autoimmune diseases.

2 Discuss the mechanisms of action, contraindications, cautions, side effects, and toxicity associated with the most commonly used immunosuppressants.

3 Develop a nursing care plan that includes all phases of the nursing process for the client receiving immunosuppressants either for an organ transplant or for the treatment of autoimmune diseases.

e-LEARNING ACTIVITIES

Student CD-ROM
- Review Questions: see questions 332–336
- Animations
- Medication Administration Checklists
- IV Therapy Checklists

evolve Website (http://evolve.elsevier.com/Lilley/pharmacology/)
- Online Chapter Worksheet • Frequently Asked Questions
- Learning Tips and Content Updates • WebLinks • Online Appendices and Supplements • Mosby/Saunders ePharmacology Update • Access to *Mosby's Drug Consult*

DRUG PROFILES

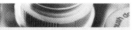

▶▶azathioprine, p. 747   glatiramer acetate, p. 749
basiliximab p. 748   ▶▶muromonab-CD3, p. 749
▶▶cyclosporine, p. 749   sirolimus, p. 749
daclizumab, p. 749

▶▶ Key drug.

GLOSSARY

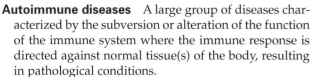

Autoimmune diseases A large group of diseases characterized by the subversion or alteration of the function of the immune system where the immune response is directed against normal tissue(s) of the body, resulting in pathological conditions.

Graft A transplanted tissue or organ.

Immune-mediated diseases A large group of diseases that result when the cells of the immune system react to a variety of situations, such as transplanted organ tissue or drug-altered cells.

Immunosuppressant (im' yoo noe sə press' ənt) An agent that decreases or prevents an immune response.

Immunosuppressive therapy A drug treatment used to suppress the immune system.

Murine antibodies (myoo' ryne) Monoclonal immunoglobulins. Monoclonal refers to a protein from a single clone of cells; all molecules of the protein are identical. Murine refers to the family Muridae, to which mice belong. An antibody is a protective protein that counters the actions of antigens, substances that cause sensitivity or an allergic response. Thus murine antibodies are protective proteins obtained from mice. Muromonab-CD3 is a murine antibody used to reverse graft rejection.

IMMUNOSUPPRESSANT AGENTS

The human body is under constant attack by invading micro-organisms, but it possesses several mechanisms with which to fight off these foreign invaders; one is the immune system. This system defends the body against invading pathogens, foreign antigens, and its own cells when they become cancerous, or neoplastic. However, this highly sophisticated system can also sometimes attack itself and cause what are known as **autoimmune diseases** or **immune-mediated diseases**. It also participates in hypersensitivity, or anaphylactic, reactions, which can be life threatening. The rejection of kidney, liver, and

TABLE 44-1

CLASSIFICATION AND MECHANISMS OF ACTION FOR AVAILABLE IMMUNOSUPPRESSANT AGENTS

Drug Names	Pharmacological Class and Mechanism of Action	Indications
azathioprine	Blocks metabolism of purines, inhibiting the synthesis of T-cell DNA, RNA, and proteins, thereby blocking immune response.	Organ rejection prevention in kidney transplantation; rheumatoid arthritis.
muromonab-CD3*	Binds to CD3 glycoprotein on T-cell receptors, which blocks antigen recognition and reverses graft rejection that is already in progress.	Treatment of acute organ rejection in kidney, liver, and heart transplantation.
cyclosporine	Inhibits activation of T-cells by blocking the production and release of the cytokine mediator IL-2.	Organ rejection prevention in bone marrow, kidney, liver, and heart transplantation; rheumatoid arthritis; psoriasis; steroid dependent and steroid resistant nephrotic syndrome. Unlabelled uses† include pancreas, lupus nephritis, and heart/lung transplantation.
glatiramer acetate	Precise mechanism unknown. Believed to somehow modify immune system processes that are associated with MS symptoms.	Reduction of relapse frequency in clients with RRMS.
tacrolimus	Inhibits T-cell activation, possibly by binding to an intracellular protein known as FKBP-12.	Organ rejection prevention in liver and kidney transplantation; active rheumatoid arthritis. Unlabelled uses† include transplantation of bone marrow, heart, pancreas, pancreatic islet cell, lung and trachea, skin, cornea, limb, and small intestine; autoimmune diseases; and severe psoriasis.
mycophenolate mofetil	Prevents proliferation of T-cells by inhibiting intracellular purine synthesis.	Organ rejection prevention in kidney, liver, and heart transplantation.
daclizumab*	Suppresses T-cell activity by blocking the binding of the cytokine receptor IL-2 to a specific receptor.	
basiliximab*	Suppresses T-cell activity by blocking the binding of the cytokine mediator IL-2 to a specific receptor.	Organ rejection prevention in kidney transplantation.
sirolimus	Inhibits T-cell activation by binding to an intracellular protein known as FKBP-12, creating a complex that subsequently binds to a cellular component known as the mTOR, which prevents cellular proliferation.	

*Note that "ab" in any drug name usually indicates that it is a monoclonal antibody synthesized using recombinant DNA technology.
†A use not approved by Health Canada but under investigation.
IL-2, interleukin-2; *MS,* multiple sclerosis; *RRMS,* relapsing-remitting multiple sclerosis; *mTOR,* mammalian target of rapamycin.

heart (whole organ) transplants is directed by the immune system as well. Thus the immune system is capable of having many beneficial and detrimental effects.

Agents that decrease or prevent an immune response, and hence suppress the immune system, are known as **immunosuppressants**. Treatment with such drugs is referred to as **immunosuppressive therapy**, and it is used to selectively eradicate certain cell lines that play a major role in the rejection of a transplanted organ. These cell lines must be targeted and selectively altered or suppressed, or organ rejection will occur. The primary immunosuppressant drugs are the corticosteroids (Chapter 32), cyclophosphamide (Chapter 46), azathioprine, cyclosporine, muromonab-CD3, tacrolimus, glatiramer acetate, daclizumab, basiliximab, and sirolimus.

Mechanism of Action and Drug Effects

All immunosuppressants have similar mechanisms of action because they all selectively suppress certain T-lymphocyte cell lines, thereby preventing their involvement in the immune response. This results in a pharmacologically immunocompromised state similar to that in a cancer client whose bone marrow and immune cells have been destroyed as the result of chemotherapy or that in a client with AIDS, whose immune cells have been destroyed by the HIV. Each agent differs in the exact way in which it suppresses certain cell lines involved in an immune response (see Table 44-1).

Indications

Immunosuppressants have many uses, which vary from agent to agent (Table 44-2). They are primarily indicated for the prevention of organ rejection. However, some are also used for other immunological illnesses such as rheumatoid arthritis and multiple sclerosis. Only muromonab-CD3 is indicated for treatment of organ rejection once rejection of a transplanted organ is underway. The four newer agents (basiliximab, daclizumab, sirolimus, and mycophenolate mofetil) are all indicated for prophylaxis. Azathioprine is used as an adjunct medication to prevent the rejection of kidney transplants and to ameliorate severe rheumatoid arthritis. Cyclosporine is the primary immunosuppressant agent used in the prevention of kidney, liver, heart, and bone marrow trans-

TABLE 44-2
SELECTED IMMUNOSUPPRESSANTS: INDICATIONS

Immunosuppressant	Indications
azathioprine	Adjunct in organ rejection prevention; rheumatoid arthritis
basiliximab	Adjunct in organ rejection prevention
cyclosporine	Organ rejection prevention and treatment; rheumatoid arthritis; nephrotic syndrome
daclizumab	Adjunct in organ rejection prevention
muromonab	Organ rejection prevention and treatment
mycophenolate mofetil	Adjunct in organ rejection prevention
sirolimus	Adjunct in organ rejection prevention
tacrolimus	Adjunct in organ rejection prevention

TABLE 44-3
IMMUNOSUPPRESSANT AGENTS: COMMON ADVERSE EFFECTS

Body System	Side/Adverse Effects
AZATHIOPRINE	
Hematological	Leukopenia, thrombocytopenia
Hepatic	Hepatotoxicity (common)
CYCLOSPORINE	
Cardiovascular	Moderate hypertension
Central nervous	Neurotoxicity, including tremors (in about 20% of clients)
Hepatic	Hepatotoxicity with cholestasis and hyperbilirubinemia
Renal	Nephrotoxicity (common and dose limiting)
Other	Hypersensitivity reactions to the vehicle, gingival hyperplasia, and hirsutism
MUROMONAB-CD3	
Cardiovascular	Chest pain, hypotension/shock
Central nervous	Pyrexia, chills, tremors
Gastrointestinal	Vomiting, nausea, diarrhea
Respiratory	Dyspnea, wheezing, pulmonary edema
Other	Flu-like symptoms, fluid retention

plant rejection. It may also have beneficial effects in the treatment of other conditions with an immunological cause, such as certain types of arthritis, psoriasis, and nephrotic syndrome.

Tacrolimus has many of the same therapeutic effects as cyclosporine but is currently indicated only for the prevention of liver and kidney transplant rejection, although it has shown promise in preventing the rejection of other transplanted organs as well.

Glatiramer acetate is the only immunosuppressant currently indicated for treatment of multiple sclerosis (MS). Specifically, it is indicated for reduction of the frequency of MS relapses (exacerbations) in a type of MS known as *relapsing-remitting multiple sclerosis* (RRMS).

Contraindications

The main contraindication for all immunosuppressants is known drug allergy. Relative contraindications, depending on the client's condition, may include renal or hepatic failure, hypertension, and concurrent radiation therapy. Pregnancy is not necessarily a contraindication to these agents, but immunosuppressants should be used in pregnant women only in urgent situations.

Side Effects and Adverse Effects

Many of the side effects of the immunosuppressants can be devastating, especially to a transplant client. Although not strictly a side effect, a heightened susceptibility to opportunistic infections is a major risk for immunosuppressed clients. Other side effects and adverse effects are specific to particular agents, and some of the most common of these are listed in Table 44-3.

Interactions

The drug interactions associated with immunosuppressant use mostly involve cyclosporine. Cyclosporine is capable of many drug interactions, several of which can be harmful. Drugs that may increase its action are diltiazem, nicardipine, verapamil, fluconazole, itraconazole, clarithromycin, allopurinol, metoclopramide, amphotericin B, cimetidine, and ketoconazole. Drugs that may decrease its effects are carbamazepine, phenobarbital, phenytoin, and rifampin. Although these are the most significant in-

teractions, there are many more of less significance. It is also not recommended that azathioprine be given with allopurinol because allopurinol inhibits azathioprine's metabolism and thereby increases its effects.

Cyclosporine can have a *rather profound interaction with grapefruit juice.* When they are taken together there is an increase in the bioavailability of cyclosporine by 20 percent to 200 percent. Grapefruit juice is sometimes given with cyclosporine deliberately to achieve therapeutic blood levels of cyclosporine with decreased doses. The manufacturer of cyclosporine does not endorse this.

Dosages

For the recommended dosages of selected immunosuppressant agents, see the table on p. 748. See Appendix B for some of the common brands available in Canada.

DRUG PROFILES

▸▸ azathioprine

Azathioprine is a chemical analogue of the physiological purines, such as adenine and guanine. It blocks T-cell proliferation by inhibiting purine synthesis, which in turn prevents DNA synthesis. Mycophenolate mofetil is another immunosuppressant with a similar mechanism. Both are used for prophylaxis of organ rejection concurrently with other immunosuppressant agents, such as cyclosporine and corticosteroids. Azathioprine is available in both an oral (PO) and a parenteral formulation as a 50-mg tablet and a 50-mg vial injection. It is contraindicated in clients who have shown a hypersensitivity to it. Pregnancy category D. Commonly recommended dosages are listed in the dosages table on p. 748.

DOSAGES Selected Immunosuppressant Agents

Agent	Pharmacological Class	Usual Dosage Range	Indications
▸▸azathioprine	Purine antagonist	**Adult and pediatric** IV/PO: 3–5 mg/kg/day to start, then 1–3 mg/kg/day maintenance	Renal transplants
		Adult PO: 1 mg/kg/day as a single or divided dose for 6–8 wk, then may increase prn by 0.5 mg/kg/day q4wk to a maximum of 2.5 mg/kg/day	Rheumatoid arthritis
basiliximab	Monoclonal antibody	**Adult and Pediatric >2 yr** IV: Bolus injection of 20 mg given 2 h pre-op; repeat same dose once 4 days post-op	Prevention of rejection of kidney transplants
▸▸cyclosporine	Polypeptide antibiotic	**Adult and pediatric** PO: 10–15 mg/kg divided within 12 h pre-op; continue same dose post-op for 1–2 wk, then reduce to a maintenance dose of 2–6 mg/kg/day IV: Dose is ⅓ PO dose: 3–5 mg/kg as a single dose within 12 h pre-op and continued daily post-op until client can be switched to PO dosing	Kidney, liver, heart transplants
		IV: 12.5–15 mg/kg divided, 24 h pre-op; maintenance 12.5 mg/kg/day divided, for 3–6 mo	Bone marrow transplant
		PO: 2.0 mg/kg/day divided; titrated up 0.5–1 mg/kg/day monthly until effect to max 5 mg/kg/day	Psoriasis
		PO: 2.0 mg/kg/day divided; increased to max 5 mg/kg/day	Rheumatoid arthritis
		Adult PO: 3.5 mg/kg/day to max 5 mg/kg/day	Nephrotic syndrome
		Pediatric PO: 4.2 mg/kg/day to max 6 mg/kg/day	
daclizumab	Monoclonal antibody	**Adult and pediatric** IV: Bolus injection of 1 mg/kg 24 h pre-op and for 4 additional post-op doses, spaced 14 days apart	Prevention of rejection of kidney transplants
glatiramer acetate	Miscellaneous biological	**Adult only** SC: 20 mg once daily	RRMS
▸▸muromonab-CD3	Monoclonal antibody	**Adult and pediatric** IV: 5 mg/day as a single bolus injection for 10–14 days	Treatment of active rejection of renal allograft transplants; treatment of active rejection of liver and heart allograft transplants resistant to conventional treatment or for which conventional treatment is contraindicated
sirolimus	Fungus-derived	**Adult and pediatric** PO: Loading dose of 6 mg on day 1, followed by maintenance dose of 2 mg/day	Prevention of rejection of kidney transplants

RRMS, Relapsing-remitting multiple sclerosis.

PHARMACOKINETICS

Half-Life	Onset	Peak	Duration
5 hr	2–4 days*	1–2 hr	Unknown

*6–8 wk for rheumatoid arthritis.

basiliximab

Basiliximab is a monoclonal antibody that functions by inhibiting the binding of the cytokine mediator interleukin-2 (IL-2) to what is known as the high-affinity IL-2 receptor. It is also used to prevent rejection of trans-planted kidneys and is generally used as part of a multidrug immunosuppressive regimen that includes cyclosporine and corticosteroids. Its only known contraindication is drug allergy. It is available only as a powder for intravenous (IV) injection in a 20-mg vial. Pregnancy category B. Dosage information appears in the dosages table above.

PHARMACOKINETICS

Half-Life	Onset	Peak	Duration
7–9 days	<1 day	3–4 days	Unknown

▸▸ *cyclosporine*

Cyclosporine is an immunosuppressant indicated for the prevention of organ rejection. It is a potent drug and the principal agent in many immunosuppressive drug regimens. Like azathioprine, it may also be used for the treatment of other immunological disorders, such as various forms of arthritis, psoriasis, and nephritic syndrome.

Cyclosporine is available in two oral formulations. Neoral is an oral formulation that immediately forms a micro-emulsion in an aqueous environment. This property allows for greater oral bioavailability and more reliable oral absorption than the older formulation of cyclosporine (Sandimmune). Neoral is available as 10-mg, 25-mg, and 100-mg soft gelatin capsules and an oral solution of 100 mg/mL. Sandimmune is available in parenteral form as a 50-mg/mL injection. Although these two products contain the same active ingredient (cyclosporine), they cannot be used interchangeably. When changing from one to the other, dosages must be adjusted to account for the greater bioavailability of Neoral, and cyclosporine blood concentration should be monitored. Cyclosporine is contraindicated in clients with a known hypersensitivity to it. It has a narrow therapeutic index and for this reason laboratory monitoring of drug levels may be used to ensure therapeutic plasma concentrations and avoid toxicity. Pregnancy category C. Commonly recommended dosages are listed in the dosages table on p. 748.

PHARMACOKINETICS

Half-Life	Onset	Peak	Duration
18 hr, high variability	3–5 hr	Unknown	Unknown

daclizumab

Daclizumab is another monoclonal antibody with a mechanism of action similar to that of basiliximab. It is used in conjunction with cyclosporine and corticosteroid therapy to prevent rejection of transplanted kidney **grafts**. Its only known contraindication is drug allergy. It is available only as a 5-mg/mL intravenous injection. Pregnancy category C. Dosage information appears in the dosages table on p. 748.

PHARMACOKINETICS

Half-Life	Onset	Peak	Duration
18 hr, high 20 days	<1 day	3–5 days	Unknown

glatiramer acetate

Glatiramer acetate is a mixture of random polymers of four different amino acids. This mixture results in a compound that is antigenically similar to myelin basic protein, which is found on the myelin sheath of nerves. The drug is believed to work by blocking T-cell autoimmune activity against this protein, which reduces the frequency of the neuromuscular exacerbations associated with multiple sclerosis. The only known contraindication is drug allergy or allergy to mannitol. It is available only in single-dose vials containing 20 mg of glatiramer acetate dissolved in mannitol. Pregnancy category B. No specific pharmacokinetic data are currently available. Dosage information appears in the dosages table on p. 748.

▸▸ *muromonab-CD3*

Muromonab-CD3 is the only agent indicated for the reversal (not just the prevention) of graft rejection. It is unique in that it is a monoclonal antibody, synthesized using recombinant DNA technology, and it is similar to the antibodies naturally produced by the body (immunoglobulin G [IgG], IgM, IgD, IgA, and IgE). It specifically targets the binding sites on the T-cells that recognize foreign invaders, such as a transplanted organ. It differs from human antibodies in that it comes from mice. These types of antibodies are commonly referred to as **murine antibodies**, hence the name muromonab. "Muro" stands for murine; "mon" for monoclonal, which means they come from a single cell clone; and "ab" for antibody. Other monoclonal antibodies used for the prevention of organ rejection are basiliximab and daclizumab. Muromonab, often called OKT3, is contraindicated in clients with hypersensitivity to murine products, history of seizures, and in those who are experiencing fluid overload. It is available only in a parenteral formulation as a 5-mg/5-mL injection. Pregnancy category C. Commonly recommended dosages are listed in the dosages table on p. 748.

PHARMACOKINETICS

Half-Life	Onset	Peak	Duration
Unknown	Minutes	~3 days	Unknown

sirolimus

Sirolimus is a macrocyclic immunosuppressive, antifungal, and antitumour agent produced by fermentation of the fungus *Streptomyces hygroscopicus*. Other macrocyclic immunosuppressive agents are cyclosporine and tacrolimus. Sirolimus and tacrolimus are structurally related and act through similar mechanisms. Sirolimus is available as an oral solution in a 1-mg/mL concentration and as a 1-mg tablet. Pregnancy category C. Commonly recommended dosages are listed in the dosages table on p. 748.

PHARMACOKINETICS

Half-Life	Onset	Peak	Duration
57–68 hr	Unknown	1–3 hr	Unknown

NURSING PROCESS

■ Assessment

Before administering any of the immunosuppressants (azathioprine, cyclosporine, or muromonab-CD3), the nurse should perform a thorough client assessment and document the findings, which may include the following data:

* Renal function (blood urea nitrogen [BUN] and creatinine levels; information about urinary function and normal patterns of elimination)
* Liver function (alkaline phosphatase, aspartate aminotransferase [AST], alanine aminotransferase [ALT], and bilirubin levels); determining whether jaundice, edema, or ascites (the accumulation of serous fluid in the peritoneum) are present.

- Cardiovascular function (baseline electrocardiogram [ECG], blood pressure, and pulse; documentation of any cardiovascular disease or history of dysrhythmias, chest pain, or hypertension)
- Central nervous system baseline assessment (motor and sensory function and history of seizure disorders)
- Respiratory assessment (any complaints of dyspnea or wheezing and documentation of any pulmonary disorder, increased airway resistance, and signs and symptoms of pulmonary edema)

See Table 44-3 for information on other systems affected by the specific agents.

Cyclosporine is contraindicated in clients with a hypersensitivity to it. Cautious use is recommended in clients with severe renal or hepatic disease and in pregnant women. Muromonab-CD3 is contraindicated in clients with a hypersensitivity to substances with a murine origin and in clients suffering from fluid overload. Cautious use is advised in pregnant women, in children under two years of age, and in children with a fever. Contraindications for basiliximab (pregnancy category B) and daclizumab (pregnancy category C) include drug allergy. Laboratory studies (e.g., hemoglobin [Hgb] level, hematocrit [Hct] values, white blood cell [WBC] and platelet counts) should be performed and the results documented before, during (monthly), and after therapy. If the leukocyte count should drop below 3.0×10^9/L the drug should be discontinued, but only after contacting the physician.

Nursing Diagnoses

Nursing diagnoses pertinent to clients receiving immunosuppressants include the following:
- Risk for injury related to physiological influence of the disease and side effects of immunosuppressants.
- Risk for infection related to altered immune status.
- Acute pain (myalgias and arthralgias) related to side effects of medications.
- Deficient knowledge related to initiation of new treatment regimen.
- Non-adherence related to undesired side effects of drug treatment.

Planning

Goals in clients receiving immunosuppressants include the following:
- Client experiences minimal complications during drug therapy.
- Client experiences maximal comfort during drug therapy.
- Client remains adherent with drug therapy and comes in for follow-up visits with the physician.
- Client states symptoms of adverse reactions to therapy and of exacerbation of illness to report to physician.

Outcome Criteria

Outcome criteria for clients receiving immunosuppressants include the following:
- Client experiences minimal side effects of immunosuppressant (e.g., myalgias, fever, nephrotoxicity, hypertension).

- Client experiences a decrease in disease-related symptoms.
- Client is adherent with follow-up visits with physician to monitor therapeutic (decreased symptomatology) and adverse reactions to medication (e.g., myalgias, arthralgias).
- Client notifies physician immediately if fever, rash, sore throat, or fatigue develops.
- Client states measures to enhance comfort while on immunosuppressant therapy, such as use of non-ASA analgesics, rest, and biofeedback.

Implementation

It is important that oral immunosuppressants are taken with food to minimize gastrointestinal (GI) upset. It is also important, considering the immunosuppressed state of clients receiving immunosuppressants, that oral forms of the drugs be used whenever possible to decrease the risk of infection associated with intramuscular (IM) injections. An oral antifungal medication (e.g., fluconazole) is usually given with these agents to treat the oral candidiasis that may occur.

Cyclosporine is now available in two oral formulations, Neoral and Sandimmune. It is important to remember that Sandimmune and Neoral are not to be used interchangeably. When given intravenously, cyclosporine should be diluted as recommended in the manufacturer guidelines and given according to the standards of care and institutional policy regarding its administration. Cyclosporine is normally diluted with normal saline (NS) or 5 percent dextrose in water (D5W) in a concentration of 50 mg of the drug to 20 to 100 mL of diluting solution, which should be infused over two to six hours using an infusion pump.

Intravenously administered muromonab is usually given over one minute, and only after the medication is withdrawn through a 0.22 low-protein–binding micron filter. A sterile needle must be used after the medication is withdrawn. During the 24 hours after administration of muromonab, clients experience *cytokine release syndrome,* thought to be a response to the release of cytokines by activated lymphocytes. Clients commonly experience temporary flu-like symptoms, but some also experience a serious shock-like reaction. This syndrome usually occurs with the initial few doses. It is usually recommended that methylprednisolone sodium succinate be administered one to four hours before the muromonab injection to minimize this reaction to the medication. Acetaminophen and antihistamines may also be given concomitantly with muromonab to reduce reactions.

Both sirolimus and tacrolimus have long half-lives (up to 68 hours) and therefore toxicity may be a concern.

Basiliximab and daclizumab are administered parenterally. Dilutional solutions and amounts should be followed as per manufacturer guidelines and the intravenous drip closely monitored. An intravenous infusion pump may help to keep the proper dosage administered.

Client teaching tips for immunosuppressants are listed in the box on p. 751.

■ Evaluation

Therapeutic responses to the immunosuppressants include no rejection of a transplanted organ or graft and no obvious immunosuppression in clients with autoimmune disorders. The nurse should also check the client for drug-specific side effects and toxicity (see Table 44-3). Blood levels of cyclosporine should be monitored, especially when switching from one product to another.

CLIENT TEACHING TIPS

The nurse should instruct clients as follows:
▲ Avoid crowds to minimize the risk of infection.
▲ Report any fever, sore throat, chills, joint pain, or fatigue to the physician, because these may indicate severe infection.
▲ (for women of childbearing age who may be sexually active) Use some form of contraception during treatment and for up to 12 weeks after the end of therapy.

Azathioprine or Muromonab-CD3

▲ If possible, you will be given all your medication orally for several days before surgery to decrease the risk of infection from injections. Take this medication with food to help decrease stomach upset.
▲ Side effects of muromonab-CD3 include chills, fever, tremors, difficulty breathing, wheezing, pulmonary edema, chest pain, vomiting, nausea, and diarrhea.

Azathioprine for Rheumatoid Arthritis

▲ It may take three to four months before this medication has its effect.

Cyclosporine for Transplant Surgery

▲ You may be given this drug, along with corticosteroids, for several days before surgery. You may also be given an oral antifungal to prevent yeast infections.
▲ Do not take St. John's wort; it may reduce the effect of the medication and lead to rejection of your transplant.
▲ You will need to take medication for the rest of your life to make your organ transplantation successful.

Oral Cyclosporine

▲ Take your medication with meals or mixed with chocolate milk to prevent stomach upset.

POINTS to REMEMBER

▼ Immunosuppressants are agents that decrease or prevent the body's immune response and include drugs such as corticosteroids, cyclophosphamide, azathioprine, methotrexate, cyclosporine, muromonab-CD3, and tacrolimus.
▼ All immunosuppressants suppress the action of various cells of the immune system.
▼ Azathioprine suppresses delayed hypersensitivity and antibody responses.
▼ Azathioprine antagonizes purine metabolism (DNA, RNA, and protein synthesis), blocks cellular metabolism, and inhibits mitosis.
▼ Cyclosporine and tacrolimus inhibit IL-2 release from T-lymphocytes (CD4) and are used in organ transplant recipients to prevent organ rejection.
▼ Regardless of the immunosuppressants, if the recipient's immune system cannot recognize the organ as being foreign, it will not mount an immune response against it.
▼ Muromonab-CD3 prevents T-cells from recognizing foreign antigens and is used in transplant recipients suffering from acute rejection of the donated organ. It is a potent immunosuppressant used to prevent acute rejection.
▼ Nursing considerations associated with the immunosuppressants include monitoring laboratory studies

(e.g., Hgb level, Hct values, WBC, and platelet count). Studies should be performed and the results documented before, during (monthly), and after therapy. Should the leukocyte count drop below $3.0 \times 10^9/L$, the drug should be discontinued.
▼ Any of these agents that are administered orally should always be taken with food to minimize GI upset. Because of the immunosuppressed state of the clients receiving immunosuppressants, oral forms of the drugs should be used whenever possible to decrease the risk of infection associated with intramuscular injections.
▼ Additional nursing considerations include the possible administration of oral antifungals to treat the oral candidiasis that occurs as a result of immunosuppression and fungal overgrowth. The nurse should inspect the oral cavity as often as necessary (at least once every shift) for any white patches on the tongue, mucous membranes, and oral pharynx. These patches may indicate oral candidiasis.
▼ Clients should be encouraged to report any fever, sore throat, chills, joint pain, or fatigue, which may indicate severe infection and immunosuppressed states. When discharged to home, checking the client's mouth for white patches is important in the identification of candidiasis.

EXAMINATION REVIEW QUESTIONS

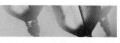

1 Cyclosporine should be used cautiously in clients with which of the following?
   a. Renal dysfunction
   b. Mild hypertension
   c. Anemia
   d. Myalgia
2 Which of the following would be a contraindication for the drug muromonab-CD3?
   a. Acute myalgia
   b. Fluid overload
   c. Severe polycythemia
   d. Treatment of pneumococcal meningitis
3 Which of the following is a common side effect of azathioprine?
   a. Bradycardia
   b. Leukocytosis
   c. Thrombocytopenia
   d. Constipation

4 Which of the following recommendations should clients taking immunosuppressants be encouraged to follow?
   a. Use oral forms of the agents to prevent the occurrence of oral candidiasis.
   b. Maintain long-term corticosteroid use just as a precaution to prevent drug side effects.
   c. Use some form of contraception during treatment and for up to 12 weeks after the end of therapy.
   d. Be given some other treatment because it may take six to nine months for a therapeutic response to occur.
5 Which of the following is a side effect most commonly associated with the administration of cyclosporine?
   a. Hepatotoxicity
   b. Neurotoxicity
   c. Polycythemia
   d. Pulmonary fibrosis

For answers see http://evolve.elsevier.com/Lilley/pharmacology/.

CRITICAL THINKING ACTIVITIES

1 K.J. is a 58-year-old heart transplant recipient who is currently taking cyclosporine to prevent his immune system from rejecting his transplanted heart. A cytomegalovirus (CMV) infection has developed, for which he is receiving ganciclovir. How does cyclosporine prevent this client's immune system from attacking his transplanted heart?
2 What type of medication may be needed with the administration of muromonab-CD3 and why?

3 Your client is about to undergo a right lung transplant. Why are intramuscular injections to be kept to a minimum during the time before his surgery?
4 What is the client teaching emphasis for oral therapy for the client undergoing a lung transplant who is about to receive an immunosuppressant?

For answers see http://evolve.elsevier.com/Lilley/pharmacology/.

BIBLIOGRAPHY

Canadian Pharmacists Association. (2003). *Therapeutic choices* (4th ed.). Ottawa, ON: Author.

Canadian Pharmacists Association. (2004). *Guide to drugs in Canada.* Toronto, ON: Dorling Kindersley.

Canadian Pharmacists Association. (2005). *Compendium of pharmaceuticals and specialties. The Canadian drug reference for health professionals.* Ottawa, ON: Author. [The subscription-based e-CPS is available at http://www.pharmacists.ca.]

Cheng, A., Williams, B.A., & Sivarajan, B.V. (Eds.). (2003). *The HSC handbook of pediatrics* (10th ed.). Toronto, ON: Elsevier.

Facts and Comparisons. (2004). *Drug facts and comparisons pocket version* (9th ed.). St Louis, MO: Wolters Kluwer Health.

Hardman, J.G., & Limbird, L.E. (2002). *Goodman and Gilman's the pharmacological basis of therapeutics* (10th ed.). New York: McGraw-Hill.

Health Canada. (2000). Potentially harmful drug interaction between St. John's wort and prescription drugs. Retrieved November 25, 2005, from http://www.hc-sc.gc.ca/ahc-asc/media/advisories-avis/2000/2000_36_e.html

Health Canada. (2005). Drug product database (DPD). Retrieved September 2, 2005, from http://www.hc-sc.gc.ca/hpb/drugs-dpd/

Katzung, B.G. (2004). *Basic and clinical pharmacology* (9th ed.). New York: McGraw-Hill.

Lacy, C.F., Armstrong, L.L., Goldman, M.P., & Lance, L.L. (2003). *Drug information handbook* (11th ed.). Hudson, OH: Lexi-Comp.

Lehne, R.A. (2004). *Pharmacology for nursing care* (5th ed.). St Louis, MO: Saunders.

Mosby. (2005). *Mosby's drug consult 2005: The comprehensive reference for generic and brand name drugs* (15th ed.). St Louis, MO: Mosby.

Skidmore-Roth, L. (2006). *Mosby's 2006 nursing drug reference* (19th ed.). St Louis, MO: Mosby.

Immunizing Agents

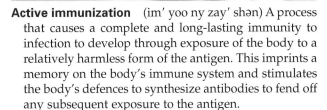

OBJECTIVES

After reading this chapter, the successful student will be able to do the following:

1 Discuss the importance of immunity as it relates to the various immunizing agents and their use in clients of all ages.

2 Identify the diseases that are prevented or treated with toxoids or vaccines.

3 Compare the mechanisms of action, indications, cautions, contraindications, side effects, toxicity, and routes of administration for various toxoids and vaccines.

4 Develop a nursing care plan that includes all phases of the nursing process related to the administration of immunizing agents.

e-LEARNING ACTIVITIES

Student CD-ROM
- Review Questions: see questions 337–340
- Animations
- Medication Administration Checklists
- IV Therapy Checklists

evolve **Web site** (http://evolve.elsevier.com/Lilley/ pharmacology/)
- Online Chapter Worksheet • Frequently Asked Questions
- Learning Tips and Content Updates • WebLinks • Online Appendices and Supplements • Mosby/Saunders ePharmacology Update • Access to *Mosby's Drug Consult*

DRUG PROFILES

diphtheria, tetanus toxoids, and acellular pertussis vaccine (adsorbed), p. 762
haemophilus influenzae type b conjugate vaccine, p. 762
▸▸hepatitis B immune globulin, p. 765
▸▸hepatitis B recombinant virus vaccine (inactivated), p. 763
▸▸immune globulin, p. 765
▸▸influenza virus vaccine, p. 763
▸▸measles, mumps, and rubella virus vaccine (live), p. 764

▸▸pneumococcal vaccine, polyvalent, p. 764
▸▸poliovirus vaccine (inactivated), p. 764
rabies immune globulin, p. 766
rabies virus vaccine (inactivated), p. 765
Rh₀(D) immune globulin, p. 765
tetanus immune globulin, p. 766
▸▸varicella virus vaccine, p. 765
varicella zoster immune globulin, p. 766

▸▸ Key drug.

GLOSSARY

Active immunization (im' yoo ny zay' shən) A process that causes a complete and long-lasting immunity to infection to develop through exposure of the body to a relatively harmless form of the antigen. This imprints a memory on the body's immune system and stimulates the body's defences to synthesize antibodies to fend off any subsequent exposure to the antigen.

Active immunizing agents Same as toxoids or vaccines (i.e., administered to host [human or animal] to stimulate host production of antibodies).

Antibody titre (tight' er) Amount of an antibody needed to react with a given volume or amount of a specific antigen.

Antiserum A serum that contains antibody or antibodies. It is usually obtained from an animal that has been immunized against a specific antigen, either by injection with the antigen or by infection with specific micro-organisms that produce the antigen.

Antitoxin An antibody against a toxin or toxoid; most often a purified antiserum obtained from animals (usually horses) by injection of a toxin or toxoid so that antibodies to the toxin (i.e., antitoxin) can be collected from the animal and used to provide artificial passive immunity to humans exposed to a given toxin (e.g., tetanus).

Antivenin An antibody or antiserum against a venom (poison produced by an animal), used to treat humans or other animals that have been envenomed (e.g., by snakebite or spider bite).

Biological antimicrobial agent   A substance of biological origin used to prevent, treat, or cure infectious diseases. These agents are often simply referred to as *biologicals*. However, that term may also be used to refer to agents of bioterrorism (e.g., anthrax spores, smallpox virus), depending on context.

Bioterrorism   The use of biological agents, especially infectious agents, as weapons for human destruction.

Booster shot   An antigen, such as a vaccine or toxoid, given to maintain an established immune response at an appropriate level. It is usually a smaller amount than the original immunization.

Herd immunity   Resistance to a disease in an entire community or population because a large proportion of its members are immune to it.

Immune response   A cascade of biochemical events that occurs in response to entry into the body of an antigen (foreign substance); key processes of the immune response include phagocytosis (literally "eating of cells") of foreign micro-organisms, as well as synthesis of antibodies that react with (by chemically binding to) molecules of specific antigens to inactivate them. Immune response centres around the blood but may also involve the lymphatic system and the reticuloendothelial system (RES; see *reticuloendothelial system*).

Immunizing biological   Toxoid or vaccine targeted against an infectious micro-organism.

Immunoglobulin   (im' yoo no glob' yoo lin) (Synonymous with immune globulin.) A glycoprotein synthesized and used by the humoral immune system to attack and kill all substances foreign to the body. More general than an antibody, an immunoglobulin is a nonspecific antibody (i.e., one that does not yet have a specific amino acid sequence that recognizes a specific antigen).

Passive immunization   A process that fights infection by bypassing the immune system. It involves giving a person serum or concentrated immune globulins obtained directly from humans or animals that directly give that person the means to fight off the invading micro-organism. The person's immune system does not have to manufacture them. This process also occurs from mother to infant when breastfeeding.

Passive immunizing agents   Agents containing antibodies that can kill or inactivate pathogens. These are directly injected into a person and provide that person with the means to fend off infection, bypassing the person's own immune system.

Recombinant   The result of combining the genetic material of two or more organisms. This is one of the key practices of biotechnology and is often used to make immunizing agents and various other medications.

Reticuloendothelial system (RES)   Specialized cells located in the liver, spleen, lymphatics and bone marrow that remove miscellaneous particles from the circulation, such as aging antibody molecules.

Toxoid   (tok' soid) A modified or inactivated (by chemicals or heat) bacterial exotoxin that is no longer toxic but can still bind and/or stimulate the formation of antitoxin; often used in the same manner as a vaccine to promote artificial active immunity in a human. It is one type of active immunizing agent.

Vaccine   A suspension of live, attenuated, or killed micro-organisms that can promote an artificially cultivated active immunity against a particular micro-organism. It is another type of active immunizing agent.

IMMUNITY AND IMMUNIZATION

Centuries ago it was noticed that people who suffered a certain disease acquired an immune tolerance to it so that, when exposed to it again, they did not suffer a second bout. This basic observation prompted scientists to investigate ways of artificially producing this tolerance. Along with this came an understanding of the way in which the normal immune system functions, knowledge important to an understanding of how immunizing agents work. Briefly, when the body first comes in contact with an invading organism (antigen), some specific information is imprinted into a cellular "memory bank" of the immune system so that the body can effectively fight, by mounting an **immune response**, any later invasion by that same organism. This cellular memory bank consists of specialized immune cells known as *memory cells*. When an antigen "presents itself" to a person's immune system by binding to B-lymphocytes (B-cells), the B-cells "differentiate" into two other types of cells. One type is the memory cells. The second type is the plasma cells, the role of which is to produce large volumes of antibodies against the antigen in question. It is because of this process that people rarely suffer twice from certain diseases such as mumps, chicken pox, and measles. Instead they have a complete and long-lasting immunity to those infections.

There are two ways of cultivating this immunity: actively and passively. In **active immunization**, the body is exposed to a relatively harmless form of an antigen (foreign invader), which imprints this information into the memory of the immune system as described and stimulates the body's defences to resist any subsequent exposure, but without actually causing full-blown infection. In **passive immunization**, serum or concentrated immune globulins obtained from humans or animals are injected into a person, directly giving that person the substance needed to fight off the invading micro-organism. This type of immunization bypasses the immune system. The major differences between active and passive immunity are summarized in Table 45-1 and discussed in greater depth in the following sections.

TABLE 45-1
ACTIVE VERSUS PASSIVE IMMUNITY

Differences	Active	Passive
Type of immunization	Toxoid or vaccine	Immune globulin or antitoxin
Mechanism of action	Causes an Ag–Ab response, similar to exposure to natural disease process	Results from direct administration of exogenous Ab; the Ab concentration will decrease over time, so if re-exposure is expected it is wise to continue passive immunizations
Indication	Minimizes or entirely avoids active infection; provides long-lasting or permanent immunity	Provides temporary protection for people who are immunodeficient, have a contraindication to active immunization, have been exposed to disease, or anticipate exposure to the disease; it does not stimulate an Ab response in the host

ACTIVE IMMUNIZATION

Toxoids and vaccines are known as **immunizing biologicals**. In general, **biological antimicrobial agents** (also simply referred to as *biologicals*) are substances such as **antitoxins**, serums, toxoids, vaccines, and similar preparations that are used to prevent, treat, or cure infectious diseases. Immunizing biologicals are toxoids or vaccines that target a particular infectious micro-organism.

Toxoids

Toxoids are antigenic (foreign) preparations or bacterial (usually gram-positive) exotoxins that are detoxified (attenuated) with chemicals or heat, rendering them nontoxic and unable to revert back to a toxic form but nonetheless highly antigenic. In other words, toxoids are diluted, changed, or altered substances (exotoxins) that are normally secreted from bacteria. When injected into a person, the person's immune system mounts an immune response by producing a specific antibody (an antitoxic antibody) against this antigen, which can then neutralize the same exotoxin upon any future exposure. Toxoids were first developed in 1923 at the Pasteur Institute by Ramon and his associates. The toxoids now available are effective against toxin-producing diseases such as diphtheria and tetanus.

Vaccines

Vaccines are suspensions of live, attenuated (weakened), or killed (inactivated) micro-organisms that can artificially promote the acquisition of active immunity against the particular organism. These slight alterations in the bacteria and viruses prevent the person injected with the substance from contracting the disease. People vaccinated with live bacteria or virus (as well as those who recover from an actual infection) enjoy lifelong immunity against that particular disease. Only partial immunity is conferred on those vaccinated with killed bacteria or virus, and for this reason they must be given periodic booster shots to maintain the protection of the immune system against infection with this bacteria or virus. One exception to this is the smallpox vaccine, because it utilizes live cowpox virus (*vaccinia* virus) instead of the more virulent smallpox virus.

Some of the first work in the development of vaccines was done in the area of smallpox immunization, starting with Lady Mary Montagu, who in 1718 introduced the Eastern practice of inoculating against the smallpox virus by applying it to the nasal membranes. In 1774 Benjamin Jesty was the first to use cowpox virus inoculations to prevent smallpox. Edward Jenner, an English physician who noticed that milkmaids who had suffered cowpox infections were rarely victims of smallpox, was the first to study the relationship of cowpox to smallpox immunity. This observation led to the development of the smallpox vaccine, which utilizes the cowpox virus. In 1796 he successfully immunized a young boy against smallpox by vaccinating him with cowpox virus obtained from a cowpox vesicle on an infected cow.

With the help of the modern version of this vaccine, smallpox has now been eradicated since 1980. Routine smallpox vaccination of Canadians was discontinued in 1972. However, in 2003 the Government of Canada updated the Canadian Smallpox Contingency Plan to allow for the possible re-emergence of smallpox (see later section on bioterrorism).

The advent of vaccines in general has dramatically changed the way we deal with public health problems. Today there are vaccines for more than 20 infectious diseases, and the past decade alone has witnessed the appearance of many new or improved vaccines.

These newer vaccines contain some extract or synthetic extract of the pathogen rather than the actual microbe and are produced by genetic engineering methods. The vaccines yielded are actually viral or bacterial antigenic preparations that cause the immune system to produce antibodies against them and hence induce immunity. Examples of viral vaccines (antigenic preparations) include hepatitis B and influenza; the latter may contain the whole virus or the split virus particle. Bacterial vaccines against meningitis (meningococcus), *Haemophilus influenzae*, and pneumococcus contain selected bacterial capsular polysaccharides (bacterial particles) that are taken from the respective microbes.

The process of attenuating or killing infectious microbes that are otherwise extremely virulent renders them safe for use in immunizing vaccines by removing that portion of them that causes infection. The advantage to such vaccines is that they have much greater antigenicity and produce more effective and longer-lasting immunity than inactivated vaccines. The attenuating or killing agent is usually a chemical such as formaldehyde or a physical mechanism such as heat. Attenuation may also be accomplished by the repeated passage of the microbe through some medium, such as a fertile hen egg or a special tissue culture. The currently available immunizing vaccines are listed in Box 45-1. Besides the individual **active immunizing agents**, there are several combinations of various vaccines and toxoids, and these are used especially in infants. Examples are the diphtheria and tetanus toxoid with pertussis vaccine (DTP) and the measles, mumps, and rubella vaccine (MMR).

The search for new and better agents will never end. A current focus of worldwide research is the development of a safe and effective vaccine against HIV, an endeavour that is proving difficult and time consuming. An immunizing biological effective against malaria is also being sought. Indeed, the ultimate goal is to develop an immunizing biological for every infectious disease.

PASSIVE IMMUNIZATION

Passive immunization bypasses the host's immune system and inoculates the person with serum containing immune globulins obtained from humans or animals. These substances give the person the means to fight off the invading organism. Passive immunization can occur naturally between a mother and the fetus or the nursing infant when the mother passes maternal antibodies directly either through the placenta to the fetus or through breast milk to the nursing infant. This is called *naturally acquired passive immunity*. *Artificially acquired passive immunity* involves injecting antibodies into the host that are acquired from an external source (e.g., horse serum antibodies) to confer temporary immunity against a particular antigen following exposure to this antigen. It differs from active immunization in that it is a comparatively transitory (short-lived) immune state and in that the antibodies are already prepared for the host—the host's immune system does not have to synthesize its own antibodies. This allows for more rapid prevention or treatment of disease. Important examples include tetanus immune globulin, hepatitis immune globulin, rabies immune globulin, and snakebite **antivenin**.

As noted in Table 45-1, passive immunization is beneficial to people rendered immunodeficient by drugs or disease. These people cannot benefit from active immunization

---

BOX 45-1

Available Immunizing Agents

Passive Immunizing Agents
Antivenin (Crotalidae) polyvalent (equine)
Antivenin, *Latrodectus mactans* (black widow spider)
Botulism antitoxin (types A, B, E)
Cytomegalovirus immune globulin (human)
Digoxin immune FAB (ovine)
Diphtheria antitoxin (equine)
Hepatitis B immune globulin (HBIG)
Immune globulin, intramuscular (human)
Immune globulin, intravenous (human)
Rabies immune globulin (human)
Respiratory syncytial virus immune globulin intravenous (RSV-IGIV)
$Rh_0(D)$ immune globulin
Tetanus immune globulin (TIG)
Varicella zoster immune globulin (VCIG)

Active Immunizing Agents
BCG vaccine (tuberculosis)
Diphtheria and tetanus toxoids, adsorbed, adult
Diphtheria, tetanus, and pertussis toxoids and poliomyelitis vaccine (DPTP)
Diphtheria and tetanus toxoids and acellular pertussis vaccine (DTaP)
Diphtheria and tetanus toxoids and poliomyelitis vaccine
Diphtheria, pertussis, and tetanus toxoids, polio vaccine, and *Haemophilus influenzae* type b

Conjugate Vaccines
Cholera vaccine
Haemophilus influenzae type b conjugate vaccine
Hepatitis A virus vaccine, inactivated
Hepatitis B virus vaccine
Hepatitis vaccines, combined
Influenza virus vaccine
Japanese encephalitis virus vaccine
Lyme disease bacterial vaccine
Measles (rubeola) virus vaccine, live, attenuated
Measles and rubella virus vaccine, live
Measles, mumps, and rubella virus vaccine, live
Meningococcal polysaccharide bacterial vaccine
Mumps virus vaccine, live
Pneumococcal bacterial vaccine, polyvalent
Poliovirus vaccine, live, oral, trivalent
Poliovirus vaccine, inactivated
Rabies virus vaccine
Rubella virus vaccine, live
Rubella and mumps virus vaccine, live
Smallpox virus vaccine[†]
Tetanus toxoid
Typhoid bacterial vaccine
Varicella virus vaccine
Yellow fever virus vaccine

[†]Not currently on the Canadian market but a supply is available in the event of bioterrorism threats.

because their immune systems are too suppressed to develop immunity in response to a toxoid or antigen. People who already have the disease targeted by the **passive immunizing agent** are also candidates for these agents, especially those with diseases that are rapidly harmful or fatal, such as rabies, tetanus, and hepatitis. The person might die before the body had time to mount an adequate immune defence against them. Although passive immunization does not stimulate an antibody response, it confers a temporary protection that is usually sufficient to keep the invading organism from killing the person.

The passive immunizing agents consist of three groups of agents: antitoxins, immune globulins, and snake and spider antivenins. Antitoxins are purified **antiserums** that are usually obtained from horses inoculated with the toxin. Immune globulins represent concentrated preparations containing predominantly **immunoglobulin G (IgG)** and are harvested from a large pool of blood donors. Antivenins are serums obtained from animals (usually horses) that have been injected with the particular venom. The serum contains immunoglobulins that can neutralize the toxic effects of the venoms.

The current published childhood immunization schedule is shown in Table 45-2. This schedule represents an overview of routine immunization for infants and children based on available evidence-based scientific knowledge. It is endorsed by the Canadian Paediatric Society, the National Advisory Committee on Immunization (NACI), and the Canadian Medical Association (CMA).

THE THREAT OF BIOTERRORISM

After the events in the United States on September 11, 2001, there were several incidents in which apparently infectious materials were mailed to government and media officials or otherwise introduced to public places. While at least one death occurred in the United States from anthrax (of unidentified source), many incidents (and all Canadian occurrences) turned out to involve ordinary inert materials. However, many governments became concerned that infectious or otherwise toxic agents could be used as weapons against human populations. This concept is referred to as **bioterrorism** (see Table 45-3 for possible bioterrorism agents). More recently, we were reminded of the reality of terrorist attacks and the need for public safety initiatives by the 2005 London bus bombings.

The Canadian government developed a Bioterrorism Package to address this issue proactively as a matter of public health. One aspect of this program is biohazard refresher courses for front-line workers such as nurses, physicians, and paramedics. In addition, the government

TABLE 45-2

ROUTINE IMMUNIZATION SCHEDULE FOR INFANTS AND CHILDREN

Age at Vaccination	DTaP	IPV	Hib	MMR	Td or dTap	Hep B (3 doses)	V	PC	MC
Birth									
2 months	X	X	X					X	X
4 months	X	X	X			Infancy or		X	X
6 months	X	X	X			pre-adolescence		X	X
12 months				X		(9–13 years)	X	X	
18 months	X	X	X	X or					or
4–6 years	X	X		X					
14–16 years					X				X

DTaP, Diphtheria, tetanus, acellular pertussis vaccine
IPV, Inactivated poliovirus vaccine
Hib, *Haemophilus influenzae* type b conjugate vaccine
MMR, Measles, mumps, and rubella vaccine
Td, Tetanus and diphtheria toxoid, adult type with reduced diphtheria toxoid
dTap, Tetanus and diphtheria toxoid, acellular pertussis, adolescent/adult type with reduced diphtheria and pertussis components
Hep B, Hepatitis B vaccine
V, Varicella
PC, Pneumococcal conjugate vaccine
MC, Meningococcal C conjugate vaccine.
Source: National Advisory Committee on Immunization (NACI)—Recommended Immunization Schedule for Infants, Children and Youth (updated March 2005).
Note: This is a general guideline for children and adolescents and may vary among provinces and territories. For more information about immunization, visit The Canadian Pediatric Society at http://www.caringforkids.cps.ca/; The Canadian Immunization Guide at http://www.phac-aspc.gc.ca/publicat/cig-gci/index.html
Notes: 1 *Haemophilus influenzae* type b (Hib) requires a series of immunizations. The exact number and timing of each may vary with the type of vaccine used.
   2 Hepatitis B requires a series of immunizations. In some jurisdictions, they may be administered at a younger age.
   3 Two-dose programs for MMR are given in all territories and provinces. Second dose MMR is given either at 18 months or 4–6 years of age. If the child is past the age at which the second MMR is recommended, the second dose can be given 1–2 months after the first.
   4 The costs of these vaccines are not covered by all provincial/territorial health plans. Parents may have to pay for them.
   5 Recommended schedule and number of doses of meningococcal vaccine depends on the age of the child.

TABLE 45-3

CATEGORY "A" (HIGH PRIORITY) POSSIBLE BIOTERRORISM AGENTS

Name of Illness	Causative Organism	Clinical Presentation	Prevention/Treatment
Anthrax	Bacterium: *Bacillus anthracis*	Inhalational form most severe and can lead to potentially fatal bacteremia.	Vaccine available. Treatable with antibiotics such as ciprofloxacin and dicloxacillin.
Smallpox	Virus: *Vaccinia*	Flu-like symptoms followed by total-body disfiguring rash.	Vaccine available and may be effective up to 3 days after exposure. Antiviral drug cidofovir possibly effective.
Botulism	Bacterium: *Clostridium botulinum*	Visual changes; dry mouth muscle weakness; progressive downward paralysis, including diaphragm.	Vaccine available only for highly exposed persons. Antitoxin effective if given early in disease; antibiotics of no benefit.
Tularemia	Bacterium: *Francisella tularensis*	Severe, potentially life-threatening respiratory illness.	Vaccine currently under review. Treatable with antibiotics such as tetracycline and ciprofloxacin.
Viral hemorrhagic fever	Viruses: Several viral causes, including Ebola, Marburg, and Lassa viruses, yellow fever virus, Argentine hemorrhagic fever virus	Bleeding from body orifices and in internal organs in severe cases; possible renal failure and coma.	No vaccines except for yellow fever virus and Argentine hemorrhagic fever virus. No current treatment other than supportive care. Prevention focuses on rodent control.
Plague	Bacterium: *Yersinia pestis*	Can occur in lungs (pneumonic plague), skin (bubonic plague—most common), or blood (septicemic plague). Death possible from respiratory failure and shock.	No vaccine currently available in Canada. Antibiotics best if given within 24 h and include gentamicin and tetracycline.

Data from Public Health Agency of Canada. Centre for Infectious Disease Prevention and Control (CIDPC) and the Centre for Surveillance Coordination, Public Health Agency of Canada, listing of category "A" possible bioterrorism agents. Available at http://www.phac-aspc.gc.ca/publicat/ccdr-rmtc/02vol28/dr2821ea.html

is stockpiling smallpox vaccine and antibiotics; improving diagnostic facilities; and increasing surveillance for possible outbreaks of suspicious disease. In Canada, the anthrax vaccine is available only to military personnel considered to be at higher risk of anthrax exposure because of the location and nature of their assigned duties and is unlikely to be used as routine vaccination.

With regard to smallpox, the Government of Canada adopted a "search and contain" strategy recommended by public health experts in Canada and around the world, including Canada's National Advisory Committee on Immunization, Canada's Council of Chief Medical Officers of Health, and the World Health Organization. This strategy begins immediately when a case of smallpox is confirmed and calls for all public health agencies to be involved in early detection. The goal is to identify, vaccinate, and isolate all contacts within a four-day window. There are also plans for rapid vaccination of local populations in the event of a suspected smallpox outbreak, with priority given to direct healthcare workers. The guidelines also identify people at higher risk for vaccine complications who should not be vaccinated unless smallpox exposure is likely or confirmed.

Anthrax

Anthrax is a bacterial infectious disease caused by spores of the bacterium *Bacillus anthracis*. In humans, infection can occur via three routes of exposure: cuta-

neous (skin; 20 percent mortality), gastrointestinal (25 to 75 percent mortality), and inhalation ($\geq$80 percent mortality). Antibiotics such as the fluoroquinolone ciprofloxacin are used to treat more severe cases such as the inhalational form. Milder cases (e.g., cutaneous, GI) are often treated with the tetracycline antibiotic doxycycline. The vaccine is developed from an attenuated strain of *B. anthracis*. It has a calculated efficacy level of 92.5 percent for protection against anthrax infection. In addition to selected military personnel, anthrax vaccination may be recommended for veterinarians and others who handle potentially infected animals, as well as workers who process imported animal hair, which is used to manufacture various commercial products. The anthrax vaccine is only available in Canada through the Special Access Programme. Anthrax has been almost entirely eliminated in Canada because of an intensive animal vaccination program and industrial safety programs.

IMMUNIZING AGENTS

Mechanism of Action and Drug Effects

Active immunizing agents consist of vaccines and toxoids that can be administered orally (PO), subcutaneously (SC), or intramuscularly (IM) and that work by stimulating that part of the immune system known as the humoral immune system. The system synthesizes substances called *immunoglobulins*—of which there are five distinct types, designated immunoglobulin M (IgM), IgG, IgA, IgE, and IgD—to attack and kill the foreign substances that invade the body. These foreign substances are called *antigens*, and the immunoglobulins are called *antibodies*.

Vaccines contain substances that trigger the formation of these antibodies against specific pathogens. They may be the actual live or attenuated (weakened) pathogen or a killed pathogen. The amount of antibodies they cause to be produced can be measured in the blood. The **antibody titre** is the amount of antibody that must be present in the blood to effectively protect the body against the particular pathogen. Sometimes the levels of these antibodies decline over time. When this happens a second dose of the vaccine is given to restore the antibody titres to a level that can protect the person against the infection. This second dose is referred to as a **booster shot**. Toxoids are altered forms of bacterial toxins that stimulate the production of antibodies in the same way as vaccines do.

Because both toxoids and vaccines rely on the immunized host to mount an immune response, the host's immune system must be intact. Therefore clients who are immunocompromised, that is, who cannot mount an immune response, such as those undergoing immunosuppressive cancer chemotherapy, those receiving immunosuppressive therapy to prevent the rejection of transplanted organs, and those with immunosuppressive diseases such as AIDS, should not receive vaccines or toxoids. Instead, their clinical situations may warrant giving them passive immunizing agents such as immune globulins.

As previously explained, passive immunizing agents are the actual antibodies (immunoglobulins) that can kill or inactivate the pathogen. The process is called "passive" because the person's immune system does not participate in the synthesis of antibodies; they are provided by the immunizing agent. However, immunity acquired in this way is not long-term, generally lasting only until the injected immunoglobulins are removed from the person's immune system by the **reticuloendothelial system (RES)**.

Vaccines and toxoids are the active immunizing agents that have been developed for the prevention of many illnesses caused by bacteria and their toxins, as well as those caused by various viruses. Antivenins, antitoxins, and immune globulins comprise the passive immunizing agents. Such agents can inactivate spider and snake venom, bacterial toxins (exotoxins), and potentially lethal viruses. Box 45-1 contains a list of the currently available immunizing agents.

Indications

Active immunization is used to prevent infection caused by bacterial toxins or viruses, and confers long-lasting or permanent immunity. If a person previously immunized against a particular pathogen is again exposed to that foreign invader, a prompt and significant increase in the person's immunoglobulin (antibody) level against that

pathogen occurs. However, an interesting phenomenon called **herd immunity** means that successful immunization of 95 percent or more of a population confers protection on the entire population. Thanks to herd immunity, people at particular risk for complications can be spared the standard vaccinations.

Passive immunizing agents consist of antivenins, antitoxins, and immune globulins. Antivenins, also known as *antisera* (singular *antiserum*), are used to prevent or minimize the effects of poisoning by the venoms. In Canada, the poison of crotalids (rattlesnakes found in northern Ontario, Manitoba, Alberta, and some parts of British Columbia) and black widow spiders can be lethal. Most healthy adults do not die from the bites of spiders or snakes if treated promptly with the appropriate antivenin. Young children and older people with health problems are particularly susceptible to the effects of venom, and should also be given antivenin.

Certain viruses are potent and even potentially lethal (e.g., hepatitis B, rabies). They can do major harm quickly before the infected person can mount an effective immune response against them. Passive immunization with the appropriate immune globulin provides the antibody needed to fend off the harmful effects of the virus. There are also immune globulins and antitoxins that provide protection against some bacterial infections such as those that cause diphtheria and tetanus.

Contraindications

Contraindications to immunizing agents include drug allergy and may also include allergy to egg products because some vaccines are derived from such products. However, in the case of a potentially fatal illness such as rabies, the corresponding agents may still need to be given, depending on the likelihood of actual rabies exposure, and any allergic reaction controlled with other medications. Some immunizing agents are best deferred until after recovery from a febrile illness or temporary immunocompromised state (e.g., following cancer chemotherapy), if possible. However, this is often a matter of clinical judgement depending on the client's condition and risk factors.

Side Effects and Adverse Effects

The undesirable effects of the various immunizing agents can range from mild and transient to more serious and even life threatening. These are listed in Table 45-4. The minor reactions can be treated with acetaminophen and rest. More severe reactions, such as fever higher than 39.4°C, should be treated with acetaminophen and sponge baths. Serum sickness sometimes occurs after repeated injections of equine-made immunizing agents. The signs and symptoms consist of edema of the face, tongue, and throat; rash; urticaria; arthritis; adenopathy; fever; flushing; itching; cough; dyspnea; cyanosis; vomiting; and cardiovascular collapse. This is best treated with analgesics, antihistamines, epinephrine, or corticosteroids. Hospitalization may be required.

TABLE 45-4
IMMUNIZING AGENTS: MINOR AND SEVERE ADVERSE EFFECTS

Body System	Side/Adverse Effects
MINOR EFFECTS	
Central nervous	Fever, adenopathy
Integumentary	Minor rash, soreness at injection site, urticaria, joint or muscle pain, cellulitis
SEVERE EFFECTS	
Central nervous	Fever >39.4°C, encephalitis, convulsions, peripheral neuropathy, anaphylactic reactions, shock, unconsciousness
Integumentary	Urticaria, rash
Respiratory	Dyspnea
Other	Cyanosis

Any serious or unusual reactions to immunizing agents should be reported to the Canadian Adverse Events Following Immunization Surveillance System (CAEFISS). This is a voluntary (except in Ontario and Québec, where reporting is mandatory) national vaccine safety surveillance program monitored by the Vaccine Safety Unit (VSU) of the Immunization and Respiratory Infections Division of the Public Health Agency of Canada. A reporting form can be printed from the Public Health Agency of Canada Web site (http://www.phac-aspc.gc.ca/dird-dimr/pdf/hc4229e.pdf). Health Canada also collaborates with the Canadian Paediatric Society (CPS), and pediatric infectious disease specialists on the Immunization Monitoring Program, ACtive (IMPACT), an active surveillance system to monitor serious adverse events following immunization, vaccination failures, and selected infectious diseases. The Public Health Agency of Canada Web site (http://www.phac-aspc.gc.ca/im/vs-sv/index.html) and the Health Canada Web site (http://www.hc-sc.gc.ca/dhp-mps/medeff/advers-react-neg/index_e.html) have extensive information describing these reporting systems and the data collected by them. Such data are used to improve the quality of immunizing agents and can even be grounds for a Health Canada recall of biological agents.

Interactions

Immunosuppressive agents such as corticosteroids and cancer chemotherapy agents block the generation of active immunity. Hepatitis B immune globulin has a drug interaction with live vaccines; defer for three months after a dose of immune globulin.

Dosages

For the recommended dosages of selected immunizing agents, see the dosages table below. See Appendix B for some of the common brands available in Canada.

DOSAGES — Selected Immunizing Agents

Agent	Pharmacologic Class	Usual Dosage Range	Indications
Active Immunizing Agents			
diphtheria, tetanus, and acellular pertussis (DTaP)	Mixed toxoid/vaccine	**Pediatric only** IM: Series of three 0.5-mL injections at 2, 4, and 6 mo	Prophylaxis against diphtheria, tetanus, and pertussis
***Haemophilus influenzae* type b conjugate vaccine**	Bacterial capsular antigenic extract vaccine	**Pediatric** **Infant 2–6 mo** IM: Series of three injections (0.5 mL each) at 2, 4, and 6 mo **For a previously unvaccinated child <7 yr** IM: Two injections about 2 mo apart. A third may be required depending on product used and age of child when immunization started	*H. influenzae* type b prophylaxis
▸▸**hepatitis B virus vaccine, recombinant**	Viral surface antigen	**Pediatric to age 10 yr** **Recombivax HB** IM: 2.5 μg at birth (depending on risk factors) then at 1 mo and 12 mo **Adolescence 11–19 yr** IM: 3 × 5 μg doses: day 0, 1 mo, and 2 mo **Adult ≥20 yr** IM: 3 × 10 μg doses: day 0, 1 mo, and 2 mo	Hepatitis B virus prophylaxis
▸▸**influenza virus vaccine**	Viral surface antigen	**Pediatric 6 mo–9 yr** IM: Single yearly dose (two doses at least 1 mo apart if receiving influenza vaccine for first time) **Adult** IM: Single yearly dose	Influenza prophylaxis
▸▸**measles, mumps, and rubella virus vaccine, live**	Live, attenuated viral vaccine	**Adult and pediatric >12 mo** SC: 0.5-mL single dose; booster at 18 mo or 4–6 yr	Prophylaxis against measles, mumps, and rubella

Continued

DOSAGES Selected Immunizing Agents—cont'd

Agent	Pharmacologic Class	Usual Dosage Range	Indications
pneumococcal polysaccharide vaccine (Pneumo 23)	Polysaccharide vaccine	*Adult and pediatric >2* IM/SC: 0.5 mL	Prevention of invasive pneumococcal infection
pneumococcal 7-valent conjugate vaccine (Prevnar)	Conjugate vaccine	*Pediatric (6 wks–9 yr)* IM: 0.5 mL	Prevention of invasive pneumococcal infection, pneumonia, otitis media caused by *S. pneumoniae*
▸▸ poliovirus vaccine, diploid cell origin, inactivated (IPV)	Inactivated viral vaccine	*Pediatric (infant)* SC: Three 0.5-mL doses: 2 mo, 4 mo, and 6 mo usually in combination with DTaP (Quadracel) or DTaP and Hib (Pentacel) *Adult* SC: Two 0.5-mL doses 1–2 mo apart, then a third dose 6–12 mo later	Polio prophylaxis
rabies virus vaccine	Inactivated viral vaccine	*Adult and pediatric* Post-exposure prophylaxis IM: 1 mL on days 0, 3, 7, 14, and 28 (with one dose of rabies immune globulin [see later] within 8 days of first vaccine dose) Pre-exposure prophylaxis for those at high risk for rabies exposure (e.g., veterinarians) IM: 1 mL IM or 0.1 mL ID on days 0, 7, and 21, q2–5yr, depending on antibody titres	Rabies prophylaxis
tetanus and diphtheria toxoids, adsorbed (Td), pediatric and adult	Mixed toxoid	*Adult and unvaccinated pediatric >7 yr* IM: 0.5 mL on day 0; second dose 2 mo later; third dose 6–12 mo later; booster 10 yr after 3rd dose	Prophylaxis against diphtheria and tetanus
▸▸ varicella virus vaccine	Live, attenuated viral vaccine	*Adult and pediatric >13 yr* SC: Two 0.5-mL doses given 4–8 wk apart *Pediatric 1–12 yr* SC: One 0.5-mL dose	Prophylaxis against varicella virus (causes chicken pox and shingles)
Passive Immunizing Agents			
▸▸ hepatitis B immune globulin	Pooled human immune globulin	*Infant (of known hepatitis B–positive mother)* IM: 0.5 mL at birth *Adult* IM: 0.06 mg/kg within 24 h after exposure	Passive hepatitis B prophylaxis
▸▸ immune globulin	Pooled human immune globulin	Dosages vary widely; refer to current manufacturer's dosage information regarding specific indications	Many indications, including primary immune deficiency syndrome, pediatric HIV, idiopathic thrombocytopenic purpura, B-cell chronic lymphocytic leukemia, bone marrow transplant
rabies immune globulin	Pooled human immune globulin	*Adult and pediatric* Single dose 20 units/kg; infiltrate as much of dose as possible into bite wound area and give remainder IM in gluteal region; do not give into same site as rabies vaccine	Rabies prophylaxis
Rh₀(D) immune globulin	Immunosuppressant globulin	*Adult female* IM (full dose): 1500 units at 28 wk gestation; 600 units within 72 h after delivery IM: 600 units after spontaneous or elective abortion of pregnancy 12 wk gestation	Postpartum antibody
tetanus immune globulin	Pooled human immune globulin	*Adult and pediatric* IM: 250 units as a single dose IM: 3000–6000 units as a single dose	Post-exposure tetanus prophylaxis Tetanus treatment

DRUG PROFILES

Some of the more commonly used vaccines, toxoids, and immunoglobulins are described in the following sections. The currently available immunizing agents are listed in Box 45-1.

ACTIVE IMMUNIZING AGENTS

diphtheria and tetanus toxoids, and acellular pertussis vaccine tetanus (adsorbed)

Diphtheria, tetanus, and pertussis are different disorders, but an injection that combines all three vaccines (DTP; also commonly called DPT) has been routinely given to children since the 1940s. Recently a new vaccine combination called diphtheria and tetanus toxoids with acellular pertussis vaccine adsorbed (DTaP) has been approved. It uses a different form of the pertussis component, known as *acellular pertussis*. Acellular pertussis consists of only a single weakened toxoid, whereas previous pertussis vaccines contained multiple toxoids. Experts hope that DTaP will prove to have fewer side effects than DTP, particularly in older clients who are more prone to them, thereby allowing adults to have a pertussis booster.

Currently DTaP is the preferred preparation for primary and booster immunization against these diseases in children six weeks to six years of age, unless the pertussis component is contraindicated. In Canada, an adolescent/adult combination of acellular pertussis vaccine with diphtheria and tetanus toxoids (dTap [Adacel]) is licensed for use in people 11 to 54 years of age. Adacel is now recommended for adolescents requiring their 14- to 16-year booster, replacing the previously used Td and TdPolio. Polio vaccine is no longer recommended with the 14- to 16-year booster. One lifetime dose of Adacel is the current recommendation of The National Advisory Committee on Immunization (NACI).

Diphtheria and pertussis are prevalent in the populations of many developing countries throughout the world, and as a result the risk of contracting one of these diseases may be high. Full immunization against these diseases is recommended both for inhabitants of these countries and for travellers to these areas. Tetanus spores are commonplace in the environment and the combination product containing only tetanus and diphtheria toxoids (Td) provides excellent protection if given every ten years. To avoid adverse reactions, Td contains less diphtheria toxoid than preparations given younger children and is used in persons seven years of age and older requiring a primary or booster immunization against tetanus for routine wound management. Emergency booster doses of Td (for adult use) are unnecessary when the wound is clean and minor (not tetanus prone) and the client has received a primary or booster immunization against tetanus within the past ten years.

Tetanus and diphtheria toxoids adsorbed (Td) for adult use are toxoids obtained from the bacteria *Clostridium tetani* and *Corynebacterium diphtheriae*. To make the agents, diphtheria and tetanus toxins are taken from these bacteria, attenuated into toxoids, and adsorbed onto aluminum hydroxide, aluminum phosphate, or potassium alum. They are given by injection to infants and children (two months to six years of age; DTaP) and older children and adults (Td) (seven years of age and older) with functioning immune systems. They pro-mote immunity to diphtheria and tetanus by inducing the production of specific antitoxins (antibodies to toxin) by the client's immune system.

These toxoids (DTaP and Td) are available only as parenteral preparations to be given as deep intramuscular injections. They are contraindicated in persons who have had a prior systemic hypersensitivity reaction or a neurological reaction to one of the ingredients. Some manufacturers state that use is contraindicated in cases of concurrent acute or active infections but not in cases of minor illness. Although there have been few, if any, studies documenting the safety of their use in pregnant women, it is generally not recommended unless there is a definite risk of exposure to pertussis. The risks and benefits need to be carefully evaluated if there is a high risk of exposure during a potential outbreak. The recommended dosages for these toxoids are given in the dosages table on p. 760.

haemophilus influenzae— type b conjugate vaccine

Haemophilus influenzae type b (Hib) vaccine is a noninfectious, bacteria-derived vaccine. It is made by extracting *H. influenzae* particles that are antigenic (cause an antigen–antibody reaction) and chemically *conjugating*, or attaching, them to a protein carrier. In Canada, acellular pertussis vaccine, adsorbed diphtheria and tetanus toxoids, inactivated polio vaccine, and *Haemophilus influenzae* type b are combined in one product (Pentacel). It is administered for the primary immunization and 18-month booster injection of all children living in Canada. NACI recommends that if other product combinations are used, all vaccines be administered on a single day. Adults and older children considered at high risk for acquiring the *H. influenzae* infection may receive a single dose of Act-HIB, Haemophilus b Conjugate Vaccine. Conditions that may predispose an individual to Hib infections are septicemia, pneumonia, cellulitis, arthritis, osteomyelitis, pericarditis, sickle cell anemia, an immunodeficiency syndrome, or Hodgkin's disease. Until recently, infections caused by Hib were the leading cause of bacterial meningitis in children three months to five years of age, and this bacterium can also cause several other serious infections in children and adults. This form of bacterial meningitis has a mortality rate of five percent. Of those who survive, 20 to 45 percent suffer serious neurological deficits.

The Hib vaccine may be combined with toxoids to make various combination products. Some examples of these combination products are listed in Table 45-5. All of these products are administered

TABLE 45-5
HIB COMBINATION PRODUCTS

Ingredients	Trade Name
Hib polysaccharide conjugate (tetanus protein conjugate) vaccine	Act-HIB
Hib polysaccharide conjugate (meningococcal protein conjugate) vaccine	PedvaxHIB
Hib oligosaccharide conjugate (diphtheria CRM197 protein conjugate) vaccine	HibTITRE

intramuscularly. These vaccines are contraindicated in clients who have had a previous hypersensitivity reaction to any one of the ingredients. It is not known whether the vaccines can cause fetal harm when administered to pregnant women or whether they can affect fertility. As a result, the administration of any of the vaccines during pregnancy is not recommended. Pregnancy category C. The recommended dosages for the Hib vaccine are given in the dosages table on p. 760.

▶▶ hepatitis B virus vaccine (inactivated)

Hepatitis B virus vaccine inactivated is a non-infectious viral vaccine containing hepatitis B surface antigen (HBsAg). It is made from yeast using **recombinant** deoxyribonucleic acid (DNA) technology. The yeast then produces this antigenic substance in mass quantities. After this it is attached to a substance known as *alum* (an adjuvant) and made into the injection that is used to vaccinate people against hepatitis B. This antigenic HBsAg is used to promote active immunity to hepatitis B infection in people, such as healthcare workers, considered at high risk for potential exposure to the hepatitis B virus or HBsAg-positive materials (e.g., blood, plasma, serum).

The vaccine is contraindicated in people who are hypersensitive to yeast. Pregnancy is not considered a contraindication. The potential for exposure to hepatitis B infection in a pregnant woman and the potential for the development of chronic infection in the neonate are both good reasons to give the vaccine. The vaccine is administered IM. In Canada, universal immunization with recombinant vaccine is recommended. There are three main formulations designed for three different populations: a pediatric formulation for neonates, infants, children, and adolescents; an adult formulation for persons older than 20 years of age; and a dialysis formulation for pre-dialysis and dialysis clients or for other immunocompromised people. It is also available in combination with hepatitis A vaccine (Twinrix). Pregnancy category C. The recommended dosages for this vaccine are given in the dosages table on p. 760.

▶▶ influenza virus vaccine

The influenza virus vaccine is used to prevent influenza. Each year before the influenza season this vaccine should be administered to high-risk persons. It is the single most important influenza control measure. Ontario, the Yukon, and the Northwest Territories provide universal influenza immunization, whereas the other provinces and territories provide the vaccine only to the highest-risk groups.

Each year a new influenza vaccine is developed by researchers. It usually contains three different influenza virus strains (usually two of type A and one type B). These strains are chosen from the hundreds of strains in the environment. Their selection is based on the latest epidemiological data that indicate which influenza viruses will most likely circulate in North America in the upcoming winter. The vaccine is made from highly purified, egg-grown viruses that have been made non-infectious (inactivated).

Influenza is characterized by abrupt onset of fever, myalgia (aching muscles), sore throat, and non-productive cough. Severe malaise may last several days. More severe illness can occur in certain populations. Older people and those with underlying health problems are at increased risk for complications from influenza infection and are more likely to require hospitalization. Increased mortality results not only from influenza and pneumonia but also from cardiopulmonary and other chronic diseases exacerbated by influenza. More than 90 percent of the deaths attributed to pneumonia and influenza occur among persons 65 years of age or older.

The effectiveness of influenza vaccine in preventing illness varies. Factors that may alter its effectiveness are the age and immunocompetence of the vaccine recipient and the degree of similarity between the predicted virus strains included in the vaccine and those that actually predominate during a given influenza season. Healthy individuals under the age of 65 have a 70 percent chance of preventing influenza when there is a good match between the vaccine and the circulating viruses.

Older people residing in nursing homes can prevent severe illness, secondary complications, and death by taking the influenza vaccine. Among frail older persons, the vaccine can prevent hospitalization and pneumonia up to 50 to 60 percent of the time and death up to 80 percent of the time. Achieving a high rate of vaccination among nursing home residents can reduce the spread of infection in a facility, thus preventing disease through herd immunity.

To summarize, influenza virus vaccine should be strongly considered in the following high-risk populations:
- Individuals 65 years of age or older
- Residents of nursing homes and other chronic-care facilities that house people of any age with chronic medical conditions
- Adults and children with chronic disorders of the pulmonary or cardiovascular systems, including children with asthma
- Adults and children who have required regular medical follow up or hospitalization during the preceding year because of chronic metabolic diseases (including diabetes mellitus), renal dysfunction,

TABLE 45-6
MEASLES VACCINE COMBINATION PRODUCTS

Product	Trade Name
Measles and rubella virus vaccine live	Moru-Viraten Berna
Measles, mumps, and rubella virus vaccine live	MMR II, Priorix

hemoglobinopathies, or immunosuppression (including immunosuppression caused by medications)

- Children and teenagers (6 months to 18 years of age) who are receiving long-term ASA therapy and therefore might be at risk for developing Reye's syndrome after influenza
- Healthcare workers
- Individuals travelling to destinations where influenza is prevalent
- Children between the ages of 6 and 23 months

Pregnant women and people with HIV should seek the advice of their physician. Pregnancy category C. The influenza vaccine should not be administered to individuals with a known hypersensitivity reaction to eggs (hives, swelling of the tongue and throat, difficult breathing, and hypotension), individuals who had an anaphylactic reaction to a previous influenza dose, or individuals who developed Guillain-Barré Syndrome, a rare paralytic disorder thought to be caused by a reaction to a previous influenza dose.

▸▸ measles, mumps, and rubella virus vaccine (live)

The measles, mumps, and rubella vaccine (MMR) is a live, attenuated virus preparation consisting of live measles (rubeola), mumps, and rubella (formerly called German measles) viruses that are weakened (attenuated). They promote active immunity to measles, mumps, and rubella by inducing the production of virus-specific IgG and IgM antibodies. The antibody response to initial vaccination resembles that caused by primary natural infection.

The measles vaccine or any of the combination products that include the virus are contraindicated in people with a history of anaphylactic, anaphylactoid, or other immediate reaction to egg ingestion. These vaccines should not be administered to pregnant women, and pregnancy should be avoided for three months after measles virus vaccination and 30 days after vaccination with a rubella-containing measles virus vaccine. This precaution is based on the theoretic risk of the live virus vaccine causing a fetal infection.

These vaccines are available only in parenteral form and should be given only by subcutaneous (SC) injection. There are two combination products containing the live measles virus vaccine, and these are listed in Table 45-6. Pregnancy category C. The recommended dosages for this vaccine are given in the dosages table on p. 761.

▸▸ pneumococcal vaccine, polyvalent and 7-valent

There are two available forms of vaccine against pneumococcal pneumonia, which also protects against any illness caused by *Streptococcus pneumoniae*. *Pneumococcus* is a common name for the bacterium *S. pneumoniae*, the causative organism of this common bacterial infection. The polyvalent type is used primarily in adults. (The term polyvalent refers to the fact that the vaccine is designed to be effective against the 23 most common strains of pneumococcus in adult cases of pneumonia.) This vaccine may also sometimes be recommended for pediatric clients at higher risk for pneumonia as a result of serious chronic illnesses, especially if immunocompromised. However, the 7-valent vaccine is routinely recommended for children two years of age and under and for high-risk children up to the age of five years. It is administered at two, four, and six months of age with a booster at twelve months of age. Its official full name is 7-valent conjugate vaccine, and it is made using a special type of protein isolated from *Corynebacterium diphtheriae*, the bacterium that causes diphtheria. It is designed to immunize against the top seven pneumococcal strains found in pediatric pneumonia cases.

Contraindications for either vaccine include known drug allergy to components of the vaccine itself, thrombocytopenia or any bleeding disorder that would contraindicate an intramuscular injection, as well as current significant febrile illnesses or immunosuppressed state as a result of drug therapy (e.g., cancer chemotherapy). The vaccine may sometimes still be given in such cases, if it is felt that withholding the vaccine poses an even greater risk to the client. Pregnancy category C for both vaccines. Dosage information appears in the dosages table on p. 761.

▸▸ poliovirus vaccine (inactivated)

The inactivated poliovirus vaccine is administered by subcutaneous injection. This is primarily because poliomyelitis, a severe side effect from the polio vaccine, can be avoided by limiting or eliminating the use of the live virus oral vaccine (OPV). The last indigenous case of poliomyelitis reported in Canada occurred in 1977. Other cases reported in Canada are as a result of wild virus importation. In 1978–1979 there were 11 reported cases and one case in 1988. Of two cases imported by an individual visiting another country, in 1993 and 1996, there was contained secondary transmission and no paralysis. The current NACI recommendations are for all children to receive four doses of IPV at ages two months, four months, and six months with a booster at 18 months and four to six years. As mentioned above, it is usually combined with acellular pertussis vaccine, adsorbed diphtheria and tetanus toxoids, and *Haemophilus influenzae* type b in a single product (Pentacel). In Canada, OPV has not been used since 1997. The United States more recently discontinued its use. Because of its ease of administration and cost, it is widely used in developing countries for mass vaccination in an attempt to eradicate polio.

IPV is available only in a parenteral form; OPV is an oral vaccine. Unlike OPV, which is a live, attenuated virus vaccine, IPV contains an inactivated form of the virus. IPV is administered subcutaneously. Pregnancy category C. The recommended dosages for this vaccine are given in the dosages table on p. 761.

▶▶ varicella virus vaccine

Licensed in Canada in 1998, the live attenuated varicella virus vaccine is used to prevent varicella (chicken pox) and herpes zoster (shingles) infections. In 2005, the National Immunization Strategy (NIS) was launched in Canada to provide universal access to varicella vaccination for all children under the age of five years not previously vaccinated. Approximately 50 percent of all cases of varicella occur in children under five years of age or in individuals with compromised immune systems such as geriatric or HIV-infected clients. It is estimated that only ten percent of children over 12 years of age are still susceptible to varicella. Only two percent of adults develop varicella infections. However, 50 percent of the deaths associated with varicella infections are in adults. Half of these are in immunocompromised clients.

The varicella vaccine is attenuated by passage of virus particles through human and embryonic guinea pig cell cultures. Varicella vaccine must be stored at 2° to 8°C in a freezer. It is administered by subcutaneous injection. It should not be given to immunodeficient clients or to clients who have received high doses of systemic steroids in the previous month. It is also recommended that salicylates be avoided for six weeks after vaccination with varicella vaccine because of the possibility of Reye's syndrome. The varicella vaccine product Varilrix should not be administered to anyone with a known hypersensitivity to neomycin. Pregnancy category C. The recommended dosages for this vaccine are given in the dosages table on p. 761.

rabies virus vaccine

Rabies immunization is not routine. However, situations requiring vaccination against the rabies virus do occur periodically in many practice settings. Rabies virus vaccine is developed using laboratory techniques involving infected human cell cultures and selected antimicrobial drugs. Rabies can infect a variety of mammals, including skunks, foxes, raccoons, bats, dogs, and cats. The virus is usually transferred to humans by an animal bite and is almost universally fatal if untreated with rabies vaccine and immune globulin (discussed later). Post-exposure prophylaxis is recommended following any bite by an animal whose rabies immunization status is unknown, unless the animal can be kept captive and observed for signs of rabies. Current recommendations call for a total of five intramuscular injections on days 0, 3, 7, 14, and 28 following the animal bite. Pre-exposure prophylaxis is recommended for persons at high risk for exposure to the rabies virus (e.g., veterinarians). The pre-exposure course consists of three injections on days 0, 7, and 21–28. Periodic booster shots are recommended approximately every two to five years, or based on the levels of the client's rabies virus antibody titres. Clients having a new bite who have been previously immunized may need to receive only two booster shots on days 0 and 3. Contraindications to rabies vaccine include a history of allergic reaction to the vaccine itself or to the drugs neomycin, gentamicin, or amphotericin B. However, given the life-threatening nature of rabies infection, treatment may still be required and supportive therapy provided (e.g., epinephrine, diphenhydramine, corticosteroids) to minimize allergic reactions. Clients with any kind of febrile illness should delay occupational pre-exposure prophylaxis treatment until their illness has subsided. Pregnancy category C. See the table on p. 761 for recommended dosages.

PASSIVE IMMUNIZING AGENTS

▶▶ hepatitis B immune globulin

Hepatitis B immune globulin (H-BIG) is used to provide passive immunity against hepatitis B infection in the post-exposure prophylaxis and treatment of persons exposed to hepatitis B virus or HBsAg-positive materials (e.g., blood, plasma, serum). It is prepared from the plasma of human donors with high titres of antibody to HBsAg. All donors are tested for the antibody to HIV to prevent transmission of the virus that causes AIDS.

H-BIG is contraindicated in persons who have exhibited hypersensitivity to it. Because of the possible devastating consequences of exposure to hepatitis B infection, pregnancy is not considered a contraindication to the use of H-BIG when there is a clear need for it. H-BIG is available only in a parenteral form that is administered intramuscularly. Pregnancy category C. The recommended dosages for hepatitis B immune globulin are given in the dosages table on p. 761.

▶▶ immune globulin

Immune globulin can be administered intramuscularly or intravenously (IV). It is used to provide passive immunity by increasing antibody titre and antigen–antibody reaction potential. The agents are available only in parenteral form and are known by the route of administration: immune globulin IM (IGIM) and immune globulin IV (IGIV). They are given to help prevent certain infectious diseases in susceptible persons or to ameliorate the diseases in those already infected. Immune globulins are pooled from the blood of at least 1000 human donors. This plasma is prepared by cold alcohol fractionation and usually washed with a detergent to destroy any harmful viruses, such as hepatitis or HIV. See Box 45-2 for Health Canada–approved uses for immune globulins. Immune globulins are contraindicated in clients hypersensitive to them. Pregnancy category C. The recommended dosages for the immune globulins are given in the dosages table on p. 761.

Rh$_0$(D) immune globulin

Rh$_0$(D) immune globulin is used to suppress the active antibody response and the formation of anti-Rh$_0$(D) in the Rh$_0$(D)-negative person exposed to Rh-positive

BOX 45-2

Health Canada–Approved Uses of Immune Globulins

AIDS
Chronic lymphocytic leukemia
Guillain-Barré syndrome (acute, progressive neuropathy)
Hemolytic disease of newborn
Hepatitis A
Idiopathic thrombocytopenic purpura
Kawasaki syndrome (acute fever and rash with swollen
 lymph nodes)
Primary and secondary immune deficiencies
Measles
Myasthenia gravis
Polyneuropathy
Pemphigus vulgaris (a rare autoimmune skin disease
 with blistering of the mouth)
Primary immunodeficiency diseases
Varicella
Staphylococcal toxic shock
Invasive group A streptococcal fasciitis with associated
 toxic shock
Respiratory syncytial virus

blood. Because an $Rh_0(D)$-negative person reacts to Rh-positive blood as if it were a foreign, "non-self" product, an immune response develops against it and an antigen–antibody reaction occurs. This can be fatal, and the administration of this immune globulin helps prevent the reaction, and hence this dire outcome. The most common use of this product is for maternal–fetal Rh incompatibility (postpartum). Only the mother is normally dosed, with the treatment objective being to prevent a harmful maternal immune response to a fetus during a future pregnancy should an Rh-negative mother become pregnant with an Rh-positive child.

$Rh_0(D)$ immune globulin is prepared from the plasma or serum of adults with a high titre of anti-$Rh_0(D)$ antibody to the red blood cell antigen $Rh_0(D)$. This product is available only in a formulation for intramuscular injection. This immune globulin is contraindicated in persons who have been previously immunized with this drug and in $Rh_0(D)$-positive/Du-positive clients. It is normally dosed postpartum but is rated as a pregnancy category C agent. The recommended dosages for $Rh_0(D)$ immune globulin are given in the dosages table on p. 761.

rabies immune globulin

Rabies immune globulin is a passive immunizing agent that is used concurrently with rabies virus vaccine following suspected exposure to the rabies virus. In humans this usually occurs following an animal bite. Rabies immune globulin is also developed from human cells that are harvested from persons who have been immunized with rabies vaccine. It is available only in a formulation for intramuscular injection. Its only contraindication is drug allergy, although the client may still

need to be dosed rather than face infection with the almost universally fatal rabies virus. The decision to dose a client in such a case would be based on the probability of rabies infection given the particular circumstances surrounding the animal bite. Pregnancy category C. Dosing guidelines are listed in the table on p. 761.

tetanus immune globulin

Tetanus immune globulin contains tetanus antitoxin antibodies that neutralize the bacterial exotoxin produced by *Clostridium tetani*, the bacterium that causes tetanus. Tetanus immune globulin is prepared from the plasma of adults hyperimmunized with the tetanus toxoid and is given as prophylaxis to people with tetanus-prone wounds. It may also be used to treat active tetanus. Its only contraindication is drug allergy. Tetanus immune globulin is available only in a formulation for intramuscular injection. Pregnancy category C. The recommended dosages for tetanus immune globulin are given in the dosages table on p. 761.

varicella zoster immune globulin

Varicella zoster immune globulin (VZIG) can be used to modify or prevent chicken pox in susceptible individuals who have had recent significant exposure to the disease. VZIG should be given as soon as possible, within 96 hours of exposure. Candidates for therapy with VZIG are those at high risk of serious disease or complications if they become infected with the varicella-zoster virus (VZV). Examples are newborn children, including premature infants with significant exposure, pregnant women, and immunocompromised adults. Healthy adults should be evaluated on a case-by-case basis. The duration of protection against infection provided by VZIG is at least three weeks.

VZIG is prepared from the plasma of normal blood donors with high antibody titres to VZV. The recommended dose of VZIG is 125 units/kg, up to a maximum of 625 units, given intramuscularly. Higher doses may be considered for immunosuppressed clients. Pregnancy category C.

NURSING PROCESS

■ Assessment

Before administering a toxoid or vaccine, the nurse should gather complete information about the client's health history, including medication history, present and past health status, previous reactions and responses to these types of agents, previous allergy test results, use of any immunosuppressants, presence of autoimmune or immunosuppressing disease or infection, and pregnancy status. In children who are to receive a vaccine or toxoid, the immunization schedule and the dose ordered by the physician must be followed. NACI, in collaboration with The Public Health Agency of Health Canada, provides the latest recommendations for adult and pediatric immunizations within Canada. These recommendations are easily accessible on the Internet at http://www.phac-aspc.gc.ca/naci-ccni/index.html. The Canadian Immunization Guide is published every four years in Canada. The most recent was written in 2002, with the seventh edition due in 2006. It is crucial for the nurse to keep current on immunization cautions and contraindications; this Web site and other published materials from NACI and Health Canada on immunization are an important source of information.

Because passive immunizing agents may precipitate serum sickness, geriatric clients and those with chronic illness or who are debilitated must be assessed carefully before treatment (i.e., vital signs, intake and output, electrocardiogram [ECG], and baseline assessment). Contraindications to the use of passive immunizing agents include hypersensitivity to them and active infections.

Contraindications to the administration of active immunizing agents include current infections (especially with the same pathogen or toxin), febrile illnesses, a history of reactions to the agent or serious side effects, and pregnancy. Clients who are already immunosuppressed (e.g., those with AIDS, geriatric clients, clients with chronic diseases or cancer, neonates) are at increased risk for experiencing serious side effects to toxoids or vaccines; therefore cautious use of these agents is called for. Varicella zoster immune globulin is contraindicated in clients with a history of severe reactions to human immune globulin and those who have had a thrombocytopenic reaction.

Some adults incorrectly assume that the vaccines they received as children will protect them for a lifetime. Some adults were never vaccinated as children, or were vaccinated with older, less effective vaccines. In addition, immunity may fade over time, and as individuals age they may become more susceptible to serious diseases caused by common infections, such as pneumococcus. The nurse should keep in mind the following with regard to adults:

- Varicella vaccine, hepatitis B vaccine (for at-risk adults), MMR, and tetanus-diphtheria vaccine are needed by all adults.
- Influenza vaccine is recommended for those age 65 years and older. Some provinces/territories in Canada offer universal influenza vaccine and all individuals between the age of two and 65 years are encouraged to receive the influenza vaccine.
- Pneumococcal vaccine is recommended for those age 65 years and older.
- The influenza vaccine is recommended for all adult healthcare workers.

The nurse should keep in mind the following with regard to teenagers and children:

- The meningococcus vaccine is part of routine vaccination in Canada and also is recommended for college students.
- The 2005 Childhood and Adolescent Immunization Schedule (see Table 45-2) from the NACI lists the age

ranges for each vaccine or series of shots. If any shots have been missed, the child's physician can assist in getting the child back on the vaccine schedule.

Nursing Diagnoses

Nursing diagnoses related to the administration of immunizing agents include the following:

- Risk for injury related to possible side effects of or allergic reactions to the immunizing agent.
- Acute pain related to local and/or systemic effects of the injection of a toxoid, vaccine, or passive immunizing agent.
- Deficient knowledge related to the use of toxoids, vaccines, or passive immunizing agents.

Planning

Goals for clients receiving immunizing agents include the following:

- Client states side effects of medication.
- Client manages minimal discomfort stemming from the administration of a toxoid, vaccine, or passive immunizing agent.
- Client returns for follow-up injections and booster injections and for follow-up visits with the physician.

Outcome Criteria

Outcome criteria related to the use of immunizing agents include the following:

- Client experience minimal side effects of or allergic reactions to the immunizing agent, such as fever, chills, myalgia, and bronchospasms.
- Client uses measures such as non-ASA analgesics or diphenhydramine (as recommended by physician) to relieve localized discomfort or to alleviate any reactions.
- Client remains adherent with therapy for prevention of illness or disease through follow-up visits with physician.
- Client states the problems to report immediately to the physician, such as fever higher than 38°C, infection, wheezing, and increasing weakness.

Implementation

When administering immunological agents, it is always important for the nurse to recheck the specific protocols concerning schedules of administration. In addition, it is always important to check and follow the manufacturer's recommendations concerning how the drug should be stored and administered, routes and site of administration (e.g., varicella zoster immune globulin is never given intravenously), dosage, precautions, and contraindications. Parents of young children must be encouraged and taught how to maintain an accurate journal of the child's immunization status with dates of immunization and the reaction(s), if any. If there is a complaint of discomfort at the injection site, warm compresses or acetaminophen may help.

Client teaching tips are presented on p. 768.

■ **Evaluation**

Therapeutic responses in clients receiving immunizing agents are the prevention or amelioration of the disease. Adverse reactions for which to monitor in clients receiving immunizing biologicals include localized swelling, redness, discomfort, and heat. The physician should be notified immediately if fever, rash, itching, or shortness of breath occur because these are the symptoms of an allergic reaction. As immunizing agents improve and newer agents are developed, it is hoped that, as with DTaP, fewer side effects, adverse drug events, and complications will occur.

A vaccine adverse event reporting system is available through the Canadian Adverse Events Following Immunization Surveillance System of the Public Health Agency of Canada.

CLIENT TEACHING TIPS

▲ If there is a local reaction (swelling, redness, or pain), you can place warm compresses on the injection site, rest (or encourage the child to rest), and take acetaminophen (or give it to the child).
▲ Notify the physician of high or prolonged fever, rash, itching, or shortness of breath after the vaccination.
▲ Keep a double record (two copies kept in separate places) of all of the medications being taken—especially all vaccinations.

▲ For more information on vaccinations, including when children should get vaccinations and what vaccinations are provided free, visit the Canadian Paediatric Society Web site (http://www.caringforkids.cps.ca/immunization/index.htm) or Health Canada's National Advisory Committee on Immunization (http://www.phac-aspc.gc.ca/im/ptimprog-progimpt/index.html).

POINTS to REMEMBER

▼ A foreign substance in the body is termed an *antigen;* the body creates a substance called an *antibody* to specifically bind to it.
▼ B-lymphocytes (B-cells), when stimulated by the binding of an antigen molecule, begin to differentiate into memory cells and plasma cells.
▼ Memory cells remember what that particular antigen looks like in case the body is exposed to the same antigen again in the future.
▼ Plasma cells manufacture the antibodies and will mass produce clones of the antibodies upon re-exposure to a particular antigen.
▼ The two types of immunity are active and passive. Different types of agents are used for each, and they are indicated for different populations.
▼ Active immunization utilizes a toxoid or a vaccine. It involves exposing the body to a relatively harmless form of the antigen (foreign invader) to imprint memory and stimulate the body's defences against any subsequent exposure. It provides long-lasting or permanent immunity. The recipient must have an active, functioning immune system.
▼ Passive immunization utilizes immune globulins, antitoxins, or antivenins. It involves taking serum or concentrated immune globulins obtained from humans or animals that, after screening and testing, are injected, directly giving the client the ability to fight off the invading micro-organism. Passive immunization provides temporary protection and does not stimulate an antibody response in the host. It is used for clients who are immunocompromised, have been exposed to the disease, or anticipate exposure to the disease.
▼ Clients who should not receive immunizing agents include those with active infections, febrile illnesses, or a history of a previous reaction to the agent. They are also usually contraindicated in pregnant women.
▼ Clients who are immunocompromised are at greater risk for suffering serious side effects from immunizing agents.
▼ Parents should keep updated records of their children's and their own immunizations.
▼ Healthcare reforms have created a need for widespread understanding of the importance of immunizations and their role in preventing disease. However, it is also critical that all risks are addressed.
▼ Although not currently recommended for public inoculation by Health Canada, vaccines for the prevention of anthrax are administered prophylactically to military personnel who are at higher risk of exposure to anthrax because of their assigned location and related duties (see p. 758).

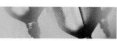

EXAMINATION REVIEW QUESTIONS

1 Contraindications to the use of passive immunizing agents include which of the following?
   a. Mild anemia
   b. Debilitated elderly
   c. Young age
   d. Polyuria
2 Which of the following is not a severe adverse effect related to immunizing agents?
   a. Dysuria
   b. Leukocytosis
   c. Anemias
   d. Fever of 39.4°C or above
3 Which of the following is a severe rare reaction to the influenza vaccine?
   a. Renal failure
   b. Cardiomegaly

   c. Hepatotoxicity
   d. Guillain-Barré syndrome
4 At what age is the DTaP vaccine first administered?
   a. 2 months
   b. 4 months
   c. 8 months
   d. 12 months
5 After the routine immunization schedule for tetanus toxoid has been completed in infancy, at what age is it recommended that the tetanus vaccine be repeated?
   a. 3 years of age
   b. 6 years of age
   c. 10 years of age
   d. Only as indicated with injury

For answers see http://evolve.elsevier.com/Lilley/pharmacology/.

CRITICAL THINKING ACTIVITIES

1 You are caring for a 56-year-old man who has recently been admitted because he is in a state of acute rejection of his transplanted heart, which he received over a year ago. This client has been on cyclosporine, azathioprine, and prednisone at home and has now had muromonab added to help stop the acute rejection. There has been an outbreak of the influenza virus at your hospital. One of your co-workers suggests vaccinating your client with the

flu vaccine that employees have been receiving. How should you respond to this co-worker?
2 Describe the schedule currently recommended for immunizations in Canada. What are the implications of not having a child properly immunized?
3 What impact have the changes to Canadian immunization schedules had on clients?

For answers see http://evolve.elsevier.com/Lilley/pharmacology/.

BIBLIOGRAPHY

Albanese, J., & Nutz, P. (2005). *Mosby's 2005 nursing drug cards.* St Louis, MO: Mosby.

Canadian Paediatric Society. (2005). Acute flaccid paralysis. Retrieved September 3, 2005, from http://www.cps.ca/english/CPSP/Studies/acute.htm

Canadian Pharmacists Association. (2003). *Therapeutic choices* (4th ed.). Ottawa, ON: Author.

Canadian Pharmacists Association. (2004). *Guide to drugs in Canada.* Toronto, ON: Dorling Kindersley.

Canadian Pharmacists Association. (2005). *Compendium of pharmaceuticals and specialties. The Canadian drug reference for health professionals.* Ottawa, ON: Author. [The subscription-based e-CPS is available at http://www.pharmacists.ca.]

Cheng, A., Williams, B.A., & Sivarajan, B.V. (Eds.). (2003). *The HSC handbook of pediatrics* (10th ed.). Toronto, ON: Elsevier.

Facts and Comparisons. (2004). *Drug facts and comparisons pocket version* (9th ed.). St Louis, MO: Wolters Kluwer Health.

Gold, R. (2002). *Your child's best shot* (2nd ed.). Ottawa, ON: Canadian Paediatric Society.

Health Canada. (2002). *Canadian immunization guide* (6th ed.). Ottawa, ON: Canadian Medical Association.

Health Canada. (2005). Drug product database (DPD). Retrieved September 3, 2005, from http://www.hc-sc.gc.ca/hpb/drugs-dpd/

Lacy, C.F., Armstrong, L.L., Goldman, M.P., & Lance, L.L. (2003). *Drug information handbook* (11th ed.). Hudson, OH: Lexi-Comp.

Mosby. (2005). *Mosby's drug consult 2005: The comprehensive reference for generic and brand name drugs* (15th ed.). St Louis, MO: Mosby.

Murray, P.R., Greenwood, D., Slack, R., & Peutherer, J. (2002). *Medical microbiology.* St Louis, MO: Mosby.

Public Health Agency of Canada. (2005). Smallpox. Retrieved September 2, 2005, from http://www.phac-aspc.gc.ca/ep-mu/smallpox_e.html

Public Health Agency of Canada. (2005). Anthrax. Retrieved September 2, 2005, from http://www.phac-aspc.gc.ca/ep-mu/anthrax_e.html

Public Health Agency of Canada. (2005). Biological threats. Retrieved September 2, 2005, from http://www.phac-aspc.gc.ca/ep-mu/faq_e.html

Public Health Agency of Canada. (2005). Vaccine safety. Canadian Adverse Events Following Immunization Surveillance System (CAEFISS). Retrieved September 2, 2005, from http://www.phac-aspc.gc.ca/im/vs-sv/index.html

Public Health Agency of Canada. (2005). Interchangeability of diphtheria, tetanus, acellular pertussis, polio, *Haemophilus influenzae* type B combination vaccines presently approved for use in Canada for children <7 years of age. *Canada Communicable Disease Report 31*(ACS-1), 1–12. Retrieved September 3, 2005, from http://www.phac-aspc.gc.ca/publicat/ccdr-rmtc/05vol31/asc-dcc-1/index.html

Public Health Agency of Canada. (2005). News release. More young Canadians have access to disease-fighting vaccines. Retrieved September 3, 2005, from http://www.phac-aspc.gc.ca/media/nr-rp/2005/2005_14_e.html

Skidmore-Roth, L. (2006). *Mosby's 2006 nursing drug reference* (19th ed.). St Louis, MO: Mosby.

Tierney, L.M., McPhee, S.J., & Papadakis, M.A. (2002). *2002 Current medical diagnosis and treatment: Adult ambulatory and inpatient management.* New York: McGraw-Hill.

Antineoplastic Agents

After reading this chapter, the successful student will be able to do the following:

1 Discuss the purpose and role of antineoplastic agents in the treatment of cancer.

2 Contrast the cell cycle in normal and malignant cells in relation to their growth and function.

3 Compare the characteristics of highly proliferating normal cells and those of cancerous or malignant cells.

4 Explain the specific differences between cell cycle–specific and cell cycle–non-specific antineoplastics.

5 Describe the common side effects of and toxic reactions to the various antineoplastic agents, including any antidotes to the toxicities.

6 Discuss the effect of the various antineoplastic agents on the normal cell cycle, including specific effects on all of the normal rapidly dividing cells found in the body, such as the cells of the hair follicle, gastrointestinal (GI) tract, GI mucosa, and bone marrow components.

7 Discuss the indications, dosages, dosage routes, cautions, contraindications, and drug interactions associated with all agents used to treat malignancies.

8 Develop a nursing care plan for clients receiving antineoplastic drugs.

ℓ-LEARNING ACTIVITIES

Student CD-ROM
- Review Questions: see questions 341–352
- Animations
- Medication Administration Checklists
- IV Therapy Checklists

evolve Web site (http://evolve.elsevier.com/Lilley/pharmacology/)
- Online Chapter Worksheet • Frequently Asked Questions
- Learning Tips and Content Updates • WebLinks • Online Appendices and Supplements • Mosby/Saunders ePharmacology Update • Access to *Mosby's Drug Consult*

DRUG PROFILES

GLOSSARY

Alkylation (al′ kə lay′ shən) A chemical reaction in which an alkyl group is transferred from an alkylating agent. When such organic reactions occur with a biologically significant cellular constituent such as DNA, they result in interference with mitosis and cell division.

Anaplasia (anaplastic) The absence of the cellular differentiation that is part of the normal cellular growth process (see *differentiation*).

Antineoplastic medications Drugs used to treat cancer. Also called *cancer drugs* and *anticancer drugs*.

Benign (bə nine′) Non-cancerous and therefore not an immediate threat to life, even though treatment eventually may be required for health or cosmetic reasons.

Bifunctional (of an alkylating agent) Composed of molecules that have two reactive alkyl groups and that are therefore able to alkylate two cancer cell DNA molecules per drug molecule.

Carcinoma (kar′ si noe′ muh) Malignant epithelial neoplasm that tends to invade surrounding tissue and to metastasize to distant regions of the body.

Cell cycle–non-specific (CCNS) (of an antineoplastic drug) Cytotoxic in any phase of the cellular growth cycle.

Cell cycle–specific (CCS) (of an antineoplastic drug) Cytotoxic only during a specific cell cycle phase.

Differentiation An important part of normal cellular growth processes; involves changes in immature cells that allow them to mature into different types of more specialized cells, each having different functions.

Dose-limiting side effects Side effects that prevent the antineoplastic agent from being given in higher doses, often limiting the effectiveness of the drug.

Emetic potential (ə me′ tik) Potential of a substance to irritate the cells of the stomach or stimulate the vomiting centre in the central nervous system (CNS), resulting in nausea and vomiting.

Growth fraction Percentage of cells in mitosis at any given time.

Intrathecal A route of drug injection through the theca of the spinal cord and into the subarachnoid space. Used to deliver certain chemotherapy medications to kill cancer cells in the central nervous system.

Leucovorin rescue (loo′ koe vor′ in) The use of leucovorin to limit and reverse the toxicity induced by the anticancer drug methotrexate. (Note: Leucovorin is also sometimes administered before or with fluorouracil to enhance the antineoplastic effect of the fluorouracil.)

Leukemia (loo kee′ mee uh) A malignant neoplasm of blood-forming tissues characterized by the diffuse replacement of bone marrow with proliferating leukocyte precursors, which, in turn, results in abnormal numbers and forms of immature white blood cells in the circulation and the infiltration of lymph nodes, spleen, and liver.

Lymphoma (lim fo′ mə) A neoplasm of lymphoid tissue that is usually malignant but in rare cases may be benign.

Malignant (mə lig′ nənt) Tending to worsen and cause death; anaplastic, invasive, and metastatic.

Metastasis (me tas′ tə sis) The process by which a cancer spreads from the original site of growth to a new and remote part of the body.

Mitosis (my toe′ sis) The process of cell reproduction occurring in somatic cells and resulting in the formation of two genetically identical daughter cells containing the diploid number of chromosomes characteristic of the species.

Mitotic index (mi to′ tik) The number of cells per unit (usually 1000) undergoing mitosis during a given time.

Mutation A permanent change in cellular genetic material (DNA) that is transmissible to future cellular generations. Mutations can transform normal cells into cancer cells.

Myelosuppression Suppression of bone marrow function, which can result in dangerously reduced numbers of red and white blood cells and platelets. Both cancer chemotherapy and radiation can cause this condition. (Also called *bone marrow suppression* [BMS] or *bone marrow depression* [BMD].)

Nadir (nay′ deer) Lowest point in any fluctuating value over time, such as the white blood cell count after it has been depressed by chemotherapy. With antineoplastic drug therapy, this term also refers to the time frame in which these drugs kill the greatest number of bone marrow cells.

Neoplasm A mass of new cells that exhibit uncontrolled cellular reproduction; tumour.

Paraneoplastic syndrome (PNS) (pair′ ə nee′ o plas′ tik) Signs and symptoms of cancer located at a distance from the tumour or its metastatic sites.

Polyfunctional (of an alkylating agent) Able to perform several alkylation reactions with cancer cell DNA molecules per single molecule of drug.

Sarcoma (sar koe′ muh) A malignant neoplasm of the connective tissues arising in fibrous, fatty, muscular, synovial, vascular, or neural tissue, often first presenting as a painless swelling.

Tumour (too′ mər or tyoo′ mər) A new growth of tissue characterized by a progressive, uncontrolled proliferation of cells. Tumours can be solid (e.g., brain tumour) or circulating (e.g., leukemia or lymphoma). Circulating tumours are also called *hematological tumours* or *hematological malignancies*.

Cancer is a broad term embracing a group of diseases that are characterized by cellular transformation (e.g., by genetic **mutation**), uncontrolled cellular growth, possible invasion into surrounding tissue, and metastasis to other tissues or organs distant from the original body site. This cellular growth differs from normal cell growth in that cancerous cells do not possess a growth control mechanism, and the resulting generations of cells usually have no positive physiological function. Cancerous cells will continue to grow and invade adjacent structures, or they may break away from the original tumour mass and travel by means of the blood or lymphatic system to establish a new clone (metastatic lesion) elsewhere in the body.

Metastasis refers to the spreading of a cancer (uncontrolled cell growth) from the original site of growth (primary lesion) to a new and remote part of the body (secondary or metastatic lesion). The terms *malignancy*, *neoplasm*, and *tumour* are often used as synonyms for cancer; however, each has a specific meaning. A **neoplasm** is a mass of new cells that exhibit uncontrolled cellular reproduction. It is another term for **tumour**. There are two types of neoplasms, or tumours: benign and malignant. A **benign** tumour is of a uniform size and shape and displays no invasive or metastatic properties. The terms non-malignant and benign suggest that such tumours may be harmless, which is true in most cases. However, a benign tumour can be lethal if it grows in vital tissue and interrupts normal function. **Malignant** neoplasms typically consist of cancerous cells that invade surrounding tissues and metastasize to other tissues and organs, where they form metastatic tumour deposits. Some of the characteristics of benign and malignant neoplasms, or tumours, are listed in Table 46-1.

Over 100 types of malignant neoplasms (cancerous tumours) affect humans. They are usually classified by their primary anatomic (organ or tissue) location and the type of cell from which the neoplasm develops. Common body sites for growth of such tumours include

- Bladder and kidney
- Colon
- Prostate gland
- Uterus
- Blood-producing tissue
- Lymphatic system
- Rectum
- Breast
- Lung
- Skin

Tissue categories for various tumour types include carcinomas, sarcomas, lymphomas, leukemias, and tumours of nervous tissue origin. Examples of these common malignant tumours are listed in Table 46-2. It is important to know the tissue of origin because this determines the type of chemotherapy used, the likely response to therapy, and the prognosis.

Carcinomas arise from epithelial tissue, which is located throughout the body. It covers or lines all body surfaces, both inside and outside the body. Examples are the skin, the mucosal lining of the entire gastrointestinal (GI)

tract, and the bronchial tree (lungs). The purpose of these epithelial tissues is to protect the body's vital organs.

Sarcomas are malignant tumours that arise primarily from connective tissues, but sometimes in epithelial cells. Connective tissue is the most abundant and widely distributed of all tissues and comprises bone, cartilage, muscle, lymphatic, and vascular structures. Its purpose is to support and protect other tissues.

Lymphomas arise from the lymphatic tissue. **Leukemias** arise from the various types of leukocytes in the blood. These two types of tumours differ from carcinomas and sarcomas in that the cancerous cells do not form solid tumours but are interspersed throughout the lymphatic or circulatory system and interfere with the normal functioning of these systems. Because they are more diffuse (spread out) than localized in one area, they are also referred to as *circulating cancers*.

The last major type of tumour, nerve or neural tissue tumours, are those arising in and affecting the cells of the central or peripheral nervous systems.

Cancers may produce signs and symptoms caused by changes in tissues remote from the tumour or its site of metastasis. This symptom complex is referred to as the **paraneoplastic syndrome (PNS)**, and some of the various disorders produced are listed in Table 46-3. The syndrome is believed to result from the effects of biologically or immunologically active substances secreted by the tumours. Some clients may also exhibit generalized symptoms, such as anorexia, weight loss, fatigue, and fever.

TABLE 46-1
TUMOUR CHARACTERISTICS: BENIGN AND MALIGNANT

Characteristics	Benign	Malignant
Potential to metastasize	No	Yes
Encapsulated	Yes	No
Similar to tissue of origin	Yes	No
Rate of growth	Slow	Unpredictable and unrestrained
Recurrence after surgical removal	Rare	Common

TABLE 46-2
TUMOUR CLASSIFICATION BASED ON SPECIFIC TISSUE OF ORIGIN

Tissue of Origin	Malignant Tissue
EPITHELIAL = CARCINOMAS	
Glands or ducts	Adenocarcinomas
Respiratory tract	Small- and large-cell carcinomas
Kidney	Renal cell carcinoma
Skin	Squamous cell, epidermoid, and basal cell carcinoma; melanoma
CONNECTIVE = SARCOMAS	
Fibrous	Fibrosarcoma
Cartilage	Chondrosarcoma
Bone	Osteogenic sarcoma (Ewing's tumour)
Blood vessels	Kaposi's sarcoma
Synovia	Synoviosarcoma
Mesothelium	Mesothelioma
LYMPHATIC = LYMPHOMAS	
Lymph tissue	Lymphomas (Hodgkin's disease and multiple myeloma)
NERVE	
Glial	Glioma
Adrenal medulla nerves	Pheochromocytoma
BLOOD	
White blood cells	Leukemia

TABLE 46-3
PARANEOPLASTIC SYNDROME ASSOCIATED WITH SOME CANCERS

Paraneoplastic Syndrome	Associated Cancer
Hypercalcemia, sensory, neuropathies, SIADH	Lung
Disseminated intravascular coagulation	Leukemia
Cushing's syndrome (increased secretion of cortisol, resulting in obesity, moon face, acne, and hypertension)	Lung, thyroid, testes, adrenal
Addison's syndrome (inadequate cortisol, resulting in exhaustion, weakness, low blood pressure, and sometimes dark pigmentation)	Adrenal, lymphomas

SIADH, Syndrome of inappropriate antidiuretic hormone secretion.

TABLE 46-4
CANCER: PROPOSED ETIOLOGICAL FACTORS

Risk Factor	Associated Cancer
ENVIRONMENT	
Radiation (ionizing)	Leukemia, breast, thyroid, lung
Radiation (ultraviolet)	Skin, melanoma
Viruses	Cervical, leukemia, liver, lymphoma, nasopharyngeal
FOOD	
Aflatoxin	Liver
Dietary factors	Colon, breast, endometrium, gallbladder
Heterocyclic amine compounds	Stomach, colon, liver
LIFESTYLE	
Alcohol	Esophagus, liver, stomach, larynx, colon, rectal, breast
Tobacco	Lung, mouth, esophagus, larynx, bladder, pancreas, kidney, cervix
MEDICAL DRUGS	
DES	Vaginal in offspring, breast, testes, ovary
Estrogens	Endometrial, breast
Alkylating agents	Leukemia, bladder
OCCUPATIONAL	
Asbestos	Lung, mesothelioma
Aniline dye	Bladder
Benzene	Leukemia
Vinyl chloride	Liver
REPRODUCTIVE HISTORY	
Late first pregnancy	Breast
No children	Ovary
Multiple sexual partners	Cervix, uterus

DES, Diethylstilbestrol.

ETIOLOGY OF CANCER

The etiology of cancer remains a mystery for the most part, and cancer researchers have made slow progress toward identifying possible causes. In recent years certain etiological factors have come to light, however, and some of these and the cancers they cause are listed in Table 46-4. Various immunological, ethnic, genetic, and age- and sex-related factors also affect vulnerability.

AGE- AND SEX-RELATED DIFFERENCES

The probability of a neoplastic disease developing generally increases with advancing age. For example, chronic lymphocytic and myelocytic leukemia, colon cancer, and lung cancer usually develop during middle and older age and are rare in young children. Exceptions are acute lymphocytic leukemia and Wilms' tumour, which decrease in incidence with age.

Except for cancers affecting the reproductive system, few cancers exhibit a sex-related difference in their incidence. Lung and urinary cancers are more common in men than in women, but this may have more to do with lifestyle factors such as smoking and exposure to environmental toxins than to sex per se. The incidence of colon, rectal, pancreatic, and skin cancers, as well as leukemia, is almost equal between the sexes.

GENETIC AND ETHNIC FACTORS

Few cancers appear to be inherited (breast, colon, and stomach cancers are exceptions). Advancements in understanding of tumour biology have helped guide therapy tremendously. Two examples of such advancements include determination of hormone receptor status and specific gene expression for various types of tumour cells. Tumour cells that are shown to express on their cell membrane surfaces either estrogen receptors (ERs) or progesterone receptors (PRs), or that express specific genes such as the HER2/neu gene, illustrate these concepts. Because they aid in the classification of a client's tumour, they also help in choosing appropriate drug therapy and predicting response to such therapy and outcome. These types of tumours also often show a familial pattern of inheritance. Burkitt's lymphoma is an example of a cancer that shows a racial pattern of inheritance. This disease, the most common non-Hodgkin's lymphoma in children, is more common in young children in Africa and in children of African descent than in non-African children. Another example of an ethnic predisposition is the high incidence of nasopharyngeal cancer in persons of Chinese descent.

ONCOGENIC VIRUSES

Extensive research has indicated that there are cancer-causing (oncogenic) viruses that can affect most mammalian species. Examples include the various cat leukemias, the

Rous* sarcoma virus in chickens, human papilloma virus (HPV), and the Shope* papilloma virus in rabbits.

The herpes viruses are common examples of oncogenic viruses. Epstein-Barr virus, a type of herpes virus, is most commonly recognized as the cause of infectious mononucleosis (commonly referred to as "mono" or the "kissing disease"). However it is also associated with the development of Burkitt's lymphoma and nasopharyngeal cancer. There also seems to be a link between the development of cervical cancer and infection with the herpes simplex type 2 virus (herpes genitalis). HPV has been linked to certain bladder cancers.

OCCUPATIONAL AND ENVIRONMENTAL CARCINOGENS

A carcinogen is any substance that can induce the development of a cancer or accelerate its growth. Many drugs that were once considered safe have proved to be carcinogenic. However, no amount of clinical testing can fully reveal all of the possible carcinogenic and mutagenic effects. Testing for carcinogenic activity is difficult and current test methods are not often satisfactory. Moreover, there can be species-related differences in carcinogenic potential with any given drug. Thus effects may not be observed in the laboratory animals on which the agent has been tested and may become obvious only when used in human subjects. Sometimes such effects become apparent before the medication is marketed. However, given the relatively small number of subjects in clinical research trials, effects may not appear until after the drug is marketed for use with the general population. If patterns of carcinogenicity begin to emerge during this period of post-marketing surveillance (or post-marketing studies), the drug may be recalled from the market, either voluntarily by the manufacturer or on mandate from Health Canada.

RADIATION

Radiation is a well-known and potent carcinogenic agent. In fact, several scientists who studied radiation or who worked on the development of the first atomic bomb were victims of cancer. For example, Enrico Fermi, a nuclear physicist who worked on the development of the atomic bomb, died of leukemia. There are two basic types of radiation: (1) ionizing, or high-energy, radiation, and (2) non-ionizing, or low-energy, radiation. Both types can be carcinogenic. Ionizing radiation is potent and can penetrate deeply into the body. It is called ionizing because it causes the formation of ions within living cells. This type of radiation (e.g., X-ray studies, radium implants) is also used to treat (irradiate) cancerous tumours. Non-ionizing radiation is much less potent and cannot penetrate deeply into the body. Sunlight and ultraviolet light are examples of this type of radiation. Both can cause skin cancer, although ultraviolet light is still used to treat various dermatological conditions such as atopic dermatitis.

IMMUNOLOGICAL FACTORS

The immune system plays an important role in the body in terms of cancer surveillance and the elimination of neoplastic cells. Neoplastic cells are believed to routinely develop in everyone, but the immune system in healthy persons recognizes them as abnormal and eliminates them by means of cell-mediated immunity (cytotoxic T-lymphocytes). Not surprisingly, there is a much higher incidence of cancer in immunocompromised people. Examples include clients undergoing cancer chemotherapy; organ transplant clients receiving immunosuppressive therapy; and clients suffering from immunological impairment or disease, including AIDS. This relationship between cancer and a suppressed immune system has also been noted in cancer clients being treated with immunotherapy consisting of interferon derivatives, the bacillus Calmette-Guérin (BCG) vaccine (used to treat bladder cancer), and lymphokines.

CELL GROWTH CYCLE

Normal cells in the body divide (proliferate) in a controlled and organized fashion, and this growth is regulated by means of various mechanisms. In contrast, cancer cells lack regulatory mechanisms and they proliferate uncontrollably, though some modulation of cancer cell proliferation may occur if blood flow to the cancer is disrupted. The growth of cancer cells may also be more constant or continuous than that of non-malignant cells. Thus an important characteristic of malignant tumours is the time it takes for the tumour to double in size. This doubling time varies greatly for various types of cancers and is directly related to and important in determining the prognosis for a particular client. Cancer treatment that cannot destroy every neoplastic cell does not prevent the regrowth of the tumour, and the time it takes for regrowth to occur depends on the doubling time of the particular cancer. For instance, Burkitt's lymphoma has an extremely short doubling time, whereas multiple myeloma has one of the longest. A cancer with a shorter doubling time may be more difficult to treat and have a poorer prognosis.

The cell growth characteristics for normal and neoplastic cells are similar. Both types of cells go through five distinct growth phase cycles: G_0, the resting phase; G_1, the first growth, or post-mitotic, phase; S, the DNA synthesis phase; G_2, the second growth, or pre-mitotic, phase; and M, the **mitosis** phase (cell reproduction). During mitosis, one cell divides into two identical daughter cells. A complete cycle from one mitosis to the next is called the *generation time* (same as doubling time), and it is different for all tumours, ranging from hours to days. The cell growth cycle and the events that occur in the various phases are summarized in Table 46-5.

The level of growth activity of a mass of tumour cells can also be characterized, and it has an important bearing

---

*Doctors P. Rous and R. Shope were early investigators of oncogenic viruses.

TABLE 46-5
CELL CYCLE PHASES

Phase	Description
G_0 Resting phase	Most normal human cells exist predominantly in this phase. Cancer cells in this phase are not susceptible to the toxic effects of cell cycle–specific drugs.
G_1 Post-mitotic phase	Enzymes necessary for DNA synthesis are produced.
S DNA synthesis phase	DNA synthesis takes place, from DNA separation to DNA replication.
G_2	RNA and specialized proteins are made.
M Mitosis phase	Divided into four phases: prophase, metaphase, anaphase, and telophase.

on the killing power of chemotherapy. The percentage of cells undergoing mitosis at any given time is called the **growth fraction** of the tumour mass. The actual number of cells that are in the M phase of the cell cycle is called the **mitotic index.** Chemotherapy is most effective when the greatest number of cells are dividing (i.e., when both the growth fraction and mitotic index are high), or what is termed *highly proliferative.* **Differentiation**, or the ability to identify the cell's origin, is also important in the treatment of neoplasms because the more differentiation there is, generally the better the response to treatments such as chemotherapy and radiation.

AN OVERVIEW OF DRUG THERAPY

Chemotherapy is a general term that can technically refer to chemical (drug) therapy for any kind of illness. However, in practice this term usually refers to the pharmacological treatment of cancer. Drugs used for cancer chemotherapy are called *antineoplastic agents,* and they can be subdivided into two main groups of agents based on where in the cellular life cycle they work. Antineoplastic drugs that are cytotoxic in any phase of the cycle are called **cell cycle–non-specific (CCNS)** agents. Those agents that are cytotoxic during a specific cell cycle phase are called **cell cycle–specific (CCS)** agents. CCNS agents are more effective against large, slowly growing tumours. CCS agents are more effective against rapidly growing tumours. Figure 46-1 shows where in the general phase of the cell cycle the primary chemotherapeutic agents kill the cancerous cells.

The ultimate goal of any anticancer regimen is to kill every neoplastic cell and produce a cure, but this goal is not achieved in most cases. One reason for this is that antineoplastic agents are usually only cytotoxic and not tumoricidal. That is, they usually only kill a portion of the cells in a tumour, such as those that are dividing, and not all the cells in the entire tumour. Other factors that affect the chances of cure and the length of survival include the can-

cer stage at the time of diagnosis, the type of neoplasm and its doubling time, the efficacy of the cancer treatment, the development of drug resistance, and the general health of the client. When total cure is not possible, the primary goal of therapy is then to control the growth of the neoplasm while maintaining the best quality of life for the client.

It must be strongly emphasized that cancer care and treatment involves many rapidly evolving medical sciences. Neoplastic disease is an intensively researched area, with the ultimate goals being to prevent cancer and prevent premature death in those diagnosed with it. Chemotherapy medications are often dosed as part of complex, specific treatment protocols that are subject to frequent revision by oncology clinicians and researchers. For these reasons the drug dosing information provided in this chapter is offered as representative of current cancer treatment, and not absolute. Furthermore, the indications listed for each specific drug are the primary Health Canada–approved indications current at the time of this writing. These, too, may change as a given drug is determined to be more (or less) effective for certain types of cancer. Also, in clinical practice clients are often treated by their supervising oncologists with one or more antineoplastic medications for "off label" uses, meaning that the drug is not currently approved for this particular use by Health Canada.

No antineoplastic agent is effective against all types of neoplasms. These drugs also have a low therapeutic index, meaning that a fine line exists between therapeutic effect and toxicity. However, one important discovery yielded by clinical experience is that a combination of agents is usually more effective than single-agent therapy. Because drug-resistant cells often develop in tumours as the result of the tumour's genetic instability, exposure to multiple drugs with multiple mechanisms and sites of action will destroy more subpopulations of such cells. The delayed onset of resistance to a particular antineoplastic agent is thus one benefit of combination drug therapy. To be most effective, however, the drugs used in such a combination regimen should possess the following characteristics:

- Some efficacy even as single drugs in the treatment of the particular type of cancer
- Different mechanisms of action so that the cytotoxic effect is maximized. This includes differences in cell cycle specificity
- Different cytotoxic properties so that each drug in the combination can be administered in a full therapeutic dose (in other words, have no or minimal overlapping toxicities)

SIDE EFFECTS AND ADVERSE EFFECTS

One major drawback to the use of antineoplastic agents is that nearly all of them cause side effects and adverse effects. Many of these effects are severe or even toxic and stem from the fact that these agents are harmful to all rapidly growing cells—both the harmful cancer cells and

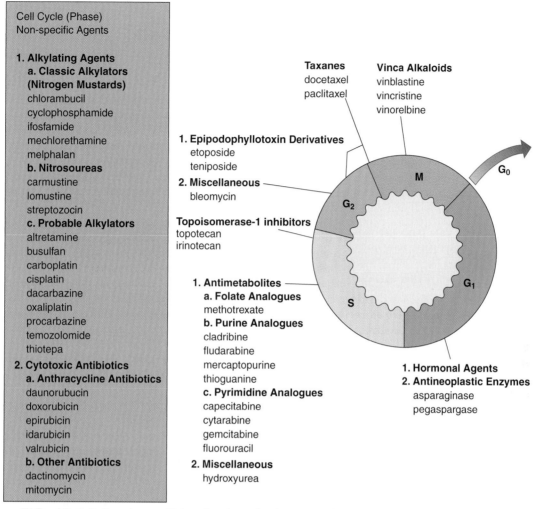

FIG. 46-1 Cell cycle specificity of antineoplastic agents. General phase of the cell cycle with corresponding action of specific antineoplastic agents to produce cancerous cell kill.

the healthy, normal human cells. Three types of such rapidly growing beneficial human cells are hair follicles, gastrointestinal cells, and bone marrow cells. Because most of today's antineoplastic agents still cannot differentiate between the cancer cells and these healthy cells, the latter are also killed, with hair loss, nausea and vomiting, and myelosuppression the undesirable consequences. As discussed later in this chapter, these effects are called **dose-limiting side effects**, because they often prevent the antineoplastic agent from being administered in sufficiently high doses to kill the entire population of cancer cells.

CONTRAINDICATIONS

Given the often fatal outcome of neoplastic diseases, most cancer drugs are only rarely considered to be absolutely contraindicated for a given client. Even if a client has a known allergic reaction to a given antineoplastic medication, the urgency of treating the client's cancer may still necessitate administering the medication and treating any allergic symptoms with supportive medications

such as antihistamines and acetaminophen. These latter medications may even be given before chemotherapy treatment.

Common relative contraindications for all cancer drugs include weakened status indicators for the client, such as low white blood cell (WBC) count, any ongoing infectious process, or severe compromise in nutritional and hydration status. These are common situations for delaying chemotherapy treatment until the client's status improves. For these reasons it can be assumed that all of the cancer drugs described in this chapter have no absolute contraindications. Clients are usually examined (including laboratory blood tests) by physicians, professional nursing staff members, and other related healthcare professionals before each chemotherapy treatment. At that time a clinical judgement is made regarding the client's fitness for receiving specific antineoplastic agents.

Because of the often severe toxicity of cancer medications, a current major focus of cancer drug research is the development of targeted drug therapy. That is, drugs that chemically recognize and act against only cancer cells, while sparing healthy cells. One example of such targeted therapy is the newer class of cancer drugs known as *monoclonal antibodies*. These are discussed in Chapter 47.

Pharmacokinetic data for antineoplastic medications are especially difficult to obtain. It is difficult to determine precise values for onset of action, peak effect, and duration of action when treating malignant tumours that often have erratic growth kinetics of their own. Response to therapy is usually determined by bedside evaluation of the client, blood sampling to determine cell counts and the presence of various enzymatic tumour markers, and imaging scans (e.g., computed tomography [CT], magnetic resonance imaging [MRI]) to assess the extent of tumour response to cancer treatment. For these reasons pharmacokinetic data are not included with the drug profiles in this chapter.

Hair follicle cells are continually in a rapidly dividing state, which results in the growth and replacement of head and body hair. Cancer drugs that affect these cells often cause the side effect known as *alopecia*, or hair loss. Many clients, especially women, may decide to purchase a wig or other type of hairpiece before alopecia is experienced (or after the side effect has occurred) or purchase various hats or scarves to disguise this side effect. Some antineoplastic agents are more disruptive or harmful to the beneficial cells of the stomach, a property known as the **emetic potential** of the drug because it represents the likelihood that a given agent will produce nausea and vomiting. Other anticancer drugs cause nausea and vomiting by stimulating the cells of the vomiting centre located in the brain. Preventing these side effects usually requires that the agent be given in doses that destroy insufficient numbers of cancer cells to have a beneficial effect for the client. **Myelosuppression**, also known as *bone marrow suppression* (BMS) or *bone marrow depression* (BMD), is another unwanted side effect of certain antineoplastics and results from the fact that certain rapidly dividing cells in the bone marrow, such as cellular precursors of granulocytes, lymphocytes, and platelets, are also destroyed. The specific hematological disorder resulting from the myelosuppression depends on the particular cell line affected. For instance, if the cells in the bone marrow that make platelets are killed, the client's platelet count will decrease and he or she will be more susceptible to bleeding. The cancer client is often at great risk for infection because of the state of immunocompromise that results from diminished WBC counts secondary to chemotherapy. For this reason such clients are often given large quantities of antibiotics, often intravenously, to prevent or treat bacterial infections. The point in time at which the bone marrow cells reach their lowest levels is the **nadir**. The time frame within which a client reaches the nadir may become shorter and the recovery time for the bone marrow may become longer with successive courses of antineoplastic treatment. The nadir varies from roughly ten to 28 days, depending on the particular cancer drug, or combinations of drugs, that are used to treat a given client. Anticipation of this nadir based on known cancer drug data can be used to guide the timing of prophylactic (preventative) administration of antibiotics and

also blood stimulants known as *biological response modifiers* (see Chapter 47).

Common specific indications for the various antineoplastic drug classes are listed in the dosages table provided for selected drugs from each class. Drug toxicity information, including the emetic potential and other common toxic effects of various antineoplastic drug classes, is provided in tables at the end of the pharmacology section of this chapter. Also included at the end of the chapter is a table containing drug-specific guidelines for the treatment of *extravasation*—unintended leakage of a chemotherapy drug into the surrounding tissues outside of the intravenous line used for administration.

CANCER DRUG NOMENCLATURE

The nomenclature (naming system) of cancer drugs can be somewhat more complex, and possibly confusing, than for other drug classes. Cancer treatment is an intensively researched area in health care. This makes for many ongoing research protocols, and often larger numbers of new drugs are approved by Health Canada for cancer treatment in any given year than are approved for other disease categories. Because of this, multiple names are often encountered for the same drug. The following discussion and Table 46-6 discuss the multiple names for various **antineoplastic medications** that may be encountered in clinical practice.

Recall from earlier chapters that medications have a chemical name, generic name, and trade name. This section introduces yet another name often encountered for medications, especially cancer drugs, in clinical practice: the investigational or protocol name. A drug's chemical name is used by the chemists who first discover and work with the drug. This is usually the first name used to identify a particular chemical compound, often before it is classified as a "drug" with known therapeutic properties. The chemical name is based on the standard chemical nomenclature recommended by the International Union of Pure and Applied Chemists (IUPAC). For this reason, it is also often referred to as the "IUPAC name." The generic name is often first assigned to a chemical compound after a pharmaceutical manufacturer has determined that it is worthy of continued clinical research because of apparent therapeutic properties. It is at this point that the chemical compound becomes an investigational drug, per se. The first evidence of such therapeutic properties often appears in the laboratory setting. For example, a research scientist may discover that a given chemical compound destroys or inhibits the growth of cancer cells in a live cell culture.

Generic names are usually shorter and less complex than chemical names, and their spelling is often at least loosely based on the chemical structural features of the drug. The trade name is a marketing name used by the manufacturer of a given drug primarily for advertising the drug to prescribers and even clients themselves. The trade name is often strategically chosen to be shorter and easier to pronounce and remember than the chemical, protocol or investigational, or generic names.

During the time before marketing that a given medication is undergoing clinical research, it is often referred to by its protocol name or investigational name. These two terms are synonymous. The protocol name can be the same as the generic name, but instead it is often a code name that consists of a combination of letters and numbers separated by one or more dashes. One of the purposes of this name is to protect the "code" of a blinded study so that neither research staff nor study clients know who is (or isn't) receiving the actual drug under investigation. This helps to distinguish real drug effects from placebo effects. Although investigational drugs for all disease classes usually have some kind of protocol name, protocol names tend to be more commonly used in client care settings for cancer drugs than for other drug classes. For this reason some common protocol or investigational names have been included in Table 46-6. Because chemical names are usually not encountered in client care, they are generally not emphasized in this table, except for occasional illustrative purposes. The following are two typical examples that illustrate these concepts:

Investigational (Protocol) Name	Generic Name	Trade Name
STI-571	imatinib	Gleevec
ZD1839	gefitinib	Iressa
5-fluorouracil*	fluorouracil	Fluoroplex Cream

*The "5" refers to the position of a fluorine atom in the cyclic ring structure of the uracil molecule.

See Table 46-6 for additional information on the naming of cancer drugs.

TABLE 46-6

COMMON NAMES FOR SELECTED ANTINEOPLASTIC AGENTS

Generic Name	Trade Names	Other Names
CELL CYCLE–NON-SPECIFIC DRUGS		
Alkylating Agents		
Classic Alkylators		
busulfan	Myleran, Bisulfex	BSF, NSC-750
chlorambucil	Leukeran	NSC-3088, WR-139013
cyclophosphamide	Cytoxan, Procytox	cyclo, CPA, CPM, CTX, CYC, CYT
ifosfamide	Ifex	IFO, NSC-10924
mechlorethamine	Mustargen	nitrogen mustard, HN2
melphalan	Alkeran	L-sarcolysin, L-phenylalanine mustard, L-PAM
Nitrosoureas		
carmustine	BiCNU, Gliadel (wafer)	BCNU, 1,3-bis(2-chloroethyl)-l-nitrosourea
lomustine	CeeNU	CCNU, cyclohexylchloroethylnitrosurea
streptozocin	Zanosar	streptozotocin, STZ, NSC-85998
Probable Alkylators		
altretamine	Hexalen	hexamethylmelamine, HMM, HXM, NSC-13875
carboplatin	Paraplatin, Paraplatin AQ	CBDCA, JM-8, NSC-241240
cisplatin	Cisplatin	Cis-Platinum; cis-diamminedichloroplatinum, DDP; CDDP; CIS; Platinum
dacarbazine	Dacarbazine	Imidazole carboxamide, dimethyl-triazeno-imidazole-carboxamide, DIC
oxaliplatin	Eloxatin	ACT-078, I-OHP, LOHP, oxalatoplatin, oxaliplatinum
procarbazine	Matulane	PCB, PCZ, N-methylhydrazine
temozolomide	Temodal	NSC-362856 TMZ, SCHS2.365
thiotepa (available in Canada through the Special Access Programme)	Thiotepa Lederle	triethylenethiophosphoramide, TSPA, TESPA
Cytotoxic Antibiotics		
Anthracyclines		
daunorubicin, conventional	Cerubidine	daunomycin, rubidomycin, DNR
daunorubicin, liposomal	DaunoXome	Vinorelbine tartrate, VRL, VNL, NVB
doxorubicin, conventional	Adriamycin	Adria, hydroxydaunomycin, hydroxyl daunorubicin, DOX
doxorubicin, liposomal	Caelyx, Myocet	Doxorubicin Hydrochloride Pegylated Liposomes
epirubicin	Pharmorubicin RDF, Pharmorubicin PFS	4'-epi-doxorubicin, NSC-256942, IMI28, epi DX
idarubicin	Idamycin	Imi 30, NSC-256439
Other Cytotoxic Antibiotics		
bleomycin	Blenoxane, Bleomycin	Bleo
dactinomycin	Cosmegen	actinomycin-D
mitomycin	Mutamycin, Mitomycin	mitomycin-C, MTC

Continued

TABLE 46-6

COMMON NAMES FOR SELECTED ANTINEOPLASTIC AGENTS—cont'd

Generic Name	Trade Names	Other Names
CELL CYCLE–SPECIFIC DRUGS		
Antimetabolites		
Folic Acid Analogue		
methotrexate	Methotrexate	MTX, amethopterin
raltitrexed	Tomudex	raltitrexed disodium, ZD-1694
Purine Analogues		
cladribine	Leustatin	2-chloro-2'-deoxyadenosine, 2-CdA, CdA, NSC-10514-F
fludarabine	Fludara	2-F-ara-AMP, Fludarabine phosphate, FAMP, NSC-312887
mercaptopurine	Purinethol	6-mercaptopurine, 6-MP, NSC 755
thioguanine	Lanvis	6-thioguanine, 6-TG, 2-amino-6-mercaptopurine
Pyrimidine Analogues		
capecitabine	Xeloda	5'-deoxy-5-fluoro-N-cytidine
cytarabine, conventional	Cytosar	ara-C, Cytosine Arabinoside, Arabinosylcytosine
cytarabine, liposomal (available only through the Special Access Programme)	DepoCyt	
gemcitabine	Gemzar	2,2-difluorodeoxycytidine, dFdC, Gemcitabine hydrochloride, difluorodeoxycytidine, LY 188011
fluorouracil	Fluorouracil Injection, Efudex Cream Fluoroplex Topical	5-fluorouracil, 5-FU
Natural Products		
Enzymes		
asparaginase (from *Escherichia coli* bacterium)	Kidrolase	L-asparaginase, Colaspase, L-ASP, Crasnitin, Elspar; NSC-106977, Porton Asparaginase
Camptothecin Analogues (from a Chinese Shrub)		
irinotecan	Camptosar	Irinotecan hydrochloride trihydrate, CPT-11
topotecan	Hycamtin	Topotecan hydrochloride, NSC-609699, NSC-609699
Epipodophyllotoxins (Mandrake Plant or Mayapple)		
etoposide	VePesid	VP-16, VP-16-213, EPEG, demethylepipodophyllotoxin-ethylidene-glucopyranoside, EPE, epipodophyllotoxin
teniposide	Vumon	VM-26, PTG
Taxanes (Yew Trees)		
paclitaxel	Taxol	NSC-125973
docetaxel	Taxotere	RP56976, NSC 628503
Vinca Alkaloids (Periwinkle plant)		
vinblastine	Vinblastine Sulphate Injection	vinca leukoblastine sulphate, VLB, VBL
vincristine	Vincristine Sulphate Injection	VCR, leurocristine, LCR
vinorelbine	Navelbine	Vinorelbine tartrate, VRL, VNL, NVB
Hormonal and Related Agents		
Androgens		
fluoxymesterone	Halotestin	NSC-12165, Androfluorene
testosterone propionate		
Anti-Androgens		
bicalutamide	Casodex	ICI 176,334
flutamide	Euflex, Novo-Flutamide, PMS-Flutamide	
nilutamide	Anandron	RU23908
Progestins		
megestrol acetate	Megace, Apo-Megestrol, Nu-Megestrol	MA, meg, megestrol acetate
medroxyprogesterone acetate	Provera, Depo-Provera, Medroxyprogesterone, Medroxy	Methylacetoxyprogesterone, Metipregnone

Continued

TABLE 46-6

COMMON NAMES FOR SELECTED ANTINEOPLASTIC AGENTS—cont'd

Generic Name	Trade Names	Other Names
Hormonal and Related Agents—cont'd		
Estrogens		
diethylstilbestrol	Stilbestrol	DES, DES, Stilbestrol, Stilboestrol
Estrogen/Nitrogen Mustard Combination		
estramustine (estradiol + nornitrogen mustard)	Emcyt	Estramustine sodium phosphate
Anti-Estrogens		
fulvestrant	Faslodex	7-alpha-[9-(4,4,5,5,5-penta fluoropentylsulphinyl) nonyl]estra-1,3,5-(10)- triene-3,17-beta-diol
tamoxifen	Nolvadex, Gen-Tamoxifen, Novo-tamoxifen, Tamofen	Tam
Adrenocorticosteroids		
dexamethasone	PHL-Dexamethasone, PMS- Dexamethasone, Ratio- Dexamethasone	
hydrocortisone	Solu-Cortef	
methylprednisolone	Medrol, Methylprednisolone, Solu-Medrol	
prednisone	Apo-Prednisone, Winpred	
Gonadotropin-Releasing Hormone Analogues		
goserelin acetate	Zoladex	Goserelin acetate, ICI-118,630
leuprolide acetate	Lupron, Lupron Depot, Eligard	Leuprorelin acetate
Aromatase Inhibitors		
anastrozole	Arimidex	IUPAC ZD1033; ICI D1033
Hormonal and Related Agents		
Aromatase Inhibitors		
letrozole	Femara	Letzazole, CGS 20267
exemestane	Aromasin	PNU 155971
Miscellaneous Cell Cycle–Specific Agent		
hydroxyurea	Hydrea	hydroxycarbamide
Miscellaneous Antineoplastics (Cell Cycle Specificity Unclear)		
imatinib	Gleevec	STI-571, imatinib mesylate
mitotane	Lysodren	o,p'-DDD
porfimer sodium	Photofrin	
Cytoprotective Agents		
amifostine	Ethyol-PWS	ethiofos, WR2721, ethanethiol, gammaphos, NSC-296961
dexrazoxane	Zinecard	2,6-Piperazinedione
leucovorin	Lederle Leucovorin Calcium	LV, calcium leucovorin, calcium folinate, leucovorin calcium, citrovorum factor, folinic acid
mesna	Mesna for injection, Uromitexan	sodium 2-mercaptoethane sulphonate
Other Toxicity Inhibitors		
allopurinol	Riva-Purinol, Purinol	
rasburicase (available in Canada through the Special Access Programme)	Elitek	
Radioactive Antineoplastics		
chromic phosphate P-32	Phosphocol P 32	
samarium SM-153 lexidronam	Quadramet	samarium-153, 153SM-EDTMP
sodium iodide I-131	Iodotope	I-131
sodium phosphate P-32	Sodium Phosphate P 32	
strontium-89 chloride	Metastron	strontium-89

ANTINEOPLASTIC DRUG CLASSES

Current pharmacological classes of antineoplastic medications include the following: cytotoxic drugs including alkylating agents and antimetabolites; cytotoxic antibiotics; natural products; hormonal and related agents; and various miscellaneous agents.

ALKYLATING AGENTS

This class is a sublass of the group of cytotoxic agents. Mustard gas and the derivatives of the nitrogen mustards were the first alkylating agents, with nitrogen mustard (mechlorethamine) the prototypical agent. It was in the 1940s that its antineoplastic activity was discovered, and since that time many analogues of the agent have been synthesized for cancer treatment.

The alkylating agents commonly used in clinical practice in Canada today consist of three categories of agents: classic alkylators (nitrogen mustards); nitrosoureas, which have a different chemical structure than the nitrogen mustards but also work by alkylation; and probable alkylators, which also have a different chemical structure than the nitrogen mustards but are known to work at least partially by alkylation. Nitrogen mustards were developed from mustard gas agents used in military operations before and during World War I. All of these antineoplastics are generally considered CCNS agents, and they are used to treat a wide spectrum of malignancies. The agents in each category are as follows:

Classic alkylators (nitrogen mustards)
- chlorambucil
- cyclophosphamide
- ifosfamide
- mechlorethamine
- melphalan

Nitrosoureas
- carmustine
- lomustine
- streptozocin

Probable alkylators
- altretamine
- busulfan
- carboplatin
- cisplatin
- dacarbazine
- oxaliplatin
- procarbazine
- temozolomide
- thiotepa

Mechanism of Action and Drug Effects

Alkylating agents are CCNS antineoplastics that are effective at any stage in the growth cycle of cancer cells and are most effective against rapidly growing cancer cells and normal body cells. These agents work by preventing the cancer cells from reproducing. Specifically, they interfere with the chemical structure of the DNA essential to the reproduction of any cell, and cause alkyl groups rather than hydrogen atoms to be attached to the nucleic acid. Recall from chemistry that alkyl groups are composed of both hydrogen and carbon atoms that are linked by covalent bonds. Examples include a methyl group ($—CH3$) and an ethyl group ($—CH2\ CH3$). This process is called **alkylation**. Two critically important molecules in cellular reproduction are the nucleic acids DNA and RNA. Recall that DNA molecules consist of two side-by-side strands, each consisting of alternating sequences of phosphate and sugar molecules. These components make up the "backbone" of the DNA strands. These two strands are cross-linked to each other by the third DNA structural element: nitrogen-containing bases (adenine [A], guanine [G], thymine [T], or cytosine[C]). These bases are bound to the sugar molecules of the DNA backbone, and two bases, linked to each other by covalent hydrogen bonds, forming the molecular bridges that link

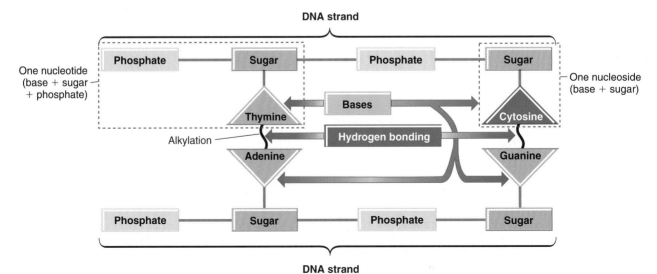

FIG. 46-2 Organization of DNA and site of action of alkylating agents.

the two DNA strands to make up its double helix structure. A nucleotide is the structural unit of DNA (and RNA) molecules and consists of one molecule each of base, sugar, and phosphate that are bound together. A nucleoside consists of a bound base molecule and sugar molecule only.

During the normal process of reproduction, the double helix can uncoil and RNA transcription can occur on each individual DNA strand. RNA strands, in turn, are involved in both protein synthesis and replication of the original DNA structure. These processes ultimately result in the creation of a new cell with the same DNA sequence, and thus the same characteristics as its parent cell.

Alkyl groups formed by the antineoplastic alkylating agents attach to DNA molecules by forming covalent bonds to the bases described earlier. The result is that abnormal chemical bonds form between the adjacent DNA strands, resulting in the formation of defective nucleic acids that are then unable to perform the normal cellular reproductive functions mentioned previously.

Alkylating agents can also be characterized by the number of alkyl groups they possess and thus the number of alkylation reactions they can perform per single molecule of drug. **Bifunctional** alkylating agents have two reactive alkyl groups that are able to alkylate two DNA molecules. There are also **polyfunctional** alkylating agents that can perform several alkylation reactions. The sites on DNA most vulnerable to this reaction are position N7 on guanine; positions 1, 3, and 7 on adenine; and position N3 on cytosine. The alkylating agents that bind to guanine appear to be the most lethal agents. Figure 46-2 shows the location along the DNA double helix where the alkylating agents work.

Indications

The most commonly used alkylating agents today are effective against a wide spectrum of malignancies, including both solid tumours and hematological cancers. Alkylating agents are often included in combination regimens because of their CCNS killing ability. The various types of cancer and the alkylating agents commonly used in their treatment are listed in the dosages table on p. 784.

Contraindications

The only usual contraindication to the use of alkylating agents is severe drug allergy.

Side Effects and Adverse Effects

Alkylating agents are capable of causing all of the dose-limiting side effects described previously (Table 46-7). The relative emetic potentials of each agent are listed in Box 46-1 on p. 786. The side effects for these agents are important because of their severity, but they can be prevented through the use of prophylactic measures. For instance, nephrotoxicity can be prevented by adequately hydrating the client with intravenously administered fluids in cases of drug extravasation. Table 46-8 gives some specific antidotes.

Interactions

Only a few alkylating agents are capable of causing significant drug interactions. The most important rule of thumb for preventing such drug interactions is to avoid administering them with any other agent capable of causing similar toxicities. For example, a major adverse effect of cisplatin is nephrotoxicity. Therefore, if possible, it should not be administered with an agent such as an aminoglycoside antibiotic (gentamicin, tobramycin, or amikacin) because of the resulting additive nephrotoxic effect, and hence the increased likelihood of renal failure. Mechlorethamine and cyclophosphamide, both of which have significant BMD effects, ideally should not be administered with radiation therapy or with other drugs that suppress the bone marrow. These two agents, as well as cisplatin, should also not be given with probenecid or sulfinpyrazone. This combination can result in hyperuricemia or gout because of competition for renal elimination between these drugs and the molecules of normal body uric acid.

TABLE 46-7
ALKYLATING AGENTS: SEVERE ADVERSE EFFECTS

Alkylating Agent	Severe Side/Adverse Effects
busulfan	Pulmonary fibrosis
carboplatin	Less nephrotoxicity and neurotoxicity but more bone marrow suppression (BMS)
cisplatin	Nephrotoxicity, peripheral neuropathy, ototoxicity
cyclophosphamide	Hemorrhagic cystitis

TABLE 46-8
ALKYLATING AGENT EXTRAVASATION: SPECIFIC ANTIDOTES

Alkylating Agent	Antidote Preparation	Method
carmustine	No specific antidote	1. Remove venipuncture needle. 2. Elevate limb and apply gentle pressure to site. 3. Apply cold compresses or ice packs wrapped in towel. Care must be taken to avoid tissue injury from excessive cold.
mechlorethamine	Mix 1.6 mL sodium thiosulphate 25% solution with 8.4 mL sterile water for injection to give 10 mL of $\frac{1}{6}$ molar solution	1. Immediately, inject 2.5 mL IV through the existing line into the same tissue as the extravasation occurred. 2. Elevate limb and apply gentle pressure to the site. 3. Apply cold compresses or ice packs wrapped in towels.

Dosages

For the recommended dosages of selected alkylating agents, see the dosages table below. See Table 46-6 for some of the common brands available in Canada.

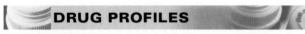

DRUG PROFILES

altretamine

Altretamine is a newer antineoplastic drug that is classified as a miscellaneous alkylating agent, although its precise mechanism of action is unclear. It is indicated for the palliative treatment of recurrent ovarian cancer, following treatment with either platinum-based or alkylating agents. It works by inhibiting DNA and RNA synthesis and has shown efficacy even in clients resistant to other alkylating agents. Contraindications include drug allergy and pre-existing severe BMD or neurological toxicity because altretamine itself can cause significant neurotoxicity. Altretamine is available only for oral use in a 50-mg gelatin capsule. Pregnancy category D. Dosage information appears in the dosages table below.

▶▶ carmustine

Carmustine is one of the three currently available nitrosoureas (carmustine, lomustine, and streptozocin). Because they act by alkylation, nitrosoureas are classified as alkylating agents. Carmustine is able to cross the blood-brain barrier and is thus useful in the treatment of primary brain tumours. It may also be used to treat Hodgkin's disease, non-Hodgkin's lymphomas, and multiple myeloma.

A newer approach to the treatment of recurrent glioblastoma multiforme (GBM, a highly malignant brain tumour) is a biodegradable wafer called a Gliadel wafer that is implanted during surgery. It contains carmustine and polifeprosan and delivers chemotherapy directly to the tumour site, minimizing drug exposure to other areas of the body. The Gliadel wafer is indicated for clients who have an operable brain tumour. It complements other standard therapies for brain cancer, such as surgery, radiation, and traditional intravenous chemotherapy.

Carmustine is contraindicated in clients with a hypersensitivity to it. It is available in a parenteral preparation as a 100-mg vial for intravenous infusion and as the 7.7-mg Gliadel wafer for neurosurgical implantation. Pregnancy category D. Commonly recommended dosages are listed in the dosages table below.

▶▶ cisplatin

Cisplatin is an antineoplastic agent that contains platinum in its chemical structure. Specifically, this structure consists of a platinum atom surrounded by two chloride atoms and two ammonia molecules. It is classified as a probable alkylating agent because it is believed to destroy cancer cells in the same way as the classic alkylating agents—by forming cross-links with DNA and thereby preventing its replication. It is considered a bifunctional alkylating agent.

Cisplatin is contraindicated in clients with drug allergy, renal insufficiency, hearing impairment, or myelosuppression. It is used for the treatment of many solid tumours, such as bladder, testicular, and ovarian tumours. It is available only in a parenteral formulation

DOSAGES Selected Alkylating Agents

Agent	Pharmacological Class	Usual Dosage Range	Indications
altretamine	Alkylating agent	PO: 6–8 mg/kg/day, divided into 4 doses, for 14–21 consecutive days for 28-day cycles	Recurrent ovarian cancer
▶▶ carmustine	Alkylating agent	IV: 200 mg/m² q6wk Implantable wafer: 8 wafers surgically implanted into resection cavity of brain tumour de-bulking area	Primary brain tumours, multiple myeloma, Hodgkin's and non-Hodgkin's lymphomas, melanoma, GI carcinoma
▶▶ cisplatin	Alkylating agent	IV: 50–270 mg/m² q3–4wk	Metastatic testicular, ovarian, bladder cancer, many other cancers
▶▶ cyclophosphamide	Alkylating agent	IV: 3–5 mg/kg 2×/wk (many other regimens as well) PO: 1–5 mg/kg/day	Lymphoma, leukemia, multiple myeloma, mycosis fungoides; breast, ovarian cancer, retinoblastoma, and many other cancers
▶▶ mechlorethamine	Alkylating agent	IV: 0.4 mg/kg, single or divided dose 0.1–0.2 mg/kg/day, no more than q3wk	Lymphoma, leukemia, mycosis fungoides, bronchogenic carcinoma, others
temozolomide	Alkylating agent	PO: 150–200 mg/m² once daily for 5 consecutive days per 28-day treatment cycle	Recurrent anaplastic astrocytoma or glioblastoma multiforme
thiotepa	Alkylating agent	IV: 0.3–0.4 mg/kg at 1–4 wk intervals Intracavity: 0.6–0.8 mg/kg/wk Intravesical ≤2 h dwell time (via bladder catheter): 30–60 mg/wk × 6, then monthly × 12 mo	Breast, ovarian, or bladder cancer, lymphoma, bone marrow transplant

as a 1-mg/mL injection for intravenous infusion. Commonly recommended dosages are listed in the dosages table on p. 784.

▸▸ cyclophosphamide

Cyclophosphamide is a nitrogen mustard derivative that was discovered during the process of research to improve mechlorethamine. It is a polyfunctional alkylating agent and is used in the treatment of cancers of the bone and lymph, as well as solid tumours. Various leukemias, Hodgkin's and non-Hodgkin's lymphomas, multiple myeloma, and some sarcomas may also respond to cyclophosphamide therapy. It is contraindicated in lactating women. It is available in both oral and parenteral formulations as 25- and 50-mg oral tablets and 200-, 500-, 1000-, and 2000-mg vials for parenteral injection. Pregnancy category D. Commonly recommended dosages are listed in the dosages table on p. 784.

▸▸ mechlorethamine

Mechlorethamine is a nitrogen analogue of sulphur mustard. It was the first alkylating antineoplastic drug discovered. Its beneficial effects in the treatment of various cancers were discovered after World War I when the agent, then known as mustard gas, was used for chemical warfare. Some of the cancers for which it is used are Hodgkin's lymphoma, other lymphomas, and chronic leukemia. It is the original prototypical alkylating agent.

Mechlorethamine is a bifunctional alkylating agent capable of forming cross-linkage between two DNA nucleotides, thereby interfering with RNA transcription and preventing cell division and protein synthesis. Mechlorethamine is available in a parenteral form only to be administered intravenously or by an intracavitary route, such as intrapleurally or intraperitoneally. It is contraindicated in cases of drug allergy and existing infectious disease. It is available as a 10-mg parenteral injection. Pregnancy category D. Commonly recommended dosages are listed in the dosages table on p. 784.

temozolomide

Temozolomide is used in the treatment of the first relapse of **anaplastic** astrocytoma, after having failed treatment with a nitrosourea and procarbazine. This tumour can occur anywhere in the central nervous system (CNS), and it is the most common type of primary (vs. metastasized) brain tumour. It is also used in the treatment of glioblastoma multiforme. Temozolomide is a pro-drug that is rapidly converted in the body to its active form. Its primary mechanism of action is alkylation by attaching methyl groups to guanine-rich sections of DNA that normally initiate the DNA replication process. Its only routine contraindication is drug allergy. It is available only in oral form as 5-, 20-, 100-, and 250-mg capsules. Pregnancy category D. Dosage information appears in the dosages table on p. 784.

thiotepa

Thiotepa, although originally used to treat various lymphomas, is now used primarily to treat certain cancers of the bladder, breast, and ovary. It is an alkylating agent structurally related to mechlorethamine and is believed to work by releasing certain free radical molecules that disrupt DNA structure. Contraindications include drug allergy and existing kidney, liver, or bone marrow damage. Thiotepa use is applied for through Health Canada and the Special Access Programme. Thiotepa is available only in a powder form as a 15-mg vial for intravenous, intracavitary, or intravesicular (bladder) administration. Pregnancy category D. Dosage information appears in the dosages table on p. 784.

ANTIMETABOLITES

Antineoplastic antimetabolites are a subclass of cytotoxic agents. These drugs are CCS agents that are structurally similar to normal cellular metabolites and work by mimicking the actions of important natural precursors that are required for the synthesis of DNA and RNA. They are effective against solid tumours such as colon, rectum, breast, stomach, lung, ovarian, liver, bladder, and pancreas cancer. They are also commonly used in circulating tumours such as leukemia.

Mechanism of Action and Drug Effects

Antimetabolites interfere with the biosynthesis of precursors essential to cellular growth by mimicking folic acid, pyrimidines, and purines, thereby interfering with the normal synthesis of nucleic acids in one of two ways: (1) by falsely substituting for purines, pyrimidines, or folic acid or (2) by inhibiting critical enzymes involved in nucleic acid or folic acid synthesis. Thus they affect DNA, RNA, and protein synthesis and, ultimately, cellular replication. Antimetabolites work in the S phase of the cell cycle, during which DNA synthesis occurs. The available antimetabolites and the metabolites they mimic are as follows:

Folic acid antagonist
- methotrexate (MTX)
- raltitrexed

Purine antagonists
- cladribine
- fludarabine (F-AMP)
- mercaptopurine (6-MP)
- thioguanine (6-TG)

Pyrimidine antagonists
- capecitabine
- cytarabine (ARA-C)
- fluorouracil (5-FU)
- gemcitabine

Folic Acid Antagonism

The antimetabolite methotrexate is an analogue of folic acid and inhibits dihydrofolate reductase, an enzyme responsible for converting folic acid to a reduced form that is normally used in the biosynthesis of other molecules. This inhibition prevents the formation of the folate, the reduced or anionic form of folic acid, that is needed for the synthesis of DNA and hence for cell reproduction. The result is that DNA is not produced and the cell dies. In practice the terms *folic acid* and *folate* are often used interchangeably.

Purine Antagonism

The purine bases present in DNA and RNA are adenine and guanine, and they are required for the synthesis of the purine nucleotides that are incorporated into the nucleic acid molecules. Mercaptopurine and fludarabine are synthetic analogues of adenine, and thioguanine is a synthetic analogue of guanine. These agents work by incorporating themselves into the metabolic pathway in lieu of these two nucleic acid bases. Once there, they interrupt the synthesis of both DNA and RNA.

Pyrimidine Antagonism

Of the pyrimidine bases, cytosine and thymine occur in the structure of DNA molecules, and cytosine and uracil are part of the structure of RNA molecules. These bases are essential for DNA and RNA synthesis. Fluorouracil is a synthetic analogue of uracil, and cytarabine is a synthetic analogue of cytosine. These agents act in a way that is similar to that of the purine antagonists, incorporating themselves into the metabolic pathway for the synthesis of DNA and RNA and thereby interrupting synthesis of both of these nucleic acids.

Indications

Antimetabolite antineoplastic agents are used for the treatment of a variety of solid tumours and some hematological cancers. They may also be used in combination chemotherapy regimens to enhance the overall cytotoxic effect. Because some of these agents are available in both oral and topical preparations, they are sometimes used for low-dose maintenance and palliative cancer therapy. The commonly used agents and their therapeutic uses are listed in the dosages table on p. 787.

Contraindications

The only usual contraindication is severe drug allergy.

Side Effects and Adverse Effects

Like all antineoplastic agents, antimetabolites cause hair loss, nausea and vomiting, and myelosuppression. The emetic potentials for some of these agents are listed in Box 46-1. Major side effects and adverse effects specific to the antimetabolite agents are listed in Table 46-9.

BOX 46-1

Relative Emetic Potential of Selected Antineoplastic Drugs

Low (<10–30%)	Moderate (30–60%)	High (60–>90%)
asparaginase	altretamine	carboplatin
bleomycin	capecitabine	carmustine
busulfan	cyclophosphamide (<750 mg/m²)	cisplatin
chlorambucil	daunorubicin (<50 mg/m²)	cyclophosphamide
cladribine	doxorubicin (20–60 mg/m²)	(750–>1500 mg/m²)
cytarabine (<1000 mg/m²)	epirubicin (<90 mg/m²)	cytarabine (>1000 mg/m²)
daunorubicin, liposomal	idarubicin	dacarbazine
docetaxel	ifosfamide (<1500 mg/m²)	dactinomycin
doxorubicin (<20 mg/m²)	imatinib	daunorubicin (>50 mg/m²)
doxorubicin, liposomal	methotrexate (250–1000 mg/m²)	doxorubicin (>60 mg/m²)
estramustine	oxaliplatin	ifosfamide (>1500 mg/m²)
etoposide	temozolomide	irinotecan
fludarabine		lomustine
fluorouracil (<1000 mg/m²)		mechlorethamine
gemcitabine		methotrexate (>1000 mg/m²)
hydroxyurea		procarbazine
melphalan		streptozocin
mercaptopurine		
methotrexate (<250 mg/m²)		
mitomycin		
paclitaxel		
teniposide		
thioguanine		
thiotepa		
topotecan		
tretinoin		
vinblastine		
vincristine		
vinorelbine		

Interactions

As is true with cancer drugs in general, the co-administration of one drug with another that causes similar toxicities may result in additive toxicities. Therefore the respective risks and benefits should be carefully weighed before therapy is initiated with either an antimetabolite or any other agent possessing a similar toxicity profile. The following are just a few examples. Because the concurrent administration of non-steroidal anti-inflammatory drugs (NSAIDs) with methotrexate may result in severe methotrexate toxicity, this combination should be avoided. In addition, cytarabine may decrease the effects of oral digoxin. Another example is that the co-administration of mercaptopurine and allopurinol may lead to additive bone marrow toxicity resulting from elevated body levels of mercaptopurine because both agents are metabolized by the same enzyme, xanthine oxidase.

Dosages

For information on the dosages of selected antimetabolite chemotherapeutic agents, see the dosages table below. See Table 46-6 for some of the common brands available in Canada.

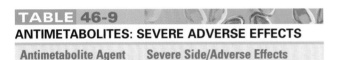

TABLE 46-9
ANTIMETABOLITES: SEVERE ADVERSE EFFECTS

Antimetabolite Agent	Severe Side/Adverse Effects
cytarabine	Liver, kidney, lung, stomach, and heart toxicities
fludarabine	Kidney and stomach toxicities
fluorouracil	
mercaptopurine	Liver and kidney toxicities
methotrexate	Liver, kidney, and stomach toxicities
thioguanine	Liver and kidney toxicities

DRUG PROFILES

FOLATE ANTAGONISTS

▶▶ methotrexate

Methotrexate is the prototypical antimetabolite antineoplastic of the folate antagonist group and is currently the only antineoplastic folate antagonist used clinically. It has proved useful for the treatment of solid tumours such as breast, head and neck, and lung cancers and for the management of acute lymphocytic

DOSAGES   Selected Antimetabolites

Agent	Pharmacological Class	Usual Dosage Range	Indications
Folate Antagonists (Analogues)			
▶▶ methotrexate	Antimetabolite	IV: Remission: 3.3 mg/m²/day; maintenance 30 mg/m²/week IM/PO: 15–30 mg/day 5 days, repeated q7d, 3–5 courses	Acute lymphocytic* leukemia Gestational choriocarcinoma (a cancer in the uterus that begins after pregnancy, birth, or abortion)
raltitrexed	Antimetabolite	IV: 3 mg/m²/every 3 weeks	Advanced colorectal cancer
Purine Antagonists (Analogues)			
cladribine	Antimetabolite	IV: 0.09 mg/kg/day by continuous infusion for 7 consecutive days	Hairy cell leukemia
fludarabine	Antimetabolite	IV: 25 mg/m²/day for 5 consecutive days; repeatable q28d	Chronic lymphocytic leukemia
▶▶ mercaptopurine	Antimetabolite	PO: 2.5 mg/kg/day once daily for several wk or more	Acute lymphocytic and acute myelocytic† leukemia
Pyrimidine Antagonists (Analogues)			
capecitabine	Antimetabolite	PO: 1250 mg/m² bid for 2 wk, followed by 1-wk rest period; this 3-wk cycle is repeatable as ordered	Colorectal and breast cancer
▶▶ cytarabine	Antimetabolite	IV: 100 mg/m²/day by continuous infusion × 7 days (other regimens as well)	Leukemias (several varieties)
fluorouracil	Antimetabolite	IV: 200–500 mg²/kg once daily for 7 days initial dose; dose varies afterward depending on client response	Colon, rectal, breast, stomach, and pancreatic cancer
gemcitabine	Antimetabolite	IV: 800–1250 mg/m² once weekly or as protocol dictates; cycle may be repeated or modified according to client tolerance	Pancreatic and non–small-cell lung cancer

* The term *lymphocytic* is synonymous in the literature with the term *lymphoblastic*.
† The term *myelocytic* is synonymous in the literature with the terms *myeloblastic* and *myelogenous*.

leukemia and non-Hodgkin's lymphomas. Methotrexate also has immunosuppressive activity because it can inhibit lymphocyte multiplication. For this reason it may be useful for the treatment of rheumatoid arthritis. Its combined immunosuppressant and anti-inflammatory properties also make it useful for the treatment of psoriasis.

Because of the severe bone marrow suppression, methotrexate should not be used in clients with pancytopenia (all cells from bone marrow are decreased). The bone marrow suppression may require dosing of **leucovorin rescue** to help "rescue" the client from these abnormalities.

Methotrexate is contraindicated in clients who have shown a hypersensitivity to it; in those with leukopenia, thrombocytopenia, or anemia; and in psoriatic clients with severe renal or hepatic disease. It is available in both oral and parenteral formulations. For oral administration it is available as a 2.5-mg tablet. It is available in a strength of 25 mg/mL for parenteral injection and in a preservative-free parenteral injection of 25 mg/mL. The preservative-free formulation is required for **intrathecal** (spinal) administration. Pregnancy category D. Commonly recommended dosages are given in the dosages table on p. 787.

raltitrexed

Raltitrexed is a quinazoline folate analogue that selectively inhibits a key enzyme (thymidylate synthase) required for the synthesis of deoxyribonucleic acid (DNA) resulting in DNA fragmentation and cell death. It is actively transported into the cells via a reduced folate carrier and then extensively metabolized to polyglutamate forms without metabolic degradation. This particular property of raltitrexed facilitates a convenient dosing schedule of an infusion every three weeks. Raltitrexed is cell-cycle phase-specific for the S phase and is also a radiation-sensitizing agent.

Raltitrexed is currently indicated for the treatment of advanced colorectal cancer. Raltitrexed is contraindicated in clients with known sensitivity and in clients with severe renal and/or hepatic impairment. It is not recommended for use in children. Caution should also be taken with clients who are immunosuppressed, in poor general health, or who had previous radiotherapy. It is available as a single dose preservative-free powder reconstituted with sterile water for 0.5 mg/mL parenteral solution. Pregnancy category D. Current recommended dosages are given in the dosages table on p. 787.

PURINE ANTAGONISTS

The currently available purine antagonists are cladribine, fludarabine, mercaptopurine, and thioguanine. Mercaptopurine and thioguanine are administered orally. The others are available in injectable form.

cladribine

Cladribine is a newer agent first marketed in the early 1990s. It is indicated for the treatment of a specific type of leukemia known as *hairy cell leukemia*, so named because of the appearance of its cancerous cells under the microscope. Its only current contraindication is drug allergy. It is available only as a 1-mg/mL solution for injection. Pregnancy category D. Dosage information is provided in the dosages table on p. 787.

fludarabine

Fludarabine was also approved by Health Canada in the early 1990s. Like cladribine, it also has a specific single indication, in this case, second-line therapy for chronic lymphocytic leukemia (CLL). Its only current contraindication is drug allergy. It is available as a 10-mg film-coated tablet and a 50-mg vial of powder for injection. Pregnancy category D. Dosage information appears in the table on p. 787.

▸▸ mercaptopurine

Mercaptopurine is used primarily for the treatment of leukemias (acute lymphoblastic and myelogenous and chronic myelocytic). It is contraindicated in clients who have shown resistance to it and in those with leukopenia, thrombocytopenia, or anemia. It is available only in oral form as a 50-mg tablet. Pregnancy category D. Commonly recommended dosages are given in the table on p. 787.

PYRIMIDINE ANTAGONISTS

The currently available antimetabolite antineoplastics that are members of the pyrimidine antagonist family are capecitabine, cytarabine, fluorouracil, and gemcitabine. They are available only in parenteral formulations, except for capecitabine, which is currently available only in tablet form.

capecitabine

Capecitabine was approved by Health Canada in 2000. Its primary indication is for metastatic breast cancer. Its only current contraindication is drug allergy. It is available in oral form as 150- and 500-mg tablets. Pregnancy category D. Dosage information appears in the dosages table on p. 787.

▸▸ cytarabine

Cytarabine is used primarily in the treatment of leukemias (acute myelocytic and lymphocytic and meningeal leukemia) and non-Hodgkin's lymphomas. As previously noted, it is available only as a parenteral agent as 100-, 500-, 1000-, and 2000-mg vials to be given by intravenous, intrathecal, or subcutaneous injection. It is also now available in a special encapsulated liposomal form of the drug for intrathecal use (10 mg/mL), used only for treating meningeal leukemia. Pregnancy category D. Commonly recommended dosages are given in the dosages table on p. 787.

fluorouracil

Fluorouracil is used in the palliative treatment of cancers of the colon, rectum, stomach, breast, and pancreas. Its only usual contraindication is drug allergy. It is available as a 50-mg/mL injection, as well as topical creams and solutions for treating skin cancer (see Chapter 55). Pregnancy category D. Dosage information appears in the dosages table on p. 787.

gemcitabine

Gemcitabine is an antineoplastic agent structurally related to cytarabine but believed to have superior antitumour activity. Gemcitabine was approved for marketing in 2001 by Health Canada. Approved indications include first-line therapy for locally advanced or metastatic cancer of the pancreas, for treatment of non–small-cell lung cancer, and for advanced bladder cancer. Its only contraindication is drug allergy. It is available only as a 20-mg/mL and 1000-mg/50-mL powder for injection. Pregnancy category D. Dosage information appears in the table on p. 787.

CYTOTOXIC ANTIBIOTICS

Cytotoxic antibiotics consist of natural substances produced by the mould *Streptomyces* as well as synthetic substances. Although they all have the ability to kill bacteria, and in some cases even viruses, they are used only for the treatment of cancer because they are too toxic for the treatment of infections. Cytotoxic antibiotics differ in toxicity, but they can all produce BMS, with the exception of bleomycin, which can cause pulmonary toxicity (pulmonary fibrosis and pneumonitis). Other severe toxicities associated with the use of cytotoxic antibiotics are heart failure (daunorubicin) and rare acute left ventricular failure (doxorubicin). The available cytotoxic antibiotics are as follows:

Anthracyclines
- daunorubicin
- doxorubicin
- epirubicin
- idarubicin
- valrubicin

Other cytotoxic antibiotics
- bleomycin
- dactinomycin
- mitomycin

Mechanism of Action and Drug Effects

Cytotoxic antibiotic antineoplastic agents are CCNS agents, although some, such as daunorubicin, are more active in the S phase. In most cases, however, the agents are active during all phases of the cell cycle. Most act either by the process of alkylation, which was previously explained for the alkylating agents, or by a process called *intercalation*, which involves inserting a drug molecule between the two strands of a DNA molecule. The agent binds to the nucleotide base pairs of the DNA helix, causing the shape of the DNA helix to change into an unstable structure. The result is the blockade of DNA, RNA, and protein synthesis. Some cytotoxic antibiotic agents can block all three, but others affect DNA synthesis only. Agents such as anthracyclines work by intercalation.

Indications

Cytotoxic antibiotics are used to treat a variety of solid tumours and some hematological malignancies. They may also be used in combination chemotherapy regimens to

TABLE 46-10 CYTOTOXIC ANTIBIOTICS: SEVERE ADVERSE EFFECTS	
Cytotoxic Antibiotic Agent	**Severe Side/ Adverse Effects**
bleomycin	Pulmonary fibrosis, pneumonitis
dactinomycin daunorubicin	Liver toxicities, extravasation
doxorubicin idarubicin	Liver and cardiovascular toxicities
mitomycin	Kidney and lung toxicities

BOX 46-2
Antidote for Doxorubicin Extravasation

1 Apply dimethylsulphoxide (DMSO) 99 percent topical solution, a free-radical scavenger, to an area double the area affected by extravasation.
2 Allow DMSO to air dry; do not cover. Repeat qid for at least seven days.
3 Elevate and rest extremity.
4 Apply cold compresses or ice pack wrapped in towel to the extravasation site for one hour. Take care to avoid tissue injury from excessive cold.

enhance the overall cytotoxic effect. Cytotoxic antibiotic antineoplastics are used to treat a wide variety of cancers, and these and the agents used to treat them are given in the dosages table on p. 790.

Contraindications

The only usual contraindication is severe drug allergy.

Side Effects and Adverse Effects

As with all of the antineoplastic agents, cytotoxic agents have the undesirable effects of hair loss, nausea and vomiting, and myelosuppression. The emetic potential of the various agents in this category is given in Box 46-1. Major side effects and adverse effects specific to these agents are listed in Table 46-10.

Toxicity and Management of Overdose

Severe cases of cardiomyopathy are associated with large cumulative doses of doxorubicin. The chances of this devastating toxicity can be decreased by routine monitoring of cardiac ejection fraction with multiple gated acquisition (MUGA) scans, cumulative dose limitations, and the use of cytoprotectant agents such as dexrazoxane. Such agents are discussed later in this chapter. Box 46-2 outlines the management of the extravasation of doxorubicin.

Interactions

The cytotoxic antibiotics that are used as chemotherapeutic agents interact with many drugs. They all tend to produce increased toxicities when used in combination with other chemotherapeutic agents or with radiation therapy. Some agents, most notably bleomycin and doxorubicin,

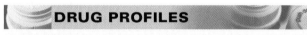

DOSAGES: Selected Cytotoxic Antibiotics

Agent	Pharmacological Class	Usual Dosage Range	Indications
Anthracycline Antibiotics			
▸▸doxorubicin, conventional	Cytotoxic antibiotic	IV: 60–75 mg/m² as a single injection given q21d	Multiple cancers, including breast, bone, leukemia, ovarian, neuroblastoma, lymphomas
doxorubicin, liposomal	Cytotoxic antibiotic	IV: 20 mg/m² q2–3wk for as long as tolerated and responsive to treatment IV: 50 mg/m² q4wk	AIDS-related Kaposi's sarcoma where client has either failed or is intolerant to other chemotherapy treatments Breast and ovarian cancer
Other Antibiotics			
bleomycin	Cytotoxic antibiotic	IV/IM/SC/intrapleural/intrarterial: 0.25–0.5 units/kg 1–2×/wk	Squamous cell carcinoma, testicular cancer, lymphomas, malignant pleural effusion, others

have been known to cause serum digoxin levels to increase. Clients receiving one of these drugs, along with digoxin, should be observed for signs of digoxin toxicity (see Chapter 21).

Dosages

For recommended dosages of selected cytotoxic antibiotics, see the dosages table above. See Table 46-6 for some of the common brands available in Canada.

DRUG PROFILES

ANTHRACYCLINE CYTOTOXIC ANTIBIOTICS

Three of the older cytotoxic antibiotics are the anthracyclines doxorubicin, daunorubicin, and idarubicin. Newer ones include valrubicin and epirubicin. They all have similar pharmacological actions in that they all work through the process of intercalation. In addition, they are effective in all phases of the cell growth cycle. These agents are used for the treatment of a wide range of cancers but are available in parenteral formulations only.

▸▸ doxorubicin

Doxorubicin is a potent and effective chemotherapeutic agent, and for this reason it is used in many combination chemotherapy regimens. It is contraindicated in clients with a known hypersensitivity to it, clients with severe myelosuppression, and clients who are at risk for severe cardiac toxicity due to having already received cumulative doses of any of the anthracycline antineoplastics. It is available in 10-, 50-, and 150-mg vials (powder) and a 2-mg/mL strength for injection.

Doxorubicin is also now available in a liposomal drug delivery system, in which the drug is encapsulated in a lipid bi-layer called a *liposome*. Liposomal encapsulation offers decreased systemic toxicity and increased duration of action. It extends the biological half-life of doxorubicin to 50 to 60 hours and increases its affinity for cancer cells. This form of doxorubicin is currently indicated for breast and ovarian cancer and for Kaposi's sarcoma, which primarily affects individuals with HIV. It is available only as a 20- and 50-mg vial

for injection. Both forms of doxorubicin are classified as pregnancy category D. Commonly used dosages are given in the dosages table above.

OTHER CYTOTOXIC ANTIBIOTICS

The other cytotoxic antibiotics have characteristics similar to those of anthracyclines. They are effective against a wide range of cancers. All are available only in parenteral formulations. These agents currently include bleomycin, dactinomycin, and mitomycin.

bleomycin

Bleomycin is active against fungi and both gram-positive and gram-negative bacteria, but because of its cytotoxicity its use as an antibiotic is prohibited. It is a CCS agent, acting primarily in the G2 and M phases. It works by inhibiting DNA synthesis and, to a lesser extent, RNA and protein synthesis.

Its only usual contraindication is drug allergy. Bleomycin doses are measured in units as opposed to milligrams. It is available as 15-unit vials, which are administered subcutaneously, intravenously, intramuscularly, or intrapleurally. Pregnancy category D. Commonly used dosages are given in the dosages table above.

MITOTIC INHIBITORS

Mitotic inhibitors consist of natural products obtained from the periwinkle plant (*Catharenthus roseus*, formerly called *Vinca rosea*) and of semi-synthetic agents obtained from the mandrake plant (also known as the *mayapple*). The periwinkle plant yields the antineoplastic alkaloids vinblastine (VLB), vincristine (VCR), and vinorelbine, also known as *vinca alkaloids*. Etoposide (VP-16) and teniposide (ETP) are semi-synthetic derivatives of epipodophyllotoxin, which is obtained from the resinous extract of the mandrake plant. Two newer plant-derived drugs include paclitaxel, from the bark of the slow-growing Western (Pacific) yew tree, and docetaxel, a semi-synthetic taxoid produced from the needles of the European yew tree. Docetaxel is pharma-

Angiogenesis Inhibitors: No Flow–No Grow

Angiogenesis (the growth of new blood vessels) occurs during fetal development, growth, wound repair, and the uterine cycle. It has four basic steps, including (1) activation of endothelial cells in existing blood vessels; (2) production of a matrix, which breaks down the extracellular matrix of surrounding tissue; (3) proliferation of endothelial cells; and (4) assembly of endothelial cells into new blood vessels. Naturally occurring endothelial growth inhibitors include angiostatin, endostatin, platelet factor 4, interferons, and several tissue inhibitors. Tumours often stimulate angiogenesis through release of growth factors. Many angiogenesis inhibitors are now in clinical trials and show promise in the treatment of melanoma and Kaposi's sarcoma, as well as ovarian, prostate, colon, and pancreatic cancers. Unlike other cytotoxic drugs, they can be used without interruption of therapy. Angiogenesis inhibitors may offer a new approach to cancer treatment with long-term maintenance rather than cure.

Data from http://www.cos.ca/; http://www.sunnybrookandwomens.on.ca/; http://www.cancer.ca/.

TABLE 46-11
MITOTIC INHIBITORS: SEVERE ADVERSE EFFECTS

Antibiotic Agent	Severe Side/Adverse Effects
etoposide	Liver and kidney toxicities
teniposide	Liver and kidney toxicities
vinblastine	Liver and kidney toxicities; neurotoxicity
vincristine	Liver toxicities; neurotoxicity

TABLE 46-12
MITOTIC INHIBITOR EXTRAVASATION

Mitotic Inhibitor Agent	Method
etoposide, teniposide, vinblastine, vincristine	1. Elevate limb and apply gentle pressure to the site. 2. Apply *warm* compresses to the site for one hour.* Take care to avoid excessive heat that may cause more tissue injury. 3. No antidote is available. A previously used antidote, hyaluronidase, is no longer available in Canada.

*Important: Corticosteroids and topical cooling appear to worsen toxicity.

cologically similar to paclitaxel. These agents and their plant sources are as follows:

Vinca alkaloids (periwinkle)
- vinblastine
- vincristine
- vinorelbine

Epipodophyllotoxin derivatives (mandrake plant)
- etoposide
- teniposide

Taxanes
- doxetaxel (European yew tree: needles)
- paclitaxel (Western yew tree: bark)

Mechanism of Action and Drug Effects

Depending on the particular agent, these plant-derived compounds can work in various phases of the cell cycle (late S phase, throughout G_2 phase, and M phase), but they all work shortly before or during mitosis, thus retarding cell division. Each subclass inhibits mitosis in a unique way. All are classified as CCS agents.

The vinca alkaloids (vincristine, vinblastine, and vinorelbine) bind to the protein tubulin during the metaphase of mitosis (M phase). This prevents the assembly of microtubules, which results in the dissolution of the mitotic spindle. Without these mitotic spindles, dividing cells cannot then multiply and divide appropriately. This inhibits cell division and DNA, RNA, and protein synthesis. Without these substances, all cells, including cancer cells, die.

The epipodophyllotoxin derivatives (etoposide and teniposide) exert their cytotoxic effects by inhibiting the enzyme topoisomerase II, which causes breaks in DNA strands. Teniposide works during the late S phase and the G_2 phase of the cell cycle whereas etoposide is more effective through interference with DNA synthesis and during the G_2 phase.

The yew tree derivatives (taxanes) paclitaxel and docetaxel both work in the late G_2 phase and M phase of the cell cycle. They work by causing the formation of nonfunctional microtubules, which halts mitosis in metaphase.

Indications

Mitotic inhibitors are used to treat a variety of solid tumours and some hematological malignancies. They are often used in combination chemotherapy regimens to enhance the overall cytotoxic effect. The commonly used agents and some of their specific therapeutic uses are listed in the dosages table on p. 793.

Contraindications

The only usual contraindication is severe drug allergy.

Side Effects and Adverse Effects

Like many of their antineoplastic counterparts in other classes, mitotic inhibitor antineoplastic agents can cause hair loss, nausea and vomiting, and myelosuppression. The emetic potential of some of the agents is given in Box 46-1. Major side effects specific to these agents are summarized in Table 46-11.

Toxicity and Management of Overdose

Most of the mitotic inhibitor antineoplastics are administered intravenously, making extravasation of the agents and its serious consequences a constant threat. (See the extravasation guidelines presented in Table 46-8.) Additional measures for the treatment of extravasation of mitotic inhibitors are given in Table 46-12.

Interactions

Many notable drug interactions are associated with the mitotic inhibitors. Etoposide competes for protein binding with warfarin and can result in increased prothrombin time due to elevated free plasma warfarin levels. When paclitaxel is given with cisplatin, it can result in increased myelosuppression due to additive toxicities. The combination of paclitaxel and ketoconazole can result in inhibited metabolism of paclitaxel and can lead to its accumulation. When teniposide is given with methotrexate, it can speed the clearance of methotrexate, resulting in decreased methotrexate duration of action and therapeutic efficacy. When vinblastine is given with methotrexate or bleomycin, it can increase the action of these two agents. Vinblastine and phenytoin co-administration can result in decreased absorption and/or increased metabolism of phenytoin, resulting in decreased phenytoin levels.

Dosages

For the recommended dosages of selected mitotic inhibitors, see the dosages table on p. 793. See Table 46-5 for some of the common brands available in Canada.

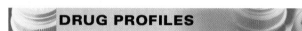

DRUG PROFILES

Mitotic inhibitors consist of three groups of agents that are derived from plant sources: vinca alkaloids (periwinkle), epipodophyllotoxin derivatives (mandrake plant), and the taxanes from various species of yew tree.

docetaxel

Docetaxel, as mentioned earlier, is obtained from the needles of the European tree. It is currently indicated for the treatment of breast cancer and non–small-cell lung cancer. Its contraindications include drug allergy and severe myelosuppression. It is available only in vials for injection in 20- and 80-mg strengths. Pregnancy category D. Common dosage recommendations are listed in the dosages table on p. 793.

▶▶ etoposide

Etoposide is a semi-synthetic epipodophyllotoxin derivative. It is believed to kill cancer cells in the late S phase and the G$_2$ phase of the cell cycle. Teniposide has a similar structure, mechanism of action, and side effect profile. Etoposide is indicated for the treatment of small-cell lung cancer and testicular cancer. Its only usual contraindication is drug allergy. It is available in an oral formulation as a 50-mg liquid-filled gelatin capsule and as a 20-mg/mL injection for intravenous infusion. Pregnancy category D. Commonly recommended dosages are listed in the dosages table on p. 793.

▶▶ paclitaxel

Paclitaxel is a natural mitotic inhibitor obtained from the bark of the Pacific yew tree. The yew is also the source of another mitotic inhibitor: docetaxel is made from the needles of the European yew tree. Paclitaxel is currently approved for the treatment of ovarian cancer, breast cancer, non–small-cell lung cancer, and Kaposi's sarcoma. However, because of its clinical effectiveness, it is also being used to treat many other types of cancer. Paclitaxel is extremely water insoluble (hydrophobic), and for this reason it is put into a solution containing oil rather than water. The particular oil is a type of castor oil called Cremophor EL, the same oil in which cyclosporin is mixed. Many clients cannot tolerate this oil, showing hypersensitivity reactions similar to anaphylactic reactions. For this reason, before clients receive paclitaxel they are premedicated with a steroid, antihistamine, and an H$_2$ antagonist (ranitidine, famotidine, or nizatidine). Paclitaxel is contraindicated in clients with drug allergy. It is available only in a 6-mg/mL injectable form. Common dosage recommendations are listed in the dosages table on p. 793. Pregnancy category D.

▶▶ vincristine

Vincristine is an alkaloid isolated from the periwinkle plant that is indicated for the treatment of acute leukemia. It is contraindicated in clients with a hypersensitivity to it and with a hereditary condition known as demyelinating Charcot-Marie-Tooth syndrome. It is available only in a parenteral formulation as a 1-mg/mL injection. Pregnancy category D. Common dosage recommendations are listed in the dosages table on p. 793.

TOPOISOMERASE-1 INHIBITORS (CAMPTOTHECINS)

Topoisomerase-1 inhibitors are a new class of chemotherapy agents. The two agents currently available in this class are topotecan and irinotecan. Both are semisynthetic analogues of the compound camptothecin, which was originally isolated in the 1960s from *Camptotheca acuminata*, a Chinese shrub. They are also referred to as camptothecins.

Mechanism of Action and Drug Effects

The camptothecins are cell cycle–specific agents and inhibit proper DNA function in the S phase by binding to the DNA-topoisomerase-1 complex. This complex normally allows DNA strands to be temporarily cleaved and then reattached (religated) in a critical step known as *religation*. The binding of the camptothecin drugs to this complex retards this religation process.

Indications

The two currently available topoisomerase-1 inhibitors are used primarily to treat ovarian and colorectal cancer. Topotecan has been shown to be effective in even metastatic cases of ovarian cancer that have failed platinum-containing regimens (i.e., cisplatin, carboplatin) and paclitaxel. Topotecan is also sometimes used to treat small-cell lung cancer.

Irinotecan is currently approved for the treatment of metastatic colorectal cancer that has recurred or progressed after standard therapy with the antimetabolite

DOSAGES Selected Mitotic Inhibitors

Agent	Pharmacological Class	Usual Dosage Range	Indications
Epipodophyllotoxin Derivative			
▸▸ etoposide	Mitotic inhibitor	IV: 50–100 mg/m²/day for 5 consecutive days PO: 2× the IV dose rounded to nearest 50 mg	Testicular and small-cell lung cancer
Taxanes			
docetaxel	Mitotic inhibitor	IV: 100 mg/m² q3wk	Breast and non–small-cell lung cancer
▸▸ paclitaxel	Mitotic inhibitor	IV: 135–175 mg/m² q3wk	Ovarian, breast, non–small-cell lung cancer; Kaposi's sarcoma
Vinca Alkaloid			
▸▸ vincristine	Mitotic inhibitor	IV: 1.4 mg/m² q1wk; usual max dose 2 mg; fatal if given intrathecally	Acute leukemia

agent fluorouracil. Irinotecan has also been shown to have significant activity against a broad range of other tumour types, including non–small-cell lung, cervical, and ovarian tumours and non-Hodgkin's lymphoma.

Contraindications

The only usual contraindication is severe drug allergy.

Side Effects and Adverse Effects

As with many antineoplastics, the main side effect demonstrated by topotecan is suppression of blood cells produced in the bone marrow. This BMS is predictable, non-cumulative, reversible, and manageable. Topotecan should not be given to clients with baseline neutrophil counts of less than 1.5×10^9/L. The most common non-hematological side effects are gastrointestinal. These include mild to moderate nausea, vomiting, and diarrhea.

Irinotecan has been associated with severe diarrhea, known as *cholinergic diarrhea*, which may occur during irinotecan infusion. Atropine treatment is recommended, unless contraindicated. Delayed diarrhea may occur two to ten days after infusion of irinotecan. This diarrhea can be severe and even life threatening. It should be treated aggressively with loperamide. Severe myelosuppression and nausea and vomiting are also possible.

Interactions

Other antineoplastics that have similar side-effect profiles should not be given concurrently with topoisomerase-1 inhibitors. Laxatives and diuretics should not be given concomitantly with irinotecan because of the potential to worsen the dehydration resulting from the severe diarrhea that can be caused with irinotecan.

Dosages

For recommended dosages of selected topoisomerase-1 inhibitors, see the dosages table on p. 794. See Table 46-6 for some of the common brands available in Canada.

DRUG PROFILES

Topoisomerase-1 inhibitors are a new class of chemotherapy agents isolated from the shrub *C. acuminata*. They are semi-synthetic derivatives of camptothecin (CPT), an alkaloid extract from plants. The two currently available are irinotecan and topotecan. These agents have shown significant activity against a broad range of tumours, from colorectal to ovarian cancers. These new agents are cell cycle–specific and are believed to act primarily during the S phase. Topotecan was approved by Health Canada in 1997 and irinotecan in 2001.

irinotecan

Irinotecan is indicated primarily for the treatment of metastatic colon or rectal cancer. It is usually given with both fluorouracil and leucovorin. Its only contraindication is drug allergy. It is available only as a 20-mg/mL injection. Pregnancy category D. Dosage information appears in the dosages table on p. 794.

topotecan

Topotecan is an effective antineoplastic agent. After initial therapy with other antineoplastics, cancer cells commonly become resistant to their effects. Topotecan has been extensively studied in the treatment of ovarian cancer and small-cell lung cancer. It produces responses even after such agents as platinum-containing regimens and paclitaxel have failed. It is contraindicated in cases of drug allergy or severe BMD. It is available only in 4-mg single-dose vials for injection. Pregnancy category D. Commonly used dosages are given in the dosages table on p. 794.

ANTINEOPLASTIC ENZYMES

Two antineoplastic enzymes are currently commercially available. A third, *Erwinia asparaginase*, is available only by special request through the Health Canada Special Access Programme for clients who

DOSAGES **Selected Topoisomerase-1 Inhibitors**

Agent	Pharmacological Class	Usual Dosage Range	Indications
irinotecan	Topoisomerase-1 inhibitor	IV: 125 mg/m² on days 1, 8, 15, 22 (many other complex regimens are used as well)	Metastatic colorectal cancer
topotecan	Topoisomerase-1 inhibitor	IV: 1.5 mg/m² once daily for 5 consecutive days on a repeatable 21-day course	Ovarian and small-cell lung cancer

have developed allergic reactions to *Escherichia coli*–based asparaginase, which is described in the following drug profile. All three agents are synthesized using cultures of certain bacteria coupled with recombinant DNA (rDNA) technology. Specifically, a critical segment of DNA (that contains the genes for producing the enzyme) is inserted into the genetic material for the bacterium, which then mass produces the enzyme as the bacteria multiply in culture. The enzyme itself is then isolated from this culture using various laboratory techniques and purified for clinical use. Commonly used dosages are given in the dosages table on p. 795.

DRUG PROFILES

▶▶ *asparaginase*

Asparaginase is used for the treatment of acute lymphocytic leukemia. Its mechanism of action is slightly different from that of traditional antineoplastics. It is an enzyme that catalyzes the conversion of the amino acid asparagine to aspartic acid and ammonia. Leukemic cells are then unable to synthesize the asparagine required for synthesis of DNA and proteins needed for cell survival. Asparaginase, when co-administered with mercaptopurine or methotrexate, can have additive hepatotoxic effects. Prednisone co-administration with asparaginase can result in additive effects on the pancreas, resulting in hyperglycemia.

Asparaginase is contraindicated in clients with drug allergy or pancreatitis. The only commercially available asparaginase product in Canada is the Kidrolase INJ PWS product manufactured by OPI S.A in France. This product is derived from the *E. coli* bacterium, and it is common for clients to develop allergic reactions to it. When this happens, one alternative is to instead use a product synthesized from an *Erwinia* sp. of bacterium. This product is not commercially available in Canada; however, it is available by special request from the Special Access Programme. Another treatment alternative is pegaspargase, also available only through the Special Access Programme, described in the following drug profile. Asparaginase is available only in a parenteral form as a 10 000-IU dosage for injection. It is currently rated as pregnancy category C, indicating a somewhat lower risk of adverse outcomes when administered during pregnancy than most antineoplastics. Common dosage recommendations are listed in the table on p. 795.

pegaspargase

Pegaspargase has a mechanism of action, indications, and contraindications similar to those of asparaginase. It is usually prescribed for clients who have developed an allergy to asparaginase, a common occurrence as mentioned earlier, especially with repeated treatment. It is available only as a 3750-unit/mL injection. Pregnancy category C. Dosage information appears in the dosages table on p. 795.

MISCELLANEOUS ANTINEOPLASTICS

The miscellaneous antineoplastic agents are those that, because of their unique structure and mechanisms of action, cannot be classified into the previously described categories. However, "miscellaneous" drugs are sometimes later reclassified as more is learned about their mechanisms of action and other characteristics. Current agents in the miscellaneous category include hydroxyurea, imatinib, mitotane, and the hormonal agents.

Indications

The miscellaneous antineoplastics are used for the treatment of a wide variety of cancers. Common agents and their therapeutic uses are listed in the dosages table on p. 796.

Side Effects and Adverse Effects

Like all antineoplastic agents, the miscellaneous agents cause hair loss, nausea and vomiting, and myelosuppression. Major side effects specific to these agents are listed in Table 46-13.

Interactions

Some important drug interactions with the miscellaneous antineoplastics are important to note. Co-administration with barbiturates, warfarin, or phenytoin can result in increased metabolism of mitotane, leading to decreased mitotane levels and decreased effectiveness. CNS depressants given with mitotane will result in additive CNS depression.

Dosages

Dosages for these agents are listed in the dosages table on p. 796. See Table 46-6 for some of the common brands available in Canada.

DOSAGES   Selected Antineoplastic Enzymes

Agent	Pharmacological Class	Usual Dosage Range	Indications
▶▶asparaginase	Antineoplastic enzyme	IM/IV: 200–1000 units/kg/day for 28 successive days, may continue for additional 14 days if remission not induced	Adult acute lymphocytic leukemia
		IM: 6000 units/m² × 3/wk for 9 doses	Pediatric acute lymphocytic leukemia
pegaspargase	Antineoplastic enzyme	IV/IM: 2500 units/m² q14d	Acute lymphocytic leukemia (usually in clients who have developed allergy to asparaginase)

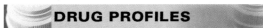

TABLE 46-13
MISCELLANEOUS AGENTS: SEVERE ADVERSE EFFECTS

Antineoplastic Agent	Severe Side/Adverse Effects
altretamine	Liver and kidney toxicities
asparaginase	Liver, kidney, metabolic, and CNS toxicities
cladribine	Hematological toxicities
hydroxyurea	CNS and renal toxicities
mitotane	GU and retinal toxicities

DRUG PROFILES

The various agents in the miscellaneous category of antineoplastics are used to treat a wide range of neoplasms. Hydroxyurea is administered orally. Imatinib and mitotane are available only in parenteral preparations.

hydroxyurea

Hydroxyurea most closely resembles the antimetabolite antineoplastics in its actions. It interferes with the synthesis of DNA by inhibiting the incorporation of thymidine into DNA. It works primarily in the S and G_1 phases of the cell cycle, making it a CCS agent. It is indicated for the treatment of squamous cell carcinoma of the head and neck. Contraindications include drug allergy and severe BMD. The drug is available only in oral formulations as a 500-mg capsule. Pregnancy category D. Common dosage recommendations are listed in the dosages table on p. 796.

imatinib

Imatinib is indicated for the treatment of chronic myeloid leukemia (CML), particularly after failure of interferon alfa therapy. It is one of the newest available antineoplastic agents, conditionally approved by Health Canada in 2001. It works by inhibiting a key enzyme (protein-tyrosine kinase) that is an important part of the CML disease process. Although its name sounds similar to that of various monoclonal antibody drugs, imatinib is not a monoclonal antibody. Its only contraindication is drug allergy. It is available only in oral form as a 100-mg capsule. Pregnancy category D. Dosage information appears in the dosages table on p. 796.

mitotane

Mitotane is an adrenal cytotoxic agent indicated specifically for the treatment of inoperable adrenal corticoid carcinoma. Its only contraindication is drug allergy. It is available only in oral form as a 500-mg tablet. Pregnancy category C. Dosage information appears in the dosages table on p. 796.

HORMONAL AGENTS

Hormonal agents are used in the treatment of a variety of neoplasms in both males and females. The rationale is that sex hormones act to accelerate the growth of many types of malignant tumour cells (e.g., certain types of breast and prostate cancer). Therefore therapy may involve administration of hormones with opposing effects (i.e., male vs. female hormones) or drugs that block the body's sex hormone receptors. These agents are used most commonly as palliative and adjuvant (that is, in addition to a primary drug) therapy. With certain types of cancer they may also be used as drugs of first choice. Some of the more common hormonal agents for female-specific neoplasms such as breast cancer are anastrazole, tamoxifen, megestrol, medroxyprogesterone, fluoxymesterone, and fulvestrant. For male-specific neoplasms such as prostate cancer, agents used include bicalutamide, flutamide, nilutamide, leuprolide, goserelin, and estramustine.

Photodynamic Agents and Radiopharmaceuticals

Antineoplastic agents that are usually administered by physicians include porfimer sodium and various radioactive pharmaceuticals (radiopharmaceuticals).

Porfimer sodium is used to treat esophageal or bronchial tumours that are present on the surface mucosa. It is also used for superficial or papillary bladder cancer. It does not destroy cancer cells on its own. Instead, it makes cells more sensitive to light. Normal cells are able to get rid of most of the agent over a couple of days, but it remains in cancer cells and skin cells. The medication is given intravenously and is followed by one or more sessions of laser light therapy to the esophageal,

DOSAGES Miscellaneous Antineoplastic Agents

Agent	Pharmacological Class	Usual Dosage Range	Indications
hydroxyurea	Miscellaneous antineoplastic agent	PO: 80 mg/kg as a single dose every third day, or 20–30 mg/kg as a single daily dose	Squamous cell carcinoma
imatinib	Miscellaneous antineoplastic agent	PO: 400–600 mg/day	Chronic myelocytic leukemia, GI stromal tumours
mitotane	Miscellaneous antineoplastic agent	PO: 2–10 g/day in divided doses	Adrenal cortical carcinoma

CASE STUDY

Breast Cancer

One of your clients is a 49-year-old woman who has just undergone a lumpectomy for treatment of breast cancer. The biopsy showed that the cancer cells from this breast tumour were estrogen receptor (ER) positive. After six weeks of radiation therapy, the client is to receive tamoxifen for approximately five years. She has no other health problems and has not gone through menopause.
- What are the side effects of tamoxifen?
- Will your client have hot flashes or any other symptoms of menopause? Explain your answer.
- What nursing measures could you share with this client to try to help relieve some of the menopausal symptoms?

For answers see http://evolve.elsevier.com/Lilley/pharmacology/.

bronchial, or bladder mucosa for direct tumour lysis and manual debridement.

Radiopharmaceuticals are drugs that have a radioactive substance in them and are used to diagnose and therapeutically treat a variety of cancers or symptoms caused by cancers. In general, a radioactive isotope targets the organ that is to be evaluated using the isotope bound to different chemical carriers. Five commonly used radiopharmaceuticals are chromic phosphate P-32 (for cancer-induced peritoneal or pleural effusions), samarium SM-153 lexidronam (bone cancer pain), sodium iodide I-131 (thyroid cancer and hyperthyroidism), sodium phosphate P-32 (various leukemias and palliative treatment of bone metastases), and strontium-89 chloride (bone cancer pain). These medications are usually administered by nuclear medicine physician specialists.

CYTOPROTECTIVE AGENTS AND MISCELLANEOUS TOXICITY INHIBITORS

Several available drugs are classified as cytoprotective agents. These medications help to reduce the toxicity of various antineoplastics. The decision whether to use them is often client specific, as is the case with chemotherapy regimens. Such decisions are generally made by the client's oncologists. All of these agents are normally administered intravenously, with the exception of allopurinol, which may also be given orally. These medications and their specific uses are summarized in the table on p. 797.

EXTRAVASATION

One of the most devastating consequences of chemotherapy is the loss of a limb or the need for skin grafting because an antineoplastic drug has extravasated into the surrounding tissue during intravenous administration. Most antineoplastic agents are administered intravenously and therefore this is a constant danger in any cancer client undergoing chemotherapy. Extravasation can result in permanent damage to nerves, tendons, and muscles, with skin grafting and even amputation needed to manage the damage. Good, attentive nursing care can prevent many of these incidents. If extravasation does occur, timely intervention can prevent the most serious consequences. There are certain basic steps involved in treating the extravasation of any drug, but specific antidotes and additional measures are required when treating the extravasation of antineoplastics.

If extravasation is suspected, administration of the agent must be stopped immediately, but the intravenous tube should be left in place and any residual drug or blood aspirated from it if possible. The requisite antidote, if one exists, must then be prepared and instilled through the existing intravenous tube, after which the needle should be removed. If the residual agent cannot be aspirated from the intravenous tube, the antidote should not be instilled through it. A sterile occlusive dressing that covers the entire area should be placed and warm or cold compresses applied, depending on the extravasated agent. The affected limb should then be elevated and allowed to rest.

NURSING PROCESS

The nursing care of clients receiving chemotherapy or antineoplastic agents presents a complex challenge to professional nurses and allied health providers. Cancer afflicts any age and gender. The nursing care of these clients often occurs in acute care and other types of settings as well,

DOSAGES   Cytoprotective Agents and Miscellaneous Toxicity Inhibitors

Agent	Pharmacological Class	Usual Dosage Range	Indications
allopurinol	Miscellaneous toxicity inhibitor	IV: 200–400 mg/m²/day PO: 600–800 mg/day	Control of hyperuricemia and prevention of uric acid nephropathy resulting from elevations in plasma and urinary uric acid levels following chemotherapy-induced cell rupture (tumour lysis syndrome)
amifostine	Cytoprotective agent	IV: 910 mg/m² once daily, starting 30 min before cisplatin dose	Reduction of cumulative renal toxicity associated with cisplatin chemotherapy
dexrazoxane	Cytoprotective agent	IV: Dose is a 10:1 ratio in mg/m² of dexrazoxane to doxorubicin, given within 30 min of doxorubicin dose (e.g., 500 mg/m² of dexrazoxane given before 50 mg/m² of doxorubicin)	Reduction of cardiomyopathy associated with cumulative doses of doxorubicin therapy in women with metastatic breast cancer who need to continue doxorubicin treatment
leucovorin	Cytoprotective agent	IV: 10 mg/m² q6h for 10 doses, beginning 24 h after start of methotrexate infusion (based on a methotrexate dose of 12–15 g/m²)	Rescue treatment ("leucovorin rescue") after high-dose methotrexate chemotherapy
mesna	Cytoprotective agent	IV: 10–12 mg/kg given at time of ifosfamide dose and again 4 and 8 h later	Prevention of hemorrhagic cystitis induced by ifosfamide
rasburicase	Miscellaneous toxicity inhibitor	IV: 0.2 mg/kg as a single daily dose for 7 days	Control of hyperuricemia and prevention of uric acid nephropathy resulting from elevations in plasma and urinary uric acid levels following chemotherapy-induced cell rupture (tumour lysis syndrome)

such as home health care, hospice care, assisted living, and long-term care. The specialty of oncology nursing has been widely accepted for many years and requires special education, certification, and skills. In 1985 a national organization for oncology nurses was formed: the Canadian Association of Nurses in Oncology (CANO). This organization provides standards of care for cancer clients and, in collaboration with the Canadian Nurses Association, offers a national oncology certification examination. Nurses who are successful in the examination receive the designation of CON(C), Certified in Oncology Nursing (Canada). For further information contact the CANO Head Office, 570 West 7th Avenue, Suite 402 Vancouver, B.C. V5Z 1B3, visit the CANO Web site at http://www.cos.ca/cano/, or contact them at 604-874-4322.

There is a great need for registered nurses to maintain current knowledge and skills related to the care of cancer clients. Oncology nursing services may be provided in hospital oncology units, hospice units, or in the home.

In Canada, hospice care began with the creation of hospital palliative care units. The first palliative care unit opened in 1974, seven years after Medicare was implemented in Canada. Hospice palliative care programs followed closely, initially as parts of larger organizations, then as volunteer-based hospice societies and organizations. Several elements distinguish hospice care from other types of nursing care. Hospice care is based on the concept that quality of care matters while the client is in the terminal phases of illness and that palliative or comfort-inducing measures are needed rather than "cures." Hospice care is generally, although not always, implemented in the home setting. Referrals and/or requests for community health care or hospice care are usually made by the primary physician but may also be made by registered nurses, hospital social workers, discharge planners, and family members or significant others. If they wish, family members or significant others may be involved in the care of the client.

Community health care is often an integral part of the care of cancer clients at various phases of the illness. It begins with a thorough assessment of the needs of the client. This plan is re-evaluated by the nurse at each visit to ensure that the client is receiving the best care possible.

Nursing actions appropriate to each antineoplastic group are presented in Table 46-14. The nurse must be aware that cancer drug regimens are constantly changing and therefore the information in the pharmacology section—as well as any information related to the nursing process—is representative and not absolute.

■ Assessment

A client should be thoroughly assessed before any antineoplastic agent is administered because these drugs act on all rapidly dividing cells, both cancerous and non-cancerous. Because bone marrow production of blood components (rapidly dividing normal cells) is impaired by

TABLE 46-14

NURSING IMPLICATIONS: ANTINEOPLASTICS*

Antineoplastic Agent	Classification	Nursing Implications
asparaginase, hydroxyurea	Miscellaneous	Administer asparaginase IV after dilution with recommended fluids (i.e., 10 000 units/ 5 mL sterile water or 0.9% NaCl with no preservatives). Administer hydroxyurea PO with extra fluids and an anti-emetic 30–60 min before.
carmustine, lomustine	Nitrosoureas	Give IV after proper dilutional guidelines have been followed, usually diluting 100 mg of drug into 3 mL of ethyl alcohol (usually provided that way), then further dilute in 27 mL of sterile water for injection, followed by further dilution in 100–500 mL of 0.9% NaCl or D5W. Give over 1 h or more. Discontinue infusion if discomfort occurs.
cisplatin†	Alkylating	Administer IV after diluting 10 mg/10mL, 50 mg/50 mL, or 100 mg/100mL sterile water for injection, then withdraw dose and dilute ½ dose with 1000 mL D5 0.3% NaCl or D5 ½ NaCl with 37.5 g mannitol. IV Cisplatin is usually administered over 3–4 h with a 0.45-micron filter. Check site for infiltration. Do not use aluminum equipment. Hydrate client with 1–2 L over 8–12 h before treatment.
cyclophosphamide	Alkylating agent	Follow instructions for mechlorethamine. Administer IV or PO with forced fluid intake because adequate hydration is needed to prevent hemorrhagic cystitis. Allopurinol may also be needed to maintain normal uric acid levels and prevent alkalinization of the urine. Administer IV after diluting to a concentration of 100 mg/5 mL of sterile NaCl; shake and let stand until clear, then may dilute more in up to 250 mL of D5W or D5NS; give via side arm at ≤100 mg/min. Always check IV site for extravasation and use 21-, 23-, or 25-gauge needle. Give as early in the morning as possible so can be eliminated before bedtime. Maintain diet low in purine, high in iron and vitamins.
fluorouracil	Antimetabolite	Administer IV undiluted through side arm; give over 1–3 min or dilute in 50–100 mL NS or D5W and give over 10–30 minutes; or in 300–500 mL (approximately 2 mg/mL) over 4 h; or add to 1 L appropriate solution and give over 24 h; or give via ambulatory pump or infuser. Administer anti-emetic therapy 30 min–1 h before therapy (as ordered) to prevent nausea. However, anti-emetics are usually not necessary when used as a single agent. Antibiotics may be needed to prevent infection. Antispasmodic may be needed to manage diarrhea. Use strict asepsis with clients. Increase fluids up to 3 L/day, unless contraindicated, to prevent dehydration. Perform mouth care with water and club soda or with soft bristle toothbrush or cotton-tipped applicator. Encourage diet high in iron and vitamins, low in fibre, and including few dairy products, especially if client is also undergoing irradiation.
mechlorethamine	Alkylating agent	Use guidelines for administering cytotoxic agent and give IV after diluting with 10 mg/ 10 mL sterile water or NaCl. Leave needle in the vial and withdraw dose. Give through side arm. Can be further diluted in 50 or 100 mL NS for infusion. With extravasation it is important to discontinue solution and apply ice pack for 6–12 h or follow hospital policy guidelines. Encourage fluid intake of up to 3 L/day to prevent formation of urate deposits in the urine. Also encourage adequate diet; special skin and mouth care; and diet low in purines (eliminate or reduce organ meats and dried beans).
methotrexate	Folic acid antagonist	Available in 2.5, 10, and 25 mg/mL for injection. Low doses (25–40 mg/m×/week) at a concentration of 5 mg/2 mL can be given through side arm of running intravenous tube over 1–2 min. Can also be administered by intramuscular injection and diluted intermittent or continuous infusion. Antacids given before PO agent may help minimize GI upset. Give anti-emetic 30–60 min before therapy. Allopurinol may be ordered to help control serum uric acid levels. Encourage fluid intake of up to 3 L/day, unless contraindicated. Leucovorin rescue is ordered within 12 h to prevent tissue damage and severe side effects of methotrexate.
paclitaxel	Mitotic inhibitor	Monitor vital signs during the first hour of IV infiltration and monitor the site for infiltration. IV solutions should follow proper dilutional guidelines and generally include 0.9% NaCl, D5W, D5NS, and D5LR to a concentration of 0.3–1.2 mg/mL. Use of an inline filter, either 0.2 or 0.22 microns, is recommended. Use only glass bottles, polypropylene, or polyolefin bags, and administration sets. Do *not* use PVC bags or sets. Premedication often includes dexamethasone, diphenhydramine, and ranitidine.
vincristine and related agents	Mitotic inhibitor	Administer antacids before PO dose to minimize GI upset. Administer IV only after diluting 10 mg/10 mL NaCl or D5W and follow administration guidelines. Administer anti-emetics 30–60 min before (as ordered).

*This table lists major classifications with examples. For additional agents in the same class, refer to specific manufacturer guidelines or discussion in chapter text.
†Caution: Do not confuse this agent's name with carboplatin. They are in the same class of agents but have different doses.
D5W, 5 percent dextrose in water; *NS,* normal saline; *D5LR,* 5 percent dextrose and lactated Ringer's solution.

antineoplastics, baseline blood counts are needed, including WBCs, neutrophils, leukocytes, red blood cell counts (RBCs), and platelets, before, during, and after drug administration. It is important for the nurse to monitor absolute neutrophil count (ANC; discussed later in this section) after administration of an antineoplastic agent because of the risk for blood counts dropping to their lowest levels. It is generally recommended that specific blood count levels be maintained to prevent severe reactions and adverse effects. Platelet levels should be above 100×10^9/L and leukocytes above 4.0×10^9/L. Other assessment parameters include appropriate radiographic tests; carcinoembryonic antigen (CEA) levels (indicates the presence of cancer with some tumours); nuclear scans; magnetic resonance imaging (MRI); and baseline hemoglobin (Hgb), hematocrit (Hct), and electrolyte levels. Other laboratory and diagnostic studies may also be necessary.

It is important for the nurse to remember that all rapidly dividing cells (both normal and cancerous) are affected by chemotherapy drugs, such as the rapidly dividing normal cells found in mucous membranes, hair follicles, and the components of bone marrow. The functioning of the body systems and the health of the tissues affected by these drugs must be monitored during treatment to avoid severe side effects or prevent complications such as the following:

- *GI mucous membranes:* stomatitis and altered bowel function with a high risk for poor appetite, nausea, vomiting (often requiring aggressive anti-emetic treatment), and diarrhea, as well as inflammation and possible ulcerations of the GI mucosa
- *Hair follicles:* loss of hair (alopecia)
- *Bone marrow components:* dangerously low (life-threatening) blood cell counts

The respiratory system should be assessed through pulmonary function studies and breath sounds. Immune status should be assessed through laboratory values such as protein levels and complete blood counts (CBCs).

In addition, the release of toxins resulting from cell death may cause systemic stimulation of the chemoreceptor trigger zone (CTZ).

Cytotoxic Antibiotics

Cytotoxic antibiotics (e.g., bleomycin, mitomycin, daunorubicin, doxorubicin) pose a greater risk for pulmonary fibrosis and/or decreased tidal volume (bleomycin) and liver toxicities. To determine the effect of the medication on the lungs, assessment may include, but is not limited to, the following: pulmonary function studies; arterial blood gases (ABGs); pCO_2 and pO_2 levels; breath sounds and breathing rate, rhythm, and depth; and X-ray examination of the chest. Side effects may not be experienced for two weeks or more after medication therapy has been initiated.

Tissue necrosis occurs when intravenous sites undergo extravasation due to infiltration; therefore frequent assessment of the intravenous site, its patency, and its status is crucial.

Reproductive history should also be assessed in both males and females because of the possibility of infertility, amenorrhea, azoospermia (absence of sperm), and possible testicular toxicity. Cardiac assessment should be made with auscultation of heart sounds, cardiac rate and rhythm, and assessment of rales in the bases of the lungs, as well as any edema in dependent areas. These drugs are contraindicated during pregnancy or lactation and in clients with systemic infections. Cautious use is recommended in clients with compromised renal, hepatic, cardiac, or bone marrow functioning.

Alkylating Agents

Alkylating agents, such as carboplatin, carmustine, cisplatin, and cyclophosphamide, are associated with peripheral neuropathy, loss of vision for light and colour, emesis, nephrotoxicity, and BMS. Baseline fluid and electrolyte levels and blood cell counts should be taken, and the presence of any numbness or tingling of extremities should be noted. Baseline assessment of the client's nutritional status is also important, with an emphasis on protein, fluid, and electrolyte levels. The use of some alkylating agents may result in hepatotoxicity; therefore liver function must be assessed. Both carmustine and cisplatin are toxic to bone marrow and pulmonary functioning, and cisplatin is also toxic to hepatic and renal functioning; therefore appropriate laboratory studies must be assessed before, during, and for months after therapy. Loss of motor function and other neurological changes (e.g., severe neuropathies) are also associated with these drugs; therefore ongoing neurological assessment is critical. Contraindications and cautions for the alkylating agents include old age, lung disease or altered pulmonary functioning, CNS disorders, seizure disorders, altered blood counts (e.g., WBCs, RBCs, platelets), or hepatic, renal, or cardiac disease. Clients with diabetes may experience worsening of pre-existing peripheral neuropathies. Some of the drug interactions include acetylsalicylic acid, NSAIDs, other antineoplastics, alcohol, vaccines, and oral anticoagulants.

Antimetabolites

Antimetabolite antineoplastics are associated with severe liver, kidney, GI tract, bladder, cardiac, and bone marrow toxicities and require thorough assessments of the affected systems and organs. Baseline fluid and electrolyte status and levels are necessary. Assessment should also include monitoring of CBC and differential blood cell counts (withhold drug if WBCs are less than 3.5×10^9/L or platelets are less than 100×10^9/L). Contraindications to these drugs include pregnancy, lactation, leukopenia, thrombocytopenia, and bladder or urinary disorders (cyclophosphamide has the severe side effect of hemorrhagic cystitis). The antimetabolites should be used cautiously in clients with alterations in bone marrow function; renal, cardiac, or hepatic dysfunction; GI abnormalities (peptic ulcer disease, ulcerative colitis, and/or stomatitis); or genitourinary abnormalities. Cautious use is recommended in clients suffering from BMS, infection, stomatitis, peptic ulcer disease, or ulcerative colitis.

Specific assessment information is important with the antimetabolite cytarabine because of the occurrence of cytarabine syndrome. This syndrome occurs usually within 6 to 12 hours after drug administration and is characterized by fever, myalgia, bone pain, nausea, vomiting, occasional chest pain, and rash. A thorough assessment of cardiac and breath sounds, with a complete nursing assessment of cardiac and respiratory systems, is warranted with the use of cytarabine, as well as with the use of all other antimetabolites that may cause cardiac and/or pulmonary toxicity. Other antimetabolites, such as fluorouracil, mercaptopurine, methotrexate, and thioguanine, also require specific assessment of related laboratory or diagnostic studies. For example, contraindications for methotrexate are hypersensitivity, leukopenia (WBCs $<3.5 \times 10^9$/L), thrombocytopenia (platelets $<100 \times 10^9$/L), anemia, psoriatic clients, alcoholism, hepatic and renal disease, and pregnancy. Additional cautions for the use of methotrexate include renal disease and lactation. Methotrexate (and other types of antineoplastics causing high volumes of cell death with release of uric acid) may also increase hyperuricemia and precipitate gout-related symptoms. If the client has had or has been exposed to chicken pox, exposure to methotrexate may cause the subsequent or residual disease process to become more generalized. A thorough medication history will allow the nurse to identify possible drug interactions with antimetabolites, such as acetylsalicylic acid, sulpha drugs, other antineoplastics, alcohol, theophylline, penicillins, oral digoxin, vaccines, oral anticoagulants, and NSAIDs (possible fatal interaction).

LEGAL and ETHICAL PRINCIPLES

Administration of Antineoplastic Agents

Regulations and standards of practice should be viewed not as extra work but as a helpful framework for safe nursing practice. To help maintain safe nursing practice and adhere to standards of nursing practice, it is important to look at the various antineoplastics with specific attention to dosage calculations and timing of dosages as ordered. Antineoplastic agents are toxic by their design. Because of the complexity and the wide variety of dosing protocols, the nurse should always be cautious with these medications and follow all standards of practice and the provincial nursing practice standards to avoid legal and/or ethical dilemmas. To help reduce errors, nursing and pharmacy personnel may design standardized, preprinted order forms or computerized order sheet sets for all antineoplastic agents. This relatively simple intervention could prevent a life-threatening medication error and maintain and uphold standards of care and nursing practice standards related to the specialty of caring for clients with cancer.

▪ Mitotic Inhibitors

Mitotic inhibitors, such as vinblastine, vincristine, etoposide, and paclitaxel, require thorough assessments of baseline fluids, electrolytes, and blood counts. Hepatic and renal toxicities are a concern and thus monitoring of liver and renal function studies is appropriate. Mitotic inhibitors are contraindicated in clients who have had chicken pox or shingles, CNS disorders and seizures (especially with the use of vinblastine and vincristine), neutropenia (neutrophils <0.50–0.70×10^9/L), platelets less than 100×10^9/L, Hgb less than 45 g/L, or reticulocytes less than 0.5 percent of red cell count. The nurse must always assess for drug–drug and drug–intravenous solution incompatibilities, especially with these drugs and other agents that are identified as irritants (irritates intravenous site and vein) or as vesicants (cell death with extravasation and necrosis with ulcerations).

Cytotoxic antibiotics, such as doxorubicin, are contraindicated in clients with cardiac disease. MUGA scans may be ordered to assess cardiac ejection fraction and evaluate the effectiveness of dexrazoxane, a cytoprotectant drug used to help decrease possible life-threatening cardiac toxicities.

▪ Topoisomerase Inhibitors

Topotecan and irinotecan (topoisomerase inhibitors) are contraindicated in clients with a history of allergies to either drug. Gemtuzumab is another agent that falls into the miscellaneous category (also identified as a monoclonal antibody) and is contraindicated in pregnancy, lactation, renal or hepatic disease, and severe BMS. Cardiac status (vital signs, lung sounds, electrocardiogram [ECG]) must be documented before treatment because of the associated cardiac toxicity.

▪ Miscellaneous

Miscellaneous antineoplastics, such as hydroxyurea, imatinib, mitotane, and the hormonal agents, are contraindicated in clients with allergies to them and in clients with BMS. Other agents, such as asparaginase and pegaspargase, are also contraindicated in clients with allergies to them. Allergic reactions with these drugs may occur later in therapy.

▪ Nursing Diagnoses

Nursing diagnoses pertinent to clients receiving antineoplastic agents include the following:
- Risk for impaired integrity of skin and oral mucous membranes related to stomatitis from drug therapy.
- Acute pain related to malignant process and GI side effects such as anorexia, nausea, and vomiting.
- Risk for self-injury related to hemodynamic side effects (e.g., BMS) of antineoplastics.
- Disturbed body image related to alopecia and/or other effects of the antineoplastic agents.
- Impaired physical mobility related to anemia-induced fatigue.

- Diarrhea related to effects of the antineoplastic agents.
- Risk for infection related to BMS and resultant neutropenia.
- Impaired skin integrity related to dermatological side effects of methotrexate, with side effects of vasculitis or photosensitivity.
- Disturbed sensory perception related to effects of the antineoplastic agent mechlorethamine.
- Disturbed body image related to disturbed gonadal functioning and growth, alopecia, and darkened skin (seen with cyclophosphamide, nitrosoureas, and other alkylating agents).
- Impaired urinary elimination (hemorrhagic cystitis, nephrotoxicity) related to cyclophosphamide treatment.
- Disturbed sensory perception (hearing loss, optic neuritis) related to ototoxicity associated with cisplatin.
- Risk for injury related to loss of reflexes, numbness of hands and feet, and ataxia stemming from neurotoxicity of cisplatin.
- Decreased cardiac output related to cardiotoxicity of cytotoxic antibiotics.
- Impaired urinary elimination related to hyperuremia, uric acid nephropathy, and neurotoxicity related to use of vinblastine and vincristine.

Planning

Goals related to the administration of antineoplastic agents, regardless of the class, include the following:
- Client regains normal or pre-chemotherapy level of oral mucosa integrity with minimal discomfort and problems stemming from stomatitis.
- Client experiences increased comfort levels during antineoplastic therapy.
- Client experiences minimal breaks in skin integrity and oral mucous membranes while receiving antineoplastics.
- Client experiences maximal comfort and minimal GI-related side effects.
- Client remains safe and free from injury.
- Client maintains an intact and healthy body image.
- Client's bowel functioning remains normal or near normal.
- Client remains free from infection.

Outcome Criteria

Outcome criteria pertinent to clients receiving antineoplastic agents include the following:
- Client states and/or demonstrates various measures to minimize alterations in mucous membranes, such as frequent mouth care with gentle sponge-type toothettes and use of non–alcohol-based mouthwash.
- Client uses non-pharmacological as well as pharmacological methods daily—including relaxation therapy, music therapy, and biofeedback—to control pain related to the neoplastic processes.
- Client demonstrates the use of various measures to enhance skin integrity, such as keeping skin clean, dry, and lubricated daily.

- Client understands the importance of daily measures to minimize risk for self-injury related to the effects of BMS, such as avoiding crowds (e.g., clients with leukopenia) and avoiding straight razors, venipuncture, and injections (e.g., clients with decreased platelets) if possible.
- Client verbalizes openly and daily any self-concept disturbances related to alopecia and other effects of the antineoplastic therapy and the neoplasm.
- Client uses non-pharmacological methods (e.g., diet, fluids, exercise) and pharmacological methods (e.g., bulk-forming laxatives) to regain normal or pre-chemotherapy bowel elimination patterns.
- Client minimizes the risk for infection by consuming a high-protein diet and avoiding crowds while blood counts are decreased.
- Client minimizes damage to the skin through the use of sunscreen and other skin protection methods and takes care to avoid skin injury (especially with methotrexate).
- Client experiences minimal auditory changes and contacts the appropriate healthcare professionals during the course of therapy for recommendations about measures to minimize these auditory changes (specific to cyclophosphamide, nitrosoureas).

COMMUNITY HEALTH POINTS

Antineoplastic Agents

- The community home care of cancer clients requires the skills of an astute, well-prepared, and experienced nurse who can react quickly to critical situations yet remain empathetic during the terminal stages of the disease.
- The community home care nurse should be certified to administer chemotherapy and to follow the specific policies established by the agency and the accepted standards of care for home health nursing.
- Documentation is a critical part of the nursing care of community home-care clients, and this should be done in accordance with the agency's policy. The nurse should document the location of the IV injection site, the details concerning the infusion of the chemotherapeutic agent, and the response of the client, along with any problems with extravasation and the actions initiated to counter the effects. Should extravasation occur, accepted nursing actions should be initiated and documented and the physician contacted. Photographs of the site should be taken, if possible, so that the degree of damage can be adequately recorded. Client and family responses to all aspects of care should also be documented.
- Antineoplastic therapy can be successfully carried out at home if the client and family members are adequately taught about the medications used, their action, side effects, toxic effects, and procedures for administration.

- Client experiences minimal disturbances in self-concept.
- Client adheres to daily activity restrictions (specifically with cyclophosphamide and nitrosoureas) but is able to maintain ADLs.
- Client states measures to prevent or minimize hemorrhagic cystitis or nephrotoxicity related to cyclophosphamide use, such as a high intake of liquids (2000 mL/day) before, during, and after chemotherapy.
- Client conserves energy throughout the day when experiencing anemia-induced fatigue and continues to participate in ADLs as much as possible.
- Client states ways to prevent or minimize the loss of reflexes, the numbness of the hands and feet, and the ataxia related to neurotoxicity (especially with cisplatin).
- Client reports any cardiac difficulty, such as shortness of breath, dysrhythmias, or chest pain, resulting from possible cardiotoxicity (related to doxorubicin) during the course of therapy.
- Client has a high intake of fluids daily (at least 2000 mL/24 h period) and maintains nutritional status within the restrictions specified by the physician to prevent or minimize hyperemia, uric acid nephropathy, or neurotoxicity with joint and back pain.

■ Implementation

Antineoplastic drugs are some of the most toxic medications given to clients. Serious complications and side effects may occur that limit the use of these drugs. Along with cancer cells, antineoplastic drugs destroy rapidly dividing cells that have a high growth fraction, such as thrombocytes, neutrophils, hair follicles, GI tract and oral mucosa, sperm-forming cells, and bone marrow components such as erythrocytes. The destruction of normal cells leads to side effects and toxicities such as infection, anemias, bleeding, alopecia, nausea, vomiting, diarrhea, stomatitis, and sterility. Because of the effects on the CTZ of the toxins that result from cell death, the destruction of cancer cells leads to nausea and vomiting and possible increases in uric acid, precipitating gout. In addition, vesicant agents are highly reactive and may result in severe local injury around any infiltrated intravenous site. They may have their own carcinogenic effect, with cancers developing in other sites. Nursing implementation is discussed here using a general approach so that the information may be applied to the use of any antineoplastic drug. The nurse should know what cells are commonly affected by the specific drug, along with its other common side effects.

BMS results from the loss of neutrophils (precipitating infection), erythrocytes (causing anemias and gross fatigue), and thrombocytes (leading to bleeding). Infection is one of the more significant side effects and cannot be emphasized enough. The onset of neutropenia, which occurs with some of the drugs, takes place rapidly; the lowest neutrophil count (nadir) usually occurs between days 10 and 14 and recovers within about three to four weeks.

However, some antineoplastics have a delayed neutropenia, and counts begin to fall within about two weeks. Their nadir is within three to four weeks, with full recovery not until about the seventh week. Checking neutrophil counts is essential to safe nursing care and for preventing infections. Normal neutrophil counts are from 2.5 to $7.0 \times 10^9/L$ /mm^3. If the neutropenia is significant (ANC $5.0 \times 10^9/L$) the physician should be contacted. Further treatment will most likely be delayed until blood cell counts return to normal. Fever is the principal early sign of infection. Therefore important measures include frequent monitoring of temperature (avoiding taking the temperature rectally to prevent tissue injury) and other parameters, such as blood pressure, pulse, respirations, and laboratory values.

Clients and family members or significant others need to be aware that they must now be their own first line of defence. Temperatures should be taken at least every four hours for fever because an increase in temperature may indicate the beginning of an infection. Minimizing exposure to contagions is critical to preventing infections. If a client is hospitalized (and some physicians avoid hospitalization because of the risk for nosocomial infections), every precaution must be taken to minimize infection. Cultures may need to be taken to identify the organism and to show sensitivity to specific antibiotics. Intravenous antibiotic empirical therapy may be used until culture reports are available. CSFs, such as G-CSF and GM-CSF, may be used to minimize neutropenia. These drugs act on the bone marrow to enhance neutrophil production and help decrease the incidence, severity, and duration of the neutropenia. Thus they may decrease the need for hospitalization and/or intravenous antibiotic therapy. Chapter 47 further discusses drug-related, as well as nursing process-related, information associated with biological response modifiers.

Clients may also need isolation to protect themselves from the infections of others. As part of protective isolation, caregivers wear gloves, mask, and gown to minimize the client's exposure to bacteria. Signs of infection that need to be documented and reported to the physician and healthcare provider include temperatures of 38°C or higher and complaints of sore throat, coughing, and flu-like symptoms. Clients taking chemotherapy should avoid vaccinations during their therapy. CBCs and differential counts should be monitored weekly; the antineoplastic agent may be withheld if WBCs are less than $3.5 \times 10^9/L$.

Thrombocytopenia and anemia may also be consequences of antineoplastic therapy and therefore the client is at risk for bleeding (from a decrease in circulating platelets) and gross fatigue (from decreased RBC production). The nurse should monitor the client for bleeding from the mouth, gums, and nose, and even after tooth brushing. Bleeding times and coagulation studies are warranted during and after therapy. It is important for the nurse to inform clients that bleeding may be increased by medications such as acetylsalicylic acid, anticoagulants,

NURSING CARE PLAN

Antineoplastic Agents

The nurse has just initiated paclitaxel chemotherapy on a 44-year-old client who has been recently diagnosed with ovarian cancer. Family members are asking many questions about paclitaxel, including what side effects to expect; how long the treatment regimen will last; and what they need to be aware of when she returns home, including problems to report to the oncologist.

ASSESSMENT	**Subjective Data**	• "What is paclitaxel?" • "How does it work?" • "What side effects can I expect with it?" • "What is the usual treatment plan?"
	Objective Data	• Newly diagnosed client with ovarian cancer • Paclitaxel infusion to begin immediately • Supportive family
NURSING DIAGNOSIS		Risk for injury (bleeding, easy bruising, infection) related to side effects of medication
PLANNING	**Goals**	• Client and family inquire about the drug and treatment plan. • Client and family will verbalize an understanding of paclitaxel before therapy is initiated.
OUTCOME CRITERIA		Client and family will report or verbalize the following during treatment: • Side effects that should be reported to healthcare provider • Action of paclitaxel • Treatment plan
IMPLEMENTATION		Client and family teaching session to include the following information: • Paclitaxel helps prevent the rapid division and growth of malignant cells by affecting certain specific structures within the cancer cell. • Treatment usually consists of intravenous infusion given over three hours every three weeks for a time specified by the oncologist. • Common side effects include slowed heartbeat. • Contraceptive measures are recommended during treatment and up to eight weeks after treatment because of adverse effects on a fetus. • Use of the following should be avoided because bleeding may occur: ASA, NSAIDs (such as ibuprofen), straight razors for shaving, and commercial mouthwashes (which often contain alcohol). • Any abnormal bleeding, such as blood in the stool or urine or easy bruising, should be reported. • Fatigue, headache, irritability, shortness of breath, and dizziness should be reported because these may indicate anemia. • Client may want to select a wig matching her hairstyle and colour now so that the wig will be available when hair is lost. The hair may be a different colour and texture when it grows back. • Client should not receive any vaccinations while on chemotherapy.
EVALUATION		Positive therapeutic outcomes include the following: • Increased response of tumour cells to the chemotherapy • Prevention of rapid division of malignant cells • Minimal side effects

and NSAIDs. These medications are contraindicated with the occurrence of thrombocytopenia. If an analgesic is needed, a drug should be selected that is not ASA or NSAID based; acetaminophen or even a narcotic may be the drug of choice.

Cautions to minimize bleeding may include the following: padding side rails, limiting intramuscular/ subcutaneous injections and/or venipunctures, and using quick methods of BP monitoring to avoid tissue trauma because overinflation of BP cuffs may lead to bruising or bleeding. The client should report any type of bleeding or ulcerations in the mouth to the healthcare provider immediately. Shaving with a straight-edge razor is discouraged. The use of electric razors is encouraged in both males and females to prevent trauma, breaks in the skin, and bleeding. Anemia may require blood transfusions or treatment with epoetin (erythropoietin), which is a hormone that stimulates RBC production. Epoetin may be managed with the client at home and may even prevent hospitalization; however, it cannot be used in clients with leukemias or myelomas.

With methotrexate, anti-emetic therapy and antacids are often needed to decrease nausea, vomiting, and GI upset. Allopurinol may be used to manage the uric acid levels (these drugs may be used with any antineoplastic that results in hyperuricemia). Alkalinization of the urine with sodium bicarbonate (pH 6.5) and adequate fluids helps to minimize hyperuricemia. The client should also be advised to do the following:

- Report black tarry stools to the healthcare provider immediately
- Report chills, sore throat, and fever to the healthcare provider
- Before initiation of therapy, decide whether to use a wig or hairpiece to cover up hair loss
- Report any bleeding, white spots, or ulcerations in the mouth (stomatitis) to the healthcare provider immediately
- Avoid foods containing citric acid and those that are hot or rough in texture
- Increase fluid intake to 2.5 to 3 L per day
- Avoid straight-edge razors
- Do not use commercial mouthwashes (irritating to mucosa)
- Use contraception during treatment and for up to about eight weeks after therapy to minimize possible teratogenic effects or fetal death
- Use sunblock when outdoors

Methotrexate, a folic acid antagonist, has toxic effects on bone marrow that may be life threatening. Leucovorin, a methotrexate antagonist, is a "rescue" (antagonist) drug used to protect the client from these potentially fatal BMS effects. A first in its class of drugs, leucovorin is usually given within one hour of methotrexate (or any folic acid antagonist agent). It is reconstituted for intravenous use and is incompatible (as are many of the intravenous antineoplastics) with many solutions within the same syringe.

Clients must be encouraged to drink at least 3 L of fluid a day. The nurse monitors creatinine clearances during therapy to detect any nephrotoxicity. The client's nutritional status may be enhanced by increasing the intake of bran, dried beans, nuts, fruits, fresh (thoroughly washed) vegetables, and asparagus because these foods are high in folic acid. This is yet another measure to minimize the possibility of methotrexate toxicity, which is essentially an overdose of a folic acid antagonist (blocking) agent. However, if GI upset and/or stomatitis is present, clients may need to decrease any sources of irritation (e.g., high-fibre food).

Chemotherapy may cause GI injury because the epithelial lining is sensitive to cytotoxic drugs. Stomatitis and diarrhea are common, but may be life threatening if severe. Stomatitis usually develops within a few days and persists for two or more weeks after treatment. However, the oral inflammation may progress to ulceration and further complications. Stomatitis may create such pain that eating, speaking, and even swallowing can be difficult. Often the healthcare provider will order an oral solution with combinations of topical anaesthetics and antifungal drugs, as well as systemic analgesics. Severe cases of stomatitis may lead to a discontinuation of antineoplastic therapy. Alcohol should be avoided and commercial mouthwashes are contraindicated. Foods high in citric acid or those that are hot or have a rough texture should be avoided. It is also recommended that hydration be part of therapy; 10 to 12 glasses of fluid per day is encouraged. Diarrhea from epithelial lining damage may lead to impaired absorption of nutrients and fluids. A diet high in fibre gives the stool a firmer consistency, and constipating foods (such as cheese) may be necessary, as well as increasing fluids, unless contraindicated, to prevent fluid volume deficits. If GI upset is associated with the drug, antacids should be administered before any oral form of the drug, after dinner, and at bedtime. Further information about antacids may be found in Chapter 49, and antidiarrheal drugs are discussed in Chapter 50.

Nausea and vomiting are commonly associated with antineoplastic drugs. The impact of cell toxins and the chemotherapy agent may stimulate the CTZ and lead to significant nausea and vomiting—possibly to the degree that the drug needs to be discontinued. The nausea and vomiting associated with these drugs is more severe than that of other emetic drugs. Severe emesis is often associated with cisplatin, dacarbazine, and nitrogen mustard; moderately severe emesis may be associated with cyclophosphamide, doxorubicin, nitrosoureas, and dactinomycin; moderate emesis occurs commonly with cytarabine, procarbazine, and high doses of methotrexate; and mild emesis is associated with etoposide, fluorouracil, hydroxyurea, bleomycin, vinblastine, vincristine, and low-dose methotrexate.

Premedication is the treatment option, and anti-emetics help to reduce the nausea and vomiting, prevent dehydration and malnutrition, and promote adherence with therapy. Anti-emetics that are usually used with the antineoplastic drugs include ondansetron or a combination of ondansetron and dexamethasone. Other anti-emetics for use with antineoplastics include metoclopramide, prochlorperazine (phenothiazine anti-emetics), and lorazepam. If these drugs are not helpful, it may be necessary to try two cannabinoid-type anti-emetics: dronabinol and nabilone. A combination of anti-emetics is generally more effective than a single drug therapy approach. Anti-emetic therapy usually begins 30 to 60 minutes before the chemotherapy and may need to be continued during therapy. A nutritious diet high in iron, protein, and vitamins is needed to help maintain an immune system that is as near normal as possible. A liquid diet with bland and non-irritating beverages is encouraged; gelatin, dry toast, and crackers may be added once the vomiting and nausea have stopped. Anti-emetic drugs and related nursing process are presented in Chapter 51.

Other significant toxicities include reproductive problems, hyperuricemia, local tissue injury (from extravasation of an intravenous drug that is either a vesicant or an irritant), other types of toxicities, carcinogenesis, and alopecia. Reversible hair loss begins seven to ten days after treatment has begun (this depends on the drug and whether there is damage to the hair follicle and other areas, glands, or tissues), and maximal effects are achieved within about two months. Although alopecia is not a danger to the client, it can be damaging to the client's self-esteem and is one of the most feared side effects of treatment. As part of planning for therapy, the client may decide to get a wig or hairpiece before hair is lost. The client should be informed that wigs and hairpieces are tax deductible as a medical expense. Some clients prefer beautifully made, fashionable head scarves and hats.

Besides informing the client about possible hair loss, it is also important for the nurse to discuss the fact that the hair lost during treatment will generally grow back different in colour and texture.

Antineoplastics also have destructive actions on the germinal epithelium of the testes (they are rapidly dividing cells). Some drugs are also teratogenic and may lead to fetal death. Women who are of childbearing age and are sexually active should protect themselves against pregnancy because of the risk of embryo death. Should pregnancy occur, termination of the pregnancy may be necessary. Some antineoplastics may cause amenorrhea because of their effect on the ovaries. Damage to the ovaries may also lead to menopausal symptoms and vaginal epithelial atrophy. Amenorrhea is reversible. Sterility in males is often irreversible, and therefore sperm banking before chemotherapy should be encouraged, if appropriate. In addition, contraceptive measures are encouraged during the chemotherapy and up to at least eight weeks after discontinuation of therapy.

Hyperuricemia occurs after cell death from chemotherapy and is especially common with the leukemias and lymphomas because of the increased percentage of cell kill. The major concern of this toxicity is the accumulation of uric acid in the kidneys. Increased fluid intake may help decrease crystal formation and, should the uric acid levels keep increasing, the high uric acid levels may be managed by allopurinol, which reduces uric acid formation. A diet low in uric acid is encouraged, and foods such as organ meats, dried beans, and peas should be avoided.

Extravasation of some of the antineoplastic drugs may lead to severe tissue damage and sloughing. Intravenous infusions of vesicant drugs should be administered via a patent intravenous infusion. The site should be monitored every hour. Extravasation of vesicants may lead to necrosis, which may be so severe that surgical interven-

tion (e.g., skin grafting) may be necessary. Should extravasation occur, the intravenous site should be assessed, the infusion stopped immediately, and the physician contacted. The intravenous catheter should be left in place because antidotes are available for some vesicants. The nurse should always check the facility policy on how extravasation of a vesicant should be managed and if antidotes may be used.

Some of the newer agents, such as gemtuzumab, require specific interventions before their administration. For antineoplastics, such as gemtuzumab, that have high incidence of allergic reactions, the physician usually orders the following protocol: diphenhydramine 50 mg orally and acetaminophen 650 to 1000 mg orally one hour before the intravenous infusion, then acetaminophen 650 to 1000 mg orally every one to four hours as needed. Gemtuzamab is also sensitive to the effects of light and should be administered via a separate intravenous line with a 1.2 micron terminal filter. The drug should be given over approximately two hours.

Doxorubicin is available in a liposomal drug delivery system, and directions for its use must be followed closely.

There are other side effects that occur with the antineoplastic agents; however, those previously listed are most common. The following additional nursing implementation guidelines are useful:

- Know that multi-drug therapy often leads to lower doses of all of the drugs used; side effects are then minimized.
- Check blood work. If neutrophils are below 5.0×10^9/L, platelets below 100×10^9/L /mm³, and/or WBCs below 4.0×10^9/L, the next scheduled chemotherapy should be cancelled.
- Check with the physician about using CSFs to minimize neutropenia and subsequent infections and hospitalizations.
- Encourage copious intake of fluids to minimize effects on the kidneys.
- Monitor intravenous sites every hour for possible infiltration.
- Report any complaints immediately to the healthcare provider, including black tarry stools, chills, fever, sore throat, bleeding, bruising, cough, dyspnea, dark or bloody urine, and ulcers or white spots in the mouth.
- Monitor renal function studies such as creatinine, blood urea nitrogen (BUN), serum uric acid, electrolytes, and creatinine clearance during and after therapy. (BUN <8.9 mmol/L, creatinine <133 μmol/L, and urinary output <30 mL/h are all indications of the need for medical intervention.)
- Monitor and report any jaundice or elevation in liver function tests (bilirubin, alkaline phosphatase, aspartate aminotransferase [AST], and alanine aminotransferase [ALT]).
- Keep epinephrine (as well as antihistamines and corticosteroids) nearby in case the client experiences an allergic or a hypersensitivity reaction.

NURSING CARE PLAN

Breast Cancer

Mrs. S., a 65-year-old woman with a recent diagnosis of estrogen-receptor–positive breast tumour, has begun antineoplastic therapy with tamoxifen citrate therapy as an adjunct to surgical therapy with a modified radical mastectomy of the left breast. Vital parameters are as follows: Hgb and Hct within normal limits, WBC 4.5 × 10⁹/L, platelets 100 × 10⁹/L, VS within normal limits. Other data pertinent to Mrs. S. include complaints of metallic taste, some nausea, and decreased energy levels with a problem some days of taking in only minimal amounts of food. No anti-emetics, antacids, vitamins, iron supplements, or nutritional supplements are being taken.

ASSESSMENT	Subjective Data	• "I just hate these hot flashes." • "Everything tastes so metallic." • "Do I really have to take this all the time?" • "I just don't feel like eating most of the time. . . nothing tastes good anymore."
	Objective Data	• Breast cancer diagnosed two months ago • 65 years old • In otherwise good health • ER-positive breast tumour • WBC 4.5 × 10⁹/L • Platelets 100 × 10⁹/L • No weight loss • Takes tamoxifen citrate as ordered • Decreased energy level but able to carry out ADLs
NURSING DIAGNOSIS		Imbalanced nutrition, less than body requirements, related to adverse and toxic effects of chemotherapy
PLANNING	Goals	Client will maintain diet of six feedings with Ensure snacks within two weeks
OUTCOME CRITERIA		Client will show improved appetite as evidenced by • Energy level • Intake of foods within the basic food groups • No weight loss • Decreased complaints of diminished appetite
IMPLEMENTATION		• Encourage use of anti-emetic 30–60 min before dosing of tamoxifen, as ordered, to prevent nausea and vomiting if a problem. • Ask client to take weekly weights at home. • Suggest antacid before medication, with physician's order, and give P.M. dose of medication after evening meal unless contraindicated. • Encourage client to try cola, gelatin, dry toast, or crackers if unable to tolerate regular food until nausea subsides. • Encourage fluid intake of at least 2–3 L/day to prevent dehydration unless contraindicated. • Encourage and give sample menus of a diet high in iron and vitamins, such as green leafy vegetables, organ meats, nutritional supplements such as Ensure, and iron or vitamin supplements as ordered. • Encourage increased activity, as tolerated, to help increase appetite. • Encourage client to keep daily journal of meals and nutritional intake. • Instruct client to call the physician should dietary intake decrease and nausea and vomiting occur.
EVALUATION		• Client will show improved nutritional status as evidenced by: • Energy level • No further weight loss • Normal lab values such as Hgb, Hct, BUN, protein levels • Dietary intake with nutritional supplements daily • Improved appetite, fewer complaints of poor taste • Client experiences minimal side effects, including little to no nausea and vomiting.

- Measure intake and output every eight hours. Alkalinization of urine may also be necessary.
Unique toxicities include the following:
- *daunorubicin:* heart damage
- *cisplatin and cyclophosphamide:* kidney damage
- *vincristine:* neurological damage or peripheral neuropathies

Antineoplastic therapy may damage DNA and lead to new malignancies different from the diagnosed primary tumour type. Each antineoplastic drug has its own peculiarities and its own set of cautions, contraindications, and nursing implementation and evaluative measures.

Cytoprotective agents are helpful in reducing certain toxicities. Examples include intravenous amifostine to reduce renal toxicity associated with cisplatin, and intravenous or oral allopurinol to reduce hyperuricemia (see the Dosages table on p. 797). Most of these cytoprotective agents must be given within specific time frames. For example, leucovorin is given every 24 hours after starting methotrexate.

Evaluation

Therapeutic responses to antineoplastic and monoclonal antibiotic therapy include a decrease in the tumour size and in the spread of malignancy and improved energy levels, ADLs, and quality of life after chemotherapy.

Laboratory studies, CEAs, blood counts, X-ray examinations, CT scans, and MRIs may be used to monitor (at intervals) tumour response to chemotherapy. It is important for the nurse to monitor clients for bleeding tendencies and the signs and symptoms of infection or anemia during and after therapy. The oral mucosa should be examined daily to identify dryness, sores, ulcerations, white patches, and bleeding of the gums. The nurse should also assess for oral discomfort and difficulty swallowing. Abnormal changes should be reported to the physician. Yellowing of the skin, abdominal pain, fever, sore throat, decreased urine production, dehydration, rapid respirations, poor skin turgor, loss of weight and appetite, skin lesions, rashes, and restlessness should also be reported immediately to the physician. The side effects of each agent are listed earlier in this chapter and in the client teaching tips box below.

CLIENT TEACHING TIPS

The nurse should instruct the client (as well as family and significant others) as follows:

▲ Report to the physician immediately any black tarry stools, chills, fever, sore throat, or shortness of breath, bleeding or easy bruising, and severe headache, fatigue, or faintness.

▲ Eat a nutritious diet, but avoid foods that are high in fibre, contain citric acid, are hot or cold, or have a rough texture.

▲ Unless you have been told otherwise, increase fluids to help prevent constipation.

▲ Take good care of your mouth, but brush gently.

▲ Examine your mouth daily, and report immediately to the nurse or physician any pain, bleeding, white spots or patches, or sores in the mouth.

▲ (For women of childbearing age who may be sexually active) Use a non-drug form of contraception during therapy and for about eight weeks after therapy, because this medication would be harmful to a fetus.

▲ Avoid taking ASA and ibuprofen, or products containing them.

▲ Expect hair loss. (Your hair will grow back, but may be a different colour or texture). You may want to purchase or rent a wig or hairpiece in advance. The Canadian Cancer Society often has wigs available, and may assist with cost for those with financial need. Contact your local chapter for more information.

▲ Avoid using alcohol and commercial mouthwash (with most anticancer drugs).

▲ Because of the risk of bleeding, do not use a straight razor.

▲ Your periods may stop, or you may become sterile. Your fertility will return to normal when the chemotherapy is finished.

▲ If your blood levels become abnormal, you may need to protect yourself from infection by avoiding crowds and anyone with a mild infection. If the condition is serious, those caring for you may need to wear gloves and masks.

▲ For more information, check out these helpful online resources: http://www.cbcn.ca/english, http://www.cos.ca/, http://www.cancer.ca, http://www.cancercare.on.ca, http://www.canceradvocacy.ca, http://www.bccancer.bc.ca, http://www.oncolink.upenn.edu.

5-fluorouracil

▲ This drug makes you particularly vulnerable to infection. Avoid crowds, and anyone with a cold or other infection. Caregivers should wear gloves and mask.

▲ Make sure to eat foods high in iron and vitamins.

Etoposide or teniposide

▲ This medication may cause infection, anemia, or bleeding disorders. Report any complaints, side effects, or changes in breathing to the physician.

Methotrexate

▲ Use sunblock when outdoors.

Doxorubicin

▲ Besides the usual side effects of chemotherapy, you may experience high blood pressure, a rapid or irregular heartbeat, and (for men) erectile dysfunction.

POINTS to REMEMBER

▼ Cancers are diseases that are characterized by uncontrolled cellular growth.

▼ Cancer may spread, or *metastasize*, from its original site to other areas within the body from the original site of growth.

▼ A neoplasm or tumour is a mass of new cells that exhibit uncontrolled cellular reproduction.

▼ Paraneoplastic syndromes consist of signs and symptoms that arise at a distance from the tumour or its sites of metastasis.

▼ Tumours that are characterized by uniform size and shape are termed *benign*. This includes tumours that show no metastatic characteristics and also show no invasiveness.

▼ Tumours composed of cancerous cells are termed *malignant*, and the neoplasm may be referred to as a *malignancy*.

▼ Malignant growths invade surrounding tissues, metastasize, and migrate to other tissues and organs, where they form metastatic tumour deposits.

▼ Tumour classification is generally by tissue of origin: epithelial (carcinoma), connective (sarcoma), lymphatic (lymphoma), and blood (leukemia).

▼ Antineoplastics are drugs that are used to treat cancer. They are either CCS agents or CCNS agents.

▼ CCS agents kill cancer cells during specific phases of the cell growth cycle. CCNS agents kill cancer cells during any phase of the cell growth cycle.

▼ Chemotherapy, or antineoplastic therapy, requires astute nursing care, with prudent actions and critical decisions. Knowledge is important for client safety and also to protect the client from the adverse effects of antineoplastics.

▼ Clients should be instructed that if the drug they are taking leads to alopecia, the hair that regrows may be a different colour and texture than it was originally. The nurse should provide information about use of wigs and scarves.

▼ Oral hygiene should be performed at least once every eight hours (sometimes more frequently) to prevent stomatitis.

▼ A holistic approach to the care of the cancer client must focus on the client's strengths and minimize the weaknesses at this time in the client's life.

▼ Clients receiving cisplatin are at risk for suffering seizures, reduced urinary output, nephrotoxicity, and neurotoxicity, and require frequent monitoring and astute nursing care to prevent or treat these problems in a timely fashion.

▼ Antimetabolite agents such as fluorouracil are contraindicated in clients with a recent history of or recent exposure to chicken pox or herpes zoster because of the risk for exacerbation of the subsequent or residual symptoms of the disease.

EXAMINATION REVIEW QUESTIONS

1 Irinotecan is most commonly used for the treatment of which of the following?
a. Estrogen receptor–positive breast tumours in Stage IV
b. Metastatic colon/rectal cancer
c. Spinal fluid involvement from breast cancer
d. Testicular cancer

2 The paraneoplastic syndrome that may occur with some cancers is most commonly characterized by which of the following?
a. Diabetes mellitus
b. Liver failure
c. Cushing's syndrome
d. Hypocalcemia

3 Your client has a history of alcohol abuse and smoking. For which cancer is the client at risk?
a. Uterine
b. Breast
c. Thyroid
d. Esophageal

4 Leucovorin may result in which of the following?
a. Rescue of bone marrow
b. Salvaging of the client's kidneys
c. Hypoglycemia
d. Hypercalcemia

5 Should mechlorethamine extravasate, which of the following would be the most appropriate nursing intervention?
a. Discontinue the IV and remove the intravenous catheter or intravenous line.
b. Apply cold compresses to the site.
c. Inject subcutaneous doses of epinephrine around the IV site every two hours.
d. Discontinue the IV fluid and leave the IV in place while you contact the physician for further orders (e.g., an antidote).

For answers see http://evolve.elsevier.com/Lilley/pharmacology/.

CRITICAL THINKING ACTIVITIES

1 Two broad categories of drugs used to treat cancer are cell cycle–specific agents and cell cycle–non-specific agents. Explain the difference between the two categories of drugs based on their mechanisms of action.

2 G.B. is a 45-year-old woman who has just been diagnosed with breast cancer. She has agreed to undergo chemotherapy and will begin a course of combination chemotherapy consisting of a CMF regimen, as follows:
- cyclophosphamide, 100 mg/m^2: orally, days 1–14
- methotrexate, 40 mg/m^2: intravenous bolus, days 1 and 8

- fluorouracil, 600 mg/m^2: intravenous bolus, days 1 and 8
- Repeat cycle every 28 days

   She weighs 61 kg and is 163 cm tall. From the body surface area (BSA) nomogram on p. 39, calculate what doses of cyclophosphamide, methotrexate, and fluorouracil she should receive.

3 Your client is experiencing stomatitis and is taking cisplatin. What kinds of food would you encourage her to avoid? Explain your answer.

For answers see http://evolve.elsevier.com/Lilley/pharmacology/.

BIBLIOGRAPHY

Albanese, J., & Nutz, P. (2004). *Mosby's 2004 nursing drug cards*. St Louis, MO: Mosby.

Anderson, P.O., Knoben, J.E., & Troutman, W.G. (2002). *Handbook of clinical drug data* (10th ed.). New York: McGraw-Hill/Appleton & Lange.

B.C. Cancer Agency. (2005). Extravasation of chemotherapy, prevention, and management of. Retrieved September 4, 2005, from http://www.bccancer.bc.ca/

B.C. Cancer Agency. (2005). Cancer drug manual. Retrieved September 3, 2005, from http://www.bccancer.bc.ca/

Canadian Association of Oncology Nurses. Retrieved September 4, 2005, from http://www.cos.ca/cano/

Cancer Care Ontario. (2005). Practice guidelines. Retrieved September 4, 2005, from http://www.cancercare.on.ca/

Canadian Hospice Palliative Care Association. (2005). Retrieved September 4, 2005, from http://www.chpca.net/

Canadian Pharmacists Association. (2003). *Therapeutic choices* (4th ed.). Ottawa, ON: Author.

Canadian Pharmacists Association. (2004). *Guide to drugs in Canada*. Toronto, ON: Dorling Kindersley.

Canadian Pharmacists Association. (2005). *Compendium of pharmaceuticals and specialties. The Canadian drug reference for health professionals*. Ottawa, ON: Author. [The subscription-based e-CPS is available at http://www.pharmacists.ca.]

Cheng, A., Williams, B.A., & Sivarajan, B.V. (Eds.). (2003). *The HSC handbook of pediatrics* (10th ed.). Toronto, ON: Elsevier.

Facts and Comparisons. (2004). *Drug facts and comparisons pocket version* (9th ed.). St Louis, MO: Wolters Kluwer Health.

Health Canada. (2005). Drug product database (DPD). Retrieved September 5, 2005, from http://www.hc-sc.gc.ca/hpb/drugs-dpd/

Katzung, B.G. (2004). *Basic and clinical pharmacology* (9th ed.). New York: McGraw-Hill.

Lacy, C.F., Armstrong, L.L., Goldman, M.P., & Lance, L.L. (2003). *Drug information handbook* (11th ed.). Hudson, OH: Lexi-Comp.

Lehne, R.A. (2004). *Pharmacology for nursing care* (5th ed.). St Louis, MO: Saunders.

McKenry, L.M., & Salerno, E. (2003). *Mosby's pharmacology in nursing—revised and updated* (21st ed.). St Louis, MO: Mosby.

Mosby. (2005). *Mosby's drug consult 2005: The comprehensive reference for generic and brand name drugs* (15th ed.). St Louis, MO: Mosby.

Skidmore-Roth, L. (2006). *Mosby's 2006 nursing drug reference* (19th ed.). St Louis, MO: Mosby.

CHAPTER

47 Immunomodulating Agents

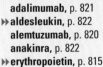
GLOSSARY

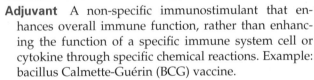

Adjuvant A non-specific immunostimulant that enhances overall immune function, rather than enhancing the function of a specific immune system cell or cytokine through specific chemical reactions. Example: bacillus Calmette-Guérin (BCG) vaccine.

B-lymphocytes (B-cells) Leukocytes of the humoral immune system that develop into plasma cells, which produce the antibodies that bind to and inactivate antigens. B-cells are one type of lymphocyte (see *T-lymphocytes*).

Biological response modifiers (BRMs) One type of immunomodulator (IM) that alters the body's response to disease, most commonly cancer. In the case of cancer, interaction between the host (client) and tumour cells is modified, usually by enhancing the natural antitumour mechanisms of the immune system, which may include alteration of host or tumour cell characteristics. BRMs may also be used to treat various autoimmune, inflammatory, and infectious diseases. Examples include cytokines (e.g., interleukin, interferons), monoclonal antibodies, and vaccines. Also called *biomodulators*. BRMs may be adjuvants, immunostimulants, or immunosuppressants (see *adjuvant*, *immunostimulant*, and *immunosuppressant* [p. 745]).

Cell-mediated immunity (CMI) Collective term for all immune responses that are mediated by T-lymphocytes

(T-cells). Also called *cellular immunity*. CMI acts in collaboration with humoral immunity.

Colony-stimulating factors (CSFs) Cytokines that regulate the growth, differentiation, and function of bone marrow stem cells.

Cytokines (site′ o kinez) The generic term for non-antibody proteins released by one cell population (e.g., activated T-cells) on contact with antigens. Cytokines act as intercellular mediators of an immune response.

Cytotoxic T-cells (site′ o tok′ sik) Differentiated T-cells that can recognize and lyse (rupture) target cells that bear antigens on their surface. These antigens are recognized by the corresponding specific antigen receptors that are expressed (displayed) on the cytotoxic T-cell surface. Also called *natural killer (NK)* cells.

Differentiation The multi-step process involved in maturation of blood cells that begins in the bone marrow with the pluripotent stem cells and ends with mature blood components such as erythrocytes, leukocytes, and platelets.

Hematopoiesis (hematopoietic) The collective term for all of the body's processes originating in the bone marrow that form various types of blood components. It includes erythropoiesis (formation of red blood cells, or erythrocytes), leukopoiesis (formation of white blood cells, or leukocytes), and thrombopoiesis (formation of platelets, or thrombocytes).

Humoral immunity (hyoo′ mər əl) The collective term for all immune responses that are mediated by B-cells, which ultimately work through the production of antibodies against specific antigens. Humoral immunity acts in collaboration with cell-mediated immunity.

Immunomodulator (IM) Collective term for any agent that specifically or non-specifically enhances or reduces immune responses. The three types of IMs are adjuvants, immunostimulants, and immunosuppressants (Chapter 44).

Immunostimulant An agent that enhances immune response through specific chemical interactions with specific immune system components. Example: interleukin-2.

Interferon (IFN) (in′ ter feer′ on) One type of cytokine that promotes resistance to viral infection in uninfected cells and can also strengthen the body's immune response against cancer cells.

Leukocytes The collective term for all subtypes of white blood cells (WBCs). Leukocytes include the granulocytes (neutrophils, eosinophils, and basophils), monocytes, and lymphocytes (B-cells and T-cells). Some monocytes also develop into tissue macrophages.

Lymphokines Cytokines that are produced by sensitized T-cells on contact with antigen particles.

Lymphokine-activated killer (LAK) cells Cytotoxic T-cells that have been further activated by interkeukin-2, resulting in a stronger and more specific response against cancer cells.

Memory cells Cells involved in the humoral immune system that remember the exact characteristics of a particular foreign invader or antigen.

Monoclonal (mon ə klone′ əl) Describing a group of identical cells or organisms derived from a single cell.

Plasma cells Cells that are derived from B-cells and that are found in the bone marrow, connective tissue, and blood. They produce antibodies.

Stem cells The general term for immature precursors of all mature blood cells. They direct the growth and differentiation of distinct cell lines.

T-helper cells Cells that promote and direct the actions of various other cells of the immune system.

T-lymphocytes (T-cells) Leukocytes of the cell-mediated immune system. Unlike B-cells, they are not involved in the production of antibodies but instead have various cell subtypes (e.g., T-helper, T-suppressor, and cytotoxic T-cells) that act through direct cell-to-cell contact or by producing cytokines that guide the functions of other immune system components (e.g., B-cells, antibodies).

T-suppressor cells Cells that regulate and limit the immune response. The opposite of T-helper cells.

Tumour antigens Chemical compounds expressed on the surfaces of tumour cells. They tell the immune system that these cells do not belong in the body, labelling the tumour cells as foreign.

OVERVIEW OF IMMUNOMODULATORS

In the past, care of clients with cancer required an understanding of three treatment modalities: surgery, radiation, and chemotherapy. Although these are highly sophisticated methods of cancer treatment, many cancer clients are still not cured. Surgery and radiation therapy are, at best, local or regional treatments. As discussed in the preceding chapter, adjuvant therapy is needed to destroy undetected distant micrometastases. The advantage of cytotoxic chemotherapy with antineoplastics is that these agents attack tumour cells throughout the body. However, this advantage is also the greatest limitation, because all normal cells are exposed to the cytotoxic drug effects as well. This accounts for the sometimes severe side effects associated with chemotherapy, which often require the administration of various other types of drugs for their control. Antineoplastic drug dosage reductions may also be required, which unfortunately will also limit their ability to cure or arrest the cancer itself.

Over the last two decades, medical technology has developed a group of agents whose primary site of action is the immune system, resulting in some new additions to the class of drugs known as **immunomodulators (IMs)**. These agents can enhance or restrict the client's immune response to disease, or even prevent disease. One class of IMs, the *immunosuppressants*, was discussed in Chapter 44. Another, the immunizing agents, was described in Chapter 45. This chapter introduces some of the newer IMs. Two broad classes of IMs are the **biological response modifiers (BRMs)** and the miscellaneous IMs. BRMs are defined as medications that therapeutically alter a client's immune response to malignant tumour cells. They make up the fourth type of cancer therapy, along with surgery, chemotherapy, and radiation. Some BRMs are also used to treat autoimmune, inflammatory, and infectious diseases. BRMs can be broadly defined as agents that modify the body's own immune response ("biological response") so that it can destroy various viruses and cancerous cells. Current subclasses of BRMs are hematopoietic agents, **interferons (IFNs)**, monoclonal antibodies, and interleukins. These operate by several different specific and non-specific mechanisms and are briefly outlined in table form later in this chapter.

The human immune system is most commonly thought of as the body's natural defence against primarily pathogenic bacteria and viruses. However, it also has effective antitumour capabilities. An intact immune system can identify cells as malignant and destroy them. In contrast to chemotherapeutic agents, a healthy immune system can distinguish between tumour cells and normal body tissues. Normal cells are recognized as "self" and are not destroyed, whereas tumour cells are recognized as "foreign" and are subject to immune system attack and destruction. It is commonly believed that people routinely develop cancerous cells in their body on a regular basis. Normally their immune system is able to eliminate these cells before they multiply to uncontrollable levels. It is only when these natural immune responses fail to keep pace with these initially microscopic cancer cell growths that a person develops a true "cancer" requiring clinical intervention.

Current BRMs work by three common mechanisms. The first enhances or restores the host's immune system defences against the tumour. The second uses agents that are directly toxic to tumour cells and cause them to lyse, or rupture. The third mechanism modifies the tumour's biology. To better understand this important class of anticancer drugs, a quick review of the immune system is beneficial.

IMMUNE SYSTEM

The immune system is an intricate biological defence network of cells that are capable of distinguishing an unlimited variety of substances as being either foreign ("non-self") or a natural part of the host or client's body ("self"). When one of these foreign substances, such as a bacteria or virus, enters the body, the cells of the immune system recognize it as being non-self and eliminate or neutralize the invader. Tumours are not truly foreign substances because they arise from cells of normal tissues whose genetic material (DNA, RNA) has somehow mutated, causing uncontrolled cell growth. However, tumour cells do express chemical compounds on their surfaces that signal the immune system that these cells are a threat to the body. These chemical markers, called **tumour antigens**, or tumour "markers," label the tumour cells as abnormal cells.

The two major components of the body's immune system are **humoral immunity**, mediated by B-cell functions (primarily through antibody production), and **cell-mediated immunity (CMI)**, which is mediated by T-cell functions. These two systems act together to recognize and destroy foreign particles and cells in the blood or other body tissues. Communication between these two divisions is vital to the success of the immune system as a whole. Attack against tumour cells by antibodies produced by the **B-lymphocytes (B-cells)** of the humoral immune system prepares those tumour cells for destruction by the **T-lymphocytes (T-cells)** of the cell-mediated immune system. This is just one example of the effective way that these two divisions of the immune system function and communicate collaboratively.

Humoral Immune System

The primary functional cells of the humoral immune system are the B-lymphocytes. They are also called *B-cells* because they originate from the bone marrow. The appearance in the body of a specific foreign substance or antigen generates a biochemical signal to B-lymphocytes. These B-cells then mature or differentiate into **plasma cells**, which in turn produce antibodies that are chemically specific for binding to and inactivating a particular antigen. The B-cells that are capable of generating a particular antibody remain dormant until the corresponding antigen is detected. The immune system in a healthy individual is genetically preprogrammed to be able to mount an antibody response against literally millions of different antigens. This process has resulted from lifetime antigen exposure from the totality of a person's ancestry, with acquired immune response capability being passed down through many generations.

Antibodies (Ab) are also known as *immunoglobulins*. Antibodies bind to antigens to form an antibody–antigen complex. The antibodies that a single plasma cell makes are all identical; therefore they are called **monoclonal** antibodies. They are made specifically to kill or neutralize the particular foreign antigen that the B-cell initially recognizes as being non-self. Some monoclonal antibodies are also synthetically prepared, using recombinant DNA (rDNA) technology, resulting in newer drug therapies. There are five major types of naturally occurring immunoglobulins (Ig) in the body: IgA, IgD, IgE, IgG, and IgM. These unique types have different structures and functions and are found in various areas of the body. As the B-lymphocytes are transformed to plasma cells, some become **memory cells**. Memory cells "remember" the exact characteristics of a particular foreign invader or antigen, allowing for a stronger and faster immune response in the event of future re-exposure to the same antigen. The cells of the humoral immune system are shown in Figure 47-1.

Cell-Mediated Immune System

The primary functional cells of the cell-mediated (as opposed to antibody-mediated) immune system are the T-lymphocytes. They are also referred to as *T-cells* because although they originate in the bone marrow like their B-cell counterparts, they mature in a mediastinal gland known as the *thymus*. There are three distinct populations of T-cells: cytotoxic T-cells, T-helper cells, and T-suppressor cells. They are differentiated by the different functions that they perform. **Cytotoxic T-cells** directly kill their targets by causing cell lysis or rupture. **T-helper cells** are considered the master controllers of the immune system. These cells direct the actions of many other components of the immune system, such as **lymphokines** and cytotoxic T-cells. Lymphokines are a subset of a broader category of blood proteins known as

cytokines. Cytokines are non-antibody proteins that serve as chemical mediators of a variety of physiological functions. Lymphokines are specifically those cytokines that are released by T-lymphocytes upon contact with antigens and serve as chemical mediators of the immune response. **T-suppressor cells** have the opposite effect on the immune system and serve to limit or control the immune response. They have the most important negative influence on antitumour actions of the immune system. Overactive T-suppressor cells may be responsible for clinically significant cancer cases by permitting tumour growth beyond immune system control. A healthy immune system has about twice as many T-helper cells as T-suppressor cells at any one time.

The cells of the cell-mediated immune system are believed to be the major cells involved in the destruction of cancer cells. The cancer-killing cells of the cellular immune system include macrophages (derived from monocytes), natural killer (NK) cells (another type of lymphocyte) and polymorphonuclear (PMN) **leukocytes** (not lymphocytes), which are also called *neutrophils*. Figure 47-2 shows the components of the cellular immune system.

Therapy with IMs combines the knowledge of several disciplines, including general biology, genetics, immunology, pharmacology, medicine, and nursing. The therapeutic effects of BRMs are as follows:

- Regulation or augmentation (enhancement) of the immune response
- Cytotoxic or cytostatic activity against cancer cells
- Inhibition of metastases, prevention of cell division, or inhibition of cell maturation

Box 47-1 lists the currently available immunomodulating agents that are used in the treatment of cancer or other illnesses that have varying levels of pathophysiology related to the immune system. They are classified according to biological effects.

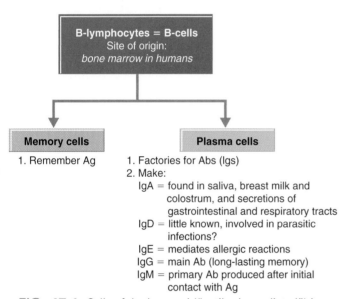

FIG. 47-1   Cells of the humoral ("antibody-mediated") immune system. *Ab*, Antibody; *Ag*, antigen; *Ig*, immunoglobulin.

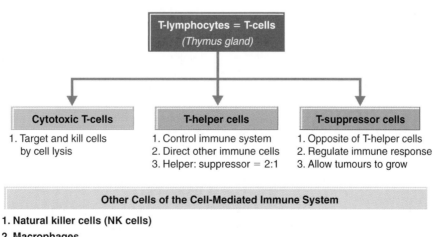

FIG. 47-2   Cells of the cellular immune system.

Immunomodulating Agents

Biological Response Modifiers
Hematopoietic Agents
Colony-Stimulating Factors
filgrastim G-CSF
pegfilgrastim

Other
darbepoetin alfa
erythropoietin

Interferons
IFN alfa-2a
IFN alfa-2b*
pegIFN alfa-2a
pegIFN alfa-2b
IFN alfacon-1
IFN beta-1a
IFN beta-1b

Monoclonal Antibodies
rituximab
trastuzumab

Interleukin Receptor Agonist and Antagonists
Agonist
aldesleukin (IL-2)

Antagonists
anakinra

Miscellaneous Immunomodulators
Tumour Necrosis Factor Receptor Antagonist
etanercept

Retinoid Receptor Agonists
tretinoin

Adjuvants (Non-specific Immunostimulants)
bacillus Calmette-Guérin (BCG) vaccine
leflunomide
mitoxantrone
thalidomide†

*Also available in combination with the antiviral drug ribavirin.
†Available only through Health Canada's Special Access Programme.
G-CSF, Granulocyte colony-stimulating factor; *IFN,* interferon; *IL,* interleukin.

HEMATOPOIETIC AGENTS

Hematopoietic agents (HAs) include several newer medications developed over the past 10 to 15 years. In this category, two erythropoietic agents (erythropoietin and darbepoetin alfa) and two **colony-stimulating factors (CSF)** (filgrastim and pegfilgrastim) are available in Canada. In the United States there is one platelet-promoting agent available (oprelvekin). All of these agents promote the synthesis of various types of major blood components by promoting the growth, **differentiation**, and function of their precursor cells in the bone marrow.

Mechanism of Action and Drug Effects

The same basic mechanism of action applies to all the HAs. They are not directly toxic to cancer cells, but they do have beneficial effects in the treatment of cancer. They decrease the duration of chemotherapy-induced anemia and neutropenia and enable higher doses of chemotherapy to be given; decrease bone marrow recovery time after bone marrow transplants or radiation; and stimulate other cells in the immune system to destroy or inhibit the growth of cancer, as well as viral- or fungal-infected, cells.

All of these agents are produced by rDNA technology, which allows them to be essentially identical to their endogenously produced counterparts in the body. These substances work by binding to receptors on the surface of cells in the bone marrow. These particular cells are called *progenitor cells* and are responsible for the production of particular cell lines (red blood cells [RBCs], white blood cells [WBCs], platelets, etc.). When an HA binds to a progenitor cell surface, the progenitor cell is stimulated to mature, proliferate (reproduce itself), differentiate (mature into its respective type of specialized blood component), and become functionally active. HAs may enhance certain functions of mature cell lines as well.

More specifically, erythropoietin is a synthetic derivative of the human hormone erythropoietin, which is produced primarily by the kidney. It promotes the synthesis of erythrocytes (RBCs) by stimulating RBC precursors. It is also called *EPO*. Darbepoetin alfa, a newer agent, is a longer-acting form of erythropoietin. Filgrastim is a CSF that stimulates precursor cells for the subset of WBCs (leukocytes) known as *granulocytes* (including basophils, eosinophils, and neutrophils). For this reason it is also commonly called *granulocyte colony-stimulating factor* (G-CSF). Pegfilgrastim is a newer, longer-acting form of filgrastim. Other interleukins are discussed later in this chapter.

Indications

There are many beneficial therapeutic uses of HAs. Because CSFs decrease the duration of low neutrophil counts (the most important of the granulocytes for fighting infection), they reduce the incidence and the duration of infections in clients who have lost bone marrow cells as a result of chemotherapy. CSFs stimulate these cells to grow and mature and thus directly oppose the detrimental bone marrow actions of chemotherapy. CSFs also enhance the functioning of mature cells of the immune system, such as macrophages and granulocytes. This results in greater ability of the body's immune system to kill cancer cells, as well as viral- and fungal-infected cells. Ultimately these CSF properties allow for higher doses of chemotherapy, resulting in the destruction of a greater number of cancer cells. EPO has a similar effect on RBCs.

The effect of HAs on the bone marrow cells also results in a decrease of the recovery time of bone marrow cells after bone marrow transplants (BMTs) and radiation therapy. Both bone marrow transplantation and radiation therapy are toxic to the bone marrow. When one or more HAs are administered as part of the drug therapy for bone marrow transplantation, bone marrow cells return to normal counts much more quickly. This helps to increase the likelihood of a successful BMT, and therefore client survival.

Contraindications

Contraindications for the HAs include drug allergy. G-CSF is also contraindicated in the presence of greater than ten percent myeloid blasts (immature tumour cells in the bone marrow) because the CSF may stimulate the growth of any myeloid tumour cells.

Side Effects and Adverse Effects

Side effects and adverse effects associated with the use of HAs are mild. The most common are fever, muscle aches, bone pain, and flushing. The common side effects and adverse effects associated with HAs are listed in Table 47-1.

Interactions

Of the currently available HAs, G-CSF (filgrastim) is the only agent that has any significant drug interactions. The most significant drug interaction with this agent occurs when myelosuppressive antineoplastic agents are given with it. G-CSF is given to enhance the production of bone marrow cells; therefore when myelosuppressive antineoplastics are given with G-CSF, they directly antagonize each other. Typically the BRM is not given within 24 hours of myelosuppressive antineoplastics. However, it is often given soon after this period to help prevent the WBC nadir from dropping to dangerous levels and also to speed its recovery. It is also recommended that filgrastim be used with caution or not given with other medications that can potentiate the myeloproliferative (bone marrow–stimulating) effects. Two examples are lithium and corticosteroids.

Dosages

For the recommended dosages of HAs, see the table on p. 816. See Appendix B for some of the common brands available in Canada.

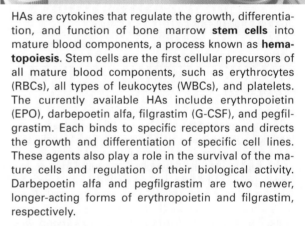

TABLE 47-1
HEMATOPOIETIC AGENTS: COMMON ADVERSE EFFECTS

Body System	Side/Adverse Effects
Cardiovascular	Hypertension (EPO), edema
Gastrointestinal	Anorexia, nausea, vomiting, diarrhea
Integumentary	Alopecia, rash
Respiratory	Cough, dyspnea, sore throat
Other	Fever, blood dyscrasias, headache, bone pain

EPO, Erythropoietin.

DRUG PROFILES

HAs are cytokines that regulate the growth, differentiation, and function of bone marrow **stem cells** into mature blood components, a process known as **hematopoiesis**. Stem cells are the first cellular precursors of all mature blood components, such as erythrocytes (RBCs), all types of leukocytes (WBCs), and platelets. The currently available HAs include erythropoietin (EPO), darbepoetin alfa, filgrastim (G-CSF), and pegfilgrastim. Each binds to specific receptors and directs the growth and differentiation of specific cell lines. These agents also play a role in the survival of the mature cells and regulation of their biological activity. Darbepoetin alfa and pegfilgrastim are two newer, longer-acting forms of erythropoietin and filgrastim, respectively.

▶▶ *erythropoietin*

Erythropoietin is a biosynthetic form of the natural hormone erythropoietin, which is normally secreted from the kidneys in response to a decrease in RBCs and many other stimuli. Erythropoietin is primarily responsible for the stimulation of erythropoiesis (formation of RBCs, or erythrocytes). It is synthetically manufactured in mass quantities by means of rDNA technology. Although not technically classified as a CSF, the actions of EPO in promoting erythrocyte synthesis are functionally similar to the leukocyte-enhancing functions of G-CSF.

Epoetin is used to correct deficiencies of endogenous EPO production common in clients with anemia resulting from end-stage renal disease, HIV infection, and cancer. The use of EPO is associated with two potentially serious adverse effects that should be closely monitored. Epoetin causes the progenitor cells in the bone marrow to manufacture large numbers of immature RBCs and to greatly speed up their maturation processes. If therapy is not stopped when the hemoglobin (Hgb) and hematocrit (Hct) reach a certain level or if they rise too quickly, hypertension and seizures can result.

The only usual contraindication to EPO use is drug allergy. It is available only in parenteral form as a 20 000-unit vial and as 1000-, 2000-, 3000-, 4000-, 5000-, 6000-, 8000-, 10 000-, and 40 000-unit single-use prefilled syringes (phosphate-buffered) for intravenous or subcutaneous injection. Pregnancy category C. Commonly recommended dosages are found in the table on p. 816.

Agent	Pharmacological Class	Usual Dosage Range	Indications
⊪erythropoietin	Human recombinant hormone (erythropoietin) analogue	IV/SC: 40 000–60 000 units 3×/wk, depending on client weight and indication	Chemotherapy-induced anemia; anemia associated with chronic renal failure
⊪filgrastim	Colony-stimulating factor	IV/SC: 5 μg/kg/day	Chemotherapy-induced leukopenia
pegfilgrastim	Long-acting colony-stimulating factor	SC: 6 mg once per chemotherapy cycle	

IL, Interleukin.

PHARMACOKINETICS

Half-Life	Onset	Peak	Duration
4–13 hr	7–10 days	5–24 hr (serum)	Variable

⊪ *filgrastim*

Filgrastim is a synthetic analogue of human G-CSF and is commonly referred to as *G-CSF.* G-CSF promotes the proliferation, differentiation, and activation of the cells that make granulocytes. The three main types of granulocytes are basophils, eosinophils, and neutrophils. They are the body's primary defence against bacterial and fungal infections. Filgrastim has the same pharmacological effects as endogenous human G-CSF, which is normally secreted by specialized leukocytes known as *monocytes,* *macrophages,* and mature *neutrophils.* Filgrastim is indicated to decrease infections (febrile neutropenia) in clients receiving myelosuppressive antineoplastics for non-myeloid (non–bone marrow) malignancies. Filgrastim is contraindicated in cases of drug hypersensitivity and in the presence of excessive myeloid blast cells (ten percent or more) in the blood or bone marrow. Filgrastim is available only in parenteral form as a 300-μg vial for intravenous or subcutaneous injection. Pregnancy category C. Commonly recommended dosages are found in the table above.

PHARMACOKINETICS

Half-Life	Onset	Peak	Duration
3.5 hr*	1 hr	2–8 hr	12–24 hr

*Highly variable.

INTERFERONS

Before the commercial use of CSFs, interferons (IFNs) were the best studied and most widely used BRMs. IFNs are proteins that have three basic properties: antiviral, antitumour, and immunomodulating. Chemically they are glycoproteins (glyco = sugar; protein = amino acid chain). There are three different groups of IFNs, each with its own antigenic and biological activity. They can be separated into alpha (α), beta (β), and gamma (γ) IFNs. They are most commonly used in the treatment of certain viral infections and certain types of cancer. They can be manufactured from genetically modified *Escherichia coli* bacteria *(E. coli)* by using rDNA technology. In addition, IFNs are also obtained from pooled human leukocytes that have been stimulated (challenged) with various natural and synthetic inducers (antigens).

Mechanism of Action and Drug Effects

IFNs are recombinantly made substances that are identical to the IFNs naturally present in the human body. Therefore they have the same properties. IFNs possess both antiviral and antineoplastic effects. They protect human cells from virus attack by enabling human cells to produce proteins (enzymes) that stop virus replication and prevent viruses from penetrating healthy cells. They prevent cancer cells from dividing and replicating and increase the activity of other cells in the immune system such as macrophages, neutrophils, and NK cells.

Their effects on cancer cells are believed to be a combination of direct inhibitory effects on DNA and protein synthesis within cancer cells (antitumour effects), along with multiple immunomodulatory effects on the host's immune system. IFNs increase the cytotoxic activity of NK cells and the phagocytic ability of macrophages. It is important to note that these characteristics of IFNs are ineffective at high doses. Unlike that of conventional cytotoxic antineoplastics, the optimal biological dose of IFNs is not necessarily the maximum dose tolerated by the client. IFNs are also believed to increase the expression of cancer cell antigens on the cell surface, which enables the immune system to recognize them more easily, specifically marking them for destruction.

Overall, IFNs have three different effects on the immune system. They can (1) restore its function if it is impaired, (2) augment (amplify) the immune system's ability to function as the body's defence, and (3) inhibit the immune system from working. This latter function may be especially useful when the immune system has become dysfunctional, as in an autoimmune disorder such as systemic lupus erythematosus (SLE). Inhibiting the dysfunctional immune system prevents further damage to the body.

Interferon: Current Health Canada–Approved Indications

Antiviral Uses (Type of Interferon)
condylomata acuminata (genital warts: HPV) (alfa-2b)
hepatitis (alfa-2a*, alfa-2b*, alfacon-1)

Antineoplastic Uses (Type of Interferon)
chronic myelogenous leukemia (alfa-2a)
follicular lymphoma (alfa-2b)
hairy-cell leukemia (alfa-2a, alfa-2b)
Kaposi's sarcoma (alfa-2a, alfa-2b)
malignant melanoma (alfa-2a, alfa-2b)

Other Immunomodulatory Uses (Type of Interferon)
multiple sclerosis (beta-1a, beta-1b)

*Including pegylated dosage forms (pegIFNs).
HPV, human papilloma virus.

TABLE 47-2

INTERFERONS: ADVERSE EFFECTS

Body System	Side/Adverse Effects
Cardiovascular	Tachycardia, cyanosis, ECG changes, rare myocardial infarction, orthostatic hypotension
Central nervous	Mild confusion, headache, depression, somnolence, irritability, poor concentration, seizures, hallucinations, paranoid psychoses
Gastrointestinal	Nausea, diarrhea, vomiting, anorexia, taste alterations, dry mouth
Hematological	Neutropenia, thrombocytopenia
Renal/hepatic	Increased BUN, creatinine, proteinuria, liver function tests (transaminases)

Indications

The beneficial actions of IFNs (antiviral, antineoplastic, and immunomodulatory) make them excellent agents for the treatment of viral infections, various cancers, and some autoimmune disorders. Box 47-2 lists the currently accepted indications for the use of IFNs.

Contraindications

Contraindications to the use of IFNs include known drug allergy and may include autoimmune disorders, concurrent use of immunosuppressant agents, AIDS-related Kaposi's sarcoma, and severe liver disease.

Side Effects and Adverse Effects

The most common side effects and adverse effects can be broadly classified as flu-like effects: fever, chills, headache, malaise, myalgia, and fatigue. The major dose-limiting side effect of IFNs is fatigue. In high doses clients become so exhausted that they are often confined to bed. Other side effects and adverse effects that can be seen with IFNs include anorexia, dizziness, nausea, vomiting, and diarrhea (Table 47-2).

Interactions

Drug interactions are seen with both IFN alfa products (2a and 2b) when used with drugs such as aminophylline that are metabolized in the liver via the cytochrome P-450 enzyme system. The combination results in decreased metabolism and increased accumulation of such drugs, which leads to drug toxicity. There is also some evidence that concomitant use of IFNs in general and antiviral agents such as zidovudine enhances the activity of both but may lead to toxic levels of zidovudine. IFNs can also interact with steroidal and non-steroidal anti-inflammatory drugs with the potential of reduced efficacy of the IFNs. Vaccines are ineffective when administered during interferon therapy. IFN gamma products can produce additive toxic effects to the bone marrow when used with other myelosuppressive agents.

Dosages

For the recommended dosages of IFNs, see the table on p. 818. See Appendix B for some of the common brands available in Canada.

DRUG PROFILES

The three major classes of IFNs include alfa, beta, and gamma (not yet available in Canada), which are sometimes also symbolized by the lowercase Greek letters α, β, and γ, respectively. The "alfa" designation is synonymous with the Greek letter "alpha," but "alfa" is now more commonly used clinically. The IFNs vary in their antigenic makeup, biological actions, and pharmacological properties. The best known IFN class is IFN alfa. IFNs can be made by using rDNA laboratory techniques with *E. coli* bacteria. Some IFNs can also be collected from pooled human leukocytes. In the body, IFNs are naturally produced by activated T-cells and by other cells in response to viral infection.

IFN products are BRMs that can be broadly classified as cytokines. Cytokines are immune system proteins that serve two essential functions: they direct the actions and communication between the cell-mediated and humoral divisions of the immune system and augment or enhance the immune response. Other cytokines include tumour necrosis factor, interleukins, and CSFs. IFNs were first found to have antiviral activity in 1957. Their beneficial effects in treating cancer were discovered much later.

With the exception of the CSFs, IFNs are the most well studied and most widely used of the BRMs. There are five IFN alfas and two IFN betas.

Currently Available Interferons

Agent	Pharmacological Class	Usual Dosage Range	Indications
▶▶ IFN alfa-2a	Immunomodulator, antiviral, antineoplastic	IM/SC: 3–36 million units daily or 3×/wk, depending on indication	Chronic hepatitis C, hairy-cell leukemia, AIDS-related Kaposi's sarcoma, chronic myelogenous leukemia
▶▶ IFN alfa-2b	Immunomodulator, antiviral, antineoplastic	IM/SC: 1–30 million units 3×/wk*	Hairy-cell leukemia, malignant melanoma, follicular lymphoma, condylomata acuminata (venereal/genital warts), AIDS-related Kaposi's sarcoma, chronic hepatitis C, chronic hepatitis B
▶▶ pegIFN alfa-2a	Immunomodulator, antiviral	SC: 180 μg weekly for 48 wk	Chronic hepatitis C
▶▶ pegIFN alfa-2b	Immunomodulator, antiviral	SC: 1 μg/kg/wk for 1 yr†	Hepatitis C Condylomata acuminata
▶▶ IFN alfacon-1	Immunomodulator, antiviral	SC: 9 μg 3×/wk for 24 wk	Chronic hepatitis C
▶▶ IFN beta-1a	Immunomodulator	IM (Avonex): 30 μg 1×/wk SC (Rebif): 44 μg 3×/wk	Multiple sclerosis
▶▶ IFN beta-1b	Immunomodulator	SC: 0.25 mg every other day	Multiple sclerosis

*May also be given by IV infusion for melanoma. Route and dose vary depending on indication.
†Dose is IFN alfa-2b 1.5 μg/kg/wk if given with ribavirin capsules (see Chapter 38).

INTERFERON ALFA PRODUCTS

▶▶ *interferon alfa-2a, interferon alfa-2b, interferon alfacon-1, peginterferon alfa-2a, peginterferon alfa-2b*

Five IFN alfa products are currently available: IFN alfa-2a, pegIFN alfa-2a, IFN alfa-2b, pegIFN alfa-2b, and IFN alfacon-1.

The most widely used IFN products are from the IFN alfa class. They are also referred to as *leukocyte interferons* because they are produced from human leukocytes. IFN alfa-2a and IFN alfa-2b are pure clones of single alpha subtypes manufactured by rDNA technology. This means that they are consistent from lot to lot. These two products differ in the sequence of two amino acids, but their therapeutic uses are similar. Two newer types of IFN alfa include pegIFN alfa-2a and pegIFN alfa-2b. The "peg" refers to the attachment of a polymer chain of the hydrocarbon polyethylene glycol (PEG). This "pegylation" process increases the size of the IFN molecule and confers upon it several advantageous properties. These include prolonged drug absorption, with increased half-life and decreased plasma clearance rate, thus prolonging its therapeutic effects. In addition, it is believed that pegylation reduces the immunogenicity of the IFN, delaying its usual recognition and destruction by the immune system because it is still a foreign substance to the body. This may also help to enhance and prolong its therapeutic effect.

Similarly, pegfilgrastim, mentioned previously in this chapter, is a pegylated form of filgrastim and has longer-acting pharmacological properties. The alfa-2a and alfa-2b IFNs both share the following indications: chronic hepatitis C, hairy-cell leukemia, and AIDS-related Kaposi's sarcoma. IFN alfa-2a is also uniquely indicated for chronic myelogenous leukemia. Additional indications unique to IFN alfa-2b include chronic hepatitis B, malignant melanoma (an often fatal form of skin cancer), follicular lymphoma (so named because its malignant cells gather in clumps called *follicles*—not to be confused with hair follicles), and condylomata acuminata, which are virally induced genital or "venereal" warts. PegIFN alfa-2b is currently indicated only for chronic hepatitis C, as is pegIFN alfa-2a. IFN alfacon-1 is a purely synthetic (i.e., non-naturally occurring) recombinant product that is currently indicated only for hepatitis C.

IFNs are contraindicated in cases of drug allergy. They are most commonly given by either intramuscular or subcutaneous injection. However, IFNs have been given by intravenous and intraperitoneal routes as well. Alfa IFNs are available only in injectable form. IFN alfa-2a is available in vials of size 9 million units (MU). PegIFN alfa-2a is only available in a 180-μg single-use vial. IFN alfa-2b is available in vials of size 6, 10, 15, 18, and 50 MU. PegIFN alfa-2b is available in concentrations of 74-, 118.4-, 177.6-, and 222-μg/mL. IFN alfacon-1 is available as a 0.03-mg/mL vial. Commonly recommended dosages are listed in the table above.

It is important to note that several IFNs are commonly dosed in the millions of units, often abbreviated "MU." For example, a dose of 10 million units might be written as "10 MU." But the prescriber's writing of "MU" can sometimes be mistaken for "mg" or "μg."

The point: If there is any question in the nurse's mind about the dose of any medication, he or she should double check with the prescriber, pharmacist, or other experienced colleague before administering the medication to the client. The benefits in terms of both client safety and the nurse's peace of mind will always be worth the inconvenience.

INTERFERON BETA PRODUCTS

▸▸ *interferon beta-1a*

IFN beta-1a and IFN beta-1b are the two currently available IFN beta products. They interact with specific cell receptors found on the surface of human cells and possess antiviral and immunomodulatory activity. Both are produced by rDNA techniques and are indicated for the treatment of relapsing multiple sclerosis to slow progression of physical disability and decrease frequency of clinical exacerbations. Drug allergy, including allergy to human albumin, is the only current contraindication. IFN beta-1a, as Rebif, is available in 11- and 30-μg/0.5 mL liquid and 11-μg powder vials for injection. It is also available as Avonex, in a 30-μg vial. IFN beta-1b is currently available only as Betaseron in a 0.3-mg vial of powder for injection. Pregnancy category C. Common dosage recommendations are listed in the table on p. 818.

MONOCLONAL ANTIBODIES

Monoclonal antibodies (MABs) are quickly becoming standards of therapy in many areas of medicine, including treatment of cancer and in organ transplantation. In cancer treatment they have advantages over traditional antineoplastics in that they can target specific cancer cells with great accuracy. This prevents the destruction of normal cells and avoids many of the side effects traditionally associated with antineoplastics. Two commercially available MABs are currently used in cancer treatment: rituximab and trastuzumab. Also available in Canada under the Special Access Programme are alemtuzumab and gemtuzumab ozogamicin. Ibritumomab tiuxetan, bevacizumab, and cetuximab are in clinical trials. Tositumomab was recently approved by Health Canada for use in follicular non-Hodgkin's lymphoma and is expected to be available in 2006. All of these agents are synthesized using rDNA technology. As mentioned in Chapter 44, the "mab" suffix in a drug name is usually an abbreviation for monoclonal antibody. Antineoplastic MABs are starting to be used with traditional antineoplastic agents to enhance the overall cytotoxic effects of cancer treatment.

Mechanism of Action, Drug Effects, and Indications

Alemtuzumab is classified as a recombinant humanized antibody that is directed against the CD52 glycoprotein that appears on the surfaces of virtually all B- and T-lymphocytes. However, it is used to treat chronic lymphocytic leukemia caused by B-cells, which is abbreviated B-CLL. It is used specifically in clients who have failed other first-line chemotherapy treatments, including alkylating agents and the antimetabolite fludarabine.

Gemtuzumab ozogamicin is unique in that it consists of a recombinant humanized antibody that is linked ("conjugated") to a cytotoxic antineoplastic antibiotic, ozogamicin, which itself is derived from calicheamicin, the natural form of the antibiotic that is isolated from a certain bacterial species. This type of drug complex is known as an *immunoconjugate*. This particular complex binds to the CD33 cell surface antigen, which is expressed on the surface of leukemia blasts (malignant immature white cells) in more than 80 percent of clients with acute myelocytic leukemia (AML). The binding of the antibody portion of the drug to the CD33 receptor leads to internalization of the drug complex by the leukemic blast. At this point the ozogamicin component is released inside the lysosomes ("suicide sacs" from biology) of the malignant cell, leading to DNA damage and cell death.

Ibritumomab tiuxetan is another immunoconjugate, consisting of the MAB ibritumomab conjugated with the metal chelator tiuxetan. It comes in kits that also include a radioactive metal isotopes (radioisotopes): either indium-111 (I-111) or yttrium-90 (Y-90). The antibody binds to the CD20 antigen that occurs on the surfaces of both normal and malignant B-lymphocytes. Once the complex is bound to the cells, the tiuxetan component serves to bind the radioisotope, which is administered as another part of the anticancer therapy. Radioactive beta-emission from the bound radioisotope induces free radical formation and cell damage in both the cell containing the drug complex and in neighbouring cells. This drug is used to treat B-cell non-Hodgkin's lymphoma. Ibritumomab tiuxetan is usually given together with the next MAB to be discussed, rituximab.

Rituximab, like ibritumomab tiuxetan, specifically binds to antigen CD20. This antigen is a protein on the membranes of both normal and malignant B-cells found in clients with non-Hodgkin's lymphoma. Antigen CD20 is expressed on more than 90 percent of B-cell non-Hodgkin's lymphomas. Once rituximab binds to these B-cells, a host immune response causes lysis of these cells.

Trastuzumab works by inhibiting the proliferation of human tumour cells that overexpress human epidermal growth factor receptor 2 (HER2) protein. This HER2 protein is overexpressed in 25 to 30 percent of cases of primary breast cancer. It is an adverse prognostic factor for early-stage breast cancer. Trastuzumab is a mediator of antibody-dependent cellular cytotoxicity (ADCC).

Adalimumab works through its specificity for human tumour necrosis factor-alpha (TNF-alpha). TNF is a naturally occurring cytokine that is involved in normal inflammatory and immune responses. In cases of rheumatoid arthritis (RA), elevated levels of TNF occur in the synovial fluid in the spaces of affected joints. In addition to preventing TNF-alpha molecules from binding to

TNF cell-surface receptors as part of the RA disease process, adalimumab also modulates the biological responses that are induced or regulated by TNF.

Contraindications

MABs are contraindicated in cases of known drug allergy and usually in clients with known active infectious processes, due to the immunosuppressive qualities of MABs. Depending on the urgency of the clinical situation, however, a given MAB may be the only viable treatment option for a seriously ill client. In such situations allergic symptoms may be controlled with supportive medications such as diphenhydramine and acetaminophen (for fever control). Many, if not most, clients receiving these potent agents do manifest acute symptoms that are comparable to classic allergy or flu-like symptoms such as fever, dyspnea, and chills. The objective is to control such symptoms as well as possible.

Side Effects and Adverse Effects

Common side effects of alemtuzumab include rash, pruritus (itching), nausea, vomiting, diarrhea, dyspnea, cough, rigors (muscle spasms), fever, fatigue, pain (especially skeletal pain), and myelosuppression.

Gemtuzumab ozogamicin has an overall lower incidence of side effects than do other drugs in this class. The most common ones include rash, herpes simplex outbreak of the skin, anorexia, constipation, diarrhea, nausea, vomiting, hypokalemia, cough, dyspnea, epistaxis (nosebleed), abdominal pain, asthenia (muscular fatigue and weakness), chills, fever, headache, and infection.

Common side effects for ibritumomab tiuxetan include nausea, myelosuppression, asthenia, infection, and chills. The most commonly reported side effects (>20 percent) for trastuzumab include fever, chills, headache, infection, nausea, vomiting, and diarrhea. Fever, chills, and headache are also commonly reported with the use of rituximab.

Potentially fatal infusion-related events can occur with rituximab. Eight deaths have been reported. Severe respiratory events, including hypoxia, pulmonary infiltrates, and adult respiratory distress syndrome, contributed to six of these deaths. Severe hypotension and/or angioedema have also preceded death in most cases. This reaction is termed *cytokine release syndrome*.

For adalimumab, the most commonly reported side effects included localized inflammatory reaction at the injection site, infectious processes such as upper respiratory and urinary tract infections, and higher rates of various malignancies. Such effects may be related to the immunosuppressive properties of this drug, and RA clients are known to have higher rates of cancer, especially those with more severe disease.

Dosages

For the recommended dosages of the antineoplastic MABs, see the table on p. 821. See Appendix B for some of the common brands available in Canada.

DRUG PROFILES

The addition of the antineoplastic MABs has revolutionized the way that certain cancers are currently treated. They are extremely specific agents that target certain tumour cells and bypass normal cells. However, they are expensive and can be toxic. They are used alone and with other traditional antineoplastic agents. All work by relatively similar antibody-driven mechanisms, but all are also directed at specific types of cancer cells. This mode of therapy truly does represent a major departure from previously established cancer therapy, which was randomly directed at generally all body cells. Although the current antineoplastic MABs can still cause significant side effects and are not precisely directed at only specific tumour cells, their scope of cell attack is certainly narrower than that of other cancer drugs, which sets the stage for even better-targeted drugs in the future. Pharmacokinetic data are not yet fully published and so are not listed for the MABs.

alemtuzumab

Alemtuzumab is available only on an individual basis through the Special Access Programme of Health Canada to treat B-CLL, prolymphocytic leukemia, and non-Hodgkin's lymphoma. Its contraindications are drug allergy; active systemic infection; and documented immunodeficiency, such as HIV-positive status. It is available only in a 30-mg/3-mL solution for injection. Pregnancy category C. Dosing information appears in the table on p. 821.

gemtuzumab ozogamicin

Gemtuzumab ozogamicin is also available only on an individual basis through Health Canada's Special Access Programme to treat leukemia. It is designed to treat AML (also called *acute myelocytic* or *myeloid leukemia*). Its only current contraindication is drug allergy. It is available only as a 5-mg vial of powder for injection. Pregnancy category D. Dosing information appears in the table on p. 821.

ibritumomab tiuxetan

Ibritumomab tiuxetan is one of the newest MABs and is currently in clinical trials in Canada, although it has been used in the United States since 2002. It is often given as part of a therapeutic regimen with rituximab to treat non-Hodgkin's lymphoma. What is unique about the drug is its radioisotope component, which promotes cell death due to radiation emission. Its only usual contraindication is drug allergy. It is available only as a 3.2-mg injection. Pregnancy category D.

▸▸ rituximab

Rituximab is one of the two currently generally available antineoplastic MABs. It binds to malignant cells, allowing the body's immune system to recognize and eliminate these cells. Rituximab has become a standard agent to treat clients with follicular low-grade non-Hodgkin's lymphoma who have failed previous therapy. Its only usual contraindication is drug allergy. It is available as a 10-mg/mL injection. Pre-medication with

DOSAGES   Monoclonal Antibodies

Agent	Pharmacological Class	Usual Dosage Range	Indications
adalimumab	Anti-TNF-alpha mono-clonal antibody	***Adult only*** SC: 40 mg every other week; concurrent use of methotrexate OK; may advance to 40 mg weekly if symptoms do not adequately respond to every-other-week dosing, but only if client does NOT receive concurrent methotrexate with this higher dose of adalimumab	Severe, progressive RA that has failed other RA therapies
alemtuzumab	Immunomodulator, monoclonal antibody	IV: 3 mg daily until adequately tolerated (by graded scale), then 10 mg daily until tolerated, then 30 mg 3×/wk (alternate days) for up to 12 wk	B-cell chronic lymphocytic leukemia
gemtuzumab ozogamicin	Immunomodulator, monoclonal antibody	IV: 9 mg/m² × 2 doses 14 days apart	Acute myeloid leukemia
▸▸rituximab	Immunomodulator, monoclonal antibody	IV: 375 mg/m² 1×/wk × 4 doses on days 1, 8, 15, and 22	Non-Hodgkin's lymphoma
trastuzumab	Immunomodulator, monoclonal antibody	IV: Loading dose, 4 mg/kg IV: Maintenance dose, 2 mg/kg/wk	Breast cancer

acetaminophen and diphenhydramine is recommended before each infusion to reduce side effects. Pregnancy category C. Common dosage recommendations are listed in the table above.

trastuzumab

Trastuzumab is the other currently generally available antineoplastic MAB. Trastuzumab kills tumour cells by mediating antibody-dependent cellular cytotoxicity. This is accomplished by inhibiting proliferation of human tumour cells that overexpress HER2 protein. This overexpression of the HER2 gene has been established as an adverse prognostic factor for early-stage breast cancer. Because of the relatively selective expression of HER2 on cancer cells, it has been an appealing target for antineoplastic therapy. The combination of trastuzumab and paclitaxel has produced encouraging results. Researchers are now investigating the combination of trastuzumab with vinorelbine, with study results showing a 71 percent response rate.

Trastuzumab has a boxed warning that administration can result in the development of ventricular dysfunction and heart failure. Clients should be monitored for signs and symptoms of heart failure and ventricular dysfunction before and during treatment. There have been over 60 post-marketing reports of serious adverse events. Hypersensitivity reactions, infusion reactions, and pulmonary events associated with the use of trastuzumab have been fatal. Its only usual contraindication is drug allergy. It is available only as a 440-mg powder for injection. Pregnancy category B. Common dosage recommendations are listed in the table above.

adalimumab

Adalimumab is a monoclonal antibody with specificity for TNF-alpha. It is indicated for severe cases of RA that have failed other RA medications, including methotrexate. However, it can be used alone or concurrently with such medications. Adalimumab is contraindicated in cases of known drug allergy and any active infectious process, whether localized or systemic, acute or chronic. The drug is currently available only in injectable form in prefilled syringes containing 40 mg (0.8 mL) of adalimumab. Pregnancy category B. Common dosage recommendations are listed in the table above.

INTERLEUKINS AND RELATED AGENTS

Interleukins are classified in the immune system as lymphokines. Lymphokines are soluble proteins that are released from activated lymphocytes such as NK cells. There are many interleukins (IL-2, IL-3, IL-4, IL-5, IL-6, and IL-11), and more are being identified as knowledge of the immune system is increased.

The sole interleukin receptor agonist currently commercially available in Canada is aldesleukin. Two interleukin receptor agonists, oprelvekin and denileukin diftitox are currently available in the United States. Aldesleukin is synthesized using rDNA technology and is patterned after corresponding natural interleukins in the body. Another drug, anakinra, is actually an IL-1 receptor antagonist. It is also a recombinant product that is patterned after its natural counterpart in the body.

Mechanism of Action and Drug Effects

Interleukins cause multiple effects within the immune system, one of which is beneficial antitumour action. Aldesleukin is produced by activated T-cells in response to macrophage-"processed" antigens and secreted IL-1. It was formerly called *T-cell growth factor* because, among other actions, it aids in the growth and differentiation of T-lymphocytes. Aldesleukin acts indirectly to stimulate or restore immune response. Aldesleukin binds to receptor sites on certain WBCs called *T-cells*, causing the T-cells to multiply. One type of cell that results from this multiplication is the **lymphokine-activated killer (LAK) cell**. The LAK cells recognize and destroy only cancer cells and ignore normal cells, avoiding some of the toxic effects of standard antineoplastics. A detailed list of aldesleukin's specific immunomodulating effects appears in Box 47-3.

Anakinra is a recombinant form of the natural human IL-1 receptor antagonist (IL-1Ra). It competitively inhibits the binding of IL-1 to its corresponding receptor sites, which are expressed in many different tissues and organs.

Indications

Aldesleukin is currently indicated for metastatic renal cell carcinoma, a malignancy that originates in the kidney tissues, and for metastatic malignant melanoma. It has been and is still under study for several other cancers, including breast, ovarian, colon, brain, head and neck, and lung cancer, as well as lymphoma, but is not yet approved by Health Canada for these malignancies. Anakinra is indicated for symptom control of rheumatoid arthritis in clients who have failed other therapy.

Contraindications

Contraindications to the administration of aldesleukin include drug allergy, organ transplants, abnormal thallium cardiac stress tests or pulmonary function tests.

For anakinra, the only usual contraindication is drug allergy.

Side Effects and Adverse Effects

Unfortunately, therapy with aldesleukin is commonly complicated by severe toxicity, caused by *capillary leak syndrome*. As the name implies, capillaries lose their ability to retain vital colloids such as albumin, protein, and other essential components of blood vessels. These substances migrate into the surrounding tissues, leading to a drop in mean arterial blood pressure. As a result of massive fluid retention (10–15 kg), respiratory distress, heart failure, dysrhythmias, and myocardial infarction can develop. Fortunately, these life-threatening problems are all reversible after discontinuation of interleukin therapy. Close client monitoring and vigorous supportive care are essential in the client receiving aldesleukin therapy. Other side effects and adverse effects are fever, chills, rash, fatigue, hepatotoxicity, myalgias, headaches, and eosinophilia.

Anakinra has a much milder side effect profile that includes local reactions at the injection site, various respiratory infections, and headache.

Interactions

Aldesleukin, when given with antihypertensives, can have additive hypotensive effects. It may also interact with psychotropic drugs. Corticosteroids co-administered with aldesleukin can reduce antitumour effectiveness. The toxic effects of aldesleukin are increased when it is administered with aminoglycosteroids, indomethacin, cytotoxic chemotherapy, methotrexate, asparaginase, and doxorubicin. No particular drug interactions have been reported to date for anakinra.

Dosages

For the recommended dosages of the interleukin agonists and antagonists, see the table below. See Appendix B for some of the common brands available in Canada.

BOX 47-3

Interleukin-2: Drug Effects

Modulating Effects
Proliferation of T-cells
Synthesis and secretion of cytokines
Increased production of B-cells (antibodies)
Proliferation and activation of natural killer (NK) cells
Proliferation and activation of lymphokine-activated killer (LAK) cells

Enhancing Effects
Killer T-cell activity
Amplified effects of these cytokines
Enhanced cytotoxic actions of NK cells and LAK cells

DRUG PROFILES

The interleukins are a natural group of cytokines in the body that were originally believed to be produced by and act primarily on leukocytes (WBCs). They are now recognized as multifunctional cytokines that are produced by a variety of cells but act at least partly within the lymphatic system.

DOSAGES **Interleukins and Related Agents**

Agent	Pharmacological Class	Usual Dosage Range	Indications
▸▸ aldesleukin	Human recombinant IL-2 analogue	IV: 600 000 units/kg (0.037 mg/kg) q8h × 14 doses	Metastatic renal-cell carcinoma, metastatic malignant melanoma
anakinra	Interleukin-1 receptor antagonist	SC: 100 mg/day	Rheumatoid arthritis

▸▸ *aldesleukin*

Aldesleukin is a human IL-2 derivative that is made by rDNA technology. It is a cytokine that is produced by lymphocytes and is therefore classified as a lymphokine. Aldesleukin is currently approved by Health Canada only for the treatment of metastatic renal cell carcinoma and metastatic malignant melanoma, despite its activity in other cancers. Aldesleukin is contraindicated in clients with hypersensitivity, abnormal thallium stress test or pulmonary function tests, and organ allografts (transplants). It is available only in parenteral form as a 22-million-unit vial for intravenous infusion. Pregnancy category C. Commonly recommended dosages are listed in the table on p. 822.

anakinra

Anakinra is an interleukin-1 receptor antagonist (IL-1Ra) that is also rDNA synthesized. It is used to help control symptoms of rheumatoid arthritis. Its only current contraindication is drug allergy. It is available only as a 150-mg/mL vial of solution for injection. Pregnancy category B. Dosage information appears in the table on p. 822.

MISCELLANEOUS IMMUNOMODULATING AGENTS

In addition to the major drug classes discussed thus far, several medications can be broadly classified as miscellaneous IMs. They work by various specific and non-specific mechanisms. A special term used for **immunostimulant** drugs that work by a non-specific mechanism is **adjuvant**. These medications, including some that are classified as adjuvants, are briefly outlined in Table 47-3.

NURSING PROCESS

■ Assessment

Before administering any of the immunomodulating agents, it is important for the nurse to rule out any contraindications, such as hypersensitivity to the drug, egg proteins, IgG, or neomycin. Cautious use with close monitoring is recommended during pregnancy and lactation; in children; and in clients with cardiac disease, angina, heart failure, chronic obstructive pulmonary disease (COPD), diabetes mellitus, bleeding disorders (hemophilia, thrombophlebitis), bone marrow depression, and convulsive disorders. In addition, baseline vital signs and an assessment of infection, level of consciousness, and mental status should be obtained and documented. Before administering any of the IFNs, the client's blood counts (i.e., CBC) should be documented, because long-term therapy with these drugs may lead to bone marrow suppression. In addition, a thorough neurological assessment and assessment of thyroid levels and baseline ECG are important because of the potential for neurotoxicity, thyroid dysfunction, and cardiotoxicity.

IL-2 is a lymphokine that is commonly ordered as an immunomodulating agent. Before administering, the nurse should assess the client for underlying diseases (e.g., cardiac disease) because these may be contraindications. Other contraindications include hypersensitivity to the drug and to proteins of *E. coli*. Interleukin-2 is not to be given at the same time with antineoplastics. Instead it is usually given no sooner than 24 hours following chemotherapy. Serum laboratory values such as CBC, platelet levels, blood urea nitrogen (BUN), creatinine,

TABLE 47-3
MISCELLANEOUS IMMUNOMODULATING AGENTS

Drug	Classification	Indications	Mechanism of Action
BCG vaccine	Live virus vaccine, adjuvant	Localized bladder cancer	Promotes local inflammation and immune response in bladder mucosa.
etanercept	TNF receptor antagonist	rheumatoid arthritis (including juvenile) and psoriatic arthritis	Blocks effects of TNF, a major inflammatory mediator in RA.
leflunomide	Antimetabolite	rheumatoid arthritis	Has anti-inflammatory effects via inhibition of cellular DNA synthesis.
mitoxantrone	Anthracycline antibiotic (also an antineoplastic agent)	Metastatic breast cancer	Inhibits cellular RNA and DNA synthesis and alters chromosome structure
thalidomide[†]	Immunostimulant	Erythremia nodosum*	Exact mechanism unclear, but may have anti-TNF properties, which counter the disease process.
tretinoin	Retinoid receptor agonist	Acute promyelocytic leukemia	Induces differentiation and maturation of leukemic cells, reducing proliferation of immature, disease-causing cells.

[†]Available through Health Canada's Special Access Programme.
*An inflammatory reaction in the subcutaneous fat, often following a bacterial infection or reaction to drugs such as oral contraceptives or sulphonamides.
BCG, Bacillus Calmette-Guérin; *TNF,* tumour necrosis factor.

The Nurse and Client Care

The nurse should never neglect or be deceptive with a client. The nurse does have the right to refuse to participate in any treatment or aspect of a client's care that violates personal ethical principles, but this refusal of care can in no way be through desertion or neglect of the client. If an ethical dilemma arises, the nurse should inform the appropriate supervisory personnel about the conflict and transfer the client to the safe care of another qualified professional. Remember that, as detailed in the Canadian Nurses Association Code of Ethics, nurses are bound by the profession to always remain ethical in the administration of their care to clients. This may include participating in the care of a client who needs the nurse's care but who may be receiving treatment or care that is not "acceptable" by the nurse's own standards or ethics.

urinalysis, aspartate aminotransferase (AST), and alkaline phosphatase should be checked before treatment and twice weekly during therapy. Neutrophil counts must also be obtained and documented.

Before aldesleukin is used, it is important for the nurse to document baseline levels of vital signs and temperature, neurological functioning, bowel status, liver and renal studies. These laboratory and baseline assessments are important because of related toxicity to the central nervous system (CNS), fever, altered mental status, hypotension, tachycardia, and impaired renal and liver functioning. Capillary leak syndrome (CLS) is also associated with these interleukin drugs; therefore it is important to document any edema and assess baseline vital signs and baseline cardiac, respiratory, renal, and liver status. The symptoms of this potentially fatal syndrome include hypotension, reduced organ perfusion, extravasation of plasma proteins and fluid, symptoms of angina, and respiratory, renal, and liver insufficiency. Because of cardiac concerns, the interleukins may not be administered to those with cardiac, pulmonary, renal, hepatic, or CNS dysfunction.

Alemtuzumab, an example of an MAB immunomodulating agent, should not be administered in any client who has an active systemic infections, is seropositive for HIV, or has known hypersensitivity to other like drugs. It is not to be used during pregnancy, and use in lactating mothers has not been established. IFN beta-1b is not to be used in clients with a history of hypersensitivity to natural or recombinant IFNs or albumin (human). Cautious use is recommended in those with neutropenia, anemia, or thrombocytopenia. General cautions include use in clients with mental health disorders, especially depression, because some suicides have been reported. Close monitoring and assessment are the key to the safe use of this drug and other drugs in this category.

Nursing Diagnoses

Nursing diagnoses related to the administration of IMs include the following:
- Acute pain related to the side effects of IMs.
- Imbalanced nutrition, less than body requirements, related to GI side effects of BRMs and IMs.
- Impaired skin integrity (rash) related to side effects of IMs.
- Risk for falls related to weakness and fatigue from the various IMs.
- Impaired gas exchange related to side effects of the various IMs.

Planning

Goals related to administration of the BRMs include the following:
- Client regains pre-chemotherapy (and as near normal as possible) nutritional status.
- Client experiences minimal weight loss during therapy.
- Client maintains or regains normal GI and genitourinary patterns.
- Client's mucous membranes maintain and/or regain intactness during therapy.
- Client is free of self-injury related to drug therapy.

Outcome Criteria

Outcome criteria related to the administration of IMs are as follows:
- Client describes nutritional needs and daily meal planning reflecting dietary needs, such as high calorie, low residue, etc.
- Client states measures to minimize GI side effects, such as eating small, frequent meals and avoiding spicy foods.
- Client is without injured tissue during therapy because of good oral hygiene daily and as needed.
- Client states ways to minimize self-injury related to weakness and fatigue resulting from IMs, such as the use of assistive devices, grab bars or rails, and help at home.

Implementation

Generally speaking, IMs should be given exactly as prescribed and within manufacturer guidelines to minimize CNS side effects. For example, IFN is usually given subcutaneously or intramuscularly and should be given at certain times, such as bedtime, to help minimize the CNS-related side effects. Acetaminophen may be needed for the commonly occurring side effects of headache, fever, and joint aches. Fluids should be increased while clients are taking these medications. During therapy the client should have CBCs drawn frequently; the dosage should be diluted with the identified dilutional substance (usually sodium chloride); and the vial of drug should be gently swirled, not shaken. Sites of self-injection include the arms, abdomen, hips, and thighs. A 27-gauge needle (generally $\frac{1}{2}$ to $\frac{5}{8}$ of an inch in length) should be used to administer the drug subcutaneously.

NURSING CARE PLAN | Neutropenia

Mr. L., a 73-year-old retired fireman, arrives at the oncologist's office with complaints of fever, fatigue, and cough. On examination of the client and assessment of his WBC levels (3.2 × 10^9/L), the physician orders an injection of filgrastim. The client asks many questions about the injection, including what to expect and if it will really help. His wife, a retired public health nurse in excellent health, is eager to help in any way and asks you, the oncology nurse, for some information.

ASSESSMENT	**Subjective Data**	• "I've been coughing for two days." • "I feel so tired and like I have the flu." • "What is this drug?"
	Objective Data	• WBCs at 3.2 × 10^9/L • Temperature 38.6°C • Pulse 110; Respiration 34 • Status after two rounds of chemotherapy • Diagnosis of liver cancer
NURSING DIAGNOSIS		Acute pain related to side effects of neutropenia (joint pain, nausea and vomiting, sores in mouth)
PLANNING	**Goals**	Client and wife will verbalize instructions and side effects before leaving the oncologist's office.
	Outcome Criteria	Before the end of this office visit, client and wife will report or verbalize the following: • Side effects of filgrastim • Symptoms that should be reported to the healthcare provider • Importance of return visits for laboratory studies
IMPLEMENTATION		Client education with written and verbal instructions includes the following points: • You may experience side effects such as nausea, vomiting, diarrhea, sores in mouth, and pain in your joints and bones. • Call us at any time if your bone or joint pain is not responding to rest and low doses of acetaminophen; we may need to order a stronger pain pill. • We will be monitoring your complete blood count and platelet counts today and about twice each week, and we may continue filgrastim treatment until the oncologist thinks your white blood cells are at a safer level. • If you require frequent injections we may teach you how to give the subcutaneous injection, if you are willing to learn the technique.
EVALUATION		Positive therapeutic outcomes include the following: • Absence of symptoms and side effects of infection • Return of WBCs to acceptable levels • Minimal side effects of filgrastim • Increased ADLs • Improved overall well-being

With CSFs, the client's response should be closely monitored. These agents may need to be discontinued if they have a limited shelf life.

Interleukins, such as filgrastim (G-CSF), should be given with single-use vials only. This agent is generally given until the absolute neutrophil count is approximately 10 × 10^9/L, after the expected chemotherapy neutrophil nadir, which is usually a two-week period. The vial should not be shaken when withdrawing solution. Aldesleukin, another interleukin, should be administered by intravenous infusion every eight hours as ordered.

Client teaching tips are presented in the box on p. 826.

■ Evaluation

Therapeutic responses to IMs include a decrease in the growth of the lesion or mass, decreased tumour size, and ease in breathing. Other therapeutic responses include improved or maintained blood counts and absence of infection, anemias, and hemorrhage. Possible side effects are presented in Tables 47-1 and 47-2.

CLIENT TEACHING TIPS

If the client is to self-administer medication, the nurse should teach self-injection techniques, explain about proper disposal of equipment, and provide an instruction sheet. The nurse should instruct the client as follows:

▲ Avoid hazardous tasks while you are taking this medication.

▲ Common side effects include fatigue, bone pain, and flu-like symptoms.

▲ Report signs of infection, such as sore throat, fever, diarrhea, and vomiting.

▲ Report immediately to your physician any side effects such as swelling, excessive fatigue, loss of appetite, and faintness.

▲ If you have pain, the doctor may prescribe a pain medication; do not take narcotic medications.

▲ (For women of childbearing age) Avoid becoming pregnant while on this medication.

▲ If you are going to give yourself injections, make sure you understand the proper technique. Follow your instruction sheet, and dispose properly of needles and syringes.

POINTS to REMEMBER

▼ Cancer treatments have traditionally involved surgery, radiation, and chemotherapy. Surgery and radiation are usually local or regional therapy. Chemotherapy is usually systemic in nature, but it often does not completely eliminate all of the cancer cells in the body. Adjuvant therapy is often used to destroy undetected distant micrometastases.

▼ The fourth type of cancer therapy is known as immunomodulator (IM) therapy. IMs modify a person's own immune system (biological response to foreign invaders) and include immunoglobulins, IFNs, CSFs, lymphokines, cytokines, and MABs.

▼ The body's own immune system is used to destroy cancerous cells. IMs may augment, restore, or modify the host defences against the tumour.

▼ The humoral and cellular immune systems act together to recognize and destroy foreign particles and cells. The humoral immune system is composed of lymphocytes known as B-cells until they are transformed into plasma cells when they come in contact with an antigen (foreign substance) and the plasma cells then manufacture antibodies to that antigen.

▼ There are five types of antibodies, also known as immunoglobulins: IgA, IgD, IgE, IgG, and IgM.

▼ IFNs enhance the activity of macrophages and NK cells.

▼ The IFNs have three basic actions: antiviral, immunomodulating, and antitumour.

▼ Lymphokines are cytokines that are released from activated lymphocytes (T-cells and NK cells), whereas CSFs are substances that regulate the growth, differentiation, and function of bone marrow stem cells, precursors of mature blood cells (platelets, granulocytes, and macrophages).

▼ New agents are being developed rapidly, such as noted with a new CSF (pegfilgrastim) and a new drug used for treatment of anemia (darbepoetin alfa).

▼ Nursing management associated with the administration of BRMs and other IMs focuses on careful asepsis, proper nutrition, oral hygiene, and the prevention of infection.

▼ Nursing care of clients receiving immonomodulating drugs often focuses on comfort because of the flu-like symptoms associated with these agents.

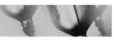

EXAMINATION REVIEW QUESTIONS

1 Which of the following best describes the action of IFNs in the management of malignant tumours?
  a. Increase the production of specific anticancer enzymes
  b. Have antiviral and antitumour properties and strengthen the immune system
  c. Stimulate the production and activation of T-lymphocytes and cytotoxic T-cells
  d. Are retrieved from healthy donors and help improve the cell-killing action of T-cells

2 Trastuzumab should be used cautiously with close monitoring in clients with which of the following?
  a. Malignant tumours
  b. Heart failure
  c. Angiomas
  d. Diabetes

3 Which of the following is an appropriate nursing intervention for the client receiving IFNs?
  a. Avoid acetaminophen products.
  b. Give the agent within one hour of reconstitution.
  c. Force fluids as ordered.
  d. Use NSAIDs and/or ASA as needed.

4 Side effects of IFN products include which of the following?
  a. Hypothermia
  b. Hypertension
  c. Myalgia
  d. Polycythemia

5 Which of the following effects are associated with IFNs?
  a. Antiviral
  b. Antifungal
  c. Antituberculous
  d. Antibiotic

For answers see http://evolve.elsevier.com/Lilley/pharmacology/.

CRITICAL THINKING ACTIVITIES

1 C.F. is to receive filgrastim after a course of carmustine and radiation for a brain tumour. C.F. weighs 60 kg. The protocol that the oncologist has given you states that the G-CSF should be dosed at 5 μg/kg. What dose should the client receive, and what vial should be used to waste as little drug as possible?

2 What is so important about the timing of the dosage of CSF in the treatment of neoplasms?

3 Many medications, especially chemotherapy, may lead to the adverse effect of bone marrow suppression of various blood cell components. What symptoms would you expect to see if your client had diminished production of platelets? RBCs? WBCs? Explain your answers.

For answers see http://evolve.elsevier.com/Lilley/pharmacology/.

BIBLIOGRAPHY

Albanese, J., & Nutz, P. (2005). *Mosby's 2005 nursing drug cards.* St Louis, MO: Mosby.

BC Cancer Agency. (2005). Cancer drug manual. Retrieved September 5, 2005, from http://www.bccancer.bc.ca/HPI/DrugDatabase/default.htm

Black, J.M., & Hawks, J.H. (2005). *Medical-surgical nursing. Clinical management for positive outcomes.* St Louis, MO: Elsevier Mosby.

Canadian Pharmacists Association. (2003). *Therapeutic choices* (4th ed.). Ottawa, ON: Author.

Canadian Pharmacists Association. (2004). *Guide to drugs in Canada.* Toronto, ON: Dorling Kindersley.

Canadian Pharmacists Association. (2005). *Compendium of pharmaceuticals and specialties. The Canadian drug reference for health professionals.* Ottawa, ON: Author. [The subscription-based e-CPS is available at http://www.pharmacists.ca.]

Cheng, A., Williams, B.A., & Sivarajan, B.V. (Eds.). (2003). *The HSC handbook of pediatrics* (10th ed.). Toronto, ON: Elsevier.

Facts and Comparisons. (2004). *Drug facts and comparisons pocket version* (9th ed.). St Louis, MO: Wolters Kluwer Health.

Hardman, J.G., & Limbird, L.E. (2002). *Goodman and Gilman's the pharmacological basis of therapeutics* (10th ed.). New York: McGraw-Hill.

Health Canada. (2005). Drug product database (DPD). Retrieved September 5, 2005, from http://www.hc-sc.gc.ca/hpb/drugs-dpd/

Katzung, B.G. (2004). *Basic and clinical pharmacology* (9th ed.). New York: McGraw-Hill.

Lacy, C.F., Armstrong, L.L., Goldman, M.P., & Lance, L.L. (2003). *Drug information handbook* (11th ed.). Hudson, OH: Lexi-Comp.

Lehne, R.A. (2004). *Pharmacology for nursing care* (5th ed.). St Louis, MO: Saunders.

McKenry, L.M., & Salerno, E. (2003). *Mosby's pharmacology in nursing– revised and updated* (21st ed.). St Louis, MO: Mosby.

Mosby. (2005). *Mosby's drug consult 2005: The comprehensive reference for generic and brand name drugs* (15th ed.). St Louis, MO: Mosby.

Skidmore-Roth, L. (2006). *Mosby's 2006 nursing drug reference* (19th ed). St Louis, MO; Mosby.

Gene Therapy and Pharmacogenomics

OBJECTIVES

After reading this chapter, the successful student will be able to do the following:

1 Understand the basic terms related to genetics and drug therapy.

2 Briefly discuss the major concepts of genetics as an evolving segment of health care, such as principles of genetic inheritance; deoxyribonucleic acid (DNA), ribonucleic acid (RNA), and their functioning; protein synthesis of DNA; and the importance of amino acids.

3 Describe the basis of the Human Genome Project and its impact on the role of genetics in health care.

4 Discuss the different gene therapies currently available for clients and those that are going through Health Canada–approved clinical trials.

5 Differentiate between the direct and indirect forms of gene therapy.

6 Identify the regulatory and ethical issues related to gene therapy, drug therapy, and the healthcare professions.

7 Briefly discuss the concept of pharmacogenomics.

e-LEARNING ACTIVITIES

Student CD-ROM
- Animations
- Medication Administration Checklists
- IV Therapy Checklists

evolve **Web site** (http://evolve.elsevier.com/Lilley/pharmacology/)
- Online Chapter Worksheet • Frequently Asked Questions
- Learning Tips and Content Updates • WebLinks • Online Appendices and Supplements • Mosby/Saunders ePharmacology Update • Access to *Mosby's Drug Consult*

GLOSSARY

Acquired disease Any disease acquired through external factors and not directly caused by a person's genes (e.g., an infectious disease, non-congenital cardiovascular diseases). Genes can be an indirect cause of an acquired disease, combined with external environmental factors (e.g., lifestyle).

Allele (a' leel) Any alternative form of a gene that can occupy a specific locus (location) on a chromosome (see

chromosome). In humans there are two alleles for each gene, one on each of 23 paired chromosomes. One unit of each pair is supplied by the mother, the other by the father. An allele may be dominant or recessive for a given genetic trait.

Chromatin Essentially a collective term for all of the chromosomal material within a given cell.

Chromosome In animal cells, a structure in the nucleus that contains a linear thread of deoxyribonucleic acid (DNA), which transmits genetic information, and is associated with ribonucleic acid (RNA) molecules.

Gene The biological unit of heredity; a segment of a DNA molecule that contains all of the molecular information required for the synthesis of a biological product such as an RNA molecule or an amino acid chain (polypeptide chain).

Gene therapy New therapeutic technologies to directly target human genes in the treatment or prevention of illness.

Genetic disease Any disorder caused by a genetic mechanism.

Genetic material DNA or RNA molecules or portions thereof.

Genetic predisposition The presence of certain factors in a person's genetic makeup (genome) that increases the likelihood of eventually developing one or more diseases, but that can also be offset by environmental factors (e.g., healthy lifestyle).

Genetics The study of the structure, function, and inheritance of genes.

Genome The complete set of genetic material of any organism. May be multiple chromosomes (groups of DNA or RNA molecules) in higher organisms, a single chromosome, as in bacteria, or a single DNA or RNA molecule, as in viruses.

Genomics The study of genomes, including their contributions to diseases and a person's genetic susceptibility to various diseases.

Genotype The alleles present at a given site (or locus) on the chromosomes of an organism (e.g., human, animal, plant), that determine a specific genetic trait for that organism (see *phenotype*).

Inherited disease Any genetic disease that results from alleles passed from parents to offspring. (Note that not all genetic diseases are inherited from parents; for example, there are chromosomal abnormalities [aberrations] that neither parent carries that can occur in the embryo.)

International Human Genome Project (IHGP) A project by an international group of scientists to describe in detail the entire genome of a human being. This project was completed ahead of schedule in 2003.

Nucleic acids Molecules of DNA or RNA. The primary molecular components of genes.

Pharmacogenomics The scientific study of the relationship between genetic factors and the nature of the body's therapeutic and toxic responses to drugs (also called *pharmacogenetics*).

Phenotype (fee′ noe type) The expression in the body of a genetic trait that results from a person's genotype (see *genotype*).

Recombinant DNA (rDNA) DNA molecules that have been artificially synthesized or modified in a laboratory setting.

Genetic processes are a highly complex part of physiology and are far from being completely understood by scientists. However, genetic research is one of the most intensely active branches of science today, involving many types of healthcare professionals, including nurses. Predicted outcomes of this research include an increasingly deeper knowledge of the genetic influences on disease, along with the development of gene-based therapies. If these predictions prove true, the practice of nursing will increasingly require an understanding of genetic concepts, health issues, and therapeutic techniques. The goal of this chapter is to introduce some of the major concepts of this complex and emerging branch of health science. In February 2000, the *National Coalition for Health Professional Education in Genetics* (NCHPEG) in the United States endorsed a set of core competencies involving ". . . the minimum knowledge, skills, and attitudes necessary for health professionals from all disciplines (medicine, nursing, allied health, public health dentistry, psychology, so-

cial work, etc.) to provide patient care that involves awareness of genetic issues and concerns." Box 48-1 lists in further detail these core competencies, which are also adhered to by nurses in Canada. Any practising nurse may be expected to develop these skills, in varying degrees, depending on the practice setting and the needs of the client population.

BASIC PRINCIPLES OF GENETIC INHERITANCE

Humans normally have 23 pairs of **chromosomes** (primarily deoxyribonucleic acid [DNA] strands) in each of their somatic cells (i.e., cells other than sperm cells or eggs, which have only 23 single unpaired chromosomes). One pair of chromosomes in each cell is called the *sex chromosomes* and is normally of the form XX for females, and XY for males. One member of each pair of chromosomes ultimately comes from the father's sperm cell and one from the mother's egg. **Alleles** are the forms of a **gene** that can vary for or against a specific genetic trait. Genetic traits can be desirable (e.g., protection against allergies) or undesirable (e.g., predisposition toward a specific disease). Alleles are said to be dominant or recessive. A person will have two alleles for every gene-coded trait (except for sex-linked traits): one allele from the mother, the other from the father. The particular combination of alleles, or **genotype**, for a given trait normally determines whether a person manifests that trait, or **phenotype**. Genetic traits that are passed on differently to male and female offspring are said to be *sex-linked traits* because they are carried on either the X or Y chromosomes. For example, hemophilia genes are carried by females but usually manifest as the bleeding disorder in males. A female would have the disorder only if she inherited an allele for the trait from both her mother and her father.

THE DISCOVERY, STRUCTURE, AND FUNCTION OF DNA

A major turning point in the current understanding of **genetics** came in 1953, when Drs. James Watson and Francis Crick first identified the chemical structures of human genetic material and named the primary biochemical compound deoxyribonucleic acid (DNA). They later received a Nobel Prize for their discovery. It is now recognized that DNA is the most important compound in the body that serves to transfer genes from parents to offspring. It exists in the nucleus of all body cells as strands of chromosomes, collectively called **chromatin**. As described in Chapter 38, DNA molecules consist of four organic bases, each with its own alphabetical designation: adenine (A), guanine (G), thymine (T), and cytosine (C). These are linked to a type of sugar molecule known as *deoxyribose*. Finally, these sugar molecules are linked to a "backbone" chain of phosphate molecules, resulting in the classic double-helix structure of two side-by-side, spiral macromolecular chains. An important related biomolecule is ribonucleic acid (RNA). RNA has a chemical structure

BOX 48-1

Core Competencies in Genetics Essential for all Healthcare Professionals

Knowledge

All health professionals should understand:

- Basic human genetics terminology
- The basic patterns of biological inheritance and variation, both within families and within populations
- How the identification of disease-associated genetic variations facilitates the development of prevention, diagnosis, and treatment options
- The importance of family history (minimum three generations) in assessing predisposition to disease
- The role of genetic factors in maintaining health and preventing disease
- The difference between clinical diagnosis of disease and identification of genetic predisposition to disease (genetic variation is not strictly correlated with disease manifestation)
- The role of behavioral, social, and environmental factors (e.g., lifestyle, socioeconomic factors, pollutants) in modifying or influencing genetics in the manifestation of disease
- The influence of ethnoculture and economics in the prevalence and diagnosis of genetic disease
- The influence of ethnicity, culture, related health beliefs, and economics on the client's ability to use genetic information and services
- The potential physical and/or psychosocial benefits, limitations, and risks of genetic information for individuals, family members, and communities
- The range of genetic approaches to treatment of disease (i.e., prevention, pharmacogenomics/prescription of drugs to match individual genetic profiles, gene-based drugs, gene therapy)
- The resources available to assist clients seeking genetic information or services, including the types of genetics professionals available and their diverse responsibilities
- The components of the genetic counseling process and the indications for referral to genetic specialists
- The indications for genetic testing and/or gene-based interventions
- The ethical, legal, and social issues related to genetic testing and recording of genetic information (e.g., privacy, the potential for genetic discrimination in health insurance and employment)
- The history of misuse of human genetic information (eugenics)

Skills

All health professionals should be able to:

- Gather genetic family history information, including an appropriate multigenerational family history
- Identify clients who would benefit from genetic services
- Explain basic concepts of probability and disease susceptibility and the influence of genetic factors on the maintenance of health and development of disease
- Seek assistance from and refer to appropriate genetics experts and peer support resources
- Obtain credible, current information about genetics for self, clients, and colleagues
- Effectively use new information technologies to obtain current information about genetics
- Educate others about client-focused policy issues

- Participate in professional and public education about genetics

The following skills delineate the components of the genetic counseling process and are not expected of all health professionals. However, health professionals should be able to facilitate the genetic counseling process and prepare clients and families for what to expect, communicate relevant information to the genetics team, and follow up with the client after genetics services have been provided. For those health professionals who choose to provide genetic counseling services to their clients, all components of the process (as delineated in the following skills) should be performed.

- Educate clients about availability of genetic testing and/or treatment for conditions commonly seen in practice
- Provide appropriate information about the potential risks, benefits, and limitations of genetic testing
- Provide clients with an appropriate informed consent process to facilitate decision making related to genetic testing
- Provide, and encourage use of, culturally appropriate, user-friendly materials to convey information about genetic concepts
- Educate clients about the range of emotional effects they and/or their family members may experience as a result of receiving genetic information
- Explain potential physical and psychosocial benefits and limitations of gene-based therapeutics for clients
- Discuss costs of genetic services, benefits and potential risks of using health insurance for payment of genetic services, and potential risks of discrimination
- Safeguard privacy and confidentiality of genetic information of clients to the extent possible
- Inform clients of potential limitations to maintaining privacy and confidentiality of genetic information

Attitudes

All health professionals should:

- Recognize philosophic, theological, cultural, and ethical perspectives influencing use of genetic information and services
- Appreciate the sensitivity of genetic information and the need for privacy and confidentiality
- Recognize the importance of delivering genetic education and counseling fairly, accurately, and without coercion or personal bias
- Appreciate the importance of sensitivity in tailoring information and services to clients' culture and knowledge and language levels
- Seek coordination and collaboration with interdisciplinary team of health professionals
- Speak out on issues that undermine clients' rights to informed decision making and voluntary action
- Recognize the limitations of their own genetics expertise
- Demonstrate a willingness to update genetics knowledge at frequent intervals
- Recognize when personal values and biases with regard to ethical, social, ethnocultural, religious, and ethnic issues may affect or interfere with care provided to clients
- Support client-focused policies

Source: The National Coalition for Health Professional Education in Genetics (NCHPEG) Web site, Feb 2000. Available at http://www.nchpeg.org.

similar to that of DNA, except that its sugar molecule is the compound ribose instead of deoxyribose and it contains the base uracil (U) in place of thymine (T). RNA more commonly occurs as a single-stranded molecule, though in some genetic processes it can also be double stranded. In double-stranded **nucleic acid** structures, the base of each strand binds (via hydrogen bonds) to the other strand in the middle space between the two strands. This binding is based on complementary base pairing determined by the chemistry of the base molecules themselves. Specifically, adenine can only bind with guanine, whereas cytosine can only bind with thymine or uracil. Figure 48-1 illustrates the location and some of the structural details of DNA molecules within the cell.

A *nucleotide* is the structural unit of DNA and consists of a single base and its attached sugar and phosphate molecules. A *nucleoside* is the same structure without the phosphate molecule. A relatively small sequence of nucleotides is called an *oligonucleotide* (the prefix *oligo-* means "a small number of").

Certain new drug therapies involve synthetic nucleoside or nucleotide analogues (see Chapters 38 and 46). One of these, in clinical trials in Canada, is the ophthalmic antiviral drug fomivirsen. Fomivirsen is an oligonucleotide with a chemical structure that is complementary to a critical part of the messenger RNA (mRNA) of the cytomegalovirus (CMV; Chapter 56); it therefore binds to this mRNA part, preventing the virus from producing specific proteins needed for its infectious reproduction. For this reason it is called an *antisense oligonucleotide* and is the first of this new class of drugs. Other types of antisense oligonucleotide drugs are anticipated

in the near future as one type of gene therapy. An organism's entire DNA structure is its **genome**. **Genomics** is the relatively new science of identifying and locating individual genes among the entire genome, along with their specific functions in both health and disease processes.

Protein Synthesis

Protein synthesis is the primary function of DNA in the nuclei of human cells. To summarize it briefly, the double strands of DNA separate, and a strand of mRNA forms on each through complementary base pairing, as described earlier. This process is called *transcription* of the DNA. These mRNA molecules leave the cell nucleus and enter the cytoplasm, where they are then "read," or translated, by a second type of RNA known as *ribosomal RNA* (rRNA). Individual sequences of three bases at a time along the mRNA molecule serve to code for specific amino acid molecules. This translation process includes molecules of a third type of RNA, *transfer RNA* (tRNA). tRNA molecules transport the corresponding amino acid molecules to the site of translation along the mRNA strand in sequence, according to the mRNA three-base codes. This in turn results in chains of multiple amino acid molecules (polypeptide chains), which are what make up protein molecules. The specificity of this code is important for proper protein synthesis.

There are countless specific amino acid sequences (polypeptides) that result in the synthesis of many thousands of types of proteins molecules. Proteins include hormones, enzymes, immunoglobulins, and numerous other biochemical molecules that regulate processes

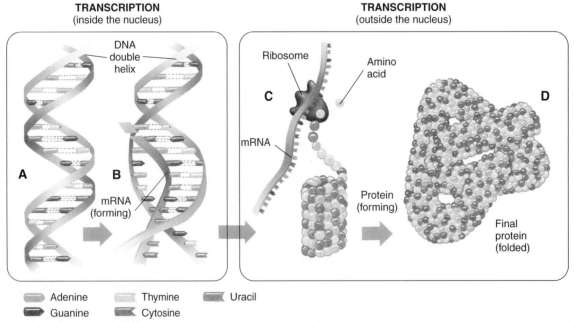

FIG. 48-1 **A,** The DNA molecule contains a sequence of genes. **B,** During transcription, the DNA code is transcribed as mRNA. **C,** During translation, the mRNA code is translated at the ribosome and the proper sequence of amino acids is assembled. The amino acid strand coils or folds as it is formed. **D,** The coiled amino acid strand folds again to form a protein molecule with a specific, complex shape. (From Thibodeau, G.A., & Patton, K.T. (2002). *The human body in health and disease* (3rd ed.). St Louis, MO: Mosby.)

throughout the body. They are involved in both healthy (normal) physiological processes and the pathophysiological processes of many diseases. The biomedical literature, which has grown exponentially, from both clinical and basic science perspectives, has identified and described many proteins that are part of disease processes. Manipulation of genetic material, as in gene therapy (see later), can theoretically modify these processes of protein synthesis and therefore help in the treatment of disease. *Proteomics* is the newest emerging genetic science, taking the discovery process one step further than genomics. It is the science of identifying the structure and functions of specific proteins in both health and disease, and it is expected to provide new drug therapies in the near future.

The Human Genome Project

In the mid-1980s, the scientific community discussed a bold project: to map the entire DNA sequence (genome) of a human being.

Officially set up in 1990, the **International Human Genome Project (IHGP)** was a worldwide research initiative. Planned to run until 2005, the project was completed ahead of schedule in 2003. Specifically, the goals of this project were to identify the estimated 30 000 genes in human DNA and determine the 3.1 *billion* base pairs (bp) that make up human DNA; to develop new tools for genetic data analysis and storage; to transfer newly developed technologies to the private sector; and to address inherent ethical, legal, and social issues.

GENE THERAPY

One emerging effect of the IHGP is the continued development of **gene therapy**. The driving force of gene therapy research is the ongoing discovery of cellular processes, including biochemical processes that occur at the molecular level. The increasing understanding of allelic variation and its role in disease susceptibility can also guide attempts at preventive therapy based on genotypic risk factors.

Gene therapy, still an experimental technique, involves treating or preventing disease by transferring exogenous (foreign) **genetic material** (DNA or RNA) into the body of a diseased person. The overall goal is to either stimulate or provide a temporary substitute for normal genetic processes in the body, such as protein synthesis, that are absent or compromised in a person with a given disease.

During gene therapy, segments of DNA are usually injected into a client's body in a process called *gene transfer*. These DNA splices are also known as **recombinant DNA (rDNA)** and must usually be inserted into some kind of vector for the gene transfer process. Current vectors being evaluated by researchers include spherical lipid compounds known as *liposomes*, free DNA splices known as *plasmids*, DNA conjugates in which DNA splices are linked (conjugated) to either protein or gold particles, and various types of viruses.

Viruses are the most widely studied rDNA vectors thus far. One commonly studied viral category is the adenoviruses, which includes the human influenza

("flu") viruses. If the desired rDNA segment can be inserted into the viral genome, the virus can then be injected into the client to intentionally infect human cells. If this planned infectious process is successful, the viral genome will be combined with the human host cell genome and produce specific proteins to counter a disease process. Ideally this would result in a permanent positive physiological change for the host. However, viruses used in this way can also induce viral disease and be immunogenic in the human host. The resulting proteins produced by such artificial methods can also be immunogenic. Even in the absence of significant virus-induced disease, the positive effects (e.g., supplemented protein synthesis) may be only temporary and therefore future treatments may be required. As a result, viruses must be carefully chosen and modified in an effort to optimize therapeutic effects while minimizing undesirable side effects. The determination of such an ideal gene transfer method remains a major challenge for gene therapy researchers. Figure 48-2 illustrates a clinical example of the potential use of gene therapy.

Many clinical trials are in progress, using various gene therapy techniques. To date no gene therapy has received Health Canada approval for routine treatment of disease. However, these techniques are anticipated to play an increasing role in client care, beginning in the current decade. Originally expected to provide treatment primarily for inherited genetic diseases, gene therapy techniques are now being researched for treatment of more common illnesses such as cancer and infectious diseases. Gene therapy may eventually be used to treat or prevent

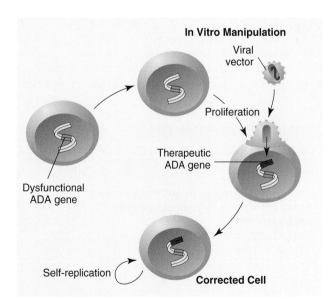

FIG. 48-2 Gene therapy to correct a deficiency of adenosine deaminase (ADA), caused by a rare genetic disorder and resulting in an immunodeficient state. The viral vector containing the therapeutic DNA gene is inserted into the client's lymphocytes. These cells can then make the ADA enzyme. (From Lewis, S.M., Heitkemper, M.M., & Dirksen, S.R. (Eds.). (2004). *Medical-surgical nursing: Assessment and management of clinical problems* (6th ed.). p. 267. St Louis, MO: Mosby.)

genetic diseases that begin before birth or relatively early in life, and **acquired diseases** that are genetically influenced (e.g., atherosclerotic heart disease, type 2 diabetes mellitus). In the more distant future *in utero* gene therapy may be used to prevent the development of serious diseases as part of prenatal care for the unborn infant.

An indirect form of gene therapy is already well established. This involves the use of rDNA vectors in the laboratory to make recombinant forms of drugs, especially biological agents such as hormones, vaccines, and antitoxins. One of the most widespread examples is the use of the *Escherichia coli* bacterial genome to manufacture a recombinant form of human insulin. The human insulin gene is inserted into the genome of the bacterial cells; the resulting culture growth artificially generates human insulin on a large scale. Though this insulin must obviously be isolated and purified from its bacterial culture source, the majority of the world's medical insulin supply has been produced by this method for well over a decade. Various other medications are already made by this method (e.g., hormonal and vaccine products), and others may be developed in the future.

Regulatory and Ethical Issues Regarding Gene Therapy

Gene therapy research is inherently complex and can also carry great risk for its recipients. Research subjects who receive gene therapy often suffer from a life-threatening illness, such as cancer, which may justify the risks involved. However, case reports of client deaths in gene therapy trials have underscored these risks and raised the awareness of client safety among researchers. The Biologics and Genetic Therapies Directorate (BGTD) of Health Canada is responsible for gene therapy research in Canada. It reviews clinical trials involving human gene transfer and schedules public forums to discuss pertinent issues. Human clinical gene therapy trials are also subject to approval under the Food and Drug Regu-

lations, as are any drug trials. The federal government also plays a significant role as a research funder through the Canadian Institutes of Health Research (CIHR) and the National Research Council's Genomics and Health Initiative. Any institution that conducts any type of research involving human subjects must have a Research Ethics Board (REB), whose purpose is to protect research subjects from unnecessary risks. The guiding requirements are outlined in Health Canada's *Tri-Council Policy Statement: Ethical Conduct for Research Involving Humans (TCPS)*. Also required for gene therapy research is an Institutional Biosafety Committee (IBC). The role of the IBC is to ensure compliance with CIHR's *Guidelines for the Handling of Recombinant DNA Molecules and Animal Viruses and Cells*.

A major ethical concern is the spectre of eugenics: the intentional breeding of human beings with traits considered particularly desirable. The prospect of manipulating genes in human germ cells (sperm and eggs), even at a pre-embryonic stage, is seen by some as opening the door to this kind of control, which many would consider abhorrent. Theoretically, even cosmetic modifications could be attempted using such techniques as a part of routine family planning. Ethical concerns such as these have resulted in Canadian gene therapy research being limited to only somatic cells. Gene therapy is therefore currently illegal in Canada in germ-line (reproductive) cells—despite fervent protests by those who believe that human germ-cell research could yield cures for many serious chronic illnesses and disabilities, such as Parkinson's disease and spinal paralysis.

PHARMACOGENOMICS

A second important branch of health science that has been stimulated by the IHGP is **pharmacogenomics**, or *pharmacogenetics*. This involves the precise determination of individual genetic factors that influence the degree of a

TABLE 48-1

CURRENT CLINICAL APPLICATIONS OF PHARMACOGENOMICS

Genetic Technique	Application
Genotyping for the presence of CYP2D6 enzyme	*Psychiatry*: helps guide prescribing of selected medications
Genotyping related to tolerance of tricyclic antidepressants*	*Psychiatry*: proactive use improves clinical outcomes and minimizes adverse reactions
Genotyping for the presence of thiopurine S-methyltransferase (TMPT) enzyme	*Oncology*: used for dosing of the cancer drug 6-mercaptopurine (6-MP) in pediatric leukemia clients
	Gastroenterology: used for observing level of enzyme activity in clients receiving the immunosuppressant drug azathioprine and 6-MP for irritable bowel disease
Genotyping for the presence of the Philadelphia chromosome	*Oncology*: identifies those clients with chronic myelogenous leukemia (CML) who can benefit from the new cancer drug imatinib
Genotyping for the presence of the HER2 proto-oncogene	*Oncology*: identifies a subset of breast cancer clients whose tumours express this gene, indicating their suitability for treatment with the cancer drug trastuzumab
Genotyping for the presence of the APOE4 gene	*Geriatrics*: identifies a subset of Alzheimer's disease clients who are less likely to respond to the drug tacrine

*Under study
CYP, Cytochrome P450 enzyme group.

person's response to medications. For example, one client may be more likely than another to benefit from (or suffer toxicity from), a certain drug, depending on the presence or absence of specific genes in his or her genome. Variations in a person's DNA sequences that give rise to such individual differences are known as *genetic polymorphisms*. Genetic polymorphisms that alter the amount or functioning of drug-metabolizing enzymes can alter the body's reactions to medications. Known examples of such effects include variations in the metabolism of certain antimalarial drugs, of the antituberculosis drug isoniazid, and of the drugs metabolized by several subtypes of cytochrome P-450 enzymes. Studying a client's genome in advance to identify these kinds of features can allow for customization of the type and dosing of any needed drug therapy. Such proactive testing is not yet a part of routine clinical practice. Dosage changes are still usually made on a trial-and-error basis. However, with increasing availability of comprehensive genetic testing, such proactively customized drug therapy is expected to become increasingly common over the next decade or two. Table 48-1 lists some current clinical applications of pharmacogenomics.

SUMMARY

Increasing scientific understanding of genetic processes is expected in many ways to revolutionize modern healthcare. The ability to artificially manipulate and transfer genetic material, while not yet a standard treatment for disease, is the topic of numerous current human clinical gene therapy trials. The spectrum of diseases that may soon be treatable by gene therapy includes **inherited diseases** that are present from birth, disabilities such as paralysis from spinal cord injuries, life-threatening illnesses such as cancer, and even chronic illnesses acquired later in life for which a person may have a **genetic predisposition**. The science of pharmacogenomics has already identified some of the genetic nuances of how different people's bodies metabolize and experience benefit or harm from drugs. Continued study in this area is expected to result in proactive customization of drug therapy to promote therapeutic benefits while minimizing or eliminating toxic effects. Genetic issues and therapeutic techniques will likely become an increasing part of nursing practice, as well as of healthcare delivery in general. As the role and impact of genetics and drug therapy increase, so will its role in the nursing process.

POINTS to REMEMBER

▲ Genetic processes are a highly complex part of physiology and are becoming an integral part of health care that holds much promise in the form of new treatments for alterations in health.

▲ The IHGP was an international project undertaken to describe in detail the entire genome of a human individual.

▲ Basic genetic inheritance begins with 23 pairs of chromosomes in each of the somatic cells, with one pair of chromosomes in each cell called the *sex chromosomes*, identified as XX for females and XY for males.

▲ Genetic traits passed on differently to male and female offspring are said to be *sex-linked traits*.

▲ Hemophilia is carried by females but usually manifests as the bleeding disorder in males.

▲ Gene therapy involves the treatment or prevention of disease by transferring exogenous (foreign) genetic material (DNA or RNA) into the body of a diseased client. Currently it is in the experimental phase, but in the future it will play an important role in client care.

EXAMINATION REVIEW QUESTIONS

1 An indirect form of gene therapy is most appropriately seen in the creation of which of the following?
   a. Stem cells
   b. Insulin
   c. Antigen substitution
   d. Platelet inhibitors or stimulators
2 Use of gene therapy may be immunogenic in the human host and should this occur it would possibly lead to which of the following?
   a. Antitoxin formation
   b. Biological vaccines
   c. Only temporary "fixes" to a disease process
   d. Cures to almost any type of antigen-related disease process
3 Which of the following is the responsibility of the BGTD?
   a. Approving all forms of clinical gene therapy
   b. Identifying all major risks to the human subjects in a specific research protocol

   c. Reviewing clinical trials involving human gene transfer and scheduling public forums
   d. Analyzing genomes and determining whether they appear mutagenic
4 Variations in a person's DNA sequences may give rise to which of the following?
   a. Genetic mutations
   b. Genome metabolism
   c. Genetic polymorphisms
   d. Genome restructuring
5 Which of the following is a commonly studied adenovirus?
   a. Hepatitis A and C
   b. Genovirum
   c. Human influenza
   d. Pallodium

CRITICAL THINKING ACTIVITIES

1 An indirect form of gene therapy is already seen in contemporary healthcare practices. Explain this statement and provide examples.

2 Explain how the use of gene therapy could also be seen as "immunogenic." How would this play out in clients? Give examples.

3 Analyze the process of the production of human insulin and present a few scenarios for how this same process could be used in other areas of healthcare practice.

For answers see http://evolve.elsevier.com/Lilley/pharmacology/.

BIBLIOGRAPHY

Canadian Institutes of Health Research. (2005). Institute of genetics. Retrieved September 6, 2005, from http://www.cihr-irsc.gc.ca/e/13147.html

Canadian Medical Association. (2005). Genomics and economics. *Canadian Medical Association Journal, 173*(4), 329.

Canadian Nurses Association. (2005). Nursing and genetics. Are you ready? *Nursing Now. Issues and trends in Canadian nursing 20,* 1–6. Retrieved September 5, 2005, from http://www.cna-nurses.ca

Evans, W.E., & McLeod, H.L. (2003). Pharmacogenomics—drug disposition, drug targets, and side effects. *New England Journal of Medicine, 348*(6), 538–549.

Goldstein, D.B. (2003). Pharmacogenetics in the laboratory and the clinic. *New England Journal of Medicine, 348*(6), 553–556.

Greco, K.E. (2003). Nursing in the genomic era: Nurturing our genetic nature. *Medsurg Nursing, 12*(5), 307–312.

HumGen. (2005). Genetic research. Retrieved September 6, 2005, from http://www.humgen.umontreal.ca/

Kasper, D.L., Braunwald, D., Faci, A., Hauser, S., Longo, D., & Jameson, J.L. (2005). *Harrison's principles of internal medicine* (16th ed.). New York: McGraw-Hill.

Kimmelman, J. (2003). Protection at the cutting edge: The case for central review of human gene transfer research. *Canadian Medical Association Journal, 169*(8), 781–782.

Lau, N.C., & Bartel, D.P. (2003). Censors of the genome. *Scientific American, 289*(2), 34–41.

Lea, D.H., & Williams, J.K. (2002). Genetic testing and screening. *American Journal of Nursing, 102*(7), 36–43.

Spahis, J. (2002). Human genetics: Constructing a family pedigree. *American Journal of Nursing, 102*(7), 44–49.

Weinshilboum, R. (2003). Inheritance and drug response. *New England Journal of Medicine, 348*(6), 529–537.

Wheelwright, J. (2003). Testing your future. *Discover, 24*(7), 33–41.

PART NINE

Drugs Affecting the Gastrointestinal System and Nutrition: Study Skills Tips

- ACTIVE QUESTIONING
- WHAT ARE THE RIGHT QUESTIONS?
- KINDS OF QUESTIONS
- QUESTIONING APPLICATION

ACTIVE QUESTIONING

One study technique cannot be overemphasized: active questioning. In the PURR study model it is critical to be able to generate questions in the Plan, Rehearsal, and Review steps. The questions you generate are essential in helping you maintain concentration as you study, improving your comprehension as you read assigned material, and developing long-term memory. Active questioning is a strategy that develops with practice; you must practise continuously.

WHAT ARE THE RIGHT QUESTIONS?

Some questions generated during the Plan step will be useful and will focus on exactly the right issues for maximum learning. On the other hand, some questions will seem logical and important when you are working with the limited amount of information available using the Plan step, but as you read the chapter you will find that they miss the mark. Do 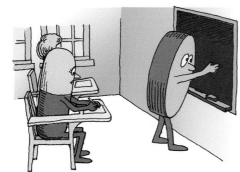 not worry about whether each question you ask is perfectly focused. As you read, rehearse, and review the material, you can and should revise questions based on your growing understanding of the material. The important point is to ask many questions to help you maintain active involvement in the learning process and anticipate questions that will appear on exams. The more questions you ask, the more effective you will become both as an active questioner and as an active learner.

KINDS OF QUESTIONS

First, you must realize that more than one kind of question can be asked. Over the years, educators have proposed many questioning hierarchies, comprising from three to eight different types of questions. Following is a simple approach that focuses on two types of questions.

Literal Questions

Literal questions are those that are answered directly and specifically by the text. When you were reading a story in elementary school and the teacher asked, "What did Sally do when she lost her movie money?" you were able to answer easily because the question asked for specific information that was stated clearly and directly in the story. If you were reading a Canadian history text and found a topic heading, "The First Prime Minister," an obvious question would be: "Who was the first prime minister?" The answer would be stated clearly and directly in the text under this heading. These are examples of literal questions. A literal question usually has a single correct response. The answer is stated directly in the text, and every reader will find the same information.

Interpretive Questions

Interpretive questions are more challenging: they require the reader to interpret, synthesize, evaluate, and analyze the material. Interpretive questions require not only knowledge of the literal information but enough understanding to select several different bits of data and put them together. In Canadian history, an interpretive question might be, "Why was Lester Pearson considered an exemplary Prime Minister?" This question requires you not only to know the facts about Pearson, but also to evaluate and judge those facts to reach a conclusion that can be supported by the literal information. Some interpretive questions have only one correct response; others have more than one correct response. The literal information can be evaluated in a number of different ways, and the answers derived by different readers will vary. Both kinds of questions are essential in the learning process.

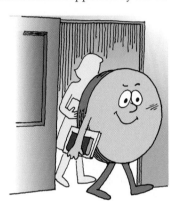

QUESTIONING APPLICATION

On the second page of Chapter 52 you will see the italicized phrase, *excessive need for or loss of*. Italicization is used to gain the reader's attention and to indicate that the italicized material is especially noteworthy. Accented material should always be considered as a potential source of questions. What is excessive need? What is excessive loss? Again, we can begin the questioning with simple, literal questions, but it is essential that interpretive questions also be asked. What do excessive need and loss have to do with the care of the client? How can we determine if there is excessive need and/or loss? What should be done to remedy excessive need or loss? These questions require that you read for broader general understanding.

At the end of each chapter there is a section entitled "Critical Thinking Activities." Even though this information is stated in question form, you should consider generating additional questions of your own. The first question in Chapter 52 is, "Explain why clients with a cardiac history need a baseline ECG and serum calcium assessment performed before initiation of calcium supplemental therapy." In answering it, some additional questions will help you focus your learning. What is serum calcium? How does calcium affect cardiac clients? Why? Is calcium supplemental therapy inappropriate for all cardiac clients? If not, what circumstances might rule out supplemental calcium? Of what signs and symptoms should the caregiver be aware if calcium supplemental therapy is being administered to a cardiac client?

The more active you become as a questioner the easier it will become to ask the kinds of questions that are necessary for your own learning.

CHAPTER

Acid-Controlling Agents 49

OBJECTIVES

After reading this chapter, the successful student will be able to do the following:

1 Discuss the physiological influence of various pathologies, such as peptic ulcer disease (PUD), gastritis, spastic colon, gastroesophageal reflux disease (GERD), and hyperacidic states on the health of clients and on their gastrointestinal (GI) tracts.

2 Compare all of the drugs used in the management of various GI disorders by their mechanism of action and classification.

3 Describe the mechanisms of action, indications, cautions, contraindications, side effects, dosages, and routes of administration associated with antacids, H_2 histamine-blocking agents (H_2 antagonists), proton pump inhibitors, and other related drugs.

4 Develop a nursing care plan, including all phases of the nursing process, related to the administration of acid-controlling agents, reflecting the antibiotic treatment for peptic ulcers and other acid-producing disorders.

e-LEARNING ACTIVITIES

Student CD-ROM
- Review Questions: see questions 357–368
- Animations
- Medication Administration Checklists
- IV Therapy Checklists

evolve **Web site** (http://evolve.elsevier.com/Lilley/pharmacology/)
- Online Chapter Worksheet • Frequently Asked Questions
- Learning Tips and Content Updates • WebLinks • Online Appendices and Supplements • Mosby/Saunders ePharmacology Update • Access to *Mosby's Drug Consult*

DRUG PROFILES

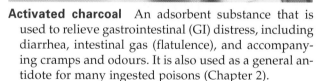

aluminum-containing
  antacids, p. 844
calcium-containing antacids,
  p. 844
▶▶cimetidine, p. 846
famotidine, p. 847

magnesium-containing
  antacids, p. 845
misoprostol, p. 850
▶▶omeprazole, p. 848
pantoprazole, p. 849
▶▶sucralfate, p. 850

▶▶ Key drug.

GLOSSARY

Activated charcoal An adsorbent substance that is used to relieve gastrointestinal (GI) distress, including diarrhea, intestinal gas (flatulence), and accompanying cramps and odours. It is also used as a general antidote for many ingested poisons (Chapter 2).

Antacids The large group of prescription and over-the-counter drugs used to correct hyperacidity of the stomach.

Antiflatulents (an' tee flat' yoo lənts) Agents used to relieve the painful symptoms associated with gas, often by reducing its surface tension, resulting in the breaking up of large, painful gas bubbles into smaller ones that are more easily expelled through the rectum. (See *simethicone*.)

Chief cells Cells that secrete the enzyme pepsinogen.

Gastric gland Highly specialized secretory gland composed of many different types of cells: parietal, chief, mucus, endocrine, and enterochromaffin.

Gastric hyperacidity The overproduction of stomach acid.

Hydrochloric acid (HCl) An acid secreted by the parietal cells in the lining of the stomach that maintains the environment of the stomach at a pH of 1 to 4.

Mucoid cell (myoo' koid) A cell whose function is to secrete mucus that serves as a protective mucous coat against the digestive properties of HCl. (Also called *surface epithelial cell.*)

Parietal cell (pə ry' ə təl) A cell responsible for producing and secreting HCl; the primary site of action for many of the drugs used to treat acid-related disorders.

Pepsin A proteolytic enzyme responsible for breaking down proteins.

Simethicone (sy meth' i kone) A substance that alters the elasticity of mucus-coated bubbles, causing them to break.

One of the conditions of the stomach requiring drug therapy is hyperacidity, or excessive acid production. Left untreated, this condition can lead to such serious conditions as ulcer disease, gastric reflux, and even esophageal cancer. **Antacids** are a large group of prescription and over-the-counter (OTC) drugs that may be used to correct this condition. Overproduction of stomach acid is also referred to as **gastric hyperacidity**.

Another condition or disorder of the gastrointestinal (GI) tract is gas. Gas can appear in the GI tract as a consequence of the normal digestive process and air swallowing, or it can result from disorders such as diverticulitis, dyspepsia (heartburn), peptic ulcers, post-operative gaseous distention, and spastic or irritable colon. **Antiflatulents** are agents that are used to relieve the painful symptoms associated with gas. Other medications for these conditions and their role in the treatment of GI-related disorders are also discussed.

ACID-RELATED PATHOPHYSIOLOGY

For a more complete understanding of the large family of drugs used to treat acid-related disorders of the stomach, a brief overview of GI system function and the role of **hydrochloric acid (HCl)** in digestion is beneficial. The stomach secretes many substances:

- HCl
- Bicarbonate
- Pepsinogen
- Intrinsic factor
- Mucus
- Prostaglandins (PGs)

Each one of these substances has a specific role in the digestive process.

The stomach, although one structure, can be divided into three functional areas. Each area is associated with specific glands. These glands are composed of different cells, which secrete different substances. Figure 49-1 shows three functional areas of the stomach and the distribution of the three different stomach glands.

The three primary glands in the stomach are the cardiac, pyloric, and gastric glands, named for their position in the stomach. The cardiac glands are located around the cardiac orifice; the gastric glands are in the fundus, over the greater part of the body of the stomach; and the pyloric glands are in the pyloric region and in the transitional zone between the pyloric and the fundic zones. The gastric glands are the largest in number and are of primary importance when discussing acid-related disorders and drug therapy.

The **gastric gland** is a highly specialized secretory gland composed of many different types of cells: parietal, chief, mucus, endocrine, and enterochromaffin. Each cell secretes a specific substance. The three primary cells are parietal cells, chief cells, and mucoid cells. These cells are depicted in Figure 49-1.

Parietal cells are responsible for producing and secreting HCl. They are the primary site of action for many of the drugs used to treat acid-related disorders. **Chief cells** secrete pepsinogen, a pro-enzyme that becomes pepsin when activated by exposure to acid. **Pepsin** breaks down proteins and is referred to as a proteolytic enzyme. **Mucoid cells** are mucus-secreting cells that are also called *surface epithelial cells.* The secreted mucus serves as a protective coat against the digestive properties of HCl.

The three cells of the gastric gland (chief, mucoid, and parietal) play an important role in the digestive process. When the balance of these three cells and their secretions is impaired, acid-related diseases occur. The most harmful of these disorders include peptic ulcer disease (PUD), and esophageal cancer; the most common is hyperacidity. Many lay terms (e.g., indigestion, sour stomach, heartburn, acid stomach) have been used to describe this condition of overproduction of HCl by the parietal cells. A commonly used technical term is *gastroesophageal reflux disease* (GERD). This refers to the tendency of excessive and acidic stomach contents to "back up," or reflux, into the lower (and even upper) esophagus. Over time this condition can lead to more serious disorders such as erosive esophagitis and Barrett's esophagus, a precancerous condition. Besides client comfort, this is one of the major reasons for aggressively treating GERD with one or more of the medications described in this section.

HCl, secreted by the parietal cells in the lining of the stomach, is the primary substance that maintains the environment of the stomach at a pH of 1 to 4. This helps to properly digest food and also serves as one of the body's defences against microbial infection. There are many stimulants of HCl secretion by the parietal cells. Some of these stimulants are normal and good. Others, such as large, fatty meals, excessive alcohol, and emotional stress, may result in hyperproduction of HCl from the parietal cells and disorders such as PUD.

Because the parietal cell is the source of HCl production, it is the primary target for many of the most effective drugs for the treatment of acid-related disorders. A closer look at how the parietal cell receives signals to produce and secrete HCl will enhance the understanding of the

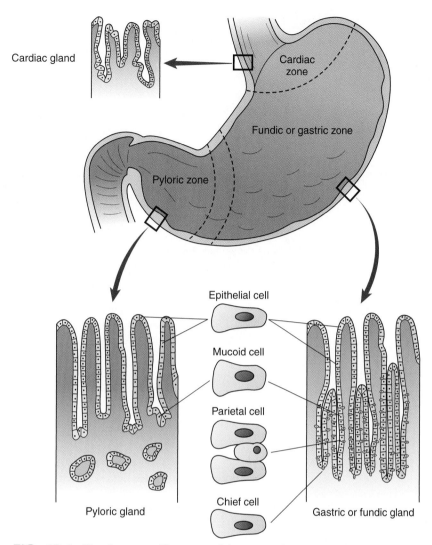

FIG. 49-1 The three specific zones of the stomach and the different glands.

mechanism of action of many of the drugs used to treat acid-related disorders.

The wall of the parietal cell has three types of receptors: acetylcholine (ACh), histamine, and gastrin. When any one of these is occupied by its corresponding chemical stimulant (which can all be considered "first messengers"), the parietal cell will produce and secrete HCl. Figure 49-2 shows the parietal cell with its three receptors. Once these receptors have become occupied, a second messenger is sent inside the cell. In the case of histamine receptors, occupation results in the production of adenylate cyclase. Adenylate cyclase converts adenosine triphosphate (ATP) to cyclic adenosine monophosphate (cAMP), which provides energy for the proton pump. The proton pump is a pump for hydrogen ions located in the parietal cell. The pump requires energy to work. If energy is present, the hydrogen–potassium–adenosine triphosphatase (ATPase) system, which drives the proton pump, will be activated and the pump will be able to produce hydrogen ions needed for the production of HCl. In the case of both ACh and gastrin receptors on the parietal

cell surfaces, the second messenger that drives the proton pump is not cAMP but is instead a calcium ion.

Ranitidine, famotidine, nizatidine, and cimetidine block hydrogen ion secretion from the parietal cells by binding to histamine₂ (H₂) receptors. For this reason these medications are classified as H₂ receptor blockers (also known as *H₂ antagonists*, the term used in this chapter). Anticholinergic drugs (Chapter 20), such as atropine block ACh receptors, also result in decreased hydrogen ion secretion from the parietal cells. There is currently no drug to block the binding of the hormone gastrin to its corresponding receptor on the parietal cell surface. However, one of the newest class of antacid gastric medications is even more powerful than the H₂ antagonists. Proton pump inhibitors (PPIs) bind directly to the H⁺/K⁺ ATPase pump mechanism itself and irreversibly inhibit this enzyme, resulting in a total inhibition of hydrogen ion secretion from the parietal cells. These medications work for up to 24 hours at a time and include omeprazole, lansoprazole, rabeprazole, pantoprazole, and esomeprazole.

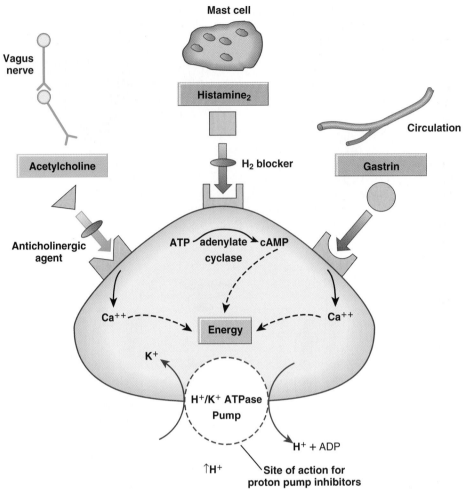

FIG. 49-2 Parietal cell stimulation and secretion.

PUD is a general term for gastric or duodenal ulcers that involve digestion of GI mucosa by the enzyme pepsin, which normally serves to break down only food proteins. Pepsin is the activated form of pepsinogen that is produced by the chief cells of the stomach in response to HCl released from the parietal cells. The sight, smell, taste, and presence of food in the stomach stimulates HCl release from the parietal cells. Because the process of ulceration is driven by the proteolytic (protein breakdown) actions of pepsin together with the caustic effects of HCl, PUD and related problems are also referred to by the more general term *acid–peptic disorders.*

In 1983 a certain gram-negative spiral bacterium, *Campylobacter pylori,* was isolated from several clients with gastritis. Over the next six years this bacterium was further studied and it was gradually understood to be implicated in the pathophysiology of PUD. At this time the official name of this bacterium was changed to *Heli-cobacter pylori* because it was felt to have more characteristics of the *Helicobacter* genus. The prevalence of *H. pylori* as measured by serum antibody tests is approximately 40 to 60 percent for clients over 60 years of age and only 10 percent for those under 30 years of age. The bacterium is found in the GI tract of roughly 90 percent of clients

with duodenal ulcers and 70 percent of those with gastric ulcers. However, the bacterium is also found in many clients who do not have PUD, suggesting that more than one factor is involved in ulceration. The bacterium is also not associated with a serious condition known as an acute perforated duodenal ulcer, again suggesting that other factors are involved in this condition.

Drug treatment of PUD generally now consists of one or more of the following: antacids to neutralize acid already present, H_2 antagonists or PPIs to inhibit further acid secretion, sucralfate to protect ulcerated areas from further damage, and antibiotics to eradicate the *H. pylori* organism. Commonly used antibiotics for this purpose include bismuth subsalicylate (Chapter 50), amoxicillin, clarithromycin, metronidazole, and tetracycline.

OVERVIEW OF ACID-CONTROLLING AGENTS

Antacids, antiflatulents, H_2 antagonists, and PPIs are some of the many commonly used drugs to treat acid-related disorders. Some of the other drugs that may be used to treat acid-related and other disorders are sucralfate, misoprostol, bismuth, anticholinergics, and tricyclic antidepressants (TCAs). Some of these agents, such as anticholinergics and TCAs, are mentioned in other chapters. Sucralfate and misoprostol are discussed in this chapter.

ANTACIDS

Antacids have been used for centuries in the treatment of clients with acid-related disorders. The ancient Greeks used crushed coral (calcium carbonate) in the first century AD to treat clients with dyspepsia. Antacids were the principal anti-ulcer treatment until the availability of the H_2 antagonists in the late 1970s. For decades the classic treatment for acid-related disorders was a combination anticholinergic/antacid regimen. H_2 antagonists, PPIs, surface protective agents, and mucus-producing PGs are rapidly replacing the anticholinergics for the treatment of acid-related GI disease. However, the antacids are still extensively used, especially on the OTC market. They are available in a variety of dosage preparations as sole antacid preparations or in multiple antacid formulations. In addition, many antacid preparations contain the antiflatulent agent **simethicone**, which reduces gas and bloating.

There are basically three forms of antacids: aluminum based, magnesium based, and calcium based. Many aluminum-based formulations also contain magnesium, which contributes to the acid-neutralizing capacity and counteracts the constipating effects of aluminum. There are multiple salts of calcium. Calcium carbonate is the most commonly used salt of calcium when calcium is used as an antacid. It is not used as often as the other antacids because its use may result in kidney stones and increased gastric acid secretion. Sodium bicarbonate is a highly soluble antacid form with a quick onset but a short duration of action. It may also cause metabolic alkalosis.

Some of the available aluminum, magnesium, and calcium salts that are used in many of the antacid formulations are listed in Box 49-1. There are far too many individual antacid products on the market to mention all formulations. Briefly, OTC antacid formulations are available as capsules, chewable tablets, effervescent granules and tablets, powders, suspensions, and tablets. This allows clients a variety of options for self-medication.

Mechanism of Action and Drug Effects

As the name implies, antacids were originally believed to work by neutralizing gastric acidity. They do nothing to prevent the overproduction of acid but neutralize it once it is in the stomach. It is now believed that, especially at low doses, antacids promote gastric mucosal defensive mechanisms. They do this by stimulating mucus, PG, and bicarbonate secretion from the cells inside the gastric glands. Mucus serves as a protective barrier against the destructive properties of HCl. Bicarbonate helps buffer the acidic properties of HCl. PGs prevent histamine from binding to its corresponding parietal cell receptors, preventing the production of adenylate cyclase. Without adenylate cyclase, no cAMP is formed and no second messenger is available to activate the proton pump.

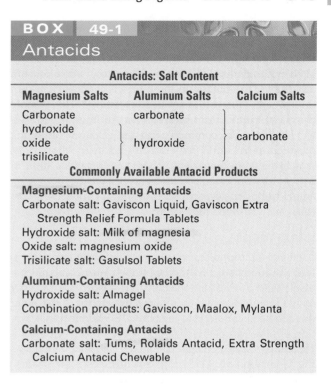

BOX 49-1
Antacids

Antacids: Salt Content		
Magnesium Salts	**Aluminum Salts**	**Calcium Salts**
Carbonate hydroxide oxide trisilicate	carbonate hydroxide	carbonate

Commonly Available Antacid Products

Magnesium-Containing Antacids
Carbonate salt: Gaviscon Liquid, Gaviscon Extra Strength Relief Formula Tablets
Hydroxide salt: Milk of magnesia
Oxide salt: magnesium oxide
Trisilicate salt: Gasulsol Tablets

Aluminum-Containing Antacids
Hydroxide salt: Almagel
Combination products: Gaviscon, Maalox, Mylanta

Calcium-Containing Antacids
Carbonate salt: Tums, Rolaids Antacid, Extra Strength Calcium Antacid Chewable

The primary drug effect of antacids is the reduction of the symptoms associated with various acid-related disorders, such as PUD and hyperacidity disorders. By raising the pH of the stomach from 1.3 to 1.6 (only 0.3 points), acid in the gastric juices will be 50 percent neutralized; if the pH is raised an entire point, from 1.3 to 2.3, a 90 percent reduction of acid will occur. This reduces the pain associated with acid-related disorders.

The ability of antacids to reduce the pain associated with acid-related disorders is thought to be a result of inhibition of the protein-digesting ability of pepsin; an increase in the resistance of the stomach lining to irritation; and an increase in the tone of the lower esophageal sphincter, which reduces reflux from the stomach.

Indications

Antacids are selected for their potential acid-neutralizing capacity and their onset of action. Antacids are indicated for the relief of symptoms associated with hyperacidity related to peptic ulcer, gastritis, gastric hyperacidity, and heartburn.

Contraindications

The only usual contraindication to antacid use is known allergy to a specific drug product. Other contraindications may include severe renal failure and GI obstruction.

Side Effects and Adverse Effects

The side effects and adverse effects of the antacids are limited. The magnesium preparations, especially milk of magnesia, can cause diarrhea. They should also be used with caution or not at all in clients with renal failure. Excretion of magnesium ions is often compromised with kidney failure. Instead, magnesium accumulates and may lead to toxicity. Both the aluminum- and calcium-containing formulations can result in constipation. For this reason many combination antacids have been formulated with agents that have counteracting side effects in an attempt to ameliorate these effects. Excessive use of these agents can result in systemic alkalosis. This is more common with sodium bicarbonate. Another adverse effect that is more common with the calcium-containing products is rebound hyperacidity, or acid rebound, in which the client experiences hyperacidity when antacid use is discontinued. Long-term self-medication with antacids may mask symptoms of serious underlying diseases such as bleeding ulcers.

Interactions

Antacids are capable of causing several drug interactions when administered with other drugs. Four basic mechanisms lead to these interactions: (1) adsorption of other drugs to antacids, which reduces the ability of the other drug to be absorbed into the body; (2) chemical inactivation of other drugs by chelation, which produces insoluble complexes; (3) increased stomach pH, which increases the absorption of basic drugs and decreases the absorption of acidic drugs; and (4) increased urinary pH, which increases the excretion of acidic drugs and decreases the excretion of basic drugs. Most drugs are either weak acids or weak bases. Therefore pH conditions, both in the GI and urinary systems, will affect the extent to which drug molecules are ionized (charged). Ionized drug molecules are generally more water soluble and therefore more likely to be excreted (at the kidney) or not absorbed (from the GI tract). Non-ionized drug molecules are more likely to be absorbed in the GI tract because they are usually more fat soluble than their ionized counterparts. This allows them to be better absorbed through the lipid-based cell membranes of the GI tract and ultimately into the bloodstream.

Medications whose effects are increased by the use of antacids include quinidine (antidysrhythmic), pseu-doephedrine (decongestant), levodopa (antiparkinson agent), valproic acid (anticonvulsant), and dicumarol (anticoagulant). Medications with decreased effects when used simultaneously with antacids include digoxin (cardiac glycoside), corticosteroids, cimetidine and ranitidine (H_2 antagonists), iron preparations, phenothiazines (antiemetics and tranquilizer), salicylates (acetylsalicylic acid), and isoniazid (INH, antituberculin agent).

Dosages

For information on dosages for selected antacid agents, see the dosages table below. See Appendix B for some of the common brands in Canada.

DRUG PROFILES

Many antacids and antacid combinations are available. One way to categorize the large family of antacid drugs is to separate them by the type of metal they contain: aluminum, calcium, or magnesium. The pregnancy category is not established, but antacids are generally considered safe for use in pregnancy if prolonged or high doses are avoided. However, it is recommended that pregnant women consult their physician before using an antacid. Most antacids are OTC drugs.

aluminum-containing antacids

The amount of antacid necessary to neutralize HCl depends on the client, the condition being treated, and the buffering capacity of the preparation used. The acid-neutralizing property of antacids varies. Examples of aluminum-containing antacids and aluminum-magnesium combination products are listed in Box 49-1.

calcium-containing antacids

Calcium-containing antacids are currently advertised as an extra source of calcium. Calcium carbonate neutralization will produce gas and possibly belching. For this reason it may be combined with an antiflatulent type of drug such as simethicone. Calcium-containing products

DOSAGES) Selected Antacid Agents*

Agent	Pharmacological Class	Usual Dosage Range	Indications
aluminum hydroxide	Aluminum-containing antacid	**Adult** PO: 600–1500 mg 3–6×/day	Hyperacidity (often the preferred antacid for use in renally compromised clients)
aluminum hydroxide and magnesium hydroxide	Combination antacid	**Adult** PO: 400–2400 mg 3–6 ×/day	Hyperacidity
calcium carbonate	Calcium-containing antacid	**Adult** PO: 0.5–1.5 g prn	Hyperacidity
magnesium hydroxide	Magnesium-containing antacid	**Adult** PO: 0.65–1.3 g prn, up to qid **Pediatric** Dose is ¼–½ adult dose	Hyperacidity (more commonly used as a laxative)

*There are many more available antacid products on the market than appear in this table. Dosages given are approximate dosages of active ingredients, keeping in mind that there may be variations among different products and different dosage forms of the same product.

have a long duration of acid action, which can cause hyperacidity rebound on abrupt discontinuation. One example of a calcium-containing antacid is calcium carbonate (Tums).

magnesium-containing antacids

Magnesium-containing antacids commonly cause a laxative effect, and frequent administration of these antacids alone often cannot be tolerated. The administration of magnesium-containing antacids is dangerous in clients with renal failure because the failing kidney cannot excrete the extra magnesium and accumulation may occur. Examples of magnesium-containing antacids are listed in Box 49-1.

Other agents that may be added in antacid combination products are antiflatulents. Flatulence is the passage of gas via the rectum, a disturbing symptom for many clients but rarely an indicator of serious disease. Gas in the upper GI tract is composed of swallowed air and is thus largely nitrogen. It is usually expelled from the body by belching. However, the composition of flatulence is determined largely by dietary intake of carbohydrates and the metabolic activity of the bacteria in the intestines. These bacteria are anaerobic and produce fermentation with the production of hydrogen (H_2), carbon dioxide (CO_2), and methane (CH_4).

Several agents have been used to bind or alter intestinal gas. **Activated charcoal** and simethicone are OTC antiflatulents and may be added to many antacid products. They are also available as sole agents. Activated charcoal appears to be effective in reducing belching and intestinal complaints caused by ingestion of indigestible carbohydrates. Simethicone alters the elasticity of mucus-coated bubbles, which causes the bubbles to break. Although simethicone is commonly used, limited data support its effectiveness.

H₂ ANTAGONISTS

H_2 antagonists are the prototypical acid secretory antagonists. These agents reduce but do not abolish stimulated acid secretion. They have become the most popular drugs for the treatment of many acid-related disorders, including PUD. This can be attributed to their efficacy, client acceptance, and excellent safety profile. There are presently four H_2 antagonists approved by Health Canada, which are listed in the drug profiles.

There is little difference among the four available H_2 antagonists from an efficacy standpoint. Their relative potencies differ, but increased potency does not necessarily confer a therapeutic advantage, provided the drugs can be administered in equipotent doses without toxicity. All four available H_2 antagonists are available OTC. The strength of the OTC dose is generally half that of the usual prescription dosage strength.

Mechanism of Action and Drug Effects

The drug effects of the H_2 antagonists are limited to specific blocking actions on the parietal cells of the gastric glands in the stomach. The parietal cells are responsible for the production of hydrogen ions and ultimately HCl. The H_2 antagonists compete with histamine for binding sites on the surface of parietal cells. The drug effects of H_2 antagonists are decreased hydrogen ion production from the parietal cells, which results in an increase in the pH of the stomach and relief of many of the symptoms associated with hyperacid-secreting conditions. The efficacy of the H_2 antagonists is related to their ability to competitively block the H_2 receptor of acid-producing parietal cells, thus rendering the cells less responsive not only to histamine but also to the stimulation of ACh and gastrin. This is shown in Figure 49-2. Up to 90 percent inhibition of vagal- and gastrin-stimulated acid secretion occurs by blocking histamine. However, complete inhibition has not been shown.

Indications

H_2 antagonists have several therapeutic uses, including GERD, PUD, erosive esophagitis, adjunct therapy in control of upper GI bleeding, and pathological gastric hypersecretory conditions such as Zollinger-Ellison syndrome. This is one form of hyperchlorhydria, or excessive gastric acidity.

Contraindications

The only usual contraindication to the use of H_2 antagonists is known drug allergy.

Side Effects and Adverse Effects

H_2 antagonists have a remarkably low incidence of side effects (less than three percent). The four available H_2 antagonists are similar in many respects but have some differences in side effect profiles. Table 49-1 lists the side effects and adverse effects seen with these agents. Central nervous system (CNS) side effects occur in less than one percent of clients taking H_2 antagonists. Cimetidine may induce erectile dysfunction and gynecomastia (breast development in males). This is the result of cimetidine inhibiting estradiol metabolism and displacement of dihydrotestosterone from peripheral androgen-binding sites. All four H_2 antagonists may increase the secretion of prolactin from the anterior pituitary.

TABLE 49-1

H₂ ANTAGONISTS: ADVERSE EFFECTS

Body System	Side/Adverse Effects
Central nervous	Headache, lethargy, confusion, depression, hallucinations (<1% total), slurred speech
Endocrine	Erectile dysfunction, increased prolactin, gynecomastia (with cimetidine)
Gastrointestinal	Diarrhea, abdominal cramps, jaundice
Genitourinary	Increased BUN, liver function tests, creatinine
Hematological	Agranulocytosis, thrombocytopenia, neutropenia, aplastic anemia
Integumentary	Urticaria, rash, alopecia, sweating, flushing, exfoliative dermatitis

BUN, Blood urea nitrogen.

DOSAGES Selected H₂ Antagonists

Agent	Pharmacological Class	Usual Dosage Range	Indications
▸▸ cimetidine		**Adult**	
		PO: 200 mg bid	Dyspepsia, heartburn
		PO: 800–1200 mg/day or divided bid	Treatment of ulcers
		PO: 300 mg bid or 400 mg at bedtime	Prophylaxis of recurrent ulcer
		PO: 1200 mg/day	GERD
		PO: 300 mg qid; do not exceed 2400 mg/day	Pathological hypersecretion
		PO: 800 mg/day or divided bid	NSAID-induced lesions and symptoms
famotidine		**Adult ≥ 12 yr**	
		PO: 10 mg 15 minutes before eating, max 20 mg	Dyspepsia, heartburn
		PO: 40 mg/day at bedtime	Ulcers
	H₂ Antagonists	PO: 20 mg at bedtime	Prevention of recurrent duodenal ulcer
		PO: 20 mg q6h	Pathological hypersecretion
		IV: 20 mg q12h	
		PO: 20 mg bid	GERD
nizatidine		**Adult**	
		PO: 75 mg bid	Dyspepsia, heartburn
		PO: 300 mg at bedtime or 150 mg bid	Ulcers
		PO: 150 mg bid	GERD
ranitidine		**Adult**	
		PO: 75 mg bid	Dyspepsia, heartburn
		PO: 150 mg bid or 300 mg at bedtime	Ulcers
		PO: 150 mg tid	Pathological hypersecretion, GERD
		PO: 150 mg qid	Erosive esophagitis
		IM/IV: 50 mg q6–8h	Any indications

Interactions

Besides the different side effect profiles of the four H₂ antagonists, differences in the drug interactions of H₂ antagonists exist. These may be of clinical importance. Cimetidine binds the hepatic cytochrome P-450 microsomal oxidase system. This is a group of enzymes in the liver that metabolize many different drugs by oxidation. By inhibiting the oxidation of drugs metabolized via this pathway, cimetidine may raise the blood concentrations of these drugs. Ranitidine has only 10 to 20 percent of the binding action of cimetidine on the P-450 system, and nizatidine and famotidine have essentially no effect. This interaction has little clinical significance for most drugs, but problems occur with medications with a narrow therapeutic-to-toxic ratio, such as theophylline, warfarin, lidocaine, and phenytoin. All H₂ antagonists may inhibit the absorption of certain drugs, such as ketoconazole, that require an acidic GI environment for gastric absorption. The absorption of H₂ antagonists may be impaired in individuals who smoke. Smoking has been shown to decrease the effectiveness of H₂ antagonists. For optimal results the H₂ antagonist should be taken one hour before antacids.

Dosages

For dosage information for the H₂ antagonists, see the dosages table above. See Appendix B for some of the common brands in Canada.

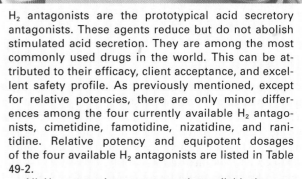

DRUG PROFILES

H₂ antagonists are the prototypical acid secretory antagonists. These agents reduce but do not abolish stimulated acid secretion. They are among the most commonly used drugs in the world. This can be attributed to their efficacy, client acceptance, and excellent safety profile. As previously mentioned, except for relative potencies, there are only minor differences among the four currently available H₂ antagonists, cimetidine, famotidine, nizatidine, and ranitidine. Relative potency and equipotent dosages of the four available H₂ antagonists are listed in Table 49-2.

All H₂ antagonists are currently available by prescription and OTC. Each agent is available orally, and all except cimetidine and nizatidine are also available parenterally. H₂ antagonists are classified as pregnancy category B agents and are contraindicated in clients with hypersensitivity.

▸▸ cimetidine

Cimetidine was the first agent in this class to be released on the market. It is the prototypical H₂ antagonist. In Canada, cimetidine is available as 200-, 300-, 400-, 600-, and 800-mg tablets and a 300-mg/5-mL oral solution. Pregnancy category B. Common dosage recommendations are listed in the dosages table above.

TABLE 49-2

H₂ ANTAGONISTS: POTENCY AND EQUIPOTENT DOSAGES

	Cimetidine	Ranitidine	Nizatidine	Famotidine
Relative potency	1	4–8	4–8	20–50
Equivalent dose (mg)	1600	300	300	40

PHARMACOKINETICS

Half-Life	Onset	Peak	Duration
2 hr	15–60 min	1–2 hr	4–8 hr

famotidine

Famotidine is another commonly used H₂ antagonist. It can be given orally or intravenously. Famotidine is available as 10-, 20-, and 40-mg tablets; 10-mg chewable tablets; a 40-mg/5-mL suspension; and a 10-mg/mL injection. Pregnancy category B. Common dosage recommendations are listed in the dosages table on p. 846.

PHARMACOKINETICS

Half-Life	Onset	Peak	Duration
2.5–3.5 hr	15–60 min	1–2 hr	6–8 hr

PROTON PUMP INHIBITORS

The newest drugs introduced for the treatment of acid-related disorders are the PPIs lansoprazole, omeprazole, rabeprazole, pantoprazole, and esomeprazole. Omeprazole was the first agent in this class of antisecretory drugs. The enzyme H⁺/K⁺ ATPase is the final step in the acid–secretory process of the parietal cell (see Figure 49-2). If there is energy present to run the pump, it will release hydrogen ions out of the parietal cell. Because hydrogen ions are protons (positively charged hydrogen atoms) the pump may also be called the *proton pump*. Anticholinergics and antihistamines (H₂ antagonists) do not completely stop the action of the pump in an individual parietal cell, whereas PPIs do so.

Mechanism of Action and Drug Effects

Gastric acid secretion occurs when histamine, gastrin, and acetylcholine are secreted. When these substances bind to specific receptors on parietal cells of the stomach, they stimulate acid secretion. Finally, the H⁺/K⁺ ATPase enzyme or the proton pump exchanges potassium for hydrogen ions. PPIs irreversibly bind to the H⁺/K⁺ ATPase enzyme preventing the movement of hydrogen ions out of the parietal cells into the stomach. Even though PPIs have potent antisecretory activity, they do not completely eliminate gastric acidity. Proton pumps are stimulated by eating and the number of proton pumps inhibited determines how efficient the PPIs are. Although H₂ antagonists may block close to 90 percent of all acid secretion, PPIs effectively block all acid secretion. Because PPIs stop over 90 percent of 24-hour acid secretion, it makes most clients achlorhydric (without acid). For acid secretion to return to normal after a PPI has been stopped, the parietal cell must synthesize new H⁺/K⁺ ATPase. PPIs are almost the ideal drugs for hypersecretion of acid. Their drug effects are confined to the parietal cell and specifically to the H⁺/K⁺ ATPase enzyme. Although there are other proton pumps in the body, the H⁺/K⁺ ATPase is distinct structurally and mechanically from other H-transporting enzymes and appears to exist only in the parietal cell. Thus the action of PPIs is limited to the inhibition of gastric acid secretion.

Indications

The ability to totally inhibit the production of acid from the parietal cells in the stomach gives the PPIs many beneficial therapeutic effects. Some concerns have been expressed regarding their chemical stability in the body. Most of these concerns pertain to long-term use of these agents in humans. There was some early concern that long-term use of PPIs might promote malignant gastric tumours. However, this initial concern about the carcinogenic potential of omeprazole and lansoprazole has subsided. These agents are now approved by Health Canada for long-term GERD maintenance therapy. These agents are currently indicated as first-line therapy for erosive esophagitis, symptomatic GERD that is poorly responsive to other medical treatment such as H₂ antagonists, short-term treatment of active duodenal ulcers and active benign gastric ulcers, gastric hypersecretory conditions (e.g., Zollinger-Ellison syndrome), and non-steroidal anti-inflammatory drug (NSAID)-induced ulcers. The only chronic therapeutic use for these agents is the maintenance of healing of erosive esophagitis and pathological hypersecretory conditions, including Zollinger-Ellison syndrome.

All of the PPIs have been approved for the treatment of clients with *H. pylori* infections. Many treatment regimens have emerged to cure *H. pylori*–induced ulcers; these are listed in Table 49-3. *H. pylori* eradication has been shown to reduce the risk of duodenal ulcer recurrence as well.

Contraindications

The only usual contraindication to the PPIs is known drug allergy.

Side Effects and Adverse Effects

Omeprazole and lansoprazole appear to be remarkably safe for short-term therapy. The frequency of adverse effects has been similar to that of placebo or H₂ antagonists. There is also some newer concern that the now popular use of these agents may predispose clients to GI infections due to reduction of the normal acid-mediated antimicrobial protection.

TABLE 49-3

CURRENT HEALTH CANADA–APPROVED REGIMENS FOR ERADICATING *HELICOBACTER PYLORI* INFECTION IN ADULTS

Suggested Treatment Regimens	Recommended Doses
A. Proton Pump Inhibitor (PPI) + amoxicillin + clarithromycin B. Proton Pump Inhibitor (PPI) + metronidazole + clarithromycin	**Proton Pump Inhibitor:** esomaprazole 40 mg bid or lansoprazole 30 mg bid or
Alternative Treatment Regimen*	omeprazole 40 mg bid
C. Proton Pump Inhibitor (PPI) + Bismuth subsalicylate + metronidazole + tetracycline (BMT)	or pantoprazole 40 mg

Treatment adherence is imperative.
Duration of therapy for adults is 7 days for all regimens.
  Some experts recommend a 14-day regimen.
Eradication rates are approximately 90 percent.
Metronidazole is appropriate for clients with
  penicillin allergies.
The alternative treatment regimen is appropriate for clients
  with clarithromycin intolerance. It may also be used
  for triple therapy failures.
	or
	rabeprazole 20 mg bid
	amoxicillin = 1 gm bid
	clarithromycin = 500 mg bid
	metronidazole = 500 mg bid **or** 250 mg qid in PPI + BMT protocol
	bismuth subsalicylate = 2 tablets qid
	tetracycline = 500 mg bid

*Tetracycline is substituted in this regimen for those clients with intolerance to clarithromycin.

DOSAGES Misoprostol, Omeprazole, Pantoprazole, and Sucralfate*

Agent	Pharmacological Class	Usual Dosage Range	Indications
misoprostol*	Antisecretory	**Adult** PO: 200 μg qid with meals and at bedtime for duration of NSAID therapy PO: 100 μg qid with meals	Gastric ulcer prophylaxis during NSAID therapy Duodenal ulcer prophylaxis during NSAID therapy†
▸▸omeprazole	Proton pump inhibitor	**Adult** PO: 20 mg/day for 4–8 wk PO: 60–120 mg/day divided	Esophagitis, duodenal ulcer Hypersecretory conditions
pantoprazole	Proton pump inhibitor	**Adult** PO/IV: 40 mg/day for 4–8 wk PO: 20 mg/day A.M.	GERD, gastric and duodenal ulcer Prevention of NSAIDs lesions
▸▸sucralfate*	Anti-ulcer agent	**Adult** PO: 1 g qid 1 hr ac	Duodenal and gastric ulcers

*Misoprostol and pantoprazole are reviewed in the following Drug Profiles section. Sucralfate is discussed in a later section of this chapter.
†Off-label use.

Interactions

There are few drug interactions with PPIs. PPIs may increase serum levels of diazepam and phenytoin. Other drug interactions include anticoagulants, sulphonylureas, antacids, diazepam, anticholinergics, and metoclopramide. There may be an increased chance for bleeding in clients who are on both a PPI and warfarin. Other possible interactions include interference with ketoconazole, ampicillin, iron salts, and digoxin absorption. The PPI may be given 30 minutes before sucralfate to avoid this interaction.

Dosages

For recommended dosages see the dosages table above. See Appendix B for some of the brands available in Canada.

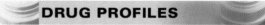

DRUG PROFILES

▸▸ omeprazole

Omeprazole is one of five PPIs. The PPIs bind to and inhibit the enzyme H^+/K^+ ATPase, which is the final common step in the acid–secretory process of the parietal cell.

The ability of omeprazole to totally prohibit the production of acid from the parietal cells in the stomach gives it many beneficial therapeutic effects. Omeprazole is indicated for acute and maintenance therapy for duodenal and gastric ulcers, NSAID-associated gastric or duodenal ulcers, *H. pylori*-associated peptic ulcer disease, acute treatment of severe GERD unresponsive to conventional therapy, endoscopically proven erosive esophagitis, and the treatment of chronic Zollinger-Ellison syndrome.

Omeprazole is available only in an oral formulation as 10-, 20-, and 40-mg gelatin capsules; 10- and 20-mg tablets; and 10- and 20-mg sustained-release tablets. It is contraindicated in clients with hypersensitivity. Pregnancy category C. Common dosage recommendations are listed in the dosages table on p. 848.

PHARMACOKINETICS

Half-Life	Onset	Peak	Duration
40 min	2 hr*	4 hr	up to 72 hr

*50–86% acid secretion reduction.

pantoprazole

Pantoprazole is currently the only PPI that is available in both an oral and an intravenous preparation. This allows pantoprazole to be used in clients who are unable to tolerate oral medications, such as intensive care clients who are intubated and cannot take oral medication. It is indicated for short-term treatment (up to eight weeks) in the healing and symptomatic relief of erosive esophagitis associated with GERD, long-term maintenance of erosive or ulcerative GERD, non-erosive reflux disease (NERD), symptomatic relief and healing of duodenal and gastric ulcers, *H. pylori*–associated peptic ulcer disease, and the treatment of chronic Zollinger-Ellison syndrome. Pantoprazole is available as 20- and 40-mg enteric-coated oral tablets and a 40-mg/mL injection. It is contraindicated in clients with a known hypersensitivity. Pregnancy category B. Common recommended dosages are listed in the dosages table on p. 848.

PHARMACOKINETICS

Half-Life	Onset	Peak	Duration
1 hr	24 hr*	2–4 hr	>24 hr

*88% decrease in acid secretion one day after initiation.

SUCRALFATE

Sucralfate is an agent used as a mucosal protective agent in the treatment of active stress ulcerations and chronically in duodenal and non-malignant gastric ulcer. It works in a manner that is totally different from that of the antacids, H_2 antagonists, and PPIs. A closer discussion of the chemical structure of sucralfate provides insight into its many actions.

Mechanism of Action and Drug Effects

Sucralfate acts locally, not systemically, binding directly to the surface of ulcers. Sucralfate has as its basic structure a sugar, sucrose. Sulphates and aluminum hydroxide groups are attached to that sugar in the place where there are normally hydroxyl groups. Once sucralfate comes into contact with the acid of the stomach, it begins to dissociate into aluminum hydroxide (an antacid) and sulphate anions. The sulphated sucrose molecules of sucralfate are attracted to and bind to the base of ulcers and erosions, forming a protective barrier over the base of this area. By binding to the exposed proteins of ulcers and erosions, su-

TABLE 49-4

SUCRALFATE: DRUG EFFECTS

Characteristic	Drug Effect
Sulphate anions	Bind to positively charged tissue proteins that are exposed at the tissue surface of an ulcer or an erosion
Weak base	Buffers the acidic pH of the stomach
Epidermal growth factor	Binds and concentrates epidermal growth factor, which accelerates the healing process
Prostaglandin synthesis	Stimulates gastric mucosal PG E_2 synthesis
Stimulation of mucus and bicarbonate	The aluminum salt stimulates the secretion of mucus and bicarbonate from the cells of the stomach to counteract the actions of hydrochloric acid

cralfate limits the access of pepsin. This enzyme normally breaks down proteins in food but can also do so in GI epithelial tissue, either causing ulcers or making them worse. This is believed to be the primary mechanism by which sucralfate heals ulcers and protects erosions. It has a multitude of other effects that may also explain its mechanism of action. The many drug effects of sucralfate are listed in Table 49-4.

Indications

Sucralfate has many attractive characteristics that make it a beneficial agent for the treatment of such disorders as stress ulcers, esophageal erosions, and PUD.

Contraindications

The only usual contraindication to sucralfate is drug allergy.

Side Effects and Adverse Effects

Sucralfate has little absorption from the gut into the blood and is chemically inert. These characteristics make it virtually devoid of systemic toxicity. The most common side effects are constipation and nausea, which appear two to three percent of the time. Dry mouth may also be seen.

Interactions

Sucralfate may impair the absorption of certain drugs, particularly tetracycline. It may also slow the absorption of ketoconazole, ampicillin, iron salts, and digoxin. This can be avoided by administering sucralfate without any other medications. This binding property of sucralfate may be used therapeutically. Sucralfate binds phosphates in the GI tract and has been used as a phosphate binder in clients with chronic renal failure.

Dosages

For recommended dosages of sucralfate, see the dosages table on p. 848. See Appendix B for some of the common brands available in Canada.

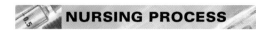

DRUG PROFILES

misoprostol

Misoprostol is a synthetic PG analogue. PGs have a wide variety of biological activities. They are believed to inhibit gastric acid secretion and exhibit cytoprotective activity. They are believed to protect the gastric mucosa from injury, possibly by enhancing the local production of mucus or bicarbonate, by promoting local cell regeneration, and by helping to maintain mucosal blood flow. Because of their inhibitory effects on gastric acid secretion and their cytoprotective properties, synthetic analogues of the "E" class of PGs have been produced. They were made with the expectation that they might be useful agents for the treatment of PUD. Misoprostol, a PG E analog, has been shown to effectively reduce the incidence of gastric ulcers in clients taking NSAIDs. The drug has been approved by Health Canada for this prophylactic use.

(Although not approved by Health Canada for the purpose, misoprostol may also be used in combination with mifepristone as a medical alternative to a surgically induced abortion. Misoprostol stimulates uterine contractility and expels the products of conception.)

Although some studies show that synthetic analogues of PGs promote the healing of duodenal ulcers, they must be used in doses that usually produce more disturbing side effects, such as abdominal cramps and diarrhea. Thus they are not believed to be as effective as the H_2 antagonists for this indication. Pregnancy category X. The commonly used dose is listed in the table on p. 848.

▶▶ sucralfate

Sucralfate is available only with a prescription in an oral formulation as a 1-g oral tablet and as a 1-g/5-mL oral solution. Sucralfate is contraindicated in clients with hypersensitivity. Pregnancy category B. The common dosage recommendation for sucralfate is 1 g 4×/day (also see the table on p. 848).

PHARMACOKINETICS

Half-Life	Onset	Peak	Duration
6–20 hr	1 hr	2–4 hr	3–6 hr

NURSING PROCESS

■ Assessment

Before administering an acid-controlling agent, the nurse should assess the client and gather information regarding the following: presence of heart failure, hypertension, sodium restrictions, and other cardiac diseases, especially if the antacid is high in sodium content; fluid imbalances; dehydration; GI obstruction; renal disease; and pregnancy. (Clients with heart failure or hypertension should use low-sodium antacids such as Maalox or Mylanta II.) Under these conditions antacids must be used cautiously. Contraindications to the use of aluminum-containing antacids include hypersensitivity

to the drug. Renal dysfunction is also a consideration before the use of antacids and other drugs (e.g., antibiotics) now used to treat ulcers.

Magnesium antacids should be used cautiously in clients who have a history of renal insufficiency and also in pregnant or lactating clients. Contraindications to the use of magnesium antacids include hypersensitivity to the medication. Calcium-containing antacids are commonly used, especially as a source of calcium. However, they carry the risk of rebound hyperacidity, milk-alkali syndrome, and changes in systemic pH, especially if the client has abnormal renal functioning. Milk-alkali syndrome is a state of hypercalcemia that can lead to calcification and renal failure. Milk-alkali syndrome and rebound hyperacidity are also problematic with the administration of antacids containing sodium bicarbonate. Sodium bicarbonate is generally not recommended as an antacid because of the high risk for systemic electrolyte disturbances and alkalosis. The sodium content of sodium bicarbonate is high and can be problematic for clients who have hypertension, heart failure, or renal insufficiency.

There are many drug interactions with antacids, because these agents affect the absorption of medications given concurrently with them.

H_2 antagonists are contraindicated in clients with known drug allergy or who have impaired renal function or liver disease. Cautious use is recommended in geriatric clients and in clients who are confused or disoriented. Omeprazole has several drug interactions, including diazepam, phenytoin, and warfarin.

PPIs are contraindicated in clients who are allergic to the particular drug, and these drugs should be used cautiously in children and in clients who are pregnant or lactating. Hepatic enzymes (alanine aminotransferase [ALT] and aspartate aminotransferase [AST]) and alkaline phosphatase should be monitored before and during treatment. Other drug interactions include anticoagulants, sulphonylureas, antacids, diazepam, anticholinergics, and metoclopramide. Sucralfate may also delay absorption of oral dosage forms of medications such as tetracyclines.

Because the treatment of PUD focuses on the use of antacids, H_2 antagonists, PPIs, sucralfate, and antibiotics, it is critical to assess the client for any possible contraindications, cautions, and drug interactions related to any of these drugs and also the antibiotics used, such as clarithromycin and amoxicillin (see Chapter 37).

■ Nursing Diagnoses

Nursing diagnoses related to the administration of acid-controlling agents include the following:
- Acute pain related to gastric hyperacidity and other GI disorders.
- Constipation related to side effects of aluminum-containing antacids and other drugs used for hyperacidity.

- Diarrhea related to side effects of magnesium-containing antacids and other drugs used for hyper-acidity.
- Deficient knowledge related to lack of information about antacids, H$_2$ antagonists, or PPIs, including their use and potential side effects.

Planning

Goals for clients receiving acid-controlling agents are as follows:
- Client has minimal to no pain during therapy with antacids or other acid-controlling agents.
- Client experiences minimal side effects while using antacids or acid-controlling agents.
- Client remains adherent to therapy.

Outcome Criteria

Outcome criteria related to the administration of acid-controlling agents include the following:
- Client experiences increased comfort as related to the use of these GI agents.
- Client states expected side effects, such as constipation and diarrhea, and when to seek further assistance regarding their management.
- Client states the importance of adherence and following administration guidelines associated with the use of acid-controlling agents to help decrease manifestations of the disease or disorder.

Implementation

When giving acid-controlling agents, the nurse should always be sure that chewable tablets are well chewed and liquid forms are thoroughly shaken before they are given to the client. All antacid agents should be administered with at least 240 mL of water to enhance absorption of the antacid in the stomach, except for newer forms that are "rapid dissolve" agents. Should constipation or diarrhea occur with single agents, the nurse should suggest a combination aluminum and magnesium product to the physician and educate the client about side effects of aluminum-only or magnesium-only products. Unless the physician has ordered otherwise, antacids should not be given within one to two hours of other medications because of their effect on the absorption of oral medications. This dosing schedule can be done safely by the nurse without interrupting safe dosing of the other medications.

Because so many H$_2$ antagonists are now available OTC, it is critical to client safety that clients are educated on proper medication use and administration. For example, cimetidine should be given with meals, and antacids (if also given) should be given one hour before or after the cimetidine. Client education should be emphasized regarding drug interactions (e.g., oral anticoagulants), side effects, and other OTC products to avoid.

Ranitidine does not need to be given with meals, and antacids should be taken one hour before or after, if also ordered. Intravenous forms should be diluted 50 mg/20 mL

normal saline (NS), D5W, 0.18 percent NS and four percent dextrose, 4.2 percent sodium bicarbonate, or LR and given at 50 mg or less over five minutes or more. Refer to appropriate sources for information on other specific agents and their intravenous administration.

Omeprazole should be taken before meals, and the capsule should be taken whole, not crushed, opened, or chewed. Omeprazole may also be given with antacids, if ordered. Like omeprazole, most of the PPIs are given short term, which should be emphasized to clients. The nurse should always double check the names and dosages of these drugs to ensure that they are not confused with similarly named agents. Intravenous pantoprazole should be given exactly as ordered and using correct dilutional fluids and no more than 40 mg/day (even oral forms). The intravenous form is helpful in cases where oral medications are not tolerated.

Nurses should realize that sucralfate is also used to bind phosphates in the GI tract in clients with renal failure.

Client teaching tips for these agents are presented in the box on p. 853.

Evaluation

Therapeutic response to the administration of antacids, antisecretory compounds, and H$_2$ antagonists includes relief of symptoms associated with the hyperacidity related to the diagnosis of peptic ulcer, gastritis, esophagitis, gastric hyperacidity, or hiatal hernia (i.e., decrease in epigastric pain, fullness, and abdominal swelling). Side effects for which to assess in clients taking antacids or antiflatulents include nausea, vomiting, abdominal pain, and diarrhea. Constipation, milk-alkali syndrome, and acid rebound are complications associated with sodium bicarbonate and calcium antacids. Therapeutic response to PPIs is similar to that listed for antacids. In addition, the client should report decreased use of any of the OTC acid-controlling drugs.

NURSING CARE PLAN | Peptic Ulcer

Dr. T., a 46-year-old university professor, has been diagnosed with gastritis and a small peptic ulcer after having an endoscopy today. Serum electrolytes were within normal limits; however, gastrin levels were elevated. The physician has encouraged a regular exercise program, stress management, a regular diet high in fibre and vegetables, and the avoidance of alcohol and nicotine (he is a non-smoker and only drinks occasionally). Along with his discharge care instructions after an endoscopy, he also received a prescription for omeprazole.

ASSESSMENT

Subjective Data

Objective Data

- Complaint of heartburn and gastric reflux with pain waking him at night
- Snacks on junk food frequently to "soak up" acid
- High-stress job
- Non-smoker; drinks alcohol occasionally
- Heartburn for six months
- Takes antacids daily
- Recent endoscopy with diagnosis of reflux and PUD with prescription for omeprazole

NURSING DIAGNOSIS

Acute pain, epigastric, related to diagnosis of reflux and hyperacidity

PLANNING

Goals

Client will experience more comfort from relief of reflux and ulcer pain within one week of treatment with medications

Outcome Criteria

Client will state the following ways to minimize discomfort associated with reflux and PUD:
- Take medications as prescribed
- Follow a proper diet
- Decrease stress
- Eliminate other factors that elevate gastric acid production

IMPLEMENTATION

Client teaching should include the following:
- The importance of testing for *Helicobacter pylori* because it is responsible for a majority of ulcers. The treatment plan generally involves antibiotic therapy. This is a departure from earlier thinking about ulcers—that they are caused by stress and an obsessive-compulsive personality.
- Always take medication as prescribed and take it before meals. Do not open, chew, or crush capsule.
- Report any severe diarrhea to the physician.
- Follow diet as recommended by physician, including the following:
  - Limit gas-producing and acidic foods (e.g., orange juice)
  - Avoid extremely spicy foods.
  - Follow diet high in fibre.
  - Drink at least 2.5 to 3 L of fluid a day.
  - Eat a balanced diet following recommendations in Canada's Food Guide.
  - Decrease food intake before bedtime to avoid reflux at night.
  - Avoid alcohol and caffeine.
- Sleep with head of bed slightly elevated for reflux disorders.
- Avoid nicotine.
- Exercise regularly at least three times a week to help decrease stress.
- Participate in relaxing activities and attend stress-reduction seminars at the hospital this month.
- Follow up with physician as ordered.
- Contact physician should gastric pain increase.

EVALUATION

Client shows a therapeutic response, evidenced by the following:
- Absence of epigastric pain
- Less belching
- Absence of abdominal fullness and swelling
- Normal stool patterns
- Less GI upset
- Lifestyle changes that help to decrease stress
- Changes in diet
- Better sleeping patterns
- Medication taken as prescribed
- Minimal side effects experienced

CLIENT TEACHING TIPS

The nurse should instruct the client as follows:

▲ Take your medication exactly as prescribed.

▲ Contact the physician immediately if you experience constipation, diarrhea, an increase in abdominal pain, or any change in symptoms.

▲ Avoid caffeine, alcohol, harsh spices, and black pepper because these may aggravate the underlying condition.

▲ If you take an over-the-counter acid medication, follow the package directions. Contact your healthcare provider if symptoms are not relieved.

Antacids

▲ Do not take any other medications within one to two hours after taking an antacid because antacids affect the absorption of many medications in the stomach. (This is particularly important if you are taking enteric-coated medications. The antacid can dissolve the coating too soon, leading to upset stomach.)

Omeprazole

▲ Take this medication before meals. Take the capsule whole; do not crush, chew, or open it. It can be taken with antacids.

Sucralfate

▲ Take this medication on an empty stomach. Don't take antacids unless your physician has told you to. If so, take them half an hour before or one hour after sucralfate.

Antiflatulents

▲ Follow manufacturer directions. Chewable forms must always be chewed thoroughly; liquid preparations should be shaken thoroughly before taking.

POINTS to REMEMBER

▼ The stomach secretes many substances (hydrochloric acid, pepsinogen, mucus, bicarbonate, intrinsic factor, and PGs).

▼ The parietal cell is responsible for the production of acid.

▼ In acid-related disorders there is an impairment in the balance among the substances secreted by the stomach.

▼ The most common impairment is hyperacidity, or the overproduction of acid. The most harmful are PUD and esophageal cancer. Antacids were used for centuries and were the mainstays of anti-ulcer therapy until the 1970s, when other agents were developed.

▼ H$_2$ antagonists are H$_2$ blockers that bind to and block histamine receptors located on parietal cells. This blockade renders these cells less responsive to stimuli and thus acid secretion.

▼ Up to 90 percent inhibition can be achieved with the H$_2$ antagonists.

▼ PPIs block the final step in the acid production pathway—H$^+$/K$^+$ ATPase—and they block acid secretion.

▼ Sucralfate is an agent for the treatment of PUD and stress-related ulcers. It is a cytoprotective agent that binds to exposed proteins of ulcers, thus limiting pepsin's proteolytic action.

▼ Misoprostol is a synthetic PG analogue and inhibits gastric acid secretion. It enhances local production of mucus or bicarbonate and helps to maintain mucosal blood flow.

▼ Cautious use of antacids is recommended in clients with heart failure, hypertension, sodium restrictions, and other cardiac diseases, especially if the antacid is high in sodium content.

▼ Other cautions to antacid use include fluid imbalances, dehydration, GI obstruction, renal disease, and pregnancy.

▼ There are many drug interactions with antacids because these agents affect the absorption of medications given concurrently with them. Interactions should always be checked before acid-controlling agents are given.

▼ Other medications should not be taken within one to two hours after an antacid is taken. The physician should be contacted if medication times need to be rescheduled.

▼ Clients taking enteric-coated medications need to know that antacids may cause premature dissolving of the enteric coating and stomach upset may occur.

▼ Magnesium-containing antacids are contraindicated in clients with renal failure and aluminum-containing antacids must be used cautiously.

▼ The recommended dosage of most antacids is usually 15 to 60 mL with water every one to three hours after meals and at bedtime.

▼ Antiflatulents are useful in the management of conditions associated with excessive gas production, such as post-operative flatus and bloating, diverticulitis, irritable or spastic colon, air swallowing associated with anxiety, and PUD.

▼ H$_2$ antagonists are used in the management of PUD by elevating the gastric pH to help neutralize the effects of hyperacidic or hypersecretory states in the GI tract.

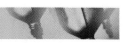

EXAMINATION REVIEW QUESTIONS

1 One of your clients, a 30-year-old business executive, is taking simethicone for excessive flatus associated with diverticulitis. Which of the following best describes the mechanism of action by which simethicone reduces flatus?
  a. It neutralizes gastric pH, thereby preventing gas.
  b. It buffers the effects of pepsin on the gastric wall.
  c. It decreases gastric acid secretion and minimizes flatus.
  d. It disperses and prevents gas formation in the stomach.

2 H_2 antagonists would most likely adversely interact with which of the following?
  a. Codeine
  b. NSAIDs
  c. Ketoconazole
  d. Acetaminophen

3 Digoxin preparations and adsorbents should not be given simultaneously because of which of the following possible interactions?
  a. Increased absorption of the digoxin
  b. Decreased absorption of the digoxin
  c. Increased absorption of the adsorbent
  d. Decreased absorption of the adsorbent

4 When used with hyperacidic disorders of the stomach, antacids are given to elevate the gastric pH to:
  a. 2.0.
  b. 4.0.
  c. 6.0.
  d. 8.0.

5 One of your clients is receiving digitalis orally and is also to receive an antacid at the same time. Which of the following is the nurse's most appropriate action, based on the pharmacokinetics of antacids?
  a. Delay the digitalis for one to two hours until the antacid is absorbed
  b. Give the antacid at least two to four hours before administering the digitalis
  c. Administer both medications as ordered and document in nurses' notes
  d. Contact the physician regarding the drug interaction and request a change in the time of dosing of the drugs

For answers see http://evolve.elsevier.com/Lilley/pharmacology/.

CRITICAL THINKING ACTIVITIES

1 What is the purpose of adding simethicone to GI agents?
2 Are there any concerns regarding the use of antacids in clients with decreased renal functioning? Explain your answer.

3 Is the following statement true or false? Explain your answer.
Antacids coat the stomach and are therefore beneficial to clients with ulcers.

For answers see http://evolve.elsevier.com/Lilley/pharmacology/.

BIBLIOGRAPHY

Albanese, J., & Nutz, P.(2005). *Mosby's 2005 nursing drug cards.* St Louis, MO: Mosby.

Alberta Medical Association. (2005). Guideline for treatment of *Helicobacter pylori* infection in adults. Retrieved September 6, 2005, from http://www.topalbertadoctors.org/

Boron, W.F., & Boulpaep, E.L. (2005). *Medical physiology. Updated edition.* St Louis, MO: Elsevier Saunders.

Canadian Pharmacists Association. (2003). *Therapeutic choices* (4th ed.). Ottawa, ON: Author.

Canadian Pharmacists Association. (2004). *Guide to drugs in Canada.* Toronto, ON: Dorling Kindersley.

Canadian Pharmacists Association. (2005). *Compendium of pharmaceuticals and specialties. The Canadian drug reference for health professionals.* Ottawa, ON: Author. [The subscription-based e-CPS is available at http://www.pharmacists.ca.]

Cheng, A., Williams, B.A., & Sivarajan, B.V. (Eds.). (2003). *The HSC handbook of pediatrics* (10th ed.). Toronto, ON: Elsevier.

Facts and Comparisons. (2004). *Drug facts and comparisons pocket version* (9th ed.). St Louis, MO: Wolters Kluwer Health.

Health Canada. (2005). Drug product database (DPD). Retrieved September 6, 2005, from http://www.hc-sc.gc.ca/hpb/drugs-dpd/

Katzung, B.G. (2004). *Basic and clinical pharmacology* (9th ed.). New York: McGraw-Hill.

Khurana, R., Fischbach, l., Chiba, N., & Veldhuyzen van Zanten, S. (2005). An update on anti-*Helicobacter pylori* treatment in children. *Canadian Journal of Gastroenterology, 19*(7), 441–445.

Lacy, C.F., Armstrong, L.L., Goldman, M.P., & Lance, L.L. (2003). *Drug information handbook* (11th ed.). Hudson, OH: Lexi-Comp.

Lehne, R.A. (2004). *Pharmacology for nursing care* (5th ed.). St Louis, MO: Saunders.

Mosby. (2005). *Mosby's drug consult 2005: The comprehensive reference for generic and brand name drugs* (15th ed.). St Louis, MO: Mosby.

Skidmore-Roth, L. (2006). *Mosby's 2006 nursing drug reference* (19th ed.). St Louis, MO: Mosby.

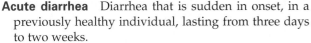

Antidiarrheals and Laxatives

OBJECTIVES

After reading this chapter, the successful student will be able to do the following:

1 Identify the various agents affecting bowel elimination, including both the agents used to manage diarrhea and those used to treat constipation.

2 Discuss the mechanisms of action, indications, cautions, contraindications, side effects, and dosages associated with the use of the various antidiarrheal and laxative agents.

3 Develop nursing care plans for clients receiving antidiarrheals and for clients receiving agents used to treat constipation.

e-LEARNING ACTIVITIES

Student CD-ROM
- Review Questions: see questions 369–374
- Animations
- Medication Administration Checklists
- IV Therapy Checklists

evolve Web site (http://evolve.elsevier.com/Lilley/pharmacology/)
- Online Chapter Worksheet • Frequently Asked Questions
- Learning Tips and Content Updates • WebLinks • Online Appendices and Supplements • Mosby/Saunders ePharmacology Update • Access to *Mosby's Drug Consult*

DRUG PROFILES

attapulgite, p. 858
bismuth subsalicylate, p. 858
▸▸ diphenoxylate with atropine, p. 858
▸▸ docusate salts, p. 864
▸▸ glycerin, p. 864
Lactobacillus acidophilus, p. 860

▸▸ lactulose, p. 864
▸▸ loperamide, p. 859
magnesium salts, p. 865
methylcellulose, p. 862
mineral oil, p. 864
polyethylene glycol, p. 865
▸▸ psyllium, p. 864
▸▸ senna, p. 865

▸▸ Key drug.

GLOSSARY

Acute diarrhea Diarrhea that is sudden in onset, in a previously healthy individual, lasting from three days to two weeks.

Adsorbent (ad sor' bent) An antidiarrheal agent that acts by coating the walls of the gastrointestinal (GI) tract, absorbing the bacteria or toxins causing the diarrhea and eliminating them with the stools.

Anticholinergic (an' tee kol' in er' jik) or **antispasmodic** (as a antidiarrheal agent) An agent that decreases the muscular tone of the intestine and thus decreases peristalsis.

Antidiarrheal Any agent that counters or combats diarrhea.

Bulk-forming laxatives Agents that absorb water into the intestine, which increases bulk, distending the bowel to initiate reflex bowel activity and promoting a bowel movement. Bulk-forming laxatives act in a manner similar to that of dietary fibre.

Cathartic Any substance that causes emptying of the bowels. Not necessarily the same as a laxative, which may be milder in its effect. Also called a *purgative*.

Chronic diarrhea Diarrhea that lasts for over three to four weeks, associated with recurring passage of diarrheal stools, fever, loss of appetite, nausea, vomiting, dehydration, weight reduction, and chronic weakness.

Constipation A condition of abnormally infrequent and difficult passage of feces through the lower GI tract.

Diarrhea The abnormal frequent passage of loose stools.

Emollient laxatives (e mol' ee ent) Agents often referred to as *stool softeners* and *lubricant laxatives*. The fecal softeners work by lowering the surface tension of fluids, resulting in more water and fat being absorbed into the stool and the intestines. The lubricant type of emollient laxatives work by lubricating the fecal material and the intestinal walls. This prevents water from leaking out of the intestines and softens and expands the stool.

Hyperosmotic laxatives Agents that produce their laxative effects by increasing fecal water content, which results in distention, increased peristalsis, and evacuation.

Intestinal flora modifiers The product obtained from bacterial cultures, most commonly *Lactobacillus* organisms.

Irritable bowel syndrome (IBS) A recurring condition of the intestinal tract involving bloating, flatulence, and often periods of diarrhea that alternate with periods of constipation.

Laxative An agent that promotes bowel evacuation by increasing the bulk of the feces, softening the stool, or lubricating the intestinal wall.

Opiate (o' pee ət) A narcotic-based agent. As antidiarrheals, opiates act by decreasing motility of the bowel and reducing the pain associated with diarrhea. They may also cause sedation and constipation.

Saline laxative (say' leen) A salt containing one or more ions that are poorly absorbed from the intestine. The salt draws water into the intestinal lumen by osmosis, causing bowel distension, which in turn promotes evacuation.

Stimulant laxative Agent that stimulates movement of the intestines by stimulating the nerves that innervate the intestines, resulting in increased peristalsis activity in the intestinal tract.

Diarrhea and the diseases commonly associated with it are among the leading causes of death and morbidity in developing nations, accounting for five to eight million deaths per year in infants and small children. Children in Canada experience approximately one to three episodes of diarrhea per year. Diarrheal disorders also have a financial impact on our society, with outpatient costs and loss of time from work because of acute infectious diarrhea. To the gastroenterologist, the "big three" symptoms of gastrointestinal (GI) disease are abdominal pain, nausea and/or vomiting, and diarrhea.

Diarrhea is defined as the abnormal frequent passage of loose stools or, more specifically, the abnormal passage of stools with increased frequency, fluidity, and weight, or with increased stool water excretion. **Acute diarrhea** refers to diarrhea that is sudden in onset in a previously healthy individual. It lasts anywhere from three days to two weeks and is self-limiting, resolving without sequelae. **Chronic diarrhea** lasts for over three to four weeks and is associated with recurring passage of diarrheal stools, fever, loss of appetite, nausea, vomiting, weight reduction, and chronic weakness.

The probable cause of diarrhea should be taken into consideration when designing a drug regimen to treat it. Causes of acute diarrhea can be drug-induced, bacterial, viral, protozoal, or nutritional. Causes of chronic diarrhea include tumours, AIDS, diabetes mellitus, hyperthyroidism, Addison's disease, and irritable bowel syndrome. Non-specific treatment is directed at the cessation of the increased stool frequency associated with

diarrhea, alleviation of abdominal cramps, prevention of dehydration from fluid and electrolyte loss, and prevention of weight loss and nutritional deficits from malabsorption.

ANTIDIARRHEALS

The agents used to treat diarrhea are called **antidiarrheals**. They are divided into different groups based on specific mechanisms of action: adsorbents and bulk-forming, anti-motility drugs (antispasmodics and opiates), bacterial replacement drugs **(intestinal flora modifiers)**, antisecretory drugs, and enzymes. The specific classes and the agents in each are listed in Table 50-1.

Mechanism of Action and Drug Effects

Antidiarrheal agents have varying mechanisms of action. It is important for the nurse to know the specific mechanism of an agent to ensure that the appropriate agent is being used (treating the underlying cause).

Adsorbents act by coating the walls of the GI tract. They remain in the intestine, bind the causative bacteria or toxin to the adsorbent surface, and eliminate it from the body through the stool.

Anticholinergics or **antispasmodics** work by decreasing peristalsis (rhythmic contractions of the GI tract) and the muscular tone of the intestine, thus slowing the movement of substances through the GI tract. They are often used in combination with adsorbents and opiates. Anticholinergics are discussed in detail in Chapter 20.

Intestinal flora modifiers are products obtained from bacterial cultures, most commonly *Lactobacillus* organisms. They make up the majority of the body's normal bacterial flora and are the organisms that are most commonly destroyed by antibiotics. Exogenously supplying these bacteria helps restore the balance of normal flora and suppress the growth of diarrhea-causing bacteria.

The primary antidiarrheal action of **opiates** is to decrease bowel motility. Opiates also reduce the pain associated with diarrhea by relieving rectal spasms. Because they increase the transit time of food through the GI tract, they permit longer contact of the intestinal

TABLE 50-1

ANTIDIARRHEALS: DRUG CATEGORIES AND SELECTED AGENTS

Category	Antidiarrheal Agents
Adsorbents and bulk-forming	Activated charcoal, aluminum hydroxide, attapulgite, bismuth subsalicylate, cholestyramine, kaolin, polycarbophil
Antispasmodics	Atropine, hyoscyamine, hyoscine
Opiates	Opium, codeine, diphenoxylate, loperamide
Intestinal flora modifiers	*Lactobacillus acidophilus*

contents with the absorptive surface of the bowel, increasing the absorption of water, electrolytes, and other nutrients from the bowel and reducing stool frequency and net volume.

Although all classes of antidiarrheal agents counteract diarrhea, other drug effects vary depending on the drug class and its specific mechanism of action. Within the class of adsorbents, bismuth subsalicylate is a form of aspirin, or acetylsalicylic acid, and therefore it has many of the same drug effects as aspirin (see Chapter 43). Activated charcoal is not only helpful in coating the walls of the GI tract and adsorbing bacteria, but is also useful in cases of overdose because of its drug-binding properties. Colestipol and cholestyramine are anion exchange resins that are prescription antidiarrheals and lipid-lowering agents. Besides binding to diarrhea-causing toxins, they have the additional benefit of decreasing cholesterol levels.

Anticholinergics have many drug effects beyond those of diarrhea relief (see Chapter 20). Some opiates are used primarily for their therapeutic effects in treating diarrhea, whereas others have analgesic properties and are used primarily to treat various types of pain. The drug effects of intestinal flora modifiers are limited to their antidiarrheal influence.

Indications

All five antidiarrheal drug families effectively combat diarrhea, although the therapeutic effects vary slightly from family to family. Because diarrhea has various causes, it is useful for the nurse to know that antidiarrheals have different mechanisms of action that allow the caregiver to pick an agent that is specific to the underlying cause of the diarrhea.

Contraindications

Contraindications for the antidiarrheals include known drug allergy and any major acute GI condition, such as intestinal obstruction or colitis, unless recommended by a physician who has examined the client and is following the client closely.

Side Effects and Adverse Effects

The side effects and adverse effects of the antidiarrheals are also specific to each drug family. Most of these potential effects are minor and not life threatening. The major side effects of specific agents in each drug class are listed in Table 50-2.

Interactions

Many drugs are absorbed from the intestines into the bloodstream, where they are delivered to their respective sites of action. Many of the antidiarrheals have the potential to alter this normal process, either by increasing or decreasing the absorption of these other drugs.

The adsorbents can decrease the effectiveness of many agents, primarily by decreasing their absorption. Examples include digoxin, clindamycin, quinidine, probenecid, and hypoglycemic agents. Oral anticoagulants are more likely to cause increased bleeding times or bruising when they are co-administered with adsorbents. This is thought to be primarily because the adsorbents may bind to vitamin K, which is needed to make certain clotting factors. Vitamin K is synthesized by the normal bacterial flora in the bowel. In addition, the toxic effects of methotrexate are more likely to occur when it is given with adsorbents.

The therapeutic effects of the anticholinergic antidiarrheals can be decreased by co-administration with

TABLE 50-2
SELECTED ANTIDIARRHEALS: ADVERSE EFFECTS

Agent	Body System	Side/Adverse Effects
ADSORBENTS		
bismuth subsalicylate	Hematological	Increased bleeding time
	Gastrointestinal	Constipation, dark stools
	Central nervous	Confusion, twitching
	Other	Hearing loss, tinnitus, metallic taste, blue gums
ANTICHOLINERGICS		
atropine, hyoscyamine, hyoscine	Genitourinary	Urinary retention and hesitancy, erectile dysfunction
	Central nervous	Headache, dizziness, confusion, anxiety, drowsiness
	Cardiovascular	Hypotension, hypertension, bradycardia, tachycardia
	Integumentary	Dry skin, rash, flushing
	Eye, ear, nose, throat	Blurred vision, photophobia, increased pressure in the eye
OPIATES		
codeine	Central nervous	Drowsiness, sedation, dizziness, lethargy
	Gastrointestinal	Nausea, vomiting, anorexia, constipation
	Respiratory	Respiratory depression
	Cardiovascular	Bradycardia, palpitations, hypotension
	Genitourinary	Urinary retention
	Integumentary	Flushing, rash, urticaria

antacids. Amantadine, tricyclic antidepressants (TCAs), monoamine oxidase inhibitors (MAOIs), and antihistamines, when given with anticholinergics, can result in increased anticholinergic effects. The opiate antidiarrheals will have additive central nervous system (CNS) depressant effects if they are given with CNS depressants, alcohol, narcotics, sedative–hypnotics, antipsychotics, and skeletal muscle relaxants.

Bismuth subsalicylate can increase bleeding times and bruising when administered with oral anticoagulants. Cholestyramine, when administered with glipizide, can result in decreased hypoglycemic effects.

Dosages

For the recommended dosages of antidiarrheal agents, see the table on p. 859. See Appendix B for some of the common brands available in Canada.

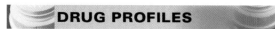

DRUG PROFILES

Drug therapy for diarrhea is dependent on the cause of the diarrhea. All antidiarrheals are orally administered agents available as suspensions, tablets, or capsules. Some antidiarrheals are over-the-counter (OTC) medications, whereas others require a prescription.

ADSORBENTS

As mentioned previously, adsorbents bind to the diarrhea-causing bacteria and pass them out with the stool. Of the adsorbent antidiarrheals, bismuth subsalicylate, attapulgite, and aluminum hydroxide are the most commonly used. These agents are all OTC medications and are classified in different pregnancy categories. They are contraindicated in children under three years of age, unless directed by a pediatrician.

attapulgite

Attapulgite has replaced the use of kaolin-pectin in the newer forms of this preparation. Kaolin is a naturally hydrated aluminum compound that is now less commonly used as an antidiarrheal agent. However, pectin, which is extracted from apples or citrus fruit, is used in many combination products. Attapulgite is also an OTC antidiarrheal. It is available as a 750-mg extra-strength caplet and 600-, 750-, and 900-mg/15-mL solutions. Pregnancy category C. Commonly recommended dosages are listed in the table on p. 859.

PHARMACOKINETICS

Half-Life	Onset	Peak	Duration
Unknown	12 hr	14–20 hr	Unknown

bismuth subsalicylate

Bismuth subsalicylate is a salicylate by chemical structure; therefore it should be used with caution in children and teenagers who have or are recovering from chicken pox or the flu because of the attendant risk of Reye's syndrome (see the Pediatric Considerations box on p. 866). It can also cause all of the side effects and adverse effects that are associated with an ASA-based product. Two alarming but harmless side effects are temporary darkening of the tongue and/or stool. Bismuth subsalicylate is available OTC as a 262-mg chewable tablet and caplet and 17.6-, 35-, and 35.2-mg/mL and 236-mg/28.4-mL suspensions. Pregnancy category D. Commonly recommended dosages are listed in the table on p. 859.

PHARMACOKINETICS

Half-Life	Onset	Peak	Duration
24–33 hr*	0.5–2 hr	2–5 hr	Variable

*For bismuth.

ANTICHOLINERGICS

The anticholinergics atropine, hyoscyamine, and hyoscine are used either alone or in combination with other antidiarrheals because they slow GI tract motility. These agents are commonly referred to as *belladonna alkaloids* and are discussed in Chapter 20. Their safety margin is not as broad as that of many of the other antidiarrheals because they can cause serious adverse effects if used inappropriately. For this reason they are available only by prescription. In Canada, belladonna is available only in combination with opium (see next section). No products with combinations of belladonna with phenobarbital, hyoscyamine, or scopolamine are available in Canada.

OPIATES

There are four opiate-related antidiarrheal agents: codeine, diphenoxylate with atropine, loperamide, and opium with belladonna. The only opiate-related antidiarrheal that is available as an OTC medication is loperamide; all others are prescription-only drugs because of the risks of respiratory depression and dependency associated with opiate use.

▸▸ diphenoxylate with atropine

Diphenoxylate is a synthetic opiate agonist that is structurally related to meperidine. It acts on smooth muscle of the intestinal tract, inhibiting GI motility and excessive GI propulsion. It has little or no analgesic activity. Diphenoxylate has been combined with subtherapeutic quantities of atropine to prevent deliberate overdosage. The amount of atropine present in the combination is too small to interfere with the constipating effect of diphenoxylate. However, when taken in large doses, the combination results in extreme anticholinergic effects (e.g., dry mouth, abdominal pain, tachycardia, blurred vision). Dependency is also a possibility in high dosages.

The combination of diphenoxylate and atropine is contraindicated in clients who have shown a hypersensitivity reaction to it, clients with jaundice, and in clients suffering from diarrhea associated with pseudomembranous colitis or toxigenic/enterotoxin bacteria. This combination antidiarrheal is available only as a tablet. Each tablet contains 2.5 mg of diphenoxylate and 0.025 mg of atropine. Pregnancy category C.

PHARMACOKINETICS*

Half-Life	Onset	Peak	Duration
2.5–4 hr	40–60 min	2–3 hr	3–4 hr

*Diphenoxylate component.

DOSAGES Selected Antidiarrheal Agents

Agent	Pharmacological Class	Usual Dosage Range	Indications
attapulgite	Adsorbent antidiarrheal	**All dosage forms** PO: One dose after each BM up to 7×/day **Maximum strength tablets (750 mg attapulgite/tab)** **Pediatric 6–12 yr** 1 tab **>12 yr–adult** 2 tabs **Concentrated liquid (600 mg attapulgite/15 mL)** **Pediatric 3–5 yr** 7.5 mL **6–12 yr** 15 mL **>12 yr–adult** 30 mL	Diarrhea
bismuth subsalicylate	Antimicrobial, antisecretory, antidiarrheal	Doses repeated q30–60 min, not to exceed 8×/day; all doses PO **Pediatric 3–5 yr** 5 mL or ⅓ tab **6–9 yr** 10 mL or ⅔ tab **10–12 yr** 15 mL or 1 tab **Adult** 30 mL or 2 tabs	Diarrhea
diphenoxylate HCl/ atropine sulphate	Antidiarrheal	**Adult** PO: 5 mg bid-qid until control of symptoms **Pediatric >2 yr** PO: 0.3–0.4 mg/kg daily in divided doses until control of symptoms	Diarrhea adjunct
Lactobacillus acidophilus	Intestinal flora modifier	**Adult only** PO: 2 caps bid–qid	Dietary supplement* Restore and maintain normal flora of intestinal tract after diarrhea
▸▸loperamide	Opiate antidiarrheal	**Pediatric 2–5 yr** PO: 1 mg tid **5–8 yr** PO: 2 mg bid **8–12 yr** PO: 2 mg tid **Adult** PO: 4 mg followed by 2 mg after each BM (not to exceed 16 mg/day)	Diarrhea

*Often used for uncomplicated diarrhea, though this is an off-label use.
BM, Bowel movement

▸▸ *loperamide*

Loperamide is a synthetic antidiarrheal that is similar to diphenoxylate. It inhibits both peristalsis in the intestinal wall and intestinal secretion, thereby decreasing the number of stools and the water content. Although the drug exhibits many characteristics of the opiate class, physical dependence to loperamide has not been reported. Because of its safety profile it is the only opiate antidiarrheal agent that is available as an OTC medication. Loperamide is contraindicated in clients who have shown a hypersensitivity reaction to it. It is also contraindicated in clients with severe ulcerative colitis, pseudomembranous colitis, and acute dysentery. Loperamide is available only in oral form as a 2-mg capsule, a 2-mg tablet, a 2-mg quick dissolve tablet, and a 0.2-mg/mL solution. It is also available as a combination product containing 2 mg of loperamide and 125 mg of antiflatulent simethicone in a caplet or chewable tablet. Pregnancy category B. Commonly recommended dosages are listed in the table above.

PHARMACOKINETICS

Half-Life	Onset	Peak	Duration
7–15 hr	1–3 hr	4 hr	40–50 hr

INTESTINAL FLORA MODIFIERS

Intestinal flora modifiers suppress the growth of diarrhea-causing bacteria and re-establish the normal flora that reside in the intestine. They are bacterial cultures that have been obtained from *Lactobacillus* organisms.

Lactobacillus acidophilus

Lactobacillus acidophilus is an acid-producing bacteria prepared in a concentrated, dried culture for oral administration. It is a normal inhabitant of the GI tract where, through the fermentation of carbohydrates (which produces lactic acid), it creates an unfavourable environment for the overgrowth of harmful fungi and bacteria. *L. acidophilus* has been used for more than 75 years in the treatment of uncomplicated diarrhea, particularly that caused by antibiotic treatment that destroys normal intestinal flora. It is available as an OTC medication in the following oral forms: capsules, tablets, enteric-coated capsules, and powder. It does not have a pregnancy category rating at this time. Commonly recommended dosages are listed in the table on p. 859.

PHARMACOKINETICS

Half-Life	Onset	Peak	Duration
Unknown	Unknown	Unknown	Unknown

LAXATIVES

Laxatives are used for the treatment of **constipation**, which is defined as a condition of abnormally infrequent and difficult passage of feces through the lower GI tract. Individuals may complain of constipation if they think they defecate too infrequently or with too much effort, if their stools are too hard or too small, if

TABLE 50-3
CAUSES OF CONSTIPATION

Causes	Examples
Adverse drug effects	Analgesics, anticholinergics, iron supplements, aluminum antacids, calcium antacids, opiates, calcium channel blockers, vinca alkaloids
Lifestyle	*Poor bowel movement habits:* Voluntary refusal to defecate resulting in constipation *Diet:* Poor fluid intake and/or low-residue (roughage) diets or excessive consumption of dairy products *Physical inactivity:* Lack of proper exercise, especially in elderly individuals *Psychological:* Anxiety, stress, hypochondria
Metabolic and endocrine disorders	Diabetes mellitus, hypothyroidism, pregnancy, hypercalcemia, hypokalemia
Neurogenic disorders	Autonomic neuropathy, intestinal pseudo-obstruction, multiple sclerosis, spinal cord lesions, Parkinson's disease, stroke

defecation is painful, or if they have a sense of incomplete evacuation. Constipation is a symptom, not a disease; it is a disorder of movement through the colon and/or rectum that can be caused by a variety of diseases or drugs. Some of the more common causes of constipation are noted in Table 50-3.

The GI tract is responsible for the digestive process, which involves (1) ingestion of dietary intake, (2) digestion of dietary intake into basic nutrients, (3) absorption of basic nutrients, and (4) storage and removal of fecal material via defecation.

Ingestion → Digestion → Absorption → Storage and removal

The usual time span between ingestion and defecation is 24 to 36 hours. The last segment of the GI tract, the large intestine (colon) is responsible for (1) forming the stool by removing excess water from the fecal material, (2) temporarily storing the stool until defecation, and (3) extracting essential vitamins from the intestinal bacteria (especially vitamin K).

The colon is 120 to 150 cm in length and is separated from the small intestine by the ileocecal valve. The colon extends into the rectum, which terminates at the anus. The rectum is the temporary storage site for the stool, which is composed of water and unabsorbed and indigestible material. Evacuation of the rectal contents is accomplished by bowel movements.

A bowel movement (defecation) is a reflex act that involves both smooth and skeletal muscles. The entry of feces into the rectum stimulates mass peristaltic movement that results in a bowel movement. However, voluntary initiation or inhibition of defecation is also possible via skeletal muscle pathways.

Treatment of constipation must involve an understanding of the whole client, with special attention given to the underlying causes for the constipation. Treatment should be individualized, taking into consideration the client's age, concerns, and expectations; duration and severity of constipation; and potential contributing factors. Treatment can be either surgical (in extreme cases) or non-surgical; non-surgical treatment can be separated into three broad categories of approach: dietary (e.g., fibre supplementation), behavioural (e.g., increased physical activity), and pharmacological. The focus in this chapter is pharmacological treatment.

Of the OTC medications, laxatives are some of the most misused. Chronic and often inappropriate use of laxatives may result in laxative dependence, produce damage to the bowel, or lead to previously non-existent intestinal problems. With the exception of the bulk-forming type, laxatives should not be used for long periods of time. All laxatives share the same general contraindications and precautions, including cautious use in the presence of acute surgical abdomen; appendicitis symptoms such as abdominal pain, nausea, and vomiting; fecal impaction (mineral oil enemas excepted); intestinal obstructions; and undiagnosed abdominal pain. They are also contraindicated in clients who have shown a hypersensitivity reaction to them.

Laxatives are divided into five major groups based on their mechanism of action: bulk-forming, emollient, hyperosmotic, saline, and stimulant laxatives. Table 50-4 lists the currently available laxative agents by their respective drug family.

Mechanism of Action and Drug Effects

All laxatives promote bowel movements, but each class of laxative has a different mechanism of action. They may act by (1) affecting fecal consistency, (2) increasing fecal movement through the colon, and/or (3) facilitating defecation through the rectum. **Bulk-forming laxatives** act in a manner similar to that of the fibre naturally contained in the diet. They absorb water into the intestine, which increases bulk and distends the bowel to initiate reflex bowel activity, thus promoting a bowel movement.

Emollient laxatives are also referred to as *stool softeners* (docusate salts) and *lubricant laxatives* (mineral oil). Fecal softeners work by lowering the surface tension of GI fluids, resulting in more water and fat being absorbed into the stool and the intestines. The lubricant type of emollient laxatives work by lubricating the fecal material and the intestinal wall and preventing absorption of water from the intestines. Instead of being absorbed, this water content in the bowel softens and expands the stool. This promotes bowel distension and reflex peristaltic actions, which ultimately lead to defecation.

Hyperosmotic laxatives work by increasing fecal water content, which results in distention, increased peristalsis, and evacuation. Their site of action is limited to the large intestine.

Saline laxatives increase osmotic pressure in the small intestine by inhibiting absorption and increasing water and electrolyte secretions, resulting in a watery stool; the increased distention promotes peristalsis and evacuation. Rectal enemas of sodium phosphate, a saline laxative, produce defecation two to five minutes after administration.

As the name implies, **stimulant laxatives** stimulate the nerves that innervate the intestines, resulting in increased peristalsis. They also increase fluid in the colon, which increases bulk and softens the stool.

The drug effects of laxatives are numerous, although their action is primarily limited to the site of the intestines and thus they have few, if any, systemic effects. Laxatives are useful in relieving constipation, in preparing for some medical procedures, and in removing unwanted substances from the body. Some of the more common indications for laxative use are as follows:

- Intestinal parasites
- Inactive colon
- Ammonia absorption in hepatic encephalopathic conditions
- Drug-induced constipation
- Constipation associated with pregnancy and/or post-obstetric period
- Reduced physical activity
- Toxic substances in the body
- Poor dietary habits
- Megacolon
- Preparation for colonic diagnostic procedures or surgery
- Facilitation of bowel movements with reduced pain in anorectal disorders

Table 50-5 lists the specific drug effects of the different classes of laxatives.

Indications

The various therapeutic uses for laxatives range from common constipation to bowel preparation before surgery.

The therapeutic effects vary by category. See Table 50-6 for specific therapeutic indications for each laxative drug class.

Contraindications

Laxatives are contraindicated in cases of known drug allergy or any acute, major GI condition, unless recommended by a physician who has examined and is following the client.

TABLE 50-4

LAXATIVES: DRUG CATEGORIES AND SELECTED AGENTS

Category	Laxative Agents
Bulk forming	psyllium, polycarbophil, methylcellulose
Emollient	docusate salts, mineral oil
Hyperosmotic	polyethylene glycol, lactulose, sorbitol, glycerin
Saline	magnesium sulphate, magnesium phosphate, magnesium citrate
Stimulant	castor oil, senna, anthraquinones

TABLE 50-5

LAXATIVES: DRUG EFFECTS

Drug Effect	Bulk	Emollient	Hyperosmotic	Saline	Stimulant
Increases peristalsis	Y	Y	Y	Y	Y
Causes increased secretion of water and electrolytes in small bowel	Y	Y	N	Y	Y
Inhibits absorption of water in small bowel	Y	Y	N	Y	Y
Increases wall permeability in small bowel	N	Y	N	N	Y
Causes wall damage in small bowel	N	Y	N	N	Y
Acts only in large bowel	N	N	Y	N	N
Increases fecal mass water	Y	Y	Y	Y	Y
Softens fecal mass	Y	Y	Y	Y	Y

TABLE 50-6
LAXATIVES: INDICATIONS

Laxative Group	Indication
Bulk forming	Acute and chronic constipation, irritable bowel syndrome, diverticulosis
Emollient	Acute and chronic constipation, softening of fecal impacts, facilitation of bowel movements in anorectal conditions
Hyperosmotic	Chronic constipation, diagnostic and surgical preparations
Saline	Constipation, removal of helminths and parasites, diagnostic and surgical bowel preparation
Stimulant	Acute constipation, diagnostic and surgical bowel preparation

TABLE 50-7
LAXATIVES: ADVERSE EFFECTS

Laxative Group	Side/Adverse Effects
Bulk forming	Impaction above strictures, fluid overload, electrolyte imbalances, gas formation, esophageal blockage, allergic reaction
Emollient	Skin rashes, decreased absorption of vitamins, lipid pneumonia, electrolyte imbalances
Hyperosmotic	Abdominal bloating, rectal irritation, electrolyte imbalances
Saline	Magnesium toxicity (with renal insufficiency), electrolyte imbalances, cramping, diarrhea, increased thirst
Stimulant	Nutrient malabsorption, skin rashes, gastric irritation, electrolyte imbalances, discoloured urine, rectal irritation

Side Effects and Adverse Effects

As is true for the drug and therapeutic effects of laxatives, the side effects and adverse effects of the various agents are specific to the laxative group. Most of the side effects from laxatives are confined to the site of the intestines; however, the overuse and misuse of laxatives lead to many unexpected and unwanted effects. The major side effects and adverse effects of the laxative agents are listed in Table 50-7.

Interactions

Many drugs are absorbed in some part of the intestine. Because laxatives alter intestinal function, they can interact with other drugs quite readily. Bulk-forming laxatives can decrease the absorption of antibiotics, digoxin, nitrofurantoin, salicylates, tetracyclines, and oral anticoagulants. Mineral oil can decrease the absorption of fat-soluble vitamins (A, D, E, and K). Hyperosmotic laxatives can cause increased CNS depression if they are given with barbiturates, general anaesthetics, opioids, and antipsychotics. Oral antibiotics can decrease the effects of lactulose. Stimulant laxatives decrease the absorption of antibiotics, digoxin, nitrofurantoin, salicylates, tetracyclines, and oral anticoagulants.

Dosages

For the recommended dosages of selected laxatives, see the table on p. 863. See Appendix B for some of the common brands available in Canada.

DRUG PROFILES

Laxatives are used to treat constipation, and this treatment must involve an understanding of the whole client. Many laxatives are available as OTC medications, whereas others require a prescription for use. The following are prototypical agents from each of the laxative groups.

BULK-FORMING LAXATIVES

Bulk-forming laxatives are composed of water-retaining (hydrophilic) natural and synthetic cellulose derivatives. Psyllium is an example of a natural bulk-forming laxative, and methylcellulose is an example of a synthetic cellulose derivative. Other bulk-forming laxatives are malt soup extract preparations and polycarbophil preparations. Bulk-forming agents increase water absorption, resulting in greater total volume (bulk) of the intestinal contents. Unlike some of the other laxatives, bulk-forming laxatives tend to produce normal, formed stools, as opposed to liquid stools. Their site of action is limited to the GI tract so there are few, if any, systemic effects. However, they should be taken with liberal amounts of water to prevent esophageal obstruction and/or fecal impaction. These laxatives are OTC medications and are classified as pregnancy category C agents. The bulk-forming laxatives are among the safest available and the only ones that are recommended for long-term use.

methylcellulose

Methylcellulose is a synthetic bulk-forming laxative that attracts water into the intestine and absorbs excess water into the stool, stimulating the intestines and increasing peristalsis. It is contraindicated in clients who have shown a hypersensitivity reaction to it and in those with GI obstruction or hepatitis. Methylcellulose is an oral agent available in powdered form that provides approximately 2 g of fibre per heaping tablespoon and a 1.8 percent oral solution. Pregnancy category B. Commonly recommended dosages are listed in the table on p. 863.

PHARMACOKINETICS

Half-Life	Onset	Peak	Duration
Unknown	12–24 hr	Unknown	Unknown

Agent	Pharmacological Class	Usual Dosage Range	Indications
▸▸docusate sodium	Fecal softener, emollient laxative	**Pediatric 3–6 yr*** PO: 20–60 mg/day divided (many products; consult product labelling) **6–12 yr*** PO: 40–120 mg/day divided **12 yr–adult*** PO: 100–200 mg/day divided	To facilitate defecation (e.g., postpartum or in any condition involving painful defecation due to hardened feces)
▸▸glycerin	Hyperosmotic laxative	**Adult and pediatric** PR only: Insert one adult, child, or infant suppository once to twice daily prn; attempt to retain × 15–30 min; suppository does not have to melt to induce BM	Constipation
▸▸lactulose	Disaccharide, hyperosmotic laxative	**Child–adolescent†** PO: 1–3 mL/kg/day divided **Adult†** PO: 15–30 mL/day	Constipation
magnesium citrate	Saline laxative	**Citrate, PO** **Pediatric <6 yr** 0.5 mL/kg (max 200 mL); may repeat q4–6h until stools clear **Pediatric 6–11 yr** 100–150 mL × 1 dose **Adult** 120–300 mL × 1 dose **Sulphate, PO** **Pediatric** 0.25 g/kg q4–6h **Adult** 10–15 g in 240 mL water	Constipation; bowel cleansing before diagnostic procedure or surgery
methylcellulose	Bulk-forming laxative	**Pediatric 6–11 yr** ½ 12 yr–adult dose **12 yr–adult** PO: 1 heaping teaspoon in 240 mL cold water daily–tid	Constipation
mineral oil	Emollient laxative	**PO** **Pediatric 6–11 yr** 5–15 mL oil or 10–25 mL Agarol Plain emulsion **12 yr–adult** 15–45 mL oil or 30–75 mL Agarol Plain at bedtime **Rectal enema** **Pediatric 2–12 yr** 60 mL PR × 1 **Adult** 120 mL PR × 1	Constipation
polyethylene glycol	Bowel evacuant	**Adult only** PO: 4 L solution, usually evening before procedure; client should fast at least 4 h before drinking solution	Bowel cleansing before diagnostic procedure or surgery
▸▸psyllium	Bulk-forming laxative	**Pediatric 6–11 yr** ½ 12 yr–adult dose **12 yr–adult** PO: 10.2 g/day divided in 240 mL water or juice	Constipation; often used as part of a daily maintenance program
▸▸senna	Stimulant/ irritant laxative	**Pediatric 2–5 yr‡** PO (granules): 2.5 mL/day bid (max 5 mL/day) PO (syrup): 3–5 mL at bedtime (max 5 mL bid) **6–12 yr‡** PO (tabs): 1–2 tabs at bedtime (max 2 tabs bid) PO (syrup): 5–10 mL at bedtime (max 10 mL bid) PO (granules): 2.5 mL at bedtime (max 5 mL bid) **Adult‡** PO (tabs): 2–4 tabs at bedtime (max 4 tabs bid) PO (syrup): 10–15 mL at bedtime (max 15 mL bid) PO (granules): 5–10 mL at bedtime (max 10 mL bid)	Constipation
tegaserod maleate	5-HT4 partial agonist	**Adult females only** PO: 6 mg twice daily before meals for 4 wk. Maximum duration of treatment is 12 wk. Treatment should be discontinued after 4 wk if no response.	Short-term treatment of constipation-predominant irritable bowel syndrome in women

*Docusate sodium available in both capsule and liquid forms. Docusate calcium available in capsule form only.
†Rectal route is sometimes used to reverse certain types of coma.
‡Many dosage forms; consult product labelling if in doubt. Most common dosage forms consist of 187 mg senna in tablet form and 1.7 mg/mL of sennosides in liquid form.

▶▶ *psyllium*

Psyllium is a natural bulk-forming laxative obtained from the dried seed of the *Plantago psyllium* plant. It has many of the characteristics of methylcellulose. Psyllium is contraindicated in clients who have shown a hypersensitivity reaction to it and in those with intestinal obstruction, undiagnosed rectal bleeding, dysphagia, or fecal impaction. Its use is also contraindicated in clients experiencing abdominal pain and/or nausea and vomiting. Psyllium is available as a variety of powdered products with strengths ranging from 0.3- to 0.6-g and 1- and 5-g as well as 525-, 600-, and 625-mg capsules. Pregnancy category B. Commonly recommended dosages are listed in the table on p. 863.

PHARMACOKINETICS

Half-Life	Onset	Peak	Duration
Unknown	12–24 hr	Unknown	Unknown

EMOLLIENT LAXATIVES

Emollient laxatives either directly lubricate the stool and the intestines, as with mineral oil, or they act as fecal softeners. By lubricating the fecal material and the intestinal walls, lubricant emollient laxatives prevent water from leaking out of the intestines, which softens and expands the stool. Stool softeners (docusate salts) work by lowering the surface tension of fluids, allowing more water and fat to be absorbed into the stool and the intestines.

▶▶ *docusate salts*

Docusate salts (calcium and sodium) are fecal softening emollient laxatives that facilitate the passage of water and lipids (fats) into the fecal mass, softening the stool. Docusate potassium salt products are not currently available. Some examples of the currently available agents in each salt form are as follows:
docusate calcium
• Stool softener DC
• Soflax C capsules
docusate sodium
• Colace capsules, liquid, syrup
• Selax
• Soflax

These agents are used to treat constipation, soften fecal impactions, and facilitate easy bowel movements in clients with hemorrhoids and other painful anorectal conditions. In addition to the docusate salt formulations, combination products are also available. Docusate is contraindicated in clients who have shown a hypersensitivity reaction to it and in those with intestinal obstruction, fecal impaction, or nausea and vomiting. Pregnancy category C. Commonly recommended dosages are listed in the table on p. 863.

PHARMACOKINETICS

Half-Life	Onset	Peak	Duration
Unknown	1–3 days	Unknown	1–3 days

mineral oil

Mineral oil eases the passage of stool by lubricating the intestines and preventing water from escaping the stool. Mineral oil is the only lubricant laxative in the emollient category. It is a mixture of liquid hydrocarbons derived from petroleum and is most commonly used to treat constipation associated with hard stools or fecal impaction.

Mineral oil is contraindicated in clients who have shown a hypersensitivity reaction to it. Its use is also contraindicated in clients with intestinal obstruction, abdominal pain, or nausea and vomiting. Mineral oil agents are available as enemas and in products for oral use. Pregnancy category B. Commonly recommended dosages are listed in the table on p. 863.

PHARMACOKINETICS

Half-Life	Onset	Peak	Duration
Unknown	6–8 hr	Unknown	Unknown

HYPEROSMOTIC LAXATIVES

The hyperosmotic laxatives glycerin, lactulose sorbitol, and polyethylene glycol (PEG) relieve constipation by increasing the water content of feces, resulting in distention, peristalsis, and evacuation. They are most commonly used to treat constipation and to evacuate the bowels before diagnostic and surgical procedures.

▶▶ *glycerin*

Glycerin promotes bowel movements by increasing osmotic pressure in the intestine, which draws fluid into the colon. Because it is a mild laxative, it is often used in children. Sorbitol, another hyperosmotic laxative, has similar properties. Glycerin is contraindicated in clients who have shown a hypersensitivity reaction to it. It is available as both adult and pediatric suppositories and as a glycerin liquid. Pregnancy category C. Commonly recommended dosages are listed in the table on p. 863.

PHARMACOKINETICS

Half-Life	Onset	Peak	Duration
30–45 min	16–36 min	1 hr	2–4 hr

▶▶ *lactulose*

Lactulose is a disaccharide sugar containing one molecule of galactose and one molecule of fructose. It is a synthetic derivative of the natural sugar lactose, which is not digested in the stomach or absorbed in the small bowel. Instead it is passed unchanged into the large intestine, where it is metabolized. This process produces lactic acid, formic acid, and acetic acid, creating a hyperosmotic environment that draws water into the colon and produces a laxative effect. This drug-induced acidic environment also reduces blood ammonia levels by forcing ammonia from the blood into the colon. This has proved helpful in treating clients with systemic encephalopathy. Lactulose is contraindicated in clients who have shown a hypersensitivity reaction to it and in clients on a low galactose diet. It is available as 10- and 20-g packets of powder for either oral or rectal use. Pregnancy category B. Commonly recommended dosages are listed in the table on p. 863.

PHARMACOKINETICS

Half-Life	Onset	Peak	Duration
Unknown	24 hr	24–48 hr	Variable

polyethylene glycol

PEG is most commonly used before diagnostic or surgical bowel procedures because it is a potent laxative that induces total cleansing of the bowel. It is usually available in a powdered dosage form that contains a balanced mixture of electrolytes that also help stimulate bowel evacuation. The powder is reconstituted to a large volume of fluid (4 L) that is then gradually drunk (250 mL every ten minutes) by the client in the late afternoon of the day before the procedure. PEG is contraindicated in clients with GI obstruction, gastric retention, bowel perforation, severe colitis, or toxic megacolon. The particular PEG that is used in the products mentioned is PEG-3350. The osmotic activity of PEG-3350, in combination with the electrolyte concentration, results in virtually no net absorption or secretion of ions or water. As a result, large volumes may be administered without significant changes in fluid and electrolyte balance. A common sample product composition is as follows (in g/L):

- PEG-3350 59
- Sodium chloride 1.46
- Potassium chloride 0.745
- Sodium bicarbonate 1.68
- Sodium sulphate 5.68

Diarrhea usually occurs within 30 to 60 minutes after ingestion; complete evacuation and cleansing of the bowel is accomplished within four hours. Pregnancy category C. Commonly recommended dosages are listed in the table on p. 863.

PHARMACOKINETICS

Half-Life	Onset	Peak	Duration
Unknown	1 hr	2–4 hr	4 hr

SALINE LAXATIVES

Saline laxatives consist of various magnesium or sodium salts. They increase osmotic pressure and draw water into the colon, producing a watery stool usually within three to six hours of ingestion. The currently available saline laxatives are listed in Box 50-1.

magnesium salts

The magnesium saline laxatives magnesium citrate, magnesium hydroxide (milk of magnesia), and magnesium sulphate (Epsom salts) are commonly used, unpleasant tasting OTC laxative preparations. They should be used with caution or not at all in clients with renal insufficiency because they can be absorbed into the systemic circulation, causing hypermagnesemia.

BOX   50-1

Saline Laxatives

Magnesium Laxatives
Sulphate
Epsom salt
Hydroxide
Milk of magnesia
Citrate
Citrate of magnesia

Sodium Laxatives
Phosphate
Fleet Phospho-Soda
Fleet enema

They are most commonly used for rapid evacuation of the bowel in preparation for endoscopic examination and to help remove unabsorbed poisons from the GI tract.

Magnesium salts are contraindicated in clients who have shown a hypersensitivity reaction to them. Their use is also contraindicated in clients with renal disease, abdominal pain, nausea and vomiting, obstruction, acute surgical abdomen, or rectal bleeding. Magnesium hydroxide is available as a 77.5-mg/mL suspension, a concentrated milk of magnesia suspension (80 mg/mL), a 385-mg chewable tablet, and 50-, 300-, and 311-mg tablets. It is also used in a variety of combination products. Other magnesium products are listed in the earlier discussion of saline laxatives. Pregnancy category B. Commonly recommended dosages are listed in the table on p. 863.

PHARMACOKINETICS

Half-Life	Onset	Peak	Duration
Unknown	0.5–3 hr	3 hr	Variable

STIMULANT LAXATIVES

Stimulant laxatives, including natural plant products and synthetic chemical agents, induce intestinal peristalsis through their irritant effect on the lining of the colon that stimulates the muscles of the colon. Plant-derived laxatives include remedies made from extracts of senna fruit or leaves, aloe, buckthorn, or rhubarb. Plant-derived laxatives are activated by bacteria in the intestine. It is thought that the resulting chemical products stimulate the cells of the intestinal wall and allow water to penetrate the intestine, which triggers elimination. The active ingredients in stimulant laxatives are known as anthraquinones. The action of the stimulant laxatives is proportional to the dose. The stimulant class is the most likely of all laxative classes to cause dependence.

▸▸ senna

Senna is an example of a commonly used OTC stimulant laxative. Senna is obtained from the dried leaves of the *Cassia acutifolia* plant. It may be used for acute constipation or bowel preparation for surgery or examination. Because of its stimulating action on the GI tract, it may cause abdominal pain. It can produce complete bowel evacuation in six to twelve hours. It is available in a variety of dosages as tablets, syrup, and granules. Pregnancy category C. Commonly recommended dosages are listed in the table on p. 863.

PHARMACOKINETICS

Half-Life	Onset	Peak	Duration
Variable	6–24 hr	24 hr	24–36 hr

DRUGS FOR IRRITABLE BOWEL SYNDROME

Irritable bowel syndrome (IBS) is a condition of chronic intestinal discomforts including cramps, diarrhea, and/or constipation. Clients usually cope with symptoms by avoiding irritating foods and/or with OTC laxatives and antidiarrheal agents. Women are affected more often than men, and the sole available prescription medication for IBS, tegaserod, is currently approved for women only. Tegaserod works through its interaction with various serotonin receptor subtypes in the intestinal tissue. It is a pregnancy Category B agent, contraindicated in cases of significant non–IBS GI history, and is available only in oral tablet form.

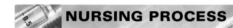

NURSING PROCESS

■ Assessment

Before administering antidiarrheal preparations, the nurse should obtain and document a thorough history of bowel patterns, general state of health, and recent history of illness or dietary changes. In addition to this assessment information, it is critical to client safety and health to rule out *Clostridium difficile* or other infectious diarrhea. The adsorbent bismuth subsalicylate should not be given to children under 16 years of age or to teenagers with chicken pox because of the risk for Reye's syndrome (see the Pediatric Considerations box at right). It should also not be given to clients who are allergic to either of the chemical ingredients (bismuth or salicylates). Caution and careful monitoring are required with the use of adsorbents in geriatric clients or in clients who have a history of decreased bleeding time, clotting disorders, recent bowel surgery, or confusion.

Anticholinergics (antispasmodics) are contraindicated in clients with a history of allergy to them and in clients with glaucoma, benign prostatic hypertrophy, urinary retention, recent bladder surgery, or cardiac history. Other contraindications include myasthenia gravis, paralytic ileus, and toxic megacolon. Cautious use is recommended in clients with a history of confusion, dizziness, hypotension, hypertension, bradycardia, tachycardia, or blurred vision.

Bulk-forming laxatives, such as psyllium preparations, are often used to treat chronic constipation and have few side effects. To ensure client safety, a thorough history of presenting symptoms and elimination patterns must be completed and documented before administering these medications. In addition, the client's intake and output ratio and serum electrolyte levels should be assessed and documented before initiating and during therapy to establish baseline values for later comparison.

■ Nursing Diagnoses

Nursing diagnoses associated with the use of antidiarrheals, laxatives, and **cathartics** include, but are not limited to, the following:
- Diarrhea related to the pathophysiology of various GI disorders.
- Risk for deficient fluid volume related to excessive loss of water and electrolytes from diarrhea.
- Risk for fall related to weakness and dizziness from possible excessive loss of fluid and electrolytes through stool.
- Deficient knowledge about OTC medications related to side effects of laxatives and cathartics.

■ Planning

Goals related to the administration of antidiarrheals, laxatives, and cathartics include the following:
- Client remains free of fluid and electrolyte disturbances related to changes in bowel patterns.

PEDIATRIC CONSIDERATIONS

Antidiarrheal Preparations

- Always check with the physician before administering antidiarrheal preparations to a child at home, and report the symptoms in case further assessment or medical management is needed.
- Dehydration and electrolyte loss occur rapidly in children because of their size and sensitivity to loss of fluid volume and electrolytes through the stool.
- Always contact the physician or pharmacist for proper dosage of antidiarrheals for any child under six years of age or if you have any doubt during discharge teaching to the family and client. Dosages are usually calculated by body weight, and the guidelines or directions provided for most OTC medications are for averaged-sized children over 12 years of age. Never hesitate to contact the physician with any concern or question regarding any medication issued for any client, especially the pediatric client.
- Immediately report to the physician abdominal distention, firm abdomen, painful abdomen, and worsening or no improvement in diarrhea 24 to 48 hours after medication administration. Measuring amounts of diarrhea by the number of diapers or number of stools per day provides important information.
- Antidiarrheal preparations should always be given cautiously to the pediatric client. If symptoms persist or dehydration occurs (e.g., no tears and decreased urine output in the child), contact the physician.
- If the client is sluggish, lethargic, or confused, or the diarrhea is bloody, contact the physician.

- Client is free from self-injury related to possible weakness and dizziness or from side effects of medications.
- Client remains adherent to medication and non-pharmacological measures.

▧ *Outcome Criteria*

Outcome criteria for the client receiving antidiarrheals, laxatives, and cathartics include, but are not limited to, the following:

- Client reports the signs and symptoms of fluid and electrolyte loss, such as weakness, lethargy, decreased urinary output, and dizziness.
- Client states measures to avoid side effects and injuries related to change in bowel patterns, changes in fluid and electrolyte status, or treatment, such as changing positions slowly.
- Client states methods of administration that enhance effective and safe use of antidiarrheals, laxatives, or cathartics, such as taking as prescribed.
- Client states non-pharmacological measures to relieve constipation, flatus, and diarrhea, such as forcing fluids, increasing fibre or bulk, or withdrawing irritating food sources from diet.

▧ Implementation

Antidiarrheals should be taken exactly as prescribed, with strict adherence to the recommended dosage. The nurse should ensure that clients are aware of their fluid intake and any dietary changes that would affect their current health status, as well as possibly exacerbate the symptoms already present. Clients should also be aware of the precipitating factors of the diarrhea and, if symptoms persist, they should know to contact a physician immediately. Bowel pattern changes, weight, fluid volume status, intake and output, and mucous membrane status should be documented before, during, and after the initiation of treatment.

Bulk-forming laxatives, such as psyllium and methylcellulose, must be administered as specified by package inserts, which is usually in the morning and evening. They should be given alone (i.e., not with food), mixed with at least 180 to 240 mL of fluid, and drunk immediately to prevent possible obstruction. Instructions for administering mineral oil agents are similar to those for other laxatives, with the additional concern of preventing aspiration in the geriatric client. Bisacodyl and cascara sagrada should be given with water only because they interact with milk, antacids, and H_2 antagonists.

Client education is important to adherence and safe, effective use of laxatives or cathartics. See the box on p. 868 for client teaching tips.

▧ Evaluation

Therapeutic responses to antidiarrheals, laxatives, and cathartics include an improvement in the GI-related signs and symptoms reported by the client, as well as improvement in bowel sounds and no abnormal findings from an assessment of the abdomen and bowel patterns. Side effects for which to monitor in clients vary according to drug classification group.

CASE STUDY ◆◆◆◆

Laxatives

One of your clients at the retirement community is complaining of constipation. As the nurse practitioner at this facility you are going to help this 75-year-old female with the changes in her bowel patterns. Initially, about two weeks ago, you suggested that she take psyllium once daily. You sent client education materials home with her at that time. As a follow-up to the initial visit, you find that she is complaining that the psyllium is "getting stuck in my throat all the time" and she goes on to tell you that she quit taking the psyllium and is taking her old Ex-Lax from years ago. Other medications include "hormone" pills (thyroid hormone).

- What role does psyllium play in helping clients with constipation compared with other laxatives?
- Why may the psyllium be getting stuck in her throat? What information would be important to share with her about this particular medication?
- What other drugs could you suggest or what information should you share with this client to help her with her constipation? Could the thyroid hormone lead to problems of constipation, or would the constipation be worsened by the psyllium? Explain your answers.

For answers see http://evolve.elsevier.com/Lilley/pharmacology/.

CASE STUDY ◆◆◆◆

Constipation

Mrs. M. is a 66-year-old retired school teacher. She enjoys good health and exercises three times a week with a senior citizens' group in a supervised arthritis swim class at the local recreation centre. She arrives at the doctor's office with complaints of "constipation" and states that for the last three months she has only one bowel movement every three days, whereas she used to have one every day. In the assessment of this client you discover that she has been taking a laxative up to twice a day and is also now feeling weak. She also states that she is experiencing "a lot of tummy cramping."

- What are at least five questions you, as the nurse, should ask Mrs. M.? Provide reasons for each question.
- What types of problems are generally related to chronic use of laxatives? Explain your answer.
- If the nurse practitioner suggested an OTC drug to help prevent constipation, what would be your choice(s) and why?

For answers see http://evolve.elsevier.com/Lilley/pharmacology/.

CLIENT TEACHING TIPS

▲ Be honest with your physician, nurse, or any other healthcare provider about dietary habits, fibre and fluid intake, and elimination patterns. It is perfectly normal not to have a bowel movement every day.

Laxatives

▲ Eat a healthy, high-fibre diet and increase your fluids. If you do this, you may not need a laxative at all.

▲ Think of laxative medication as short term. If you take it too long, your bowel may lose tone, and you may become unable to have normal bowel movements without medication.

▲ Do not take a laxative or cathartic if you are experiencing nausea, vomiting, and/or abdominal pain.

▲ Do not crush or chew tablets, especially if they are enteric coated. Swallow whole with a full or almost full glass of water.

▲ If you are taking a bulk-forming laxative such as psyllium or methylcellulose, take it as directed by the manufacturer with at least a full glass of water.

▲ Contact your physician if you experience severe abdominal pain, muscle weakness, cramps, or dizziness, which may indicate possible fluid or electrolyte loss.

Antidiarrheals

▲ Take the medication exactly as prescribed.

▲ Record how often you have bowel movements, as well as their consistency and approximate amount to make it easier to evaluate whether the medication is helping you.

POINTS to REMEMBER

▼ Diarrhea is a leading cause of morbidity and mortality in developing countries.

▼ Diarrhea accounts for up to eight million deaths worldwide per year in infants and children.

▼ Diarrhea often results in loss of time and productivity at work and has an enormous financial impact.

▼ Drug therapy for diarrhea includes adsorbents, anticholinergics, opiates, and intestinal flora modifiers.

▼ Most acute diarrhea is self-limiting, subsiding in three days to two weeks.

▼ Fluid and electrolyte replacement is vital while a client is experiencing diarrhea.

▼ Clients should be encouraged to check and recheck dosage instructions before taking medication and note any drug–food and drug–drug interactions.

▼ Anticholinergics (antispasmodics) work by decreasing GI peristalsis due to their parasympathetic blocking effects. Side effects include urinary retention, headache, confusion, dry skin, rash, and blurred vision.

▼ Adsorbents work by coating the walls of the GI tract. They remain in the intestine, bind the causative bacteria or toxin to the adsorbent surface, and eliminate it from the body through the stool. They may increase bleeding and cause constipation, dark stools, and black tongue.

▼ Intestinal flora modifiers are also used to manage diarrhea and consist of bacterial cultures of *Lactobacillus*. They supply normal intestinal flora destroyed by infection or antibiotics and suppress the growth of diarrhea-causing bacteria.

▼ Opiates are also used as antidiarrheals and help to decrease bowel motility and thus permit longer contact of intestinal contents with the absorptive surface of the bowel. Opiates also help to reduce the pain associated with rectal spasms.

▼ Laxatives and cathartics may cause fluid and electrolyte loss.

▼ Clients must be made aware of the abuse potential and the problems associated with the misuse of laxatives.

▼ Clients should be encouraged to keep a log of daily elimination patterns and any problems related to laxative use.

▼ Stool softeners and bulk-forming agents are often preferred in the treatment of constipation because they are not as problematic with regard to fluid and electrolyte loss.

▼ All antidiarrheals and laxatives must be kept out of the reach of children because they may be toxic to a child.

▼ Clients taking either antidiarrheals or laxatives should report immediately abdominal distention, firm abdomen, pain, worsening (or no improvement) of diarrhea, and GI-related signs and symptoms.

▼ Long-term use of laxatives may lead to dependence. However, bulk-forming laxatives are not habit-forming.

▼ The nurse should always check for possible drug–drug and drug–food interactions with antidiarrheals and laxatives.

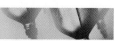

EXAMINATION REVIEW QUESTIONS

1 Which of the following is a PEG-3550 agent?
   a. Fleet Phospho-Soda
   b. CoLyte solution
   c. Pepto-Bismol
   d. docusate sodium

2 What is the major concern regarding the administration of oral methylcellulose?
   a. Dehydration
   b. Polycythemia
   c. Inducing heart failure
   d. Possible obstruction

3 Which of the following medications is most problematic in geriatric clients? Be sure to choose the response that contains the correct drug and related rationale.
   a. Metamucil; common side effects of hypovolemia and hypokalemia
   b. Laxatives; side effects of fluid and/or volume depletion and potential electrolyte imbalances

   c. Fleet enema; major toxicities of hyperkalemia and hypermagnesemia
   d. Entrocel; common toxicities of abdominal cramping and emesis

4 Methylcellulose is classified as a
   a. Potent laxative
   b. Glycerin osmotic
   c. Hypertonic osmotic
   d. Bulk-forming laxative

5 Which of the following is a side effect associated with diphenoxylate?
   a. Dysphagia
   b. Epigastric pain
   c. Anticholinergic side effects
   d. CNS overstimulation

For answers see http://evolve.elsevier.com/Lilley/pharmacology/.

CRITICAL THINKING ACTIVITIES

1 You need to explain to a group of geriatric clients the importance of seeking treatment for diarrhea. During your discussion with the group the following questions were posed to you:
   • "What are some non-drug therapies I can use once I have begun to recover from diarrhea caused by a virus or the flu?"
   • "If I have eaten something bad, does it matter if I take something to stop the diarrhea?"

Answer these questions for the geriatric population and provide a rationale for each response.

2 A mother calls the clinic because her four-month-old daughter has had diarrhea for about eight hours. What would you recommend and why?

3 Why is it important that geriatric clients are monitored closely while taking any type of bowel preparation for diagnostic studies such as a colonoscopy? Explain your answer.

For answers see http://evolve.elsevier.com/Lilley/pharmacology/.

BIBLIOGRAPHY

Albanese, J., & Nutz, P. (2005). *Mosby's 2005 nursing drug cards.* St Louis, MO: Mosby.

Canadian Pharmacists Association. (2003). *Therapeutic choices* (4th ed.). Ottawa, ON: Author.

Canadian Pharmacists Association. (2004). *Guide to drugs in Canada.* Toronto, ON: Dorling Kindersley.

Canadian Pharmacists Association. (2005). *Compendium of pharmaceuticals and specialties. The Canadian drug reference for health professionals.* Ottawa, ON: Author. [The subscription-based e-CPS is available at http://www.pharmacists.ca.]

Cheng, A., Williams, B.A., & Sivarajan, B.V. (Eds.). (2003). *The HSC handbook of pediatrics* (10th ed.). Toronto, ON: Elsevier.

Facts and Comparisons. (2004). *Drug facts and comparisons pocket version* (9th ed.). St Louis, MO: Wolters Kluwer Health.

Health Canada. (2005). Drug product database (DPD). Retrieved September 8, 2005, from http://www.hc-sc.gc.ca/hpb/drugs-dpd/

Lacy, C.F., Armstrong, L.L., Goldman, M.P., & Lance, L.L. (2003). *Drug information handbook* (11th ed.). Hudson, OH: Lexi-Comp.

Lehne, R.A. (2004). *Pharmacology for nursing care* (5th ed.). St Louis, MO: Saunders.

Mosby. (2005). *Mosby's drug consult 2005: The comprehensive reference for generic and brand name drugs* (15th ed). St. Louis, MO: Mosby.

Skidmore-Roth, L. (2006). *Mosby's 2006 nursing drug reference* (19th ed.). St Louis, MO: Mosby.

51 Anti-Emetic and Antinausea Agents

OBJECTIVES

After reading this chapter, the successful student will be able to do the following:

1 Discuss the pathophysiology of nausea and vomiting, including specific precipitating factors and/or diseases.

2 Identify the various anti-emetic and antinausea drugs and their drug classification groupings.

3 Identify the mechanisms of action, indications for use, contraindications, cautions, and drug interactions associated with the various categories of anti-emetic and antinausea agents.

4 Develop a nursing care plan as related to the nursing process in the administration of anti-emetic and antinausea agents.

e-LEARNING ACTIVITIES

Student CD-ROM
- Review Questions: see questions 375–386
- Animations
- Medication Administration Checklists
- IV Therapy Checklists

evolve Web site (http://evolve.elsevier.com/Lilley/pharmacology/)
- Online Chapter Worksheet • Frequently Asked Questions
- Learning Tips and Content Updates • WebLinks • Online Appendices and Supplements • Mosby/Saunders ePharmacology Update • Access to *Mosby's Drug Consult*

DRUG PROFILES

dronabinol, p. 876
droperidol, p. 875
granisetron, p. 875
‣‣meclizine, p. 875

‣‣metoclopramide, p. 875
‣‣ondansetron, p. 875
‣‣prochlorperazine, p. 875
scopolamine, p. 874

‣‣ Key drug.

GLOSSARY

Anti-emetic agent (an' tee ə met' ik) A drug given to relieve nausea and vomiting.

Chemoreceptor trigger zone (CTZ) The area in the brain that is involved with the sensation of nausea and the action of vomiting.

Emesis (em' ə sis) The forcible emptying or expulsion of gastric and, occasionally, intestinal contents through the mouth; vomiting.

Nausea Sensation often leading to the urge to vomit.

Neuroleptic agent (nyur' o lep' tik) (as an anti-emetic) A drug that prevents nausea and vomiting by blocking dopamine receptors on the CTZ. Also an older name for antipsychotic drugs.

Pro-kinetic agent (pro' ki net' ik) A drug that stimulates peristaltic movement in the gastrointestinal (GI) tract.

Serotonin blocker (ser' o toe' nin) An agent that prevents nausea and vomiting by blocking serotonin receptors located in the GI tract, the CTZ, and the vomiting centre.

Tetrahydrocannabinol (THC) (tet' ruh hy' droe kə nab' i nol) A major psychoactive substance in marijuana. Non-intoxicating doses have been used experimentally to treat glaucoma and to relieve nausea and increase the appetite in clients receiving cancer chemotherapy.

Vomiting centre (VC) The area in the brain that is involved in stimulating the physiological events that lead to nausea and vomiting.

NAUSEA AND VOMITING

Nausea and vomiting are two gastrointestinal (GI) disorders that not only can be extremely unpleasant but also can lead to more serious complications if not treated promptly. **Nausea** is an unpleasant feeling that often precedes vomiting. If it does not subside spontaneously or is not relieved by medication, it can lead to vomiting. Vomiting, which is also called **emesis,** is the forcible emptying or expulsion of gastric and, occasionally, intestinal contents through the mouth. A variety of stimuli can induce nausea and vomiting, including foul odours or tastes, unpleasant sights, irritation of the stomach or intestines, and certain drugs (antibiotics or antineoplastic agents).

Much research on the nature of nausea and vomiting has been conducted over the past decade, resulting in a better understanding of the physiology of these phenomena. The **vomiting centre (VC)** is an area in the brain that is responsible for initiating the necessary physiological events that lead to nausea and, eventually, vomiting. Several pathways transmit stimuli to the VC and the **chemoreceptor trigger zone (CTZ)**, another area in the brain involved in the causation of nausea and vomiting. These pathways communicate with the CTZ and VC by means of neurotransmitters and thereby alert these areas of the brain to the existence of nauseating substances (nauseous stimuli) that need to be expelled from the body. Once the VC and CTZ are stimulated, they initiate the events that stimulate the vomiting reflex. The neurotransmitters involved in this process and their respective receptors are listed in Table 51-1. The various pathways and the areas of the body that send the signals to the VC via these pathways are illustrated in Figure 51-1.

ANTI-EMETIC AGENTS

The drugs used to relieve nausea and vomiting are called **anti-emetic agents.** The discovery of new agents coupled with a better understanding of the way in which the older drugs work has had a dramatic impact on the way in which nausea and vomiting are now treated. There are six categories of anti-emetics, all working at some site in the vomiting pathway, but with varying mechanisms of action. Combining agents from different categories can increase effectiveness by blocking more than just one of the pathways. Some of the more commonly used anti-emetics in the different categories are listed in Table 51-2, and the sites where they work in the vomiting pathway are shown in Figure 51-2.

Mechanism of Action and Drug Effects

The numerous drugs used to prevent or treat nausea and vomiting have many different mechanisms of action. Most work by blocking just one of the vomiting pathways, as shown in Figure 51-2, and in doing so block the stimulus that induces vomiting. The mechanisms of action of the drugs in the six anti-emetic drug categories are summarized in Table 51-3.

Anticholinergics act by binding to and blocking acetylcholine (ACh) receptors on the vestibular nuclei, which are located in the labyrinth (cochlea and vestibule portions of the inner ear). By preventing ACh from binding to these receptors, these agents prevent nauseous stimuli originating from this area from being transmitted to the CTZ. Anticholinergics also block receptors located in the reticular formation and by doing so prevent ACh from binding to these receptors so that nauseous stimuli originating from this area cannot be transmitted to the VC. *Antihistamines* (histamine$_1$ [H$_1$] receptor blockers) act similarly to inhibit vestibular stimulation. They inhibit ACh by binding to H$_1$ receptors, thereby preventing cholinergic stimulation in both the vestibular and reticular systems. Nausea and vomiting occur when these areas of the brain are stimulated.

Neuroleptic agents prevent nausea and vomiting by blocking dopamine receptors on the CTZ. Many of the neuroleptics also have anticholinergic actions.

TABLE 51-1

NEUROTRANSMITTERS INVOLVED IN NAUSEA AND VOMITING

Neurotransmitter	Site in the Vomiting Pathway
Acetylcholine (ACh)	VC in brain; vestibular and labyrinth pathways in inner ear
Dopamine (D$_2$)	GI tract and CTZ in brain
Histamine (H$_1$)	VC in brain; vestibular and labyrinth pathways in inner ear
Prostaglandins (PGs)	GI tract
Serotonin (5-HT3)	GI tract; CTZ and VC in brain

VC, Vomiting centre; *CTZ,* chemoreceptor trigger zone.

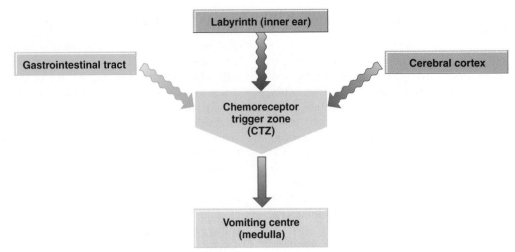

FIG. 51-1 The various pathways and areas in the body sending signals to the vomiting centre.

TABLE 51-2
ANTI-EMETIC AGENTS: COMMON DRUG CATEGORIES

Anti-Emetic Category	Anti-Emetic Agents
Anticholinergic agents (ACh blockers)	scopolamine
Antihistamine agents (H₁ receptor blockers)	dimenhydrinate, diphenhydramine, meclizine, promethazine
Neuroleptic agents	chlorpromazine, perphenazine, prochlorperazine, promethazine, trimeprazine
Pro-kinetic agents	metoclopramide
Serotonin blockers	dolasetron, granisetron, ondansetron
Tetrahydrocannabinoids	dronabinol, nabilone

ACh, Acetylcholine.

Pro-kinetic agents, in particular metoclopramide, block dopamine in the CTZ, which causes it to be desensitized to the impulses it receives from the GI tract. However, their primary action is to stimulate peristalsis in the GI tract. This enhances both emptying of stomach contents into the duodenum and intestinal movements.

Serotonin blockers work by blocking serotonin receptors located in the GI tract, CTZ, and VC. There are many subtypes of serotonin receptors, and these various receptors are located throughout the body (central nervous system [CNS], smooth muscles, platelets, and GI tract). The subtype of receptor involved in the mediation of nausea and vomiting is the 5-hydroxytryptamine 3 (5-HT3) receptor. These receptors are the site of action for the serotonin blockers such as ondansetron and granisetron.

Tetrahydrocannabinol (THC) is the major psychoactive substance in marijuana. In the form of the drug dronabinol it is occasionally used as an anti-emetic because of its inhibitory effects on the reticular formation, thalamus,

and cerebral cortex. These effects cause an alteration in mood and the body's perception of its surroundings, which may be beneficial in relieving nausea and vomiting. Although this particular category of anti-emetics is less commonly used, there are occasionally unusual cases of nausea and vomiting that respond well to THCs. Examples include that associated with clients being treated for cancer or acquired immunodeficiency syndrome (AIDS).

The drug effects of the anti-emetic agents are related to their mechanisms of action. All these agents act by blocking receptors that, when occupied by neurotransmitters, stimulate various vomiting pathways. These receptors are located in areas throughout the CNS, as well as in other areas of the body. For this reason anti-emetics may have drug effects other than anti-emetic ones. For instance, by blocking ACh and histamine receptors throughout the CNS and the GI tract, anticholinergic drugs and antihistamines may also cause drowsiness, drying of secretions, and prevention of smooth muscle spasms. In addition, neuroleptic agents calm the CNS, an effect beneficial in treating the symptoms of various psychotic disorders (anxiety, tension, and agitation).

Indications

The therapeutic uses of the anti-emetic agents vary depending on the category of agents. There are, however, many indications for drugs in each category. These agents have a variety of therapeutic uses because of the wide distribution of dopamine, ACh, and serotonin receptors throughout the body. Most anti-emetics act on these receptors to produce a specific physiological response. The specific indications for each class of anti-emetic agents are listed in Table 51-4.

Contraindications

For contraindications of the anti-emetic agents, see the individual drug profiles starting on p. 874.

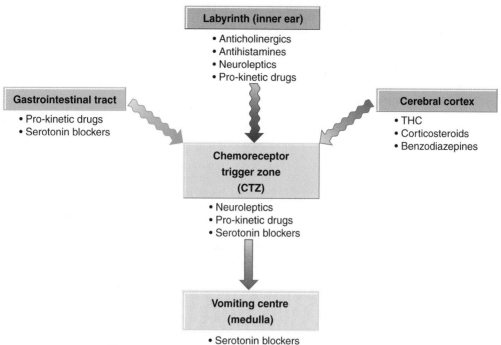

FIG. 51-2 Sites of action of selected antinausea drugs.

TABLE 51-3
ANTI-EMETIC AGENTS: MECHANISMS OF ACTION

Anti-Emetic Category	Mechanism of Action
Anticholinergic agents	Block ACh receptors in the vestibular nuclei and reticular formation
Antihistamine agents	Block H_1 receptors, thereby preventing ACh from binding to receptors in the vestibular nuclei
Neuroleptic agents	Block dopamine in the CTZ and may also block ACh
Pro-kinetic agents	Block dopamine in the CTZ or stimulate ACh receptors in the GI tract
Serotonin blockers	Block serotonin receptors in the GI tract, CTZ, and VC
Tetrahydrocannabinoids	Have inhibitory effects on the reticular formation, thalamus, and cerebral cortex

TABLE 51-4
ANTINAUSEA AGENTS: INDICATIONS

Antinausea Category	Indications
Anticholinergic agents	Motion sickness, secretion reduction before surgery, nausea and vomiting
Antihistamine agents	Motion sickness, non-productive cough, sedation, rhinitis, allergy symptoms, nausea and vomiting
Neuroleptic agents	Psychotic disorders (mania, schizophrenia, anxiety), intractable hiccups, nausea and vomiting
Pro-kinetic agents	Delayed gastric emptying, gastroesophageal reflux, nausea and vomiting
Serotonin blockers	Nausea and vomiting associated with cancer chemotherapy, postoperative nausea and vomiting
Tetrahydrocannabinoids	Nausea and vomiting associated with cancer chemotherapy, anorexia associated with weight loss in AIDS clients

Side Effects and Adverse Effects

Most of the side effects and adverse effects of the anti-emetics stem from their non-selective blockade of receptors. For example, antihistamines not only bind to H_1 receptors and prevent ACh from binding to receptors in the vestibular nuclei, but they also bind to histamine receptors located elsewhere in the body, thus, for instance, causing secretions to become dry. Some of the more common side effects associated with the various categories of anti-emetics are listed in Table 51-5.

Interactions

The drug interactions associated with the anti-emetic agents are also specific to the individual categories of agents. Anticholinergic anti-emetics have additive drying effects when given with antihistamines and

TABLE 51-5

ANTINAUSEA AGENTS: ADVERSE EFFECTS

Body System	Side/Adverse Effects
ANTICHOLINERGICS	
Central nervous	Dizziness, drowsiness, disorientation
Ears, eyes, nose, throat	Blurred vision, dilated pupils, dry mouth
Genitourinary	Difficult urination, constipation
Integumentary	Rash, erythema
ANTIHISTAMINES	
Central nervous	Dizziness, drowsiness, confusion
Ears, eyes, nose, throat	Blurred vision, dilated pupils, dry mouth
Genitourinary	Urinary retention
NEUROLEPTIC AGENTS	
Cardiovascular	Orthostatic hypotension, ECG changes, tachycardia
Central nervous	Extrapyramidal symptoms, pseudoparkinsonism, akathisia, dystonia, tardive dyskinesia, headache
Ears, eyes, nose, throat	Blurred vision, dry eyes
Genitourinary	Urinary retention
Gastrointestinal	Dry mouth, nausea and vomiting, anorexia, constipation
PRO-KINETIC AGENTS	
Cardiovascular	Hypotension, supraventricular tachycardia
Central nervous	Sedation, fatigue, restlessness, headache, dystonia
Gastrointestinal	Dry mouth, nausea and vomiting, diarrhea
SEROTONIN BLOCKERS	
Central nervous	Headache
Gastrointestinal	Diarrhea, transient increased AST and ALT levels
Other	Rash, bronchospasm
TETRAHYDROCANNABINOIDS	
Central nervous	Drowsiness, dizziness, anxiety, confusion, euphoria
Ears, eyes, nose, throat	Visual disturbances
Gastrointestinal	Dry mouth

ECG, Electrocardiogram; *AST,* aspartate aminotransferase; *ALT,* alanine aminotransferase.

antidepressants. Antihistamine anti-emetics, when given with barbiturates, opioids, hypnotics, tricyclic antidepressants (TCAs), and alcohol, can increase CNS depression. Neuroleptic anti-emetics, when given with levodopa, may cancel the beneficial effects of levodopa. Increased CNS depression can be seen when alcohol or other CNS depressants are given with neuroleptic agents. Quinidine and neuroleptic agents may result in increased adverse cardiac effects. Pro-kinetic agents, when given with alcohol, can result in additive CNS depression. Anticholinergics and analgesics can block the motility effects of metoclopramide. Serotonin blockers and THCs have no significant drug interactions.

Dosages

For the recommended dosages of selected anti-emetic agents, see the dosages table on pp. 876 and 877. See Appendix B for some of the common brands available in Canada.

DRUG PROFILES

The various anti-emetics have many different therapeutic uses, but the ultimate goals of such therapy are to minimize or prevent fluid and electrolyte disturbances, to minimize deterioration in nutritional status, and to blunt the memory of the nausea and vomiting experience (especially with cancer chemotherapy). Most of the anti-emetics act by blocking receptors within the CNS, but some work directly in the GI tract. As well as the six main classes of anti-emetic agents, corticosteroids (dexamethasone) and anxiolytics (lorazepam) may also be used to treat nausea and vomiting. In combination therapies, these latter agents, as well as THC, are beneficial in preventing the nausea and vomiting caused by cancer chemotherapy. Chemotherapy-induced nausea and vomiting (CINV) and post-operative nausea and vomiting (PONV) can be especially difficult to treat and result in devastating adverse effects. The serotonin blockers have proven to be effective in preventing CINV and PONV.

ANTICHOLINERGICS

scopolamine

Scopolamine is the primary anticholinergic drug used as an anti-emetic. It has potent effects on the vestibular nuclei, which are located in the inner ear and represent the area of the brain that controls balance. It works by blocking the binding of ACh to the cholinergic receptors in this region, thereby correcting an imbalance between the neurotransmitters ACh and norepinephrine. These effects make scopolamine one of the most commonly used drugs for the treatment and prevention of the nausea and vomiting associated with motion sickness.

Scopolamine is contraindicated in clients with a known hypersensitivity to it and in clients with glaucoma. Scopolamine is available in many dosage formulations. The most commonly used formulation is the 72-hour transdermal patch, which releases a total of 1 mg of the agent. It is also available as a 10-mg tablet, and as 0.4- and 0.6-mg/mL as well as 20-mg/mL parenteral injections. Pregnancy category C. Commonly recommended dosages are listed in the table on p. 876.

PHARMACOKINETICS

Half-Life	Onset	Peak	Duration
Unknown	1–2 hr	6–8 hr	8 hr

ANTIHISTAMINES

Antihistamine anti-emetics are some of the most commonly used and safest anti-emetics. Some of the popular antihistamines are promethazine, meclizine, dimenhydrinate, and diphenhydramine. Many of them are available OTC.

▸▸ *meclizine*

Meclizine is available as a 25-mg chewable tablet. It is most commonly used to treat the dizziness, vertigo, and nausea and vomiting associated with motion sickness. Contraindications include hypersensitivity. Pregnancy category B. Commonly recommended dosages are listed in the table on p. 876.

PHARMACOKINETICS

Half-Life	Onset	Peak	Duration
6 hr	1 hr	Variable	8–24 hr

NEUROLEPTIC AGENTS

Prochlorperazine, chlorpromazine, perphenazine, promethazine, and trifluoperazine are anti-emetics in the neuroleptic class. Many of these agents are used to treat psychotic disorders such as mania and schizophrenia, their associated anxiety, intractable hiccups, and nausea and vomiting. Droperidol is another drug commonly used for its neuroleptic (anti-anxiety) and anti-emetic properties.

droperidol

Droperidol, not to be confused with dronabinol (see later), is actually classified as a general anaesthetic and can be used as an adjunct during surgery. However, it is more commonly used to prevent nausea and vomiting during or after surgery or invasive diagnostic procedures. It also has neuroleptic (tranquilizing) effects to reduce client anxiety during such procedures. Its only listed contraindication is drug allergy. It is available only in injectable form in a 2.5-mg/mL strength. Pregnancy category C.

PHARMACOKINETICS

Half-Life	Onset	Peak	Duration
2.3 hr	3–10 min	30 min	2–4 hr

▸▸ *prochlorperazine*

Prochlorperazine is contraindicated in clients with a hypersensitivity to phenothiazines, those in a coma, and those suffering from seizures, encephalopathy, renal or liver disorders, or bone marrow depression. It is available in many dosage formulations: 10-mg suppositories; a 5-mg/mL parenteral injection; and 5- and 10-mg tablets. Pregnancy category C. Commonly used dosages are listed in the table on p. 876.

PHARMACOKINETICS

For oral tablet

Half-Life	Onset	Peak	Duration
6–8 hr	30–40 min	2–4 hr	3–4 hr

PRO-KINETIC AGENTS

Pro-kinetic agents promote the movement of substances through the GI tract and increase GI motility. The pro-kinetic agent that is also used to prevent nausea and vomiting is metoclopramide. Janssen-Ortho stopped marketing cisapride in Canada as of May 30, 2000. As of December 31, 1999, the use of cisapride was associated with 341 reports of heart rhythm abnormalities, including 80 reports of death in the United States. In Canada, there were 44 reports of cardiac abnormalities and ten deaths. For these reasons, cisapride is currently available only through Health Canada's Special Access Programme and the drug manufacturer.

▸▸ *metoclopramide*

Metoclopramide is the oldest and most commonly used pro-kinetic agent. It is available only by prescription because it can cause some severe side effects if not used correctly. Metoclopramide is used for the treatment of delayed gastric emptying and gastroesophageal reflux and also as an anti-emetic. It is contraindicated in clients with gastrointestinal hemorrhage, pheochromocytoma, or GI obstruction, and also in clients with a hypersensitivity to it or to procaine or procainamide. Metoclopramide is available in both oral and parenteral formulations as 5- and 10-mg tablets and a 5-mg/mL parenteral injection. Pregnancy category B. Commonly used dosages are listed in the table on p. 876.

PHARMACOKINETICS

Half-Life	Onset	Peak	Duration
PO: 3–5 hr	PO: 30–60 min	PO: 45–90 min	PO: 3–4 hr

SEROTONIN BLOCKERS

The serotonin blockers are also called *5-HT3 receptor blockers* because they block the 5-HT3 receptors in the GI tract, CTZ, and vomiting centre. The chemical name for serotonin is 5-hydroxytryptamine (5-HT). Because of their specific actions, these agents cause few adverse effects. They are indicated for the prevention of nausea and vomiting associated with cancer chemotherapy and also for the prevention of post-operative or radiation-induced nausea and vomiting. Currently there are three agents in this category: dolasetron, granisetron, and ondansetron.

granisetron

Granisetron is the second serotonin antagonist anti-emetic, approved by Health Canada for this use in 2004. It is more potent than ondansetron, requiring fewer doses for comparable effectiveness. It is available only by prescription and is contraindicated in cases of drug allergy. Only two dosage forms are currently available: a 1-mg film-coated tablet and a 1-mg/mL injection. Pregnancy category B. Commonly used dosages are listed in the table on p. 876.

PHARMACOKINETICS

Half-Life	Onset	Peak	Duration
6 hr	1–3 min	Unknown	Up to 24 hr

▸▸ *ondansetron*

Ondansetron is a commonly used serotonin blocker. It is a prescription-only drug available orally or intravenously. Its only contraindication is hypersensitivity. Ondansetron is available as a 2-mg/mL parenteral injection, 4- and 8-mg tablets, a 4-mg/5-mL oral solution, and 4- and 8-mg oral disintegrating tablets (ODT).

DOSAGES Selected Anti-Emetic and Antinausea Agents

Agent	Pharmacological Class	Usual Dosage Range	Indications
Anticholinergic Agent			
scopolamine	Anticholinergic, belladonna alkaloid	Apply 1 patch (1 mg) to hairless area behind ear q3d (starting at least 4 h before travel)	Motion sickness prophylaxis
Antihistamine Agent			
▶▶**meclizine**	Anticholinergic, antihistamine	**Adult** PO: 25–50 mg 1 h before travel and repeated daily during travel	Motion sickness prophylaxis
		25–100 mg/day, divided once daily–qid	Vertigo
		50 mg 2–12 h prior to treatment	Radiation sickness
Neuroleptic Agent			
▶▶**prochlorperazine**	Phenothiazine	**Pediatric:** PO/Rectal: **9–14 kg:** 2.5 mg once daily–bid (max 7.5 mg/day) **14–18 kg:** 2.5 mg bid–tid (max 10 mg/day) **18–39 kg:** 2.5 mg tid or 5 mg bid (max 15 mg/day) IM: 0.13 mg/kg, one dose is usually sufficient **Adult** PO/Rectal: 5–10 mg tid–qid IM: 5–10 mg q3–4h (max 40 mg/day)	Anti-emetic
Pro-Kinetic Agent			
▶▶**metoclopramide**	Dopamine antagonist	**Adult** IV: 1–2 mg/kg (30 min before chemotherapy; repeat q2h × 2 doses, then q3h × 3 doses)	Chemotherapy anti-emetic
		IM: 10–20 mg × 1 dose near end of surgery	Prevention of postoperative nausea and vomiting
Serotonin Blockers			
granisetron	Antiserotonergic	**Adult and pediatric ≥2 yr** IV: 10 μg/kg × 1 dose 30 min before chemotherapy, once daily on chemotherapy days PO: 2 mg 1 h before chemotherapy or 1 mg 1 h before and 1 mg 12 h post-chemotherapy	Chemotherapy anti-emetic

Continued

Pregnancy category B. Commonly used dosages are listed in the table above.

PHARMACOKINETICS

Half-Life	Onset	Peak	Duration
IV: 3–5.5 hr	IV: 15–30 min	IV: 1–1.5 hr	IV: 6–12 hr

TETRAHYDROCANNABINOIDS
dronabinol

Dronabinol is a synthetic derivative of the major active substance in marijuana. Also available in Canada is the cannabinoid nabilone, a synthetic form of THC, approved for nausea and vomiting associated with chemotherapy. In April 2005, Canada became the first country to approve Sativex, a cannabis-based drug, for the adjunctive treatment of neuropathic MS-related pain. It is available as a solution supplied in small vials as a buccal spray. Dronabinol was officially approved by Health Canada in 2000 for the treatment of the nausea and vomiting related to cancer chemotherapy. It is generally used as a second-line agent after treatment with other anti-emetics has failed. It is also used to stimulate appetite and weight gain in clients with AIDS. Dronabinol is contraindicated in clients with drug allergy and in the treatment of nausea and vomiting stemming from any cause other than cancer chemotherapy or in those with a history of psychotic disorders. It is available as 2.5-, 5-, and 10-mg capsules. Pregnancy category B. Commonly used dosages are listed in the table above.

PHARMACOKINETICS

Half-Life	Onset	Peak	Duration
25–36 hr	30–60 min	2–4 hr	4–6 hr

▣ NURSING PROCESS

■ Assessment

Before administering any antinausea or anti-emetic agent, a thorough nursing assessment of the client should be completed, including a complete nausea and vomiting

DOSAGES Selected Anti-Emetic and Antinausea Agents—cont'd

Agent	Pharmacological Class	Usual Dosage Range	Indications
Serotonin Blockers—cont'd			
▶▶ondansetron	Antiserotonergic	**Pediatric 4–12 yr** PO: 4 mg tid, after chemotherapy, × up to 5 days **Pediatric 4–12 yr** IV: 3–5 mg/m² over 15 min, immediately before chemotherapy, then oral as above **Adult** PO: 8 mg tid up to 5 days after the initial 24 h IV dose IV: 8 mg over 15 min, given 30 min before chemotherapy, followed by 1 mg/h continuous infusion up to 24 h, or one dose of 32 mg over 15 min, given 30 min before chemotherapy	Chemotherapy anti-emetic
		PO: 16 mg 1 h before surgery IV: 4 mg over 2–5 min × 1 dose (second dose not shown to be effective in clients who fail first dose)	Post-operative nausea
Tetrahydrocannabinoids			
dronabinol	Marijuana-derived anti-emetic	**Adult** PO: Initially, 5 mg/m² 1–3 h before chemotherapy, then q2–4h after chemotherapy up to 4–6×/day; this dose may, if needed, be increased in 2.5-mg/m² increments to a max dose of 15 mg/m²	Chemotherapy anti-emetic
		PO: 2.5–5 mg bid before lunch and before or after dinner, or 2.5 mg as single P.M. or bedtime dose for clients intolerant of 5-mg doses	Appetite stimulation in HIV/AIDS
nabilone	Marijuana-derived anti-emetic	**Adult** PO: 1–2 mg bid; first dose night before chemotherapy, the second dose 1–3 h before chemotherapy. May be given × 24 h to max of 6 mg, divided	Management of severe nausea and vomiting associated with chemotherapy
Sativex	Marijuana-derived anti-emetic	**Adult >18 yr** Buccal spray: dosage adjusted to need	Pain related to multiple sclerosis

history; past and present medical history; and past and present medication history, including OTC, natural health products (including herbals), prescription drugs, and use of social drugs. Precipitating factors, weight loss, baseline vital signs, and laboratory findings (such as electrolyte levels and fluid volume status) should also be assessed and the findings documented. Intake and output also needs to be assessed, especially any changes, as well as skin turgor, mucous membranes, and capillary refill.

The anticholinergic agent scopolamine is contraindicated in clients with a hypersensitivity to it and in those with glaucoma. Cautious use with careful and close monitoring is recommended in clients suffering from blurred vision, dizziness, or benign prostatic hyperplasia (BPH). The effects of antihistamines and antidepressants are enhanced when these agents are used with anticholinergic anti-emetics; therefore, the nurse should find out whether the client is taking these other agents.

Antihistamines such as meclizine are often the most commonly used and safest anti-emetics. Meclizine is contraindicated in clients with a hypersensitivity to it, those in

shock, and lactating women. Cautious use is recommended in clients suffering from BPH, dizziness, confusion, or blurred vision. Barbiturates, opioids, hypnotics, TCAs, and alcohol cause increased CNS depression when used with antihistamines; therefore the client should be asked about the use of these agents and about alcohol consumption.

Neuroleptic agents such as prochlorperazine are contraindicated in clients with a hypersensitivity to them and in those suffering from coma, seizures, encephalopathy, or bone marrow depression. Cautious use is encouraged in clients with hypotension, cardiac dysrhythmias, BPH, or a CNS disorder. The effect of levodopa is decreased or absent in clients with Parkinson's disease taking neuroleptic agents. An increase in adverse cardiac effects occurs when quinidine and neuroleptic agents are taken simultaneously.

Pro-kinetic agents (e.g., metoclopramide) are often reserved for the treatment of the nausea and vomiting associated with chemotherapy and radiation therapy. Contraindications include hypersensitivity to the agent or to procaine or procainamide, seizure disorders, pheochromocytoma, breast cancer, and GI obstruction. Cautious use is recommended in pregnant or lactating women and in clients with heart failure or GI hemorrhage. Their action is decreased when they are used with anticholinergics or opiates. Increased sedation may also occur when pro-kinetic agents are used with alcohol and other CNS depressants.

Ondansetron, a serotonin blocker, increases tolerance to chemotherapy because of its effective antinausea properties. It is contraindicated in clients with a hypersensitivity to it, and cautious use is recommended in pregnant or lactating women, children, and geriatric clients. Before its use, the client should be asked about the nature of the nausea and vomiting caused by chemotherapy and the findings should be documented. Granisetron is the second serotonin antagonist anti-emetic and is more potent than ondansetron. Granisetron is contraindicated in those with drug allergies to the serotonin blockers.

The THC agent dronabinol is generally used only in clients who are undergoing chemotherapy and experiencing the attendant nausea and vomiting. It may sometimes be used as an appetite stimulant in AIDS clients. As with all of these drugs, it is essential to document nausea and vomiting, specifically duration and precipitating factors. A thorough nursing history and assessment must also be done before the start of therapy.

The newer marijuana-derived anti-emetic nabilone is used in clients experiencing nausea and vomiting from chemotherapy. Another new drug derived from marijuana, Sativex, is used for pain related to multiple sclerosis. A thorough nursing history and assessment of current cannabinoid use and the effects achieved should be documented.

■ Nursing Diagnoses

Nursing diagnoses appropriate to clients receiving antinausea medications include the following:
- Risk for self-injury related to side effects of the medication.
- Risk for falls related to weakness and dizziness from vomiting.
- Impaired physical mobility related to weakness from fluid and electrolyte disturbances secondary to vomiting.

■ Planning

Goals for clients receiving antinausea medications include the following:
- Client remains free of injury from nausea, vomiting, or medication therapy.
- Client manages the side effects or identifies when to seek medical care for them.
- Client regains normal fluid volume status and electrolyte levels.
- Client regains normal levels of activity.

■ *Outcome Criteria*

Outcome criteria for clients receiving antinausea medications include the following:
- Client states measures to implement to prevent injury, such as assistance while ill, rising slowly, and changing positions slowly.

- Client states side effects of the medication to report to the physician, such as severe sedation, confusion, or lethargy.
- Client states measures to implement to prevent further fluid volume deficits, such as use of oral fluids, clear liquids, or chilled gelatin.
- Client increases activity day by day by 10 to 15 minutes.

The timeframe for goals and outcome criteria must be individualized for all clients.

■ Implementation

It is important that undiluted forms of diphenhydramine be administered intravenously at a rate of 25 mg/min. Intramuscular forms should be administered in large muscles, such as the gluteus maximus, and the sites should be rotated. Agents used to prevent nausea and vomiting in clients undergoing chemotherapy should be administered before the chemotherapy.

When metoclopramide is given orally, it should be given 30 minutes before meals and at bedtime. If given intravenously, it should be given slowly over one to two minutes. Parenteral infusions should not be given over less than 15 minutes. In addition, solutions for parenteral dosage should be kept for only 48 hours and protected from light. Metoclopramide should not be given in combination with any other medications, such as phenothiazines, which together would cause extrapyramidal reactions.

The scopolamine transdermal patch should be applied behind the ear at least four hours before the anti-emetic effect is desired. The area behind the ear should be cleansed and dried before its application.

Ondansetron should be diluted in 50 mL of either 5 percent dextrose in water (D5W) or 0.9 percent NaCl solution, or in amounts specified by hospital policy or in the manufacturer's guidelines. Individual doses of ondansetron are generally given over at least 15 minutes for parenteral dosages. Granisetron, a newer anti-emetic, provides 24-hour protection against chemotherapy-induced

CASE STUDY

Chemotherapy

Ms. S., a 68-year-old retired seamstress, has begun outpatient chemotherapy for a recent diagnosis of breast cancer. She has recovered well from a right modified mastectomy with well-healed incisions and is now physically and emotionally ready for her three-month regimen of chemotherapy. Her pre-meds consist of a variety of medications, including granisetron. Her home medication list includes oral ondansetron.
- What is the mechanism of action of granisetron that makes it effective in the management of chemotherapy-induced nausea and vomiting?
- What important points should you emphasize to Ms. S. about ondansetron?
- What role would dronabinol play in the management of nausea and vomiting in clients receiving antineoplastics?

For answers see http://evolve.elsevier.com/Lilley/pharmacology/.

nausea and vomiting. In adult clients, the agent is administered intravenously over five minutes, starting half an hour before the chemotherapy session. Dronabinol should be administered one to three hours before chemotherapy and may be taken at home before the appointment at the oncologist's office.

Client teaching tips for antinausea agents are presented in the box below.

■ Evaluation

The therapeutic effects of antinausea drugs range from a decrease in to the elimination of complaints of nausea and vomiting and no complications, such as fluid and electrolyte imbalances and weight loss. The client should also be monitored for adverse effects such as GI upset, drowsiness, lethargy, weakness, extrapyramidal reactions, and orthostatic hypotension.

CLIENT TEACHING TIPS

▲ This medication may cause drowsiness. Avoid driving or performing any hazardous tasks while on this medication.
▲ Don't take alcohol or sedatives with this medication; the combination can be dangerous.

Ondansetron

▲ This medication may cause a headache; if so, you can take a simple painkiller.

Dronabinol

▲ This drug may lower your blood pressure and make you feel dizzy. To avoid fainting, change positions slowly.

Sativex

▲ Direct the spray under the tongue or on the inside of the cheeks.

▲ Start with a small dose; if this does not relieve your pain, gradually increase the dose until it does, or up to the level your physician has prescribed. Lower the dose if you start having side effects.
▲ This drug contains alcohol, so don't drink alcohol while taking it.
▲ Use reliable contraception while taking this drug and for at least three months after.

Scopolamine Patch

▲ Wash hands thoroughly before and after applying the patch.
▲ Apply the patch to non-irritated areas behind the ear.
▲ If you're using the patch repeatedly, rotate positions.

POINTS to REMEMBER

▼ Anti-emetics work to help control vomiting, or emesis, and are also helpful in relieving or preventing nausea.
▼ The categories of anti-emetics are anticholinergics, antihistamines, neuroleptic agents, pro-kinetic agents, serotonin blockers, and tetrahydrocannabinoids.
▼ Anti-emetics are used to prevent motion sickness, reduce secretions before surgery, treat delayed gastric emptying, and prevent post-operative nausea and vomiting. They are also used in the management of many other conditions.
▼ Anticholinergics work by blocking ACh receptors in the vestibular nuclei and reticular formation. This blockade prevents areas in the brain from being stimulated by nauseous stimuli.
▼ Antihistamines work by blocking H_1 receptors, which has the same effect as the anticholinergics.
▼ Neuroleptic anti-emetics block dopamine receptors in the CTZ and may also block ACh receptors.
▼ Pro-kinetic agents also block dopamine receptors in the CTZ.
▼ The serotonin-blocking agents may be highly effective anti-emetics. They are most commonly used for the

prevention of chemotherapy-induced nausea and vomiting and work by blocking 5-HT3 receptors in the GI tract, CTZ, and VC.
▼ Anti-emetics are often administered half an hour to three hours before a chemotherapy agent is administered and may also be given during the chemotherapeutic treatment.
▼ Most anti-emetics cause drowsiness.
▼ Ondansetron and similar agents are successful in treating chemotherapy-induced nausea and vomiting.
▼ Dronabinol (synthetic THC) therapy is used to prevent chemotherapy-induced nausea and vomiting and is associated with postural hypotension.
▼ Sativex (a synthetic THC) is available as a buccal spray and is used for pain associated with multiple sclerosis.
▼ Clients taking anti-emetics should be cautioned that drowsiness and hypotension may occur and therefore they should avoid driving and using heavy machinery while taking these medications.
▼ Parameters reflecting hydration status should be monitored, such as input and output, skin turgor, and vital signs.

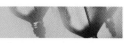

EXAMINATION REVIEW QUESTIONS

1 Anticholinergic agents work by which of the following mechanisms?
  a. Blocking THC molecules in the blood
  b. Antagonistic to ACh receptors in the vestibular nuclei
  c. Blocking dopamine receptors in the stomach
  d. Antagonistic to epinephrine in the cerebrum
2 Anti-emetics have which of the following actions?
  a. Increase oral secretions only in preoperative preparations
  b. Decrease cerebellum-related vomiting
  c. Treat delayed gastric emptying
  d. Decrease vestibular motion
3 Anti-emetics used with chemotherapy work mainly by which of the following actions?
  a. Anticholinergic
  b. Antiserotonergic

  c. Anti-epileptic
  d. Antihistaminic
4 As a nurse practitioner, when suggesting a protocol for motion sickness, why would you not recommend prokinetic drugs? They:
  a. are only for post-operative nausea.
  b. cause vestibular stimulation.
  c. are used mainly to decrease chemotherapy-related nausea.
  d. are anti-emetics by increasing GI motility.
5 What is the mechanism of action of ondansetron and granisetron?
  a. Block serotonin
  b. Inhibit acetylcholine
  c. Block dopamine receptors
  d. Inhibit effects on reticular formation, thalamus, and cerebral cortex

For answers see http://evolve.elsevier.com/Lilley/pharmacology/.

CRITICAL THINKING ACTIVITIES

1 Explain how ondansetron decreases the nausea and vomiting associated with chemotherapy. Compare its effectiveness to prochlorperazine for treatment of chemotherapy-induced nausea and vomiting.
2 Explain the mechanism(s) behind chemotherapy-induced nausea and vomiting.

3 Diphenhydramine, ondansetron, and granisetron are anti-emetic agents. Which drug(s) can be administered pre-operatively to prevent post-operative nausea and vomiting?

For answers see http://evolve.elsevier.com/Lilley/pharmacology/.

BIBLIOGRAPHY

Albanese, J., & Nutz, P. (2005). *Mosby's 2005 nursing drug cards.* St Louis, MO: Mosby.

Anderson, P.O., Knoben, J.E., & Troutman, W.G. (2002). *Handbook of clinical drug data* (10th ed.). New York: McGraw-Hill/Appleton & Lange.

Canadian Pharmacists Association. (2003). *Therapeutic choices* (4th ed.). Ottawa, ON: Author.

Canadian Pharmacists Association. (2004). *Guide to drugs in Canada.* Toronto, ON: Dorling Kindersley.

Canadian Pharmacists Association. (2005). *Compendium of pharmaceuticals and specialties. The Canadian drug reference for health professionals.* Ottawa, ON: Author. [The subscription-based e-CPS is available at http://www.pharmacists.ca.]

Cheng, A., Williams, B.A., & Sivarajan, B.V. (Eds.). (2003). *The HSC handbook of pediatrics* (10th ed.). Toronto, ON: Elsevier.

Committee on Injury, Violence, and Poison Prevention. (2003). Poison treatment in the home. *Pediatrics, 112*(5), 1182–1185.

Facts and Comparisons. (2004). *Drug facts and comparisons pocket version* (9th ed.). St Louis, MO: Wolters Kluwer Health.

Health Canada. (2000). "Dear health care provider"—Prepulsid (Cisapride). Retrieved September 8, 2005 from http://www.hc-sc.gc.ca/dhp-mps/medeff/advisoriesavis/prof/2000/prepulsid_hpc-cps_html

Health Canada. (2005). Approval of Sativex with conditions fact sheet. Retrieved November 26, 2005 from http://www.hc-sc.gc.ca/dhp-mps/prodpharma/notices-avis/conditions/sativex_factsheet_e.html

Health Canada. (2005). Drug product database (DPD). Retrieved September 8, 2005, from http://www.hc-sc.gc.ca/hpb/drugs-dpd/

Lacy, C.F., Armstrong, L.L., Goldman, M.P., & Lance, L.L. (2003). *Drug information handbook* (11th ed.). Hudson, OH: Lexi-Comp.

Lehne, R.A. (2004). *Pharmacology for nursing care* (5th ed.). St Louis, MO: Saunders.

Mosby. (2005). *Mosby's drug consult 2005: The comprehensive reference for generic and brand name drugs* (15th ed.). St Louis, MO: Mosby.

Skidmore-Roth, L. (2006). *Mosby's 2006 nursing drug reference* (19th ed.). St Louis, MO: Mosby.

CHAPTER

52

Vitamins and Minerals

GLOSSARY

Beriberi (ber′ ee ber′ ee) A disease of the peripheral nerves caused by an inability to assimilate thiamine. Symptoms are fatigue, diarrhea, loss of appetite, weight loss, and disturbed nerve function, causing paralysis and wasting of limbs, edema, and heart failure.

Coenzyme (ko en′ zime) A non-protein substance that combines with a protein molecule to form the active enzyme.

Enzyme (en′ zime) A specialized protein that catalyzes chemical reactions in organic matter.

Fat-soluble vitamin A vitamin that can be dissolved in fat. These vitamins can be stored in large amounts in the liver and fatty tissues, thus daily ingestion of these vitamins is not necessary to maintain good health. Because they are not water soluble, overdose states known as hypervitaminosis are more likely because fat-soluble vitamins are not excreted as readily via the urinary system.

Mineral An inorganic substance that is ingested and attaches to enzymes or other organic molecules. Minerals play a vital role in regulating many body functions, some functioning as coenzymes.

Pellagra (pə lag′ ruh) A disease resulting from a niacin or a metabolic defect that interferes with the conversion of tryptophan to niacin. It is characterized by scaly dermatitis, glossitis (inflamed tongue), inflammation of the mucous membranes, diarrhea, and mental disturbances.

Rhodopsin (ro dop′ sin) The purple-pigmented compound in the rods of the retina, formed by a protein, opsin, and a derivative of vitamin A, retinol.

Rickets A condition caused by a vitamin D deficiency. Symptoms include soft, pliable bones, causing such deformities as bow-legs and knock knees; nodular enlargement on the ends and sides of the bones; muscle pain; enlarged skull; chest deformities; spinal curvature; enlargement of the liver and spleen; profuse sweating; and general tenderness of the body when touched.

Scurvy A condition resulting from an ascorbic acid (vitamin C) deficiency. It is characterized by weakness, anemia, edema, spongy gums, mucocutaneous hemorrhages, and hardening of leg muscles.

Tocopherols (to kof′ ər olz) Biologically active chemicals that make up vitamin E compounds.

Vitamin An organic compound essential in small quantities for normal physiological and metabolic functioning of the body.

Water-soluble vitamin A vitamin that can be dissolved in water. Unlike their fat-soluble counterparts, water-soluble vitamins are not stored in the body for long periods because they are readily excreted through the urinary system. Therefore daily ingestion of these vitamins through proper diet alone or with specific vitamin supplements is necessary for good health.

Vitamins and minerals are essential in our life whether we are conscientious in our food choices or consume whatever we desire. In Canada, vitamins and minerals are considered natural health products (NHPs) and are governed under the Natural Health Products Regulations. Laws in Canada require detailed nutritional information to be listed on any packaged food product. Standard labelling requirements are established to ensure consumers can make informed choices. Under most circumstances, daily requirements of vitamins and minerals are met by ingestion of fluids and regular, balanced meals. Ingesting food helps us maintain adequate stores of essential vitamins and minerals and serves to preserve the intestinal mass and structure, provide chemicals for hormones and enzymes, and prevent harmful overgrowth of bacteria.

Various life events can occur that create an excessive need for or loss of nutrients, vitamins, minerals, electrolytes, and fluids, requiring replacement or supplementation. Excessive vitamin and mineral needs can occur with almost any illness and are typically seen in burn victims and persons with AIDS. Excessive loss of vitamins and minerals may be the result of poor dietary intake, an inability to swallow after cancer chemotherapy or radiation, or a mental illness disorder such as anorexia nervosa. Poor dietary absorption attributable to many types of gastrointestinal (GI) disorders or alcoholism can also contribute to inadequate intake that may require vitamin and mineral supplementation.

For the body to grow and maintain itself, it needs the essential building blocks provided by carbohydrates, fats, and proteins. Vitamins and minerals are needed to efficiently utilize these nutrients. **Vitamins** are organic molecules needed in small quantities for normal metabolism and other biochemical functions such as growth or repair of tissue. They attach to enzymes or coenzymes and help them activate anabolic (tissue-building) processes in the body. Minerals are as important as vitamins. **Minerals** are inorganic elements or salts found naturally in the earth. Like vitamins, mineral ions bind with enzymes or other organic molecules and help regulate many body functions. For example, the collagen, hormone, and enzyme synthesis that is needed to heal wounds requires vitamins and minerals.

Although vitamins and minerals are essential to life, there are instances when we are unable to acquire these essential compounds through diet or when a normal diet cannot meet the increased demand for them. In such cases vitamin and mineral supplementation is necessary. This chapter discusses both vitamins and minerals and their therapeutic effects. Because of some of their relatively distinct properties and functions in the body related to blood formation, the mineral iron and the vitamin folic acid (vitamin B_9) are discussed separately in Chapter 54.

OVERVIEW OF VITAMINS

As previously mentioned, vitamins are organic molecules needed in small amounts in the body to carry on normal metabolism. **Enzymes** are proteins secreted by cells; they act as catalysts to induce chemical changes in other substances, but they themselves remain chemically unchanged by the process. A **coenzyme** is a substance that enhances or is necessary for the action of enzymes. Vitamins and minerals function primarily as coenzymes in various metabolic pathways throughout the body. Many enzymes are totally useless without the appropriate vitamins that chemically bind with them and cause them to function properly. For example, coenzyme A (CoA) is an important carrier molecule associated with the citric acid cycle, one of the body's major energy-producing metabolic reactions. However, it requires pantothenic acid (vitamin B_5) to complete its function in the citric acid cycle.

Vitamin sources occur naturally in both plant and animal foods. Generally, natural source vitamins are derived from fruits, vegetables, and other food sources; synthetic imitations are created in the laboratory and replicate only one of perhaps dozens of beneficial nutrients.

The human body requires vitamins in specific minimum amounts on a daily basis and can obtain them from both plant and animal food sources. Non-dietary supplemental amounts of vitamin B complex and vitamin K are obtained from the synthesis of these vitamins by normal bacterial flora in the GI tract. In addition, vitamin D can be synthesized by the skin with the proper precursors when exposed to sunlight. An insufficient diet will cause various nutrition-related vitamin deficiencies. As a result of extensive food content studies, in 1942, Canada's Official Food Rules were published, developed by the Nutrition Division of the federal government in collaboration with the Canadian Council on Nutrition. Based on six food groups, a list of Recommended Daily Allowances (RDAs) of essential nutrients was identified. In 1944, the RDAs became Canada's Food Rules. There have since been six revisions of these RDAs, with the latest revision occurring in 1992. Currently the RDAs are being phased out and replaced by a more comprehensive set of dietary standards known as Dietary Reference Intakes (DRIs) that will serve as standards for both the United States and Canada. The DRIs are established by Canadian and American scientists through a review process overseen by an independent non-government association, the Food and Nutrition Board of the National Academy of Sciences (FNBNAS). The most current DRIs were published by FNBNAS from 1998 to 2000. Whereas the RDAs represent minimum nutrient requirements, the DRIs are being designed to represent optimal nutrient requirements for good health. Finally, percentage daily values (DVs) are the values that appear on the mandatory labels of commercial food products and indicate what percentage of the DRI for a specific nutrient is met by a single serving of the food product. See Table 52-1 for the latest DRI values.

Vitamins are classified as either fat or water soluble. **Water-soluble vitamins** can be dissolved in water; **fat-soluble vitamins** are dissolvable in fat. Because water-soluble vitamins (B-complex group and vitamin C) cannot be stored in the body in large amounts over long periods, daily intake is required to prevent the development of deficiencies. Conversely, fat-soluble vitamins (vitamins A, D, E, and K) do not need to be taken daily because they are stored in the liver and fatty tissues in large amounts. Deficiency in these vitamins occurs only after prolonged deprivation from an adequate supply or from disorders that prevent their absorption. Table 52-2 lists the fat-soluble and water-soluble vitamins.

One controversial topic related to vitamins is that of nutrient "megadosing," both as a strategy for health promotion and maintenance and for treating various illnesses. Some cancer clients are electing to use supplemental megadosing of specific nutrients in hopes of strengthening their body's response to more conventional cancer treatments such as surgery, radiation, and chemotherapy. Megadosing is considered to be doses of a nutrient that are ten or more times the customary recommended amount. A related term, orthomolecular medicine, is the use of vitamins, minerals, and amino acids to create optimum nutritional content and balance in the body. Probably the best-known authority of orthomolecular medicine in Canada is researcher and physician Dr. Abram Hoffer, who endorses the use of nutritional medicine for a wide variety of conditions, including depression, hypertension, schizophrenia, cancer, and other mental and physiological disorders. Nobel Prize–winning chemist Linus Pauling claimed that megadoses of vitamin C (at more than 100 times the Canadian RDA) could prevent or cure the common cold. Many studies since have refuted this claim. Even more controversial was the claim that vitamin C could prevent or cure cancer. Many careful studies since have not supported this claim either.

There are some situations where nutrient megadosing is known to be helpful, including the following:

- When concurrent long-term drug therapy depletes vitamin stores or otherwise interferes with the function of a vitamin. A common clinical example is the use of vitamin B_6 (pyridoxine) supplementation in patients receiving the drug isoniazid (INH) for tuberculosis (TB; Chapter 39).
- For malabsorption syndromes such as those seen in patients with severe colitis and cystic fibrosis.
- For the treatment of pernicious anemia, which results from vitamin B_{12} (cyanocobalamin) deficiency. The GI tract uses a fairly complex mechanism to drive cyanocobalamin absorption. When this process is compromised (e.g., by disease), megadoses of cyanocobalamin can bypass this absorption mechanism by allowing a small amount of the vitamin to diffuse through the intestinal mucosa on its own.
- When the vitamin acts as a drug when megadosed. The most common example is niacin (vitamin B_3, also called *nicotinic acid*). At doses of up to 20 mg daily it functions as a vitamin, but at doses 50 to 100 times higher it reduces blood levels of both tryglycerides and low-density lipoprotein (LDL) cholesterol, thus acting more as a drug than a vitamin (Chapter 28).

Benefits from megadoses of other vitamins are not as well established.

There are some situations where nutrient megadosing is known to be harmful. For example, any excess of one or more nutrients can result in deficiencies of other nutrients due to chemical "competition" for sites of absorption through the intestinal mucosa. This is more likely to be the case with mineral megadosing, such as with calcium, copper, iron, and zinc, and is less likely to result from vitamin megadosing.

Megadosing can lead to toxic hypervitaminosis states, especially with the fat-soluble vitamins A, D, and K. Vitamin E appears safer though, even at doses ten to twenty times the recommended DV. Hypervitaminosis is much less likely to occur with the water-soluble vitamins (B-complex and C) because they are readily excreted through the urinary system. However, it is known that megadosing with vitamin B_6 (pyridoxine) at 50 to 100 times the DV can cause nerve damage.

Persons with an illness may be the least able to tolerate nutrient megadosing, even though megadosing regimens are often prescribed for them. For example, megadosing may be more of a strain for a GI tract that is already

TABLE 52-1

DIETARY REFERENCE INTAKES (DRIs) LISTED AS RECOMMENDED DAILY DIETARY ALLOWANCES (RDAs) (NOW ALSO CALLED ADEQUATE INTAKES [AIs])

These units designed for basic health maintenance of at least 97–98 percent of healthy people living in the United States (and apply to Canada as well).

Life Stage/Gender	Age	Protein (g/day)	Carbohydrate (g/day)	Fat (g/day)	Fat-Soluble Vitamins			
					Vitamin A (μg/day)*	Vitamin D (μg/day)†	Vitamin E‡ (mg/day)	Vitamin K (μg/day)
Infants	0–6 mo	9.1	60	31	400	5	4	2
	7–12 mo	13.5	95	30	500	5	5	2.5
Children	1–3 yr	13	130	30–40	300	5	6	30
	4–8 yr	19	130	25–35	400	5	7	55
Males	9–13 yr	34	130	25–35	600	5	11	60
	14–18 yr	52	130	25–35	900	5	15	75
	19–30 yr	56	130	20–35	900	5	15	120
	31–50 yr	56	130	20–35	900	5	15	120
	50–70 yr	56	130	20–35	900	10	15	120
	>70 yr	56	130	20–35	900	15	15	120
Females	9–13 yr	34	130	25–35	600	5	11	60
	14–18 yr	46	130	25–35	700	5	15	75
	19–30 yr	46	130	20–35	700	5	15	90
	31–50 yr	46	130	20–35	700	5	15	90
	50–70 yr	46	130	20–35	700	10	15	90
	>70 yr	46	130	20–35	700	15	15	90
Pregnancy	≤18 yr	71	175	20–35	750	5	15	75
	19–30 yr	71	175	20–35	770	5	15	90
	31–50 yr	71	175	20–35	770	5	15	90
Lactation	≤18 yr	71	210	20–35	1200	5	19	75
	19–30 yr	71	210	20–35	1300	5	19	90
	31–50 yr	71	210	20–35	1300	5	19	90

Reprinted with permission from Dietary Reference Intakes for Energy, Carbohydrate, Fiber, Fat, Fatty Acids, Cholesterol, Protein, and Amino Acids (Macronutrients) © 2002 by the National Academy of Sciences, courtesy of the National Academies Press, Washington, D.C.
*Measured in retinol activity equivalents (RAEs); 1 RAE = 1 μg retinol = 12 μg beta-carotene = 24 μg alpha-carotene = 24 μg beta-cryptoxanthin.
†As calciferol; 1 μg calciferol = 40 international units (IU) of vitamin D. The DRI values assume lack of adequate sunlight exposure.
‡Vitamin E is also known as alpha-tocopherol.
Reference sources for the entire table are from the following reports of the Food and Nutrition Board, National Academy of Sciences. All tables can be found online, linked from the Institute of Medicine Web site at http://www.iom.edu/.
Specific reference tables:
1. Dietary Reference Intakes for Energy, Carbohydrate, Fiber, Fat, Fatty Acids, Cholesterol, Protein, and Amino Acids (2002).
2. Dietary Reference Intakes for Calcium, Phosphorus, Magnesium, Vitamin D, and Fluoride (1997).
3. Dietary Reference Intakes for Thiamin, Riboflavin, Niacin, Vitamin B₆, Folate, Vitamin B₁₂, Pantothenic Acid, Biotin, and Choline (1998).
4. Dietary Reference Intakes for Vitamin C, Vitamin E, Selenium, and Carotenoids (2000).
5. Dietary Reference Intakes for Vitamin A, Vitamin K, Arsenic, Boron, Chromium, Copper, Iodine, Iron, Manganese, Molybdenum, Nickel, Silicon, Vanadium, and Zinc (2001).

weakened by illness. Megadosing can even interfere with other treatments for illness, such as drug therapy. For example, in cancer clients, many chemotherapy drugs, as well as radiation treatments, work to destroy cancer cells through oxidation processes. Nutritional supplementation with antioxidants may hinder such treatment mechanisms.

Clients should be advised to share with their healthcare provider any unusual nutritional regimens that they plan to try, especially if they have a serious illness.

FAT-SOLUBLE VITAMINS

The fat-soluble vitamins are A, D, E, and K. As a group they share the following characteristics:
- Present in both plant and animal foods
- Stored primarily in the liver
- Exhibit slow metabolism or breakdown
- Excreted via the feces
- Can become toxic if excessive amounts are consumed (a condition known as *hypervitaminosis*)

			Water-Soluble Vitamins						Minerals			
Vitamin C (Ascorbic Acid, mg/day)	Thiamine (Vitamin B_1, mg/day)	Riboflavin (Vitamin B_2, mg/day)	Niacin (Nicotinic Acid or Vitamin B_3, mg/day)	Pyridoxine (Vitamin B_6, mg/day)	Folic Acid (Folate or Vitamin B_9, μg/day)	Cyanocobalamin (Vitamin B_{12}, μg/day)	Calcium (mg/day)	Phosphorus (mg/day)	Magnesium (mg/day)	Iron (mg/day)	Zinc (mg/day)	Iodine (μg/day)
40	0.2	0.3	2	0.1	65	0.4	210	100	30	0.27	2	110
50	0.3	0.4	4	0.3	80	0.5	270	275	75	11	3	130
15	0.5	0.5	6	0.5	150	0.9	500	460	80	7	3	90
25	0.6	0.6	8	0.6	200	1.2	800	500	130	10	5	90
45	0.9	0.9	12	1.0	300	1.8	1300	1250	240	8	8	120
75	1.2	1.3	16	1.3	400	2.4	1300	1250	410	11	11	150
90	1.2	1.3	16	1.3	400	2.4	1000	700	400	8	11	150
90	1.2	1.3	16	1.3	400	2.4	1000	700	420	8	11	150
90	1.2	1.3	16	1.7	400	2.4	1200	700	420	8	11	150
90	1.2	1.3	16	1.7	400	2.4	1200	700	420	8	11	150
45	0.9	0.9	12	1.0	300	1.8	1300	1250	240	8	8	120
65	1.0	1.0	14	1.2	400	2.4	1300	1250	360	15	9	150
75	1.1	1.1	14	1.3	400	2.4	1000	700	310	18	8	150
75	1.1	1.1	14	1.3	400	2.4	1000	700	320	18	8	150
75	1.1	1.1	14	1.5	400	2.4	1200	700	320	8	8	150
75	1.1	1.1	14	1.5	400	2.4	1200	700	320	8	8	150
80	1.4	1.4	18	1.9	600	2.6	1300	1250	400	27	12	220
85	1.4	1.4	18	1.9	600	2.6	1000	700	350	27	11	220
85	1.4	1.4	18	1.9	600	2.6	1000	700	360	27	11	220
115	1.4	1.6	17	2.0	500	2.8	1300	1250	360	10	13	290
120	1.4	1.6	17	2.0	500	2.8	1000	700	310	9	12	290
120	1.4	1.6	17	2.0	500	2.8	1000	700	320	9	12	290

TABLE 52-2

FAT- AND WATER-SOLUBLE VITAMINS

Fat-Soluble		Water-Soluble	
Designation	Name	Designation	Name
vitamin A	retinol	vitamin B_1	thiamine
vitamin D	D_3, cholecalciferol	vitamin B_2	riboflavin
	D_2, ergocalciferol	vitamin B_3	niacin
	dihydrotachysterol	vitamin B_5	pantothenic acid
vitamin E	tocopherols	vitamin B_6	pyridoxine
vitamin K	K_1, phytonadione	vitamin B_9	folic acid
	K_2, menaquinone	vitamin B_{12}	cyanocobalamin
		biotin	
		vitamin C	ascorbic acid

VITAMIN A

Vitamin A (retinol) is derived from animal fats such as those found in dairy products (butter and milk), eggs, meat, liver, and fish liver oils. The vitamin A stored in animal tissues is derived from carotenes, which are found in plants (green and yellow vegetables and yellow fruits).

There are over 600 naturally occurring carotenoid compounds in plant-based foods. Of these, 40 to 50 occur commonly in the human diet. Beta-carotene is the most prevalent of these, followed by alpha-carotene and cryptoxanthin. These are known as *provitamin A carotenoids* because they are all metabolized to various forms of vitamin A in the body. One molecule of beta-carotene is metabolized in the body to two molecules of the aldehyde compound retinaldehyde, the name of which is often shortened to retinal. Some of this retinal is used in its essential role in vision. However, some of it is also reduced to the alcohol compound retinol mentioned earlier. The term *vitamin A*, in the strictest sense, refers to this compound. The remainder of the retinal may be oxidized to the carboxylic acid compound retinoic acid. Unlike retinal, retinoic acid has no direct role in vision, but it is essential for normal cell growth and differentiation and the development of the physical shapes of the body's many parts—a process known as *morphogenesis*.

The sources of vitamin A as discussed are outlined as follows:

Vitamin A (retinol) → animal source (dairy products; meat, especially liver) or → metabolized from provitamins

Retinal → metabolized from provitamins

Retinoic acid → metabolized from provitamins

Provitamin A (carotenoids) → plant source (green and yellow/orange vegetables, yellow/orange fruit)

Mechanism of Action and Drug Effects

Vitamin A is an exogenous substance because it must be obtained from either plants or animals. Vitamin A is required for the growth and development of bones and teeth and is also necessary for maintaining other processes, including reproduction, integrity of mucosal and epithelial surfaces, and cholesterol and steroid synthesis. It is essential for night vision and for normal vision because it is part of one of the major retinal pigments. Vitamin A is converted to the aldehyde, *cis* retinal, which combines with opsin to form **rhodopsin**, the visual pigment that is required for normal "rod vision" in the retina. This is the vision that results from stimulation (by light) of the retinal visual cells known as *rods*, resulting in black-and-white vision and peripheral vision. It is the predominant operative vision at night, when colours of objects are not as visible. Other retinal cells known as *cones* are chiefly involved in colour and central vision (see Chapter 56).

Indications

Therapeutic uses for vitamin A are listed in Box 52-1. Supplements of vitamin A may be used to satisfy normal body requirements or an increased demand such as in infants and pregnant and nursing women. A normal diet

---

BOX 52-1
Vitamin A: Indications

Dietary Supplement
Infants
Pregnant women
Nursing women

Deficiency States
Hyperkeratosis of the skin
Night blindness
Retarded infant growth
Xerophthalmia

Skin Conditions
Acne (vitamin A derivatives)
Keratosis follicularis
Psoriasis

---

should provide adequate amounts of vitamin A, but in cases of excessive need or inadequate dietary intake, vitamin A supplementation is indicated to avoid problems associated with deficiency. Symptoms of vitamin A deficiency include night blindness, xerophthalmia (dry eyes), keratomalacia (softening of the cornea), hyperkeratosis of both the stratum corneum (outermost layer) of the skin and the sclera (outermost layer of eyeball), retarded infant growth, generalized weakness, and increased susceptibility of mucous membranes to infection.

Vitamin A-related compounds such as isotretinoin are also used to treat various forms of acne (see Chapter 55).

Contraindications

The only usual contraindications to vitamin A supplementation include known allergy to the individual vitamin product, known current state of hypervitaminosis, and excessive supplementation beyond recommended guidelines, especially during pregnancy.

Side Effects and Adverse Effects

There are few acute side effects and adverse effects associated with normal vitamin A ingestion. Only after long-term, excessive ingestion of vitamin A do symptoms appear. Side effects and adverse effects are usually noticed in bones, mucous membranes, the liver, and the skin. Table 52-3 lists some of the symptoms of long-term, excessive ingestion of vitamin A.

Toxicity and Management of Overdose

The major toxic effects of vitamin A result from ingestion of excessive amounts, which occurs most commonly in children. A few hours after administration of an excess dose of vitamin A (>25 000 units/kg) headache, irritability, drowsiness, vertigo, delirium, coma, vomiting, and/or diarrhea may occur. In infants, excessive amounts of vitamin A can cause an increase in cranial pressure, resulting in symptoms such as bulging fontanelles, headache, exophthalmos (bulging eyeballs), visual disturbances, and papilledema. Papilledema is the presence of edematous fluid, often including blood, in the optic disk—the portion of the eye in the back of the retina, where nerve fibres converge to form the optic nerve.

Over several weeks to months a generalized peeling of the skin and erythema (skin reddening), bone demineralization, brittle nails, enlarged liver and spleen,

---

TABLE 52-3
VITAMIN A: ADVERSE EFFECTS

Body System	Side/Adverse Effects
Central nervous	Headache, increased intracranial pressure, lethargy, malaise
Gastrointestinal	Nausea, vomiting, anorexia, abdominal pain, jaundice
Integumentary	Drying of skin, pruritus, increased pigmentation, night sweats
Metabolic	Hypomenorrhea, hypercalcemia
Hematological	Hypoplastic anemia, leukopenia
Musculoskeletal	Arthralgia, retarded growth, bone pain

and hair loss may occur. These symptoms seem to disappear a few days after discontinuation of the drug, which is the only treatment necessary in situations of overdose.

Interactions

Vitamin A is absorbed to a lesser extent with the simultaneous use of lubricant laxatives, neomycin, and cholestyramine. In addition, the use of isotretinoin concurrently with vitamin A supplementation can result in additive effects and possibly toxicity.

Dosages

For the RDAs for vitamin A, see Table 52-1. For the recommended dosages for vitamin A, see the table on p. 889.

DRUG PROFILES

There are three forms of vitamin A: retinol, retinyl palmitate, and retinyl acetate. Medications containing vitamin A may require a prescription, but many OTC products, such as multivitamins, are also available. All vitamin A products are classified as pregnancy category A agents and are contraindicated in clients who have a hypersensitivity to vitamin A and in those with oral malabsorption syndromes.

vitamin A

Vitamin A, also known as *retinol, retinyl palmitate*, and *retinyl acetate*, is available orally as 10 000- and 50 000-unit capsules, a 10 000-unit tablet, and 5000-unit drops. Doses for vitamin A can be expressed in international units (IU) or microgram retinol equivalents (RE); one IU is approximately equal to 0.3 μg of retinol equivalents (RE) from animal foods and about 3.6 μg of beta-carotene from plant foods. Currently the IU and RE standards are being replaced by a newer standard of vitamin A measurement: the retinol activity equivalent (RAE). One RAE is approximately equal to the following:

    1 μg of retinol (either dietary or supplemental)
    2 μg of supplemental beta-carotene
    12 μg of dietary beta-carotene
    24 μg of dietary carotenoids

Current RDAs are listed in Table 52-1 and common dosages are given in the table on p. 889.

PHARMACOKINETICS

Half-Life	Onset	Peak	Duration
50–100 days*	42 days†	3–5 hr	Unknown

*Rate of elimination of hepatic reserves upon eating a retinol-free diet.
†Follicular hyperkeratosis resolution with 300 μg/day of retinol.

VITAMIN D

Vitamin D, also called the *sunshine vitamin*, is responsible for the proper utilization of calcium and phosphorus in the body. The term *vitamin D* designates a group of analogue steroid structural chemicals with vitamin D activity. The two most important members of the vitamin D family are vitamin D_2 (ergocalciferol) and vitamin D_3 (cholecalciferol). They have different sites of origin but similar functions in the body. Ergocalciferol (vitamin D_2) is plant vitamin D and

is therefore obtained through dietary sources. The natural form of vitamin D produced in the skin by ultraviolet irradiation (sun), 7-dehydrocholesterol, is referred to as *cholecalciferol* (vitamin D_3). This endogenous synthesis of vitamin D_3 usually produces sufficient amounts to meet daily requirements. Chemically the two vitamin D compounds are different, but physiologically they produce the same effect.

Vitamin D_2 = ergocalciferol = plant vitamin D

Vitamin D_3 = cholecalciferol = human vitamin D

Vitamin D then is obtained through both endogenous synthesis and through foods containing D_2. Some foods contain the vitamin naturally, such as liver, eggs, butter, fish oil, and fish (especially salmon, sardine, herring). Milk, bread, and cereal are also fortified with Vitamin D.

Mechanism of Action and Drug Effects

The basic function of vitamin D is to regulate the absorption and subsequent utilization of calcium and phosphorus. It is also necessary for the normal calcification of bone. Vitamin D, in coordination with parathyroid hormone and calcitonin, regulates serum calcium levels by increasing calcium absorption from the small intestine and extracting calcium from the bone when needed. As ergocalciferol and cholecalciferol, vitamin D is inactive and requires transformation into active metabolites for biological activity. Both vitamin D_2 and vitamin D_3 are biotransformed primarily in the liver by the actions of the parathyroid hormone. The resulting compound, calcifediol, is then transported to the kidney, where it is converted to calcitriol, which is believed to be the most physiologically active vitamin D analogue. Calcitriol promotes the intestinal absorption of calcium and phosphorus and the deposition of calcium and phosphorus into the structure of teeth and bones.

The drug effects of vitamin D are similar to those of vitamin A and essentially all vitamin and mineral compounds. It is used as a supplement to satisfy normal daily requirements or an increased demand, as in infants and pregnant and nursing women.

Indications

Vitamin D can be used either to supplement the present daily intake of vitamin D or to treat a deficiency of vitamin D. In the case of supplementation it is given as a prophylactic measure to prevent deficiency-related problems. Vitamin D is also used therapeutically to treat conditions resulting from long-term insufficiency, such as infantile **rickets**, tetany (involuntary sustained muscular contractions), and osteomalacia (softening of bones). Vitamin D can also help promote the absorption of phosphorus and calcium. For this reason its use is important in preventing osteoporosis. Because of vitamin D's role in the regulation of calcium and phosphorus, it may be used to correct deficiencies of these two elements. Box 52-2 lists the therapeutic indications for vitamin D.

Contraindications

The only usual contraindications to vitamin D supplements are known allergy to a given vitamin product, or known hypervitaminosis D state.

DOSAGES **Selected Vitamins**

Agent	Pharmacological Class	Usual Dosage Range	Indications
Vitamin D–Active Compounds			
alfacalcidol	Fat-soluble	**Adult and pediatric** PO/IV: 1.0 μg/day with food; increase 0.5 μg every 2–4 wk followed by 0.25–1.0 μg/day	Hypocalcemia and osteodystrophy in hemodialysis clients
calcitriol	Fat-soluble	**Adult** PO/IV: 0.25 μg/day; increase by 0.25 μg q4–6wk as necessary followed by 0.5–1.0 μg/day **Pediatric** PO/IV: 0.01–0.02 μg/kg/day followed by 0.01–0.05 μg/kg/day PO/IV: 0.010–0.025 μg/kg/day followed by 0.0046–0.015 μg/kg/day IV/PO: 0.03–0.05 μg/kg/day; if no improvement in 2 wk, then increase dose by 25%; followed by 0.014–0.04 μg/kg/day	Hypocalcemia and osteodystrophy in clients receiving regular hemodialysis X–linked hypophosphatemic rickets Vitamin D dependent rickets Hypoparathyroidism
dihydrotachysterol	Fat-soluble	PO: 0.75–2.5 mg/day several days, followed by 0.25 mg weekly to 1 mg/day based on serum calcium levels	Hypoparathyroidism Acute, chronic, and latent post-operative tetany
ergocalciferol	Fat-soluble	**Adult** PO: 12 000–500 000 units/day **Adult and pediatric** PO: 50 000–200 000 units/day **Adult and pediatric** PO: 5000 units/day	Rickets Hypoparathyroidism Vitamin D deficiency
Vitamin B–Active Compounds			
vitamin B_1 (thiamine HCL)	Water-soluble, B-complex group	**Adult** PO/IM/IV: 5–30 mg/day **Infant/child** PO/IM/IV: 10–50 mg/day	Nutritional supplement; alcohol-induced deficiency Nutritional supplement; nutritional deficiency
vitamin B_{12}	Water-soluble, B-complex group	**Adult** IM/SC: 30–100 μg/day × 5–10 days, then 100–200 μg/mo PO: 1000–2000 μg/day then 1000 μg/day **Pediatric** IM/SC: 100 μg/day to 1–5 mg, then 60 μg/mo	Deficiency; anemia
vitamin B_2	Water-soluble, B-complex group	**Adult** PO: 5–30 mg/day divided **Pediatric** 3–10 mg/day divided	Deficiency
vitamin B_3	Water-soluble, B-complex group	**Adult** PO: 300–500 mg/day **Pediatric** PO: 100–300 mg divided **Niacin** PO: 1.5–6 g/day divided bid–qid	Deficiency (pellagra) Hyperlipidemia
vitamin B_6	Water-soluble, B-complex group	**Adult** PO/IV/IM/SC: 2.5–10 mg/day then 2–5 mg/day for several wk (use multivitamin product) **Pediatric** PO/IV/IM/SC: 5–25 mg/day for 3 wk, then 1.5–2.5 mg/day (use a pediatric multivitamin product) **Adult** PO/IV: 10–50 mg/day **Pediatric** 1–2 mg/kg/day	Dietary deficiency Prevention of drug-induced neuritis (e.g., isoniazid for TB)

Continued

DOSAGES   Selected Vitamins—cont'd

Agent	Pharmacological Class	Usual Dosage Range	Indications
Vitamins A, C, E, and K			
vitamin A	Fat-soluble	**Adult and pediatric >8 yr** PO: Up to 500 000 units/day × 3 days, then 50 000 units/day × 2 wk, then 10 000–20 000 units/day for up to 2 mo **Pediatric 1–8 yr** PO: 5000–10 000 units/kg/day for 5 days, then 17 000–35 000 units/day for 14 days	Deficiency
vitamin C	Water-soluble	**Adult** PO/IV/IM/SC: 100–250 mg once to twice daily × 2–3 wk **Pediatric** PO/IV/IM/SC: 100–300 mg/day divided	Deficiency (scurvy)
vitamin E	Fat-soluble	**Adult** PO: 60–75 units/day	Nutritional supplement
vitamin K	Fat-soluble	**Adult** IM/SC: 2.5–10 mg single dose, repeat in 8 h **Pediatric** IM/SC: 2.5–10 mg single dose, repeat in 6–8 h **Infant** IM/SC: 1–2 mg, repeat in 4–8 h	Deficiency; warfarin-induced hypoprothrombinemia
		Pediatric IM: 0.5–1 mg single dose within 6 h of birth	Hemorrhagic disease of newborn infant

---

BOX 52-2

Vitamin D: Therapeutic Indications

- Dietary supplement
- Hypocalcemia
- Hypoparathyroidism
- Hypophosphatemia
- Osteodystrophy
- Osteomalacia
- Osteoporosis
- Pseudohypoparathyroidism
- Rickets
- Tetany (acute, chronic, or post-operative)

TABLE 52-4

VITAMIN D: ADVERSE EFFECTS

Body System	Side/Adverse Effects
Cardiovascular	Hypertension, dysrhythmias
Central nervous	Fatigue, weakness, drowsiness, headache, tinnitus, ataxia (loss of muscular coordination)
Gastrointestinal	Nausea, vomiting, anorexia, cramps, metallic taste, dry mouth, constipation
Genitourinary	Polyuria, albuminuria, increased BUN
Musculoskeletal	Decreased bone growth, bone pain, muscle pain

Side Effects and Adverse Effects

As with vitamin A, few acute side effects and adverse effects are associated with normal vitamin D ingestion. Only after long-term, excessive ingestion of vitamin D do symptoms appear. Such effects are usually noticed in the GI tract or the central nervous system (CNS) and are listed in Table 52-4.

Toxicity and Management of Overdose

The major toxic effects from ingesting excessive amounts of vitamin D occur most commonly in children. Discontinuation of vitamin D and reduced calcium intake reverse the toxic state. The amount of vitamin D considered to be too much varies considerably among individuals but is generally thought to be 1.25 to 2.5 mg of ergocalciferol daily in adults and 25 μg daily in infants and children.

The toxic effects of vitamin D are those associated with hypertension, such as weakness, fatigue, headache, anorexia, dry mouth, metallic taste, nausea, vomiting, abdominal cramps, ataxia (loss of muscular coordination), and bone pain. If not recognized and treated, these symptoms can progress to impairment of renal function and osteoporosis.

Interactions

Reduced absorption of vitamin D occurs with the simultaneous use of lubricant laxatives and cholestyramine. Clients taking digitalis preparations can develop cardiac dysrhythmias as a result of vitamin D intake.

Dosages

For the RDAs for vitamin D, see Table 52-1. For the recommended dosages for vitamin D, see the table on p. 888. See Appendix B for some of the common brands available in Canada.

DRUG PROFILES

There are five forms of vitamin D: alfacalcidol, calcitriol, cholecalciferol, dihydrotachysterol, and ergocalciferol. Vitamin D is available in OTC medications, such as a multivitamin product, or by prescription. Although various pharmaceutical manufacturers may list their individual vitamin D products as pregnancy category C, these products are generally considered to be category A or B as long as the client is not dosed higher than the RDA of vitamin D for a pregnant woman. Contraindications to vitamin D products include known drug product allergy and clients who have hypercalcemia, renal dysfunction, or hyperphosphatemia.

calcitriol

Calcitriol is the 1,25-dihydroxylated form of cholecalciferol (vitamin D_3). It is a vitamin D analogue used for the management of hypocalcemia in clients with chronic renal failure who are undergoing hemodialysis. It is also used in the treatment of hypoparathyroidism and pseudohypoparathyroidism, vitamin D–dependent rickets, hypophosphatemia, and hypocalcemia in premature infants. It is available orally as 0.25- and 0.5-μg capsules and a 1-μg/mL oral solution and parenterally as a 1-μg/mL injection. Commonly recommended dosages are listed in the table on p. 888.

PHARMACOKINETICS

Half-Life	Onset	Peak	Duration
3–6 hr	<3 hr	3–6 hr	3–5 days

dihydrotachysterol

Dihydrotachysterol is a vitamin D analogue that is administered orally once daily for the treatment of any of the previously mentioned conditions. Intramuscular use is indicated for clients with GI, liver, or biliary disease associated with malabsorption of vitamin D analogues. It is available orally as a 0.125-mg capsule. Commonly recommended dosages are listed in the table on p. 888.

PHARMACOKINETICS

Half-Life	Onset	Peak	Duration
Unknown	Unknown	Unknown	Unknown

ergocalciferol

Ergocalciferol is vitamin D_2. Its use is indicated for clients with GI, liver, or biliary disease associated with malabsorption of vitamin D analogues. It is available orally and parenterally. One milligram provides 40 000 units of vitamin D activity. Oral agents include a 50 000–unit capsule and a 8288-unit/mL oral solution. Commonly recommended dosages are listed in the table on p. 888.

PHARMACOKINETICS

Half-Life	Onset	Peak	Duration
19 days*	30 days†	Unknown	Months to years

*Biological half-life.
†Therapeutic effects.

VITAMIN E

Four biologically active chemicals called **tocopherols** (alpha, beta, gamma, and delta) make up the vitamin E compounds. Alpha-tocopherol is the most biologically active natural form of vitamin E. Dietary plant sources of vitamin E are fruits, grains, cereals, vegetables, oils, and wheat germ. Animal sources are eggs, meats, and fish. The exact biological function of vitamin E is unknown, but it is believed to act as an antioxidant.

Vitamin E = alpha-tocopherol → plant and animal sources

Mechanism of Action and Drug Effects

Although vitamin E may be a powerful biological antioxidant and an essential component of the diet, its exact nutritional function has not been fully demonstrated. The only significant deficiency syndrome for vitamin E has been recognized in premature infants. In this situation vitamin E deficiency may result in irritability, edema, thrombosis, and hemolytic anemia.

The drug effects of vitamin E are not as well defined as those of the other fat-soluble vitamins. It is believed to protect polyunsaturated fatty acids, a component of cellular membranes. It has also been shown to hinder the deterioration of substances such as vitamin A and ascorbic acid (vitamin C), two substances that are highly oxygen sensitive and readily oxidized, thus acting as an antioxidant.

Indications

Vitamin E is most commonly used as a dietary supplement to augment present daily intake or to treat a deficiency. Those at greatest risk of complications from vitamin E deficiency are premature infants. Vitamin E has recently received much attention as an antioxidant. Preventing the oxidation of various substances prevents the formation of toxic chemicals within the body, some of which are believed to cause cancer. There is a popular but unproved theory that vitamin E has beneficial effects for clients with cancer, heart disease, premenstrual syndrome (PMS), and sexual dysfunction.

Contraindications

Contraindications for vitamin E include known allergy to a specific vitamin E product.

TABLE 52-5

VITAMIN E: ADVERSE EFFECTS

Body System	Side/Adverse Effects
Central nervous	Fatigue, headache, blurred vision
Gastrointestinal	Nausea, diarrhea, flatulence
Genitourinary	Increased BUN, increased serum creatinine
Musculoskeletal	Weakness

Side Effects and Adverse Effects

As with vitamin D, few acute side effects and adverse effects are associated with normal vitamin E ingestion because it is relatively non-toxic. Side effects and adverse effects are usually noticed in the GI tract or CNS and are listed in Table 52-5.

Dosages

For the RDAs for vitamin E, see Table 52-1. For the recommended dosages for vitamin E, see the table on p. 889.

DRUG PROFILES

vitamin E

Vitamin E is available as an OTC medication. It has four forms: alpha-, beta-, gamma-, and delta-tocopherol. It is available in many multivitamin preparations and is also available by prescription. Vitamin E products are usually contraindicated only in cases of known drug allergy.

Vitamin E activity is generally expressed in international units (IU). One IU of vitamin E equals the biological activity of the following:

> 1 mg of dl-alpha-tocopheryl acetate
> 1.12 mg of dl-alpha-tocopheryl acid succinate
> 735 μg of d-alpha-tocopheryl acetate
> 830 μg of d-alpha-tocopheryl acid succinate
> 670 μg of d-alpha-tocopherol

Vitamin E is available for oral use in capsules of various strengths, one aqueous oral liquid, and topical creams and ointments.

PHARMACOKINETICS

Half-Life	Onset	Peak	Duration
Variable	Unknown	Unknown	Variable

VITAMIN K

Vitamin K is the last of the four fat-soluble vitamins (A, D, E, and K). There are three types of vitamin K: phytonadione (vitamin K_1), menaquinone (vitamin K_2), and menadione (vitamin K_3). The primary dietary sources of vitamin K_1 are green leafy vegetables (e.g., cabbage, spinach), meats, and milk. The body does not store large amounts of vitamin K; however, vitamin K_2 is synthesized by the intestinal flora, thus providing an endogenous supply.

> Vitamin K_1 = phytonadione → green leafy vegetables
> (exogenous)
>
> Vitamin K_2 = menaquinone → intestinal flora
> (endogenous)

Vitamin K is essential for the synthesis of blood coagulation factors, which takes place in the liver. Vitamin K-dependent blood coagulation factors are factors II, VII, IX, and X. Other names for these clotting factors are as follows:

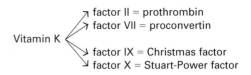

> factor II = prothrombin
> factor VII = proconvertin
> factor IX = Christmas factor
> factor X = Stuart-Power factor

Mechanism of Action and Drug Effects

Vitamin K activity is essential for effective blood clotting because it facilitates the hepatic biosynthesis of factor II (prothrombin), factor VII (proconvertin), factor IX (Christmas factor), and factor X (Stuart-Power factor). Vitamin K deficiency results in coagulation disorders caused by hypoprothrombinemia.

The drug effects of vitamin K are limited to its action on the vitamin K-dependent clotting factors produced in the liver (II, VII, IX, and X). Coagulation defects affecting these clotting factors can be corrected with administration of vitamin K. Vitamin K deficiency is rare because intestinal flora are able to synthesize sufficient amounts. If a deficiency develops, it can be corrected with vitamin K supplementation.

Indications

Vitamin K is indicated for dietary supplementation and for treating deficiency states. Although rare, deficiency states can develop with inadequate dietary intake or broad-spectrum inhibition of the intestinal flora resulting from the administration of broad-spectrum antibiotics. Deficiency states can also be seen in newborns because of malabsorption attributable to inadequate amounts of bile or selected drugs. For this reason infants born in hospitals are often given a prophylactic intramuscular dose of vitamin K on arrival in the nursery. Vitamin K deficiency can also result from the administration and pharmacological action of specific anticoagulants that inhibit hepatic vitamin K activity. Coumarin- and indanedione-derivative anticoagulants thin the blood by inhibiting vitamin K-dependent clotting factors in the liver. Administration of vitamin K overrides the mechanism by which the anticoagulants inhibit production of vitamin K-dependent clotting factors.

Contraindications

The only usual contraindication to treatment with vitamin K is known drug allergy.

Side Effects and Adverse Effects

Vitamin K is relatively non-toxic and thus causes few side effects and adverse effects. Severe hypersensitivity or anaphylaxis reactions have occurred rarely during or immediately after intravenous administration. Side effects and adverse effects are usually related to injection site reactions and hypersensitivity. See Table 52-6 for a list of such major effects by body system.

Toxicity and Management of Overdose

Toxicity is primarily limited to use in the newborn. Hemolysis of red blood cells (RBCs) can occur, especially in infants with low levels of glucose-6-phosphate dehydrogenase (G6PD). In this case, replacement with blood products is indicated.

TABLE 52-6

VITAMIN K: ADVERSE EFFECTS

Body System	Side/Adverse Effects
Central nervous	Headache, brain damage (large doses)
Gastrointestinal	Altered sensations of taste, decreased liver function tests
Hematological	Hemolytic anemia, hemoglobinuria, hyperbilirubinemia
Integumentary	Rash, urticaria, anaphylaxis

Dosages

The dose of phytonadione is 0.5 to 1 mg as a single intramuscular dose for infants within one hour after delivery and 2.5 to 10 mg administered parenterally as an intramuscular or a subcutaneous injection for adults and children. Oral vitamin K is only available through the Special Access Programme (Health Canada). For the recommended dosages for vitamin K, see the table on p. 889.

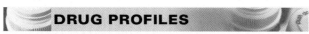

DRUG PROFILES

vitamin K₁

The most commonly used form of vitamin K is phytonadione (vitamin K₁). Phytonadione is available by prescription only in parenteral form. It is a category C agent. Phytonadione is contraindicated in clients who have shown a hypersensitivity reaction to it. Its use is also contraindicated during the last few weeks of pregnancy and in clients with severe hepatic disease. Phytonadione is available parenterally as 2-mg/mL and 10-mg/mL injections for intravenous, subcutaneous, or intramuscular use.

PHARMACOKINETICS

Half-Life	Onset	Peak	Duration
Unknown	Variable	1–2 hr	Unknown

WATER-SOLUBLE VITAMINS

The water-soluble vitamins include the vitamin B complex and vitamin C (ascorbic acid). They are present in a variety of plant and animal food sources. The vitamin B complex is a group of ten vitamins that are often found together in food, although they are chemically dissimilar and have different metabolic functions. Because the B vitamins were originally isolated from the same sources, primarily liver and yeast, they were grouped together as B-complex vitamins. Vitamin C (ascorbic acid), the other principal water-soluble vitamin, is concentrated more heavily in different food sources (primarily citrus fruits) than the B-complex vitamins and thus is not classified as part of the B complex. The numeric subscripts associated with various B vitamins reflect the sequential order in which they were discovered. In clinical practice some B

BOX 52-3

Water-Soluble Vitamins: Alternate Names

Vitamin B complex	Vitamin B₁ = thiamine Vitamin B₂ = riboflavin Vitamin B₃ = niacin/niacinamide Vitamin B₅ = pantothenic acid Vitamin B₆ = pyridoxine Vitamin B₉ = folic acid Vitamin B₁₂ = cyanocobalamin, hydroxocobalamin
Vitamin C	= ascorbic acid

vitamins are more often referred to by their "common" name, while others are more often referred to by their numeric designation. For example, "vitamin B_{12}" is used more often in clinical practice than its corresponding common name, "cyanocobalamin." However, "folic acid" is rarely referred to as "vitamin B_9," though this would also be correct. The most commonly used B complex vitamins, as well as vitamin C, are listed in Box 52-3. Both folic acid (vitamin B_9) and cyanocobalamin (vitamin B_{12}) are distinguished by their special role in hematopoiesis. For this reason they are both described further in a separate chapter (Chapter 54).

Water-soluble vitamins are a chemically diverse group sharing only the characteristic of being dissolvable in water. Like fat-soluble vitamins, they act primarily as coenzymes or oxidation-reduction agents in important metabolic pathways. Unlike fat-soluble vitamins, water-soluble vitamins are not stored in the body in appreciable amounts. Their water-soluble properties promote urinary excretion and reduce their half-life in the body. Therefore dietary intake must be adequate and regular or deficiency states will develop. Because these vitamins are water soluble, excess amounts are excreted in the urine. The body excretes what it does not need, which makes toxic reactions to water-soluble vitamins rare.

VITAMIN B₁

Vitamin B_1 (thiamine) is present in a wide variety of foods, especially whole grains, liver, and beans. A deficiency of vitamin B_1 results in the classic disease **beriberi** or Wernicke's encephalopathy (cerebral beriberi). Common findings in beriberi include brain lesions, polyneuropathy of peripheral nerves, serous effusions (abnormal collections of fluids in body tissues), and cardiac anatomic changes. Vitamin deficiency can result from poor diet, extended fever, hyperthyroidism, liver disease, alcoholism, malabsorption, or pregnancy and breastfeeding.

Mechanism of Action and Drug Effects

Thiamine is an essential precursor for the formation of thiamine pyrophosphate. When it is combined with adenosine triphosphate (ATP) the result is thiamine pyrophosphate coenzyme, which is required for carbohydrate metabolism. In addition to carbohydrate metabolism, several other metabolic pathways require thiamine to function, including the Krebs cycle. The Krebs cycle is also known as the citric acid or tricarboxylic cycle, and is a series of reactions that provides the main source of energy in the body and is the end toward which carbohydrate, fat, and protein metabolism all point.

The drug effects of vitamin B_1 are multiple. The integrity of the peripheral nervous system, cardiovascular system, and the GI tract are all heavily dependent on thiamine.

Indications

The beneficial drug effects and the essential role of thiamine in so many metabolic pathways make it useful in treating a variety of disorders, including thiamine deficiency and metabolic disorders. It is also used as a dietary supplement. Some of the deficiency states treated by thiamine are beriberi, Wernicke's encephalopathy syndrome, peripheral neuritis associated with **pellagra**, and neuritis of pregnancy. Thiamine has also been proposed as an oral insect repellant, but studies do not support this use.

Thiamine is used as a dietary supplement in cases of malabsorption such as those induced by alcoholism, cirrhosis, or GI disease. Thiamine may be useful in preventing deficiency in clients with these diseases. Some metabolic disorders that benefit from thiamine treatment are subacute necrotizing encephalomyelopathy (Leigh's disease; a serious neurological disorder of infancy and childhood), maple syrup urine disease (an inherited disorder of the ability to metabolize amino acids; so called because the urine has a sweetish smell), and lactic acidosis associated with pyruvate carboxylase enzyme deficiency and hyper-beta-alaninemia.

Other areas in which thiamine may have therapeutic value are the management of poor appetite, ulcerative colitis, chronic diarrhea, and cerebellar syndrome or ataxia (impaired muscular coordination).

Contraindications

The only usual contraindication to any of the B-complex vitamins is known allergy to a specific vitamin product.

Side Effects and Adverse Effects

Adverse effects are rare but include hypersensitivity reactions, nausea, restlessness, pulmonary edema, pruritus, urticaria, weakness, sweating, angioedema, cyanosis (bluish skin due to deficient oxygenation), hemorrhage into the gastrointestinal tract, and cardiovascular collapse. Administration by intramuscular injection can produce local tenderness, and intravenous injections can produce anaphylaxis.

Interactions

Thiamine is incompatible with alkaline- and sulphite-containing solutions.

Dosages

The RDAs for thiamine are 0.3 to 1 mg for infants and children, 1.1 mg for women, and 1.2 to 1.5 mg for men. However, people may need a higher intake if they eat raw fish or a high-carbohydrate diet or exercise heavily. The usual dose for treating beriberi is 10 to 20 mg intramuscularly three times daily for two weeks, with the addition of a multivitamin with 5 to 10 mg of thiamine for one month. See also Table 52-1. For the recommended dosages for vitamin B_1, see the table on p. 888.

DRUG PROFILES

thiamine

Thiamine is contraindicated only in individuals with a history of a hypersensitivity reaction. Thiamine is available orally as 50- and 500-mg tablets, 100-mg capsules, a 670-mg/1.25-mL powder, and parenterally as 100- and 500-mg/mL injections. Pregnancy category A.

PHARMACOKINETICS

Half-Life	Onset	Peak	Duration
Unknown	Unknown	Unknown	24 hr

VITAMIN B₂

Vitamin B_2 (riboflavin) is found in leafy green vegetables, eggs, nuts, meats, and yeast. Riboflavin serves several important functions. In the body, riboflavin is converted into two coenzymes (flavin mononucleotide [FMN] and flavin adenine dinucleotide [FAD]) that are essential for tissue respiration. Another B vitamin, vitamin B_6 (pyridoxine), requires riboflavin for activation. It is also needed to convert tryptophan into niacin and to maintain erythrocyte integrity. A deficiency of riboflavin results in cutaneous, oral, and corneal changes that include seborrheic dermatitis, keratitis (inflammation of the cornea), and cheilosis (chapped or fissured lips). Alcoholism is a major cause of riboflavin deficiency.

Mechanism of Action and Drug Effects

As previously mentioned, vitamin B_2 is an important precursor for the synthesis of FMN and FAD that are required in tissue respiration pathways. Riboflavin also plays an important part in transfer reactions, especially in carbohydrate catabolism.

The drug effects of riboflavin are mainly limited to replacement therapy for deficiency states. Deficiency is rare and does not usually occur in healthy people. However, deficiency may occur as a result of malnutrition or intestinal malabsorption or because of alcoholism or other diseases or infections.

Indications

Riboflavin is primarily used as a dietary supplement and to treat deficiency states. Although few disorders result because of a deficiency of riboflavin, supplementation is sufficient treatment for those disorders. Clients who may suffer from riboflavin deficiency are those with long-standing infections, liver disease, alcoholism, malignancy, and those taking probenecid. Riboflavin supplementation may be beneficial in treating microcytic anemia, acne, migraine headache, congenital methemoglobinemia (presence in the blood of an abnormal, non-functional hemoglobin [Hgb] pigment), muscle cramps; and Gopalan's syndrome, a symptom of suspected riboflavin [and possibly pantothenic acid (vitamin B₅)] deficiency that involves a sensation of tingling in the extremities. For this reason, it is also called "burning feet syndrome."

Contraindications

The only usual contraindication to riboflavin is known allergy to a given vitamin product.

Side Effects and Adverse Effects

Riboflavin is a safe and effective vitamin; to date, no side effects or toxic effects have been reported. Riboflavin will discolour urine to a yellow-orange.

Dosages

For the RDAs for riboflavin, see Table 52-1. Commonly recommended dosages for riboflavin are listed in the table on p. 888.

DRUG PROFILES

riboflavin

Riboflavin (vitamin B₂) is needed for normal respiratory reactions. It is a safe, non-toxic water-soluble vitamin with almost no adverse effects. It is available orally as 50- and 100-mg tablets and 100-mg capsules. It is also available as a 50-mg/mL parenteral form for intramuscular and intravenous use. Pregnancy category A.

PHARMACOKINETICS

Half-Life	Onset	Peak	Duration
66–84 min	Unknown	Unknown	24 hr

VITAMIN B₃

Vitamin B₃ (niacin) can be synthesized from tryptophan, an essential amino acid obtained from protein digestion. Niacin is present in meats, beans, yeast, liver, and wheat germ. Once in the body, niacin is converted to nicotinamide (also called *niacinamide*), which is then converted into two coenzymes, nicotinamide adenine dinucleotide (NAD) and nicotinamide adenine dinucleotide phosphate (NADP). These coenzymes are needed for glycogenolysis, tissue respiration, and lipid, protein, and purine metabolism (Figure 52-1).

A dietary deficiency of niacin will produce the classic symptoms of pellagra:
* *Mental:* various psychotic symptoms
* *Neurological:* neurasthenic syndrome
* *Cutaneous:* crusting, erythema, and desquamation
* *Mucous membrane:* oral, vaginal, and urethral lesions
* *GI:* diarrhea or bloody diarrhea

Niacin is also an antihyperlipidemic agent. It lowers serum cholesterol and triglyceride levels by reducing very-low-density lipoprotein (VLDL) synthesis. The principal carrier of cholesterol in the blood is LDL. Because VLDL is the precursor to LDL, reducing VLDL will result in reduction of LDL and, consequently, harmful plaque-forming, artery-narrowing cholesterol.

Mechanism of Action and Drug Effects

Generally speaking, the metabolic actions of niacin (vitamin B₃) are not due to niacin in the ingested form but rather to its metabolic product, nicotinamide. However, niacin itself does have a pharmacological role in the reduction of serum cholesterol. The doses of niacin required for this pharmacological effect are substantially higher than those required for its nutritional and metabolic effects (compare niacin doses between the dosages table on p. 888 and Table 52-1). The body is also able to produce a small amount of niacin from dietary tryptophan, an amino acid occurring in dietary proteins and some commercially available nutritional supplements. As previously mentioned, nicotinamide is required for numerous metabolic reactions, including those involved in carbohydrate, protein, and lipid metabolism, as well as tissue respiration (Figure 52-1).

The drug effects of niacin result from the production of NAD and NADP.

Indications

Niacin is indicated for the prevention and treatment of pellagra, a condition caused by a deficiency of vitamin B₃ that is most commonly the result of malabsorption.

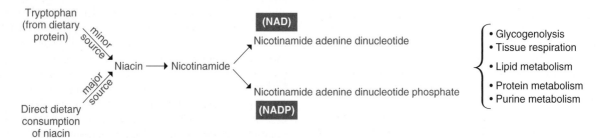

FIG. 52-1 Niacin, once in the body, is converted to NAD and NADP, which are coenzymes needed for many metabolic processes.

Niacin is also an antihyperlipidemic agent that reduces VLDL synthesis, resulting in lower serum cholesterol and triglyceride levels.

Contraindications

Niacin, unlike certain other B-complex vitamins, does have a few additional contraindications besides drug allergy. These include liver disease, diabetes mellitus, hyperuricemia and a history of gouty arthritis, severe hypotension, arterial hemorrhage, and active peptic ulcer disease.

Side Effects and Adverse Effects

The most frequent side effects associated with the use of niacin are flushing, pruritus, and gastrointestinal distress. These usually subside with continual use. They are most frequently seen when larger doses of niacin are used in the treatment of hyperlipidemia. Table 52-7 lists side effects and adverse effects by body system.

Dosages

For the RDAs for niacin, see Table 52-1. Commonly recommended dosages for niacin are listed in the table on p. 888.

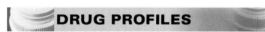

DRUG PROFILES

niacin

Niacin (vitamin B₃) is used to treat pellagra and hyperlipidemia. Its use should be monitored closely in clients who have a history of coronary artery disease, gallbladder disease, jaundice, liver disease, or arterial bleeding. Niacin is available orally as an immediate-release capsule and tablets, a sustained-release capsule, a powder, and a 100-mg/mL injection. Pregnancy category A.

PHARMACOKINETICS

Half-Life	Onset	Peak	Duration
20–60 min	Variable	Serum: 45 min	Variable

TABLE 52-7
NIACIN: ADVERSE EFFECTS

Body System	Side/Adverse Effects
Cardiovascular	Postural hypotension, dysrhythmias, atrial fibrillation
Central nervous	Headache, dizziness, anxiety, sensation of warmth
Gastrointestinal	Nausea, vomiting, bloating, flatulence, heartburn, diarrhea, peptic ulcer
Genitourinary	Hyperuricemia
Hepatic	Abnormal liver function tests, hepatitis
Integumentary	Flushing, dry skin, rash, pruritus, keratosis
Metabolic	Decreased glucose tolerance

VITAMIN B₆

Vitamin B₆ (pyridoxine) is composed of three compounds: pyridoxine, pyridoxal, and pyridoxamine. Plant sources that contain pyridoxine include whole grains, wheat germ, nuts, and yeast. Fish and organ meats contain both pyridoxal and pyridoxamine.

Pyridoxine is taken up by RBCs, where it is converted into the coenzyme pyridoxal phosphate, which is necessary for many metabolic functions such as protein, carbohydrate, and lipid utilization in the body. It also plays an important part in the conversion of tryptophan to niacin or serotonin.

Deficiency of vitamin B₆ can lead to a type of anemia known as *sideroblastic anemia*, neurological disturbances, seborrheic dermatitis, cheilosis, and xanthurenic aciduria (formation of xanthine crystals or "stones" in urine). It may also result in epileptiform convulsions, especially in neonates and infants; hypochromic microcytic anemia; and glossitis (inflamed tongue) and stomatitis (inflamed oral mucosa). Inadequate intake or poor absorption of pyridoxine causes the development of these conditions. Vitamin B₆ deficiency may occur as a result of uremia, alcoholism, cirrhosis, hyperthyroidism, malabsorption syndromes, and heart failure. It may also be induced by various drugs, such as isoniazid, cycloserine, ethionamide, hydralazine, penicillamine, and pyrazinamide.

Mechanism of Action and Drug Effects

Pyridoxine, pyridoxal, and pyridoxamine are all converted to the active forms of vitamin B₆, pyridoxal phosphate and pyridoxamine phosphate. They act as coenzymes in a wide variety of reactions, including the transamination of amino acids and the conversion of tryptophan to niacin. They are also essential in the synthesis of gamma-aminobutyric acid (GABA), an inhibitory neurotransmitter in the CNS. They are important in the synthesis of heme and the maintenance of the hematopoietic system. Pyridoxine deficiency principally affects the peripheral nerves, skin, mucous membranes, and the hematopoietic system.

The drug effects of pyridoxine are the result of the two coenzymes pyridoxal phosphate and pyridoxamine phosphate.

Indications

Pyridoxine is used to prevent and treat vitamin B₆ deficiency. Although deficiency of vitamin B₆ is rare, it can occur in conditions of inadequate intake or poor absorption of pyridoxine, from therapy with certain medications including isoniazid (for TB), hydralazine (mushrooms of the genus *Gyromitra*), and oral contraceptives. Seizures that are unresponsive to usual therapy, morning sickness during pregnancy, and various metabolic disorders may respond to pyridoxine therapy. Unlabelled uses for pyridoxine include PMS and nausea and vomiting of pregnancy but more study is required to determine if there is a benefit.

Contraindications

The only usual contraindication to pyridoxine use is drug allergy.

Side Effects and Adverse Effects

Side effects and adverse effects with pyridoxine use are rare and usually do not occur with normal doses; high doses and chronic usage may produce the effects listed in Table 52-8. Toxic effects are a result of large doses sustained for several months. Neurotoxicity is the most likely result, but this will subside upon discontinuation of the pyridoxine.

Interactions

Pyridoxine exhibits several significant interactions with selected drugs. Pyridoxine will reduce the activity of levodopa; this effect is not evident when levodopa is combined with carbidopa. Drugs that reduce absorption of pyridoxine include isoniazid and oral contraceptives.

Dosages

For the RDAs for vitamin B$_6$, see Table 52-1. Commonly recommended dosages for vitamin B$_6$ are listed in the table on p. 888.

DRUG PROFILES

pyridoxine

Pyridoxine is a water-soluble B-complex vitamin composed of three components: pyridoxine, pyridoxal, and pyridoxamine. It has several vital roles in the body but is primarily responsible for the integrity of peripheral nerves, skin, mucous membranes, and the hematopoietic system. Pyridoxine is available orally as 8.3-, 10-, 20-, 25-, 50-, 100-, and 250-mg tablets; a 100-mg capsule; a 200-mg slow-release tablet; a 800-mg/mL powder; and a 100-mg/mL injection. Pregnancy category A.

PHARMACOKINETICS

Half-Life	Onset	Peak	Duration
15–20 days	Unknown	Unknown	Unknown

TABLE 52-8

PYRIDOXINE: ADVERSE EFFECTS

Body System	Side/Adverse Effects
Central nervous	Paraesthesia, flushing, warmth, headache, lethargy
Integumentary	Pain or stinging at injection site

VITAMIN B$_{12}$

Vitamin B$_{12}$ (cyanocobalamin) is a cobalt-containing, water-soluble B-complex vitamin. It is synthesized by micro-organisms and is present in the body as two different coenzymes: adenosylcobalamin and methylcobalamin. Cyanocobalamin is a required coenzyme for many metabolic pathways, including fat and carbohydrate metabolism and protein synthesis. It is also required for growth, cell replication, hematopoiesis, and nucleoprotein and myelin synthesis (Figure 52-2).

Cyanocobalamin is present in foods of animal origin, particularly liver, kidney, fish and shellfish, meat, and dairy foods. Plants contain only minimal amounts of cyanocobalamin, unlike the other B vitamins. Vitamin B$_{12}$ deficiency results in GI lesions, neurological symptoms that can result in degenerative CNS lesions, and megaloblastic anemia. The major cause of cyanocobalamin deficiency is malabsorption. Other possible but less likely causes are poor diet, chronic alcoholism, and chronic hemorrhage.

Mechanism of Action and Drug Effects

Humans must have an exogenous source of cyanocobalamin because it is required for nucleoprotein and myelin synthesis, cell reproduction, normal growth, and the maintenance of normal erythropoiesis. The cells that have the greatest requirement for vitamin B$_{12}$ are those that divide rapidly, such as epithelial cells, bone marrow, and myeloid cells.

Reduced sulfhydryl (SH) groups are required to metabolize fats and carbohydrates and to synthesize protein. Cyanocobalamin is involved in maintaining SH groups in the reduced form that is required by many SH-activated enzyme systems. Cyanocobalamin deficiency can lead to neurological damage that begins with an inability to produce myelin and is followed by gradual degeneration of the axon and nerve head.

Cyanocobalamin activity is identical to the activity of the anti-pernicious anemia factor present in liver extract called the *extrinsic factor* or *Castle's factor*. The oral absorption of cyanocobalamin (extrinsic factor) requires the presence of the intrinsic factor, which is a glycoprotein secreted by gastric parietal cells. A complex is formed between the two factors, which is then absorbed by the intestines. This is depicted in Figure 52-3.

Indications

Cyanocobalamin is used to treat deficiency states that develop because of an insufficient intake of the vitamin. It is also included in a multivitamin formulation that is used as a dietary supplement. As previously mentioned,

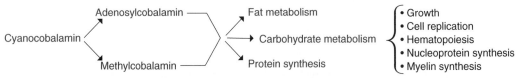

FIG. 52-2 Cyanocobalamin is a required coenzyme for many body processes.

deficiency states are most often the result of malabsorption or poor dietary intake. Poor dietary intake is most common in vegetarians because the primary source of cyanocobalamin is foods of animal origin.

The most common manifestation of untreated cyanocobalamin deficiency is pernicious anemia. The use of vitamin B_{12} to treat pernicious anemia and other megaloblastic anemias results in a rapid conversion of a megaloblastic bone marrow to a normoblastic bone marrow. The preferred route of administration of vitamin B_{12} in treating megaloblastic anemias is by deep intramuscular injection. If not treated, deficiency states can lead to megaloblastic anemia and irreversible neurological damage. Cyanocobalamin is also useful in the treatment of pernicious anemia caused by an endogenous lack of intrinsic factor.

Contraindications

The only usual contraindication to administration of extrinsic cyanocobalamin (vitamin B_{12}) is known drug product allergy. This may include sensitivity to the chemical element cobalt, which is part of the structure of cyanocobalamin, as this chemical name implies. Other contraindications include hereditary optic nerve atrophy (Leber's disease).

Side Effects and Adverse Effects

Vitamin B_{12} is non-toxic and large doses must be ingested to produce adverse effects, which include itching, transitory diarrhea, and fever. Other side effects and adverse effects are listed by body system in Table 52-9.

Interactions

Use with anticonvulsants, aminoglycosides, most antibiotics, or long-acting potassium preparations and excessive alcohol intake decreases the oral absorption of vitamin B_{12}. In addition, it has been suggested that chloramphenicol antagonizes the hematological response of vitamin B_{12}.

Dosages

For RDAs for vitamin B_{12}, see Table 52-1. Commonly recommended dosages for vitamin B_{12} are listed in the table on p. 888.

DRUG PROFILES

cyanocobalamin

Cyanocobalamin (vitamin B_{12}) is a water-soluble B-complex vitamin required for maintaining body fat and carbohydrate metabolism and protein synthesis. It is also needed for growth, cell replication, blood cell production, and the integrity of normal nerve function. Cyanocobalamin is available both as OTC preparations and by prescription. Most of the OTC cyanocobalamin-containing products are multivitamin preparations, whereas many of the sole cyanocobalamin-containing products contain large doses for parenteral injection and are available by prescription only. Cyanocobalamin is available orally as 100-, 250-, 500-, and 1000-μg tablets, a 1000-μg capsule, and 1000-μg lozenges. It is also available as liquid drops with 1000-μg/drop and 50- and 1000-μg/5-mL liquid and for injection as 1000- and 5000-μg/mL solutions. Pregnancy category A.

PHARMACOKINETICS

Half-Life	Onset	Peak	Duration
6 days	Unknown	Plasma: 8–12 hr	Unknown

TABLE 52-9

CYANOCOBALAMIN: ADVERSE EFFECTS

Body System	Side/Adverse Effects
Central nervous	Flushing, optic nerve atrophy
Gastrointestinal	Diarrhea
Integumentary	Itching, rash, pain at injection site
Metabolic	Hypokalemia

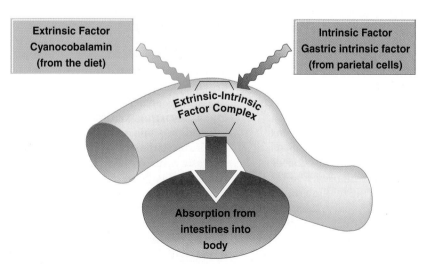

FIG. 52-3 The oral absorption of cyanocobalamin requires the presence of the intrinsic factor secreted by gastric parietal cells.

VITAMIN C

Vitamin C (ascorbic acid) is a water-soluble vitamin present in citrus fruits and juices, tomatoes, green pepper, cabbage, cherries, strawberries, mangoes, and liver. It can be synthesized for use as a drug and is used in many therapeutic situations. Prolonged ascorbic acid deficiency results in the nutritional disease **scurvy**, which is characterized by gingivitis and bleeding gums, loss of teeth, anemia, subcutaneous hemorrhage, bone lesions, and delayed healing of soft tissues and bones. Scurvy was recognized for several centuries, especially among sailors; in 1795 the British navy ordered the eating of limes to prevent the disease.

Mechanism of Action and Drug Effects

Vitamin C is reversibly oxidized to dehydroascorbic acid in the body, and it acts in oxidation-reduction reactions. It is required for several important metabolic activities, including collagen synthesis and the maintenance of connective tissue; tissue repair; maintenance of bone, teeth, and capillaries; and folic acid metabolism (specifically, the conversion of folic acid into its active metabolite). Accordingly, it is essential for erythropoiesis. Vitamin C enhances the absorption of iron and is required for the synthesis of lipids, proteins, and steroids. It has also been shown to aid in cellular respiration and resistance to infections.

Indications

Vitamin C is used to treat diseases associated with vitamin C deficiency and as a dietary supplement with the use of total parenteral nutrition. It is most beneficial in clients who require larger daily requirements because of pregnancy, lactation, hyperthyroidism, fever, stress, infection, trauma, burns, smoking, exposure to cold temperatures, and the consumption of certain drugs (e.g., salicylates). Because vitamin C is an acid it can also be used as a urinary acidifier. The benefits of other uses of vitamin C are less well documented. For example, taking vitamin C to prevent or treat the common cold is common practice. However, most large controlled studies have shown that ascorbic acid has little or no value as a prophylactic for the common cold.

Contraindications

The only usual contraindication for vitamin C use is known allergy to a specific vitamin product.

Side Effects and Adverse Effects

Vitamin C is usually non-toxic unless excessive dosages are consumed. Megadoses can produce nausea, vomiting, headache, and abdominal cramps, and will acidify the urine, resulting in the formation of cystine, oxalate, and urate renal stones. Furthermore, individuals who discontinue taking excessive daily doses of ascorbic acid can suffer from scurvy-like symptoms.

Interactions

Ascorbic acid has the potential to interact with many classes of drugs. However, clinical experience concerning many interactions is inconclusive. For example, it has been reported that ascorbic acid can decrease the effectiveness of oral anticoagulants. This does not always happen, but practitioners should be aware of this possibility. Co-administration with acid-labile drugs such as penicillin G or erythromycin should be avoided. As previously mentioned, megadoses of vitamin C can acidify the urine, which can enhance the excretion of basic drugs and delay the excretion of acidic drugs.

Dosages

The RDAs for vitamin C are listed in Table 52-1. Commonly recommended dosages for vitamin C are listed in the table on p. 889.

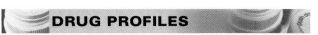

DRUG PROFILES

ascorbic acid

Ascorbic acid (vitamin C) is a water-soluble vitamin required for the prevention and treatment of scurvy. As previously explained, it is also required for erythropoiesis and the synthesis of lipids, protein, and steroids. Ascorbic acid is available both in OTC preparations such as multivitamin products and by prescription. Ascorbic acid is available in many oral dosage forms, including tablets (125-, 250-, 500-, 1000-, and 4000-mg), timed-release tablets (1000- and 1500-mg), chewable tablets (40-, 100-, 250-, 500-, and 1000-mg), a 500-mg capsule, various crystals and powders for making an oral solution, various premixed oral solutions (0.3 mg/mL), and 250- and 500-mg/mL solutions for injection. Pregnancy category A.

PHARMACOKINETICS

Half-Life	Onset	Peak	Duration
Unknown	Unknown	Unknown	Unknown

MINERALS

Minerals are essential nutrients that are classified as inorganic compounds. They act as building blocks for many body structures and thus are necessary for a variety of physiological functions. They are also needed for intracellular and extracellular body fluid electrolytes. Iron is essential for the production of Hgb, which is necessary for oxygen transport throughout the body (Chapter 54). Minerals are required for muscle contraction, nerve transmission, and the makeup of essential enzymes.

Mineral compounds are composed of various metallic and non-metallic elements that are chemically combined with ionic bonds. When these compounds are dissolved in water they separate (dissociate) into positively charged metallic cations and electrolytes or negatively charged non-metallic anions and electrolytes (Figure 52-4).

Ingestion of mineral nutrients provides essential elements necessary for vital bodily functions. Elements that are required in larger amounts are called *macrominerals;* those required in smaller amounts are called *microminerals* or *trace elements.* Table 52-10 classifies nutrient elements as either macrominerals or microminerals and as metal or non-metal.

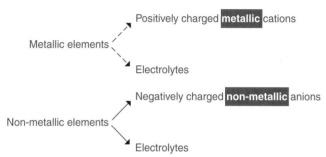

FIG. 52-4 When mineral compounds are dissolved in water, they separate into positively charged metabolic cations or negatively charged non-metallic anions and electrolytes.

TABLE 52-10
MINERAL ELEMENTS

Element	Symbol	Type	Ionic/Electrolyte Form
MACROMINERALS			
Calcium*	Ca	Metal	Ca^{12} calcium cation
Chlorine	Cl	Non-metal	Cl^{-1} chloride anion
Magnesium*	Mg	Metal	Mg^{+2} magnesium cation
Phosphorus*	P	Non-metal	PO_4^{-3} phosphate anion
Potassium	K	Metal	K^{+1} potassium cation
Sodium	Na	Metal	Na^{+1} sodium cation
Sulphur	S	Non-metal	SO_4^{-2} sulphate anion
MICROMINERALS			
Chromium	Cr	Metal	Cr^{-3} chromium cation
Cobalt	Co	Metal	Co^{+2} cobalt cation
Copper	Cu	Metal	Cu^{+2} copper cation
Fluorine	F	Non-metal	F^{-1} fluoride anion
Iodine*	I	Non-metal	I^{-1} iodide anion
Iron*	Fe	Metal	Fe^{+2} ferrous cation
Manganese	Mn	Metal	Mn^{+2} manganese cation
Molybdenum	Mo	Metal	Mo^{+6} molybdenum cation
Selenium*	Se	Metal	Se^{+14} selenium cation
Zinc*	Zn	Metal	Zn^{+2} zinc cation

*Mineral elements that have a current recommended daily allowance (RDA).

CALCIUM

Calcium is the most abundant mineral element in the human body, accounting for approximately two percent of the total body weight. The highest concentration of calcium is in bones and teeth. Calcium is widely distributed in many foods, especially milk and dairy products. Calcium requirements are high for growing children and for women who are pregnant or breastfeeding. The efficient absorption of calcium requires adequate amounts of vitamin D.

Calcium deficiency results in hypocalcemia and affects many bodily functions. Causes of calcium deficiency include inadequate calcium intake and/or insufficient vitamin D to facilitate absorption; hypoparathyroidism; and malabsorption syndrome, especially in older people. Disorders related to calcium deficiency include infantile rickets, adult osteomalacia, muscle cramps, osteoporosis (especially in post-menopausal females), hypothyroidism, and renal dysfunction. Table 52-11 lists the possible causes of calcium deficiency and the resulting disorders.

Calcium is essential for the normal maintenance and function of the nervous, muscular, and skeletal systems and for cell membrane and capillary permeability. It is an important catalyst in many enzymatic reactions and is essential in many physiological processes, including transmission of nerve impulses, renal function, respiration, blood coagulation, and contraction of cardiac, smooth, and skeletal muscles. Calcium also plays a regulatory role in the release and storage of neurotransmitters and hormones, in white blood cell (WBC) and hormone activity, in the uptake and binding of amino acids, and in intestinal absorption of cyanocobalamin (vitamin B_{12}) and gastrin secretion. The roles of calcium in normal physiological processes are summarized in Table 52-12.

Mechanism of Action and Drug Effects

Calcium participates in a variety of essential physiological functions and is a building block for body structures. Specifically, calcium is involved with the proper development and maintenance of teeth and skeletal bones. It is an important catalyst in many of the coagulation pathways in the blood. Calcium acts as a cofactor in clotting reactions involving the intrinsic and extrinsic pathways of thromboplastin. It is also a cofactor in the conversion of prothrombin to thrombin by thromboplastin and the conversion of fibrinogen to fibrin.

TABLE 52-11
CALCIUM DEFICIENCY: CAUSES AND DISORDERS

Cause	Disorder
Inadequate intake	Infantile rickets
Insufficient vitamin D	Adult osteomalacia
Hypoparathyroidism	Muscle cramps
Malabsorption syndrome	Osteoporosis

TABLE 52-12
PHYSIOLOGICAL PROCESSES REQUIRING CALCIUM

Role	Area Influenced
Normal maintenance and function	Nervous system
	Muscular system
	Skeletal system
	Cell membranes
	Capillary permeability
Physiological processes	Transmission of nerve impulses
	Contraction of cardiac, smooth, and skeletal muscles
	Renal function
	Respiration
	Blood coagulation
Regulatory	Release and storage of neurotransmitters and hormones
	Uptake and binding of amino acids
	Cyanocobalamin (vitamin B_{12}) absorption
	Gastrin secretion

TABLE 52-13
CALCIUM SALTS: CALCIUM CONTENT

Calcium Salt	Calcium Content (per gram)
Phosphate tribasic	400 mg
Carbonate	400 mg
Phosphate dibasic anhydrous	290 mg
Chloride	270 mg
Acetate	253 mg
Phosphate dibasic dihydrate	230 mg
Citrate	211 mg
Glycerophosphate	191 mg
Lactate	130 mg
Gluconate	90 mg
Glucoheponate	82 mg
Glubionate	64 mg

Indications

Calcium salts are used as a source of calcium cations for the treatment or prevention of calcium depletion in clients for whom dietary measures are inadequate. Many conditions may be associated with calcium deficiency:

- Achlorhydria (absence of hydrochloric acid from gastric juice)
- Alkalosis
- Chronic diarrhea
- Hyperphosphatemia
- Hypoparathyroidism
- Menopause
- Pancreatitis
- Pregnancy and lactation
- PMS
- Renal failure
- Sprue (primary intestinal malabsorption)
- Steatorrhea (passage of fat in feces)
- Vitamin D deficiency

Calcium is also used to treat various manifestations of established deficiency states, including adult osteomalacia, hypothyroidism, infantile rickets or tetany, muscle cramps, osteoporosis, and renal insufficiency. In addition, calcium is used as a dietary supplement for women during pregnancy and lactation.

There are over 12 different selected calcium salts available for treatment or nutritional supplementation. Each calcium salt contains a different amount of elemental calcium per gram of calcium salt. Table 52-13 lists the available salts and their associated calcium contents.

Contraindications

Contraindications for administration of exogenous calcium include hypercalcemia, ventricular fibrillation of the heart, and known allergy to a specific calcium drug product.

Side Effects and Adverse Effects

Although adverse effects and toxicity are rare, hypercalcemia can occur. Symptoms include anorexia, nausea, vomiting, and constipation. In addition, when calcium salts are administered by intramuscular or subcutaneous injection, mild to severe local reactions may occur, including burning, necrosis and sloughing of tissue, cellulitis, and soft tissue calcification. Venous irritation may occur with intravenous administration. Other side effects and adverse effects associated with both oral and parenteral use of calcium salts are listed in Table 52-14.

Toxicity and Management of Overdose

Chronic and excessive calcium intake can result in severe hypercalcemia, which can cause cardiac irregularities, delirium, and coma. Management of acute hypercalcemia may require hemodialysis, whereas milder cases will respond to discontinuation of calcium intake.

Interactions

Calcium salts will chelate (bind) with tetracyclines to produce an insoluble complex. If hypercalcemia is present in clients taking digitalis preparations, serious cardiac dysrhythmias can occur.

Dosages

For the RDAs for calcium, see Table 52-1.

DRUG PROFILES

calcium

Calcium salts are minerals that are used primarily in the treatment or prevention of calcium depletion in clients in whom dietary measures are inadequate. Many calcium salts are available, all with a different content of elemental calcium per gram of salt. Calcium is available in both oral and parenteral forms. There are numerous dosages and names of calcium preparations. Consult manufacturer instructions for recommended dosages.

TABLE 52-14
CALCIUM SALTS: ADVERSE EFFECTS

Body System	Side/Adverse Effects
Gastrointestinal	Constipation, obstruction, nausea, vomiting, flatulence, gastric irritation
Genitourinary	Renal dysfunction, renal stones, renal failure
Metabolic	Hypercalcemia, metabolic alkalosis

The calcium salts are available in capsules, powders, oral suspensions, tablets, chewable tablets, film-coated tablets, oral solutions, and parenteral injections. The pharmacokinetics of calcium are highly variable and depend on individual client physiology and the characteristics of the specific drug product used. Pregnancy category C.

MAGNESIUM

Magnesium is one of the principal cations present in the intracellular fluid. It is an essential part of many enzyme systems associated with energy metabolism. Magnesium deficiency (hypomagnesemia) is usually caused by (1) malabsorption, especially in the presence of high calcium intake; (2) alcoholism; (3) long-term intravenous feeding; (4) diuretics; and (5) metabolic disorders, including hyperthyroidism and diabetic ketoacidosis. Symptoms associated with hypomagnesemia include cardiovascular disturbances, neuromuscular impairment, and mental disturbances. Dietary intake from vegetables and other foods will usually prevent magnesium deficiency. However, magnesium is required in greater amounts in individuals with diets high in protein-rich foods, calcium, and phosphorus.

Mechanism of Action and Drug Effects

The precise mechanism for magnesium has not been fully determined. Magnesium is a known cofactor for many enzyme systems. It is required for muscle contraction and nerve physiology. Magnesium produces an anticonvulsant effect by inhibiting neuromuscular transmission for selected convulsive states.

Indications

Magnesium is used to treat magnesium deficiency and as a nutritional supplement in total parenteral nutrition (TPN) and multivitamin preparations. It is used as an anticonvulsant in magnesium deficiency–induced seizures; for complications of pregnancy, including pre-eclampsia and eclampsia; as a tocolytic agent for inhibition of uterine contractions in premature labour; in pediatric acute nephropathy; for various cardiac dysrhythmias; and for short-term treatment of constipation.

Contraindications

Contraindications to magnesium administration include known drug product allergy, heart block, renal failure, adrenal gland failure (Addison's disease), and hepatitis.

Side Effects and Adverse Effects

Adverse effects of magnesium are due to hypermagnesia, which results in tendon reflex loss, difficult bowel movements, CNS depression, respiratory distress and heart block, and hypothermia.

Toxicity and Management of Overdose

Toxic effects are extensions of symptoms caused by hypermagnesia, a major cause of which is the long-term use of magnesium products (especially antacids in clients with renal dysfunction). Severe hypermagnesia is treated with a calcium salt administered intravenously.

Interactions

The use of magnesium with neuromuscular blocking agents and CNS depressants produces additive effects.

Dosages

The RDA for magnesium is 6 to 10 mg for infants and children, 10 to 15 mg for women, and 10 to 12 mg for men. The usual dose of magnesium for treating convulsant conditions is 4 to 5 g intravenously or intramuscularly, repeated as required. For the RDAs for magnesium, see Table 52-1.

DRUG PROFILES

magnesium

Magnesium is a mineral that has a variety of dosage forms and uses. It is an essential part of many enzyme systems. When absent or diminished in the body, cardiovascular, neuromuscular, and mental disturbances can occur. Magnesium sulphate is the most common form of magnesium used as a mineral replacement. It is available in parenteral form as a 200- and 500-mg/mL injection. Pregnancy category B.

PHOSPHORUS

Phosphorus is widely distributed in foods and thus a dietary deficiency is rare. Deficiency states are usually non-dietary and are primarily due to malabsorption, extensive diarrhea or vomiting, hyperthyroidism, hepatic disease, and long-term use of aluminum or calcium antacids.

Mechanism of Action and Drug Effects

Phosphorus in the form of the phosphate group and/or anion (PO_4^{-3}) is a required precursor for the synthesis of essential body chemicals. In addition, the mineral is an important building block for body structures. Phosphorus is required as a structural unit for the synthesis of nucleic acid and the adenosine phosphate compounds (adenosine monophosphate [AMP], adenosine diphosphate [ADP], and adenosine triphosphate [ATP]) responsible for cellular energy transfer. It is also necessary for the development and maintenance of the skeletal system and teeth. The skeletal bones contain up to 85 percent of the phosphorus content of the body. In addition, phosophorus is required for the proper utilization of many B-complex vitamins, and it is an essential component of physiological buffering systems.

Indications

Phosphorus is used to treat deficiency states and as a dietary supplement in many multivitamin formulations.

Contraindications

Contraindications to phosphorus or phosphate administration include hyperphosphatemia and hypocalcemia.

Side Effects and Adverse Effects

Adverse effects are usually associated with phosphorus replacement products. Effects include diarrhea, nausea, vomiting, and other GI disturbances. Other side effects include confusion, weakness, and breathing difficulties.

Toxicity and Management of Overdose

Toxic reactions to phosphorus are extremely rare and are usually restricted to the ingestion of the pure element.

Interactions

Antacids can reduce the oral absorption of phosphorus.

Dosages

For the RDAs for phosphorus, see Table 52-1.

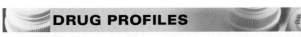

DRUG PROFILES

phosphorus

Phosphorus is a mineral that is essential to well-being. It is needed to make energy in the form of ADP and ATP for all bodily processes. Fortunately it is present in a variety of foods and drinks, and a true dietary deficiency is rare. Phosphorus is present in a large number of drug formulations and appears as a phosphate salt (PO_4).

Phosphorus should be used with caution in clients with renal impairment. It is available in both oral and parenteral formulations. Oral phosphorus is available as an oral liquid and tablets. The parenteral form is potassium phosphate. Recommended dosages vary depending on the indication.

zinc

The metallic element zinc is often taken orally as a mineral supplement and is available as a sulphate salt for this purpose. Normally a dietary trace element, zinc plays a crucial role in the enzymatic metabolic reactions of both proteins and carbohydrates. This serves to make it especially important for normal tissue growth and repair. It therefore also has a major role in wound repair. It is available in many combinations with vitamins and minerals and as a 10-mg oral OTC capsule. There is also a zinc lozenge available.

NURSING PROCESS

■ Assessment

Before administering vitamins, the nurse must assess clients for nutritional disorders with an evaluation of baseline Hgb, hematocrit (Hct), WBC and RBC counts, and protein and albumin levels. A daily journal of dietary intake and a history of dietary patterns and meals must also be documented. To test for vitamin A deficiency, a baseline assessment of the client's vision, including night vision, and an examination of the appearance of the skin and mucous membranes must be done. Serum laboratory values of vitamin A that are less than 0.7 μmol/L indicate a deficiency. Interactions of vitamin A with the drug isotretinoin may lead to toxicity, with manifestations such as headache, nausea, vomiting, elevated liver enzymes, and dry, cracked skin.

Vitamin D is contraindicated in clients with hypercalcemia or hypervitaminosis D. Cautious use with close and careful monitoring is recommended in clients with arteriosclerosis, hyperphosphatemia, renal or cardiac dysfunction, and hypersensitivity to vitamin D. Baseline assessment should include a status assessment of the client's skeletal formation and a baseline serum calcium level. Serum calcium levels less than 2.25 mmol/L indicate possible vitamin D deficiency. In addition, the nurse should monitor baseline levels of inorganic phosphorus and serum citrate. Drug interactions may occur with antacids, high doses of calcium preparations, thiazide diuretics, and products high in vitamin D.

Before administering vitamin E, clients should be assessed for hypoprothrombinemia secondary to vitamin E deficiency. Vitamin E will aggravate this condition and result in hematological problems such as bleeding. Baseline assessment data include a check of skin integrity and determination of the presence or absence of edema and any muscle weakness.

Vitamin B_1 (thiamine) hypersensitivity may cause skin rash and wheezing. Because it is rare that only one vitamin B_1 deficiency occurs, deficiencies of all forms of vitamin B_1 must be ruled out. Baseline assessments of vital signs, mental status, and urinary thiamine levels must be done. When dietary intake is inadequate, little or no thiamine is excreted in the urine. When the diet contains an excess of the minimal requirement, the excess is excreted in the urine as intact thiamine or as pyrimidine.

Vitamin C is contraindicated in clients with cystinuria, oxalosis, or a history of gout or urate kidney stones. In clients with sickle cell anemia, large doses of vitamin C may precipitate a sickle cell crisis. Diabetic clients may experience abnormal glucose levels when taking large doses of vitamin C.

There are few contraindications to the administration of trace elements. However, baseline assessments of nutritional status and specific nutrition-related laboratory studies (Hgb, Hct, RBC and WBC counts; trace elemental laboratory values) should be ordered by the physician and documented before initiation of therapy. Trace elements should be administered as ordered and only after researching the element or mineral, reviewing laboratory studies, and consulting specific manufacturer guidelines. Cautious use is recommended in any client with liver or biliary disease.

Before calcium and magnesium are administered, the client's current levels should be obtained and recorded. Calcium is contraindicated in clients who are hypercalcemic and have digitalis toxicity, ventricular fibrillation, or renal calculi. Cautious use is recommended in clients who are pregnant or breastfeeding, in children, in clients with renal or respiratory disease or failure, and in clients taking digitalis. Calcium interacts with digitalis, calcium channel blockers, amphotericin, cephalothin, digoxin, digitoxin, epinephrine, tetracycline, sodium warfarin, phosphate, and sodium bicarbonate. A baseline electrocardiogram (ECG) is often necessary with clients who have cardiac disease. If decreased QT and T wave inversion are observed, calcium is often discontinued or given in reduced dosages.

Magnesium is contraindicated in clients with hypersensitivity to it, and cautious use is recommended in clients with severe renal disease, GI bleeding, diarrhea, and possible intestinal obstruction. Magnesium interacts with tetracyclines, anticholinergics, iron salts, cimetidine, corticosteroids, and chlordiazepoxide.

COMMUNITY HEALTH POINTS

Vitamin–Drug Interactions

Many prescribed medications have an adverse effect on various vitamins within the body or may affect their metabolism. Antibiotics often interfere with the absorption of folic acid, vitamin B_{12}, and vitamin K. Anticonvulsants often interfere with the absorption of folic acid, vitamin B_{12}, and vitamin D. Oral contraceptives, hydralazine, and isoniazid (INH) interfere with the absorption of vitamin B_6. Oral contraceptives may also deplete folic acid. Oral hypoglycemics are known to interfere with the absorption of vitamin B_{12}.

The nurse must ensure that clients who are taking any of these medications are aware that their vitamin levels may be altered or that there may be other vitamin–drug interactions.

Nursing Diagnoses

Nursing diagnoses related to the use of vitamins and minerals include, but are not limited to, the following:
- Disturbed sensory perception (visual) related to night blindness from vitamin A deficiency.
- Acute pain related to bone or skeletal deformities resulting from vitamin D deficiency.
- Impaired physical mobility related to poorly developed muscles from vitamin D deficiency.
- Diarrhea related to vitamin E side effects.
- Impaired physical mobility related to vitamin E deficiency.
- Disturbed thought processes related to vitamin B_1 deficiency.
- Impaired physical mobility related to fatigue from poor nutrition and B vitamin deficiencies.
- Acute pain in joints related to disease from vitamin C deficiency.
- Impaired tissue integrity related to vitamin C deficiency and subsequent decreased healing.

Planning

Goals related to the use of vitamins and minerals are as follows:
- Client maintains sensory and perceptual integrity during therapy.

CASE STUDY

Magnesium Sulphate Therapy

D.C., a 68-year-old female, was admitted to a small community hospital (100 beds with a six-bed intensive care unit and critical care unit) for exacerbation of heart failure. After two days of diuretic treatment with furosemide, the physician ordered serum potassium and magnesium levels, which came back with the serum magnesium level at 0.45 mmol/L. The physician ordered magnesium sulphate 500 mg q6h 2 doses, with the first dose stat. The night supervisor has to retrieve the medication because the pharmacy is closed. She returns to your unit with the medication. Because you are aware of many medication errors with magnesium sulphate you are extra cautious in checking and double checking the order.
- What are the normal serum levels for magnesium?
- What are some of the indications for magnesium sulphate as a medication? Think of the mineral's (a) anticonvulsant properties, (b) tocolytic properties, (c) antidysrhythmic properties, (d) electrolyte replacement properties.
- Think back to your basic anatomy and physiology education and provide a rationale for the use of magnesium sulphate in clients with heart failure.
- What are some manifestations of overdosage with magnesium sulphate?

For answers see http://evolve.elsevier.com/Lilley/pharmacology/.

- Client experiences minimal complaints related to vitamin and mineral therapy.
- Client maintains skin integrity.
- Client regains and maintains activity level considered normal for him or her.

■ *Outcome Criteria*

Outcome criteria related to the use of vitamins and minerals include the following:

- Client openly verbalizes fears and anxieties about possible visual changes.

NURSING CARE PLAN | Magnesium Sulphate Therapy

D.G. is a 49-year-old heart failure client on the cardiac care unit who has been admitted for exacerbation of the disease. After initial treatment with furosemide intravenously (IV) and digoxin, the physician ordered serum potassium and magnesium levels. D.G.'s magnesium levels came back low, and the physician ordered magnesium sulphate 500 mg intravenously 2 doses.

ASSESSMENT	**Subjective Data**	• "The doctor says my magnesium levels are low. What type of drug am I going to receive, and what are its side effects?" • "I rarely take any medications. Is this a safe medication?" • "What will it do to me?"
	Objective Data	• Client admitted for diagnosis or exacerbation of heart failure • Low serum magnesium levels upon admission to critical care unit • Intravenous therapy ordered with infusion of magnesium • Asking questions about magnesium sulphate therapy • Anxious about treatment and not used to taking medications
NURSING DIAGNOSIS		Risk for injury related to potential side effects of CNS depressants
	Goals	At the end of the teaching session, client will verbalize an understanding of treatment with magnesium sulphate.
	Outcome Criteria	Client will verbalize the following during teaching session: • Reason for use of magnesium • Common side effects
IMPLEMENTATION		Inform the client of the following: • Magnesium sulphate therapy is used to return magnesium to within normal levels and to prevent problems with heartbeat. It is also sometimes used to prevent seizures. • Common side effects include sweating, slowed reflexes, flushing, drop in blood pressure, and breathing problems. Monitor the client closely for the following: • Vital signs q15min after intravenous dosing with a check of temperature, pulse, BP, and respirations • Input and output q4h with at least 120 mL/4 h and at least 30 mL/h; if less, contact the physician • Mental status • Respiratory status with a focus on respiratory rate, character, and rhythm • Hypermagnesemia (too much magnesium), which is manifested by depressed patellar (knee jerk) reflex, flushing, confusion, weakness, drop in body temperature, and shortness of breath Keep calcium gluconate on hand to reverse symptoms should toxicity occur.
EVALUATION		• Positive therapeutic outcome: elevated magnesium levels to within normal limits. • Evaluate for adverse effects such as depressed reflexes, confusion, sweating, dyspnea, hypothermia, decreased BP, and decreased respiratory functioning.

- Client keeps skin clean and dry to moist (as needed) to maintain skin integrity and prevent infection.
- Client increases activities of daily living as warranted and as tolerated.
- Client returns to pre-illness levels of function.

■ Implementation

Before administering vitamin A, the nurse should check and document the client's diet and signs and symptoms of hypervitaminosis and hypercarotenemia (excess vitamin A).

Vitamin D should be given with concurrent evaluations of renal function and serum calcium levels, especially at the beginning of therapy. The nurse should assess growth measurements in children before starting therapy, and all clients should be assessed for signs of toxicity, such as constipation, anorexia, nausea, vomiting, metallic taste, and dry mouth. Clients taking vitamin D should be closely monitored and should maintain regular visits to the physician for review of diet and calcium therapy.

Vitamin B_1 (thiamine) therapy is usually administered in an oral preparation, but parenteral forms are also available. Niacin should be administered with milk or food to decrease GI upset. Oral forms of niacin are preferred. If administered intravenously, pyridoxine should be given at a rate of 50 mg/min and may be given with most intravenous fluids. Cyanocobalamin should be administered orally with meals to increase its absorption. Ascorbic acid should be administered orally, if possible; if administered intravenously it should be given at a rate no greater than 100 mg/min. The oral effervescent forms should be dissolved in at least 180 mL of fluid, such as water or juice.

When vitamin C is prescribed for acidification of the urine, it is important for the nurse to frequently assess urinary pH. If vitamin C is administered intravenously, it should be given as a continuous infusion (not to exceed 100 mg/min) as an additive to intravenous solutions. Oral effervescent tablets should be dissolved thoroughly in water before administration.

Because of venous irritation, calcium should be given via an intravenous infusion pump when given intravenously. The nurse should also monitor closely for hypercalcemia. Intravenous calcium should be given slowly (<1 mL/min for adults) to avoid cardiac dysrhythmias and cardiac arrest, and the client should be kept recum-

bent for 15 minutes after the infusion. Should extravasation occur, the nurse should discontinue the infusion immediately. The physician may order the infusion with 1 percent procaine or other antidote to reduce vasospasm and dilute the effects of calcium on surrounding tissue. The nurse should follow institutional guidelines regarding treatment of calcium extravasation. Oral calcium supplements should be given one to three hours after meals.

Magnesium should be administered according to manufacturer guidelines and as ordered. Because different dosages result in different effects, the nurse should always recheck the order, dosage, and intended use and therapeutic effects. Calcium gluconate should be easily accessible for use as an antidote to magnesium toxicity.

For client teaching tips related to vitamins, minerals, and trace elements, see the box below.

■ Evaluation

Therapeutic responses to vitamin A therapy include restoration of normal vision and intact skin. Effects of deficiency may include lethargy, night blindness, skin and corneal changes, and, in infancy, failure to thrive.

Therapeutic responses to vitamin D include improved bone growth and formation and an intact skeleton with decreased or no pain. Side effects include constipation, anorexia, metallic taste, and dry mouth.

Therapeutic responses to vitamin E include improved muscle strength, improved skin integrity, and alpha tocopherol levels within normal limits. Side effects include blurred vision, dizziness, drowsiness, breast enlargement, and flu-like symptoms.

Therapeutic response to vitamin B_1 (thiamine) includes improved mental status with less confusion. Therapeutic responses to riboflavin, niacin, pyridoxine, and cyanocobalamin include improved skin integrity; normal vision; improved mental status; and normal RBC, Hgb, and Hct levels. Therapeutic responses to vitamin C include improved capillary intactness, skin and mucous membrane integrity, healing, and energy and mental state. An adverse reaction associated with vitamin C is precipitate formation in the urine with possible stone formation. Side effects for the B vitamins and ascorbic acid are included in the discussion and tables pertinent to each vitamin.

Therapeutic responses to trace elements include resolution of the deficient state and associated signs and symptoms, depending on the specific element or mineral.

CLIENT TEACHING TIPS

The nurse should provide information and counselling to clients about dietary sources for any vitamins or minerals in which they are deficient. Clients who have had a gastrectomy or ileal resection or who have pernicious anemia should be informed of the necessity for Vitamin B$_{12}$ in their diet.

The nurse should instruct the client as follows:

Vitamin A

▲ Vitamin A is found in egg yolks, butter, milk, liver, kidney, cream, cheese, and fortified margarine. Carotene, which the body uses to make vitamin A, is found in leafy green vegetables and yellow and orange fruits and vegetables.

Vitamin D

▲ Foods high in vitamin D include egg yolks, vitamin D–fortified milk, fish liver oils, whole grain cereals, wheat germ, liver, and vegetable oils.

▲ (unless medically contraindicated) Get some sunshine, but be careful not to overdo it: use sunscreen and a wide-brimmed hat.

Vitamin E

▲ Foods high in vitamin E include vegetable oils, wheat germ, whole grain cereals, egg yolks, and liver.

Vitamin B

▲ Vitamin B is found in many different foods. Thiamine is found in enriched cereals or whole grains, pork,

nuts, fish, organ and muscle meats, poultry, rice bran, and green vegetables. Riboflavin is found in milk and other dairy products, meats, eggs, fish, poultry, and enriched grains and cereals. Niacin is found in meats, eggs, whole grain and enriched cereals, breads, flour, and milk and other dairy products. Pyridoxine is found in meats, poultry, fish, eggs, whole grains, sweet potatoes, lima beans, and bananas.

Vitamin C

▲ You may experience a slight increase in daily urination; if you take more than 1 g per day, you may get diarrhea.

▲ You can get vitamin C from foods such as citrus fruits, tomatoes, strawberries, cantaloupe, and raw peppers.

Trace Elements (e.g., zinc, copper, magnesium, iodine, chromium)

▲ Take the medication as prescribed.

▲ Call the physician if any unusual reactions occur.

Calcium

▲ Foods high in calcium include milk and other dairy products, shellfish, and dark green leafy vegetables.

▲ Limit foods high in oxalate and zinc, such as nuts, legumes, chocolate, spinach, and soy products, and avoid bran, because these foods decrease the absorption of calcium.

▲ If you are prescribed antibiotics, make sure the physician knows you are taking calcium. Calcium decreases the effects of some antibiotics.

POINTS to REMEMBER

▼ The OTC use of vitamins and minerals may lead to serious problems and side effects; therefore a physician should be consulted before supplements are taken.

▼ Nurses must incorporate the nutritional status of each client into the nursing care plan to provide comprehensive care during medication therapy.

▼ The nurse's participation in health promotion and wellness includes providing information about dietary needs and the body's need for vitamins and minerals.

▼ Client education as related to vitamin and mineral replacement must focus on dietary sources of the spe-

cific nutrient, drug and food interactions, and side effects. Clients must be instructed about when it is necessary to contact the physician.

▼ Vitamins and minerals can be dangerous to the client if given without concern and caution for the client's overall condition and underlying disease processes.

▼ It should never be assumed that because the drug is a vitamin or a mineral it does not have adverse reactions or toxicity. Most vitamins and minerals can become toxic.

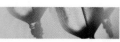

EXAMINATION REVIEW QUESTIONS

1 Which of the following may occur if intravenous calcium is given too rapidly?
a. Ototoxicity
b. Liver failure
c. Renal shutdown
d. Cardiac dysrhythmias

2 Calcium products chelate with which of the following?
a. Penicillins
b. Oxafloxins
c. Aminoglycosides
d. Tetracyclines

3 Which of the following are high in thiamine?
a. Strawberries
b. Poultry

c. Organ meats
d. Greens

4 Foods high in vitamin E include which of the following?
a. Liver
b. Citrus fruits
c. Poultry
d. Pork

5 The best sources of carotene include which of the following?
a. Yellow fruits and vegetables
b. Pork
c. Orange-coloured candied yams
d. Bran

For answers see http://evolve.elsevier.com/Lilley/pharmacology/.

CRITICAL THINKING ACTIVITIES

1 Explain why clients with a cardiac history need a baseline ECG and serum calcium assessment performed before initiation of calcium supplemental therapy.

2 Your client is experiencing constipation and abdominal pain since beginning calcium therapy. Your assessment reveals a distended abdomen and diminished bowel

sounds. What could be occurring, and what should your nursing actions be at this time?

3 Ms. W. takes 2500 mg of calcium carbonate daily in the form of an OTC calcium supplement. How much elemental calcium is Ms. W. actually taking?

For answers see http://evolve.elsevier.com/Lilley/pharmacology/.

BIBLIOGRAPHY

Albanese, J., & Nutz, P. (2005). *Mosby's 2005 nursing drug cards.* St Louis, MO: Mosby.

Canadian Pharmacists Association. (2003). *Therapeutic choices* (4th ed.). Ottawa, ON: Author.

Canadian Pharmacists Association. (2004). *Guide to drugs in Canada.* Toronto, ON: Dorling Kindersley.

Canadian Pharmacists Association. (2005). *Compendium of pharmaceuticals and specialties. The Canadian drug reference for health professionals.* Ottawa, ON: Author. [The subscription-based e-CPS is available at http://www.pharmacists.ca.]

Cheng, A., Williams, B.A., & Sivarajan, B.V. (Eds.). (2003). *The HSC handbook of pediatrics* (10th ed.). Toronto, ON: Elsevier.

Facts and Comparisons. (2004). *Drug facts and comparisons pocket version* (9th ed.). St Louis, MO: Wolters Kluwer Health.

Hardman, J.G., & Limbird, L.E. (2002). *Goodman and Gilman's the pharmacological basis of therapeutics* (10th ed.). New York: McGraw-Hill.

Health Canada. (2005). Drug product database (DPD). Retrieved September 8, 2005, from http://www.hc-sc.gc.ca/hpb/drugs-dpd/

Health Canada. (2004). Canada food guides from 1942 to 1992. Retrieved September 8, 2005, from http://www.hc-sc.gc.ca/

Health Canada. (2004). Dietary reference intakes. Retrieved September 8, 2005, from http://www.hc-sc.gc.ca/fn-an/nutrition/reference/index_e.html

P. Turner, R. E., & Ross, D. (2003). *Discovering nutrition.* Boston, MA: Jones and Bartlett.

Kasper, D.L., Braunwald, D., Faci, A., Hauser, S., Longo, D., & Jameson, J.L. (2005). *Harrison's principles of internal medicine* (16th ed.). New York: McGraw-Hill.

Katz, D. (2005). *Nutrition in clinical practice: A comprehensive, evidence-based manual for the practitioner* (2nd ed.). Philadelphia: Lippincott Williams & Wilkins.

Katzung, B.G. (2004). *Basic and clinical pharmacology* (9th ed.). New York: McGraw-Hill.

Lacy, C.F., Armstrong, L.L., Goldman, M.P., & Lance, L.L. (2003). *Drug information handbook* (11th ed.). Hudson, OH: Lexi-Comp.

Lehne, R.A. (2004). *Pharmacology for nursing care* (5th ed.). St Louis, MO: Saunders.

McKenry, L.M., & Salerno, E. (2003). *Mosby's pharmacology in nursing—revised and updated* (21st ed.). St Louis, MO: Mosby.

Mosby. (2005). *Mosby's drug consult 2005: The comprehensive reference for generic and brand name drugs* (15th ed.). St Louis, MO: Mosby.

Skidmore-Roth, L. (2006). *Mosby's 2006 nursing drug reference* (19th ed.). St Louis, MO: Mosby.

53 Nutritional Supplements

OBJECTIVES

After reading this chapter, the successful student will be able to do the following:

1 Describe the pathophysiology and diseases that lead to the need for nutritional supplements.

2 Discuss the various enteral and parenteral supplements, including each of their ingredients.

3 Describe the nurse's role in the process of initiating and maintaining continuous or intermittent enteral feedings, total parenteral nutrition (TPN), and other forms of nutritional supplementation.

4 Compare the various enteral feeding tubes, including specific uses and the special needs of clients requiring this nutritional support.

5 Discuss the mechanisms of action, cautions, contraindications, and nursing implications associated with enteral and parenteral nutritional supplements.

6 Develop a nursing care plan that includes all phases of the nursing process for clients receiving enteral and parenteral supplemental feedings.

7 Discuss the various laboratory values related to nutritional deficits or any form of altered nutritional status.

ℯ-LEARNING ACTIVITIES

Student CD-ROM
- Review Questions: see question 392
- Animations
- Medication Administration Checklists
- IV Therapy Checklists

evolve Web site (http://evolve.elsevier.com/Lilley/pharmacology/)
- Online Chapter Worksheet • Frequently Asked Questions
- Learning Tips and Content Updates • WebLinks • Online Appendices and Supplements • Mosby/Saunders ePharmacology Update • Access to *Mosby's Drug Consult*

DRUG PROFILES

amino acids, p. 914
carbohydrate formulation, p. 912
carbohydrates, p. 914

fat formulation, p. 912
fats, p. 914
lipid emulsions, p. 914
protein formulation, p. 912

GLOSSARY

Anabolism (ə nab′ ə liz′ əm) Constructive metabolism characterized by the conversion of simple substances into the more complex compounds of living matter.

Casein The principal protein of milk and the basis for curd and cheese.

Catabolism (kə tab′ ə liz′ əm) A complex metabolic process in which energy is liberated for use in work, energy storage, or heat production by the destruction of complex substances by living cells to form simple compounds.

Dumping syndrome A complex bodily reaction to the rapid entry of concentrated nutrients into the jejunum of the small intestine. The client may experience nausea, weakness, sweating, palpitations, syncope, sensations of warmth, and diarrhea. Most commonly occurs with eating following partial gastrectomy or with enteral feedings that are administered too rapidly into the stomach or jejunum via a feeding tube.

Enteral nutrition (en′ ter əl) The provision of food or nutrients via the gastrointestinal tract, either naturally by eating or through a feeding tube in clients unable to eat.

Essential amino acids   Those amino acids that cannot be manufactured by the body.

Essential fatty acid deficiency   A condition that develops if fatty acids that the body cannot produce are not present in dietary or nutritional supplements.

Hyperalimentation   (hy' per al' ə men tay' shən) Same as parenteral nutrition.

Malnutrition   Any disorder of nutrition.

Multivitamin infusion (MVI)   A concentrated solution containing several common vitamins and used as part of an intravenous (parenteral) nutrition source.

Non-essential amino acids   Those amino acids that the body can produce without extracting from dietary intake.

Nutrient   A substance that provides nourishment and affects the nutritive and metabolic processes of the body.

Nutritional supplements   A means of providing adequate nutritional support to meet the body's nutritional needs.

Nutritional support   Support for the body's nutritional needs; can be natural (i.e., normal eating) or artificial (e.g., tube feeding, intravenous feeding).

Parenteral nutrition   (pə ren' tər əl) The administration of nutrients by a route other than through the alimentary canal, such as intravenously.

Semi-essential amino acids   Those amino acids that can be produced by the body but not in sufficient amounts in infants and children.

Total parenteral nutrition (TPN)   Same as parenteral nutrition.

Whey   The thin serum of milk remaining after the casein and fat have been removed. It contains proteins, lactose, water-soluble vitamins, and minerals.

The integrity and normal function of all cells within the body require a constant supply of nutrients. **Nutrients** are dietary products that undergo chemical changes when ingested (metabolized) and cause tissue to be enhanced and energy to be liberated. Nutrients are required for cell growth and division; enzyme activity; protein, carbohydrate, and fat synthesis; muscle contraction; neurohormonal secretion (e.g., vasopressin, gastrin); wound repair; immune competence; gut integrity; and numerous other essential cellular functions. Providing for these nutritional needs is known as **nutritional support**. Adequate nutritional support is needed to prevent the breakdown of tissue proteins for use as an energy supply to sustain essential organ systems. This is what happens during starvation. **Malnutrition** can decrease organ size and impair the function of organ systems (e.g., cardiac, respiratory, gastrointestinal [GI], hepatic, renal). Nutritional supplements are a means of providing adequate nutritional support to meet the body's nutritional needs.

Malnutrition is a condition in which the body's essential need for nutrients is not met by nutrient intake. The purpose of nutritional support is the successful prevention, recognition, and management of malnutrition. **Nutritional supplements** are dietary products used to provide nutritional support. Nutritional supplement products can be administered to clients in a variety of

ways. They vary in their amounts and the chemical complexity of carbohydrate, protein, and fat. Specific products can also vary in electrolyte, vitamin, and mineral content and in osmolality (concentration of dissolved substances in the solution—see Chapter 26). These nutrients may be given in a digested form, a partially digested form, or an undigested form. Nutritional supplements can also be tailored for specific disease states.

A wide variety of nutritional supplements is needed because of the wide variety of conditions for which clients require nutritional support. Clients' nutrient requirements vary according to age, sex, size or weight, physical activity, pre-existing medical conditions, and current medical or surgical treatment.

Nutritional supplements are classified according to the method of administration, as either enteral or parenteral. **Enteral nutrition** is the provision of food or nutrients via the GI tract. **Parenteral nutrition** is the delivery of nutrients directly into the circulation by means of intravenous infusion. The selection of enteral or parenteral nutrition and the specific nutritional composition of the product depend on the client profile and the clinical situation.

Nutritional support
↗ Enteral nutrition → Gastrointestinal tract
↘ Parenteral nutrition → Circulation

ENTERAL NUTRITION

Enteral nutrition is the provision of food or nutrients through the GI tract. The most common and least invasive route of administration is oral consumption—eating and drinking. A feeding tube is used in the other five routes (Figure 53-1). The six routes of enteral nutrition delivery are listed in Table 53-1. Clients who may benefit from a feeding tube include those with abnormal esophageal or stomach peristalsis, altered anatomy secondary to surgery, depressed consciousness, or impaired digestive capacity. Nutrients may be administered via the enteral or parenteral routes depending on the clinical

TABLE 53-1
ROUTES OF ENTERAL NUTRITION DELIVERY

Route	Description
Gastrostomy	Feeding tube surgically inserted directly into the stomach
Jejunostomy	Feeding tube surgically inserted into the jejunum
Nasoduodenal	Feeding tube placed from the nose to the duodenum
Nasojejunal	Feeding tube placed from the nose to the jejunum
Nasogastric	Feeding tube placed from the nose to the stomach
Oral	Nutritional supplements delivered by mouth

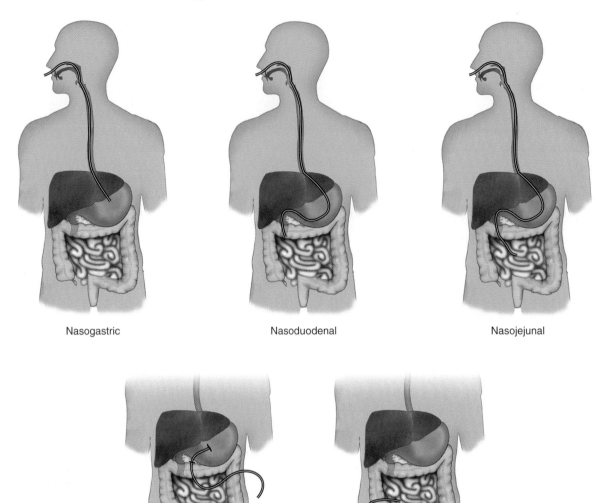

Nasogastric   Nasoduodenal   Nasojejunal

Gastrostomy   Jejunostomy

FIG. 53-1 Tube feeding routes. (From Beare, P.G., & Myers, J.L. (1998). *Adult health nursing* (3rd ed.). St Louis, MO: Mosby.)

situation. Many processes occur from the beginning of the digestive system in the mouth to the end of the digestive system in the anus. These processes have evolved over time to most effectively digest dietary nutrients. For this reason the enteral route is considered to be superior and should therefore be used whenever possible.

Approximately 100 different enteral formulations are available. The enteral supplements have been divided into four basic groups: elemental, polymeric, modular, and altered amino acid. These are described in Box 53-1.

Mechanism of Action and Drug Effects

The enteral formula groups provide the basic building blocks for **anabolism**. Different combinations and amounts of these agents are used based on the individual client's anabolic needs. After the body receives and absorbs these nutrients, it must process them into living matter. Enteral nutrition supplies complete dietary needs through the GI tract by the normal oral route or by feeding tube.

Indications

Enteral nutrition can be used to supplement an oral diet that is currently insufficient for a client's nutrient needs or used solely to meet all of the client's nutrient needs. It is used for clients who are unable to consume or digest normal foods, who have accelerated catabolic status, or who are undernourished because of disease. Box 53-2 lists the main types of enteral nutrition supplements and their indications.

Contraindications

The only usual contraindication to nutritional supplements of any kind is known drug allergy to a specific product or genetic disease that renders a client unable to digest certain types of nutrients.

BOX 53-1
Enteral Formulations

Atered Amino Acid Formulations

Amin-Aid
Hepatic-Aid
Lonalac
Stresstein
Travasorb Renal
Traum-Aid HBC

Contents: varying amounts of specific amino acids

Indications: clients with problems due to genetically altered metabolism

Elemental Formulations

Peptamen
Vital HN
Vivonex Plus
Vivonex TEN

Contents: dipeptides, tripeptides, or crystalline amino acids, glucose oligosaccharides, and vegetable oil or MCTs

Comments: minimum digestion; residue is minimal

Indications: partial bowel obstruction, irritable bowel disease, radiation enteritis, bowel fistulas, and short bowel syndrome

Modular Formulations

Carbohydrate
Moducal
Polycose

Contents: single nutrient formulas (protein, carbohydrate, or fat)

Fat
MCT Oil
Microlipid

Indications: can be added to a monomeric or polymeric formulation to provide a more individual specialized nutrient formulation

Protein
Casec
ProMod
Propac
Stresstein

Polymeric Formulations

Complete
Ensure
Ensure-Plus
Isocal
Osmolite
Portagen
Precision LR
Sustacal

Contents: complex nutrients (proteins, carbohydrates, and fat)

Indications: preferred over elemental for clients with fully functional GI tracts and few specialized nutrient requirements because hyperosmolarity of elemental formulas causes more GI problems

MCT, Medium-chain triglyceride.

BOX 53-2
Enteral Nutrition Supplements: Therapeutic Effects

Complete Nutritional Formulations
- Unable to consume or digest normal foods
- Accelerated catabolic status
- Undernourished because of disease

Incomplete Nutritional Formulations
- Genetic metabolic enzyme deficiency
- Hepatic or renal impairment

Infant Nutritional Formulations
- Sole nutritional intake for premature and full-term infants
- Supplemental nutritional intake for older infants receiving solid foods
- Supplemental nutrition for breastfed infants

Interactions

Various nutrients can interact with drugs to produce significant food–drug interactions. With some exceptions, food usually delays the absorption of drugs when administered simultaneously. Chemical inactivation with high gastric acid content or prolonged emptying time can result in decreased effects of cephalosporins, erythromycin, and penicillins when given with nutritional supplements. An increased absorption rate resulting in increased therapeutic effects can be seen when adrenal steroids or vitamins A and D are given with nutritional supplements. Decreased antibiotic effects of tetracycline are seen when it is given with nutritional supplements as a result of chemical inactivation that occurs when this drug complexes with calcium.

Dosages

Because nutrient requirements vary greatly, dosages are individualized according to client needs.

DRUG PROFILES

Enteral nutrition can be provided by a variety of supplements. Individual client characteristics determine the appropriate enteral supplement. There are four basic types of enteral formulations: elemental, polymeric, modular, and altered amino acid.

ELEMENTAL FORMULATIONS

Elemental formulations are enteral supplements that contain dipeptides, tripeptides, or crystalline amino acids. Minimal digestion is required. These agents are indicated in clients with partial bowel obstruction, irritable bowel disease, radiation enteritis, bowel fistulas, and short bowel syndrome. They are contraindicated in clients who have had hypersensitivity reactions to them. Elemental formulation supplements are available without a prescription and have no pregnancy category.

Side Effects and Adverse Effects

The most common side effect of nutritional supplements is GI intolerance leading to diarrhea. Infant nutritional formulations are most commonly associated with allergies and digestive intolerance. The other nutritional supplements are most commonly associated with osmotic diarrhea. Rapid feeding or bolus doses can result in **dumping syndrome**, which produces intestinal disturbances. In addition, tube feeding can often result in aspiration.

POLYMERIC FORMULATIONS

Polymeric formulations are enteral supplements that contain complex nutrients derived from proteins, carbohydrates, and fat. The polymeric formulations are some of the most commonly used enteral formulations because they most closely resemble normal dietary intake. They are preferred over elemental formulations in clients with fully functional GI tracts who have no specialized nutrient needs. They are also less hyperosmolar (i.e., less concentrated) than elemental formulations and therefore cause fewer GI problems. They are contraindicated in clients who have had hypersensitivity reactions to them. They are available without a prescription and have no pregnancy category.

Ensure is a commonly used enteral supplement in this category. It is lactose free and is also available in a higher caloric formula called Ensure-Plus. Other polymeric formulations include Isocal, Magnacal, Meritene, Osmolite, Portagen, and Sustacal. These agents contain complex nutrients such as **casein** and soy protein for protein, corn syrup and maltodextrins for carbohydrates, and vegetable oil or milk fat for fat. They are available in liquid formulations only.

MODULAR FORMULATIONS

carbohydrate formulation

Moducal and Polycose are examples of commonly used enteral supplements from the carbohydrate modular formulation category. Both supply carbohydrates only. They are intended to be used as an addition to monomeric or polymeric formulations to provide a more individual specialized nutrient formulation. They are available in liquid formulations only. These products are available without a prescription, have no pregnancy category, and are contraindicated only if a client has had a hypersensitivity reaction to them.

fat formulation

Microlipid and MCT Oil are the formulations available in the fat category. Microlipid is a fat supplement supplying solely fats. It is a concentrated source of calories and contains 4.5 kcal/mL. These agents are used to help individualize nutrient formulations. They may be used in malabsorption and other GI disorders and in clients with pancreatitis. They are available in liquid formulations only. These products are available without a prescription, have no pregnancy category, and are contraindicated only if a client has had a hypersensitivity reaction to them.

protein formulation

Casec, ProMod, and Propac are examples of protein modular formulations. They are used to increase and provide additional proteins to enhance clients' protein intake. They are derived from a variety of sources such as **whey**, casein, egg whites, and amino acids. All of the available products are dried powders that have to be reconstituted with water. They may sometimes be reconstituted by placing them in enteral feedings that are already in liquid form. They are indicated for clients with increased protein needs. They are contraindicated

in clients who have had hypersensitivity reactions to them. Protein formulation supplements are available without a prescription and have no pregnancy category.

ALTERED AMINO ACID FORMULATIONS

Amin-Aid is one of the many amino acid formulation nutritional supplements available. Many of the nutritional supplements in this category are also listed as modular formulations because they can be used as both single-nutrient formulas and as nutrition formulations for clients with genetic errors of metabolism. Amino acid formulations are used most commonly in clients who have metabolic disorders such as phenylketonuria, homocystinuria, and maple syrup urine disease. They are also used to supply nutritional support to clients with such illnesses as renal impairment, eclampsia, heart failure, or liver failure.

PARENTERAL NUTRITION

Parenteral nutritional supplementation (intravenous administration) is the preferred method for clients who are unable to tolerate and maintain adequate enteral or oral intake. Instead of administering partially digested nutrients into the GI tract, totally digested vitamins, minerals, amino acids, dextrose, and so on are administered intravenously directly into the circulatory system. This effectively bypasses the entire GI system, eliminating the need for absorption, metabolism, and excretion. Parenteral nutrition is also called **total parenteral nutrition (TPN)** or **hyperalimentation**. It is generally accepted that TPN should be considered only when oral or enteral support is impossible or when the GI absorptive or functional capacity is not sufficient to meet the nutritional needs of the client.

TPN can supply all of the calories, carbohydrates, amino acids, fats, trace elements, vitamins, minerals, and other essential nutrients needed for growth, weight gain, wound healing, convalescence, immunocompetence, and other health-sustaining functions.

TPN can be administered either through a peripheral vein or a central vein. Each route of delivery of TPN has specific requirements and limitations (see Table 53-2).

PERIPHERAL TOTAL PARENTERAL NUTRITION

In peripheral TPN, nutrients are delivered to the client's circulatory system through a peripheral vein. The long-term administration of nutritional supplements via a peripheral vein may lead to phlebitis and ultimately the loss of a limb. Peripheral TPN should be considered a temporary measure to provide adequate nutrient needs in clients with mild deficits or who are restricted from oral intake and have slightly elevated metabolic rates.

Peripheral TPN is most valuable in clients who do not have large nutritional needs, can tolerate moderately

TABLE 53-2
PERIPHERAL AND CENTRAL PARENTERAL NUTRITION: CHARACTERISTICS

Considerations	Characteristics	
	Peripheral	Central
Goal of nutritional therapy (total vs. supplemental)	Supplemental (total if moderate to low needs)	Total
Length of therapy	Short (<5 days)	Long (>7–10 days)
Osmolarity	Isotonic (<900 mOsm/L)	Hypertonic (2000 mOsm/L)
Fluid tolerance	Must be high	Can be fluid restricted
Dextrose	<5–12.5%	10–50%
Amino acids	3–5%	3–7%
Fats	10–20%	10–20%
Calories/day	<2000 kcal/day	> 2000 kcal/day

TABLE 53-3
AMINO ACIDS: RECOMMENDED DOSAGE GUIDELINES

Healthy		Undernourished or Traumatized
Adult	Infant/Child	
0.9 g/kg	1.4–2.2 g/kg	Up to 2 g/kg

large fluid loads, and need nutritional supplements only temporarily. Peripheral TPN may be used alone or in combination with oral nutritional supplements to provide the necessary fat, carbohydrate, and protein needed by the client to maintain health. The recent addition of peripherally inserted central catheters (PICC) has provided the opportunity for longer term administration of nutritional therapy. The PICC is a long flexible catheter inserted into a peripheral vein that is then threaded so that its tip is positioned in a central location such as the superior vena cava.

Mechanism of Action and Drug Effects

Peripheral TPN provides the basic nutrient building blocks for anabolism. Different combinations and amounts of these agents are used based on the individual client's anabolic needs. After the body receives these nutrients, it must process them into living matter.

Indications

Peripheral TPN is used to supplement nutrients for clients who cannot take in enough orally or to provide entire daily nutrition. Peripheral TPN is meant only as a temporary means (less than two weeks) of delivering TPN.
Peripheral TPN may be indicated
- When procedures restrict oral feedings
- When radiation or cancer chemotherapy causes anorexia
- When GI illnesses prevent oral food ingestion
- After any type of surgery
- When nutritional deficits are minimal but oral nutrition will not be started for more than five days

Contraindications

The only usual contraindication to nutritional supplements of any kind is known drug allergy to a specific product or genetic disease that renders a client unable to digest certain types of nutrients.

Side Effects and Adverse Effects

The most devastating adverse effect of peripheral TPN is phlebitis, which is a vein irritation or inflammation of a vein. If it is severe enough and not treated appropriately, phlebitis can lead to the loss of a limb. However, this is rare. Another potential adverse effect is fluid overload. Peripheral TPN is limited to lower dextrose-concentrated solutions, generally less than 10 percent, to avoid sclerosing of the vein. Larger amounts of nutritional supplements are needed with lower concentrated solutions to meet a client's daily nutritional requirements. Some clients, such as those with renal or heart failure, cannot tolerate large fluid volume. In these clients, peripheral TPN may be contraindicated or used cautiously only if absolutely necessary.

Dosages

Dosage requirements vary from client to client. Age, sex, weight, and numerous other factors must be considered for proper administration of TPN. Guidelines for amino acids appear in Table 53-3.

DRUG PROFILES

The individual components of peripheral and central TPN are the same. The difference lies in the concentrations and amounts of the components delivered per volume of nutritional supplement. The four basic components of peripheral or central TPN are amino acids, carbohydrates, lipids, and trace elements and electrolytes. Most of the electrolyte components are discussed in Chapter 26.

AMINO ACIDS

Amino acids have many roles in the maintenance of normal nutritional status. The primary role is protein synthesis, or anabolism. Adequate amino acids in nutritional supplements reduce the breakdown of proteins (**catabolism**) and also help to promote normal growth and wound healing.
Amino acids are commonly classified as essential or non-essential according to whether they can or cannot be produced by the body. **Non-essential amino acids** are those that the body produces and are therefore not needed in dietary intake. The body is able to manufacture from nutritional nitrogen sources all but eight of the available amino acids. **Essential amino acids** are those amino acids that cannot be produced by the body. Therefore they must be included in daily dietary

Amino Acids: Classification

Essential	Non-Essential	Semi-Essential
Isoleucine	Alanine	Arginine
Leucine	Asparagine	Histidine
Lysine	Aspartic acid	
Methionine	Cysteine	
Phenylalanine	Glutamine	
Threonine	Glutamic acid	
Tryptophan	Glycine	
Valine	Proline	
	Serine	
	Tyrosine	

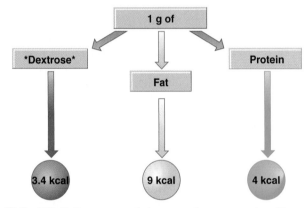

FIG. 53-2 One gram of dextrose, fat, or protein will provide varying amounts of energy as calories.

intake. Amino acids are used as building blocks for protein that is needed for normal growth and development. Two amino acids, histidine and arginine, are not manufactured by the body in large enough quantities during rapid growth periods such as infancy or childhood. Thus they are referred to as **semi-essential amino acids.** Box 53-3 lists the amino acids according to their categories.

amino acids

Amino acid crystalline solutions (Aminosyn 3 percent, 5 percent, and 10 percent and Primene 10 percent) can be used in either peripheral or central TPN. The two currently available amino acid solutions differ only in their respective concentrations. The dosage of these solutions varies depending on the client's weight and requirements. These drugs have no restrictions regarding pregnancy and have no contraindications to use. Recommended dosages for healthy and traumatized clients are listed in Table 53-2.

carbohydrates

In nutritional support, carbohydrates are usually supplied to clients through dextrose. Under normal circumstances both carbohydrates and lipids are used as calorie sources (Figure 53-2). Concentrations of dextrose in TPN are important considerations. In peripheral TPN, dextrose concentrations are kept below 10 percent to decrease the possibility of phlebitis. In central TPN,

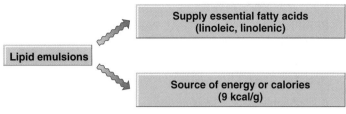

FIG. 53-3 Lipid emulsions supply essential fatty acids and energy.

dextrose concentrations can range from 10 to 50 percent but are commonly 25 to 35 percent. Because dextrose is a sugar, supplemental insulin may be given simultaneously in nutritional supplements. A balanced nutritional supplement that contains dextrose and lipids for caloric sources decreases the need for large amounts of insulin.

fats

The average North American diet contains 40 percent fat. This means that of the total calories supplied, 40 to 50 percent of the calories are obtained through fat grams. The ideal diet contains 30 percent fat. Intravenous fat emulsions serve two functions: they supply essential fatty acids and they are a source of energy or calories. As with the amino acids, certain fatty acids are essential because the body cannot produce them. Linoleic acid cannot be synthesized by the body. It is needed to produce linolenic and arachidonic acid. If these fatty acids are not present in dietary or nutritional supplements, an **essential fatty acid deficiency** may develop. Clinical signs of essential fatty acid deficiency are hair loss, scaly dermatitis, growth retardation, reduced wound healing, decreased platelets, and fatty liver (Figure 53-3).

lipid emulsions

The currently available lipid emulsions, Intralipid and Liposyn II, are available as either 10 percent or 20 percent emulsions. They differ in fat origin. Intralipid is made from soybean oil; Liposyn is made from both soybean and safflower oil.

Fat emulsions should be calibrated to deliver no more than 60 percent of the total daily caloric intake. Fat emulsions are most beneficial when combined with dextrose solutions. The use of fat to meet caloric needs prevents potentially harmful conditions—such as hyperglycemia, hyperinsulinemia, and hyperosmolarity—that can occur when a client's entire caloric needs are being met solely by dextrose. A healthy diet contains 30 percent fat, 40 percent protein, and 30 percent carbohydrate.

TRACE ELEMENTS

Trace element solutions are available individually or in many different combinations. The following are considered trace elements:

- Chromium
- Copper
- Iodine
- Manganese

- Molybdenum
- Selenium
- Zinc

Other combination trace element formulations are listed in Box 53-4. Specific dosages and frequencies depend on the individual client's requirements. Vitamins and minerals may also be added accordingly. A common multivitamin combination is **multivitamin infusion (MVI)**.

CENTRAL TOTAL PARENTERAL NUTRITION

In central TPN, a large central vein is used to deliver nutrients directly into the client's circulation. Usually the subclavian or internal jugular vein is used. Central TPN is generally indicated for clients who require nutritional supplements for a prolonged period, usually more than seven to ten days. It can also be used in the home care setting. There are a variety of indications for central TPN. The disadvantages of central TPN are the risks associated with venous catheter insertion and use and maintenance of the central vein.

Mechanism of Action and Drug Effects

Central TPN is used to supply nutrients to clients who cannot ingest nutrients by mouth and cannot meet required daily nutritional needs by the enteral or peripheral parenteral routes. Like peripheral TPN, central TPN provides the basic building blocks for anabolism. However, TPN solutions for central intravenous infusion may be more concentrated, especially in terms of carbohydrate content, and may contain as much as 70 percent dextrose. Different combinations and amounts of liquid nutrients are used, based on the individual client's anabolic needs. After the body receives these nutrients, it must process them into living matter. Central TPN works by delivering these essential nutrients directly into the circulation via a central vein. It provides the fat, carbohydrate, and protein that the client needs to maintain health.

Indications

TPN delivers total dietary nutrients to clients who require nutritional supplementation. Clients may benefit from central TPN when they

- Have large nutritional requirements (metabolic stress or hypermetabolism)

- Need nutritional support for prolonged periods (more than seven to ten days)
- Are unable to tolerate large fluid loads

Contraindications

The only usual contraindication for TPN is when the client has a functional GI tract that does not justify the use and risks of TPN.

Side Effects and Adverse Effects

The most common side effects and adverse effects of central TPN are those surrounding the use of the central vein. Complications can arise from the insertion of the infusion line, as well as the use and maintenance of the central vein. There is a greater potential than with peripheral TPN for infection, more serious catheter-induced trauma and related events, and other technical or mechanical problems. There are larger and more concentrated volumes of nutritional supplements being delivered with central TPN and therefore a greater chance for metabolic complications such as hyperglycemia.

Dosages

Administration is individualized according to client needs.

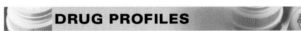

DRUG PROFILES

The same formulations used in peripheral TPN are used in central TPN. Often the concentrations of fluids administered through the central vein are much higher than those used in peripheral nutrition supplements.

NURSING PROCESS

◼ Assessment

Before any nutritional supplementation, the nurse should measure weight and height and conduct a thorough nutritional assessment with a dietary history and weekly and daily food intakes. Consultation with a registered dietician is crucial to identify the nutrients missing in a particular client's diet. After completing the assessment the nurse may need to contact the physician about the need for a consult on either an inpatient or outpatient basis. Laboratory studies, including total protein, albumin, blood urea nitrogen (BUN), red blood cells (RBCs), white blood cells (WBCs), vitamin B_{12}, cholesterol, and hemoglobin (Hgb), are needed. Other laboratory studies may include cholesterol, electrolytes, total lymphocyte count, serum transferrin, iron levels, urine creatinine clearance, lipid profile, and urinalysis (to assess protein loss). Anthropometric measurements and weights also provide much-needed data. The data collected help the physician and other members of the healthcare team select the appropriate nutritional supplements for the client.

Before beginning an enteral nutritional supplement of elemental formulation such as Vivonex, the nurse must determine if the client has a history of allergic reaction to its contents. Polymeric formulations, such as Ensure, are contraindicated in clients with a hypersensitivity to any of their ingredients. Modular formulations such as Centrality, fat formulations such as Microlipid, and protein formulations such as Hepatic-Aid are also contraindicated in clients with known hypersensitivity. Altered amino acid formulas are contraindicated in clients who have a known hyper-sensitivity to the formulation. Enteral feedings are generally contraindicated in clients who are capable of oral intake or who have intestinal obstruction, severe vomiting, or esophageal fistulas.

Casec, ProMod, and Propac are protein formulations that are reconstituted with water for enteral feedings. They are contraindicated in clients with allergies to whey, egg whites, and the product.

Nursing Diagnoses

Nursing diagnoses appropriate for the client receiving enteral or parenteral nutritional supplementation are as follows:

- Diarrhea related to a decreased tolerance to enteral feedings and their ingredients.
- Ineffective airway clearance related to possible aspiration of enteral feedings.
- Deficient fluid volume related to nutritional status.
- Risk for infection related to parenteral infusions and the loss of skin integrity.
- Ineffective individual therapeutic management related to lack of information.

Planning

Goals related to the use of nutritional supplements are as follows:

- Client remains free of complications.
- Client regains near-normal to normal bowel patterns.
- Client remains free of injury during nutritional support.
- Client remains free of infection.
- Client regains normal fluid volume status.
- Client remains adherent and makes return visits to the physician as needed.

Outcome Criteria

Outcome criteria are as follows:

- Client identifies measures to decrease diarrhea, such as use of drug and non-drug therapies.
- Client (or caregiver) demonstrates adequate technique for enteral tube feedings to decrease risk of aspiration, with emphasis on elevated head of bed and checking tube placement.
- Client states measures to minimize risk of infection at TPN site, such as making sure site is changed as ordered and assessed for redness, swelling, or drainage.
- Client begins to show adequate fluid volume status with improved turgor, improved urinary output, and a return to normal laboratory values.
- Client states symptoms to report to the physician, such as increased lethargy, fever, and shortness of breath.

Implementation

A physician's order must be complete and dated before beginning enteral and/or parenteral nutrition supplementation.

Enteral

In general, monitoring the status of the client during and after enteral feedings is crucial to safe and prudent nursing care. Tinting solutions with blue food colouring helps the nurse to detect aspiration in the tube-feeding substance. Gastric residual volumes should be obtained and documented before each feeding and before each medication is administered. The tube feeding should be stopped and the stomach contents aspirated to detect any residual. If the volume is more than that from two hours of continuous feeding, the nurse should return the aspirate, hold the feeding, and contact the physician.

For intermittent bolus feedings, if the residual amount is greater than 50 percent of the volume previously infused, the nurse should return the aspirate, withhold the feeding, and contact the physician. Reduced feeding volume will probably be ordered by the physician.

The head of the bed should always remain elevated during tube feedings to decrease the risk of aspiration. The process of medication administration through a nasogastric tube is reviewed in Chapter 9.

Newer tubes for nasogastric and enteral feeding are thinner (Nos. 5 through 10 French) and more pliable for better client tolerance. However, the smaller-diameter tubes make checking for gastric aspiration more difficult. If the attempt is unsuccessful, the nurse should instill air and auscultate over the gastric area. Air sounds in the stomach denote accurate placement. The external end of the tube should be placed in water to test for air bubbles, which signify incorrect placement.

To prevent clogging of the feeding tube with formula, it is often helpful to flush the tube with 30 mL of cranberry juice (per policy), followed by 10 mL of water. The juice may help break up the formula residue and unclog certain tubes. Percutaneous enteral gastrostomy (PEG) tubes are also now commonly used in certain situations but do require surgical insertion (often done under moderate sedation) by a gastroenterologist.

Physician-ordered enteral feeding infusion rates and concentration should be followed carefully. Usually the initial rate is 50 mL/h at one-half strength, but this can be increased per client tolerance to a rate of 25 mL/h at three-quarter strength concentration. Although more rapid feeding increases the risk of hyperglycemia or dumping syndrome, the nurse should continue to increase the client's intake because 1000 mL to 2000 mL of the milk-based formula (1 kcal/mL) is needed to provide adequate calories and recommended daily allowances (RDAs) of vitamins and minerals. Tube-feeding formulas should always be at room temperature.

If all the necessary steps to decrease or prevent diarrhea have failed, antidiarrheal medications may be needed.

NURSING CARE PLAN	**Total Parenteral Nutrition**	

Ms. D. is about to receive TPN with fat emulsions of Intralipid 10 percent for management of weight loss and cachexia (malnutrition and wasting) related to long-term treatment of breast cancer. This is her first treatment with TPN, and she has many questions, especially about the fat emulsions. She asks, "Are these safe to go into my circulation?" and "Are you sure these won't hurt me?"

ASSESSMENT

Subjective Data — Client reports the following:
- Weight loss 4.5 kg in 3 wk
- Decreased appetite and energy
- Increased fatigue

Objective Data
- Diagnosis of breast cancer
- Treatment with chemotherapy (long-term)
- Weight loss

NURSING DIAGNOSIS

Deficient knowledge related to lack of experience with a new treatment regimen

PLANNING

Goals — Client will verbalize understanding of purpose of TPN—especially Intralipid therapy—by the end of one treatment.

Outcome Criteria — Before the end of the infusion, client will do the following:
- State the purpose of Intralipid treatment
- Verbalize the side effects of the treatment
- State the therapeutic benefit of treatment with Intralipid

IMPLEMENTATION

Client education will include the following information about Intralipid 10 percent:
- This fat emulsion provides neutral triglycerides, primarily unsaturated fatty acids that are needed for energy and heat production.
- It is used for increasing caloric intake and to prevent fatty acid deficiency.
- The therapeutic effects of this treatment include higher fatty acid levels, weight gain, and more energy.

EVALUATION

Positive therapeutic outcomes include the following:
- Increase in weight
- Fatty acids at adequate levels
- Increased energy levels

Side effects include the following:
- Headache
- Drowsiness
- Nausea
- Vomiting
- Dyspnea
- Altered liver function

TPN, Total parenteral nutrition.

Lactose-free solutions are available and should be used with clients who are lactose intolerant. Clients who suffer from this condition experience cramping, diarrhea, abdominal bloating, and flatulence with the ingestion of lactose.

■ *TPN*

Infusions of TPN should be assessed every hour. The entire system and the condition of the client should be included in this assessment. It is good practice to examine the client first and then check the TPN insertion site and the tubing at the site of connection to the infusion pump. Patency should be assessed every hour as well.

Tubing should be changed every 24 hours to prevent infection. It is recommended that tubing changes occur daily with the beginning of each new infusion. A 0.22-micron filter is used to trap bacteria, including *Pseudomonas* spp. The client's temperature should be recorded every four hours. Any increase in temperature should be reported to the physician immediately because it may be the first sign of infection.

The client should also be checked frequently for signs and symptoms of hyperglycemia, such as headache, dehydration, and weakness. Intravenous feeding rates should never be accelerated to increase plasma volume because the rapid increase of dextrose solution may precipitate hyperglycemia. Insulin replacement may be needed; therefore glucometer readings are important for immediate recognition and treatment of hyperglycemia.

Hypoglycemia is manifested by cold, clammy skin, dizziness, tachycardia, and tingling of the extremities. If TPN is discontinued abruptly, rebound hypoglycemia may occur. Hypoglycemia associated with TPN may be prevented by gradual reduction of the intravenous feeding rate to allow the pancreas time to adapt to the changing blood glucose levels. If TPN must be discontinued immediately, hypoglycemia can be prevented with infusion of 5 to 10 percent glucose.

Fluid overload may occur with TPN, manifested by weak pulse, hypertension, tachycardia, confusion, decreased urine output, and pitting edema. This can be prevented by maintaining intravenous feeding rates and assessing the intravenous infusion every hour. If signs of overload occur, the nurse should slow the infusion rate, remain with the client, and contact the physician immediately. A continual assessment of the client and vital signs is also necessary at this time.

Client teaching tips for nutritional supplements are found in the box below.

■ **Evaluation**

Therapeutic responses to nutritional supplementation include improved well-being, energy, strength, and performance of activities of daily living; an increase in weight; and laboratory studies that reflect improved nutritional status. Specific laboratory values may include some of the following: albumin, total protein, hemoglobin, hematocrit, RBC and WBC levels, BUN, electrolytes, blood glucose and insulin levels, and iron values. Regular evaluation is very important to meet nutritional needs as closely as possible.

CLIENT TEACHING TIPS

Enteral

Because clients are often discharged while on tube feedings, the client and family should begin preparation for this procedure at least one week before discharge. The client should have written and oral instructions. Individualized client teaching about the procedure and care of the tube requires at least six hours. More instructional time is needed if the tube is to be inserted and removed at night only.

The nurse should instruct the client and family as follows:
▲ Coughing, choking, difficulty in speaking, or turning bluish means the tube is incorrectly placed.
▲ Keep the physician's number handy as well as numbers for other resources in case you need immediate help.
▲ You can call Ross Laboratories (1-800-227-5767) with questions.
▲ Contact the physician if diarrhea, nausea, vomiting, fever, or any other unusual symptoms occur.

TPN

Clients on home TPN will need some support from home healthcare. The client and family need practice to acquire the necessary skill. All procedures for storage, cleansing and care of site, dressing changes, irrigation of the catheter, pump function and care; and changing of the bag, filters, and tubing should also be demonstrated and practised well before the client is discharged. Procedures for glucometer use and periodic checking of urine glucose should also be demonstrated and practised.

The nurse should instruct the client and family as follows:
▲ Weigh yourself daily at the same time wearing the same clothing.
▲ Record how much fluid you take in and how much urine you pass.
▲ Check glucose levels at home. Make sure you understand how to use the glucometer and how to check urine glucose.
▲ If any of the following occur, stop the infusion and call the physician immediately:
  • Fever or chills
  • Cough, chest pain, or difficulty breathing
  • Restlessness or nervousness
  • Fainting
  • Rapid heartbeat
  • Nausea or vomiting
  • Greatly increased urination or constant thirst
  • High glucose readings

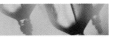

POINTS to REMEMBER

▼ A thorough nutritional assessment is essential for adequate intervention for the malnourished client. A consultation with a registered dietitian or nutritionist is helpful.

▼ There are various enteral feedings with different nutritional content, including some that are lactose-free.

▼ Enteral feedings may result in complications such as hyperglycemia, dumping syndrome, and aspiration of feeding.

▼ TPN is often administered through a central vein catheter because of the hyperosmolarity of substances used.

▼ Parenteral feedings may result in air embolism, hyperglycemia, or hypoglycemia. If discontinued abruptly, infection and fluid volume overload may result.

▼ Cautious and astute nursing care with enteral or parenteral nutritional supplementation may prevent or decrease the occurrence of associated complications.

EXAMINATION REVIEW QUESTIONS

1 The route of enteral nutritional delivery with a basic nasogastric feeding tube would be through which of the following?
   a. Surgical placement into the stomach
   b. Placement from the nose into the jejunum
   c. Surgical insertion directly into the jejunum
   d. Placement from the nose into the stomach

2 Which of the following is an indication for elemental formulations such as Vivonex Plus?
   a. Severe metabolic disorders
   b. Cardiomyopathy
   c. Radiation enteritis
   d. Hyperosmolar diarrhea

3 Central TPN is associated with which of the following characteristics?
   a. Is used only for <10 days
   b. Provides more than 2000 kcal/day

   c. Has about 10 percent fat
   d. Is isotonic, or <600 mOsm/L

4 What type of therapy may be ordered to help with the long-term nutritional needs of a client with cachexia related to cancer?
   a. Peripheral TPN with <5% glucose
   b. Oral Ensure six times a day
   c. Nasogastric tube feedings around the clock with regular dextrose
   d. Central TPN with up to 50% dextrose

5 Lipid emulsions supply which of the following?
   a. Safflower or soybean oil
   b. 15 g protein per 500 mL
   c. Linoleic and other essential fatty acids
   d. Albumin and hismonal

For answers see http://evolve.elsevier.com/Lilley/pharmacology/.

CRITICAL THINKING ACTIVITIES

1 Which nursing actions will help address the nursing diagnosis of diarrhea as related to enteral feedings?
2 What outcome criteria will address the nursing diagnosis of deficient fluid volume related to imbalanced nutrition?

3 What is the concern relating to abrupt withdrawal of a 10 percent glucose TPN solution? Explain your answer.

For answers see http://evolve.elsevier.com/Lilley/pharmacology/.

BIBLIOGRAPHY

Albanese, J., & Nutz, P. (2004). *Mosby's 2004 nursing drug cards.* St Louis, MO: Mosby.

Facts and Comparisons. (2004). *Drug facts and comparisons pocket version* (9th ed.). St Louis, MO: Wolters Kluwer Health.

Johns Hopkins Hospital, Gunn V.L., & Nechyba, C. (2002). *The Harriet Lane handbook* (16th ed.). St Louis, MO: Mosby.

Lacy, C.F., Armstrong, L.L., Goldman, M.P., & Lance, L.L. (2003). *Drug information handbook* (11th ed.). Hudson, OH: Lexi-Comp.

Mosby. (2005). *Mosby's drug consult 2005: The comprehensive reference for generic and brand name drugs* (15th ed.). St Louis, MO: Mosby.

Skidmore-Roth, L. (2006). *Mosby's 2006 nursing drug reference* (19th ed.). St Louis, MO: Mosby.

Miscellaneous Therapeutics: Hematological, Dermatological, Ophthalmic, and Otic Agents: Study Skills Tips

- TIME MANAGEMENT   • PURR   • REPEAT THE STEPS

TIME MANAGEMENT

As you plan your study time for Part Ten, it should be clear that Chapter 56 will take significantly more time to complete than the other chapters. Do not let the length of the chapter overwhelm you. Apply the principles of time management to this chapter and you will succeed. The most important aspect of time management to apply to this chapter is the use of clear goal statements and action plan steps to help you achieve the goals.

Goal Statements

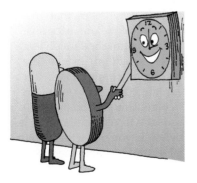

Remember the criteria for goal statements. First, they must be realistic. The statements must be things you know you can accomplish. Second, they must be specific to the task. "I will study the chapter" is not a very specific goal. Specify what you expect to accomplish. "I will master the 28 terms in the chapter glossary" is a more specific goal statement. Third, there must be a time limit. How long will you spend in achieving this goal? Set a time limit for the completion of each activity. Finally, goal statements must be measurable. In the example of studying the glossary, including the number of terms contained in Chapter 56 helps clarify the goal.

Action Planning

The second segment of time management is the use of action planning. An action plan is a series of smaller, specific activities that you will accomplish to meet your goal statements. Your goal is to master the 28 terms. What will you do to meet that goal?

Action Steps Example

1 I will spend one hour making vocabulary drill cards for the terms found in the glossary in Chapter 56 from 3:00 to 4:00 pm on Monday.
2 I will spend 15 minutes in rehearsal and review of these cards every day until the exam on this chapter is over.
3 Each time I cannot define and explain a term I will put an "x" on the card to identify it as a term needing more review.
4 I will spend one hour the night before the exam doing a comprehensive review of the terms in Chapter 56, with special emphasis on those cards that have one or more x marks.

Action steps help ensure that you are spending your study time actively focusing on what you need to learn.

PURR

Prepare Example

Chapter 56, Objective 3: "Discuss the mechanisms of action, indications, side effects, cautions, and contraindications of ophthalmic preparations."

- Question 1. What does *ophthalmic* mean? (Literal question [LQ])

- Question 2. What are ophthalmic preparations? (LQ)
- Question 3. What is the mechanism of action of ophthalmic preparations? (LQ)
- Question 4. Is there more than one mechanism of action? (LQ)
- Question 5. If there is more than one mechanism of action, how are the mechanisms similar and how are they different? (Interpretive Question)

These questions are only suggestions of generated questions based on the chapter objectives. Many more questions can be asked about Objective 3. These questions are an essential part of the study process. Questions help make you an active reader and an active learner. The more questions you generate the easier it will be to understand the chapter.

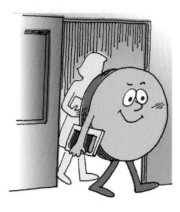

Outline Example

1 *Looking through the chapter, decide how much material is appropriate for a single reading session.* The section headed "Antiglaucoma Drugs" is probably too much material. Looking at the chapter headings, this section could be broken down into six blocks of material. Block one would cover the introductory material under the main heading, as well as the material under the heading "Parasympathomimetics." Block two would be the material under the heading "Sympathomimetics." The next four blocks would be "Beta-Adrenergic Blockers," "Carbonic Anhydrase Inhibitors," "Osmotic Diuretics," and "Prostaglandin Agonists."

2 *Apply the Prepare step to each block.* Beginning with the first block, generate some questions to guide your reading. Remember that it is important to ask both questions that will focus on literal information and questions that will help you interpret, evaluate, and analyze as you read.

3 *Read the material.* As soon as you have completed the self-questioning over the first block of material, read the block immediately. Read for understanding, and, as you read, remember the questions you generated. This approach will help your concentration and comprehension.

4 *Take a short break.* Once you have completed the reading of this section of the chapter, give your mind a chance to reflect and consolidate the learning. Limit the time you allow for a break and use the time for something pleasurable. Give yourself five or ten minutes to read the newspaper, get a snack, or just take a short walk.

5 *Rehearse.* Before going on to the next section of the chapter it is important to spend a few minutes in rehearsal. Using the questions from Step 2, go back over the material you read and try to respond to those questions. When you find yourself unable to answer a question, put a mark in the text beside the heading that caused the difficulty and move on. The mark will serve as a reminder for future review. At this point, the objective is not complete mastery of the material. The objective is to see what you have learned so that you can move smoothly into the next section. Breaking a chapter into blocks is useful, but it is imperative to make links between sections as you study.

6 *Review.* After completing two or three major sections of the chapter, it is time to review. Start at the beginning of the chapter. Ask your questions. Try to answer them. If you cannot formulate a clear answer, then some rereading is necessary. Also, pay attention to the marks you made during the rehearsal step. Those marks indicate areas that you have already identified as needing review. When rereading, remember that the object is to read only as much of the material as needed to be able to respond to self-generated questions. There simply is not enough time to read the entire chapter a second or third time.

REPEAT THE STEPS

Prepare, read for understanding, take a short break, and then rehearse the material just read. It may seem that this process takes an excessive amount of time and involves a lot of repetition, but in the long run it will produce better learning. The time spent in Prepare, Understand, and Rehearsal will reduce the time needed to review. Frequent review as you move through the chapter will make the final review at exam time proceed more quickly and enable you to achieve mastery of the material.

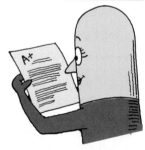

CHAPTER 54

Blood-Forming Agents

GLOSSARY

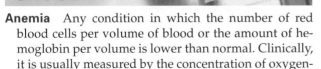

Anemia Any condition in which the number of red blood cells per volume of blood or the amount of hemoglobin per volume is lower than normal. Clinically, it is usually measured by the concentration of oxygen-carrying material in a designated volume of blood.

Cytoplasmic maturation defects (sy' toe plaz' mik) A cause of anemia in which red blood cells fail to mature properly as a result of abnormal Hgb synthesis, which can be due to deficient iron or globin.

Erythrocyte (ə rith' ro site) Another name for red blood cell (RBC).

Erythropoiesis (ə rith' ro poy ee' sis) The process of erythrocyte production involving the maturation of a nucleated precursor into a hemoglobin (Hgb)-filled, nucleus-free erythrocyte that is regulated by erythropoietin, a hormone produced by the kidney.

Globin (glo' bin) A protein chain of which there are four different structural chains: alpha₁ and alpha₂, and beta₁ and beta₂.

Heme (heem) The pigmented, iron-containing, nonprotein portion of the Hgb molecule.

Hemoglobin (Hgb) (hee' mo glo' bin) A complex protein-iron compound in the blood that carries oxygen to the cells from the lungs and carbon dioxide away from the cells to the lungs.

Hypochromic (hy' po kro' mik) Having less than normal colour. The term usually describes an RBC and characterizes anemias associated with decreased synthesis of Hgb.

Macrocytic (mak' ro site' ik) having larger-than-normal cells.

Microcytic (myk' ro site' ik) having smaller-than-normal cells.

Nuclear maturation defects A cause of anemia in which red blood cells fail to mature properly due to defects in DNA or protein synthesis, which may be caused by a deficiency of Vitamin B₁₂ or folate.

Normochromic Of normal colour. The term usually describes an RBC and characterizes anemias associated with decreased DNA or protein synthesis.

Pernicious anemia A blood disorder characterized by a low number of RBCs.

Reticulocyte (rə tik' yu lo site) An immature erythrocyte characterized by a meshlike pattern of threads and particles at the former site of the nucleus.

Spherocyte (sfer' o site) Small, globular, completely hemoglobinated erythrocyte without the usual central pallor.

HEMATOPOIESIS

The formation of new blood cells is one of the primary functions of bones. Bones are also responsible for support, protection, movement, and mineral storage. They provide a framework for the body that acts as a support and also serves to protect delicate internal organs. Bones in coordination with muscles help the body to move, and major reservoirs of minerals, such as calcium and phosphorus, are stored in bone. The focus of this chapter is the process of red blood cell (RBC), or **erythrocyte**, formation. Hematopoiesis, the process of blood cell formation (RBCs, white blood cells [WBCs], and platelets), takes place in the myeloid tissue. This specialized tissue is located primarily in the ends, or epiphyses, of certain long bones; in the flat bones of the skull; in the pelvis; and in the sternum and ribs.

When RBCs are manufactured in the bone marrow by myeloid tissue, they are released into the circulation as immature RBCs called **reticulocytes**. Once in the circula-

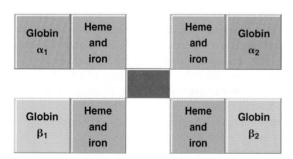

FIG. 54-1 Schematic structure of a hemoglobin molecule.

tion, reticulocytes undergo a 24- to 36-hour maturation process to become mature, fully functional RBCs. Once in the circulation they have a life span of about 120 days.

It is important to know the structural components of the RBC to understand how anemia develops and why certain drugs are used to correct it. Over one-third of an RBC is made of hemoglobin. **Hemoglobin (Hgb)** is composed of two parts: heme and globin. **Heme** is a red pigment; each molecule of heme contains one atom of iron. **Globin** is a protein chain that consists of four structurally different parts or globulins: alpha$_1$ and alpha$_2$, and beta$_1$ and beta$_2$ ($\alpha_1 + \alpha_2$ and $\beta_1 + \beta_2$). Together one molecule of heme and one protein chain of globin make one Hgb molecule (Figure 54-1).

TYPES OF ANEMIA

Anemia is defined as any condition in which the concentration of RBCs or of hemoglobin in the blood is lower than normal. Anemias are classified into four main types based on underlying causes. Knowledge of the etiologies of anemias will help you to understand the therapies used to treat them. Anemias can be caused by maturation defects—the failure of enough RBCs to develop properly—or they can be secondary to increased destruction of RBCs. Two types of maturation defects cause anemias: cytoplasmic maturation defects and nuclear maturation defects. Factors responsible for increased destruction can be either intrinsic or extrinsic (Figure 54-2). Some common causes of iron-deficiency anemia are blood loss, surgery, childbirth, gastrointestinal (GI) bleeding, and hemorrhoids.

RBCs in anemias associated with **cytoplasmic maturation defects** appear **hypochromic** (lighter red than normal) and **microcytic** (smaller than normal) on blood smear. All cytoplasmic maturation anemias occur as a result of abnormal Hgb synthesis. Because Hgb is synthesized from both iron and globin, a deficiency in either one can lead to a Hgb deficiency (Figure 54-3).

Anemias associated with immature RBC **nuclear maturation defects** occur secondary to defects in DNA or protein synthesis problems. DNA and protein require vitamin B$_{12}$ and folate to be present in normal amounts for their proper production. If either of these two vitamins is

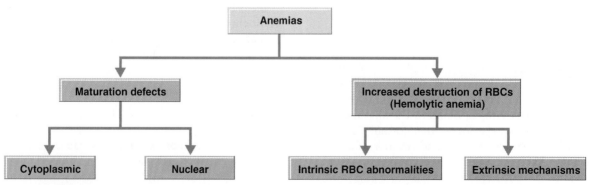

FIG. 54-2 Underlying causes of anemia are maturation defects and factors secondary to increased destruction.

absent or deficient, anemias secondary to nuclear maturation defects may develop (Figure 54-4). RBCs in such anemias appear to be **normochromic** (normal in colour) and **macrocytic** (larger than normal) on blood smear.

Anemias secondary to increased RBC destruction can occur because of abnormalities in the RBCs themselves (intrinsic factors) as a result of factors outside (extrinsic) the RBCs. The erythrocytes in anemias attributable to RBC destruction are **spherocytes** and appear to be fragmented when observed on blood smear. Intrinsic RBC abnormalities are usually the result of a genetic defect. Some examples are sickle-cell anemia, hereditary spherocytosis, and glucose-6-phosphate dehydrogenase (G6PD) deficiency. Extrinsic mechanisms for increased RBC destruction are not attributable to abnormalities in the RBC itself. Examples of extrinsic mechanisms are drug-induced antibodies that target and destroy RBCs, septic shock that produces disseminated intravascular coagulation (DIC), and mechanical forces such as intra-aortic balloon pumps and ventricular assist devices that directly damage RBCs (Figure 54-5).

IRON

Iron is an essential mineral for the proper function of all biological systems in the body. It is an oxygen carrier in Hgb and myoglobin, is used for tissue respiration, and is used in many enzyme reactions in the body. Although iron is stored in many sites throughout the body (liver, spleen, and bone marrow), it is the principal nutritional deficiency in Canada, resulting in anemia. Children and women, especially pregnant women, require the greatest amount of iron, and are most likely to develop iron-deficiency anemia.

Dietary sources for iron are meats and certain vegetables and grains. This form of iron must be converted by gastric juices before it can actually be absorbed. Other foods such as orange juice, veal, fish, and ascorbic acid may help with iron absorption. Conversely, eggs, corn, beans, and many cereal products containing phytates may impair iron absorption. Iron-fortified cereal and meat are available as well as formulas for breastfed and formula-fed infants.

Supplemental iron contained in multivitamins plus iron or iron supplements alone are indicated for the treatment

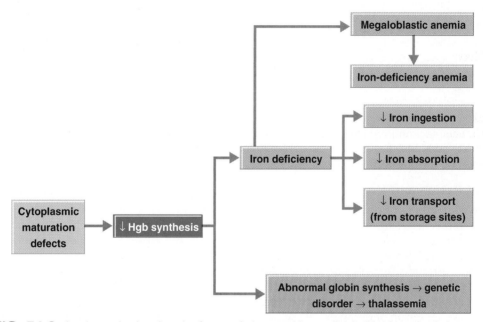

FIG. 54-3 A schematic showing the forms of abnormal hemoglobin (Hgb) synthesis in cytoplasmic maturation anemia.

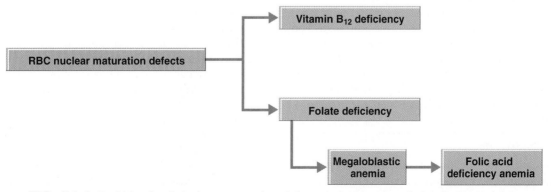

FIG. 54-4 Red blood cell nuclear maturation defects occur because of vitamin B_{12} or folate deficiencies.

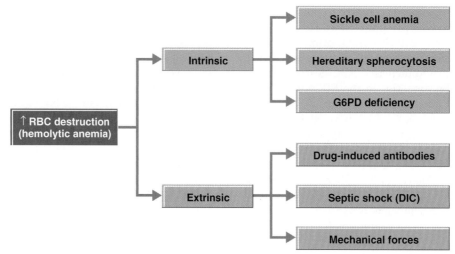

FIG. 54-5 Increased red blood cell destruction occurs as a result of intrinsic and extrinsic factors. *DIC,* Disseminated intravascular coagulation; *G6PD,* glucose-6-phosphate dehydrogenase.

TABLE 54-1
FERROUS SALTS: IRON CONTENT

Ferrous Salts	Iron Content
Ferrous fumarate	33% iron or 330 mg/g
Ferrous gluconate	11.6% iron or 116 mg/g
Ferrous sulphate	20% iron or 200 mg/g
Ferrous sulphate (desiccated, dried, or exsiccated)	30% iron or 300 mg/g

TABLE 54-2
IRON PREPARATIONS: ADVERSE EFFECTS

Body System	Side/Adverse Effects
Gastrointestinal	Nausea, constipation, epigastric pain, black and red tarry stools, vomiting, diarrhea, dyspepsia
Integumentary	Temporarily discolored tooth enamel and eyes, pain upon injection

of iron-deficiency anemia. Iron preparations are available as ferrous salts. See Table 54-1 for a list of the currently available iron salts and their respective iron content.

Mechanism of Action and Drug Effects

Iron is a required component of a number of enzyme systems in the body and is necessary for energy transfer in the cytochrome oxidase and xanthine oxidase enzyme systems. It is present in Hgb and myoglobin, which are necessary for transport and utilization of oxygen. Administration of iron corrects iron-deficiency states such as anemia, dysphagia (painful swallowing), dystrophy of the nails and skin, and fissuring of the angles of the lips.

Indications

Iron preparations are used to prevent and treat iron-deficiency syndromes. The symptoms associated with iron-deficiency anemia can be alleviated by the administration of iron. In all cases an underlying cause should be identified. After identification of the cause, treatment should attempt to correct the cause rather than simply alleviate the symptoms. Iron supplementation is also used in epoetin therapy (Chapter 47) because it is essential for the production of RBCs.

Contraindications

Contraindications to the use of iron products include known drug allergy, hemolytic anemia, hemosiderosis (abnormal accumulation of the protein hemosiderin), hemochromatosis (a disorder of iron metabolism involving

increased absorption of iron), and any anemia not associated with iron deficiency.

Side Effects and Adverse Effects

The most common side effects and adverse effects associated with iron preparations are nausea, vomiting, diarrhea, constipation, stomach cramps, and stomach pain. Excess iron intake can lead to accumulation and iron toxicity (see Table 54-2).

Toxicity and Management of Overdose

Iron overdose is a leading cause of pediatric poisoning deaths reported to Canadian poison control centres. Many iron supplements are enteric coated and resemble candy. Toxicity from iron ingestion results from a combination of the corrosive effects on the GI mucosa and the metabolic and hemodynamic effects caused by the presence of excessive elemental iron.

Treatment is founded on good symptomatic and supportive measures, including suction and maintenance of airway, correction of acidosis, and control of shock and dehydration with intravenous fluids or blood, oxygen, and vasopressor. Abdominal radiographs may be helpful because iron preparations are radiopaque and may be visualized on X-ray film. Serum iron concentrations may be helpful in establishing severity of ingestion. A serum iron concentration of 54 μmol/L places the client at serious risk of toxicity. Consultation with a poison control centre is recommended. Because many of the iron products are extended-release formulations that release contents in the

DOSAGES   Selected Iron Preparations and Folic Acid

Agent	Pharmacological Class	Usual Dosage Range	Indications
▸▸ferrous fumarate	Oral iron salt	**Pediatric** **Infant–6 mo** 0.25 mL tid (15 mg/day elemental iron) **6 mo–2 yr** 0.75 mL tid (45 mg/day elemental iron) **2–6 yr** 2.5 mL hs (50 mg/day elemental iron) **>6 yr** 5 mL hs (100 mg/day elemental iron) **>12 yr–adult** 1 capsule at bedtime (100 mg elemental iron)	Iron deficiency
▸▸folic acid	Vitamin B–complex group; water-soluble B-vitamin	**Pediatric** PO/IV/IM/SC: 0.1–0.4 mg/day **Adult** PO/IV/IM/SC: Up to 1 mg/day PO/IV/IM/SC: 3–15 mg/day	Folate deficiency; nutritional supplement; pregnancy supplement Tropical sprue
iron dextran	Parenteral iron salt	**Pediatric** IM/IV: *<5 kg:* 25 mg/day elemental iron (0.5 mL/day); *5–10 kg:* 50 mg/day elemental iron (1 mL/day) **Adult** IM/IV: 100 mg/day elemental iron (2 mL/day)	Iron deficiency when oral iron is unsatisfactory

intestines rather than the stomach, whole gut irrigation using a polyethylene glycol solution is generally believed to be a superior and more effective approach to decontaminating the bowel. Possible surgical removal of intake iron tablets may also be considered. In clients with severe symptoms of iron intoxication such as coma, shock, or seizures, chelation therapy with deferoxamine should be initiated.

Interactions

The absorption of iron can be enhanced when it is given with ascorbic acid or decreased when it is given with antacids. Iron preparations can decrease the absorption of thyroid drugs, biphosphonates, tetracycline, levodopa, methyldopa, and quinolone antibiotics.

Dosages

For the recommended dosages of iron preparations, see the table above. See Appendix B for some of the common brands available in Canada.

▎ DRUG PROFILES

Iron preparations are available by prescription and OTC. They are classified as pregnancy category A agents except iron dextran, which is a pregnancy category C agent. They are contraindicated in clients who have shown a hypersensitivity reaction to them. Their use is also contraindicated in clients with ulcerative colitis and regional enteritis, hemosiderosis and hemochromatosis, peptic ulcer disease (PUD), hemolytic anemia, cirrhosis, gastritis, and esophagitis. At the initiation of and throughout therapy, Hgb and hematocrit (Hct) should be monitored. These laboratory values, as well as client's symptomatic response, should help guide therapy.

▸▸ *ferrous fumarate*

The ferrous fumarate iron salts contain the largest amount of iron per gram of salt consumed. Ferrous sulphate and ferrous gluconate are two other forms of iron that are commonly used. Ferrous fumarate is 33 percent elemental iron; therefore a 300-mg tablet of ferrous fumarate provides 100 mg of elemental iron. Ferrous fumarate is available only as an oral preparation in the following forms: an 18-mg extended-release tablet, a 300-mg/5-mL suspension, and a 300-mg tablet. Pregnancy category A. Commonly recommended dosages for iron salts are listed in the table above.

PHARMACOKINETICS

Half-Life	Onset	Peak	Duration
6 hr	3–10 days*	Unknown	Variable

*Increased reticulocyte values.

iron dextran

Iron dextran is a colloidal solution of iron (as ferric hydroxide) and dextran. Ferrlecit is another parenteral formulation of iron that has recently been approved for iron-deficiency anemia. It is intended for intravenous use. Anaphylactic reactions to iron dextran, including fatal anaphylaxis, have been reported in 0.2 to 0.3 percent of clients. Because of this, a test dose of 25 mg (0.5 mL) of iron dextran should be administered by the chosen route and appropriate method of administration before injection. Although anaphylactic reactions usually occur within a few moments after the test dose, it is recommended that a period of at least one hour elapses before the remaining portion of the initial dose is given. Individual doses of 2 mL or less may be given daily until the calculated total amount required has been reached. The product Dexiron is given undiluted at a gradual rate not to exceed 50 mg (1 mL)/min. Iron dextran is available as a 50-mg/mL parenteral injection for either intravenous or intramuscular use. Pregnancy category C. Commonly recommended dosages for iron salts are listed in the table on p. 927.

PHARMACOKINETICS

Half-Life	Onset	Peak	Duration
5–20 hr	Unknown	IM: 24–48 hr	≤3 wk

FOLIC ACID

Folic acid is a water-soluble B-complex vitamin. It is converted in the body to tetrahydrofolic acid, which is then used for normal **erythropoiesis** and to produce nucleoproteins such as DNA and RNA. The human body requires oral intake of folic acid. Dietary sources of folic acid are dried beans, peas, oranges, and green vegetables.

Folic acid is primarily used to prevent and treat folic acid deficiency. Folic acid should not be used to treat anemias until the underlying cause and type of anemia have been determined. The potential risk involved in administering folic acid without first determining the cause is that folic acid will correct the hematological changes of anemia but will mask pernicious anemia symptoms. **Pernicious anemia** is a blood disorder characterized by a low number of RBCs. It requires specific treatment other than folic acid. If pernicious anemia is masked, underlying neurological damage progresses. Pernicious anemia is sometimes the result of a dietary deficiency of vitamin B$_{12}$, which is used in the formation of new RBCs. In many cases it results from the failure of the stomach lining to produce intrinsic factor. Intrinsic factor allows vitamin B$_{12}$ to be absorbed.

Several conditions can lead to folic acid deficiency. However, because folic acid is absorbed in the upper duodenum, malabsorption syndromes are the most common cause of deficiency.

Mechanism of Action and Drug Effects

Dietary ingestion of folate is required for the production of nucleoproteins such as DNA and RNA. It is also essential for normal erythropoiesis. Folic acid is not active in the ingested form. It must first be converted to tetrahydrofolic acid, which is a cofactor for reactions in the biosynthesis of purines and thymidylates of nucleic acids.

Indications

Anemias caused by folic acid deficiency can be treated by exogenous supplementation of folic acid. There is also much evidence to support the use of folic acid in the prevention of fetal neural tube defects such as spina bifida, anencephaly, and encephalocele. It is recommended that administration begin at least three months before pregnancy and continue through the first three months of pregnancy to reduce the risk of neural tube defects. Indications for folic acid include the following:

- Megaloblastic anemia
- Tropical sprue
- Prophylaxis of fetal neural tube defects in pregnant women

Megaloblastic anemia is most often due to poor dietary intake and is most commonly seen in infancy, childhood, and pregnancy.

Contraindications

Contraindications to the use of folic acid include known drug product allergy and any anemia not related to folic acid deficiency (e.g., pernicious anemia).

Side Effects and Adverse Effects

Side effects and adverse effects associated with folic acid use are rare. Allergic reaction or yellow discoloration of urine may occur.

Interactions

No significant drug interactions are reported with folic acid.

Dosages

For recommended dosages of folic acid, see the table on p. 927.

DRUG PROFILES

Folic acid is a water-soluble B-complex vitamin that is used primarily in the treatment and prevention of folic acid deficiency and anemias caused by folic acid deficiency. It is essential in the body for the production of normal RBCs and nucleoproteins such as DNA and RNA.

▶▶ *folic acid*

Folic acid is available as an OTC medication in multivitamin preparations and by prescription as a single agent. It is contraindicated in clients who have shown a hypersensitivity reaction to it and in clients with anemias other than megaloblastic or macrocytic anemia, such as vitamin B$_{12}$ deficiency anemia, and uncorrected pernicious anemia. Folic acid is available as an oral formulation in 0.8-mg capsules and 0.4-, 1-, 5-, and 25-mg tablets and as a 5-mg/mL parenteral injection. Pregnancy category A. Commonly recommended dosages for folic acid are listed in the table on p. 927.

PHARMACOKINETICS

Half-Life	Onset	Peak	Duration
Unknown	Unknown	60–90 min	Unknown

OTHER BLOOD-FORMING AGENTS

Other agents that may be used in the prevention and treatment of anemia are cyanocobalamin (vitamin B$_{12}$) and erythropoietin. Cyanocobalamin is discussed in detail in Chapter 52, and erythropoietin is discussed in Chapter 47.

NURSING PROCESS

■ **Assessment**

Before administering any blood-forming agent, it is important for the nurse to assess for contraindications to use, such as hypersensitivity reactions, colitis, enteritis, possible hemochromatosis, PUD, hemolytic anemia, and cirrhosis. Long-term use of hematopoietic agents for treatment of anemia should be approached cautiously and underlying cause(s) identified when possible. Laboratory studies such as Hgb, Hct, reticulocytes, bilirubin levels, and baseline levels of folate and/or B-complex vitamins should be obtained and documented before initiation of drug treatment. A nutritional assessment should also be performed, with concentration on the amount of iron intake in the client's diet (a nutritional consult may be necessary) and a 24-hour recall of all food intake with serving sizes.

The major contraindication to folic acid is hypersensitivity to it or any derivative of it. Drug interactions with folic acid include chloramphenicol, phenobarbital, hydantoins, and methotrexate. Chemical incompatibilities (in syringe) include calcium, chlorpromazine, iron sulphate, B-complex vitamin with vitamin C in solution or syringe, and dextrose 40 percent concentrations.

Iron dextran is contraindicated in hypersensitivity and in all anemias with the exception of iron-deficiency anemia. It is also contraindicated in clients with liver disease. Cautious use and careful monitoring is recommended in clients with acute renal disease, asthma, and rheumatoid arthritis; in pregnant or lactating women; and in infants under four months of age. Iron dextran is incompatible in the syringe with many other parenterally administered medications. It also interacts with chloramphenicol and oral iron products (increased toxicity).

Ferrous salts are contraindicated in clients with ulcerative colitis and other GI disorders, PUD, and liver disease (such as cirrhosis). Drug interactions include levodopa, methyldopa, penicillamine, and tetracycline; absorption of each of these agents may be decreased. In particular, tetracycline chelates (binds) to the ferrous salts and renders the antibiotic ineffective. Vitamin C increases the absorption of ferrous fumarate.

Folic acid is contraindicated in clients with anemias other than megaloblastic or macrocytic anemia and with vitamin B_{12} deficiency-related anemias. Drug interactions include methotrexate, triamterene, and sulphonamides (all of which lead to decreased action of the folic acid), as well as phenytoin, estrogens, and glucocorticoids (all of which lead to increased need for folic acid).

Vitamin B_{12} interacts with alcohol, colchicine (an antigout drug), para-aminosalicylic acid, certain anticonvulsants, and some antibiotics. Treatment of vitamin B_{12} deficiencies is critical to prevent possibly irreversible neurological damage. Therefore assessment of underlying symptoms before initiating drug therapy is essential for effective treatment (whether it is vitamin B or iron deficiency states). A thorough dietary history is also important with B_{12} deficiencies, and clients should be questioned about their intake of foods high in vitamin B_{12}, such as organ meats, clams, oysters, seafood, non-fat dry milk, and fermented cheeses. Inadequate intake of these foods may contribute to the client's deficiency.

Nursing Diagnoses

Nursing diagnoses associated with the use of blood-forming agents include, but are not limited to, the following:
* Activity intolerance related to fatigue and lethargy associated with anemias.
* Risk for injury related to side effects of iron products.
* Deficient knowledge related to limited exposure to use of medication.
* Imbalanced nutrition, less than body requirements, related to disease process.

Planning

Goals for the client receiving blood-forming agents include, but are not limited to, the following:
* Client maintains normal level of activity as ordered.
* Client remains free of self-injury related to anemia or use of iron products.
* Client discusses side effects and rationale for use.
* Client attains normal nutritional status through use of pharmacological and non-pharmacological measures.

Outcome Criteria

Outcome criteria related to the administration of blood-forming agents include the following:
* Client is able to tolerate gradual increase in activity as ordered (e.g., performing activities of daily living, walking ten minutes per day with increases as tolerated) while taking blood-forming agents.
* Client uses measures to minimize occurrence of side effects of blood-forming agents, such as taking with food.
* Client takes medication exactly as prescribed to enhance its efficacy.
* Client states symptoms to report associated with increased symptomatology related to disease process or to adverse reactions to medications, such as abdominal distention, cramping, nausea, and vomiting.
* Client keeps daily journal of dietary intake to share with healthcare provider.
* Client uses examples of a balanced diet for daily menu planning.

Implementation

Liquid oral forms of iron products should be diluted per manufacturer instructions and taken through a plastic straw to avoid discoloration of tooth enamel. Oral forms should be given with juice (but not antacids or milk) between meals for maximal absorption; however, should GI distress occur, the iron should be taken with meals.

Iron dextran should be administered only after all oral iron preparations have been discontinued and only after a test dose of iron dextran has been ordered (usually 25 mg [0.5 mL] by preferred route with remaining dose given one hour later). Intramuscularly administered iron should be administered deep in a large muscle mass using the Z-track method and a 23-gauge 1½-inch needle. Intravenous iron dextran should be given after the intravenous line is flushed with 10 mL of normal saline (NS). Intravenous iron dextran may be given with 50 to 250 mL of NS. The label on the intravenous solution bag should be carefully read to be sure that there are no drug interactions to the iron dextran. Epinephrine and resuscitative equipment should always be available in case of anaphylactic reaction (to iron or any drug). In addition, it may be necessary for the client to remain recumbent 30 minutes after the intravenous injection to prevent orthostatic hypotension. Change in positioning should be slow and purposeful.

GERIATRIC CONSIDERATIONS

Iron Intake in Older Adults

- Instructions on how to take oral forms of iron are crucial to safe administration. Clients should not make changes in the medication regimen such as doubling doses or discontinuing without a physician's order.
- Geriatric clients should be instructed on food sources high in iron and how to include them in their menu planning. Instructions on how to steam vegetables and not overcook foods would also be helpful to ensure that foods do not lose folic acid compounds.
- Clients should be instructed to take oral iron with meals to help minimize GI distress.
- Geriatric clients should be encouraged, when appropriate, to use community resources (e.g., Meals on Wheels, senior citizen community centres, public recreation centres). A list of resources for meals, such as churches in the community that have geriatric care programs, should be provided. This may help improve nutritional intake.

Ferrous salts are best given between meals for maximal absorption, but often need to be taken with food or meals to decrease GI upset. At least one to two hours should be allowed between iron and the intake of milk or antacids. The medication should be stored in a light-resistant airtight container. Clients should be cautioned to avoid reclining positions for 15 to 30 minutes to avoid esophageal irritation or corrosion and to be careful not to change positions quickly, which could precipitate orthostatic changes in blood pressure. It is important that clients are reminded that any iron product may cause the stools to turn black or dark green.

Folic acid should be given with food. If ordered intravenously, it may be administered undiluted if the dosage is 5 mg or less and over one minute. Folic acid is also often added to total parenteral nutrition solutions and other intravenous solutions.

Client teaching tips for blood-forming agents are presented in the box below.

■ Evaluation

Therapeutic responses to iron products include improved nutritional status, increased weight, increased activity tolerance and well-being, and absence of fatigue. Side effects include nausea, constipation, epigastric pain, black and tarry stools, and vomiting. Toxic signs include nausea, diarrhea (green, tarry stools), hematemesis, pallor, cyanosis, shock, and coma. With the use of vitamin B_{12}, clients who have heart failure or cardiac disorders should be closely monitored for worsening of heart failure or pulmonary edema.

CLIENT TEACHING TIPS

The nurse should instruct the client as follows:

Iron

▲ Take the recommended amount. Excessive doses can be poisonous.

▲ Don't crush tablets. Swallow whole with at least half a glass of water.

▲ Don't substitute one iron product for another, because each product contains different forms of the iron salt in different amounts.

▲ Don't lie down for 15 to 30 minutes after taking iron to avoid irritating or corroding the esophagus.

▲ Continue to eat foods high in iron, such as meat, dark green leafy vegetables, dried beans and seeds, dried fruits, and eggs.

Vitamin B_{12}

▲ If you have pernicious anemia, you will need to take vitamin B_{12} for life.

▲ Oral forms can be taken with fluids and/or meals to help disguise the taste.

▲ Eat a well-balanced diet, including foods high in vitamin B_{12}, such as egg yolks, fish, organ meats, oysters, dairy products, and clams.

▲ If you have pernicious anemia, your immune system is compromised, and you should try to avoid people with an infection.

POINTS to REMEMBER

▼ Iron and vitamin B_{12} are important in the treatment of many disorders and diseases (e.g., malignancies) to achieve RBC and Hgb formation that is as adequate as possible and to help prevent nutritional deficits that can affect all body systems, especially the immune system.

▼ Blood-forming agents are often used in the treatment of pernicious anemias, malabsorption syndromes,

hemolytic anemias, hemorrhage, and renal and liver diseases.

▼ The client must have a thorough assessment, including a head-to-toe nursing assessment, dietary history, and list of medications (including OTC agents) to rule out any major nutritional deficits. Baseline values in nutritional disorders should also be documented.

▼ Iron dextran, if given intramuscularly, should be administered by Z-track method.
▼ A physician should be consulted before any vitamin B_{12} or iron products are administered.
▼ Oral iron products are not interchangeable.
▼ Oral iron products may lead to GI and esophageal irritation.

▼ Foods high in vitamin B_{12} include egg yolks, fish, organ meats, dairy products, and oysters. Foods high in iron include red meat, dark green vegetables, dried beans, and dried fruits.

EXAMINATION REVIEW QUESTIONS

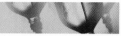

1 Which of the following should NOT be administered at the same time with liquid oral forms of iron products?
a. Vitamin B_{12}
b. NaCl
c. Milk
d. Apple juice
2 Treatment of anaphylaxis in reaction to iron supplementation includes use of which of the following?
a. digoxin
b. furosemide
c. phenylephrine
d. epinephrine
3 Which of the following is an interaction with or contraindication to the use of folic acid?
a. Anuria
b. Normal saline

c. Pernicious anemia
d. Pregnancy
4 Which of the following interact(s) with vitamin B_{12}?
a. Vitamin C
b. Zinc
c. Vitamin E
d. colchicine
5 Which of the following is a food that is high in iron?
a. Dairy products
b. Dried beans
c. Fish
d. Poultry

For answers see http://evolve.elsevier.com/Lilley/pharmacology/.

CRITICAL THINKING ACTIVITIES

1 In your clinical area, take a 24-hour dietary intake history of one of your assigned clients. Analyze the iron content of the person's intake while hospitalized. In addition, note the medications ordered to identify any supplemental vitamins or iron tablets and to identify any drug interactions. Also note any laboratory values, such as RBC, Hgb, Hct, bilirubin levels, and reticulocyte levels.

2 Discuss the importance of monitoring reticulocyte counts, Hgb, and Hct levels once oral iron therapy has been initiated.
3 Discuss tips you should share with a client who is taking oral iron supplements.

For answers see http://evolve.elsevier.com/Lilley/pharmacology/.

BIBLIOGRAPHY

Albanese, J., & Nutz, P. (2005). *Mosby's 2005 nursing drug cards.* St Louis, MO: Mosby.

Anderson, P.O., Knoben, J.E., & Troutman, W.G. (2002). *Handbook of clinical drug data* (10th ed.). New York: McGraw-Hill/Appleton & Lange.

Canadian Pharmacists Association. (2003). *Therapeutic choices* (4th ed.). Ottawa, ON: Author.

Canadian Pharmacists Association. (2004). *Guide to drugs in Canada.* Toronto, ON: Dorling Kindersley.

Canadian Pharmacists Association. (2005). *Compendium of pharmaceuticals and specialties. The Canadian drug reference for health professionals.* Ottawa, ON: Author. [The subscription-based e-CPS is available at http://www.pharmacists.ca.]

Cheng, A., Williams, B.A., & Sivarajan, B.V. (Eds.). (2003). *The HSC handbook of pediatrics* (10th ed.). Toronto, ON: Elsevier.

Health Canada. (2005). Drug product database (DPD). Retrieved September 9, 2005, from http://www.hc-sc.gc.ca/hpb/drugs-dpd/

Lehne, R.A. (2004). *Pharmacology for nursing care* (5th ed.). St Louis, MO: Saunders.

Mosby. (2005). *Mosby's drug consult 2005: The comprehensive reference for generic and brand name drugs* (15th ed.). St Louis, MO: Mosby.

Skidmore-Roth, L. (2006). *Mosby's 2006 nursing drug reference* (19th ed.). St Louis, MO: Mosby.

CHAPTER

55 Dermatological Agents

OBJECTIVES

After reading this chapter, the successful student will be able to do the following:

1 Discuss the normal anatomy, physiology, and functions of the skin.

2 Describe the different skin disorders, infections, and conditions commonly affecting the skin.

3 Identify the various dermatological agents used to treat skin disorders, infections, and infestations and describe their classifications.

4 Discuss the mechanisms of action, indications, contraindications, cautions, and side effects associated with the various dermatological agents.

5 Develop a nursing care plan that includes all phases of the nursing process for clients receiving dermatological agents.

e-LEARNING ACTIVITIES

Student CD-ROM
- Review Questions: see questions 395–396
- Animations
- Medication Administration Checklists
- IV Therapy Checklists

evolve **Web site** (http://evolve.elsevier.com/Lilley/pharmacology/pharmacology/)
- Online Chapter Worksheet • Frequently Asked Questions
- Learning Tips and Content Updates • WebLinks • Online Appendices and Supplements • Mosby/Saunders ePharmacology Update • Access to *Mosby's Drug Consult*

DRUG PROFILES

▶▶ bacitracin, p. 935
▶▶ benzoyl peroxide, p. 935
▶▶ clotrimazole, p. 937
▶▶ erythromycin, p. 936
    finasteride, p. 940
    fluorouracil, p. 940
▶▶ isotretinoin, p. 936
▶▶ lindane, p. 940

    miconazole, p. 937
    minoxidil, p. 940
    neomycin and polymyxin B, p. 935
    pimecrolimus, p. 941
▶▶ silver sulfadiazine, p. 940
    tretinoin, p. 936

▶▶ Key drug.

GLOSSARY

Actinic keratosis (ak tin' ik ker' ə toe' sis) A slowly developing, localized thickening of the outer layers of the skin resulting from long-term, prolonged exposure to the sun. Also called *solar keratosis*.

Carbuncle A necrotizing infection of skin and subcutaneous tissue caused by multiple furuncles (boils). It is usually caused by the bacterium *Staphylococcus aureus*.

Cellulitis An acute, diffuse, spreading infection involving the skin, subcutaneous tissue, and sometimes muscle as well. It is usually caused by a wound infected with *Streptococcus* or *Staphylococcus* spp.

Dermatological agent (der' mə to loj' ik əl) A drug used to treat reactions or disorders of the skin.

Dermatophyte Any of common groups of fungi that infect skin, hair, and nails. These fungi are most commonly from the genera *Microsporum*, *Epidermophyton*, and *Trichophyton*.

Dermis (der' mis) The layer of the skin just below the epidermis, consisting of papillary and reticular layers and containing blood and lymphatic vessels, nerves and nerve endings, glands, and hair follicles.

Epidermis (ep' i der' mis) The superficial, avascular layers of the skin, made up of an outer, dead, cornified portion and a deeper, living, cellular portion.

Folliculitis Inflammation of a follicle, usually a hair follicle. A follicle is defined as any sac or pouchlike cavity.

Furuncle A painful skin nodule caused by a staphylococcal infection that enters skin through the hair follicles. Also called a *boil*.

Impetigo A pus-generating, contagious skin infection, usually caused by staphylococci or streptococci. It usually occurs on the face and is most commonly seen in children.

Keratolytic (ker′ ə toe lit′ ik) A drug that promotes loosening and shedding of the outer layer of the skin.

Pediculicide (pə dik′ yoo li side) A drug that kills lice.

Pediculosis (pə dik′ yoo loe′ sis) An infestation with lice of the family Pediculidae.

Scabicide (ska′ bi side) Any one of a large group of drugs that destroy the itch mite *Sarcoptes scabiei*.

Scabies (skay′ bez) A contagious disease caused by *S. scabiei*, the itch mite, characterized by intense itching of the skin and injury to the skin (excoriation) resulting from scratching.

Tinea (tin′ ee uh) A group of fungal skin diseases caused by dermatophytes of several kinds and characterized by itching, scaling, and, sometimes, painful lesions. *Tinea* is a general term for infections of various dermatophytes that occur on several sites. Also called *ringworm*.

SKIN

The largest organ of the body is the skin. It covers the body and serves several functions, most of which we take for granted. It serves as a protective barrier for the internal organs. Without the skin, harmful external forces such as micro-organisms and chemicals would gain access to

and damage or destroy many of our delicate internal organs. Part of this protection includes its ability to maintain a surface pH of 4.5 to 5.5. This weakly acidic environment discourages the growth of micro-organisms that grow at a more alkaline pH of 6 to 7.5, explaining why infected skin usually has a higher pH than non-infected skin. The skin also has the ability to sense changes in temperature (hot or cold), pressure, or pain—information that is then transmitted along nerve endings. The temperature of the environment changes constantly and can be extremely hot or cold. Despite this, the body maintains an almost constant internal temperature in most environments, thanks in large part to the skin, which plays a major role in the regulation of body temperature. Heat loss and conservation are regulated in coordination with the blood vessels that supply blood to the skin and by means of perspiration. The skin is also able to excrete fluid and electrolytes through sweat glands. In addition, it stores fat, synthesizes vitamin D, and provides a site for drug absorption.

The skin is made up of two layers: the dermis and the epidermis (Figure 55-1). The outer skin layer, or **epidermis**, is composed of five layers. From the outermost to innermost layer, these are the stratum corneum, stratum lucidum, stratum granulosum, stratum spinosum, and the stratum germinativum (sometimes called stratum basale). The respective functions of these layers are described in Table 55-1. None of these layers has a direct

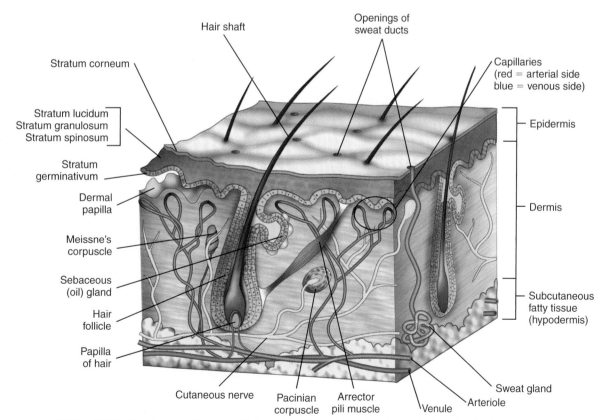

FIG. 55-1 A microscopic view of the skin. The epidermis, shown in longitudinal section, is raised at one corner to reveal the ridges in the dermis. (Modified from Thibodeau, G.A., & Patton, K.T. (2003). *Anatomy and physiology* (5th ed.). St Louis, MO: Mosby.)

TABLE 55-1
EPIDERMAL LAYERS

Layer	Description
Stratum corneum ("horny layer," so named because keratin is the same protein that makes up the horns of animals)	Outermost layer consisting of dead skin cells that are made of a converted water-repellent protein known as *keratin*; it is the protective layer for the entire body. After it is desquamated or shed, it is replaced by new cells from below.
Stratum lucidum ("clear layer")	Layer where keratin is formed; it is translucent and contains flat cells. Represents the transition from the stratum granulosum and stratum corneum. Usually only visible in thick epidermis such as on the palms of the hands and soles of the feet.
Stratum granulosum ("granular layer")	Cells die in this layer; granulated cells are located here, giving this layer the appearance for which it is named.
Stratum spinosum ("prickle cell layer")	Cells that divide in the statum germinativum accumulate desmosomes (intercellular junctions) on their outer surface which provide the characteristic prickles.
Stratum germinativum or stratum basale ("germinative layer")	New skin cells are made in this layer; it contains melanocytes, which produce melanin, the pigment that gives skin its colour. The melanocytes extend in between epidermal cells and reach into the more superficial stratum spinosum. Melanin enters into the keratinocytes and protects them from the destructive effect of ultraviolet radiation.

TABLE 55-2
EXOCRINE GLANDS OF THE SKIN

Gland	Function
Sebaceous antiseptic	Large lipid-containing cells that produce oil or film that covers the epidermis; protects and lubricates skin and is water repellent and antiseptic
Eccrine	Sweat glands that are located throughout the skin surface; help regulate body temperature and prevent skin dryness
Apocrine	Mainly in axilla, genital organs, and breast areas; emit an odour; believed to be scent or sex glands

blood supply of its own. Instead, its nourishment is provided through diffusion from the dermis below.

The **dermis** lies between the epidermis and subcutaneous fat and differs from the epidermis in many ways. It is approximately 40 times thicker than the epidermis. Traversing the dermis is a rich supply of blood vessels, nerves, lymphatic tissue, elastic tissue, and connective tissue, which provide extra support and nourishment to the skin. Also contained in this layer are the exocrine glands—the eccrine, apocrine, and sebaceous glands—and the hair follicles. The functions of the various types of exocrine glands are explained in Table 55-2.

Below the dermis is a layer of loose connective tissue called the *hypodermis*. It helps make the skin flexible. It is also here that the subcutaneous fat tissue is located, which provides thermal insulation and cushioning or padding. It is also the source of nutrition for the skin.

DERMATOLOGICAL AGENTS

Reactions or disorders of the skin are common and numerous. The drugs used to treat these disorders can be administered directly to the site and are called **dermatological agents**. There are many such agents available in a multitude of formulations, some of the more common of which are as follows:
- Aerosol foam
- Aerosol spray
- Bar (similar to soap)
- Cream
- Gel/jelly
- Lotion
- Oil
- Ointment
- Paste
- Powder
- Tape (not available in Canada)

Each formulation has certain characteristics that make it suitable for specific indications (Table 55-3).

There are also many categories of dermatological agents. Some of the most common ones are as follows:
- Antibacterial agents
- Antifungal agents
- Anti-inflammatory agents
- Antineoplastics
- Antipruritic agents (for itching)
- Antiviral agents
- Burn drugs
- Debriding agents (promote wound healing)
- Emollients (skin softener)
- Keratolytics (cause softening and peeling of the stratum corneum)
- Local anaesthetics
- Topical vasodilators

Because there are so many available agents, the scope of this chapter is limited to some of the most commonly used medications.

TOPICAL ANTI-INFECTIVES

The topical anti-infectives are antibacterial, acne, antifungal, and antiviral drugs that, as the name implies, are applied topically. The systemically administered anti-infective agents are discussed in detail in Part Seven, where their specific pharmacological characteristics are also described.

TABLE 55-3
DERMATOLOGICAL FORMULATIONS: CHARACTERISTICS AND EXAMPLES

Formulation	Characteristics	Examples
Aerosol foam	Can cover large area; useful for drug delivery into a body cavity (e.g., vagina, rectum) or hair areas	Proctofoam, contraceptive foams
Aerosol spray	Spreads thin liquid or powder film; covers large areas; useful when skin is tender to touch (e.g., burns)	Solarcaine, Tinactin
Cream	Contains water and can be removed with water; not greasy or occlusive; usually white semi-solid; good for moist areas	hydrocortisone cream, Benadryl cream, Triaderm
Gel/jelly	Contains water and possibly alcohol; easily removed and good lubricator; usually clear, semi-solid substance; useful when lubricant properties are desirable	K-Y jelly
Lotion	Contains water, alcohol, and solvents; may be a suspension, emulsion, or solution; good for large or hairy areas	Calamine lotion, Lubriderm lotion
Oil	Contains little if any water; occlusive, liquid; not removable with water	Aveeno bath treatment
Ointment	Contains no water; not removable with water; occlusive, greasy, and semi-solid; desirable for dry lesions because of occlusiveness	petrolatum (Vaseline), zinc oxide ointment, A & D ointment, Triaderm
Paste	Similar properties to those of the ointments; contains more powder than ointments; excellent protectant properties	zinc oxide paste
Powder	Slight lubricating properties; may be shaken on affected area; promotes drying of area where applied	Tinactin powder, Desenex powder
Tape	Most occlusive formulation; consistent topical drug delivery; useful when small, straight areas require drug application	Not available in Canada

Those with available topical dosage forms are discussed here. Although they have many of the same properties as the systemic forms, there are some differences in terms of their toxicities and side effects. The drugs used to treat dermatological parasitic infections, the pediculicides and scabicides, as well as the drugs commonly used to treat acne, are also covered in this section.

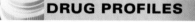

DRUG PROFILES

ANTIBACTERIAL AGENTS

Common skin disorders caused by various bacteria are **folliculitis, impetigo, furuncles, carbuncles,** and **cellulitis.** The bacteria responsible are most commonly *Streptococcus pyogenes* and *Staphylococcus aureus.* Dermatological antibacterial agents are used to treat or prevent these skin infections, and the most commonly used agents are bacitracin, polymyxin, and neomycin.

▶▶ bacitracin

Bacitracin is a polypeptide antibiotic that is applied topically for the treatment or prevention of local skin infections caused by susceptible aerobic and anaerobic gram-positive organisms such as staphylococci, streptococci, anaerobic cocci, corynebacteria, and clostridia. It works by inhibiting bacterial cell wall synthesis, which leads to cell death. It can be either bactericidal or bacteriostatic, depending on the causative organism.

Bacitracin's antimicrobial spectrum is broadened when it is used in combination with other topical antibiotics, and there are several such combination products available. Most contain neomycin and polymyxin B (see later). Bacitracin usually has a low order of toxicity

when applied topically. Rash and allergic anaphylactoid reactions have occurred. If itching, burning, inflammation, or other signs of sensitivity occur, bacitracin should be discontinued. Ointment formulations of the agent are most commonly used, but powders and aerosols are also available. As a single-agent product, bacitracin is available as a 500-unit/g ointment that is usually applied to the affected area one to three times daily.

neomycin and polymyxin B

Neomycin and polymyxin B are two additional broad-spectrum antibiotics that are available as the popular non-prescription product known as Neosporin. Neosporin cream is a combination of these two agents with gramicidin, whereas Neosporin ointment also contains bacitracin. Several brand-name and generic combinations of these topical antibiotics are available, and all are commonly used as topical antiseptics for minor skin wounds. More serious wounds may also require prescription topical and/or systemic (oral or intravenous) antibiotics.

ACNE AGENTS

Other antibacterial agents are used to treat acne, the skin infection commonly caused by *Propionibacterium acnes.* These agents include benzoyl peroxide, clindamycin, erythromycin, tetracycline, isotretinoin, and the vitamin A acid known as *retinoic acid.* Many other agents are also used in the treatment and prevention of acne.

▶▶ benzoyl peroxide

The micro-organism that most commonly causes acne, *P. acnes,* is an anaerobic bacterium that needs an environment poor in oxygen to grow. Benzoyl peroxide is effective in combatting such infection because it slowly and continuously liberates active oxygen in the skin, causing antibacterial, antiseptic, drying, and keratolytic actions. These actions create an environment unfavourable for the continued growth of the *P. acnes* bacteria, and they soon die. Drugs such as benzoyl peroxide that soften scales and loosen the outer horny layer of the skin are referred to as **keratolytics**.

Benzoyl peroxide generally produces signs of improvement within four to six weeks. Side effects are infrequent and rarely a problem. Most are confined to the skin and involve peeling skin, red skin, or a sensation of warmth. Blistering or swelling of the skin is generally considered an allergic reaction to the product and is an indication to stop treatment.

Benzoyl peroxide is available in multiple topical dosage forms including a cleansing bar, liquid, lotion, mask, cream, gel, and cleanser. Dosage strengths range from 2.5 percent to 20 percent. It is usually applied topically one to four times daily, depending on the dosage form and prescriber's instructions. Pregnancy category C.

▶▶ *erythromycin*

Erythromycin is a macrolide antibiotic used for the topical treatment of acne vulgaris, a common form of acne. It usually only stops the growth of the acne-causing bacteria (bacteriostatic), but it may kill bacteria either when given in high concentrations or when a particular strain of organism is highly susceptible. It exerts its antibacterial effects by inhibiting protein synthesis in susceptible organisms. Erythromycin topical preparations are applied to the cleansed affected areas each morning and evening. Skin reactions are the most common side effect and consist of erythema, desquamation, tenderness, dryness, pruritus, burning, oiliness, and acne. Erythromycin is available topically in a solution or gel, in strengths ranging from 2 to 4 percent. It is contraindicated in clients with known hypersensitivity to it. Pregnancy category B or C, depending on specific product.

▶▶ *isotretinoin*

Isotretinoin is an oral product indicated for the treatment of severe recalcitrant cystic acne. Isotretinoin inhibits sebaceous gland activity and has antikeratinizing (anti-skin hardening) and anti-inflammatory effects. Isotretinoin is one of relatively few medications that are classified as pregnancy category X agents. This means that it is a proven human teratogen (a chemical known to induce birth defects). It is imperative that female clients of childbearing age be counselled and agree not to become pregnant during use. It is recommended that at least two contraceptive methods be used by sexually active women during and for one month after completion of therapy with isotretinoin. It is available as 10- and 40-mg capsules. It is contraindicated in clients who are pregnant or have hypersensitivity to it.

tretinoin

Tretinoin is a derivative of vitamin A that is used to treat acne and ameliorate the dermatological changes (e.g., fine wrinkling, mottled hyperpigmentation, roughness) associated with photodamage (sun damage). The drug appears to act as an irritant on the skin, in particular the follicular epithelium. Specifically, it stimulates the turnover of epidermal cells, which results in skin peeling. While this is occurring, the free fatty acid levels of the skin are reduced and horny cells of the outer epidermis cannot then adhere to one another. Without fatty acids and horny cells, acne and its comedo, or pimple, cannot exist.

Topically administered tretinoin has been shown to enhance the repair of skin damaged by ultraviolet radiation, or sunlight. It does this by increasing the formation of fibroblasts and collagen, both of which are needed to rebuild skin. The drug may also reduce collagen degradation by inhibiting the enzyme collagenase, which breaks down collagen.

As with erythromycin, tretinoin's main side effects are local inflammatory reactions, which are reversible when therapy is discontinued. Some of the most common side effects are excessively red and edematous blisters, crusted skin, and temporary alterations in skin pigmentation. Tretinoin is available in many topical formulations, including creams, gels, and a liquid, in strengths ranging from 0.02 to 0.1 percent. Because of its potential to cause severe irritation and peeling, it may initially be applied once every two or three days, often starting with a lower-strength product.

One of the newer tretinoin dosage forms is Retin-A Micro, which has been approved for the treatment of acne vulgaris. This newer acne treatment is formulated with tretinoin inside a synthetic polymer called a *Microsponge system*. This system is made of round microscopic particles of synthetic polymer. These microspheres act as a reservoir for tretinoin, allowing the skin to absorb small amounts of the drug over time. Retin-A Micro is currently available only as a 0.1 percent gel. All topical forms of tretinoin are rated pregnancy category C. They are not to be confused with the oral capsule form of tretinoin mentioned in Chapter 47 that is used to treat leukemia and is rated pregnancy category D.

Another agent in the retinoid family is tazarotene. Tazarotene is a receptor-selective retinoid. It is thought to normalize epidermal differentiation, reducing the influx of inflammatory cells into the skin. Synthetic retinoids are vitamin A analogues and are thought to play a role in skin cell differentiation and proliferation. It is available as a 0.05 percent and 0.1 percent gel and is approved for the treatment of stable plaque psoriasis and mild to moderately severe facial acne vulgaris. Tazarone is also a pregnancy category X agent, requiring appropriate counselling for female clients, as described earlier.

ANTIFUNGAL AGENTS

A few fungi produce keratinolytic enzymes, which allows them to live on the skin. Topical fungal infections are primarily caused by *Candida* spp. (candidiasis), **dermatophytes**, and *Malassezia furfur* (tinea versicolor). These fungi exist in moist, warm environments, especially in dark areas such as the feet or groin.

Candidal infections are most commonly caused by *Candida albicans*, a yeast-like opportunistic fungus present in the normal flora of the mouth, vagina, and intestinal tract. Two significant factors that commonly predispose a person to a candidal infection are broad-spectrum antibiotic therapy, which promotes an overgrowth of non-susceptible organisms in the natural body florae, and immunodeficiency disorders such as those that occur in clients with cancer, AIDS, or organ transplants. Because these infections favour warm, moist areas of the skin and mucous membranes, they most commonly occur orally (e.g., thrush in infants), vaginally, and cutaneously in such sites as beneath the breasts and in diapered areas. They may also cause nail infections.

Dermatophytes are a group of three closely related genera consisting of *Epidermophyton* spp., *Microsporum* spp., and *Trichophyton* spp. that use the keratin found on the skin to feed their growth. They produce superficial mycotic (fungal) infections of keratinized tissue (hair, skin, and nails). Infections caused by dermatophytes are collectively called **tinea**, or *ringworm*, infections. The name *ringworm* comes from the fact that the infection often assumes a circular pattern at the site of infection. The tinea infections are further identified by the body location where they occur: tinea pedis (foot), tinea cruris (groin), tinea corporis (body), and tinea capitis (scalp). Tinea infections are also known as *athlete's foot* or *jock itch*.

Fungi usually invade the stratum corneum, which is the dead layer of desquamated (shed) cells. Inflammation occurs when the fungi invade this layer; sensitivity (e.g., itching) occurs when they penetrate the epidermis and dermis.

Many of the fungi that cause topical infections are difficult to eradicate. They are slow growing, and antifungal therapy may be required for periods ranging from several weeks to as long as one year. However, many topical antifungal drugs are available for the treatment of both dermatophyte infections and those caused by yeast and yeast-like fungi. Some of these agents, their dosage forms, and their uses are listed in Table 55-4.

The most commonly reported side effects of topical antifungals are local irritation, pruritus, a burning sensation, and scaling. Ciclopirox and clotrimazole are classified as pregnancy category B agents, and econazole and ketoconazole and miconazole are classified as pregnancy category C agents. Hypersensitivity is the one contraindication to the use of any of these agents.

▸▸ *clotrimazole*

Clotrimazole is available both OTC and with a prescription. It is available as a cream for the treatment of dermatophytoses (e.g., athlete's foot), superficial mycoses, and cutaneous candidiasis. Similar topical preparations are also available for intravaginal administration in the treatment of vulvovaginal candidiasis, commonly called a *yeast infection,* and vaginal trichomoniasis. Pregnancy category B.

miconazole

Miconazole is a topical antifungal agent that is available in several OTC and prescription products. It inhibits the growth of several fungi, including dermatophytes and yeast, as well as gram-positive bacteria, and is commonly used to treat dermatophytoses, superficial mycoses, cutaneous candidiasis, and vulvovaginal candidiasis. It is present in many OTC remedies for athlete's foot, jock itch, and yeast infections.

For the treatment of athlete's foot, jock itch, ringworm, and other susceptible fungal infections, miconazole should be applied sparingly to the cleansed, dry, infected area twice daily, in the morning and evening. For the treatment of yeast infections, one 400-mg ovule suppository should be inserted in the vagina once daily at bedtime for three consecutive days or 100 mg (one suppository or 5 g of the 2 percent cream) should be administered intravaginally once daily at bedtime for seven days.

The most common side effects of topically administered miconazole are vulvovaginal burning and itching, pelvic cramps and rash, urticaria, stinging, and contact dermatitis. It is available in a variety of topical formulations: a 2-percent aerosol spray and powder, a 2-percent cream, a 2-percent vaginal cream, and a 100-, 200-, and 400-mg vaginal suppository. It is also now available as a 1200-mg vaginal suppository for one-time dosing. Pregnancy category C.

ANTIVIRAL AGENTS

As noted in Chapter 38, viral infections are difficult to treat because they live in the body's own healthy cells and use their cell mechanisms to reproduce. The same holds true for topical viral infections. Infections caused by herpes simplex types 1 and 2 are particularly serious and are becoming more common. The only topical antiviral agent currently available to treat such viral infections

TABLE 55-4
TOPICAL ANTIFUNGAL AGENTS

Agent	Dosage Forms	Uses	Legal Status
butenafine	1% cream	Tinea pedis	OTC
butoconazole	2% vaginal cream	Candidiasis	Rx
ciclopirox olamine	1% cream and lotion, 80 mg/gm solution (for nails), 1.5% shampoo	Candidiasis, dermatophytoses, tinea versicolor	Rx
clioquinol	3% cream	Dermatophytoses	OTC
clotrimazole	1% vaginal cream, 200- and 500-mg vaginal tabs	Candidiasis	OTC
clotrimazole	1% topical cream	Candidiasis; dermatophytoses; tinea vesicolor	OTC
clotrimazole	1%, 2%, 10% cream	Candidiasis	OTC
econazole	1% cream	Candidiasis, dermatophytoses	Rx
econazole	150-mg vaginal ovule	Candidiasis	Rx
ketoconazole	2% cream and shampoo	Candidiasis, dermatophytoses, tinea versicolor	Rx
miconazole	2% cream, powder spray	Candidiasis, dermatophytoses, tinea versicolor	OTC
miconazole	2% cream	Candidiasis, dermatophytoses, tinea versicolor	OTC
miconazole	100-, 400-, and 1200-mg vaginal ovules	Candidiasis	OTC
naftifine	1% cream and gel	Dermatophytoses	OTC
nystatin	Cream, ointment, powder	Candidiasis	Rx
nystatin	Vaginal cream, tab	Candidiasis	Rx
oxiconazole	1% cream	Dermatophytoses	OTC
terbinafine	1% cream and spray	Dermatophytoses	Rx
tolnaftate	1% cream, solution, gel, powder, swab, and spray	Dermatophytoses	OTC
undecylenic acid	Powder, liquid, ointment, spray	Dermatophytoses	OTC

Rx, Currently available by prescription only.

is acyclovir. Systemic (as opposed to topical) antiviral agents may also be used as described in Chapter 38.

Acyclovir works by inhibiting the viral enzymes necessary for deoxyribonucleic acid (DNA) synthesis. It is applied topically for the treatment of initial and recurrent herpes simplex infections in immunocompromised clients. However, often these topical infections can be prevented or treated more efficaciously with systemically administered antiviral agents. Topically applied antiviral agents do not cure viral skin infections but do appear to decrease the healing time and associated pain. They should be applied as soon as possible during a skin outbreak.

Acyclovir is available as a 5 percent topical ointment. It is applied four to six times daily, for one week. A finger cot or rubber glove should be worn for the application of the ointment to prevent the spread of infection. The most common side effects are stinging and itching. Acyclovir is contraindicated in clients with hypersensitivity to it. It is classified as a pregnancy category C agent.

TOPICAL ANAESTHETIC, ANTIPRURITIC, AND ANTI-INFLAMMATORY AGENTS

Topical anaesthetic agents are drugs used to numb the skin. They accomplish this by inhibiting the conduction of nerve impulses from sensory nerves, thereby reducing or eliminating the pain or pruritus associated with insect bites, sunburn, and plant allergies such as poison ivy, as well as many other uncomfortable skin disorders. They are also used to numb the skin before a painful injection. Topical anaesthetics are available as ointments, creams, sprays, liquids, and jellies and are discussed in Chapter 11.

Topical antipruritic (anti-itching) agents contain antihistamines or corticosteroids. Many exert a combined anaesthetic and antipruritic action when applied topically. The antihistamines and their therapeutic effects are covered in Chapter 35. New recommendations for the use of topical antihistamines state that they should not be used for chicken pox or widespread poison ivy or over a large body surface area because of systemic absorption and the risk of toxicity.

Topical anti-inflammatory agents are most commonly corticosteroids, and they are generally indicated for the relief of inflammatory and pruritic dermatoses. Topical corticosteroids provide anti-inflammatory, antipruritic, and vasoconstricting actions, but have few of the undesirable systemic side effects associated with systemic corticosteroids.

The many different available dosage forms of the various corticosteroids vary in their relative potency, and this often guides their selection for treating various conditions. For instance, fluorinated corticosteroids are used for the treatment of dermatological disorders such as psoriasis. The vehicle in which the corticosteroid is contained

TABLE 55-5
TOPICAL CORTICOSTEROIDS*

Range of Potency	Corticosteroid
Most potent	betamethasone dipropionate (cream and ointment), clobetasol 17-propionate, halobetasol propionate
Potent	amcinonide, betamethasone dipropionate (lotion), betamethasone valerate (0.1% cream, ointment, and lotion), desoximetasone (0.25% cream and ointment), diflucortolone diacetate, fluocinolone acetonide, halcinonide, mometasone furoate
Moderately Potent	clobetasone 17-butyrate, desonide, desoximetasone (0.5% cream and gel), flumethasone pivalate, hydrocortisone valerate, prednicarbate, triamcinolone acetonide
Weak	hydrocortisone, hydrocortisone valerate, methylprednisolone, methylprednisolone acetate

*Skin penetration and thus potency is enhanced by the vehicle containing the steroid. In decreasing order of effectiveness are ointments, gels, creams, and lotions.

also has the effect of altering its vasoconstrictor properties and therapeutic efficacy. Ointments are generally the most penetrating, followed next by gels, creams, and lotions. Propylene glycol also enhances the penetration of the corticosteroid and its vasoconstrictor effects. Most corticosteroids are available in many topical formulations, thus offering a variety of options. The currently available topical corticosteroids, along with their respective potencies, are listed in Table 55-5.

Side effects of these agents include skin reactions such as acne eruptions, allergic contact dermatitis, burning sensations, dryness, itching, striae (striations or "striping"), hypopigmentation, purpura (hemorrhaging into the skin), hirsutism (usually facial), folliculitis, round and swollen face, and alopecia (usually of the scalp). Another side effect is the opportunistic overgrowth of bacterial, fungal, or viral flora as a result of the immunosuppressive effects of this class of drugs. The usual adult dosage of these drugs is one or two applications daily, as directed. Less potent topical corticosteroids are used for children following the same schedule. Corticosteroids are classified as pregnancy category C agents and are contraindicated in clients with hypersensitivity to them. Many of these drugs are available orally as well as topically. The same drug should not be given both orally and topically; this combined use can lead to toxicity.

MISCELLANEOUS DERMATOLOGICAL AGENTS

There are many other topically applied drugs. Those discussed here are the topical ectoparasiticidal (scabicides and pediculicides), hair growth, antineoplastic, and anti-infective drugs. Many of these agents are available both

NATURAL HEALTH THERAPIES

ALOE (Aloe vera L.)

Overview
The dried leaves of the aloe plant contain anthranoids, which give aloe a laxative effect when taken orally. The topical application of the plant has been known for years to help aid in wound healing.

Common Uses
Wound healing, constipation

Adverse Effects
Diarrhea, nephritis, abdominal pain, dermatitis when used topically

Potential Drug Interactions
Digoxin, antidysrhythmics, diuretics, corticosteroids

Contraindications
Contraindicated in clients who are menstruating or have renal disease.

OTC and by prescription. Aloe vera herbal preparations (see Natural Health Therapies box above) are also available OTC.

DRUG PROFILES

TOPICAL ECTOPARASITICIDAL DRUGS

Ectoparasites are insects that live on the outer surface of the body, and the drugs that are used to kill them are called *ectoparasiticidal drugs*. Lice are transmitted from person to person by close contact with infested people, clothing, combs, or towels. A parasitic infestation on the skin with lice is called **pediculosis**, and such infestations go by one of three different names, depending on the location of the infestation:
- Pediculosis pubis—pubic lice or "crabs," caused by *Phthirus pubis*
- Pediculosis corporis—body lice, caused by *Pediculus humanus corporis*
- Pediculosis capitis—head lice, caused by *Pediculus humanus capitis*

Common findings in infested persons include itching; eggs of the lice (called *nits*) attached to the hair shafts; lice on the skin or clothes; and in the case of pubic lice, sky blue macules (discoloured skin patches) on the inner thighs or lower abdomen. Pediculoses are treated with a class of drugs called **pediculicides**. Examples include pyrethrins, permethrin 1 percent, and lindane. OTC preparations of pyrethrins (e.g., Lice Killing Shampoo), permethrin (e.g., Nix Creme Rinse), and lindane (e.g., Hexit Shampoo) are all available without a prescription. These products require a second treatment seven to ten days after the initial application. A second common parasitic skin infection known as **scabies** is caused by the itch mite *Sarcoptes scabiei*. Scabies is transmitted from person to person by close contact, such as by sleeping next to an infested person. The scabies mite causes irritation and itching by boring into the horny layers of skin located in cracks and folds. Itching seems to occur most commonly in the evening. The drugs used to treat these infestations are called **scabicides**.

Treatment of these parasitic infestations should begin with identification of the source of infestation to prevent reinfestation. Next, the clothing and personal articles of the infested person should be decontaminated. This is best accomplished by washing them in hot, soapy water or by dry cleaning them. All close contacts of the person should also be treated to prevent reinfestation.

Crotamiton is also an ectoparasiticidal drug.

▶▶ lindane

Lindane is a chlorinated hydrocarbon originally developed as an agricultural insecticide. It is both a **scabicide** and a pediculicide because it is effective in treating both scabies and pediculosis. It is available in two topical formulations: a 1 percent lotion and a 1 percent shampoo.

For the treatment of pubic or body lice, the cream or lotion is applied in a sufficient quantity to cover the skin and hair of the infested and surrounding areas. It is left on for 12 hours and then thoroughly washed off. A second application is seldom needed. Head lice can be treated with lindane shampoo, which should be worked into the hair with just enough water to obtain a good lather and left on for four minutes. The hair should then be rinsed and dried, after which the nits (eggs) should be combed from the hair shafts. The treatment for scabies is similar. It involves the application of lindane over the entire body, from the neck down. It is left on for 8 to 12 hours and washed off. Side effects of lindane are an eczematous skin rash and, rarely, central nervous system (CNS) toxicity. The latter is more common in young children and in cases of overuse. The Canadian Paediatric Society has recommended that topical lindane not be used on infants and children under the age of six years.

TOPICAL HAIR GROWTH DRUGS

minoxidil

Minoxidil is a vasodilating drug that is administered systemically to control hypertension (see Chapter 24). Topically it has the same vasodilating effect, but when used in this way it is applied to the scalp to stimulate hair growth. The vasodilation it causes is one possible explanation for how it stimulates hair growth. It may also act at the level of the hair follicle, possibly stimulating hair follicle growth directly.

Minoxidil can be used in men suffering from baldness or hair thinning. It is not approved by Health Canada for use in women. Treatment involves administering the agent to the affected (balding and anticipated balding) area twice daily, usually morning and evening. It generally takes four months before results are seen. Systemic absorption of the topically applied minoxidil may occur, with possible side effects including tachycardia, fluid retention, and weight gain. Local effects may include skin irritation, but the drug should not be applied to skin that is already irritated, nor should it be used concurrently with other topical medications applied to the same site. Topically administered minoxidil is available as a 2 percent solution. Six squirts using the

pump-spray delivers 1 mL (20 mg) of the agent. The maximum recommended daily topical dose is 2 mL. Pregnancy category C.

SYSTEMIC HAIR GROWTH DRUGS

finasteride

Finasteride is a lower strength version of the medication used to treat benign prostatic hyperplasia, described in Chapter 34. It is currently the only available oral medication indicated for treating male pattern baldness (alopecia). It works by inhibiting the enzyme 5-alpha-reductase. This enzyme normally catalyzes the conversion of testosterone to 5-alpha-dihydrotestosterone, which somehow promotes hair loss as one of its effects. It must be remembered that only the lower-strength finasteride, available in a 1-mg tablet, is indicated for treatment of hair loss (in men only). The higher-strength 5-mg finasteride tablet is used for benign enlarged prostate. The usual dose of finasteride for baldness is 1 mg daily on a continuous basis. Withdrawal of treatment is associated with reversal of any hair-growth benefits within 12 months. It is recommended by the manufacturer that pregnant women, or even women who may become pregnant, not handle broken finasteride tablets because of teratogenic data from animal studies.

TOPICAL ANTINEOPLASTIC DRUGS

fluorouracil

Basal cell carcinomas and various premalignant skin lesions may be treated with the topically applied antineoplastic drug fluorouracil. It acts by destroying rapidly growing cells, such as premalignant and malignant cells. It is also used topically in the treatment of premalignant solar or **actinic keratosis** and superficial basal cell carcinomas of the skin when surgical and other techniques are not feasible.

Unlike systemic administration of the agent (see Chapter 46), topical use of fluorouracil usually has minimal side effects, generally limited to local inflammatory reactions such as dermatitis, stomatitis, and photosensitivity. Major adverse effects of fluorouracil topical therapy are swelling, scaling, pain, pruritus, burning, soreness, tenderness, suppuration, scarring, and hyperpigmentation.

Fluorouracil is available as a 1 percent and a 5 percent topical cream. It can be applied with a non-metallic applicator or gloved fingers. The 1 percent fluorouracil cream should be used for the treatment of multiple actinic keratoses of the head and neck. It should be applied twice daily to the lesions. Superficial basal cell carcinoma may be treated with 5 percent fluorouracil, administered twice daily for at least two to four weeks.

OTHER TOPICAL ANTI-INFECTIVE DRUGS

▶▶ silver sulfadiazine

One of the concerns with burn victims is infection at the burn site, but there are two problems posed by the use of either topically or systemically administered anti-infective agents in this setting. Because increased systemic absorption of a drug can occur in compromised skin areas such as burns, topical burn agents that are too potent or toxic can cause dangerous systemic effects. This is especially true for larger burned areas, because the larger the surface area the greater the absorption. On the other hand, because the blood supply to burned areas is often drastically reduced, systemically administered antibiotics often cannot reach the site in effective quantities. Therefore the only way to ensure the agents reach the burn site is topical application. Some of the commonly used agents that have proved both effective and safe in the prevention or treatment of infections in burns are silver sulfadiazine, mafenide, and nitrofurazone.

Silver sulfadiazine is a synthetic anti-infective agent produced when silver nitrate reacts with the chemical sulfadiazine. It appears to act on the cell membrane and cell wall of susceptible bacteria and is used as an adjunct in the prevention and treatment of infection in second- and third-degree burns. The side effects of silver sulfadiazine are similar to those of other topical drugs and include pain, burning, and itching. This medication should not be used in clients who are allergic to sulphonamide drugs. It is available only as a 1 percent cream and should be applied topically to cleansed, debrided, burned areas once or twice daily using a sterile-gloved hand.

TOPICAL IMMUNOMODULATORS
pimecrolimus

The latest dermatological drug is currently the only drug in a brand new class of medications. Pimecrolimus is available in a cream form for use in treating atopic dermatitis. This drug works through a mechanism similar to that of the anti–transplant-rejection drug tacrolimus, which was discussed in Chapter 44 on immunosuppressant agents.

NURSING PROCESS

▉ Assessment

Before using any of the dermatological preparations, the nurse should rule out the presence of the many conditions that may be a contraindication, such as known hypersensitivity. It is important for the nurse to always check to make sure that the client has no drug allergies and no previous sensitivity to antimicrobials or benzoyl- or peroxide-containing drugs. Topical antibacterial agents are associated with a broad risk of reactions because of the generalized sensitivity of clients to the same antibiotic even when in a different dosage form. In other words, if a client has an allergy to a particular antibacterial agent used systemically, that agent should not be used topically either. The nurse should always be sure that if culture and sensitivity testing has been ordered, the appropriate specimen has been collected before the first application of the antibacterial or other type of dermatological agent.

Before administering any type of topical medication, such as an antimicrobial, a steroid, or an anti-acne agent, the nurse should consider the concentration of the medication, length of exposure to the skin, condition of the skin, size of the area affected, and hydration status of the skin, because all have a significant effect on the action of the medication.

The skin, and in particular the area affected, must be inspected thoroughly under an adequate light source and the area palpated with a gloved hand, especially with dark-skinned clients, because often an erythematous area may not be visible but may be palpated as an area of warmth. With oral tretinoin, liver function studies should be assessed, and with lindane it is important for the source of the scabies infection to be assessed and identified. In addition, with the use of silver sulfadiazine, any problems related to ototoxicity and nephrotoxicity should be assessed. All findings should be thoroughly documented and reflect a systematic and bilateral assessment of all areas of the body.

The client's overall health status and hygiene practices should also be assessed, including whether the client has suffered any trauma or whether his or her immune system is suppressed. Exudate or drainage material should also be obtained for culture studies before therapy is initiated if ordered by the prescriber. The nurse should also remember that the skin of the very young and the very old is often more permeable to some of the dermatological preparations and has more risk of absorption from the skin into systemic circulation. Contraindications to the use of some of the topical agents may include pus, debris, abrasions, and/or breaks in the skin. Natural health products, such as topical aloe, may be used to increase healing, but assessment of any cautious use or contraindications is needed (see the Natural Health Therapies box on p. 939).

▉ Nursing Diagnoses

Nursing diagnoses pertinent to the use of dermatological preparations include the following:
- Impaired skin integrity related to disease or disorder, causing a break in skin barrier.
- Acute pain related to the skin condition or adverse reactions to the topical preparation.
- Deficient knowledge related to lack of experience with and exposure to use of topical agents.
- Ineffective therapeutic regimen related to lack of information about importance of adherence.

▉ Planning

Goals related to the administration of dermatological preparations include the following:
- Client's skin remains intact and healed in appearance and integrity.
- Client remains adherent with therapy.
- Client remains free of injury to skin while on therapy.
- Client experiences minimal to no complications of therapy.

▉ *Outcome Criteria*

Outcome criteria related to the administration of dermatological agents include the following:
- Client's skin improves daily (e.g., there is less redness, drainage, discomfort, itching, rash).
- Client has fewer complaints about localized skin discomfort (e.g., pain, itching).

- Client demonstrates how to apply medication as prescribed.
- Client states the rationale for treatment, the side effects of the dermatological preparation, and symptoms to report.
- Client remains adherent with the medication therapy.

Implementation

Generally speaking, before applying any topical medication the nurse should cleanse the affected site of any debris and residual medication, making sure to follow any specific directions, such as removing water- or alcohol- based topicals with soap and water and using Standard Precautions (see Box 9–1). The nurse should wear gloves, not only to prevent contamination from secretions but also to prevent absorption of the medication through his or her skin. Lotions should be stored according to the manufacturer's recommendations and shaken well before use. Creams and ointments are often applied with a sterile cotton-tipped applicator or tongue blade. Any dressings should be applied as ordered with special attention to directions concerning occlusive, wet, or wet-to-dry dressings. Information should be documented about the site of application, including drainage (colour and

---

TABLE 55-6

DERMATOLOGICAL AGENTS: NURSING IMPLICATIONS

Classification	Specific Agents	Nursing Implications
Acne products (keratolytics)	benzoyl peroxide, tretinoin	With benzoyl peroxide. effects are seen in 4–6 wk. Apply sparingly using lotion, bar, gel, or cream. Tretinoin is applied each night at bedtime; apply after cleansing and allow 30 min to dry; no rubbing. Apply only enough to cover the affected area lightly. If applied to wet skin there may be increased redness or drying. Avoid weather extremes and UV radiation; wear sunscreen during therapy because of increased sensitivity. Avoid abrasive cleansers and other keratolytic products because of possible toxicity to the skin. Follow directions closely when using the new Micro-sponge System with Retin-A Micro.
Antifungals	clotrimazole, ketoconazole, miconazole, nystatin	May apply any of these liberally to clean, dry, affected skin area. Occlusive dressings are not recommended unless ordered. Avoid contact with eyes. Encourage good hygiene: keep area clean, dry, and exposed to air; keep dry with powders to prevent maceration if needed. Notify healthcare provider if sore throat, fever, or skin rash occurs (may indicate overgrowth of organisms).
Anti-infectives and antibiotics	bacitracin, clindamycin, erythromycin, neomycin, tetracycline	Bacitracin is odourless and non-staining. Neomycin may cause sensitization and photosensitivity when used with topical gentamicin. Apply thin film of clindamycin and assess for allergy to drug and other antibiotics. Erythromycin is applied using cotton balls or topical applicator as ordered. Tetracycline is applied until area is moistened. Avoid eyes and mucous membranes because of alcohol content and related irritation. Allergic reactions indicated by burning, redness, swelling, and stinging.
Anti-inflammatories (corticosteroids)	betamethasone valerate, fluocinolone acetonide, fluocinonide, hydrocortisone, methylprednisolone	All of these help stabilize cell membranes, and the ointment bases and glycol enhance the penetration of the agent into the skin. They usually are applied bid, and application technique depends on site. Be careful with occlusive dressings because this can lead to follicle infections, heat retention, or systemic effects. Note that occlusive dressings are often ordered because of photosensitivity to area. Avoid sunlight on affected areas because burns may occur.
Antiparasitics	lindane	With lindane, leave shampoo on for 4 min, then rinse and use nit comb to remove nits (eggs) from the hair shafts. Cream and lotions are usually left on for 12 h, then washed off. Pubic lice are treated by applying for 12 h, then washing off.
Antivirals	acyclovir	Cream or ointment to be applied using a finger cot or gloved hand to prevent contamination; avoid contact with eyes. With genital lesions, loose covering or clothing over lesion is recommended to prevent further irritation to site. Client should avoid sexual activity if active lesions; may be transmitted even if the person is asymptomatic. Condom use is encouraged depending on location of lesion. Apply 1.25-cm ribbon of ointment to about a 10-cm area. Begin treatment when symptoms arise.
Burn products	silver sulfadiazine	Apply as a 1% cream only to clean, debrided wounds with gloved hands; apply 3 to 5 cm thick; keep continuously covered. Daily cleansing and debriding are important. If applied to extensive areas, adverse systemic reactions may occur similar to those seen with sulphonamide. Reapply every 24 h.

amount), swelling, temperature, odour, colour, pain, or other sensations, as well as the type of treatment rendered and the response.

The manufacturer's guidelines regarding the use of any of the dermatological preparations should always be followed because each medication has a different type of base solution and specific application procedures may be required for different dosage forms. It is also important to follow any instructions or orders regarding other treatments to the affected area, such as use of an occlusive or wet dressing. Medicated areas may also need to be protected from exposure to air or sunlight. Strict adherence to the proper method of application and dosage of any dermatological preparation is important to its effectiveness. Doubling up on dosing if a dose is missed is not recommended.

After completing the application of the medication the nurse should properly dispose of all contaminated dressings; remove gloves, and wash hands. The privacy, comfort, and safety of the client must be maintained at all times, as with any procedure. See Table 55-6 for the nursing implications pertinent to each group of dermatological agents.

Client teaching tips for dermatological agents are presented in the box below.

■ Evaluation

Therapeutic responses to the various dermatological preparations include improved condition of skin and healing of lesions or wounds; a decrease in the size of the lesions with eventual resolution; and a decrease in swelling, redness, weeping, itching, and burning of the area. The physician should be notified if a therapeutic response is not noted within an appropriate time (for some agents, possibly 48 to 72 hours; for acne agents, often no response is seen for one to two months). Side effects for which to monitor include an increased severity of symptoms such as increased redness, swelling, pain, and drainage; fever; or any other unusual adverse reactions. Side effects may range from slight irritation of the site where the topical agent has been applied to an allergic reaction to toxic systemic effects. The nurse should always research each agent thoroughly so that side effects and toxic effects can be understood and monitored during therapy.

CLIENT TEACHING TIPS

The nurse should have the client demonstrate the application technique and instruct the client as follows:
▲ Keep your skin clean and dry.
▲ Maintain adequate general hygiene and diet during therapy for skin disorder.
▲ Apply medication only as ordered and follow instructions carefully.
▲ Avoid exposure to sunlight, unless it is indicated.
▲ If you need to apply a dressing after the medication has been applied, follow the physician's instructions or the manufacturer's guidelines.
▲ Notify your physician of any unusual or adverse reactions.
▲ Using the medication regularly as ordered is crucial to its effectiveness.

Antifungals
▲ Fungal infections are difficult to treat and often require prolonged therapy. If you don't see immediate results, be patient and keep using the medication as ordered.

Finasteride
▲ Women who could possibly be pregnant should not handle crushed or broken tablets. Even a slight exposure could cause abnormalities in a male fetus.

Isotretinoin
▲ (for women) This drug is known to cause birth defects in fetuses. If you are sexually active you must use contraception during treatment and for at least one month afterward. At least two contraceptive methods are recommended.

POINTS to REMEMBER

▼ Dermatological agents are used to treat topical infections.

▼ Common skin disorders caused by bacteria are folliculitis, impetigo, furuncles, carbuncles, and cellulitis.

▼ The bacterium most commonly responsible for acne is *Propionibacterium acnes*.

▼ The fungi that are responsible for causing topical fungal infections are *Candida*, dermatophytes, and *Malassezia furfur*.

▼ The most common topical fungal infections are candidal infections such as yeast infections.

▼ One of the most common topical viral infections is herpes simplex types 1 and 2.

▼ Topical anaesthetics are used to numb the skin.

▼ Indications for topical anaesthetics include insect bites, sunburn, poison ivy, and before painful injections.

▼ Corticosteroids are some of the most widely used topical drugs that are indicated for relief of topical inflammatory and pruritic disorders.

▼ Beneficial effects of corticosteroids include anti-inflammatory, antipruritic, and vasoconstrictor actions.

▼ Topical antineoplastics are used to treat basal cell carcinomas and various skin lesions that are believed to be premalignant.

▼ Adverse and toxic reactions to dermatological agents can and do occur; therefore these agents should be administered cautiously and the physician's orders and manufacturer's guidelines followed.

▼ Client education about the medication, its administration, and its effectiveness is important to ensure adherence.

EXAMINATION REVIEW QUESTIONS

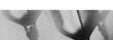

1 Which of the following drugs is considered to be one of the most potent topical corticosteroids?
  a. betamethasone valerate 0.1 percent
  b. desonide
  c. hydrocortisone valerate
  d. betamethasone dipropionate 0.05 percent

2 Skin penetration and potency of topical agents is often enhanced by which of the following?
  a. Application to a clean and dry area
  b. Use of only water-based gel
  c. Vigorous and thick application
  d. Vehicle containing the steroid

3 Allergic reactions to topical bacitracin and similar anti-infectives include which of the following?
  a. Petechia
  b. Hair loss
  c. Redness
  d. Ototoxicity

4 Client teaching about lindane should include which of the following statements?
  a. Apply at least 1.25 cm of ointment five times per day.
  b. Creams or lotions are usually left on for 12 hours.
  c. Therapeutic results may take up to four months after treatments begin.
  d. Use gloves or a tongue blade to apply a thin film, as ordered.

5 Which of the following is one of the most common reactions or side effects to tretinoin?
  a. Inflammation
  b. Antiparasitic
  c. Anthelmintic
  d. Emesis

For answers see http://evolve.elsevier.com/Lilley/pharmacology/.

CRITICAL THINKING ACTIVITIES

1 Develop a teaching plan for a 29-year-old mother who has a six-year-old child newly diagnosed with head lice. Include an emphasis on how to prevent future episodes and contaminating others.

2 Would you consider tretinoin therapy beneficial for all clients? Why or why not? Support your answer.

3 Discuss the major functions of the epidermis that make its intactness so important to homeostasis.

For answers see http://evolve.elsevier.com/Lilley/pharmacology/.

BIBLIOGRAPHY

Albanese, J., & Nutz, P. (2005). *Mosby's 2005 nursing drug cards.* St Louis, MO: Mosby.

Canadian Pharmacists Association. (2003). *Therapeutic choices* (4th ed.). Ottawa, ON: Author.

Canadian Pharmacists Association. (2004). *Guide to drugs in Canada.* Toronto, ON: Dorling Kindersley.

Canadian Pharmacists Association. (2005). *Compendium of pharmaceuticals and specialties. The Canadian drug reference for health professionals.* Ottawa, ON: Author. [The subscription-based e-CPS is available at http://www.pharmacists.ca.]

Cheng, A., Williams, B.A., & Sivarajan, B.V. (Eds.). (2003). *The HSC handbook of pediatrics* (10th ed.). Toronto, ON: Elsevier.

Facts and Comparisons. (2004). *Drug facts and comparisons pocket version* (9th ed.). St Louis, MO: Wolters Kluwer Health.

Health Canada. (2005). Drug product database (DPD). Retrieved September 10, 2005, from http://www.hc-sc.gc.ca/hpb/drugs-dpd/

Infectious Diseases and Immunization Committee, Canadian Paediatric Society. (2004). Head lice infestations: A clinical update. *Paediatrics & Child Health, 9*(9), 647–651.

Indian and Inuit Health Committee, Canadian Paediatric Society. (2001). Scabies management. *Paediatrics & Child Health, 6*(110), 775–777.

Lacy, C.F., Armstrong, L.L., Goldman, M.P., & Lance, L.L. (2003). *Drug information handbook* (11th ed.). Hudson, OH: Lexi-Comp.

McKenry, L.M., & Salerno, E. (2003). *Mosby's pharmacology in nursing–revised and updated* (21st ed.). St Louis, MO: Mosby.

Mosby. (2005). *Mosby's drug consult 2005: The comprehensive reference for generic and brand name drugs* (15th ed.). St Louis, MO: Mosby.

Skidmore-Roth, L. (2006). *Mosby's 2006 nursing drug reference* (19th ed.). St Louis, MO: Mosby.

Weinstein, G.D., Koo, J.Y., & Krueger, G.G. (2003). Tazarotene cream in the treatment of psoriasis: Two multicenter, double-blind, randomized, vehicle-controlled studies of the safety and efficacy of tazarotene creams 0.05% and 0.1% applied once daily for 12 weeks. *Journal of the American Academy of Dermatology, 48,* 760–767.

56 Ophthalmic Agents

OBJECTIVES

After reading this chapter, the successful student will be able to do the following:

1 Discuss the anatomy and physiology of the structures of the eye and how it is influenced by glaucoma and other disorders of the eye.

2 List the various ophthalmic agents and their classifications.

3 Discuss the mechanisms of action, indications, side effects, cautions, and contraindications of ophthalmic preparations.

4 Develop a nursing care plan related to the nursing process for clients receiving ophthalmic agents.

e-LEARNING ACTIVITIES

Student CD-ROM
- Review Questions: see questions 397–398
- Animations
- Medication Administration Checklists
- IV Therapy Checklists

evolve **Web site** (http://evolve.elsevier.com/Lilley/pharmacology/)
- Online Chapter Worksheet • Frequently Asked Questions
- Learning Tips and Content Updates • WebLinks • Online Appendices and Supplements • Mosby/Saunders ePharmacology Update • Access to *Mosby's Drug Consult*

DRUG PROFILES

acetazolamide, p. 958	▶▶ciprofloxacin, p. 963
acetylcholine, p. 953	cromolyn, p. 967
apraclonidine, p. 955	cyclopentolate, p. 967
▶▶artificial tears, p. 967	▶▶dexamethasone, p. 965
▶▶atropine sulfate, p. 967	▶▶dipivefrin, p. 955
▶▶bacitracin, p. 962	▶▶dorzolamide, p. 958
▶▶betaxolol, p. 956	▶▶erythromycin, p. 962
brinzolamide, p. 958	fluorescein, p. 967
chloramphenicol, p. 963	flurbiprofen, p. 965

ganciclovir, p. 963	mannitol, p. 959
▶▶gentamicin, p. 961	▶▶pilocarpine, p. 954
hyperosmolar sodium chloride, p. 968	▶▶sulfacetamide, p. 963
	tetracaine, p. 967
ketorolac, p. 966	▶▶timolol, p. 956
▶▶latanoprost, p. 960	trifluridine p. 963

▶▶ Key drug.

GLOSSARY

Accommodation The state or process of adapting or adjusting one thing or set of things to another. In ophthalmology, accommodation refers to the adjustment of the eye to variation in distance; the elasticity of the lens allows it to change shape and focusing power.

Angle-closure glaucoma (glaw ko' muh) Glaucoma that occurs if the pupil in an eye with a narrow angle between the iris and cornea dilates markedly, causing the folded iris to block the exit of aqueous humor through the canal of Schlemm. When acute, can cause rapid loss of eyesight due to elevated intra-ocular pressure. Also called *closed-angle glaucoma, narrow-angle glaucoma, congestive glaucoma,* and *pupillary closure glaucoma.*

Anterior chamber   The bubble-like portion of the front of the eye between the iris and the cornea.

Aqueous humor   (ay' kwee əs hyoo' mər) The clear, watery fluid circulating in the anterior and posterior chambers of the eye.

Canal of Schlemm   A tiny circular vein at the angle of the anterior chamber of the eye that connects with the pectinate villi, draining the aqueous humor and funneling it into the bloodstream. Also called *Schlemm's canal*.

Cataract   (kat' ə rakt) An abnormal progressive condition of the lens of the eye, characterized by loss of transparency. A grey-white opacity can be seen within the lens. If cataracts are untreated, sight is eventually lost. At onset, vision is blurred, then bright lights glare diffusely and distortion and double vision may develop.

Ciliary muscle   The circular muscle between the anterior and posterior chambers behind the iris. It acts to change the shape of the lens in visual accommodation and is controlled by the parasympathetic nervous system (PSNS) through the oculomotor cranial nerve (CN-III). The structure that contains and supports this muscle is called the *ciliary body*.

Cones   Photoreceptive (light-receiving) cells in the retina of the eye that enable a person to visualize colours and that play a large role in central (straight-ahead) vision.

Cornea   (kor' nee ə) The convex, transparent anterior part of the eye. It is non-vascular and allows light to pass through it to the lens.

Cycloplegia   (sy' klo plee' jyuh) Paralysis of the ciliary muscles, which prevents the accommodation of the lens to variations in distance. Certain ophthalmic drugs are used to induce cycloplegia to allow examination of the eye.

Cycloplegics   (sy' klo plee' jiks) Drugs that paralyze the ciliary muscles of the eye.

Dilator muscle   (dy' layt ər) A muscle that contracts the iris of the eye and dilates the pupil. It is composed of radiating fibres, like spokes of a wheel, that converge from the circumference of the iris toward the centre. The sympathetic nervous system controls this muscle. Also called *dilator pupillae*.

Glaucoma   (glaw ko' muh) An abnormal condition of elevated pressure within an eye because of obstruction of the outflow of aqueous humor.

Lens   The transparent, crystalline, curved structure of the eye that is located directly behind the iris and the pupil and attached to the ciliary body by ligaments.

Lysozyme   (ly' so zyme) An enzyme with antiseptic actions that destroys some foreign organisms. It is normally present in tears, saliva, sweat, and breast milk.

Miotics   (my o' tiks) Drugs that constrict the pupil.

Mydriatics   (mid ree a' tics) Drugs that dilate the pupil.

Open-angle glaucoma   (glaw ko' muh) A type of glaucoma that is often bilateral, develops slowly, and is genetically determined. Pathological changes in the tissues in or near the canal of Schlemm create the obstruction that prevents outflow of aqueous humor, but the angle between the iris and cornea is not closed off as in angle-closure glaucoma (see *angle-closure glaucoma*). It occurs more commonly than angle-closure glaucoma. Open-angle glaucoma is also called *chronic glaucoma*, *wide-angle glaucoma*, and *simple glaucoma*.

Ophthalmoscopic examination   (off thal' mə skop' ik) An eye examination using an *ophthalmoscope*, a device that includes a light, a mirror with a single hole through which the examiner may look, and a dial holding several lenses of varying strengths.

Posterior chamber   The part of the eye behind the iris but in front of the vitreous body. Includes the lens and its suspensory ligaments, as well as aqueous humor.

Pupil   A circular opening in the iris of the eye, located slightly to the nasal side of the centre of the iris. The pupil lies behind the anterior chamber of the eye and the cornea and in front of the lens. Its diameter changes with contraction and relaxation of the muscular fibres of the iris as the eye responds to changes in light, emotional states, and other kinds of stimulation. The pupil is the window of the eye through which light passes to the lens and the retina.

Rods   The tiny cylindrical photoreceptive elements arranged perpendicularly to the surface of the retina. Rods are especially sensitive in low-intensity light and are responsible for black-and-white and peripheral vision.

Sphincter muscle   (sfingk' ter) A circular band of muscle fibres that constricts a passage or closes a natural opening in the body, such as the sphincter pupillae. The sphincter pupillae is a muscle that expands the iris, narrowing the diameter of the pupil of the eye. The PSNS controls this muscle.

Tears   Watery saline or alkaline fluid secreted by the lacrimal glands to moisten the conjunctiva (see Figure 56-1). It is isotonic and contains an enzyme called *lysozyme*. Tears are also called *dacrya*.

Uvea   (yoo' vee uh) The fibrous tunic beneath the sclera that includes the iris, the ciliary body, and the choroid of the eye (see Figure 56-1). Also called *tunica vasculosa bulbi* or *uveal tract*.

Vitreous humor   (vit' ree əs) A transparent, semi-gelatinous substance contained in a thin membrane filling the cavity behind the crystalline lens of the eye. Also called the *corpus vitreum* or *vitreous body*.

STRUCTURE OF THE EYE

To thoroughly understand the agents used to treat disorders of the eye, it is necessary to understand the structure and normal function of the eye. The eye is the organ responsible for the sense of sight. Figure 56-1 illustrates the structures of the eye, all of which are needed for accurate eyesight. Each eyeball is nearly spherical and approximately $2\frac{1}{2}$ cm in diameter. Each eye is recessed into a skull cavity, one of the frontal orbits of the skull. The exposed

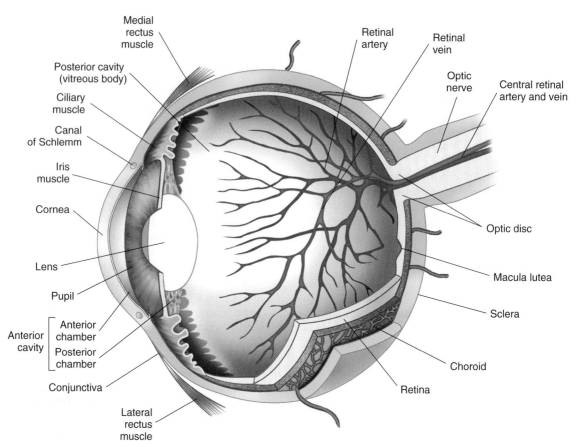

FIG. 56-1 A horizontal section through the left eyeball, looking from the top down. (Modified from Thibodeau, G.A., & Patton, K.T. (2003). *Anatomy and physiology* (5th ed.). St Louis, MO: Mosby.)

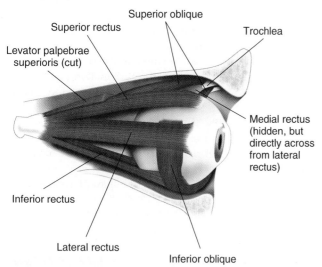

FIG. 56-2 Extrinsic muscles of the right eye. Lateral view. (Modified from Thibodeau, G.A., & Patton, K.T. (2003). *Anatomy and physiology* (5th ed.). St Louis, MO: Mosby.)

Each eye is held in place and moved by six muscles that are controlled by cranial nerves. These muscles include the rectus and oblique muscles. There are four types of rectus muscles: inferior, superior, medial, and lateral. There are two types of oblique muscles: inferior and superior. These muscles are shown in Figure 56-2. (The medial rectus muscle, directly across from the lateral rectus muscle, is hidden from view.) There are several other important structures that are either part of or adjacent to the eye.

- *Eyebrow:* Rows of short hair above (superior) the upper eyelids. The eyebrow protects the eye from direct light, falling dust or other small particles, and perspiration coming from the forehead.
- *Eyelid:* The layer of muscle and skin lined by the conjunctiva. The eyelid is movable and can open or close. It protects the eye when closed and allows for vision when open. The eyelid is raised by contraction of the levator palpebrae superioris muscle, which sits above the superior rectus muscle (see Figure 56-2).
- *Eyelashes:* Two or three rows of hairs that are located on the edge (margin) of the eyelids. They help prevent small particles from falling into the eye when it is open.
- *Palpebral fissure:* The space between the upper and lower eyelids when the eyelids are open.

anterior (front) portion of the eye is covered by three layers: the protective external layer (**cornea** and sclera), middle layer (choroid, iris, and ciliary body), and the internal layer (light-sensitive retina). All of these layers are protected by the eyelid, an external protection device.

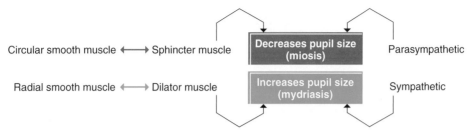

FIG. 56-3 Different nervous systems control pupil size.

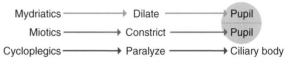

FIG. 56-4 Drug classes and their effects on pupil size.

- *Sclera:* A tough white coat of fibrous tissue that surrounds the entire eyeball except for the cornea; it helps to maintain the shape of the eye. Commonly called the *white of the eye.*
- *Choroid:* One of the middle-layer structures of the eyeball, which contains the blood vessels that supply the eye.
- *Conjunctiva:* The mucous membrane that lines the eyelids and covers the exposed surface of the eyeball.
- *Iris:* The coloured (pigmented) muscular apparatus behind the cornea.
- *Pupil:* The variable-sized opening in the centre of the iris that allows light to enter into the eyeball when the eyelids are open.
- *Medial canthus:* The site of union near the nose for the upper and lower eyelids.
- *Lacrimal caruncle:* A small, red, rounded elevation covered by modified skin at the medial angle of the eye.
- *Lateral canthus:* The site of union away from the nose for the upper and lower eyelids.

LACRIMAL GLANDS

The eye is kept moist and healthy by an intricate network of connected canals, ducts, and sacs that work together. The lacrimal glands produce tears that bathe and cleanse the exposed anterior portion of the eye. **Tears** are composed of an isotonic, aqueous solution that contains an enzyme called **lysozyme**, which acts as an antibacterial to help prevent eye infections.

LAYERS OF THE EYE

The fibrous outer layer of the eye has two parts: the sclera and the cornea. The sclera is a tough, fibrous layer that protects and maintains the shape of the eye. The cornea is a non-vascular transparent portion of the outer layer that allows light to enter the eye. It is located at the extreme front of the eye and is continuous with the sclera. It is pain sensitive and obtains nutrition from the **aqueous humor**, the clear watery fluid that circulates in the anterior and posterior chambers of the eye.

The vascular middle layer of the eye is composed of the anterior iris, ciliary body, and posterior choroid. These three structures are collectively called the **uvea**. The iris gives colour to the eye and has an adjustable-sized opening in the centre called the **pupil**. The main function of the iris is to regulate the amount of light that enters the eye by causing the size of the pupil to vary. Pupil size is controlled by a circular smooth muscle called the **sphincter muscle** and a radial smooth muscle called the **dilator muscle**. The circular muscle decreases pupil size and the radial muscle increases pupil size. The parasympathetic nervous system (PSNS) innervates the sphincter muscles, whereas the sympathetic nervous system (SNS) controls the dilator muscle (Figure 56-3).

The anterior portion of the retina and choroid becomes the ciliary body, which produces aqueous humor. The aqueous humor is removed from the **anterior chamber** via the **canal of Schlemm**. The choroid is a thin dark layer that lines most of the internal side of the sclera. The function of the choroid is to absorb light and prevent its reflection out of the eye.

The **lens** is the transparent crystalline structure of the eye, located directly behind the iris and the pupil. It has a biconvex (oval) shape and is held in place by ligaments that are attached to the ciliary body. Accordingly the lens divides the interior of the eyeball into posterior (back) and anterior (forward) chambers. The larger chamber behind the lens is filled with a jelly-like fluid called the **vitreous humor**.

The transparent lens is composed of uniform layers of protein fibres that are encased by a clear connective tissue capsule. A loss of lens transparency results in a visual condition called a **cataract**. Before light images reach the retina, they are focused into a sharp image by the biconvex lens of the eye. The elasticity of the lens enables it to change its shape and focusing power. This process is called **accommodation** and is facilitated by the ciliary body. Paralysis of accommodation is called **cycloplegia**.

Mydriatics (e.g., atropine) are drugs that dilate the pupil. Agents that constrict the pupil (e.g., acetylcholine, pilocarpine) are called **miotics**. Drugs that paralyze the ciliary body (e.g., atropine, cyclopentolate) are called **cycloplegics**, but they also have mydriatic properties (Figure 56-4).

The retinal layer of the eye is a thin delicate layer that contains light-sensitive receptors. It is internal relative to the choroid and is attached to the optic nerve near its centre. The basic function of the retina is image formation

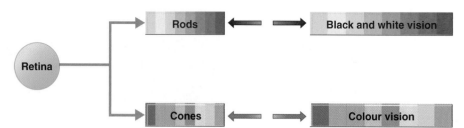

FIG. 56-5 Function of rods and cones in relation to colour vision.

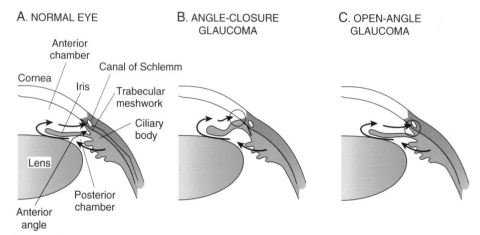

FIG. 56-6 Main structures of the eye and an enlargement of the canal of Schlemm showing an aqueous flow. **A,** Normal eye. **B,** In angle-closure glaucoma, the closure of the anterior angle prevents aqueous humor from exiting through the canal of Schlemm, leading to increased intra-ocular pressure. **C,** In open-angle glaucoma, the anterior angle remains open, but the canal of Schlemm is obstructed by tissue abnormalities. (Modified from McKenry, L.M., & Salerno, E. (2003). *Mosby's pharmacology in nursing–revised and updated* (21st ed.). St Louis, MO: Mosby.)

via light-sensitive receptors called **rods** and **cones.** Both types of photoreceptors are located near the surface of the retina. Rods produce black and white vision, including shades of grey, especially in low light, and cones are responsible for colour vision (Figure 56-5). Additionally, rods are more active in providing peripheral (to the side) vision, whereas cones are more active in central (straight-ahead) vision. The function of the attached optic nerve is to connect the retina with the visual centre of the brain, located within the occipital lobe that extends above and behind the cerebellum.

This chapter focuses on the drugs used to treat disorders of the eye, which can be divided into three major groups: antiglaucoma agents, mydriatic and cycloplegic agents, and anti-infective and anti-inflammatory agents. In addition to the three principal types of drugs are several miscellaneous types of eye products, including enzymes, irrigating solutions, eye washes, and hyperosmolar preparations.

ANTIGLAUCOMA DRUGS

The aqueous humor is a nourishing liquid that is produced by the ciliary body and flows from the **posterior chamber** (behind the iris) to the anterior chamber (in front of the iris). It is removed via the canal of Schlemm, which is located adjacent to the union of the sclera and cornea in the anterior chamber. When the normal flow and drainage of aqueous humor is inhibited, a serious ocular condition called **glaucoma** occurs. Figure 56-6 illustrates the main structures of the eye and an enlargement of the canal of Schlemm showing aqueous flow.

Glaucoma is an eye disorder characterized by excessive intra-ocular pressure (IOP) created by abnormally elevated levels of aqueous humor. This occurs when the aqueous humor is not drained through the canal of Schlemm as quickly as it is formed by the ciliary body. The accumulated aqueous humor creates a backward pressure that pushes the vitreous humor against the retina. Continued pressure on the retina destroys its neurons, leading to impaired vision and eventual blindness (Figure 56-7). Unfortunately, glaucoma is often without early symptoms and therefore many people are not diagnosed until some permanent sight loss has occurred. An estimated 300 000 Canadians have glaucoma, the second most common cause of blindness in Canada. The incidence of glaucoma is three times as high among Blacks as whites. In addition, it has been shown that Blacks and whites may respond differently to particular surgical treatments for glaucoma. Glaucoma is classified according to underlying cause. The three main

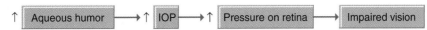

FIG. 56-7 How increased aqueous humor can result in impaired vision. *IOP,* Intra-ocular pressure.

↑ Aqueous humor → ↑ IOP → ↑ Pressure on retina → Impaired vision

TABLE 56-1

GLAUCOMA: TYPES AND CHARACTERISTICS

	Chronic Open-Angle	Acute Angle-Closure
Nature of angle	Large	Narrow
Most common age of onset and race	>50 yr Black	>50 yr white
Major symptoms	Blurred vision, occasional headaches	Blurred vision, severe headaches, eye pain
Treatment	Topical or systemic drugs, surgery	Topical or systemic drugs, surgery

TABLE 56-2

ANTIGLAUCOMA DRUG EFFECTS ON AQUEOUS HUMOR

Drug Class	Increased Drainage	Decreased Production
MIOTICS		
Direct-acting parasympathomimetic	+++	0
OTHERS		
Sympathomimetic	++	+++
Beta-blockers	+	+++
Carbonic anhydrase inhibitors	0	+++
Osmotic diuretics	+++	0
Prostaglandin agonist	+++	0

categories are primary, secondary, and congenital glaucoma (Table 56-1).

Effective treatment of glaucoma involves reducing IOP by either increasing the drainage of aqueous humor or decreasing its production. Some drugs may do both. Effective drug therapy can delay and possibly even prevent the development of glaucoma. Drugs used to reduce IOP include the following:

- Beta-blockers
- Carbonic anhydrase inhibitors
- Osmotic diuretics
- Parasympathomimetics, direct-acting
- Prostaglandins
- Sympathomimetics

See Table 56-2 for a comparison of drug effects on aqueous humor flow.

PARASYMPATHOMIMETICS

The direct-acting parasympathomimetic drugs work to mimic the PSNS neurotransmitter acetylcholine (ACh). In the eye they cause miosis (pupillary constriction). For this reason they are also called *miotics*. They lower IOP by an average of 20 to 30 percent. Examples of ophthalmic drugs that fall into this drug category include acetylcholine, carbachol, and pilocarpine.

Mechanism of Action and Drug Effects

The direct-acting miotics are able to directly stimulate PSNS receptors because their structures closely resemble that of the PSNS neurotransmitter ACh. Direct-acting miotics are administered topically to the eye. This route of administration drastically limits systemic absorption of the drug by keeping the cholinergic effects localized. The cholinergic response produced by these drugs causes pupillary contraction (miosis), which leads to a reduction

of IOP secondary to an increased outflow of aqueous humor (Figure 56-8).

ACh is the endogenous mediator of nerve impulses in the PSNS. It stimulates cholinergic receptors. This results in several effects in the eye: miosis, vasodilation, contraction of **ciliary muscles**, and reduced IOP (see Figure 56-9). The action of ACh is short lived. It is rapidly hydrolyzed by cholinesterases (AChE and pseudocholinesterase) to choline and acetic acid. Direct-acting miotics have effects similar to those of ACh, but their actions are more prolonged (Figure 56-10).

The drug effects of direct-acting miotics alter various eye muscles, IOP, aqueous humor flow, and vasodilation of blood vessels in and around the eye. The drug effects that alter the muscles of the eye result in contraction of the iris sphincter, which produces constriction of the pupil (miosis) and contraction of the ciliary muscle, resulting in spasm (paralysis) of visual accommodation by the lens.

Drug-induced pressure alterations within the eye act to reduce IOP in both normal and glaucomatous eyes. They do this by facilitating aqueous humor outflow by causing contraction of the ciliary muscle, thus widening the area from which this fluid escapes. IOP is also reduced by constriction of the pupil, which causes the iris to stretch and thus relieves blockage of the area where the fluid leaves the inner eye. This effect is less pronounced in individuals with dark eyes (brown or hazel) than in those with light eyes (blue) because the pigment absorbs the drugs and dark eyes have more pigment.

Miotic agents also cause vasodilation of blood vessels of the conjunctiva, iris, and ciliary body, resulting in increased permeability of the blood–aqueous barrier—an anatomic mechanism that normally prevents exchange of fluids between eye chambers and the blood. This effect may lead to vascular congestion and ocular inflammation.

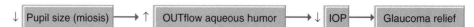

FIG. 56-8 The therapeutic effects of direct-acting parasympathomimetics on glaucoma. *IOP,* Intra-ocular pressure.

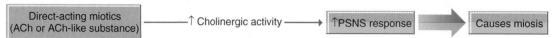

FIG. 56-9 Cholinergic response of miosis to parasympathomimetics. *ACh,* Acetylcholine; *PSNS,* parasympathetic nervous system.

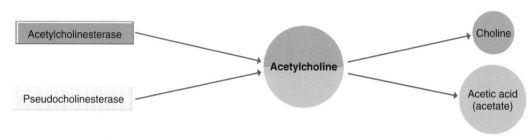

FIG. 56-10 Metabolism of acetylcholine by endogenous enzymes.

Indications

The direct-acting miotics are used for **open-angle glaucoma**, **angle-closure glaucoma**, ocular surgery, convergent strabismus (condition where one eye points toward the other ["cross-eye"]), and ophthalmologic examinations. The miotics are used topically on the eye to reduce elevated IOP by contraction of the ciliary muscle and widening of the exit route of the aqueous humor. Acute (congestive) angle-closure glaucoma may be relieved temporarily by pilocarpine or occasionally by carbachol to acutely decrease extremely high IOP.

Some of the miotic drugs may be used for ocular surgery. Pilocarpine, carbachol, and acetylcholine are used to reduce IOP and to protect the lens by causing miosis before certain types of laser surgery on the iris. Miotics may be used to counteract the mydriatic effects (dilation effects) of sympathomimetic agents such as phenylephrine used for **ophthalmoscopic examinations**. Table 56-3 lists the miotic drugs and their indications.

Contraindications

Contraindications of miotics include known drug allergy and any serious active eye disorder with which induction of miosis might be harmful. An ophthalmologist will usually make this judgement.

Side Effects and Adverse Effects

Most of the side effects and adverse effects associated with the use of the cholinergic drugs (miotics) are local and limited to the eye. Some systemic effects can occur, however, especially if sufficient amounts of drug pass into the bloodstream (see Table 56-4).

The most common ocular side effects are blurred vision, accommodative spasms, and temporary stinging on instillation. Other undesirable effects include conjunctivitis, lacrimation (watering eyes), twitching eyelids, poor low-light vision, and pain. Prolonged use can result in iris cysts, lens opacities, and, rarely, retinal detachment.

Systemic effects are caused by PSNS stimulation. The most common include bronchodilation, nausea, vomiting, salivation, sweating, gastrointestinal (GI) stimulation, and urinary incontinence.

Toxicity and Management of Overdose

Occasionally toxic effects may develop after the use of topically applied miotic drugs. Toxicity produced by miotics is an extension of their systemic effects and is more common with prolonged use of high doses. Excessive PSNS effects are treated with 0.4 to 2 mg of atropine administered intravenously or intramuscularly for adults and 0.04 to 0.08 mg/kg administered intravenously or intramuscularly for children. If required, repeat doses can be given every five minutes intravenously and every 15 minutes intramuscularly.

Interactions

Direct-acting miotics are capable of interactions with several categories of drugs. The miotic drugs, when given with topical epinephrine, timolol, and carbonic anhydrase inhibitors, have additive lowering effects on IOP.

TABLE 56-3
MIOTICS: INDICATIONS

Miotic Agent	Indications
acetylcholine	Complete and rapid miosis after cataract lens extraction, penetrating keratopathy (corneal graft), or iridectomy (excision of a portion of the iris)
carbachol	Open-angle glaucoma
pilocarpine	Open-angle glaucoma, secondary glaucoma after iridectomy, cycloplegic reversal, symptoms of xerophthalmia (dry eyes) in Sjögren's syndrome

TABLE 56-4
MIOTICS: ADVERSE EFFECTS

Body System	Side/Adverse Effects
Cardiovascular	Hypotension, bradycardia, or tachycardia
Central nervous	Headache
Eye, ear, nose, throat	Visual blurring, myopia (nearsightedness), ciliary spasm, brow pain
Gastrointestinal	Nausea, vomiting, abdominal cramps, diarrhea
Respiratory	May precipitate asthma attacks

DOSAGES Autonomic Nervous System Ophthalmic Agents

Agent	Pharmacological Class	Usual Dosage Range	Indications
Selected Miotics (Parasympathomimetics)			
acetylcholine	Direct-acting	>0.5 to 2 mL pre-op	Surgical miosis
▶▶**pilocarpine**	Direct-acting	Solution: 1–2 drops qid Gel: 0.5 inch into lower conjunctival sac at bedtime (use any other eye drops at least 5 min before gel)	Chronic open-angle and angle-closure glaucoma; acute angle-closure glaucoma; pre- and post-op intra-ocular hypertension; reversal of drug-induced mydriasis
Selected Sympathomimetics			
apraclonidine	Direct-acting	0.5% solution: 1–2 drops tid 1% solution: 1 drop in eye pre-op	Short-term adjunctive therapy for glaucoma not controlled with other drugs Anterior segment laser surgery
▶▶**dipivefrin**	Direct-acting	1 drop q12h	Chronic open-angle glaucoma, ocular hypertension
Selected Beta-Blockers			
▶▶**betaxolol**	Direct-acting	1–2 drops bid	Chronic open-angle glaucoma; ocular hypertension
▶▶**timolol**	Direct-acting	Solution: 1 drop bid Gel-forming solution: 1 drop/day	Open-angle glaucoma; ocular hypertension

Systemic cholinesterase inhibitors have additive effects when given with mitotic drugs.

Dosages

For recommended dosages of miotic agents, see the dosages table above. See Appendix B for some of the common brands available in Canada.

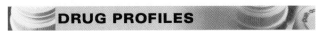

DRUG PROFILES

DIRECT-ACTING MIOTICS (DIRECT-ACTING OPHTHALMIC PARASYMPATHOMIMETICS)

Direct-acting miotics have a variety of uses. The principal use is that of relief of symptoms caused by glaucoma and increased IOP. The three most commonly used direct-acting miotics are acetylcholine, carbachol, and pilocarpine. These drugs have actions similar to those of ACh. Because the safe use of miotics in pregnancy has not been established, many of the miotics are classified as pregnancy category C agents.

Direct-acting miotic drugs are contraindicated in clients who have shown a hypersensitivity reaction to them, those with acute inflammatory conditions in the anterior chamber, and those with pupillary block glaucoma.

acetylcholine

Acetylcholine is a direct-acting parasympathomimetic agent that is used to produce miosis during ophthalmic surgery. It is a pharmaceutical form of the naturally occurring neurotransmitter in the body. It has quick onset and may begin to work almost immediately. When used for ophthalmic indications, acetylcholine is administered directly into the anterior chamber of the eye before and after securing one or more sutures. It is available as a 10- and 20-mg powder for intra-ocular use only. Commonly recommended dosages for acetylcholine are listed in the dosages table on p. 953.

PHARMACOKINETICS

Half-Life	Onset	Peak	Duration
Short	Instant	Instant	10 min

▸▸ *pilocarpine*

Pilocarpine is a direct-acting parasympathomimetic agent that is used as a miotic in the treatment of glaucoma. Pilocarpine is available in many different formulations and strengths.

Pilocarpine is available as 1 percent, 2 percent, 4 percent, and 6 percent ophthalmic solutions. Commonly recommended dosages for pilocarpine are listed in the dosages table on p. 953.

PHARMACOKINETICS

Half-Life	Onset	Peak	Duration
Unknown	10–30 min	75 min	4–8 hr

SYMPATHOMIMETICS

Sympathomimetic drugs such as brimonidine, apraclonidine, dipivefrin, and epinephrine are used for the treatment of glaucoma and ocular hypertension. Dipivefrin is a pro-drug of epinephrine. When instilled into the eye it is hydrolyzed to epinephrine. Its advantage over epinephrine is that it has enhanced lipophilicity (fat solubility) and can better penetrate into the tissues of the anterior chamber of the eye. Per weight, dipivefrin is 4 to 11 times as potent as epinephrine in reducing IOP and 5 to 12 times as potent in pupil dilation (mydriasis). Apraclonidine and brimonidine are structurally and pharmacologically related to clonidine. Apraclonidine is relatively selective for alpha$_2$ receptors.

Because these drugs are sympathomimetic agents, they mimic the sympathetic neurotransmitters norepinephrine and epinephrine and stimulate the dilator muscle to contract. This stimulation results in increased pupil size (mydriasis, illustrated in Figure 56-11). Dilation is seen within minutes of instillation of the ophthalmic drops and lasts for several hours, during which time the IOP is reduced. This occurs secondary to either enhanced outflow or decreased production of aqueous humor, which is also a drug-related effect.

Mechanism of Action and Drug Effects

These agents reduce IOP in clients with normal IOP and in clients with elevated IOP, such as those with glaucoma. Dipivefrin 0.1 percent reduces mean IOP by approximately 15 to 25 percent. The exact mechanism by which the sympathomimetic drugs lower IOP is unknown. They are believed to work by stimulating both alpha$_2$ and beta$_2$ receptors, causing the dilator muscle to contract, resulting in mydriasis. During mydriasis there is an increase in aqueous humor outflow, resulting in a decrease in IOP (Figure 56-12). These effects appear to be dose dependent.

Apraclonidine reduces IOP by 23 to 39 percent. By stimulating alpha$_2$ and beta$_2$ receptors, apraclonidine prevents constriction of the blood vessels of the eye and reduces pressure, resulting in reduced aqueous humor formation. Brimonidine works in a similar fashion to apraclonidine.

Dipivefrin is a more lipophilic agent and therefore has more localized effects in the eye. However, both dipivefrin and epinephrine can cause drug effects outside the eye. Because these two drugs mimic the effects of the SNS neurotransmitters, they can cause increased cardiovascular effects such as increased heart rate or blood pressure.

Indications

Both epinephrine and dipivefrin may be used to reduce elevated IOP in the treatment of chronic, open-angle glaucoma, either as initial therapy or as chronic therapy.

Apraclonidine is primarily used to inhibit perioperative IOP increases. Increases in IOP during ophthalmic

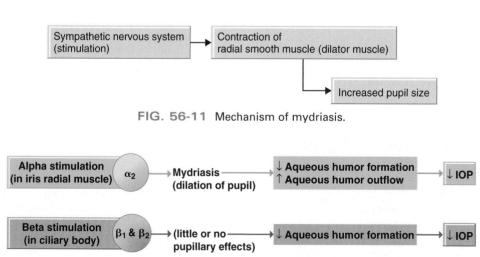

FIG. 56-11 Mechanism of mydriasis.

FIG. 56-12 Ocular effects of alpha (α) and beta (β) stimulation.

surgery are usually mediated via increased catecholamine stimulation of the SNS. Apraclonidine stimulates the alpha$_2$ receptors, which oppose these effects, and thus corrects the surgery-induced changes in IOP. Brimonidine is used to lower IOP in clients with open-angle glaucoma or ocular hypertension.

Contraindications

Contraindications for the sympathomimetic ophthalmics include drug allergy and any active, severe ophthalmic problem, which might be aggravated by the effects of these drugs.

Side Effects and Adverse Effects

The side effects and adverse effects of the sympathomimetic mydriatics are primarily limited to ocular effects; however, systemic effects are possible. Ocular side effects are transient and most commonly consist of burning, eye pain, and lacrimation. Other ocular effects are conjunctival hyperemia, localized melanin deposits in the conjunctiva, and released pigment granules from the iris.

Systemic effects are rare but include cardiovascular effects such as extrasystoles, tachycardia, and hypertension. Headache and faintness may also occur.

Toxicity and Management of Overdose

Rare toxic reactions are primarily the result of an extension of the therapeutic and adverse effects of these drugs. The most significant are cardiac dysrhythmias. Discontinuation of the drugs usually alleviates the toxic symptoms.

Interactions

With sufficient topical absorption, sympathomimetic mydriatics have the potential to react with other drugs. Cardiac dysrhythmias are potentiated when mydriatic drugs are given with halogenated anaesthetics, cardiac glycosides, thyroid hormones, or tricyclic antidepressants.

Dosages

For recommended dosages of sympathomimetic agents, see the dosages table on p. 953. See Appendix B for some of the common brands available in Canada.

DRUG PROFILES

Sympathomimetic ophthalmic agents include dipivefrin, epinephrine, apraclonidine, and brimonidine. Brimonidine works similarly to apraclonidine by stimulating primarily alpha$_2$ receptors. Dipivefrin and epinephrine are believed to work by stimulating both alpha$_2$ and beta$_2$ receptors. This stimulation causes the dilator muscle to contract and results in mydriasis. Both alpha and beta receptor stimulation result in reduced IOP by reducing aqueous humor formation. Alpha receptor stimulation is also known to reduce IOP by enhancing aqueous humor outflow through the canal of Schlemm.

Both epinephrine and apraclonidine are classified as pregnancy category C agents. Because of the lipophilicity and limited systemic absorption of dipivefrin, it is classified as a pregnancy category B agent. Brimonidine is also classified as a pregnancy category B agent. These drugs are available only by prescription.

apraclonidine

Apraclonidine is structurally and pharmacologically related to the alpha$_2$ stimulant clonidine. Apraclonidine 1 percent is primarily used to inhibit perioperative IOP increases and in Canada it is restricted to post-laser treatment in clients with glaucoma. Apraclonidine 0.5 percent is used as a short-term adjunctive in lowering intra-ocular pressure for glaucoma. Apraclonidine stimulates alpha$_2$ receptors, which inhibits increases in IOP that occur during ophthalmic surgery. Its use in the treatment of open-angle glaucoma remains to be established. Apraclonidine is currently available as a 0.5 percent and a 1 percent ophthalmic solution. Commonly recommended dosages for apraclonidine are listed in the dosages table on p. 953.

PHARMACOKINETICS

Half-Life	Onset	Peak	Duration
8 hr	1 hr	3–5 hr	12 hr

▸▸ dipivefrin

Dipivefrin is a synthetic sympathomimetic miotic drug. It is a pro-drug of epinephrine. The pro-drug has little or no pharmacological activity until hydrolyzed in the eye to two forms of epinephrine. These chemical alterations allow epinephrine to penetrate into the anterior chamber of the eye. The decrease in IOP is apparently the result of aqueous humor fluid outflow from the anterior chamber of the eye. Dipivefrin is available as a 0.1 percent ophthalmic solution. Commonly recommended dosages for dipivefrin are listed in the dosages table on p. 953.

PHARMACOKINETICS

Half-Life	Onset	Peak	Duration
1–3 hr	30 min	1 hr	12 hr

BETA-ADRENERGIC BLOCKERS

The antiglaucoma beta-adrenergic blockers that reduce IOP include selective beta$_1$- and non-selective beta$_1$- and beta$_2$-blockers. These drugs are believed to work by reducing IOP through reducing aqueous humor formation and increasing its outflow. The most commonly used drugs in this drug class are listed in Table 56-5.

TABLE 56-5

**GLAUCOMA THERAPY:
BETA-ADRENERGIC BLOCKERS**

Class	Beta-Blockers
Selective beta-blocker (beta$_1$)	betaxolol
Non-selective beta-blocker (beta$_1$ and beta$_2$)	levobunolol, timolol

Mechanism of Action and Drug Effects

The ophthalmic beta-blockers reduce both elevated and normal IOP. They do this without affecting pupillary size, accommodation, or night vision. They appear to reduce IOP by reducing aqueous humor formation. In addition, timolol may produce a minimal increase in aqueous outflow.

The drug effects of the ophthalmic beta-blockers are primarily limited to ocular effects; however, occasional systemic effects may occur.

The systemic effects are primarily those associated with the adrenergic blockers as discussed in Chapter 18, specifically systemic pulmonary and cardiovascular effects. Because these drugs are administered topically, few if any systemic effects are expected. These agents have not been shown to affect glucose metabolism as do some of the systemic adrenergic blockers.

Indications

Ophthalmic beta-blockers are used to reduce elevated IOP in various conditions, including chronic open-angle glaucoma and ocular hypertension. They may also be used alone or in combination with a topical miotic (e.g., pilocarpine), topical dipivefrin, and/or systemic carbonic anhydrase inhibitors (CAIs). When used in combination, these agents may have an additive IOP-lowering effect. They may also be used to treat some forms of angle-closure glaucoma.

Contraindications

Contraindications of ophthalmic beta-blockers include known drug allergy and any ocular condition where beta-receptor blockade might do harm.

Side Effects and Adverse Effects

The side effects and adverse effects of antiglaucoma beta-blockers are primarily limited to ocular effects and limited systemic effects. The most common ocular effects are transient burning and discomfort. Other effects include blurred vision, pain, photophobia, lacrimation, blepharitis (inflammation of the eyelids), keratitis (inflammation of the cornea), and decreased corneal sensitivity. The potential but uncommon systemic effects produced by ophthalmic beta-blockers include headache, dizziness, cardiac irregularities, and bronchospasm.

Toxicity and Management of Overdose

Toxic reactions to beta-blockers are rare and primarily involve the cardiovascular system. Symptoms include bradycardia, cardiac failure, hypotension, and bronchospasms. Treatment involves discontinuation of the drug and symptomatic treatment.

Interactions

With sufficient topical absorption, beta-blockers can react with several categories of drugs. Ophthalmic beta-blockers may have additive therapeutic and adverse effects when given with systemically administered beta-blockers. This occurs when high doses of ophthalmic beta-blockers are used and significant systemic absorption occurs. Verapamil, when used with ophthalmic beta-blockers, can have additive adverse effects, resulting in asystole (cardiac arrest).

Dosages

For recommended dosages of beta-adrenergic blockers, see the dosages table on p. 953. See Appendix B for some of the common brands available in Canada.

DRUG PROFILES

The currently available ophthalmic beta-blocking drugs are betaxolol, levobunolol, and timolol. The action of these drugs is reduction of IOP by decreased aqueous humor formation and increased outflow of aqueous humor.

These ophthalmic drugs are classified as pregnancy category C agents and are contraindicated in clients with bronchial asthma, cardiac failure, cardiogenic shock, obstructive breathing disorders, second- or third-degree atrioventricular (AV) block, or sinus bradycardia. They are also contraindicated in clients who have shown a hypersensitivity reaction to them. They are all available only by prescription.

▶▶ *betaxolol*

Betaxolol is a beta$_1$-selective beta-blocker. It is structurally related to the systemic adrenergic beta-receptor blocker metoprolol that is used primarily for cardiovascular disorders. Betaxolol is one of the most potent and selective beta-blocking agents. Its ability to decrease aqueous humor formation and consequently IOP has made it an excellent agent for the treatment of ocular disorders such as open-angle glaucoma and ocular hypertension.

Betaxolol is available as a 0.5 percent ophthalmic solution and a 0.25 percent ophthalmic suspension. Commonly recommended dosages for betaxolol are listed in the dosages table on p. 953.

PHARMACOKINETICS

Half-Life	Onset	Peak	Duration
Unknown	0.5 hr	2 hr	≥12 hr

▶▶ *timolol*

Timolol may differ slightly from the other ophthalmic beta-blockers in that it may increase the outflow of aqueous humor as well as reducing its formation. The drug acts at both beta$_1$ and beta$_2$ receptors and is indicated for the treatment of open-angle glaucoma and ocular hypertension. It is available in 0.25 percent and 0.5 percent ophthalmic solutions. Timolol is also available in a gel-forming solution (with preservatives) in strengths of 0.25 percent and 0.5 percent. These gel-forming products are longer acting and allow for once-daily dosing, a convenience over the twice-daily dosing that many clients require with the other timolol formulations. Many studies for all types of medications have demonstrated that once-daily dosing improves client adherence with drug therapy. Commonly recommended dosages for timolol are listed in the dosages table on p. 953.

PHARMACOKINETICS

Half-Life	Onset	Peak	Duration
Unknown	15–30 min	1–2 hr	12–24 hr

CARBONIC ANHYDRASE INHIBITORS

CAIs include acetazolamide, brinzolamide, dorzolamide, and methazolamide. Brinzolamide and dorzolamide are available only as ophthalmic topical preparations. However, the other two are available in tablet or capsule form for oral use in treating glaucoma. Other indications for acetazolamide, the prototype CAI, include acute mountain sickness that occurs in mountain climbers at high altitudes, edema due to heart failure, drug-induced edema, and certain types of epilepsy. The other CAIs are indicated solely for glaucoma. All four CAIs are able to decrease IOP. Their specific ophthalmic uses include treatment for open-angle, secondary, and angle-closure glaucoma and ocular hypertension.

Historically, acetazolamide has been the most widely used of the CAIs.

Mechanism of Action and Drug Effects

These agents work by inhibiting the enzyme carbonic anhydrase, which exists throughout the body and is involved in acid-base balance. In the eye, however, the inhibition of this enzyme results in decreased IOP through reduced aqueous humor formation. Systemic effects of CAIs, especially when administered orally, include increased renal excretion of water, bicarbonate, and potassium and urinary alkalinization through decreased excretion of ammonia.

Indications

CAIs are used primarily in the treatment of glaucoma. Because they decrease IOP by reducing aqueous humor formation, they are excellent therapeutic agents in the treatment of such ocular disorders as open-angle, secondary, and angle-closure glaucoma before ocular surgery.

Contraindications

As with any medication, contraindications for the CAIs include known prior allergic or other severe adverse drug reaction. Relative contraindications to the CAIs, especially with systemic use, include hyponatremia, hypokalemia, hyperchloremic acidosis, major kidney or liver disease, and adrenocortical (adrenal gland) failure.

Side Effects and Adverse Effects

Because some of the CAIs are administered orally, they can produce systemic side effects and adverse effects. Table 56-6 lists the most common such effects associated

TABLE 56-6

CARBONIC ANHYDRASE INHIBITORS: ADVERSE EFFECTS

Body System	Side/Adverse Effects
Central nervous	Dizziness, drowsiness, headache, confusion, paraesthesia, seizures
Eyes, ears, nose, throat	Transient myopia, tinnitus
Gastrointestinal	Anorexia, vomiting, diarrhea
Genitourinary	Polyuria, hematuria
Integumentary	Urticaria, rare photosensitivity
Metabolic	Acidotic states and electrolyte imbalance with long-term therapy

with CAIs. Clients with sulpha allergies may develop cross-sensitivities to the CAIs.

Toxicity and Management of Overdose

Toxicity associated with the use of CAIs is rare. The mechanism by which these agents work predisposes the client to possible acidotic states and electrolyte imbalances. These toxic reactions generally require only supportive care. This may include the restoration of electrolytes, especially potassium, and the administration of bicarbonate to correct the CAI-induced acidotic state.

Interactions

The systemic use of CAIs can result in several significant drug interactions. CAIs can cause hypokalemia and increase the likelihood of digitalis toxicity. Hypokalemia is also more likely to occur when they are co-administered with corticosteroids and diuretics. CAIs increase renal excretion of lithium and decrease lithium's effects. CAIs increase the drug effects of basic drugs as a result of decreased renal excretion.

Dosages

For recommended dosages of selected CAIs, see the dosages table on p. 958. See Appendix B for some of the common brands available in Canada.

DRUG PROFILES

CAIs are the first class of ophthalmic drugs discussed thus far that can be given orally as well as topically. Currently available CAI products include acetazolamide, brinzolamide, dorzolamide, and methazolamide. Brinzolamide and dorzolamide are available only as ophthalmic drops, whereas the other two are generally used in orally administered tablet or capsule form to treat glaucoma.

All CAIs are classified as pregnancy category C agents and are contraindicated in clients with a history of hypersensitivity reactions to them or in clients with chronic non-congestive angle-closure glaucoma, marked kidney or liver disease, hyperchloremic acidosis, low sodium

DOSAGES Selected Classes of Ophthalmic Agents

Agent	Pharmacological Class	Usual Dosage Range	Indications
Carbonic Anhydrase Inhibitors			
acetazolamide	Carbonic anhydrase inhibitor	PO (tab): 250–1000 mg/day (doses 250 mg divided); 250 mg q4h (short-term acute therapy only)	Chronic open-angle glaucoma; secondary glaucoma and pre-op treatment of acute angle-closure glaucoma
brinzolamide	Carbonic anhydrase inhibitor	One drop bid–tid	Open-angle glaucoma; ocular hypertension
⏩dorzolamide	Carbonic anhydrase inhibitor	One drop tid	Open-angle glaucoma; ocular hypertension
Osmotic Diuretics			
mannitol	Osmotic diuretic	IV: 1.5–2 g/kg over at least 30 min; for pre-op use give 1–1.5 h before surgery	Acute reduction of elevated IOP
Prostaglandin Agonist			
⏩latanoprost	Prostaglandin agonist	One drop/day in evening	Open-angle glaucoma and ocular hypertension; chronic angle-closure glaucoma in iridotomy clients (creating an opening in the iris to relieve IOP) or laser iridoplasty (another operation to provide a bypass of the drainage angle)

IOP, Intra-ocular pressure.

and potassium serum levels, and adrenal gland failure. All CAIs are available only by prescription. The prototype CAI, acetazolamide, is also used as an adjunct anticonvulsant and for treatment of acute mountain sickness. Their ophthalmic uses include open-angle, secondary, and angle-closure glaucoma.

acetazolamide

Acetazolamide is a CAI that is used in the treatment of chronic open-angle glaucoma, secondary glaucoma, and the preoperative treatment of acute angle-closure glaucoma. It is also used for edema associated with heart failure and drug-induced edema. It is available orally as a 500-mg sustained-release capsule and 250-mg tablet. Commonly recommended dosages of acetazolamide for the treatment of glaucoma are listed in the dosages table above.

PHARMACOKINETICS

Half-Life	Onset	Peak	Duration
2.5–6 hr	1–1.5 hr	2–4 hr	8–12 hr

brinzolamide

Brinzolamide is a newer ophthalmic CAI with indications and dosage identical to and pharmacokinetics comparable to dorzolamide. The only notable difference is that it is available in a 1 percent ophthalmic topical suspension. Dosages appear in the dosages table above.

⏩ dorzolamide

Dorzolamide is solely indicated for elevated IOP associated with either ocular hypertension or open-angle glaucoma. It is currently available only as a 2 percent

ophthalmic topical solution. Dosages appear in the dosages table above.

PHARMACOKINETICS

Half-Life	Onset	Peak	Duration
3–4 mo*	Rapid	Variable	Variable

*Due to red blood cell distribution in plasma.

OSMOTIC DIURETICS

Osmotic agents may be administered either intravenously, orally, or topically to reduce IOP. In Canada, the osmotic diuretic most commonly used for this purpose is mannitol.

Mechanism of Action and Drug Effects

Mannitol creates ocular hypotension by producing an osmotic gradient. This causes the blood to become hypertonic in the presence of both intra-ocular and spinal fluids. The gradient forces the water from the aqueous and vitreous humors into the bloodstream, causing a reduction of volume of intra-ocular fluid, which results in a decrease in IOP (Figure 56-13).

Intracranial pressure is also reduced because of the shifting of excess fluid into the bloodstream from cerebrospinal fluid compartments. In the kidney, osmotic diuretics promote diuresis by increasing the osmolarity of the glomerular filtrate, which results in the inhibition of tubular reabsorption and an increase in the renal excretion of electrolytes (Chapter 26).

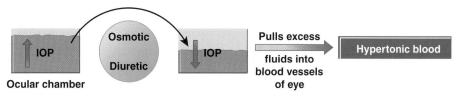

FIG. 56-13 Mechanism and ocular effects of osmotic diuretics.

TABLE 56-7

OSMOTIC DIURETICS (MANNITOL): ADVERSE EFFECTS

Body System	Side/Adverse Effects
Cardiovascular	Edema, thrombophlebitis, hypotension, hypertension, tachycardia, angina-like chest pains, fever, chills
Central nervous	Dizziness, headache, convulsions, rebound increased intracranial pressure, confusion
Electrolytes	Fluid-electrolyte imbalances, acidosis, electrolyte loss, dehydration
Eyes, ears, nose, throat	Loss of hearing, blurred vision, nasal congestion
Gastrointestinal	Nausea, vomiting, dry mouth, diarrhea
Genitourinary	Marked diuresis, urinary retention, thirst

Indications

The therapeutic effectiveness of the osmotic diuretics is the result of the production of hypertonic blood, which causes fluid extraction from various areas. In the brain this is beneficial for the treatment of cerebral edema associated with altitude sickness and other causes such as head trauma. When fluid from the enclosed space of the skull is reduced, pressure is relieved and mountain sickness symptoms subside. In glaucoma, aqueous humor and vitreous humor are extracted from the anterior chamber of the eye and forced into the bloodstream. This reduces IOP. The primary osmotic agent used in ocular disorders is mannitol. It is used primarily to treat acute glaucoma episodes and may be used before or after ocular surgery to reduce IOP.

Contraindications

Mannitol is contraindicated in clients with pronounced anuria, acute pulmonary edema, cardiac decompensation, and severe dehydration. It is also contraindicated in clients who have shown a hypersensitivity to it.

Side Effects and Adverse Effects

The most frequent reactions to mannitol are nausea, vomiting, and headache. The most significant adverse effects are fluid and electrolyte imbalance. Other effects are possible irritation and thrombosis at the injection site. For a list of other possible side effects and adverse effects asso-

ciated with the use of osmotic diuretics such as mannitol, see Table 56-7.

Toxicity and Management of Overdose

Toxic reactions are primarily a result of the hyperosmolarity of the blood. The most significant toxic reactions include hypovolemia (secondary to diuresis), cardiac dysrhythmias, and hyperosmolar non-ketotic coma. Treatment involves discontinuation of the drug and treatment of symptoms with fluids and electrolytes.

Interactions

Increased lithium excretion caused by mannitol is the only significant drug interaction that has been reported.

Dosages

For recommended dosages of mannitol, see the dosages table on p. 958. See Appendix B for some of the common brands available in Canada.

DRUG PROFILES

mannitol

Mannitol is used only by intravenous infusion to reduce elevated IOP when the pressure cannot be lowered by other treatments. Mannitol has been shown to be effective in the treatment of acute episodes of angle-closure, absolute, or secondary glaucoma and for lowering IOP before intra-ocular surgery. Mannitol does not penetrate the eye and may be used when irritation is present. It is available as 10 percent, 20 percent, and 25 percent parenteral injections. It is classified as pregnancy category C. Commonly recommended dosages for mannitol are listed in the dosages table on p. 958.

PHARMACOKINETICS

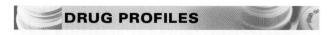

Half-Life	Onset	Peak	Duration
15–100 min	30–60 min	1 hr	6–8 hr

PROSTAGLANDIN AGONISTS

Latanoprost is the most popular of four agents in this newer class of ophthalmic agents used to treat glaucoma. The other three agents are travoprost, bimatoprost, and unoprostone isopropyl. They are all classified as prostaglandin agonists (PAs).

Mechanism of Action and Drug Effects

Latanoprost is a pro-drug of a naturally occurring prostaglandin known as prostaglandin F_2-alpha. When this ester pro-drug is administered, it is converted by hydrolysis (with water from ocular fluids) to F_2-alpha, which in turn reduces IOP. Prostaglandins reduce IOP primarily by increasing the outflow of aqueous fluid, not by decreasing its production. They are believed to increase the outflow of aqueous fluid by increasing uveoscleral outflow in addition to the usual exit through the trabecular meshwork, a filter-like structure within the eye.

A single dose of ocular PAs lowers IOP for 20 to 24 hours, allowing a single daily dosage regimen. One exception is unoprostone isopropyl, which is administered twice daily.

The drug effects of PAs are primarily limited to their effects on the eye. Their primary therapeutic effect is decreased IOP in open-angle glaucoma and ocular hypertension.

Indications

PAs are used in the treatment of glaucoma.

Contraindications

The only usual contraindication to the use of PAs is known drug allergy.

Side Effects and Adverse Effects

PAs are generally well tolerated. Adverse effects reported in clinical trials included foreign body sensation, punctate epithelial keratopathy (dotted appearance of cornea), stinging, conjunctival hyperemia ("bloodshot" eyes), blurred vision, itching, and burning. In controlled clinical trials the incidence of these adverse effects was similar to those seen in clients treated with timolol. Systemic effects occur in a small percentage of clients and include skin reactions, upper respiratory infections, and headache. There is one unique side effect associated with all PAs. In some people with hazel, green, or bluish-brown eye colour, eye colour will permanently turn brown, even if they stop using the medication. This side effect appears to be cosmetic with no known ill effects on the eye. For example, about 3 to 10 percent of clients treated with latanoprost have shown increased iris pigmentation after three to four and a half months of treatment. This iris colour change does not affect IOP readings.

Interactions

Concurrent administration of latanoprost with any other eye drops containing the preservative thimerosal may result in precipitation. It is recommended that the two medications be administered at least five minutes apart.

Dosages

For recommended dosages of latanoprost, see the table on p. 958. See Appendix B for some of the common brands available in Canada.

DRUG PROFILES

▸▸ *latanoprost*

Latanoprost is believed to reduce IOP in glaucoma by increasing aqueous humor outflow. Latanoprost has several positive features, including a single daily dosage regimen, a mechanism of action that enhances the IOP-lowering effect of other agents, and a low incidence of systemic adverse effects. Latanoprost is available as a 0.005 percent (50 μg/mL) ophthalmic solution and is contraindicated in clients who have had a hypersensitivity reaction to it. Pregnancy category C. Dosage information appears in the table on p. 958.

OCULAR ANTI-INFECTIVE DRUGS

Topical anti-infectives used for treating ocular infections include a wide range of antibacterial and antiviral drugs. Many of these drugs are also available for systemic administration. While eye infections can be treated systemically by any available antibiotic appropriate to the particular pathogen, the antibiotic of choice is often administered topically to avoid development of resistant strains and possible sensitization to common systemic anti-infectives.

However, caution should be used when deciding whether to administer a topical anti-infective ophthalmic drug. In general, prophylactic use of anti-infective drugs is useless, wasteful, and potentially dangerous. Many of the inflammatory diseases seen in ophthalmology are caused by viruses or other microbes that are not susceptible to any currently available anti-infective agents. The use of these agents in such situations is unwarranted.

Topically applied anti-infective drugs can cause sensitivity reactions involving stinging, itching, angioneurotic edema, urticaria, and dermatitis. These drugs may also interfere with growth of the normal bacterial flora of the eye, which may encourage growth of other more harmful organisms.

The choice of a particular ophthalmic anti-infective drug should be based on the following:
- Clinical experience
- Sensitivity and characteristics of the organisms most likely to cause the infection
- The disease itself
- Sensitivity and response of the client
- Laboratory results (cultures and sensitivities)

Some common eye infections that may require antibiotic therapy are listed in Table 56-8.

Mechanism of Action and Drug Effects

The drugs used to treat infections of the eye work in a variety of ways to destroy the invading organism. The antimicrobial effects on susceptible organisms are primarily caused by inhibition of cell wall synthesis, inhibition of

TABLE 56-8
COMMON OCULAR INFECTIONS

Infection	Description
Blepharitis	Inflammation of the eyelids.
Conjunctivitis	Inflammation of the conjunctiva, which is the mucous membrane lining the back of the lids and the front of the eye except the cornea. It may be bacterial or viral in nature and is often associated with common colds. When caused by *Haemophilus* organisms it is commonly called "pink eye." It is highly contagious but usually self-limiting.
Hordeolum (sty)	Acute localized infection of the eyelash follicles and the glands of the anterior lid; results in the formation of a small abscess or cyst.
Keratitis	Inflammation of the cornea often caused by bacterial infection. Herpes simplex keratitis is caused by viral infection.
Uveitis	Infection of the uveal tract or the vascular layer of the eye, which includes the iris, ciliary body, and choroid.
Endophthalmitis	Inflammation of the inner eye structure caused by bacteria.

protein synthesis, or alteration of cell membrane permeability. Specific mechanisms of action can be found for the individual classes of anti-infectives in Chapter 37.

The drug effects of the agents used to treat ocular infections are focused on the micro-organism invading the eye. Some anti-infectives destroy the causative organism (bactericidal), whereas others simply inhibit the organism's growth (bacteriostatic), allowing the body's immune system to fight the infection. Whatever the case, the final drug effect is elimination of the infecting organism.

Indications

Indications for ocular anti-infectives are known or suspected infection with one or more specific micro-organisms.

Contraindications

Contraindications of anti-infectives include known drug allergy or other severe prior adverse drug reaction.

Side Effects and Adverse Effects

The most common side effects and adverse effects of ocular antibiotics are local and transient inflammation, burning, stinging, and drug hypersensitivity. Other effects, toxicities, and drug interactions are specific for the individual anti-infectives and are therefore mentioned in the drug profiles.

Interactions

Ophthalmic agents undergo little if any systemic absorption. For this reason there are few drug interactions for this category of agents. One possible interaction is the concurrent use of corticosteroids (e.g., dexamethasone).

When used with ophthalmic antibiotics, the immunosuppression that may occur may make it more difficult to rid the eye of infection.

Dosages

For recommended dosages of ocular anti-infectives, see the dosages table on p. 962. See Appendix B for some of the common brands available in Canada.

DRUG PROFILES

A variety of infections can occur in the eye; many are self-limiting (i.e., the body's own immune system fights them). These infections seldom result in harm. However, some infections require the use of ocular anti-infectives. The most commonly used anti-infectives from the main anti-infective drug classes are discussed here.

AMINOGLYCOSIDES

Aminoglycosides are potent anti-infectives that destroy bacteria by interfering with protein synthesis in bacterial cells. They bind to ribosomal subunits, eventually leading to bacteria death. Because aminoglycosides kill bacteria, they are classified as bactericidal.

The three aminoglycosides used to treat ocular infections are gentamicin, neomycin, and tobramycin. They are classified as pregnancy category C agents and are contraindicated in clients who have shown a hypersensitivity reaction to them and in clients with vaccinia, varicella, mycobacterial or fungal infections of the eye, or epithelial herpes simplex keratitis.

Side effects and adverse effects include swollen eyelids, mydriasis, and local erythema. Toxic reactions are rare because of poor topical absorption. A possible toxic reaction is the overgrowth of non-susceptible organisms, which can lead to eye infections that are resistant to treatment.

▸ *gentamicin*

Gentamicin is effective against a wide variety of gram-negative and gram-positive organisms. It is particularly useful against *Pseudomonas*, *Proteus*, and *Klebsiella* organisms.

Staphylococci and streptococci that have developed resistance to other antibiotics are effectively destroyed by gentamicin. Gentamicin is available as an ophthalmic ointment and a solution. It is also available in combination with betamethasone as a suspension and an ointment. It is available as a 0.3 percent ophthalmic ointment and a 0.3 percent ophthalmic solution. Commonly recommended dosages are listed in the dosages table on p. 962.

PHARMACOKINETICS

Half-Life	Onset	Peak	Duration
Unknown	Variable	Immediate	6–12 hr

MACROLIDES

The antibacterial erythromycin is a bacteriostatic drug. In normal concentrations it inhibits the growth of an organism but does not destroy it. Erythromycin relies on the body's defence mechanisms to destroy the bacteria;

DOSAGES **Selected Ocular Anti-Infectives**

Agent	Pharmacological Class	Usual Dosage Range	Indications
Antibacterial Agents			
▸▸ bacitracin			
▸▸ bacitracin/polymyxin B			
▸▸ bacitracin/polymyxin B/ neomycin	Miscellaneous antibiotic	Varies; refer to package insert of specific product	Ocular infections
chloramphenicol			
▸▸ ciprofloxacin	Quinolone		
▸▸ erythromycin	Macrolide		
▸▸ gentamicin	Aminoglycoside	2 drops in conjunctival sac tid–qid	Superficial bacterial infections of conjunctiva, cornea, eyelids, tear ducts, and skin adjacent to eye
▸▸ sulfacetamide	Sulphonamide	Solution: 1–2 drops q1–4h Ointment: 1 cm ribbon into lower conjunctival sacs tid–qid	Ocular infections
Antiviral Agents			
idoxuridine		1% solution: Initially: 1 gtt q1h during the day, q2h during the night until definite improvement is noted (usually within 7 days) Following improvement: 1 gtt q2h during the day and q4h at night. Continue 3–7 days after healing is complete. Alternate dosing schedule: 1 gtt q min for 5 min; repeat q4h, day and night	Viral ocular infections: HSV type 1- and type 2-induced keratitis, keratoconjunctivitis
ganciclovir	DNA antimetabolite (nucleoside analogue)	1 surgical implant, which releases drug over 5–8 mo (inserted by ophthalmologist)	Viral ocular infections: CMV retinitis in clients with AIDS (first-line therapy)
trifluridine		Initially 1 drop q2h while awake (max 9 drops/day); may later decrease to 5 drops/day	Viral ocular infections: HSV type 1- and type 2-induced keratitis, keratoconjunctivitis

CMV, Cytomegalovirus; *HSV,* herpes simplex virus.

however, in high concentrations it becomes bactericidal. It is indicated for the treatment of neonatal conjunctivitis caused by *Chlamydia trachomatis* and for the prevention of eye infections in newborns that may be caused by *Neisseria gonorrhoeae* or other susceptible organisms.

The most commonly used agent in this antibiotic category is erythromycin ophthalmic ointment. Eye irritation is the only rare adverse reaction reported with this anti-infective.

▸▸ *erythromycin*

Erythromycin is a macrolide antibiotic indicated for the treatment of various ophthalmic infections. It is available only as a 0.5 percent strength ophthalmic ointment. It is classified as a pregnancy category B agent and is contraindicated in clients who have shown a hypersensitivity reaction to it and in clients with epithelial herpes, varicella, mycobacterial or fungal infections, or epithelial herpes simplex keratitis. Commonly recommended dosages are listed in the dosages table above.

PHARMACOKINETICS

Half-Life	Onset	Peak	Duration
Unknown	Variable	Immediate	Variable

POLYPEPTIDES

Bacitracin and polymyxin B are polypeptide antibiotics. These drugs are rarely used systemically because of their potent nephrotoxic effects. They are bactericidal anti-infectives that inhibit protein synthesis in susceptible organisms, which leads to cell death. They are most commonly used in the treatment of surface infections caused by gram-positive bacteria.

Polypeptides are often used in combination with other antibiotics to broaden their spectrum of activity.

Neosporin ophthalmic solution is a combination of gramicidin, neomycin, and polymyxin. Bacitracin is preferable to neomycin for topical use because fewer organisms are resistant to it, allergic reactions occur less often, and sensitization is avoided.

▸▸ *bacitracin*

Bacitracin is an ophthalmic anti-infective drug used to treat various eye infections. It is available as a single-ingredient product for topical use and as a combination product with polymyxin (Polysporin) or neomycin and polymyxin (Diosporin ointment) for ophthalmic use. These combinations were developed to make bacitracin a broader-spectrum antibiotic. Polysporin is available as drops and an ointment whereas Diosporin is available as an ointment only. Commonly recommended dosages are listed in the dosages table on p. 962.

PHARMACOKINETICS

Half-Life	Onset	Peak	Duration
Unknown	Variable	Immediate	Variable

QUINOLONES

Quinolone antibiotics are effective broad-spectrum antibiotics. They are discussed in detail in Chapter 37. They are bactericidal, destroying a wide spectrum of organisms that are often difficult to treat. There are currently two ophthalmic quinolones available: ciprofloxacin and ofloxacin.

Quinolones are all classified as pregnancy category C agents and are contraindicated in clients who have shown a hypersensitivity reaction to them. Significant side effects and adverse effects include corneal precipitates during treatment for bacterial keratitis. Other reactions include corneal staining and infiltrates. Toxic reactions are limited because of poor topical absorption. Those that occur are usually taste disorders and nausea. There are no significant drug interactions.

▸▸ *ciprofloxacin*

Ciprofloxacin is a synthetic quinolone antibiotic. It is available only by prescription. Although it is available in many systemic formulations, it is currently available for ophthalmic use as both a 0.3 percent ophthalmic solution and an ophthalmic ointment. Ciprofloxacin is indicated in the treatment of bacterial keratitis and conjunctivitis caused by susceptible gram-positive and gram-negative bacteria. One notable adverse reaction to ophthalmic ciprofloxacin has been the appearance on the corneal surface of a white, crystalline precipitate occurring within any corneal lesions. This has occurred in about 17 percent of clients, and within one to seven days of starting therapy. However, all cases to date have been self-limiting, have not required drug discontinuation, and have not adversely affected clinical outcome. Also available is a combination with hydrocortisone. Commonly recommended dosages are listed in the dosages table on p. 962.

PHARMACOKINETICS

Half-Life	Onset	Peak	Duration
1–2 hr	Variable	Immediate	Variable

SULPHONAMIDES

Sulphonamides are synthetic bacteriostatic antibiotics that work by blocking the synthesis of folic acid in susceptible bacteria. Sulfacetamide sodium is the sole sulphonamide used to treat conjunctivitis and other ocular infections.

The side effects and adverse effects are primarily limited to local reactions and include local irritation and stinging. Sulphonamide use can result in the overgrowth of non-susceptible organisms. No significant topical toxic effects have been reported with its use. This ocular anti-infective is classified as a pregnancy category C agent and is contraindicated in infants younger than two months of age and in clients with varicella, vaccinia, viral disease, mycobacterial and fungal infections of the eye, or epithelial herpes simplex keratitis. It is also contraindicated in clients who have shown a hypersensitivity reaction to it.

▸▸ *sulfacetamide*

Sulfacetamide is the most commonly used ophthalmic sulphonamide antibacterial agent. It is available as a 10 percent ophthalmic solution and a 10 percent ophthalmic ointment. It is also used in combination with prednisolone. Commonly recommended dosages are listed in the dosages table on p. 962.

PHARMACOKINETICS

Half-Life	Onset	Peak	Duration
Unknown	Variable	Immediate	Variable

MISCELLANEOUS OCULAR ANTI-INFECTIVE AGENTS

chloramphenicol

Chloramphenicol is a commonly used bacteriostatic anti-infective that works by preventing peptide bond formation and protein synthesis in a wide variety of gram-positive and gram-negative organisms. This anti-infective has been available for many years and remains effective for susceptible organisms. It is extremely useful in the treatment of superficial ocular infections. Side effects with the ophthalmic use of chloramphenicol are usually rare. As with most of the other ophthalmic anti-infectives, the most common side effects and adverse effects are burning and stinging upon instillation. Irreversible aplastic anemia has not been reported with the ophthalmic preparation of this drug, as is the case with systemic dosage forms (Chapter 37). It is available as a 0.5 percent solution and a 1 percent ointment. Commonly recommended dosages are listed in the dosages table on p. 962.

PHARMACOKINETICS

Half-Life	Onset	Peak	Duration
Unknown	Variable	Immediate	Variable

ANTIVIRALS

There are three currently available antiviral ophthalmic agents: idoxuridine, ganciclovir and trifluridine. Dosages for these agents appear in the dosages table on p. 962.

ganciclovir

Ganciclovir is used in the form of an implant to treat ocular cytomegalovirus (CMV) infection, one of the many possible opportunistic infections associated with HIV and AIDS. The implant releases ganciclovir to the site of disease in the eye in which it is implanted. The implant must be surgically placed in the posterior of the eye, which allows diffusion of the drug locally to the site of infection over a period of months. Implantation normally takes less than one hour, requires only local anaesthesia, and is conducted in an outpatient setting.

trifluridine

Recall from biochemistry that the chemical bases associated with DNA and RNA structure are classified as pyrimidines and purines and that a nucleoside is a base with its attached sugar molecule from the DNA or RNA "backbone" chain (a nucleotide is a nucleoside plus its associated phosphate molecule in the "backbone" chain). Trifluridine is a pyrimidine nucleoside. Trifluridine inhibits viral replication because its metabolites block viral DNA synthesis by inhibiting viral DNA polymerase, an enzyme needed for DNA synthesis. This antiviral ophthalmic drug is used against ocular infections (keratitis and keratoconjunctivitis) caused by types 1 and 2 of the herpes simplex virus (HSV). It is classified as a pregnancy category C agent and contraindicated in clients who have shown a hypersensitivity reaction to it. Significant side effects and adverse effects include secondary glaucoma, corneal punctate defects, uveitis, and stromal edema (edema in the tough, fibrous, transparent portion of the cornea known as the *stroma*). The drug exhibits no appreciable topical absorption, and no significant drug interactions have been reported.

ANTI-INFLAMMATORY OPHTHALMIC AGENTS

Many of the same anti-inflammatory drug classes that are used systemically may also be used ophthalmically to treat various ocular inflammatory disorders and surgery-related pain and inflammation. Both non-steroidal anti-inflammatory drugs (NSAIDs) and corticosteroids are used ophthalmically as listed in Box 56-1.

Mechanism of Action and Drug Effects

Corticosteroids and NSAIDs both act to reduce inflammatory responses that arise from the body's metabolic pathway (series of biochemical reactions) for the naturally occurring biochemical arachidonic acid. Each of these two drug classes acts at different enzymatic sites of this complex metabolic pathway, as illustrated in Figure 56-14.

When tissues are damaged, their cell membranes release phospholipids. These phospholipids are then broken down by several different enzymes within the arachidonic acid metabolic pathway. Phospholipase is one of the first enzymes involved, and it is the enzyme that is inhibited by corticosteroids. A second enzyme, cyclo-oxygenase, occurs farther down the pathway and is the site of action of the NSAIDs. Both drug actions reduce the production of various inflammatory mediators, such as leukotrienes, prostaglandins, and thromboxanes. This in turn reduces pain, erythema, and other inflammatory processes.

Indications

Corticosteroids and NSAIDs are applied topically for the symptomatic relief of many ophthalmic inflammatory conditions. They may be used to treat corneal, conjuncti-

---

BOX 56-1

Ophthalmic Anti-Inflammatory Agents

NSAIDs	Corticosteroids
diclofenac	dexamethasone
flurbiprofen	fluorometholone
ketorolac	medrysone
	prednisolone
	rimexolone

---

val, and scleral injuries from chemical, radiation, or thermal burns or penetration of foreign bodies. They are used during the acute phase of the injury process to prevent fibrosis and scarring, which results in visual impairment. They should not be used for minor abrasions or wounds because they may suppress the eye's ability to resist bacterial, viral, or fungal infections. This immunosuppressant effect is more notable in corticosteroids than in NSAIDs. Consequently, NSAIDs are considered less toxic and are preferred as initial topical therapy.

Corticosteroids and NSAIDs may also be used prophylactically after ocular surgery, such as cataract extraction, glaucoma surgery, and corneal transplants, to prevent inflammation and scarring. NSAIDs are also used in the symptomatic treatment of seasonal allergic conjunctivitis. They may also be used prophylactically before ocular surgery to prevent or reduce intra-operative miosis that may occur secondary to surgery-induced trauma.

Contraindications

The only usual contraindication to the use of ophthalmic corticosteroids and NSAIDs is known drug allergy.

Side Effects and Adverse Effects

The most common adverse effect of corticosteroids is transient burning or stinging on application. Because NSAIDs have the potential to cause increased bleeding, clients should be monitored closely. The extended use of corticosteroids may result in cataracts, increased IOP, and optic nerve damage.

Dosages

For recommended dosages of corticosteroid agents, see the dosages table on p. 966. See Appendix B for some of the common brands available in Canada.

DRUG PROFILES

Corticosteroids and NSAIDs that are used to treat ophthalmic inflammatory disorders are discussed in Chapter 32 and Chapter 43, respectively. Ophthalmic formulations share many of the characteristics of their systemic counterparts. However, the ophthalmic derivatives have limited systemic absorption. Thus the majority of therapeutic and toxic effects are limited to the eye.

With the exception of diclofenac, which is classified as a pregnancy category B agent, NSAIDs are classified

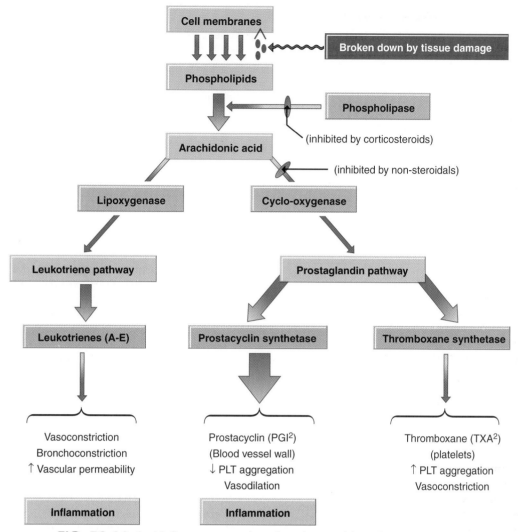

FIG. 56-14 Anti-inflammatory action of corticosteroids and non-steroidals.

as pregnancy category C agents. They are contraindicated in clients who have shown a hypersensitivity reaction to them and in clients with epithelial herpes simplex keratitis. They are all available only by prescription as ophthalmic solutions.

Corticosteroid ophthalmic preparations are indicated for many of the same conditions as NSAIDs, with a few exceptions. Corticosteroids are classified as pregnancy category C agents and are contraindicated in clients with fungal and viral ocular infections and acute epithelial herpes simplex keratitis. Systemic reactions as a result of ophthalmic absorption and drug interactions with the ophthalmic corticosteroids are rare.

▶▶ dexamethasone

Dexamethasone is a synthetic corticosteroid that has many systemic and ophthalmic formulations. It is used to treat inflammation of the eye, eyelids, conjunctiva, and cornea, and it may also be used in the treatment of uveitis, iridocyclitis (inflammation of both the iris and the ciliary body), allergic conditions, and burns, and in the removal of foreign bodies. Dexamethasone is available as a

0.1 percent ophthalmic ointment, a 0.1 percent suspension, and a 1 percent solution. It is also contained in many combination formulations with various antibiotics. Other ophthalmic corticosteroid products with properties and uses similar to dexamethasone are fluorometholone, prednisolone, and rimexolone. Commonly recommended dosages are listed in the dosages table on p. 966.

PHARMACOKINETICS

Half-Life	Onset	Peak	Duration
Unknown	Variable	Immediate	Variable

flurbiprofen

Flurbiprofen is an NSAID that is used to treat inflammatory ophthalmic conditions, such as post-operative inflammation after a cataract extraction. It is also used to inhibit intra-operative miosis, which may be induced by operative trauma and tissue injury. It is available as a 0.03 percent ophthalmic solution. Commonly recommended dosages are listed in the dosages table on p. 966.

DOSAGES Topical Ocular Anti-Inflammatory Agents

Agent	Pharmacological Class	Usual Dosage Range	Indications
▸▸ dexamethasone	Corticosteroid	Solution (suspension): 1–2 drops into conjunctival sac up to q1h as initial therapy (usually tid–qid) Ointment: Apply thin coating bid–qid	Ocular inflammatory conditions (herpes zoster keratitis, iritis, many others); corneal injury
flurbiprofen	NSAID	1 drop q30min beginning 2 h pre-op	Inhibition of intra-operative miosis
ketorolac	NSAID	1 drop qid	Ocular itching; inflammation after cataract removal
tetracaine	Topical local anaesthetic	1–2 drops pre-procedure	Ocular procedures

PHARMACOKINETICS

Half-Life	Onset	Peak	Duration
Unknown	30 min	90 min	>2 hr

ketorolac

Ketorolac is an NSAID that is available in both oral and injectable formulations for systemic use. The ophthalmic formulation is used to reduce certain manifestations of ocular inflammation caused by trauma, such as ocular surgery, and inflammation secondary to external agents, such as allergens and bacteria. Ketorolac is contraindicated in clients who have exhibited hypersensitivity to it. It is available as 0.4 percent and 0.5 percent ophthalmic solutions. Another ophthalmic NSAID product with properties and uses similar to flurbiprofen is diclofenac. Commonly recommended dosages are listed in the dosages table above.

PHARMACOKINETICS

Half-Life	Onset	Peak	Duration
Unknown	Rapid	Immediate	4–6 hr

TOPICAL ANAESTHETICS

Topical anaesthetic ophthalmic drugs are used to prevent eye pain. This is beneficial during surgery, ophthalmic examinations, removal of foreign bodies, and any other painful procedure or condition. The currently available topical anaesthetics used for ophthalmic purposes are benoxinate and tetracaine. Anaesthetic drugs are discussed in depth in Chapter 11.

Mechanism of Action and Drug Effects

Local anaesthetics stabilize the membranes of nerves, resulting in a decrease in the movement of ions into and out of the nerve endings. Without a change in the concentrations of these ions, a nerve impulse cannot be started or transmitted. Pain and many other sensory impulses are transmitted via nerves. When nerves are stabilized, as they are after application of topical anaesthetics, they cannot transmit signals about painful stimuli to the brain. Usually the application of topical anaesthetic drugs to the eye results in local anaesthesia in less than 30 seconds.

Indications

Ophthalmic anaesthetic drugs are used to produce ocular anaesthesia for short corneal and conjunctival procedures. They prevent pain during the following procedures:

- Contact lens fitting
- Tonometry (an external measuring technique involving a puff of air used to estimate IOP)
- Minor conjunctival surgery
- Paracentesis (surgical puncture of the eye to remove fluid for diagnostic or therapeutic reasons)
- Gonioscopy (an examination technique for measuring the angle of the anterior chamber of the eye and for demonstrating ocular rotation and motility)
- Eye examinations of painful injuries
- Irrigation of painful injuries
- Removal of foreign bodies
- Removal of sutures
- Corneal scraping for diagnostic purposes
- Any other uncomfortable short procedure

Contraindications

Contraindications to local ophthalmic anaesthetics include known drug allergy. These medications are recommended only for short-term use and are not recommended for self-administration.

Side Effects and Adverse Effects

Side effects and adverse effects are rare with ophthalmic anaesthetic agents and are usually limited to local effects such as stinging, burning, redness, and lacrimation. Some of the more common side effects and adverse effects are allergic contact dermatitis, softening and erosion of corneal epithelium, pupillary dilation, cycloplegia, conjunctival congestion and hemorrhage, and stromal edema. Systemic toxicity is rare but may involve central nervous system (CNS) stimulation, followed by CNS and cardiovascular depression.

Interactions

Because of limited systemic absorption and short duration of action, ophthalmic anaesthetic agents have no significant drug interactions.

Dosages

Dosage information for tetracaine is provided in the dosages table on p. 966. See Appendix B for some of the common brands available in Canada.

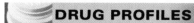 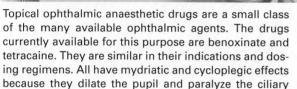

DRUG PROFILES

Topical ophthalmic anaesthetic drugs are a small class of the many available ophthalmic agents. The drugs currently available for this purpose are benoxinate and tetracaine. They are similar in their indications and dosing regimens. All have mydriatic and cycloplegic effects because they dilate the pupil and paralyze the ciliary muscle, which prevents accommodation of vision.

tetracaine

Tetracaine is a local anaesthetic of the ester type. It is applied as an eye drop to numb the eye for various ophthalmic procedures. Tetracaine begins to work in about 25 seconds and lasts for about 30 minutes. Additional drops are applied as needed. It is currently available only as a 0.5 percent ophthalmic solution.

PHARMACOKINETICS

Half-Life	Onset	Peak	Duration
Short	<30 sec	1–5 min	15–20 min

ANTI-ALLERGIC AGENTS

▸▸ artificial tears

An array of OTC products is available to use as lubrication or moisture for the eyes. This is often helpful to clients with dry or otherwise irritated eyes. Artificial tears are isotonic and contain buffers for pH control. In addition, they contain preservatives for microbial control and may contain viscosity agents for extended ocular activity. Selected OTC brand names include Moisture Eyes, Murine, Akwa Tears, Isopto Tears, Visine True Tears, Refresh Tears, and Tears Plus. There are many similar products on the market available both as a solution (eye drop) and as a lubrication ointment. They are often dosed to client comfort as needed.

OPHTHALMIC ANTIHISTAMINES

Three topical ophthalmic antihistamine solutions are currently available: levocabastine, olopatadine, and emedastine difumarate. All are prescription medications and all are used to treat symptoms of allergic conjunctivitis ("hay fever"), which can be seasonal or non-seasonal. Levocabastine has the simplest dosing regimen at one drop in each affected eye twice daily. Olopatadine usually requires one to two drops twice daily, and emedastine difumarate is dosed at one drop up to four times daily.

OPHTHALMIC MAST CELL STABILIZERS AND DECONGESTANTS

cromolyn

Cromolyn sodium is an anti-allergic agent that inhibits the release of inflammation-producing mediators from sensitized inflammatory cells called *mast cells*. It is used in the treatment of vernal keratoconjunctivitis (springtime inflammation of the cornea and conjunctiva). The usual dose for children over five years of age and adults is two drops in each eye, four times daily at regular intervals. The only other mast cell stabilizer with similar effects is nedocromil. Other ophthalmic decongestants are ketotifen fumarate, Iodoxamide tromethamine, and levocabastine.

OPHTHALMIC DIAGNOSTIC AND OTHER ANTI-INFLAMMATORY AGENTS

Cycloplegic Mydriatics

▸▸ atropine sulphate

Atropine sulphate solution 1 percent and ophthalmic ointment 1 percent are used as mydriatic and cycloplegic agents. They dilate the pupil (mydriasis) and paralyze the ciliary muscle (cycloplegic refraction), which prevents accommodation. Such drug action may be needed for either eye examination or uveal tract inflammatory states that benefit from pupillary dilation. The usual dose for uveitis (inflammation of the choroid, iris, or ciliary body) in children and adults is one to two drops of 1-percent solution or 0.3 to 0.5 cm of ointment (1 percent) two to three times daily. The adult dose for refraction is one drop of 1 percent solution one hour before the procedure.

cyclopentolate

Cyclopentolate solution, 0.5 percent and 1 percent, is used primarily as a diagnostic mydriatic and cycloplegic drug. Unlike atropine, it is not normally used to treat uveitis. The usual dose for adults or children is one to two drops (0.5 percent or 1 percent). This is repeated in five to ten minutes if needed. Infants require one drop of the 0.5 percent solution. The drug effects usually subside within 24 hours. Other cycloplegic mydriatics are homatropine and tropicamide. Both are topical ophthalmic solutions with indications similar to atropine and cyclopentolate, except that tropicamide, like cyclopentolate, is generally used for diagnostic purposes only and not for inflammatory states.

phenylephrine

Phenylephrine, a sympathomimetic, causes both vasoconstriction of ocular blood vessels and mydriasis. Other ophthalmic vasoconstrictors with properties similar to phenylephrine are tetrahydrozoline, oxymetazoline, and naphazoline. All are ophthalmic solutions (eye drops) and available without prescription. Dosage ranges from one to two drops, three to four times daily, depending on the manufacturer's recommendations for each specific formulation and strength.

fluorescein

Fluorescein sodium is an ophthalmic diagnostic dye used to identify corneal defects and to locate foreign objects in the eye. It is also used in fitting hard contact lenses. After the instillation of fluorescein, various defects are highlighted:

- Corneal defects are coloured bright green.
- Conjunctival lesions are coloured yellow-orange.
- Foreign objects have a green halo around them.
- A contact lens that touches the cornea will appear black with ultraviolet light.

Fluorescein is available in a 10 percent and a 25 percent injectable form, as a 2 percent ophthalmic solution, and as 1-mg diagnostic strips. It is also available in combination with a local anaesthetic, benoxinate hydrochloride. Dosing and drug administration is usually carried out by an ophthalmologist.

hyperosmolar sodium chloride

Hyperosmolar sodium chloride preparations are used to decrease corneal edema caused by osmotic pressure. These agents produce an osmotic gradient that draws fluid out of the cornea. One to two drops of either the 5 percent solution or the 5 percent ointment is applied every three to four hours.

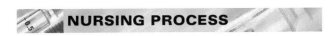

NURSING PROCESS

Assessment

Before administering an ophthalmic agent per the physician's orders, the nurse should perform a baseline assessment of the eye and its structures to help document specific data about possible causes of the eye disorder and to measure the success of the treatment. Any redness, swelling, pain, tearing, eye discharge, decrease in visual acuity, or other unusual symptoms should be noted, documented, and reported to the client's physician. Hypersensitivity to the specific medication and any other drug- or disorder-related contraindications and cautions should also be noted and documented. Baseline vital signs and a visual acuity test (e.g., Snellen chart) should be assessed and documented before, during, and after drug treatment.

Specific contraindications and cautions to the use of each specific ophthalmic agent are as follows:

- Parasympathomimetics are usually contraindicated in clients with bradycardia, hyperthyroidism, coronary artery disease, GI or urinary obstructive problems or disease, peptic ulcers, epilepsy or convulsive disorders, parkinsonism, and asthma. Cautious use and careful monitoring are recommended in clients who are pregnant or have hypertension or bronchial asthma. Baseline vital signs and an assessment of the respiratory system should be obtained and documented, with any abnormal findings reported to the healthcare provider.
- Contraindications to sympathomimetic ophthalmic agents include allergic reaction to the drugs and narrow-angle glaucoma. Cautious use is recommended in clients who are pregnant and/or breastfeeding.
- Beta-adrenergic blockers are contraindicated in clients who are allergic to these agents and in those who have chronic obstructive pulmonary disease (COPD), asthma, heart block, right pump failure, and congenital glaucoma.
- CAIs should be administered cautiously in clients who have adrenocortical insufficiency because they are at higher risk for associated fluid and electrolyte disturbances. Cross-allergies are possible in individuals sensitive to sulphonamide drugs, such as thiazide di-

uretics and oral sulphonylureas and sulphonamide antibiotics. CAIs are contraindicated in clients with hyponatremia or hypokalemia or renal or liver dysfunction. In addition, it is important for the nurse to question the client about current medications because of the possibility of interactions with amphetamines, quinidine, mecamylamine, and methenamine. Baseline vital signs and an assessment of the client's vision, IOP, serum electrolytes, urinalysis, platelets and complete blood cell count (CBC) are also recommended before initiation of drug therapy.

- The osmotic agent mannitol may cause dehydration in geriatric clients because of rapid fluid shifts and subsequent diuretic action.
- Ophthalmic antibiotic drops and ointments are contraindicated in clients who are allergic to the medication, and cautious use is recommended in clients who are pregnant or have antibiotic hypersensitivity. Each drug also carries its own contraindications or cautions. See Chapter 37 for information on the various antibiotic agents and classes.
- Mydriatic agents, such as atropine, are contraindicated in clients with a history of severe reactions to them and should be used extremely cautiously in clients who have primary glaucoma. The dilation of the pupil results in narrowing of the canal of Schlemm and restriction of the drainage of intra-ocular fluids, which increases IOP and may precipitate an acute glaucoma attack. It is important for the nurse to obtain and document baseline vital signs and vision status.
- Contraindications and cautions to sympathomimetics include coronary heart disease, angina, tachycardia, and hypertension.
- Antiviral agents are contraindicated during pregnancy.
- Topical anaesthetics have few contraindications.
- Topical corticosteroid ophthalmic agents are contraindicated in clients with bacterial eye infections or minor corneal abrasions. Ophthalmic corticosteroids may increase the incidence of fungal infections of the eye and are to be used only as directed with the advice of a physician.
- Anti-inflammatory agents may mask allergic reactions or hypersensitivity to other ophthalmic agents.
- Artificial tears and lubricants are safe and have no major contraindications or cautions to their use.

Nursing Diagnoses

Nursing diagnoses associated with the use of ophthalmic agents include the following:

- Risk for infection related to eye disorder or due to possible non-adherence to therapy.
- Risk for self-injury to the eye related to improper use of medication.
- Acute pain related to eye disorder, infection, and/or inflammatory eye condition.
- Disturbed sensory perception related to eye disorder and side effects of medication.
- Deficient knowledge related to lack of information about medication and disorder.

Planning

Goals related to the administration of ophthalmic medications include the following:
- Client remains free of signs and symptoms of infection of the eye.
- Client remains adherent to therapy.
- Client remains free from self-injury related to side-effects of therapy.
- Client is without eye pain related to eye disorder.
- Client regains normal visual patterns or pre-infection or pre-disorder vision.

Outcome Criteria

Outcome criteria for the client receiving ophthalmic agents include the following:
- Client states the signs and symptoms of infection of the eye, such as eye pain, drainage, redness, and decreased activity, and reports them immediately to the physician.
- Client states how medication is to be taken.
- Client minimizes self-injury by creating a safe environment and using assistance at home while experiencing decreased vision.
- Client minimizes eye pain related to the eye disorder by using compresses or non-ASA analgesics as ordered.
- Client shows improvement in visual acuity by increased tolerance to reading and ability to participate in activities of daily living.

Implementation

Because it is important to administer only clean solutions, the nurse should shake the medication container before each use and avoid touching the eye with the tip of the dropper or container to prevent contamination of the product. Any excess medication must be removed promptly and pressure must be applied to the inner canthus for one minute (or whatever is ordered or suggested) to avoid systemic symptoms or side effects. Ointments should be applied as a thin layer (as should all ophthalmic medications) and administered to the conjunctival sac. To

---

NURSING CARE PLAN | Glaucoma

Ms. B., 82, is at the physician's office today for instructions about self-administration of pilocarpine. She is healthy and all senses are intact. Her motor and cognition skills are intact with no deficits noted. She is eager to learn and has many questions regarding her glaucoma and associated care. She lives alone, but her 21-year-old niece helps her out quite a bit and has come with her today to learn how to help with this medication.

ASSESSMENT	Subjective Data	• Complaint of blurred vision, decreased vision acuity, and difficulty with close-up vision • Frequent headaches and eye pain • States, "I live all alone but I do pretty good."
	Objective Data	• 82-year-old woman who is having annual eye examination • Increased IOP • Good health otherwise and without significant medical problems
NURSING DIAGNOSIS		Deficient knowledge related to technique for administration of pilocarpine
PLANNING	Goals	Client will remain adherent and have therapeutic response to pilocarpine technique within one day of therapy
	Outcome Criteria	Client will demonstrate proper instillation technique before leaving physician's office
IMPLEMENTATION		Client teaching should include the following instructions on inserting pilocarpine: • Wash your hands. • Pull down lower lid of eye. • Drop pilocarpine into lower conjunctival sac. • Apply gentle pressure to the top of the nose where it meets the corner of the eye for 30 to 60 seconds • Teach a significant other, friend, or relative how to insert medication, just in case you have any difficulty with the medication.
EVALUATION		Client will show therapeutic response to medication regimen as evidenced by: • Decreased IOP • Decreased headaches and eye pain

TABLE 56-9

OPHTHALMIC AGENTS: NURSING IMPLICATIONS

Drug Group	Drug Examples	Nursing Implications
Beta-adrenergic blocking agents	timolol	Use nasolacrimal pressure to prevent possible systemic absorption as with all other topical ophthalmic solutions or ointments; monitor for bradycardia, heart block, and wheezing.
Carbonic anhydrase inhibitors	acetazolamide brinzolamide dorzolamide methazolamide	Administer as ordered and with meals if necessary to decrease GI upset; fluid volume should be monitored carefully; monitor affected eye closely for therapeutic effects; check for drug interactions.
Osmotic agents	mannitol	Mannitol may result in digitalis toxicity when given concurrently; if crystallized, may dissolve in warm water; adequate hydration is important—up to 2000 mL/day.
Mydriatics and cycloplegics	atropine cyclopentolate	Atropine: Monitor for side effects such as irregular pulse, confusion, dry mouth, and fever; causes blurred vision and photosensitivity, so sunglasses should be worn outside until effect is gone. Cyclopentolate: Use with caution and give as ordered; same nursing management as with atropine.
Sympathomimetics	epinephrine phenylephrine tetrahydrozoline	Monitor for serious side effects that may occur if systemically absorbed, such as tachycardia and elevated BP. With corticosteroid agents, report blurred vision or visual disturbances, eye pain, ptosis (lid drooping), or enlarged pupils.
Anti-infectives/ Anti-inflammatories		Prophylactic use is potentially dangerous and is not recommended; may cause local reactions such as redness, itching, edema, and dermatitis; follow instructions for instillation.
Antibacterials	chloramphenicol erythromycin gentamicin neomycin sulphonamides tobramycin	With chloramphenicol, monitor for drop in CBC, fever, sore throat, and unusual bleeding. With erythromycin, make sure to administer as ordered and apply only a thin ointment strip. Gentamicin and similar agents should be given as ordered. With neomycin combination agents, be sure to follow instructions. Cleanse eye with use of sulphonamide agents such as sulfacetamide because they will be inhibited by purulent drainage or exudate; discard any darkened solution; may cause mild pain on instillation.
Antivirals	idoxuridine trifluridine	Notify physician if the client complains of blurred vision, visual disturbances, or photosensitivity if not present before therapy; notify the physician about any blurred vision, eye irritations, or visual changes not previously experienced; apply as ordered and, if ointment, apply only a thin strip; always instill drops and ointments into the conjunctival sac.
Topical anaesthetics	benoxinate tetracaine	These are not recommended for long-term use because they could lead to possible irreversible eye damage; eye should be patched until injury heals; CNS excitation and subsequent depression are potential systemic side effects if absorbed.
Artificial tears	Lacri-Lube, Optilube, and HypoTears are ointment forms	Instill as directed.
Anti-allergics	cromolyn sodium	Instill as ordered; therapeutic effects in 4 wk if given regularly.
Enzyme preparations	chymotrypsin	May result in post-operative glaucoma for about 1 wk, which can be reversed with parasympathomimetics.
Hyperosmolar preparations	sodium chloride ointment	Apply as ordered.
Non-steroidal anti-inflammatories	diclofenac flurbiprofen ketorolac	Use only as prescribed; solutions preferred for eye infections because ointments often decrease healing.
Ophthalmic surgery aids		Used to protect the eye from damage; to be given exactly as ordered.
Prostaglandin preparations	latanoprost	Instill as ordered; lowers IOP for 20–24 h with single dose; well tolerated; clients with hazel-coloured eyes may experience permanent iris colour change to brown, but this is not harmful to the client.

facilitate the installation of drops, the nurse should have the client look up to the ceiling during administration. If more than one medication is ordered by the physician, they must be administered in the proper order. The nurse should refer to an appropriate authoritative drug resource or handbook for specific instructions and guidelines.

Atropine is an antidote for miotics and should be available in case it is needed. Other agents and associated nursing implications are presented in Table 56-9.

Directions for antiviral ophthalmic preparations should be followed closely. Topical anaesthetics should be administered as ordered for use in foreign body removal or treatment of eye injury. Repeated and continuous use should be avoided because of the risk for delayed wound healing, corneal perforation, permanent corneal opacification, and visual loss. When topical anaesthetics are used, the eye should be patched to prevent further injury resulting from the loss of the blink reflex.

With latanoprost, there is one unusual side effect to emphasize during client education: this drug permanently turns hazel, green, and bluish-brown eye colour to brown eye colour. There is no known injury to the eye associated with this colour change.

OTC tear solutions may be suggested by the healthcare provider.

Client teaching tips for ophthalmic agents are presented below.

■ Evaluation

Therapeutic responses to miotics include decreased aqueous humor of the eye with resultant decreased IOP and decreased signs, symptoms, and long-term effects associated with glaucoma. Possible side effects are included in the discussion of client education.

Beta-adrenergic blockers, such as timolol maleate optic solution, have been therapeutic if there is a resultant decrease in IOP. Possible side effects include weakness, depression, anxiety, nausea, confusion, eye irritation, rash, bradycardia, hypotension, and dysrhythmias.

Therapeutic responses to antibiotic and antiviral ophthalmic agents include elimination of the infection and resolution of symptoms.

Therapeutic responses to ophthalmic anaesthetic topical agents include healing of the eye without permanent damage and a decrease in symptoms associated with the damage. Side effects include CNS excitation if systemically absorbed, causing blurred vision, dizziness, tremors, nervousness, and restlessness. Drowsiness, dyspnea, and cardiac dysrhythmias may occur secondary to CNS depression.

A therapeutic response to anti-inflammatory ophthalmic solutions is a decrease in allergic reactions such as itching, tearing, redness, and eye discharge. Potential complications of this agent include hypersensitivity to it and chemosis (swelling of the conjunctiva).

CASE STUDY

Glaucoma

Ms. R., an 89-year-old client with open-angle glaucoma, arrives at the physician's office for her usual checkup. During the visit the ophthalmologist checks her IOP, which is elevated from her last checkup six weeks ago. During their discussion, Ms. R. tells the physician that she just has problems getting the eye drops in and so she often just doesn't take the medicine. The physician has now decided to change her miotic drops to an oral agent, acetazolamide 250 mg tid.
- Why is acetazolamide effective against glaucoma?
- What is a rationale for switching Ms. R. to the oral agent?
- What specific client teaching tips should be shared with Ms. R. in written and oral forms?

For answers see http://evolve.elsevier.com/Lilley/pharmacology/.

CLIENT TEACHING TIPS

Clients taking eye drops should have a demonstration on the proper technique for instilling them and for applying pressure to the inner canthus. They should show by return demonstration that they have mastered the technique. The nurse should instruct the client as follows:
▲ Avoid touching any eye surface with the eye dropper to keep it sterile.

Parasympathomimetics
▲ Long-term therapy is usually necessary. To prevent eye damage, you need to take your medication regularly.

Sympathomimetics
▲ Report any stinging, burning, itching, watering, or puffiness of the eye.

Beta-Adrenergic Blockers
▲ Apply pressure to the inner canthus for one full minute after administration.
▲ Report to your physician any blurred vision, difficulty breathing, wheezing, sweating, flushing, or loss of sight.

CAIs
▲ While taking this medication, eat foods high in potassium, such as bananas, potatoes, soy products, dried fruit, and apricots.
▲ Reduce your salt intake.
▲ Drink at least eight glasses of fluid a day to reduce the risk of kidney stones.
▲ Record your weight daily.

▲ Report to your physician any swelling, excessive thirst, dry mouth, muscle spasm, unusual weakness, confusion, lethargy, numbness, twitching, or irregular heartbeat.

Mannitol

▲ Drink at least eight glasses of fluid a day.

Atropine

▲ If you experience a dry mouth or racing heart, skip your next dose and contact your physician.

▲ This medication will likely make you more sensitive to sunlight; sunglasses help ease the discomfort.

Topical Anaesthetics

▲ Don't rub or touch the eye while it is numb because of possible eye damage.

▲ Wear a patch to protect your eye while it is numb, because you do not have the protection of your normal blink reflex.

Anti-Infective and Anti-Inflammatory Solutions

▲ Take as prescribed and carefully follow instructions.

▲ Report to your physician any increase in eye pain, discharge, or fever.

Corticosteroids

▲ Take this medication cautiously and do not overuse it.

▲ Do not stop taking this medication without consulting the physician because of the possibility of adverse reactions.

▲ Mix suspensions well before use.

▲ Stinging after putting in the drops is normal.

▲ Do not wear contact lenses while taking this medication.

Cromolyn

▲ Do not wear contact lenses while taking this medication.

POINTS to REMEMBER

▼ Glaucoma is a disorder of the eye caused by inhibition of the normal flow and drainage of aqueous humor; its treatment helps to reduce IOP either by increasing aqueous humor drainage or decreasing its production.

▼ Drugs that increase aqueous humor drainage are direct-acting parasympathomimetics, sympathomimetics, beta-blockers, osmotic diuretics, and prostaglandin agonists.

▼ A large proportion of the inflammatory diseases of the eye are caused by viruses, and there are many ocular anti-infectives used to treat bacterial, viral, and fungal infections of the eye.

▼ Common ocular infections include conjunctivitis, hordeolum (sty), keratitis, uveitis, and endophthalmitis.

▼ Anti-inflammatory ophthalmic agents include agents such as corticosteroids and are used to inhibit inflammatory response to mechanical, chemical, or immunological agents.

▼ Topical anaesthetics are used to prevent pain to the eye and are beneficial during surgery, ophthalmic examinations, and the removal of foreign bodies.

▼ All ophthalmic preparations need to be administered exactly as ordered and into the conjunctival sac; safe and accurate application or instillation technique must be used while avoiding contact of the dropper or tube to the eye to prevent contamination of the drug.

▼ Clients should report any increase in symptoms, such as eye pain or drainage, to the physician immediately.

EXAMINATION REVIEW QUESTIONS

1 Acute angle-closure glaucoma is characterized by which of the following?
 a. Rapid loss of vision
 b. Higher risk in clients of Asian descent
 c. Higher risk in white clients
 d. Mydriasis

2 Treatment for chronic open-angle glaucoma includes which of the following?
 a. Surgical mydriasis
 b. Complete elimination of any infections
 c. Cauterization of the lens
 d. Topical or systemic drugs

3 Ophthalmic agents should be given using which technique?
 a. Tip the bottle over the iris and squeeze out 5 mL.
 b. Monitor for severe systemic reactions such as an immediate blockage.

 c. Administer the agent in the conjunctival sac.
 d. Always apply pressure to the inner canthus for 20–30 minutes after administration of the drug.

4 Miotics help glaucoma by which of the following actions?
 a. Decreasing intracranial pressure
 b. Pupillary constriction
 c. Increasing tearing ability
 d. Pupillary dilation

5 Which of the following is a side effect of pilocarpine ophthalmic drops?
 a. Bradycardia
 b. Hypertension
 c. Headache
 d. Biliary spasm

CRITICAL THINKING ACTIVITIES

1 Describe the process of glaucoma and explain the value of treatment to preserve vision.

2 Develop a teaching plan for the geriatric client who is already vision-impaired and needs instructions for the daily administration of antiglaucoma ophthalmic drops.

3 Your client has developed an infection and inflammation of the eye. What is the importance of using only the antibiotic agent before initiation of a corticosteroid ointment?

For answers see http://evolve.elsevier.com/Lilley/pharmacology/.

BIBLIOGRAPHY

Albanese, J., & Nutz, P. (2005). *Mosby's 2005 nursing drug cards.* St Louis, MO: Mosby.

Boron, W.F., & Boulap, E.L. (2005). *Medical physiology. Updated edition.* Philadelphia: Elsevier Saunders.

Canadian Pharmacists Association. (2003). *Therapeutic choices* (4th ed.). Ottawa, ON: Author.

Canadian Pharmacists Association. (2004). *Guide to drugs in Canada.* Toronto, ON: Dorling Kindersley.

Canadian Pharmacists Association. (2005). *Compendium of pharmaceuticals and specialties. The Canadian drug reference for health professionals.* Ottawa, ON: Author. [The subscription-based e-CPS is available at http://www.pharmacists.ca.]

Cheng, A., Williams, B.A., & Sivarajan, B.V. (Eds.). (2003). *The HSC handbook of pediatrics* (10th ed.). Toronto, ON: Elsevier.

Eliola, R., & Stokes, J. (2000). Monograph series on aging-related diseases: XI. Glaucoma. *Chronic Diseases in Canada* 19(4). Retrieved September 10, 2005, from http://www.phac-aspc.gc.ca/publicat/cdic-mcc/19-4/d_e.html

Facts and Comparisons. (2004). *Drug facts and comparisons pocket version* (9th ed.). St Louis, MO: Wolters Kluwer Health.

Hardman, J.G., & Limbird, L.E. (2002). *Goodman and Gilman's the pharmacological basis of therapeutics* (10th ed.). New York: McGraw-Hill.

Health Canada. (2005). Drug product database (DPD). Retrieved September 11, 2005, from http://www.hc-sc.gc.ca/hpb/drugs-dpd/

Katzung, B.G. (2004). *Basic and clinical pharmacology* (9th ed.). New York: McGraw-Hill.

Lacy, C.F., Armstrong, L.L., Goldman, M.P., & Lance, L.L. (2003). *Drug information handbook* (11th ed.). Hudson, OH: Lexi-Comp.

Lehne, R.A. (2004). *Pharmacology for nursing care* (5th ed.). St Louis, MO: Saunders.

McKenry, L.M., & Salerno, E. (2003). *Mosby's pharmacology in nursing–revised and updated* (21st ed.). St Louis, MO: Mosby.

Mosby. (2005). *Mosby's drug consult 2005: The comprehensive reference for generic and brand name drugs* (15th ed.). St Louis, MO: Mosby.

Skidmore-Roth, L. (2006). *Mosby's 2006 nursing drug reference* (19th ed.). St Louis, MO: Mosby.

57 Otic Agents

OBJECTIVES

After reading this chapter, the successful student will be able to do the following:

1 Describe the anatomy of the ear and the purposes of each structure.

2 Cite the two categories of ear disorders and the disorders in each and explain their causes.

3 List the various types of otic preparations.

4 Discuss the mechanisms of action, dosage, cautions, contraindications, and specific application techniques related to otic agents.

5 Discuss the nursing process as it relates to the administration of otic preparations.

6 Develop a nursing care plan that includes all phases of the nursing process as it relates to the administration of otic preparations.

e-LEARNING ACTIVITIES

Student CD-ROM
- Review Questions: see questions 399–400
- Animations
- Medication Administration Checklists
- IV Therapy Checklists

evolve Web site (http://evolve.elsevier.com/Lilley/pharmacology/)
- Online Chapter Worksheet • Frequently Asked Questions
- Learning Tips and Content Updates • WebLinks • Online Appendices and Supplements • Mosby/Saunders ePharmacology Update • Access to *Mosby's Drug Consult*

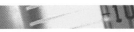

DRUG PROFILES

chloramphenicol, p. 976   ▸▸ urea hydrogen peroxide,
▸▸ lidocaine, p. 976   p. 976

▸▸ Key drug.

GLOSSARY

Cerumen (se roo' men) A yellowish or brownish waxy excretion produced by vestigial (evolutionary remnant) apocrine sweat glands in the external ear canal. Also called *earwax*.

Otic agents (o' tik) Drugs applied locally to treat inflammation of the external ear canal or to remove excess cerumen (earwax). Also called *otics*.

Otitis media (o ty' tis mee' dee uh) Inflammation or infection of the middle ear, a common affliction of childhood. It is often preceded by an upper respiratory tract infection.

Tragus (tray' gus) plural: tragi (tray' jy) The cartilaginous projection anterior to the external opening of the ear.

Wax emulsifiers (e mul' si fy erz) Products that loosen and help in the removal of cerumen.

The ear is made up of three parts: the outer, middle, and inner ear. The outer, or external, ear is composed of the pinna (outer projecting part of the ear) and the external auditory meatus, also called the external acoustic meatus. Synonyms for the pinna are *auricle* and *ala*. The middle ear is composed of the tympanic cavity, the mastoid appendages (malleus, incus, and stapes), and the auditory, or eustachian, tube. The inner ear is composed of such structures as the cochlea and semicircular canals. The ear and its associated structures are illustrated in Figure 57-1.

The disorders of the ear can be categorized according to the portion of the ear affected. Those of the outer and middle ear are the disorders usually treated with the agents discussed in this chapter. In general the most common disorders of these portions of the ear are bacterial

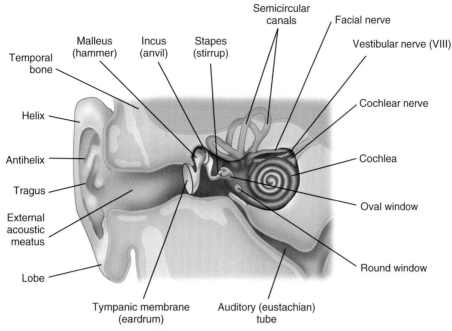

Semicircular
canals

Facial nerve

Vestibular nerve (VIII)

Malleus
(hammer)

Incus
(anvil)

Stapes
(stirrup)

Temporal
bone

Cochlear nerve

Helix

Antihelix

Cochlea

Tragus

External
acoustic
meatus

Oval window

Lobe

Round window

Tympanic membrane
(eardrum)

Auditory (eustachian)
tube

FIG. 57-1   Structure of the ear.

and fungal infections, inflammatory disorders that cause pain and earwax accumulation. Such disorders tend to be self-limiting, and if treatment is needed it is generally successful. However, if problems persist or are left untreated, more serious problems such as hearing loss may result.

External ear disorders are generally the result of physical trauma to the ear and consist of disorders such as lacerations or scrapes to the skin and localized infection of the hair follicles resulting in the development of a boil (furunculosis). These are examples of self-limiting disorders. They are often minor and heal with time. Other more serious disorders may initially appear to be minor but, if left untreated, can become more serious. Such "minor" irritations are dermatitis of the ear, itching, local redness, weeping, or drainage. These may be the result of inflammation caused by seborrhea, psoriasis, or contact dermatitis. They may also be the first signs of a more serious underlying disease process such as head trauma. Drainage, pain, and dizziness warrant prompt medical care.

By far the most common middle ear disorder is infection caused by various micro-organisms, a condition commonly called **otitis media**. This disorder most often afflicts children and usually occurs after an upper respiratory tract infection. It may also occur in adults, but it is then generally associated with trauma to the middle ear stemming from trauma to the tympanic membrane, often from foreign objects or water sports. Otitis media is more common in high-humidity climates.

Common symptoms of middle ear disorders such as otitis media are pain, fever, malaise, pressure, a sensation of fullness in the ears, and hearing loss. If left untreated, tinnitus (ringing in the ears), nausea, vertigo, and mastoiditis may occur. Hearing deficits and even hearing loss

may result if appropriate and prompt therapy is not started.

TREATMENT OF EAR DISORDERS

Some of the minor ailments that affect the outer ear can be treated with OTC medications, but persistent, painful conditions always require a physician's care. Middle ear disorders are rarely treated with OTC medications unless they are prescribed by a physician after referral. The drugs commonly used to treat the relatively minor disorders of the external and middle ear are called **otic agents** and are topically applied. They are listed as follows:

- Antibiotics
- Anti-inflammatory agents
- Local analgesics
- Local anaesthetics
- Steroids
- Wax emulsifiers

More serious problems than those previously mentioned may require treatment with potent, systemically administered medications such as antimicrobial agents, analgesics, anti-inflammatory drugs, and antihistamines. These medications have been discussed in earlier chapters.

ANTIBACTERIAL OTIC AGENTS

Many of the antibacterial agents that are given systemically also come in topical formulations that are applied to the external ear. Chloramphenicol and gentamicin are two such agents that are commonly used. Several antibacterial agents are also combined with steroids to take advantage of their additional anti-inflammatory, antipruritic, and anti-allergic drug effects. The antimicrobial drugs used as otic agents are

TABLE 57-1
STEROID AND ANTIBIOTIC COMBINATIONS FOR OTIC USE

Steroid (percentage concentration)	Antibiotics (dose/10 mL bottle)
hydrocortisone (1%) solution	3.5 mg of neomycin and 10 000 units of polymyxin B
hydrocortisone (1%) suspension	3.5 mg of neomycin and 10 000 units of polymyxin B
hydrocortisone (1%)	2 mg ciprofloxacin

effective in the treatment of mastoidectomy infections and infections of the external auditory canal. However, middle ear infections such as otitis media generally require treatment with systemically administered antibiotics.

DRUG PROFILES

chloramphenicol

Chloramphenicol has the advantage of possessing a broad spectrum of activity. It is effective against *Staphylococcus aureus*, *Escherichia coli*, *Pseudomonas aeruginosa*, *Enterobacter aerogenes*, *Haemophilus influenzae*, and many other bacteria. It can cause adverse effects similar to those caused by many of the topically applied antibiotics. These include burning, redness, rash, swelling, and other signs of topical irritation. Chloramphenicol is available as a suspension in combination with hydrocortisone acetate that is usually instilled in the ear. Each mL contains 2 mg chloramphenicol and 10 mg hydrocortisone acetate. Two to three drops three times daily is the recommended dosage for both adults and children.

ANTIBIOTIC AND STEROID COMBINATION PRODUCTS

The steroid most commonly used in combination with antibiotics is hydrocortisone, which is added to reduce the inflammation and itching associated with ear infections. The antibiotics contained in the most popular combination products are listed in Table 57-1. These products are most commonly used for the treatment of bacterial infections of the external auditory canal caused by susceptible bacteria such as *S. aureus*, *E. coli*, *Klebsiella* spp., and others.

MISCELLANEOUS OTIC AGENTS

A wide variety of products are used to treat bacterial infections, inflammation, and other minor or superficial problems of the external ear. An additional problem is the accumulation and eventual impaction of earwax, or **cerumen**, which can be the cause of many of these symptoms. Products that soften and help to eliminate earwax are re-

ferred to as **wax emulsifiers** and are discussed with the miscellaneous agents.

DRUG PROFILES

LOCAL ANAESTHETIC AGENTS

Some otic combination products contain local anaesthetic agents. Many common ear disorders are associated with some degree of pain and inflammation, and the numbing effect of local anaesthetic agents makes them beneficial for pain relief. The same characteristics of the local anaesthetics that were discussed in Chapter 11 apply to the topical local anaesthetics used in these preparations.

▶▶ lidocaine

One combination product that contains a local anaesthetic is Lidosporin ear drops. This preparation contains the local anaesthetic lidocaine HCL, and polymyxin B sulphate. It is used for the relief and prevention of infection of susceptible organisms, pain and itching associated with external otitis ("swimmer's ear"), otitis media (if the tympanic membrane is perforated), and furunculosis.

Lidocaine is a local anaesthetic of the amide type. It stabilizes the neuronal membrane, preventing the production and initiation of nerve impulses. Side effects to this agent are rare and consist mostly of localized allergic reactions. They are typically seen after prolonged or repeated use.

WAX EMULSIFERS

Wax, or cerumen, is a natural product of the ear and is produced by modified sweat glands in the auditory canal. However, it can occasionally build up and become impacted, resulting in pain and temporary deafness. A number of OTC ear remedies loosen and help remove such impacted cerumen. Often the simple application of olive or almond oil is sufficient to soften wax.

▶▶ urea hydrogen peroxide

The only wax removal system is urea hydrogen peroxide. This combination of agents works together to loosen and help remove cerumen.

Hydrogen peroxide when exposed to moisture such as that on the skin or the mouth releases oxygen. This release of oxygen imparts a weak antibacterial action to the otic agent. In addition, the effervescence resulting from the release of oxygen has the mechanical effect of removing cerumen from inaccessible spaces such as the ear canal. The urea acts as a rehydrating or softening agent to facilitate easier cerumen removal.

NURSING PROCESS

■ Assessment

Before administering any of the otic preparations, the nurse should ensure that the client's baseline hearing or auditory status is evaluated and the findings are documented. There should also be a thorough evaluation of the client's symptoms, and any other related medical information should be elicited. Any drug and food allergies should be noted and documented. The nurse must understand the specific indication for, or the intended use of, the medication so that it can be given exactly as ordered. This understanding should extend to the specific administration technique used. An understanding of the anatomy of the ear is also important, especially as it relates to clients in different age groups. Contraindications to the use of otic preparations include a hypersensitivity to any of the ingredients, whether an antibacterial, steroidal (hydrocortisone), or triple antibiotic-type agent (e.g., neomycin sulfate, polymyxin B). Perforated eardrum(s) may also be a contraindication to the use of these agents.

Nursing Diagnoses

Nursing diagnoses related to clients receiving otic agents include the following:
- Impaired verbal communication related to hearing loss stemming from damage from long-term ear disorders.
- Risk for injury related to symptoms of the ear disorder and possible vestibular dysfunction.
- Risk for infection related to inadequate treatment.
- Disturbed sensory perception related to complications from an ear infection.
- Deficient knowledge related to lack of experience with otic drugs and their method of administration.

Planning

Goals pertaining to clients receiving otic agents include the following:
- Client regains normal patterns of hearing and communicating.
- Client is free of discomfort and symptoms related to the ear disorder.
- Client remains free of or experiences minimal signs and symptoms of ear infection with the course of treatment.
- Client is free of adverse reactions or side effects.
- Client is free of complications associated with medication therapy.

Outcome Criteria

Outcome criteria for clients receiving otic agents include the following:
- Client openly verbalizes feelings related to problems with communication (decreased hearing).
- Client reports to the physician immediately any increased hearing loss, fever, or increased ear pain, redness, or swelling of the ear canal.
- Client demonstrates accurate medication administration techniques.

Implementation

Ear drops should be instilled only after the ear has been thoroughly cleansed, all cerumen removed (by irrigation if necessary or if ordered), and the dropper cleaned with alcohol. Ear drops should be warmed to approximately body temperature before instillation. Solution that is too cold may cause a "vestibular" type of reaction, with vomiting and dizziness. If the solution has been refrigerated, allow it to warm to room temperature. Do not warm further; higher temperatures may affect the potency of these solutions. Generally speaking, the corticosteroid, antibiotic, corticosteroid–antibiotic combination agents, wax emulsifiers, and ear-drying agents should all be administered according to these same guidelines. In adults, ear drops should be administered while holding the pinna *up* and back, whereas in children younger than three years of age, the pinna should be held down and back. Time should be allowed for adequate coverage of the ear. It may also help to gently massage the **tragus**, the cartilaginous projection in front of the ear canal (Figure 57-1).

See the box on p. 978 for client teaching tips.

Evaluation

The therapeutic effects of the otic preparations include less pain, redness, and swelling in the ear; a reduction in fever and the white blood cell counts; and negative culture findings if the previous culture has yielded positive findings. The ear canal should be monitored for the occurrence of rash and/or any signs of local irritation such as redness and heat at the site.

NURSING CARE PLAN | Otitis Media

Karen, an 11-year-old with otitis media, has been placed on cefaclor 250 mg tid. She has tolerated cefaclor in the past, but her grandmother brought her into the physician's office and needs instructions for administration of the medicine because Karen's mother is out of town. Use of hydrogen peroxide has been recommended as well.

ASSESSMENT	Subjective Data Objective Data	• "I don't remember much about how to take this medicine." • Successful therapy before with cefaclor • Grandmother caregiver for now; mother is out of town
NURSING DIAGNOSIS		Deficient knowledge related to needs for information about cefaclor and other otic drug administration

Continued

NURSING CARE PLAN

Otitis Media—cont'd

PLANNING	**Goals**	Client and grandmother verbalize instructions associated with taking cefaclor before leaving physician's office.
	Outcome Criteria	Before leaving the physician's office, client and grandmother do the following:

- State dosing times and amounts
- State side effects of medication
- State side effects to report to the physician
- Demonstrate adequate technique for instilling hydrogen peroxide as ordered

IMPLEMENTATION

Client education should include the following information:

- It is important to take the medication exactly as prescribed and until all medication is gone.
- Eating yogourt while on antibiotics will help maintain normal bacteria in the intestines and decrease diarrhea.
- Contact the physician should you experience sore throat, bleeding, easy bruising, or joint pain.
- Common side effects include diarrhea and loss of appetite. Other possible side effects include headache, dizziness, nausea, vomiting, and rash.
- Use hydrogen peroxide daily.

The client and her grandmother should be taught how to administer hydrogen peroxide properly.

EVALUATION

- Client will display the following therapeutic responses to cefaclor:
  - Decreased ear pain
  - Decreased fever
- Client will experience minimal side effects, such as diarrhea.
- Client's ear pain will decrease with adequate response to cefaclor and with daily use of hydrogen peroxide.

CLIENT TEACHING TIPS

The nurse should explain how ear drops work and demonstrate the proper technique for instilling them. The nurse should instruct the client or caregiver as follows:

▲ Do not touch the dropper to the ear.
▲ Some people become dizzy after putting in ear drops, so you may want to lie down to put them in.
▲ Remain lying on your side (with the affected ear up) for about five minutes after putting in drops. If you prefer, you can put a small cotton ball into the ear canal to keep the drops there, but be careful not to force or jam the cotton into the ear canal.
▲ Administer ear drops at body temperature. You can warm the bottle by running warm (not hot) water over it, but be careful not to get water in the bottle or to damage the label so that the directions are unreadable. Don't overheat, which can reduce the effectiveness of the medication.
▲ In children older than three years of age and in adults, it is important to hold the outer ear *up* and back while putting in ear drops. In children three years of age or younger, the ear should be gently pulled *down* and back. Gently massage the area around the ear (the tragus) to help the drops get to the ear canal.
▲ Show family members how to instill ear drops in case you need help.
▲ You may temporarily lose hearing because of the treatment or the infection. But if hearing loss continues, contact your physician.

POINTS to REMEMBER

▼ Otic agents include the following ingredients, either by themselves or mixed together (depending on physician's order): corticosteroids, antibacterials, and other anti-inflammatory agents.

▼ Most disorders of the ear are self-limiting, but treatment is important to prevent complications to the area and/or systemic complications.

▼ Many of the anti-infective agents are combined with corticosteroids, in solution, to take advantage of their additional anti-inflammatory, antipruritic, and anti-allergic drug effects.

▼ Local anaesthetic otic agents are associated with some degree of discomfort and inflammation upon application; lidocaine is an example.

▼ Wax, or cerumen, is a natural product of the ear and is normally produced by modified sweat glands in the auditory canal; emulsifying otic agents (such as urea hydrogen peroxide) loosen and help remove this wax.

▼ Single agents and combination products are used to treat many ear conditions, and the nurse must know the indications and specific information about the drug(s) to ensure their safe use.

▼ Otitis media occurs at a higher rate in high-humidity climates.

EXAMINATION REVIEW QUESTIONS

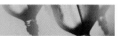

1 Untreated otitis media may lead to which of the following?
 a. Minor ear infection reoccurrences
 b. Mastoiditis
 c. Fungal infection
 d. Decreased cerumen production

2 Which of the following most accurately describes the action of lidocaine?
 a. Softens cerumen
 b. Decreases itching and inflammation
 c. Has antifungal effects
 d. Area is anaesthetized to decrease pain

3 Ear drops should be administered using which of the following techniques?
 a. Warm the solution to 41°C before using.
 b. Administer with the client properly positioned so that the unaffected ear is accessible.

 c. Put drops on a cotton-tipped applicator for insertion to the inner ear.
 d. Apply to the affected ear after careful cleansing.

4 Which of the following is recommended after application of ear drops?
 a. There are no special actions.
 b. Stuff the ear with a moderate amount of cotton.
 c. Put the client on bed rest for four to six hours.
 d. Keep the affected ear up for three to five minutes.

5 Which of the following is the most likely allergic reaction to an otic solution?
 a. Minor redness
 b. Inflammation and discomfort
 c. Outer ear deformity
 d. Severe fungal infections

For answers see http://evolve.elsevier.com/Lilley/pharmacology/.

CRITICAL THINKING ACTIVITIES

1 Develop a client teaching plan for the caregiver who will be administering antibacterial and steroidal otic drops to a three-year-old child.

2 Your pediatric client's mother tells you that she does not understand why ear infections require treatment with an-

tibiotics. She states, "We used home remedies when I was growing up." What information would you share with the client's mother and why?

3 What is the indication for a wax emulsifier? Explain your answer.

For answers see http://evolve.elsevier.com/Lilley/pharmacology/.

BIBLIOGRAPHY

Albanese, J., & Nutz, P. (2005). *Mosby's 2005 nursing drug cards.* St Louis, MO: Mosby.

Canadian Pharmacists Association. (2003). *Therapeutic choices* (4th ed.). Ottawa, ON: Author.

Canadian Pharmacists Association. (2004). *Guide to drugs in Canada.* Toronto, ON: Dorling Kindersley.

Canadian Pharmacists Association. (2005). *Compendium of pharmaceuticals and specialties. The Canadian drug reference for health professionals.* Ottawa, ON: Author. [The subscription-based e-CPS is available at http://www.pharmacists.ca.]

Cheng, A., Williams, B.A., & Sivarajan, B.V. (Eds.). (2003). *The HSC handbook of pediatrics* (10th ed.). Toronto, ON: Elsevier.

Facts and Comparisons. (2004). *Drug facts and comparisons pocket version* (9th ed.). St Louis, MO: Wolters Kluwer Health.

Hardman, J.G., & Limbird, L.E. (2002). *Goodman and Gilman's the pharmacological basis of therapeutics* (10th ed.). New York: McGraw-Hill.

Health Canada. (2005). Drug product database (DPD). Retrieved September 11, 2005, from http://www.hc-sc.gc.ca/hpb/drugs-dpd/

Katzung, B.G. (2004). *Basic and clinical pharmacology* (9th ed.). New York: McGraw-Hill.

Lehne, R.A. (2004). *Pharmacology for nursing care* (5th ed.). St Louis, MO: Saunders.

Mosby. (2005). *Mosby's drug consult 2005: The comprehensive reference for generic and brand name drugs* (15th ed.). St Louis, MO: Mosby.

Skidmore-Roth, L. (2006). *Mosby's 2006 nursing drug reference* (19th ed.). St Louis, MO: Mosby.

Pharmaceutical Abbreviations

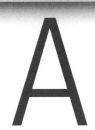

A

Abbreviation	Translation
DRUG DOSAGE	
cc	Cubic centimetre (equivalent to 1 ml)
g or Gm	Gram
gtt	Drop
L	Litre
m	Minim
mEq	Milliequivalent
min	Minute
mL	Millilitre
no	Number
qs	Quantity sufficient, as much as needed
ss	One half
tbsp	Tablespoon
tsp	Teaspoon
μg or mcg	Microgram
DRUG ROUTE	
AD	Right ear
AS	Left ear
AU	Both ears
ID	Intradermal
IM	Intramuscular
IV	Intravenous
NG	Nasogastric
PO	Per orally (by mouth)
SC	Subcutaneous
SL	Sublingual

Abbreviation	Translation
DRUG ADMINISTRATION	
ac	Before meals
ad lib	As desired, freely
bid	Twice a day
h or hr	Hour
noct	Night
NPO	Nothing by mouth
pc	After meals
prn	When needed
qh	Every hour
qid	Four times a day
qod	Every other day
Rx	Prescribe/take
stat	Immediately
tid	Three times a day

Some Common Drug Brands Available in Canada

Generic Name [Brand Name]

CHAPTER 10: ANALGESIC AGENTS

acetaminophen [Tylenol]
acetaminophen 300 mg/caffeine 15 mg/codeine 8 mg [Tylenol No. 1]
acetaminophen 300 mg/caffeine 15 mg/codeine 15 mg [Tylenol No. 2]
acetaminophen 300 mg/caffeine 15 mg/codeine 30 mg [Tylenol No. 3]
acetaminophen 300 mg/codeine 60 mg [Tylenol No. 4]
acetaminophen 500 mg/caffeine 15 mg/codeine 8 mg [Tylenol No. 1 Forte]
acetaminophen 325 mg/oxycodone HCl 5 mg [Percocet]
acetaminophen 325 mg/oxycodone HCl 2.5 mg [Percocet-Demi]
buprenorphine hydrochloride [Subutex]
butorphanol tartrate [Apo-butorphanol]
codeine sulphate; codeine monophosphate [Codeine Contin]
codeine phosphate [codeine]
fentanyl [Duragesic]
fentanyl citrate [Fentanyl Citrate]
meperidine hydrochloride [Pethidine]
methadone hydrochloride [Metadol]
morphine sulphate [Kadian; M.O.S.; MS Contin]
naloxone hydrochloride dihydrate [Naloxone HCl inj]
naltrexone hydrochloride [ReVia]
pentazocine [Talwin]
propoxyphene napsylate [Darvon-N]

CHAPTER 11: GENERAL AND LOCAL ANAESTHETICS

alfentanil hydrochloride [Alfenta]
atracurium besylate [Tracrium]
atropine sulphate [Atropine; Isopto Atropine]

benzocaine [Anbesol Gel; Dermoplast, Lanacane]
bupivacaine hydrochloride [Marcaine, Sensorcaine]
chloroprocaine hydrochloride [Nesacaine-CE]
desflurane [Suprane]
diazepam [Diastat; Diazemuls; Valium, Vivol]
dibucaine hydrochloride/esculin/framycetin sulphate/hydrocortisone [Proctosedyl]
doxacurium chloride [Nuromax]
dyclonine hydrochloride [Sucrets]
enflurane [Enflurane]
fentanyl [Duragesic]
fentanyl citrate [Fentanyl Citrate]
glycopyrrolate [Glycopyrrolate Injection]
halothane [halothane]
isoflurane [Forane]
ketamine hydrochloride [Ketalar]
lidocaine [Betacaine, Xylocaine, Lidodan Ointment]
lidocaine hydrochloride [Lidocaine Parenteral, Lidodan Endotracheal, Xylocard]
lorazepam [Ativan]
mepivacaine [Carbocaine]
midazolam [Apo-Midazolam]
mivacurium chloride [Mivacron]
morphine sulphate [Kadian, M-Eslon, M.O.S. Sulphate, MS Contin]
nitrous oxide ["laughing gas"]
pentobarbital [Nembutal]
pramoxine hydrochloride/calamine [Caladryl]
pramoxine hydrochloride/hydrocortisone acetate/zinc sulphate monohydrate [Anugesic-HC]
prilocaine/lidocaine [EMLA Cream, EMLA Patch]
promethazine hydrochloride [Phenergan]
propofol [Diprivan]
rocuronium bromide [Zemuron]
ropivacaine [Naropin]
scopolamine [Transderm-V]
sevoflurane [Sevorane AF]

succinylcholine chloride [Quelicin]
sufentanil citrate [Sufenta]
tetracaine hydrochloride [Ametop, Pontocaine]
thiopental sodium [Pentothal]

CHAPTER 12: CENTRAL NERVOUS SYSTEM DEPRESSANTS AND MUSCLE RELAXANTS

alprazolam [Xanax]
baclofen [Lioresal Oral, Apo-Baclofen]
bromazepam [Lectopam]
chlordiazepoxide hydrochloride [Apo-chlordiazepoxide]
chlorzoxazone/acetaminophen [Acetazone Forte, Parafon Forte]
clobazam [Apo-Clobazam]
clonazepam [Rivotril]
clorazepate dipotassium [Apo-Clorazepate, Novo-Clopate]
cyclobenzaprine hydrochloride [PHL-Cyclobenzaprine, Riva-Cycloprine]
dantrolene sodium [Dantrium Capsules; Dantrium Intravenous]
flurazepam hydrochloride [Apo-Flurazepam]
lorazepam [Ativan]
methocarbamol [Robaxin, Robaxin-750]
midazolam [Midazolam Injection]
nitrazepam [Mogadon]
orphenadrine citrate [Norflex]
orphenadrine citrate/ASA/caffeine [Norgesic]
oxazepam [Novoxapam, Oxpam]
pentobarbital sodium [Nembutal Sodium]
temazepam [Apo-Temazepam; Restoril]
tizanidine hydrochloride [Zanaflex]
triazolam [Halcion, Apo-Triazo]
zopiclone [Rhovane, Imovane]

CHAPTER 13: ANTI-EPILEPTIC AGENTS

carbamazepine [**Tegretol, Tegretol CR**]
clonazepam [**Rivotril**]
clorazepate dipotassium [**Novo-Clopate**]
ethosuximide [**Zarontin**]
fosphenytoin sodium [**Cerebyx**]
gabapentin [**Neurontin**]
lamotrigine [**Lamictal**]
levetiracetam [**Keppra**]
oxcarbazepine [**Trileptal**]
phenobarbital [**PMS-Phenobarbital**]
phenytoin sodium [**Dilantin Capsules, Dilantin Infatabs**]
primidone [**Apo-Primidone**]
topiramate [**Topamax**]
valproic acid [**Depakene, Epival**]

CHAPTER 14: ANTIPARKINSONIAN AGENTS

amantadine hydrochloride [**Symmetrel**]
benztropine mesylate [**PMS-Benztropine, APO Benztropine Mesylate, Benztropine Omega**]
biperiden hydrochloride [**Akineton**]
bromocriptine mesylate [**Parlodel**]
diphenhydramine hydrochloride [**Benadryl Preparations**]
entacapone [**Comtan**]
ethopropazine hydrochloride [**Parsitan**]
levodopa/benserazide hydrochloride [**Prolopa**]
levodopa-carbidopa [**Sinemet, Sinemet CR**]
pergolide mesylate [**Permax**]
pramipexole dihydrchloride [**Mirapex**]
ropinirole hydrochloride [**Requip**]
selegiline [**Nu-Selegiline, Anipryl**]
trihexyphenidyl [**PMS Trihexy-phenidyl, Trihexyphen**]

CHAPTER 15: PSYCHOTHERAPEUTIC AGENTS

alprazolam [**Xanax**]
amitriptyline hydrochloride [**PMS-Levazine, Etrafon, Novo-Tryptan, Elavil**]
bupropion hydrochloride [**Zyban, Wellbutrin SR**]
buspirone hydrochloride [**BuSpar**]
chlordiazepoxide hydrochloride [**Apo-Chlordiazepoxide**]
chlorpromazine [**Largactil**]
citalopram HBr [**Celexa**]
clozapine [**Clozaril**]
diazepam [**Diazemuls**]
diazepam rectal delivery system [**Diastat**]

escitalopram [**Cipralex**]
fluoxetine hydrochloride [**Apo-Fluoxetine, Prozac**]
fluphenazine decanoate [**Modecate**]
fluvoxamine maleate [**Luvox**]
haloperidol [**Apo-Haloperidol, Haldol, Novo-Peridol**]
hydroxyzine hydrochloride [**Atarax**]
lithium carbonate [**Carbolith, Duralith, Lithane**]
lithium citrate [**Lithium**]
lorazepam [**Ativan**]
loxapine hydrochloride [**Loxapine, Loxapac IM**]
mirtazapine [**Remeron, Remeron RD**]
nortriptyline hydrochloride [**Aventyl**]
olanzapine [**Zyprexa, Zyprexa Zydis, Zyprexa IntraMuscular**]
paroxetine hydrochloride [**Paxil, Paxil CR**]
phenelzine sulphate [**Nardil**]
quetiapine fumarate [**Seroquel**]
risperidone [**Risperdal Consta, Risperdal M-Tab**]
risperidone tartrate [**Risperdal Oral Solution**]
sertraline hydrochloride [**Zoloft**]
thiothixene [**Navane**]
tranylcypromine sulphate [**Parnate**]
trazodone hydrochloride [**Desyrel**]
venlafaxine hydrochloride [**Effexor XR**]

CHAPTER 16: CENTRAL NERVOUS SYSTEM STIMULANT AGENTS

almotriptan malate [**Axert**]
caffeine [**Wake Ups Tablets, Destim, Pep-Back Tablets**]
dextroamphetamine sulphate [**Dexedrine**]
diethylpropion hydrochloride [**Tenuate**]
eletriptan HBr [**Relpax**]
methylphenidate hydrochloride [**Concerta, Ritalin SR**]
modafinil [**Alertec**]
naratriptan hydrochloride [**Amerge**]
orlistat [**Xenical**]
rizatriptan benzoate [**Maxalt**]
sibutramine hydrochloride monohydrate [**Meridia**]
sumatriptan succinate [**Imitrex DF Tablets**]
zolmitriptan [**Zomig**]

CHAPTER 17: ADRENERGIC AGENTS

dobutamine hydrochloride [**Dobutrex, Dobutamine Hydrochloride Injection**]

dopamine hydrochloride/dextrose [**Dopamine Hydrochloride Injection, Intropin Injection**]
ephinephrine [**Epipen**]
epinephrine hydrochloride [**Adrenalin, Vaponefrin**]
formoterol fumerate [**Foradil**]
formoterol fumurate dihydrate [**Oxeze Turbohaler**]
isoproterenol hydrochloride [**Isoproterenol hydrochloride Injection**]
midodrine hydrochloride [**Amatine**]
norepinephrine bitartrate [**Levophed**]
phenylephrine hydrochloride [**Mydfrin, Neo-Synephrine Parenteral**]
pseudoephedrine hydrochloride [**Pseudofrin, Sudafed**]
salbutamol [**Ventolin Nebules P.F., Ventodisk**]
salbutamol sulphate [**Airomir**]
salmeterol xinafoate [**Serevent Inhalation Aerosol, Serevent Diskus, Serevent Diskhaler Disk**]
terbutaline sulphate [**Bricanyl Turbuhaler**]
tetrahydrozoline hydrochloride [**Visine Original Eye Drops**]

CHAPTER 18: ADRENERGIC-BLOCKING AGENTS

acebutolol hydrochloride [**Monitan, Rhotral, Sectral**]
atenolol [**Tenormin**]
atenolol/chlorthalidone [**Tenoretic**]
betaxolol hydrochloride [**Betaxolol, Betoptic S**]
bisoprolol fumarate [**Monocor**]
carvedilol [**Coreg**]
ergotamine tartrate/caffeine [**Cafergot**]
esmolol hydrochloride [**Brevibloc**]
labetalol hydrochloride [**Trandate**]
metoprolol tartrate [**Betaloc, Betaloc Durules, Lopresor**]
nadolol [**Corgard**]
oxprenolol hydrochloride [**Trasicor**]
phentolamine mesylate [**Rogitine**]
pindolol [**Visken**]
pindolol/hydrochlorothiazide [**Viskazide**]
prazosin hydrochloride [**Apo-Prazo, Minipress**]
propranolol hydrochloride [**Inderal-LA**]
sotalol hydrochloride [**Rhoxal-Sotalol, Sotamol, Rylosol**]
timolol maleate [**Timoptic**]

CHAPTER 19: CHOLINERGIC AGENTS

bethanechol chloride [**Duvoid**]
donepezil hydrochloride [**Aricept**]
galantamine HBr [**Reminyl**]
memantine [**Ebixa**]
physostigmine (available only under the Special Access Programme)
pyridostigmine bromide [**Mestinon**]
rivastigmine hydrogen tartrate [**Exelon**]

CHAPTER 20: CHOLINERGIC-BLOCKING AGENTS

atropine sulphate [**Isopto Atropine**]
benztropine mesylate [**PMS-Benztropine, Benztropine Omega**]
dicyclomine hydrochloride [**Bentylol**]
flavoxate hydrochloride [**PMS-Flavoxate, Urispas**]
glycopyrrolate bromide [**Glycopyrrolate Injection**]
imipramine hydrochloride [**Tofranil**]
oxybutynin [**Oxytrol**]
oxybutynin chloride [**Ditropan, Ditropan XL**]
propantheline bromide [**Pro-Banthine**]
scopolamine [**Transderm-V**]
tolterodine L-tartrate [**Detrol, Detrol LA**]
trihexyphenidyl hydrochloride [**Apo-Trihex**]

CHAPTER 21: POSITIVE INOTROPIC AGENTS

digoxin [**Lanoxin**]
digoxin immune Fab [**Digibind**]
milrinone lactate [**Apo-Milrinone Injectable**]

CHAPTER 22: ANTIDYSRHYTHMIC AGENTS

adenosine [**Adenocard**]
amiodarone hydrochloride [**Cordarone**]
atenolol [**Tenormin**]
bretylium tosylate [**bretylium tosylate**]
diltiazem [**Cardizem, Tiazac**]
disopyramide [**Rythmodan**]
disopyramide phosphate [**Rythmodan LA**]
esmolol hydrochloride [**Brevibloc**]
flecainide acetate [**Tambocor**]
lidocaine hydrochloride [**Lidocaine Parenteral**]
metoprolol tartrate [**Betaloc, Lopresor**]
mexiletine hydrochloride [**Novo-Mexiletine**]

procainamide hydrochloride [**Apo-Procainamide, Procan SR**]
propafenone hydrochloride [**Rythmol**]
propranolol hydrochloride [**Novo-Pranol, Inderal-LA**]
quinidine bisulphate [**Biquin Durules**]
sotalol hydrochloride [**Rhoxal-Sotalol, Sotamol, Rylosol**]
verapamil hydrochloride [**Covera, Isoptin SR, Nu-Verap**]

CHAPTER 23: ANTI-ANGINAL AGENTS

amlodipine besylate [**Norvasc**]
atenolol [**Tenormin**]
diltiazem hydrochloride [**Cardizem, Nu-Diltiaz, Tiazac**]
felodipine [**Plendil, Renedil**]
isosorbide dinitrate [**Apo-ISDN, Novo-Sorbide, Coronex**]
isosorbide-5-mononitrate [**Imdur**]
metoprolol tartrate [**Betaloc, Lopresor**]
nifedipine [**Adalat XL, Apo-Nifed**]
nimodipine [**Nimotop**]
nitroglycerin [**Minitran, Nitro-Dur, Nitrostat, Nitrol**]
verapamil hydrochloride [**Covera, Isoptin SR, Nu-Verap**]

CHAPTER 24: ANTIHYPERTENSIVE AGENTS

benazepril hydrochloride [**Lotensin**]
bosentan [**Tracleer**]
candesartan cilexetil [**Atacand**]
candesartan cilexil/hydrochlorothiazide [**Atacand Plus**]
captopril [**Capoten**]
carvedilol [**Coreg**]
cilazapril monohydrate [**Inhibace**]
cilazapril monohydrate/hydrochlorothiazide [**Inhibace Plus**]
clonidine hydrochloride [**Catapres, Dixarit**]
doxazosin mesylate [**Cardura**]
enalapril maleate [**Vasotec**]
enalapril maleate/hydrochlorothiazide [**Vaseretic**]
epoprostenol sodium [**Flolan**]
eprosartan mesylate [**Teveten**]
eprosartan mesylate/hydrochlorothiazide [**Teveten Plus**]
fosinopril sodium [**Monopril, Novo-Fosinopril**]
hydralazine hydrochloride [**Apresoline, Nu-Hydral**]
irbesartan [**Avapro**]
irbesartan/hydrochlorothiazide [**Avalide**]
lisinopril [**Prinivil, Zestril**]
lisinopril/hydrochlorothiazide [**Prinzide, Zestoretic**]
losartan potassium [**Cozaar**]

losartan potassium/hydrochlorothiazide [**Hyzaar**]
minoxidil [**Loniten**]
perindopril erbumine [**Coversyl**]
prazosin hydrochloride [**Apo-Prazo, Nu-Prazo, Minipress**]
quinapril hydrochloride [**Accupril**]
quinapril hydrochloride/hydrochlorothiazide [**Accuretic**]
ramipril [**Altace**]
sodium nitroprusside [**Nipride**]
tamsulosin hydrochloride [**Flomax**]
terazosin hydrochloride [**Hytrin**]
trandolapril [**Mavik**]
trandolapril/verapamil hydrochloride [**Tarka**]
treprostinil sodium [**Remodulin**]
valsartan [**Diovan**]
valsartan/hydrochlorothiazide [**Diovan-HCT**]

CHAPTER 25: DIURETIC AGENTS

acetazolamide [**Apo-Acetazolamide, Acetazolam**]
amiloride hydrochloride [**Apo-Amiloride, Midamor, Moduret**]
bumetanide [**Burinex**]
ethacrynic acid [**Edecrin**]
furosemide [**Lasix**]
hydrochlorothiazide [**Apo-Hydro, Novo-Hydrazide**]
mannitol [**Osmitrol**]
metolazone [**Zaroxolyn**]
spironolactone [**Aldactone**]
spironolactone/hydrochlorothiazide [**Aldactazide**]
triamterene/hydrochlorthiazide [**Nu-Triazide**]

CHAPTER 26: FLUIDS AND ELECTROLYTES

albumin [**Albuminar-25, Plasbumin-25, Plasbumin-5**]
dextran 40 [**Gentran 40**]
hetastarch [**Hextend**]
potassium salts [**PO forms: acetate, bicarbonate, chloride, citrate, and gluconate salts; IV forms: acetate, chloride, and phosphate**]
sodium chloride [**table salt, NaCl**]
sodium polystyrene sulphonate [**Kayexalate**]

CHAPTER 27: COAGULATION MODIFIER AGENTS

abciximab [**Reopro**]
acetylsalicylic acid [**ASA, Aspirin**]
alteplase [**Activase Rt-PA**]
clopidogrel bisulphate [**Plavix**]

dalteparin sodium [**Fragmin**]
desmopressin acetate [**DDAVP**]
enoxaparin sodium [**Lovenox**]
eptifibatide [**Integrilin**]
heparin sodium [**Hepalean,
    Hepalean-Lok, Heparin Leo**]
nadroparin calcium [**Fraxiparine**]
pentoxifylline [**Trental**]
streptokinase [**Streptase**]
ticlopidine hydrochloride [**Ticlid**]
tinzaparin sodium [**Innohep**]
tirofiban hydrochloride [**Aggrastat**]
warfarin sodium [**Coumadin**]

CHAPTER 28: ANTILIPEMIC AGENTS

atorvastatin [**Lipitor**]
bezafibrate [**Bezalip**]
cholestyramine resin [**PHL
    Cholestyramine, Novo-Cholamine**]
colestipol hydrochloride [**Colestid**]
ezetimibe [**Ezetrol**]
fenofibrate [**Apo-Fenofibrate,
    Nu-Fenofibrate**]
fenofibrate microcoated [**Lipidil Supra**]
fluvastatin sodium [**Lescol**]
gemfibrozil [**Lopid**]
lovastatin [**Mevacor**]
niacin [**nicotinic acid, vitamin B₃**]
pravastatin sodium [**Pravachol**]
rosuvastatin calcium [**Crestor**]
simvastatin [**Zocor**]

CHAPTER 29: PITUITARY AGENTS

cosyntropin [**Cortrosyn**]
cosyntropin/zinc hydroxide
    [**Synacthen Depot**]
desmopressin acetate [**DDAVP,
    Octostim**]
octreotide acetate [**Sandostatin,
    Sandostatin LAR**]
somatropin [**Humatrope, Nutropin,
    Nutropin AQ, Saizen, Serostim**]
vasopressin [**Pressyn AR**]

CHAPTER 30: THYROID AND ANTITHYROID AGENTS

dessicated thyroid [**thyroid hormone**]
levothyroxine sodium [**Eltroxin,
    Synthroid**]
liothyronine sodium [**Cytomel**]
methimazole [**Apo-Methimazole**]
propylthiouracil [**Propyl-Thyracil**]

CHAPTER 31: ANTIDIABETIC AGENTS

acarbose [**Prandase**]
chlorpropamide [**Novo-Propamide**]
gliclazide [**Diamicron, Diamicron MR**]
glimepiride [**Amaryl**]
glyburide [**Diabeta**]
insulin aspart [**NovoRapid**]
insulin delivery device [**Novolin GE
    Penfill Injection**]
insulin doser [**Innovo**]
insulin glargine [**Lantus**]
insulin lente [**Humulin-L**]
insulin lente (pork) [**Hypurin Regular
    Insulin Pork**]
insulin lispro [**Humalog**]
insulin lispro/insulin lispro protamine
    [**Humalog Mix 25**]
insulin NPH (human biosynthetic)
    [**Humulin-N, Novolin GE NPH**]
insulin regular (human biosynthetic)
    [**Humulin-R, Novolin GE Toronto**]
insulin regular (human biosynthetic)/
    insulin NPH (human biosynthetic)
    [**Novolin GE 50/50 and other
    combinations 10/90, 20/80, 30/70,
    40/60; Humulin 70/30, 80/20**]
insulin NPH (pork) [**Hypurin regular
    insulin pork**]
insulin zinc suspension [**Humulin-L,
    Novolin GE Toronto inj**]
insulin ultralente (human
    biosynthetic) [**Humulin-U**]
metformin hydrochloride
    [**Glucophage**]
metformin hydrochloride XR
    [**Glumetza**]
nateglinide [**Starlix**]
orlistat [**Xenical**]
pioglitazone hydrochloride [**Actos**]
repaglinide [**GlucoNorm**]
rosiglitazone maleate [**Avandia**]
rosiglitazone maleate/metformin
    hydrochloride [**Avandamet**]
tolbutamide [**Apo-Tolbutamide**]

CHAPTER 32: ADRENAL AGENTS

dexamethasone [**Apo-Dexamethasone,
    Dexasone, Maxidex**]
fludrocortisone acetate [**Florinef**]
hydrocortisone sodium succinate
    [**Solu-Cortef**]
methylprednisolone sodium succinate
    [**Solu-Medrol**]
prednisone [**Apo-Prednisone, Winpred**]

CHAPTER 33: WOMEN'S HEALTH AGENTS

HORMONE REPLACEMENT THERAPY

conjugated estrogens [**C.E.S.,
    Congest, PMS Conjugated
    Estrogens, Premarin**]
conjugated estrogens/
    medroxyprogesterone acetate
    [**Premplus**]
diethylstilbestrol [**Stilbestrol**]
esterified estrogens [**Neo-Estrone**]
estradiol [**Estrace**]
estradiol/norethindrone acetate
    [**Estracomb**]
estradiol transdermal [**Estraderm,
    Estradot, Climara, Vivelle**]
estradiol vaginal dosage forms
    [**Vagifem, Estring**]
estradiol valerate [**Delestrogen, PMS-
    Estradiol Valerate**]
estradiol valerate/testosterone
    enanthate [**Neo Pause**]
estropipate [**Ogen**]
medroxyprogesterone [**Depo-Provera**]
megestrol acetate [**Megace, Megace
    OS**]
norethindrone [**Micronor**]
norethindrone acetate/ethinyl
    estradiol [**FemHRT**]
progesterone [**Crinone, Prometrium**]

CONTRACEPTIVES

ethinyl estradiol/drospirenone [**Yasmin
    21, Yasmin 28**]
etonogestrel/ethinyl estradiol
    [**NuvaRing**]
levonorgestrel [**Plan B**]
levonorgesterol/ethinyl estradiol,
    monophasic class [**Alesse 21, Alesse
    28, Min-Ovral 21, Min-Ovral 28**]
levonorgesterol/ethinyl estradiol,
    triphasic class [**Triphasil 21, Triphasil
    28, Triquilar 21, Triquilar 28**]
medroxyprogesterone acetate [**Depo-
    Provera**]
norelgestromin/ethinyl estradiol [**Evra**]
norethindrone/ethinyl estradiol,
    monophasic class [**Brevicon 0.5/35,
    Brevicon 1/35, Ortho 1/35, Ortho
    0.5/35**]
norethindrone/ethinyl estradiol,
    biphasic class [**Synphasic**]
norethindrone/ethinyl estradiol,
    triphasic class [**Ortho 7/7/7**]
norgestrel/ethinyl estradiol [**Lo-
    Femenal 21, Ovral 21, Ovral 28**]

OSTEOPOROSIS DRUG THERAPIES

alendronate sodium trihydrate **[Fosamax]**

calcitonin, salmon **[Calcimar, Miacalcin NS]**

clodronate disodium **[Bonefos, Ostac]**

etidronate disodium **[Didronel]**

raloxifene **[Evista]**

risedronate sodium **[Actonel]**

tamoxifen **[Nolvadex-D, Tamofen]**

teriparatide **[Forteo]**

FERTILITY AGENTS

choriogonadotropin alfa **[Ovidrel]**

clomiphene citrate **[Clomid, Serophene]**

follitropin alfa **[Gonal-F]**

follitropin beta **[Puregon]**

human chorionic gonadotropin **[Pregnyl, Profasi HP]**

menotropins **[Repronex]**

urofollitropin **[Bravelle]**

UTERINE-ACTIVE DRUGS (FOR LABOUR AND POSTPARTUM)

carboprost tromethamine **[Hemabate]**

dinoprostone **[Prostin E$_2$, Prepidil, Cervidil]**

ergonovine maleate **[ergonovine maleate injection]**

misoprostol **[Apo-Misoprostol]**

oxytocin

CHAPTER 34: MEN'S HEALTH AGENTS

ANDROGENS AND ANABOLIC STEROIDS

bicalutamide **[Casodex]**

danazol **[Cyclomen]**

doxazosin **[Cardura]**

dutasteride **[Avodart]**

finasteride **[Propecia, Proscar]**

flutamide **[Euflex]**

goserelin **[Zoladex]**

leuprolide acetate **[Eligard, Lupron]**

nandrolone decanoate **[Deca-Durabolin]**

nilutamide **[Anandron]**

tamsulosin hydrochloride **[Flomax]**

terazosin hydrochloride **[Hytrin]**

testosterone cypionate testosterone, transdermal **[Androderm, AndroGel]**

vardenafil **[Levitra]**

ERECTILE-DYSFUNCTION AGENTS

alprostadil **[MUSE]**

sildenafil citrate **[Viagra]**

CHAPTER 35: ANTIHISTAMINES, DECONGESTANTS, ANTITUSSIVES, AND EXPECTORANTS

ANTIHISTAMINES

Azatadine maleate **[Optimine]**

azatadine maleate/pseudoephineprine sulphate **[Trinalin Repetabs]**

brompheniramine maleate/phenylephrine hydrochloride **[Dimetapp]**

cetirizine hydrochloride **[Reactine]**

chlorpheniramine maleate **[Chlor-Tripolon, Novo-Pheniram]**

clemastine **[Tavist]**

cyproheptadine hydrochloride **[Euro-Cyproheptadine]**

desloratadine **[Aerius, Aerius Kids]**

dimenhydrinate **[Gravol]**

diphenhydramine hydrochloride **[Benadryl]**

fexofenadine hydrochloride **[Allegra]**

fexofenadine hydrochloride/pseudoephedrine hydrochloride **[Allegra-D]**

hydroxyzine hydrochloride **[Atarax]**

loratadine **[Claritin]**

loratadine/pseudoephedrine sulphate **[Claritin Allergy + Sinus, Liberator]**

meclizine hydrochloride **[Bonamine]**

promethazine **[Phenergan]**

DECONGESTANTS

beclomethasone dipropionate **[Qvar, Gen-Beclo AQ-AEM SUS, Ratio-Beclomethasone AQ]**

budesonide **[Pulmicort Turbuhaler, Rhinocort Aqua, Rhinocort Turbuhaler]**

ephedrine **[Rhino-Vaccin]**

flunisolide **[Rhinalar]**

fluticasone propionate **[Flonase]**

ipratropium bromide **[Atrovent HFA, Atrovent]**

oxymetazoline hydrochloride **[Afrin]**

phenylephrine hydrochloride/pheniramine maleate **[Dristan Decongestant Nasal Mist]**

pseudoephedrine hydrochloride **[Sudafed Decongestant Extra Strength, Sudafed Decongestant 12 Hour]**

triamcinolone acetonide **[Nasacort]**

ANTITUSSIVES

codeine (as part of a combination product) **[Dimetane-Expectorant-C, Dimetapp-C, CoActifed, Robitussin AC]**

dextromethorphan (as part of a combination product) **[Balminil DM, Benylin DM-E, Dimetapp DM, Robitussin-DM]**

EXPECTORANTS

guaifenesin (a.k.a. glyceryl guaiacolate) **[Bismutal, Robitussin]**

potassium iodide/guaifenesin/pyrilamine maleate/theophylline **[ratio-Theo-Bronc]**

CHAPTER 36: BRONCHODILATORS AND OTHER RESPIRATORY AGENTS

aminophylline **[Aminophylline, Phyllocontin]**

beclomethasone dipropionate **[Qvar, Rivanase]**

budesonide **[Pulmicort Nebuamp, Pulmicort Turbuhaler, Rhinocort Aqua, Rhinocort Turbuhaler]**

budesonide/formoterol fumarate dihydrate **[Symbicort Turbuhaler]**

cromolyn sodium **[Intal Inhaler, Intal Spincaps, Nalcrom]**

ephedrine hydrochloride **[Abundance Ephedrine Hydrochloride]**

epinephrine **[Adrenalin Chloride]**

fenoterol hydrobromide **[Berotec]**

fenoterol hydrobromide/ipratropium bromide **[Duovent UDV]**

flunisolide **[Rhinalar Nasal Mist]**

fluticasone propionate **[Flonase, Flovent, Flovent Diskus]**

fluticasone propionate/salmeterol xinafoate **[Advair Diskus inhaler]**

formoterol fumarate **[Oxeze, Foradil]**

hydrocortisone **[Solu-Cortef]**

ipratropium bromide **[Atrovent]**

isoproterenol hydrochloride

methylprednisolone **[Solu-Medrol]**

montelukast sodium **[Singulair]**

nedocromil sodium **[Alocril, Tilade]**

salbutamol **[Airomir, Apo-Salvent, Ventolin, Ventodisk]**

salbutamol/ipratropium bromide **[Combivent]**

terbutaline sulphate **[Bricanyl Turbohaler]**

theophylline **[Theolair, Uniphyl SRT]**

triamcinolone acetonide **[Nasacort]**

zafirlukast **[Accolate]**

CHAPTER 37: ANTIBIOTICS

amikacin **[Amikin]**

amoxicillin **[PHL-Amoxicillin, Moxilean]**

amoxicillin/clavulanic acid **[Apo-Amoxi-Clav, Clavulin]**

ampicillin **[Novo-Ampicillin]**

azithromycin [**Zithromax**]
cefazolin sodium
cefepime [**Maxipime**]
cefixime [**Suprax**]
cefoxitin sodium [**Cefoxitin for Injection**]
ceftazidime [**Fortaz**]
ceftriaxone [**Rocephin**]
cefuroxime sodium [**Zinacef**]
cefuroxime axetil [**Ceftin**]
cephalexin [**Apo-Cephalex, Keflex, Novo-Lexin**]
ciprofloxacin [**Cipro XL, Cipro Oral Suspension**]
clarithromycin [**Biaxin, Biaxin XL**]
clindamycin [**Apo-Clindamycin, Dalacin C, Gen-Clindamycin**]
cloxacillin sodium [**Apo-Cloxi, Novo-Cloxin, Nu-Cloxi**]
dapsone demeclocycline hydrochloride [**Declomycin**]
doxycycline hyclate [**Doxycin, Vibra-Tabs**]
ertapenem [**Invanz**]
erythromycin [**Apo-Erythro E-C, PCE Tab, Erythro-Base Tab, Erybid, Eryc**]
erythromycin estolate [**Novo-Rythro Estolate**]
erythromycin ethylsuccinate [**Apo-Erythro E.S. Tab, EES 600, Novo-Rythro Ethylsuccinate, EES 200 Granules**]
erythromycin lactobionate IV [**Erythrocin**]
erythromycin stearate PO [**Nu-Erythromycin-S, Erythromycine, Erythro-500**]
gatifloxacin [**Tequin**]
gentamicin sulphate [**PMS Gentamicin, Ratio-Gentamicin**]
imipenem/cilastatin [**Primaxin**]
levofloxacin [**Levaquin**]
linezolid [**Zyvoxam**]
meropenem [**Merrem**]
metronidazole [**Flagyl**]
moxifloxacin [**Avelox**]
nitrofurantoin [**Apo-Nitrofurantoin, MacroBid, Novo-Furantoin**]
norfloxacin [**Apo-Norflox**]
ofloxacin [**Apo-Oflox**]
penicillin G potassium [**Penicillin G Potassium**]
penicillin V potassium [**Apo-Pen VK, Novo-Pen-VK**]
piperacillin sodium [**Piperacillin**]
piperacillin/tazobactam [**Tazocin**]
quinupristin/dalfopristin [**Synercid**]
sulfamethoxazole/trimethoprim [**Apo-Sulfatrim, Novo-Trimel, Septra Injection**]
sulfisoxazole [**Apo-Sulfisoxazole**]
sulfisoxazole acetyl/erythromycin ethylsuccinate [**Pediazole**]
ticarcillin disodium/clavulanate potassium [**Timentin**]

tobramycin [**TOBI**]
vancomycin [**Vancocin**]

CHAPTER 38: ANTIVIRAL AGENTS

abacavir [**Ziagen**]
abacavir/lamivudine/zidovudine [**Trizivir**]
acyclovir [**Zovirax**]
amantadine hydrochloride [**Symmetrel**]
amprenavir [**Agenerase**]
atazanavir [**Reyataz**]
delavirdine mesylate [**Rescriptor**]
didanosine [**Videx, Videx EC**]
efavirenz [**Sustiva**]
enfuvirtide [**Fuzeon**]
famciclovir [**Famvir**]
ganciclovir [**Cytovene**]
indinavir [**Crixivan**]
lamivudine [**Heptovir, 3TC**]
lamivudine/zidovudine [**Combivir**]
lopinavir/ritonavir [**Kaletra**]
nelfinavir [**Viracept**]
nevirapine [**Viramune**]
oseltamivir [**Tamiflu**]
ribavirin [**Virazole**]
ritonavir [**Norvir**]
saquinavir [**Invirase**]
stavudine [**Zerit**]
tenofovir disoproxil [**Viread**]
valacyclovir [**Valtrex**]
valganciclovir [**Valcyte**]
zalcitabine [**Hivid**]
zanamivir [**Relenza**]
zidovudine [**Retrovir (AZT)**]

CHAPTER 39: ANTITUBERCULOUS AGENTS

ethambutol hydrochloride [**Etibi**]
isoniazid [**Isotamine**]
pyrazinamide [**Tebrazid**]
rifabutin [**Mycobutin**]
rifampin [**Rifadin, Rofact**]
rifampin/isoniazid/pyrazinamide [**Rifater**]
streptomycin

CHAPTER 40: ANTIFUNGAL AGENTS

amphotericin B [**Fungizone, Amphotec, Abelcet**]
amphotericin B (liposomal) [**AmBisome**]
caspofungin [**Cancidas**]
clotrimazole [**Canesten, Clotrimaderm**]
fluconazole [**Diflucan**]
griseofulvin [**Fulvicin**]
itraconazole [**Sporanox**]
ketoconazole [**Ketoderm, Nizoral**]

miconazole nitrate [**Micatin, Micozole, Monistat**]
nystatin [**Candistatin, Mycostatin, Ratio-Nystatin**]
terbinafine hydrochloride [**Lamisil**]
voriconazole [**Vfend**]

CHAPTER 41: ANTIMALARIAL, ANTIPROTOZOAL, AND ANTHELMINTIC AGENTS

ANTIMALARIALS
atovaquone/proguanil hydrochloride [**Malarone**]
chloroquine diphosphate [**Novo-Chloroquine**]
doxycycline [**Doxycin, Vibra-Tabs**]
hydroxychloroquine sulphate [**Plaquenil**]
mefloquine [**Lariam**]
primaquine
pyrimethamine [**Daraprim**]
trimethoprim [**Apo-Trimethoprim**]

ANTIPROTOZOALS
atovaquone [**Mepron**]
chloroquine [**Novo-Chloroquine**]
metronidazole [**Flagyl, Florazole ER**]
paromomycin [**Humatin**]
pentamidine isethionate [**Pentamidine Isethionate for Injection**]
pyrimethamine [**Daraprim**]

ANTHELMINTICS
mebendazole [**Vermox**]
praziquantel [**Biltricide**]

CHAPTER 42: ANTISEPTIC AND DISINFECTANT AGENTS

acetic acid (vinegar)
benzalkonium chloride [**Amazing Nok Out**]
benzoic acid
benzoyl peroxide [**Acetoxyl, Benoxyl, Benzac AC Gel 10%, Panoxyl**]
boric acid
carbolic acid (phenol) [**Chloraseptic**]
cetylpyridinium chloride/alcohol anhydrous [**Green Antiseptic MWH & Gargle**]
cetylpyridinium chloride/sodium fluoride [**Cepacol Mouthwash with Fluoride**]
chlorhexidine gluconate [**Apo-Chlorhexidine Oral Rinse**]
formaldehyde [**Vapophene**]
gentian violet (crystal violet) [**Gentian, Gentiane Violet**]

glutaraldehyde [**BM-28 Plus Activated 2% Glutaradehyde**]

hexachlorophene [**Phisohex**]

hydrogen peroxide [**Hydrogen Peroxide USP**]

iodine [**Iodine Tincture**]

isopropyl alcohol [**Isopropanol 99, Alcogel, Loris, Dermorapid, Ecocare 350**]

povidone-iodine [**Swabplus Povidine-Iodine, Rougier Swab Povidine Iodine Swabs, Swabsticks, Povidine Iodine Solution, Betadine**]

sodium hypochlorite [**Clorox, Dakin's Solution 0.5% Modified, Exsept 0.114%, Hygeol 1%, Javex 5 Bleach**]

CHAPTER 43: ANTI-INFLAMMATORY, ANTIRHEUMATIC, AND RELATED AGENTS

ANTI-INFLAMMATORY AGENTS

acetylsalicylic acid [**ASA; Aspirin, Aspergum, Bufferin, many product names**]

acetylsalicylic acid/butalbital/caffeine [**Fiorinal**]

celecoxib [**Celebrex**]

diclofenac potassium [**Voltaren Rapide, Novo-Difenac-K**]

diclofenac sodium [**Pennsaid Topical Solution, Voltaren-SR**]

diflunisal [**Apo-Diflunisal**]

etodolac [**Apo-Etodolac**]

flurbiprofen [**Ansaid, Froben**]

ibuprofen [**Motrin IB, Advil**]

indomethacin [**Rhodacine**]

ketoprofen [**Anafen**]

ketorolac tromethamine [**Nu-Ketorolac, Toradol**]

magnesium salicylate [**Herbogesic, Kneerelief Tablets**]

mefenamic acid [**Apo-Mefenamic**]

meloxicam [**Mobicox**]

nabumetone [**Gen-Nabumetone, Apo-Nabumetone, Sandoz Nabumetone**]

naproxen sodium [**Naprosyn**]

oxaprozin [**Daypro**]

piroxicam [**Apo-Piroxicam**]

sodium salicylate [**Dodd's Tablets, Natrum Salicylicum**]

sulindac [**Apo-Sulin, Novo-Sundac**]

ANTI-GOUT AGENTS

allopurinol [**Zyloprim, Alloprin**]

colchicine [**Colchicinum, Pekana-Colchicinum**]

probenecid [**Benuryl**]

sulfinpyrazone [**Apo-Sulfinpyrazone**]

ANTI-ARTHRITIC AGENTS

Auranofin [**Ridaura**]

Etanercept [**Enbrel**]

gold sodium thiomalate [**Sodium Aurothiomalate Injection, Myochrisine**]

ketorolac tromethamine [**Nu-Ketorolac, Toradol**]

leflunomide [**Arava**]

methotrexate

CHAPTER 44: IMMUNO-SUPPRESSANT AGENTS

azathioprine [**Imuran**]

basiliximab [**Simulect**]

cyclosporine [**Apo-Cyclosporin, Neoral, Sandimmune**]

daclizumab [**Zenapax**]

glatiramer acetate [**Copaxone**]

muromonab-CD3 [**Orthoclone OKT3**]

mycophenolate mofetil [**CellCept**]

sirolimus [**Rapamune**]

tacrolimus [**Prograf, Protopic**]

CHAPTER 45: IMMUNIZING AGENTS

acellular pertussis vaccine/adsorbed diphtheria and tetanus toxoids/inactivated polio vaccine/*Haemophilus influenzae* type b [**Pentacel**]

acellular pertussis vaccine/diphtheria and tetanus toxoids (dTap) [**Adacel**]

Haemophilus influenzae type b conjugate vaccine [**Act-HIB**]

hepatitis B immune globulin [**HyperHep B S/D**]

hepatitis B surface antigen (recombinant) [**Engerix-B, Recombivax HB**]

hepatitis B surface antigen inactivated/hepatitis A vaccine inactivated [**Twinrix**]

Hib polysaccharide conjugate (tetanus protein conjugate) vaccine [**Act-HIB**]

immune globulin [**Gammagard S/D, Gamimune N 5%, Iveegam Immuno, Gamunex, Atgam**]

influenza virus vaccine [**Fluzone Trivalent Subvirion, Fluviral**]

measles and rubella virus vaccine live [**Moru-Viraten Berna**]

measles, mumps, and rubella vaccine (MMR) [**M-M-R II, Priorix**]

pneumococcal vaccine, 7-valent [**Prevnar**]

pneumococcal vaccine, polyvalent [**Pneumovax-23 (5 dose) (1 dose)**]

poliovirus vaccine trivalent (inactivated) diploid cell origin, inactivated [**IPV**]

rabies immune globulin human [**Imogam Rabies Pasteurized, HyperRab S/D**]

rabies virus vaccine inactivated (human diploid-cell culture [**Imovax Rabies Vaccine Inactivated**]

rabies vaccine (purified chick embryo cell culture) [**RabAvert**]

RhO(D) immune globulin [**WinRho SDF**]

tetanus and diphtheria toxoids, adsorbed (Td), pediatric and adult [**TD Adsorbed**]

tetanus immune globulin (human) [**Hypertet S/D**]

varicella virus vaccine, live attenuated [**Varivax III, Varilrix**]

varicella zoster immune globulin human [**Varizig**]

CHAPTER 46: ANTINEOPLASTIC AGENTS

See Table 46-6 for drugs in the various antineoplastic classes.

CHAPTER 47: IMMUNOMODULATING AGENTS

adalimumab [**Humira**]

aldesleukin [**Proleukin**]

alemtuzumab (available only through Special Access Programme) [**Campath**]

anakinra [**Kineret**]

BCG vaccine [**BCG Vaccine (Freeze-Dried), Oncotice**]

epoetin alfa (EPO) (erythropoietin) [**Eprex**]etanercept [**Enbrel**]

filgrastim (G-CSF) [**Neupogen**]

gemtuzumab ozogamicin (available only through Special Access Programme) [**Mylotarg**]

ibritumomab tiuxetan [**Zevalin**]

interferon alfa-2a [**Pegasys**]

interferon alfa-2b [**Intron A**]

interferon alfacon-1 [**Infergen**]

interferon beta-1a [**Avonex, Rebif**]

interferon beta-1b [**Betaseron**]

leflunomide [**Arava**]

mitoxantrone [**Mitoxantrone Injection USP**]

pegfilgrastim [**Neulasta**]

peginterferon alfa-2a [**Pegasys**]

peginterferon alfa-2a/ribavirin [**Pegasys RBV**]

peginterferon alfa-2b [**Unitron-PEG**]

rituximab [**Rituxan**]

thalidomide (available only through the Special Access Programme) [**Thalomid**]

trastuzumab [**Herceptin Vials**]

tretinoin [**Vesanoid-Cap**]
vinorelbine [**Navelbine, Vinorelbine Tartrate for Injection**]

CHAPTER 49: ACID-CONTROLLING AGENTS

aluminum hydroxide/magnesium hydroxide [**Almagel, Diovol Plus Supension, Mylanta**]
calcium carbonate [**Calmicid, Extra Strength Calcium Antacid Chewable, Rolaids Antacid, TUMS Dual Action, many others**]
cimetidine [**Apo-Cimetidine**]
esomeprazole [**Nexium**]
famotidine [**Pepcid Tablets, Pepcid AC**]
lansoprazole [**Prevacid Fastab, Prevacid-SRC**]
magnesium carbonate salt/alginic acid [**Gaviscon Heartburn Relief, Gaviscon Heartburn Relief Extra Strength Tablets**]
magnesium hydroxide [**Milk of Magnesia**]
magnesium oxide [**Magnesium Oxide Tab**]
magnesium trisilicate/aluminum hydroxide [**Gasulsol Tablets**]
misoprostol [**Apro-Misoprostol**]
misoprostol/diclofenac sodium [**Arthrotec**]
nizatidine [**Axid, Apo-Nizatidine, Gen-Nizatidine**]
omeprazole [**Losec**]
pantoprazole [**Pantoloc, Panto IV**]
rabeprazole sodium [**Pariet**]
ranitidine [**Zantac**]
sucralfate [**Sulcrate**]

CHAPTER 50: ANTIDIARRHEALS AND LAXATIVES

ANTIDIARRHEALS

activated charcoal [**Acti-Charcoal, Charac-50, Charactol-50**]
aluminum hydroxide [**Amphojel**]
atropine sulphate [**Isopto Atropine 1%**]
attapulgite, activated [**Children's Kaopectate, Fowler's, Kaopectate**]
bismuth subsalicylate [**Pepto-Bismol**]
calcium polycarbophil [**Equalactin, Prodiem Bulk Fibre Therapy**]
cholestyramine resin [**PHL-Cholestyramine**]
codeine phosphate [**Ratio-Codeine**]
diphenoxylate hydrochloride/atropine sulphate [**Lomotil**]
hyoscyamine sulphate [**Levsin, Hyoscyaminum**]
kaolin [**Alumina Silicata**]

lactobacillus acidophilus [**Baktera, Lacidofil**]
loperamide hydrochloride [**Apo-Loperamide, Diarrhea Relief, Imodium Quick Dissolve**]
loperamide hydrochloride/ simethicone [**Imodium Advanced**]
meperidine hydrochloride [**Demerol**]
opium/belladonna [**PMS-opium and Belladona Sup**]
scopolamine n-butylbromide [**Hyoscine Butylbromide**]

LAXATIVES

bisacodyl [**Carter's Little Pills, Dulcolax**]
cascara sagrada [Cascara Sagrada]
docusate calcium [**Apo-Docusate Calcium, Calax, Soflax C**]
docusate sodium [**Correctol Stool Softener, Colace, Selax, Soflax**]
glycerine [**Glycerine, Glycerin Suppository**]
lactulose [**Ratio-Lactulose, Euro-Lac**]
magnesium citrate [**Citro-Mag**]
magnesium hydroxide [**Milk of Magnesia**]
magnesium phosphate dibasic [**Magnesium Phosphate, Phosphate De Magnesium H8**]
magnesium sulphate [**Epsom Salts**]
methylcellulose [**Entrocel Solution**]
mineral oil [**Fleet Enema Mineral Oil**]
mineral oil/glycerine [**Agarol Plain**]
mineral salts in combination [**Colyte, Klean-Prep, PegLyte**]
calcium polycarbophil [**Equalactin, Prodiem Bulk Fibre Therapy**]
plantago seed [**Metamucil, Psyllium**]
sodium phosphate [**Fleet Enema**]
senna [**Senokot**]
sorbitol
tegaserod maleate [**Zelnorm**]

CHAPTER 51: ANTI-EMETIC AND ANTINAUSEA AGENTS

cannibis-sativa extract [**Sativex**]
cisapride (available only through the Special Access Programme) [**Propulsid**]
dolasetron mesylate [**Anzemet**]
dronabinol [**Marinol**]
droperidol [**Droperidol Injection**]
granisetron [**Kytril**]
meclizine hydrochloride [**Bonamine**]
metoclopramide hydrochloride [**Apo-Metoclop, Metoclopramide Omega**]
nabilone [**Cesamet**]
ondansetron [**Zofran, Zofran ODT**]
prochlorperazine [**Stemetil**]
scopolamine [**Transderm-V**]

CHAPTER 52: VITAMINS AND MINERALS

alfacalcidol [**One-Alpha**]
calcitriol (vitamin D) [**Rocaltrol, Calcijex**]
nicotinic acid [**vitamin B complex**]
vitamin A [**Arginax, Nutrol A**]
vitamin B_2 [**Riboflavin Tab**]
vitamin B_6 (pyridoxine)
vitamin B_{12} [**cyanocobalamin**]
vitamin C [**Natural Source Ascorbic Acid, Chewable Vitamin C**]
vitamin D cholecaliferol
vitamin D_2 ergocalciferol [**Drisdol, D-Forte, Ostoforte**]
vitamin E (DL-alpha tocopheryl acetate) [**Vitamin E capsules**]
vitamin K oral (available only through the Special Access Programme)
vitamin K_1 [**Vitamin K_1 Inj**]
thiamine hydrochloride [**Vitamin B_1Tab**]

CHAPTER 54: BLOOD-FORMING AGENTS

Vitamin B_{12} (cyanocobalamin) [**Liquid Vitamin B_{12}, Vitamin B_{12} Sterile Injection, Prime**]
epoetin alfa (erythropoietin) [**Eprex**]
ferrous fumarate [**Palafer**]
ferrous gluconate [**Novo-Ferrogluc Tab**]
ferrous sulphate [**Ferodan**]
folic acid [**Folic Acid Tab**]
iron (iron dextran complex) [**Dexiron, Infufer**]

CHAPTER 55: DERMATOLOGIC AGENTS

ANTIBACTERIALS

bacitracin [**Baciguent First Aid Ointment**]
benzoyl peroxide [**Acetoxyl 2.5 Gel, Clear Acne Treatment, Benoxyl Benzac, many others**]
erythromycin, combinations [**Erysol, Stievamycin Preparations**]
isotretinoin [**Accutane, Clarus**]
neomycin sulphate
polymyxin B combination with other antibiotics [**Polysporin**]
tazarotene [**Tazorac**]
tretinoin [**Renova Crm, Rejuva-A-Crm, Retin-A**]

ANTIFUNGALS

butenafine hydrochloride [**Dr. Scholl's Athlete's Foot Cream**]
butoconazole nitrate [**Gynazole.1**]
ciclopirox olamine [**Loprox**]

clioquinol/hydrocortisone [**Vioform Hydrocortisone Cream**]

clotrimazole [**Canesten, Clotrimaderm**]

econazole nitrate [**Ecostatin**]

ketoconazole [**Nizoral**]

miconazole nitrate [**Micatin, Monistat 3, Monistat 7**]

naftifine hydrochloride [**Naftin**]

nystatin [**Nyaderm, Mycostatin, Ratio-Nystatin**]

oxiconazole [**Oxizole**]

tazarotene [**Tazorac**]

terbinafine hydrochloride [**Lamisil**]

tolnaftate [**Tinactin, Fungicure Gel, Swabplus**]

undecylenic acid [**Desenex, Fungicure Liquid**]

ANTIVIRALS

acyclovir [**Zovirax**]

MISCELLANEOUS AGENTS

amcinonide [**Cyclocort**]

betamethasone dipropionate [**Diprolene Glycol, Diprosone**]

betamethasone valerate [**Betaderm, Prevex B**]

betamethasone valerate/gentamicin [**Valisone G**]

clobetasol 17-propionate [**Dermovate**]

clobetasone 17-butyrate [**Eumovate**]

crotamiton [**Eurax**]

desonide [**Desocort, Tridesilon**]

desoximetasone [**Topicort**]

diflucortolone diacetate [**Sterile Diflucortone Diacetate**]

diflucortolone valerate [**Nerisone**]

finasteride [**Propecia**]

flumethasone pivalate/clioquinol [**Locacorten Vioform Cream**]

fluocinolone acetonide [**Derma-Smoothe FS, Fluoderm, Synalar**]

fluorouracil [**Efudex, Fluoroplex**]

halcinonide [**Halog**]

halobetasol propionate [**Ultravate**]

hydrocortisone [**Cortate, Cortoderm, Prevex HC**]

hydrocortisone valerate [**Westcort**]

lindane [**Hexit Lotion, Hexit Shampoo**]

mafenide [**Sulfamylon Cream**]

methylprednisolone acetate [**Medrol**]

minoxidil [**Rogaine**]

mometasone furoate [**Elocom**]

nitrofurazone [**Furacin**]

permethrin [**Nix**]

pimecrolimus [**Elidel**]

piperonyl butoxide, pyrethrins [**Lice Killing Shampoo, R & C**]

prednicarbate [**Dermatop**]

silver sulfadiazine [**Flamazine, Dermazin**]

triamcinolone acetonide [**Aristocort R, Triaderm**]

CHAPTER 56: OPHTHALMIC AGENTS

acetazolamide [**Acetazolam**]

acetylcholine chloride [**Miochol-E, Miogan**]

apraclonidine [**Iopidine**]

artificial tears [**Bausch & Lomb Moisture Eyes, Murine, Akwa Tears, Isopto Tears, Visine Advance True Tears, Refresh Tears, and Tears Plus**]

atropine sulphate [**Dioptic's Atropine Solution 1, Atropine, Isopto Atropine 1, Minims Atropine Sulphate 1**]

bacitracin [**Baciguent**]

bacitracin/polymyxin B [**Polysporin Sterile Ophthalmic Ointment**]

bacitracin zinc/polymyxin B sulphate/neomycin [**Diosporin, Neosporin Ointment**]

bacitracin zinc/hydrocortisone/neomycin sulphate/polymyxin B [**Sandoz Cortimyxin**]

betaxolol [**Betaxolol, Betoptic S**]

bimatoprost [**Lumigan**]

brimonidine tartrate [**Alphagan**]

brinzolamide [**Azopt**]

chloramphenicol [**AK-Chlor, Chloroptic, Pentamycetin**]

ciprofloxacin hydrochloride [**Ciloxan**]

cromolyn sodium [**Opticrom**]

cyclopentolate hydrochloride [**Minims Cyclopentolate Hydrochloride, Cyclogyl, AK-Pentolate**]

dexamethasone [**Maxidex**]

dexamethasone sodium phosphate [**AK-Dex**]

dexamethasone sodium metasulphobenzoate/framycetin sulphate/gramicidin [**Sofracort Sterile Ear/Eye Drops**]

diclofenac sodium [**Voltaren Ophtha**]

dipivefrin [**Propine Liq**]

dorzolamide [**Trusopt**]

emedastine difumarate [**Emadine**]

epinephrine racemic [**Epifrin**]

erythromycin [**AK Mycin**]

fluorescein sodium [**Fluorets**]

fluorescein sodium/proxymetacain hydrochloride [**Fluoracaine**]

fluorometholone acetate [**Flarex**]

flurbiprofen sodium [**Ocufen**]

gramicidin/polymyxin B sulphate [**Polysporin Eye and Ear Drops Sterile**]

gramicidin/neomycin/polymyxin B sulphate [**Neosporin Eye-Ear Solution**]

ganciclovir [**Vitrasert**]

gentamicin [**Alcomicin, Garamycin, Garasone**]

gentamicin/betamethasone [**Garasone**]

homatropine [**Isopto Homatropine**]

hyperosmolar sodium chloride preparations [**Muro 128**]

idoxuridine [**Herplex, Herplex-D**]

ketorolac tromethamine [**Acular**]

ketotifen fumarate [**Zaditor**]

latanoprost [**Xalatan**]

levobunolol hydrochloride [**Betagan**]

levocabastine [**Livostin**]

lodoxamide tromethamine [**Alomide**]

mannitol [**Osmitrol**]

methazolamide [**Apo-Methazolamide**]

naphazoline hydrochloride [**Albalon, Clear Eyes**]

nedocromil sodium [**Alocril**]

olopatadine [**Patanol**]

oxymetazoline hydrochloride [**Clariti Eye Allergy Relief**]

phenylephrine hydrochloride [**AK-Dilate**]

pilocarpine [**Isopto Carpine, Akarpine, Diocarpine**]

prednisolone acetate [**AK Tate**]

rimexolone [**Vexol**]

sulfacetamide sodium [**AK Sulf, Bleph 10, Cetamide ONT**]

sulfacetamide sodium/prednisolone acetate [**Blephamide, Dioptimyd**]

tetracaine hydrochloride [**Minims Tetracaine Hydrochloride, Pontocaine, Viractin**]

tetrahydrozoline hydrochlorine [**Visine Allergy**]

timolol [**Timoptic, Timoptic-XE**]

trifluridine [**Viroptic**]

tropicamide [**Mydriacyl**]

CHAPTER 57: OTIC AGENTS

cefaclor [**Ceclor**]

chloramphenicol/hydrocortisone acetate [**Pentamycetin/HC**]

hydrocortisone/ciprofloxacin [**Cipro HC Otic Suspension**]

hydrocortisone/neomycin/polymyxin B [**Sandoz Cortimyxin**]

hydrogen peroxide

lidocaine HCl/polymyxin B sulphate [**Lidosporin ear drops**]

urea hydrogen peroxide [**Murine Ear Wax Removal System/Murine Ear Drops**]

Data sources:

Canadian Pharmacists Association. (2005). *Compendium of pharmaceuticals and specialties. The Canadian drug reference for health professionals.* Ottawa, ON: Author.

Council for Continuing Pharmaceutical Education. (2005). Drugs List. Accessed December 6, 2005, at http://www.ccpe-cfpc.com/en/drug_lists/drug_list_b.pdf

Health Canada. (2006). Drug product database (DPD). Retrieved March 28, 2006, from http://www.hc-sc.gc.ca/hpb/drugs-dpd/

Glossary Terms with Page Numbers

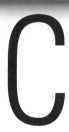

Beta-lactamase inhibitor, p. 627
Beta-lactams, p. 627
Bifunctional, p. 783
Bioavailability, p. 20
Biogenic amine hypothesis (BAH), p. 243
Biological antimicrobial agent, p. 755
Biological response modifiers (BRMs), p. 812
Bioterrorism, p. 757
Bipolar disorder (BPD), p. 237
Blinded investigational drug study, p. 52
B-lymphocytes (B-cells), p. 812
Booster shot, p. 759
Bronchial asthma, p. 595
Bronchodilators, p. 598
Bulk-forming laxatives, p. 861

C

Canada Health Act, p. 52
Canal of Schlemm, p. 949
Cancer pain, p. 148
Carbuncle, p. 935
Carcinoma, p. 773
Cardiac glycoside, p. 346
Cardiac output, p. 397
Cardioprotective, p. 309
Cardioselective beta-blockers, p. 309
Casein, p. 912
Catabolism, p. 568, 913
Cataract, p. 949
Catechol O-methyltransferase (COMT) inhibitors, p. 226
Catecholamines, p. 290
Cathartic, p. 866
Cell cycle–non-specific (CCNS), p. 776
Cell cycle–specific (CCS), p. 776
Cell-mediated immunity (CMI), p. 656, 812
Cellulitis, p. 935
Central nervous system (CNS stimulants), p. 274
Central pain, p. 148
Centrally acting adrenergic agents, p. 401
Cerumen, p. 976
Chemical name, p. 18
Chemoreceptor trigger zone (CTZ), p. 871
Chief cells, p. 840
Cholesterol, p. 478
Cholinergic agents, p. 320
Cholinergic-blocking agent, p. 330
Cholinesterase, p. 320
Chorea, p. 222
Chromatin, p. 830
Chromosome, p. 830
Chronic bronchitis, p. 595
Chronic diarrhea, p. 856
Chronic pain, p. 146
Chronic salicylate intoxication, p. 730
Chronic stable angina, p. 380
Chronotropic agent, p. 346

Chylomicrons, p. 478
Ciliary muscle, p. 951
Clot specific, p. 467
Coenzyme, p. 882
Collecting duct, p. 423
Colloid, p. 438
Colloid oncotic pressure (COP), p. 438
Colony-stimulating factors (CSFs), p. 814
Community-acquired infection, p. 715
Compendium of Monographs, p. 79
Competitive antagonist., p. 331
Cones, p. 950
Constipation, p. 860
Contraindication, p. 28
Controlled Drug and Substances Act (CDSA), p. 49
Conventional medicine, p. 79
Convulsion, p. 205
Cornea, p. 948
Coronary arteries, p. 380
Coronary artery disease (CAD), p. 380
Corpus luteum, p. 545
Cortex, p. 535
Corticosteroids, p. 535, 586
Crystalloids, p. 440
Cushing's syndrome, p. 536
Cycloplegia, p. 949
Cytochrome P-450, p. 24
Cytokines, p. 813
Cytoplasmic maturation defect, p. 924
Cytotoxic T-cells, p. 813

D

Decongestant, p. 580
Deep vein thrombosis (DVT), p. 456
Dehydration, p. 439
Deoxyribonucleic acid (DNA), p. 655
Depression, p. 237
Dermatological agent, p. 934
Dermatophyte, p. 936
Dermis, p. 934
Diabetes mellitus, p. 516
Diabetic ketoacidosis (DKA), p. 517
Diarrhea, p. 856
Differentiation, p. 776, 814
Dilator muscle, p. 949
Direct-acting cholinergic agonists, p. 320
Disease-modifying antirheumatic drugs (DMARDs), p. 736
Disinfectant, p. 716
Dissolution, p. 19
Distal convoluted tubule, p. 423
Diuretic, p. 423
Done nomogram, p. 730
Dopamine hypothesis, p. 254
Dopaminergic agents, p. 224
Dopaminergic receptors, p. 290
Dose-limiting side effects, p. 777
Double-blind, placebo-controlled study, p. 52
Dromotropic agent, p. 346

Drug, p. 18
Drug actions, p. 19
Drug effect, p. 27
Drug Identification Number (DIN), p. 52
Drug-induced teratogenesis, p. 32
Drug interaction, p. 30
Drug polymorphism, p. 55
Dumping syndrome, p. 911
Duration of action, p. 27
Dyskinesia, p. 222
Dysregulation hypothesis, p. 244
Dysrhythmia, p. 310, 360
Dysthymic disorder or dysthymia, p. 237
Dystonia, p. 222

E

Echinocandin, p. 690
Edema, p. 439
Effective refractory period (ERP), p. 362
Efferent arteriole, p. 423
Ejection fraction, p. 346
Embolus, p. 456
Emesis, p. 871
Emetic potential, p. 778
Emollient laxatives, p. 861
Emphysema, p. 595
Empirical therapy, p. 580, 621
Endocrine gland, p. 545
Endogenous, p. 224
Endometrium, p. 545
Enteral nutrition, p. 909
Enuresis, p. 90
Enzyme, p. 20, 882
Epidermis, p. 933
Epilepsy, p. 205
Epinephrine, p. 535
Ergosterol, p. 690
Erythrocyte, p. 924
Erythrocytic phase, p. 701
Erythropoiesis, p. 928
Erythropoietic effect, p. 568
Essential amino acids, p. 913
Essential fatty acid deficiency, p. 914
Essential hypertension, p. 409
Estrogens, p. 545
Exoerythrocytic phase, p. 701
Exogenous, p. 224
Exogenous lipids, p. 478
Expectorant, p. 580
Extracellular fluid (ECF), p. 438
Extravasation, p. 306
Extravascular fluid (EVF), p. 438

F

Fallopian tube, p. 545
Fast channels, sodium channels, p. 361
Fat-soluble vitamin, p. 883
Fibrin, p. 454
Fibrinogen, p. 461
Fibrinolysis, p. 455

Disorders Index

Page numbers followed by "f" denote figures; those followed by "t" denote tables; those followed by "b" denote boxes.

General Index

Page numbers followed by "f" denote figures; those followed by "t" denote tables; and those followed by "b" denote boxes.

Special Features

Special Features—cont'd